Psychiatric and mental health nursing

Psychiatric and mental health nursing

The craft of caring

Third edition

Edited by
Mary Chambers

Professor of Mental Health Nursing,
Director, Centre for Public Engagement
Associate Editor, Health Expectations

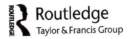
Routledge
Taylor & Francis Group

First published 2017
by Routledge
2 Park Square, Milton Park, Abingdon, Oxon OX14 4RN

and by Routledge
711 Third Avenue, New York, NY 10017

Routledge is an imprint of the Taylor & Francis Group, an Informa business

© 2017 Taylor & Francis Group

British Library Cataloguing-in-Publication Data
A catalogue record for this book is available from the British Library

Library of Congress Cataloging in Publication Data
A catalogue record for this book is available from the Library of Congress

ISBN: 978-1-4822-2195-4 (pbk)

Typeset in Minion Pro
by Datapage India (Pvt.) Ltd.

Contents

Section 5:
Services and support for those with mental health distress

Section 6:
Opportunities and challenges for mental health nursing in the twenty-first century

List of contributors

Chapter 1

Ben Thomas, PhD, MSc, BSc (Hons), RGN, RMN, DipN (Lond), RNT, CertHE, FRCN
Mental Health, Learning Disability and Dementia Care Professional Officer
Department of Health
Visiting Professor
South Bank University
Honorary Senior Fellow
Kingston University and St George's
University of London
London, UK

Chapter 2

Vince J. Mitchell, PhD, RN, MA, PGCertAP
Associate Lecturer
The Open University
UK

Chapter 3

Rosie Stenhouse, PhD, MSc (Res), BSc, RMN, PGCertHET
Lecturer in Nursing Studies
University of Edinburgh
Edinburgh, UK

Chrys Muirhead is a mental health writer, activist and campaigner, who worked in the voluntary sector and NHS inpatient and community settings as a mental health nurse for 10 years before embarking on an academic career.

Chapter 4

Liam Clarke, PhD, Dip Med Phil, Dip Theol, BA, MA, MSc
Teaching Fellow
University of Brighton
Brighton, UK

Phil Ruthen is a writer, poet and survivor researcher.

Chapter 5

Tim Thornton, PhD, MPhil, MA (Cantab)
Professor of Philosophy and Mental Health
University of Central Lancashire
Preston, UK

David Crepaz-Keay, DProf
Head of Empowerment and Social Inclusion
Mental Health Foundation for People with Learning Disabilities
London, UK

Sebastian Birch
Mental health nursing student
St George's, University of London
London, UK

Jan Verhaegh, DTh, MA (Philosophy and Mental Health)
Board member of European Network of (ex-)Users and Survivors of Psychiatry (ENUSP) and Autism Europe

Chapter 6

Hugh McKenna, CBE, PhD, BSc (Hons), RMN, RGN, RNT, DipN (Lond), AdvDipEd, FFN RCSI, FEANS, FRCN, FAAN
Pro Vice Chancellor
University of Ulster
Coleraine, UK

Chapter 7

Joanne McDonnell, Registered Mental Health Nurse, Master of Research in Health Science
Senior Nurse for Mental Health and Learning Disabilities
NHS England
Warrington, UK

Chapter 8

Kay Jansen, DNP, RN, PMHCNS-BC, CNE
Terminology Manager, International Classification for Nursing Practice (ICNP®) Programme
eHealth Programme, International Council of Nurses
College of Nursing, University of Wisconsin-Milwaukee
Milwaukee WI, USA

Amy Coenen, PhD, RN, FAAN
Director, International Classification for Nursing Practice (ICNP®) Programme, International Council of Nurses
College of Nursing, University of Wisconsin-Milwaukee
Milwaukee WI, USA

Nicholas R. Hardiker, PhD, RN, FACMI
Director, eHealth Programme, International Council of Nurses
School of Nursing, Midwifery, Social Work & Social Sciences, University of Salford
Manchester, UK

Chapter 9

Sarah Gibson, BA (Hons), MA (Oxon)
Service User Researcher
St George's, University of London
London, UK

John Swinton, PhD, BD, RMN, RNMH
Professor in Practical Theology and Pastoral Care
School of Divinity, Religious Studies and Philosophy, University of Aberdeen
Aberdeen, UK

Chapter 10

John R. Cutcliffe, PhD, RMN, RGN, RN, BSc (Hons)Nrsg
'Blanke' Endowed Chair in Nursing Research and Professor
Director, Centre for Nursing Research, Wright State University
Ohio, USA
Adjunct Professor, University of Ottawa, Canada
Adjunct Professor, University of Coimbra, Portugal
Adjunct Professor, University of Malta
CEO, Cutcliffe Consulting

Katherine Owen is a service user.

Chapter 11

Jan Fook, PhD, FAcSS
Professor of Higher Education Pedagogy and Director, International Centre for Higher Education Educational Research, Leeds Trinity University
Leeds, UK

Jane Royes, BSW
Social Work Continuing Professional Development Officer
London, UK

Anthony White, BSc, Grad Dip
Case manager, Inner South
Community Health Service
Melbourne, Australia

Chapter 12

David Kingdon, MD, FRCPsych
Professor of Mental Health Care Delivery
University of Southampton
Southampton, UK

Shanaya Rathod, MD, MRCPsych
Director of Research & Development
and Consultant Adult Psychiatrist
Southern Health NHS Foundation Trust
Southampton, UK

Carolyn Asher is a patient, carer and
Public Involvement and Engagement
Coordinator and Service User
Research Assistant for Southern
Health NHS Foundation Trust at
the Research and Development
Department, Southampton, UK.

Chapter 13

Tony Warne, PhD, MBA, RMN
Professor in Mental Health Care
University of Salford
Manchester, UK

**Sue McAndrew, PhD, MSc, BSc, CPN
Cert RMN**
Reader (Mental Health)
University of Salford
Manchester, UK

Fiona Jones is a survivor activist, a
member of Comensus (service user/
carer group, University of Central
Lancashire) and an associate board
member of the International Institute
for Special Needs Offenders.

Chapter 14

Paul Fallon, RMN, BA (Hons), MSc, PhD
Lecturer, University of Salford
Manchester, UK
Senior Practitioner for Nursing
Cromwell House Community Mental
Health Centre
Salford, UK

G~ is a service user.

Chapter 15

Catherine Gamble
Head of Nursing and Consultant Nurse
South West London and St George's
Mental Health Care Trust
London, UK

Christine Lewis is a family member.

**John Baker, PhD, MPhil, MSc,
BNurs (Hons)**
Professor
School of Health Care, Faculty of
Medicine and Health, University of
Leeds
Leeds, UK

**Ruth Allen, MSW, CQSW,
Postgraduate Diploma in Applied
Systemic Theory, EdD**
Director of Social Work
South West London and St George's
Mental Health Care Trust
London, UK

Chapter 16

**Keith Waters, RMN, Dip Nursing
(London)**
Clinical Advisor, Suicide
Prevention, East Midlands Health
Science Network
Honorary Research Fellow (Self-Harm/
Suicide Prevention) and Director of
Centre for Self-Harm and Suicide
Prevention
Centre for Research and
Development, Derbyshire Healthcare
NHS Foundation Trust
Derby, UK

**Alys Cole-King, MB, BCh, DGM,
MSc, FRCPsych**
Consultant Liaison Psychiatrist, Betsi
Cadwaladr Health Board, Glan Clwyd
Hospital
Clinical Director, Connecting with
People
Bodelwyddan, UK

Chapter 17

Fiona Nolan, RMN, BA, PhD
Deputy Director of Nursing and
Research
University College London and
Camden and Islington NHS
Foundation Trust
London, UK

The Late Caren Watson was a service
user.

Mary Ellen Khoo, RMN, BSc
Research Nurse
Camden and Islington NHS
Foundation Trust
London, UK

Chapter 18

Helen Leigh-Phippard, BA (Hons), PhD
Service User Member, Carer and User
Group (CUSER)
University of Brighton
Brighton, UK

**Alec Grant, BA (Hons), MA, PhD,
Cert Res Meth, PGCTLHE, FHEA,
RMN, ENB650Cert**
Reader in Narrative Mental Health
School of Health Sciences, University
of Brighton
Eastbourne, UK

Chapter 19

Kati Turner
Service user researcher
St George's, University of London
London, UK

Chapter 20

**Eimear Muir-Cochrane, BSc (Hons),
RN, Grad Dip Adult Ed, MNS, PhD,
FACMHN, Credentialled MHN**
Professor, Chair of Nursing (Mental
Health)
Flinders University
Adelaide, Australia

**Deb O'Kane, RMN, ENB603, RN, Grad
DipCN, MN, Grad Cert Ed (Higher Ed)**
Lecturer
Flinders University
Adelaide, Australia

**Kylie Harrison, Certificate 1V in
Mental Health,** is a Community Peer
Worker, writer, comedian and poet.

Chapter 21

**Ian Beech, RMN, RGN, PhD, MA,
BA (Hons), PGCE**
Academic Manager for Mental Health
Faculty of Life Sciences and Education,
University of South Wales
Pontypridd, UK

Chapter 22

Jane Bunclark, RGN, RMN, MA, MSc
Consultant Nurse for Self-Harm/Head
of Nursing for Mood, Anxiety and
Personality Disorder
South London and Maudsley NHS
Foundation Trust
London, UK

Louise Stone is a recovered service user.

Chapter 23

Vanessa Gordon
Formerly Senior Head of Patient Safety, Mental Health, Learning Disability and Offender Health, Domain 5, Patient Safety
NHS England

Karen James, BSc (Hons), MSc, PhD
Post-doctoral researcher
Kingston University and St George's University of London, Joint Faculty of Health, Social Care and Education
London, UK

Marion Janner, OBE, is the founder of Star Wards, London, UK.

Kirsten Windfuhr, BA, MA, PhD
Associate Director of Quality and Development
Healthcare Quality Improvement Partnership (HQIP)
Manchester, UK

Isabelle M. Hunt, PhD
Research Fellow
Confidential Inquiry into Suicide and Homicide by People with Mental Illness, Manchester University
Manchester, UK

Chapter 24

Janet Wood, MA, BSc, PG Dip CBT, PGCEA, RGN, RMN
Senior Lecturer, Mental Health Nursing

Niall McLaughlin, BSc, RMN
Senior Lecturer, Mental Health Nursing
Canterbury Christ Church University
Canterbury, UK

Warwick Owen has worked with a number of education and health and social care providers delivering teaching and consultancy based on his experience of mental health and mental health services.

Chapter 25

Joy A. Duxbury, PhD, MA, BSc, RMN
Professor of Mental Health Nursing
University of Central Lancashire
Preston, UK

Fiona Jones is a service user researcher.

Chapter 26

Sally Hardy, EdD, MSc, ACHEP, BSc (Hons), DPNS, RMN, RN
Head of Department for Mental Health and Learning Disabilities
Professor of Mental Health and Practice Innovation
School of Health and Social Care, London South Bank University
London, UK
Adjunct Professor for Mental Health Nursing
Monash University
Melbourne, Australia

Chapter 27

Christopher Alec Gordon, RMN, BSc (Hons), MSc
Operational Services Manager – Eating Disorders (Adults) and Personality Disorder
Somerset Partnership NHS Foundation Trust
Yeovil, UK

Chapter 28

Cheryl Forchuk, RN, BA, BScN, MScN, PhD
Distinguished University Professor
University of Western Ontario
Assistant Director and Scientist
Lawson Health Research Institute
London ON, Canada

Elsabeth Jensen, RN, BA, BScN, MSN, PhD
Associate Professor
School of Nursing, York University
Toronto ON, Canada
Scientist
Lawson Health Research Institute
London ON, Canada

Natalie Farquhar
Nursing student
University of Western Ontario
London ON, Canada

Chapter 29

Roxane Agnew-Davies, MA (Hons), MSc, PhD
Director, Domestic Violence Training Ltd
Honorary Research Fellow
School of Social and Community Medicine, University of Bristol
Bristol, UK

Phoebe has used mental health and health services since her teenage years, following her repeated experiences of sexual and physical abuse by a paedophile ring.

Chapter 30

Gillian Todd, RMN, MSc
Independent Trainer
London, UK

Rosemary Marston is a recovered service user.

Chapter 31

Philip A. Cooper
Nurse Consultant
Dual Diagnosis, 5 Boroughs Partnership NHS Foundation Trust
Warrington, UK

Graham Naughton is a service user with a diagnosis of psychosis with accompanying mood disorder, who has experience of using a variety of substances and is now 2 years substance free.

Chapter 32

Agnes Higgins, PhD, MSc, BNS, RPN, RGN, RNT
Professor in Mental Health
School of Nursing and Midwifery, Trinity College Dublin
Dublin, Ireland

Liz Brosnan, PhD, MA
Post-doctoral researcher
Centre for Disability Law and Policy, NUIGalway
Galway, Ireland

Chapter 33

Julia Wood, Registered Nurse, PhD
Senior Researcher
Faculty of Health Social Care and Education, Kingston and St George's University of London
Dementia Navigator Team Leader (Specialist Practitioner)
Camden and Islington NHS Foundation Trust, UK
London, UK

Jacquie Nunn has cared for her husband Tony since his Alzheimer's diagnosis in 2010, and her professional background is in teaching and teacher education.

Chapter 34

Angus Forsyth, RMN, RGN, ENB 650, BA, MSc, Prof Doc
Senior Lecturer in Mental Health Nursing
Northumbria University
Newcastle, UK

Marion Janner, OBE, is the founder of Star Wards, London, UK.

Chapter 35

Julie Repper, PhD, MPhil, BA (Hons), RMN, RGN
Recovery Lead – Nottinghamshire Healthcare Foundation Trust
Programme Director – ImROC (Implementing Recovery through Organisational Change)
Nottingham, UK

Rachel Perkins, BA (Hons), MPhil (Clinical Psychology), PhD, OBE
Senior Consultant, ImROC (Implementing Recovery through Organisational Change)
London, UK

Chapter 36

Jess Holley, PhD
Research Associate
Centre for Mental Health, Imperial College London
London, UK

Dean Pearsey is a teacher of English as a foreign language and an aspiring novelist, whose latest work revolves around his own road to recovery.

Chapter 37

Martin Ward, RMN, Dip Nurs, RNT, Cert Ed, NEBSS Dip, MPhil
Visiting Senior Lecturer
Department of Mental Health,
Faculty of Health Sciences,
University of Malta
Msida, Malta

Chapter 38

Anthony J. O'Brien, RN, BA, MPhil (Hons), PhD, FNZCMHN
Senior Lecturer
School of Nursing, Faculty of Medical and Health Sciences, University of Auckland
Nurse Specialist
Liaison Psychiatry, Auckland District Health Board
Auckland, New Zealand

Ruth DeSouza, Dip Nurs, Grad Dip Counselling, MA, PhD
Stream Leader, Research, Policy and Evaluation
Centre for Culture, Ethnicity & Health
Melbourne, Australia

Maria Baker, MPhil Nursing, PGDip Mental Health Nursing, Grad Dip Maori Development
Ngapuhi nui tonu (Maori – Northern Tribe of New Zealand)
Workforce Innovation Manager
Te Rau Matatini Ltd (National Maori Health Workforce Development Organisation)
Wellington, New Zealand

Chapter 39

Elizabeth Hughes, PhD, BSc (Hons), Dip HE, RN (Mental Health)
Professor
University of Huddersfield and South West Yorkshire Partnership NHS Foundation Trust
Huddersfield, UK

Bobby Swift is a patient, carer, and public involvement representative for Northumbria University at Newcastle, UK.

Chapter 40

Lina Gega, PhD, BA (Hons), BN (Hons), RMN, ENB650
Reader in Mental Health
University of York
York, UK

Carolyn Asher is a patient, carer and Public Involvement and Engagement Coordinator and Service User Research Assistant for Southern Health NHS Foundation Trust at the Research and Development Department, Southampton, UK.

Chapter 41

Simon Proudlock
Consultant Psychologist
Berkshire Healthcare NHS Foundation Trust and Independent Practice
Reading, UK

Sonia Sanghvi has been battling with her mental health for nearly 15 years, and has spent time under a community mental health team, as an inpatient, and supported by a crisis resolution home treatment team.

Chapter 42

Angela Cotton, PhD, BSc, RMN
Lecturer in Mental Health Nursing
University of Salford
Manchester, UK

Dina Poursanidou, PhD
Researcher
Institute of Psychiatry, King's College, University of London
London, UK

Chapter 43

Antony Froggett, BA, MA, UKCP
Registered Psychotherapist, Member of Institute of Group Analysis

Chapter 44

Mary E. Campbell, RN, MSN, CNS-BC
Adjunct Professor
Dalhousie School of Nursing
Faculty Member
Atlantic Contemplative Centre
Meditation Instructor and Senior Teacher
Shambhala International
Halifax NS, Canada

Laura Burke is a drama therapist, mental health advocate, peer support worker and theatre artist, and a psychiatric survivor.

Chapter 45

Henrietta Mbeah-Bankas, MSc, BSc (Hons) RN (Mental Health), PGCert (Leadership in Health)
Professional Advisor, Early Intervention in Psychosis/Psychiatric Liaison and Crisis
Health Education England, Tower Hamlets Early Detection of Psychosis Service
London, UK

Chapter 46

Julie Taylor, MA Systemic Practice, RMN
Nurse Consultant
Newcastle and North Tyneside Crisis Resolution and Home Treatment Service
Newcastle upon Tyne, UK

Mrs M is a service user.

Mr M is a carer.

Miss M is a carer.

Chapter 47

Carl Holvey, MRPharmS, DipClinPharm, DBA, Ipresc
Lead Clinical and Deputy Chief Pharmacist
South West London and St George's NHS Trust
London, UK

Nikola Nikolić, MPharm, DipClinPharm, CertPsychTher
Senior Clinical Pharmacist
North West Dublin Mental Health Services
Dublin, Ireland

Chapter 48

Rebecca M. Burgess-Dawson, MSc, PGCert RMN (TCH, V300), FHEA
Clinical Lead (Mental Health)
Health Education England
Leeds, UK

Steve Hemingway, PhD, MA, PGDE, BA (Hons), RMN (V300), FHEA
Senior Lecturer in Mental Health
University of Huddersfield
Huddersfield, UK

Chapter 49

Georgina Wakefield runs Spotlight on Schizophrenia and is an honorary lecturer at the Institute of Psychiatry, King's College London, UK.

Gary Hickey, PhD Health Studies, BA (Hons) Public Administration
Public and Patient Involvement Lead
Centre for Public Engagement,
Kingston University and St George's, University of London
London, UK

Chapter 50

Douglas Hamandishe
Care Planning Lead Nurse and Technology Lead
South West London and St George's Mental Health NHS Trust
London, UK

Daniel Barrett
Co-production Practitioner and Prosper Lead
South West London and St George's Mental Health NHS Trust
London, UK

Chapter 51

Martin Atchison, BSc (Hons), RMN Dip
Deputy Director
Meriden Family Programme,
Birmingham and Solihull Mental Health NHS Foundation Trust, UK

Jeanette Partridge, Cert Ed, is a carer.

Jo Twiss, BA (Hons), is a service user.

Chapter 52

Kate Chartres, RN (MH), BSc Hons
Nurse Consultant
Sunderland Psychiatric Liaison Team,
Northumberland Tyne and Wear NHS Foundation Trust
Sunderland, UK

Rikke Albert, RNMH, BA (Hons), MSc
Nurse Consultant
Tower Hamlets Mental Health Liaison/RAID, East London NHS Foundation Trust
Honorary Lecturer
City University
London, UK

Sarah Eales, RN, BNurs, PGDip, FHEA, PhD
Senior Lecturer in Mental Health Nursing
Bournemouth University
Bournemouth, UK

Angela Warren, BEd (Hons), Carer and Service User Coordinator at Bournemouth University), is a service user who has had experience of psychiatric inpatient admissions and a range of psychological therapies which contributed to her recovery and led to her return to full-time work.

Chapter 53

Angela Simpson, RMN, BA, MA, PGCE, PhD
Head of Nursing, Midwifery and Professional Education
University of York
York, UK

Rob Allison, RMN MSc, PGCAP
Senior Lecturer in Mental Health and Leader of BSc Nursing Programme
University of York
York, UK

Ruth Lambley, BSc, MA, is an expert by experience.

Chapter 54

Christopher Dzikiti, MSc, MSc, BSc (Hons), Dip in Nursing
Strategic Case Manager
NHS England
London, UK

Rebecca Lingard, MSc, BA, Dip in Nursing
Modern Matron
East London NHS Foundation Trust
London, UK

Chapter 55

Denis Ryan, PhD, BSc, RPN, RGN, Dip Prof Studies, Cert BT, CAC
Professor of Counselling and Psychotherapy
Irish College of Humanities and Applied Sciences
Limerick, Ireland

Jane Alexander, PhD, MA Couns Psych, BA (Hons), PGCE
Deputy Director of Academic Affairs
Irish College of Humanities and Applied Sciences
Limerick, Ireland

Chapter 56

Paul Veitch, RN, MSc
Nurse Consultant
St Nicholas Hospital, Northumberland, Tyne and Wear NHS Foundation Trust
Newcastle upon Tyne, UK

Lisa Strong, RMN, MSc
Clinical Nurse Specialist
St Nicholas Hospital, Northumberland, Tyne and Wear NHS Foundation Trust
Newcastle upon Tyne, UK

Nicola Armstrong has been contributing to service improvement from a service user and carer perspective for over 23 years, and is currently Service Improvement Facilitator at Northumberland, Tyne and Wear NHS Foundation Trust, Newcastle upon Tyne, UK.

Chapter 57

Simon Clarke, DClinPsy, PGCert, BSc, Cert Ed
Lecturer/Senior Lecturer in Psychology
Department of Psychology,
Nottingham Trent University
Nottingham, UK

Simon Clarke has lived experience of psychosis and using mental health services and is a former member and leader of Christ Church Deal (CCD) therapeutic community.

Gary Winship, PhD, MA, RMN, Dip Gp Psych, Dip Add
Associate Professor
University of Nottingham
Nottingham, UK

Jenelle Clarke, PhD, MA, BA
Research Fellow
Business School, University of Nottingham
Nottingham, UK

Nick Manning, PhD, DPhil, MA, MPhil, BA
Professor of Sociology
King's College London
London, UK

Chapter 58

Steven Pryjmachuk, PhD, MSc, PGDipEd, BA (Hons), RN (Mental Health), RNT CPsychol SFHEA
Professor of Mental Health Nursing Education
University of Manchester
Manchester, UK

Hannah Welsby has lived experience as a user of mental health services for young people.

Chapter 59

Gemma Trainor, PhD, MA
Lecturer
Kings College London
London, UK

'Aiden' is a service user with a long-term history of eating disorder and self-harm, who has accessed a variety of services since the age of 13 and is now employed in a mental health setting.

Rebecca McPhillips, PhD
Senior Research Assistant
MHSCT Research & Innovation,
Manchester Royal Infirmary
Manchester, UK

Chapter 60

Chris Knifton, SBStJ, MA, MSc, MSc, LLB (Hons), BSc (Hons), PGCertHE, FAETC, Dip AROM, Dip Counselling & Psychotherapy, Dip SW, RNLD, FHEA
Faculty of Health and Life Sciences

Dementia Lead, Senior Lecturer
Dementia, Learning Disability and Mental Health
De Montfort University
Leicester, UK
Admiral Nurse
Dementia UK

Richard Postance, BSc (Hons), RNLD
Senior Lecturer, Learning Disability
De Montfort University
Leicester, UK

Dorothy Hemel is the mother of a 43-year-old son with learning disabilities and autism.

Chapter 61

Hugh Palmer, MSc, BSc (Hons), RGN, RMN, Cert Ed
UKCP Registered Systemic Psychotherapist

Chapter 62

Joy Bray
has worked in mental health for over 40 years as a clinician, lecturer and researcher, and is now semi-retired, working as a trainer in Mental Health First Aid and teaching mental health in the university sector and NHS.

Jeannette Harding who has experience of using mental health services, has been involved in the service user movement locally and nationally, and currently works as a mental health trainer and researcher.

Chapter 63

Michael McKeown, PhD, BA (Hons), DPSN (Thorn), RGN, RMN
Reader in Democratic Mental Health
School of Nursing, University of Central Lancashire
Preston, UK

Fiona Edgar
Service User Researcher
Community Futures
Preston, UK

Ian Callaghan, BA (Oxon), MB BS, PGCert
Chair
National Secure Care Recovery & Outcomes Network, Rethink Mental Illness
London, UK

Chapter 64

Helen Pusey, PhD, MSc, PGDE, BA (Hons), RMN
Lecturer
University of Manchester
Manchester, UK

John Keady, PhD, RMN, RNT
Professor of Mental Health Nursing and Older People
University of Manchester/Greater Manchester West Mental Health NHS Foundation Trust
Manchester, UK

Chapter 65

Ann Jackson, RMN, BA (Hons), MA
Independent and Associate Consultant
City University
London, UK

Jessica Worner
Peer Support Practice Manager
Service User Involvement Directorate,
Together for Mental Wellbeing
London, UK

Chapter 66

Nicholas Procter, PhD, MBA, Grad Dip Adult Ed, BA, RN
Professor
School of Nursing and Midwifery, University of South Australia
Adelaide, Australia

Monika Ferguson, PhD, GradCertSuicidePreveSt, BPsych (Hons)
Research Associate
School of Nursing and Midwifery, University of South Australia
Adelaide, Australia

Amy Baker, PhD, BHSc (Hons) (OccTh), B App Sc (OccTh)
Lecturer
School of Health Sciences, University of South Australia
Adelaide, Australia

Asma Babakarkhil, BBus, BA
Former Strategic Partnerships Officer
University of South Australia
Adelaide, Australia

Chapter 67

Michael Hazelton, PhD, MA, BA, RN
Professor of Mental Health Nursing
University of Newcastle
Newcastle, Australia

Peter Morrall, PhD, MSc, BA (Hons), PGCE, RGN, RMN, RNMH
Associate Professor in Health Sociology
University of Leeds
Leeds, UK

Chapter 68

Dawn Freshwater, PhD, BA (Hons), FRCN, RN, RNT
Senior Deputy Vice Chancellor and Registrar
University of Western Australia
Perth, Australia

Chapter 69

Louise E. Howard, RMN, MSc, BSc (Hons), LPE
Senior Lecturer, Mental Health Nursing
Kingston University and St George's University of London
London, UK

Chapter 70

Thomas J. Currid, RMN, RNT, BSc (Hons), PGCE, MA, PG Dip (CBT)
Programme Lead
University of Essex
Colchester, UK

Carl Chandra, DIPSW, BA (Hons), PG Cert (Practice Education), PGCHE, MA
Senior Lecturer
University of West London
London, UK

Chapter 71

Mary Chambers, BEd, PhD, RN, ENB650, RNT
Professor of Mental Health Nursing
Director, Centre for Public Engagement
Faculty for Health, Social Care and Education, Kingston University and St George's, University of London
London, UK

Sarah Markham, BA (Hons), MA (Cantab), PhD
Visiting Researcher
King's Clinical Trials Unit, IoPPN, King's College London
London, UK

Chapter 72

Maritta Välimäki, PhD, RN
Professor
Department of Nursing Science, University of Turku
Nursing Director
Turku University Hospital
Turku, Finland

Chapter 73

Patrick Callaghan RN, BSc, MSc, PhD, CPsychol FHEA
Professor of Mental Health Nursing
School of Health Sciences, University of Nottingham
Nottingham, UK

Debbie Butler
Mental Health Service User Consultant
East Midlands
Nottingham, UK

Preface

This third edition of what has become a well-established textbook is published at a time of considerable change. Change is inevitable due to advances in science and technology, demography altering as we live longer, changes in healthcare philosophy and the delivery of healthcare services moving from paternalism to partnerships. This last difference is particularly evident in mental health care, with its increasing emphasis on recovery and service-user involvement.

The political landscape across Europe and beyond is also changing with many countries experiencing major unrest and global recession. Such conditions have implications for the mental health and well-being of citizens, further adding to the social, economic and healthcare pressures of many countries, especially those of the developing world.

With respect to the United Kingdom, there has been an emphasis on austerity, which has resulted in the re-configuration of a number of society's benefits and services including health care. These measures have caused the closure of some services and the merging of others, despite a governmental commitment to protected funding. Of late, there has been considerable media attention given to the shortage of inpatient beds especially for young people. This has resulted in many young people being admitted to services hundreds of miles away from home. The media have also been highlighting the increased incidence of self-harm again amongst young people including school children.

The nature and delivery of health care features on the agenda of every government despite, not infrequently, election promises suggesting there will be no change. Recently, mental health appears to have greater prominence on the British government's agenda, for example, in the *No Health without Mental Health* (2011) strategy and the *Five Year Forward View* (2014). However, despite this, there are many contradictions when it comes to the nature of, and access to, services. One example is the introduction of new roles in an effort to make care more readily available where and when necessary, against the backdrop of shortage of trained staff, especially doctors and nurses.

Mental health nursing as a profession is not immune to these changes and currently questions are being asked about the nature and value of mental health nursing and the future education and training of registered mental health nurses. Some of these questions are coming from the profession itself. This textbook, by virtue of its breadth and depth provides an opportunity to explore what registered mental health nurses do and highlight their value.

Efforts have been made to retain the integrity of the first two editions of this textbook whilst at the same time addressing some of the more contemporary issues surrounding mental health nursing. For example, it includes new content on the nature of nursing knowledge, the role of nursing classification in care planning, the increasingly important role of technology in health care and the need for a metric to indicate the contribution of mental health nursing to service user recovery.

Service-user involvement featured in the last edition of *Psychiatric and Mental Health Nursing* and the trend continues in this edition. Each chapter has input from service users, either as authors, co-authors, personal stories or in the form of a commentary. This approach has ensured a strong service-user voice throughout the text and has highlighted some challenging issues that require exploration. For some chapters, such as collaborative care planning, there is evidence of the creative tensions that can exist between the mental health nurse and service user: 'Who Owns the Care Plan'? With its strong emphasis on service-user involvement, this new edition of *Psychiatric and Mental Health Nursing* will provide the opportunity for critical reflection and questioning approaches to the craft of caring.

In keeping with previous editions, the book is comprehensive and broad, reflecting the diverse nature of mental health nursing and the range of activities undertaken. Although there are a number of changes to this edition, it retains many of the sections and features from the second edition. It still takes a multi-disciplinary approach with contributions from leading experts in the field including those actively involved in clinical practice. Each chapter has between three and eight reflective points enabling the reader to consider their own practice or to explore challenging issues related to practice, with most commenting on the craft of caring.

This edition of the book is divided into six sections. It begins with **Section 1: Aspects of mental health nursing** setting the scene by looking at the nature of mental health nursing with the remaining chapters addressing key elements. Chapter 3 focuses on the importance of developing and maintaining therapeutic relationships, which is the crux of mental health nursing. An understanding of how nursing knowledge is generated and how nursing is classified is increasingly important and discussed in detail within Chapters 5 and 8. Mental illness and mental health care are highly politicized areas, raising a number of ethical issues which are addressed in Chapters 2 and 4. Promoting evidence-informed practice and building practice from research are discussed in Chapters 6 and 7. Clinical supervision and critical reflection, vital for enhancing clinical competency and personal development, are considered in Chapters 10 and 11. Spirituality, which plays a key role in holistic mental health nursing, is considered in Chapter 9.

Section 2: The foundations of mental health nursing begins with Chapter 12 looking at the classification of mental illness. Following this, the importance of assessment and its different aspects are considered in Chapters 13, 14, and 15. Assessing risk of suicide is the focus of Chapter 16, with engagement and observation of those at risk of suicide discussed in Chapter 17. Freedom and consent is explored in Chapter 18 and the section concludes with Chapter 19 asking what it means to have a diagnosis of mental illness.

Section 3: Caring for those experiencing mental health distress encourages the reader to consider many of the challenging situations experienced by mental health service users with each chapter in the section including a service user perspective. The section starts with two of the most common mental health problems: Chapter 20 looks at depression and Chapter 21 considers anxiety. Self-harm and suicide are the focus of Chapters 22 and 23, with Chapter 24 discussing schizophrenia, Chapter 25 looking at the care and support for those who are extremely distressed and disturbed and Chapter 26 focusing on the person who experiences bipolar disorder. How to support those with a personality disorder is considered in Chapter 27 and those with disturbing voices, ideas and beliefs are discussed in Chapter 28. Chapter 29 pays attention to individuals who have experience of sexual abuse while Chapter 30 looks at those with an eating disorder and Chapter 31 explores mental health and substance misuse problems. Sexuality and gender is the basis of Chapter 32 and, finally, dementia is discussed in Chapter 33.

Section 4: Care planning and approaches to therapeutic practice explores a range of approaches from the more general to the specialist, beginning with the admission of a person in acute distress in Chapter 34. What the recovery approach really means is explored in Chapter 35 and the recovery approach and risk is looked at in Chapter 36. Using the care programme approach is considered in Chapter 37 and culturally safe care in Chapter 38. The remainder of this section considers more specific interventions. For example, motivational interviewing in Chapter 39, cognitive behaviour therapy in Chapter 40, and solution focused approaches in Chapter 41. Psychodynamic interventions are the focus of Chapters 42 and 43. Mindfulness forms the basis of Chapter 44, with early interventions the focus of Chapter 45. Chapter 46 explores crisis assessment and resolution. This section concludes with Chapter 47 addressing psychopharmacology and mental health and Chapter 48 considering psychopharmacology in clinical practice.

Section 5: Services and support for those with mental health distress considers individual and generic support services available to those experiencing mental health issues. Chapter 49 covers what it means to be a carer for someone with a mental health problem, followed by collaborative care planning with service users and carers in Chapter 50. Family involvement and support networks are the focus of Chapter 51 and liaison services in Chapter 52. Care settings are covered in Chapter 53, concentrating on acute care, and Chapter 54 on intensive care. Mental health nursing in the community is the basis of Chapter 55 and assertive outreach is explored in Chapter 56, along with therapeutic communities in Chapter 57. Services specifically for children and young people are discussed in Chapter 58 and group treatment for adolescents in Chapter 59. Bereavement and grief counselling form the discussion for Chapter 61 and the nurse's role in the administration of ECT is the focus of Chapter 62. The remaining chapters look at services more generally. For example, Chapter 60 looks at services for individuals with both a learning disability and a mental health issue. Those who require secure forms of care are discussed in Chapter 63, while services for older people with mental health problems are considered in Chapter 64. Chapter 65 covers women's services, and services for refugees and asylum seekers are discussed in Chapter 66.

Finally, **Section 6: Opportunities and challenges for mental health nursing in the twenty-first century** focuses on some challenging issues in contemporary mental health nursing and considers the way forward. The section begins by looking at mental health, the law and human rights in Chapter 67, followed by the political landscape of mental health care in Chapter 68. Physical health care and mental health promotion are topical and challenging issues in mental health care and are considered respectively in Chapters 69 and 70. At governmental level much is made of the parity of esteem between physical and mental health care. However, the reality speaks for itself with those experiencing severe and enduring mental illness have a life expectancy between 10 and 20 years less than the general population. The importance of developing a metric in mental health nursing is the focus of Chapter 71, with healthcare technology and mental health discussed in Chapter 72. This section concludes with Chapter 73's consideration of mental health nursing in the twenty-first century.

I wish to thank everyone who has contributed to the completion of this book; without your commitment, diligence, patience and support it would not have been possible. It has been a huge pleasure and honour working with each and every one of you. I would also like to thank Holly Elson for her help with chapter management and, finally, a thank you to Naomi Wilkinson, Jennifer Blaise, and Grace McInnes from Routledge and our copy-editor Kathleen McCully and project manager Nora Naughton, from NPM, who have encouraged, supported and guided me throughout this journey and to whom I am extremely grateful.

Mary Chambers
Professor of Mental Health Nursing
Director, Centre for Public Engagement
Associate Editor, Health Expectations

Section 1

Aspects of mental health nursing

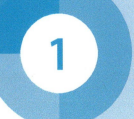

1 The nature of mental health nursing

BEN THOMAS

LEARNING OUTCOMES

- To know what values-based practice means and its importance in mental health nursing.
- To be able to describe recent government policies relating to mental health and their implications for mental health nursing.
- To understand the wider context of nursing and the application of the 6 Cs (*Compassion in practice*) to mental health nursing.
- To be able to identify the difference between competence and capability and their development in mental health nursing.
- To be aware of the national reviews of mental health nursing and the changing nature of the profession.
- To understand some recent developments and future directions for mental health nursing.

SUMMARY OF KEY POINTS

- Mental health nurses have a key role to play in implementing the major developments and changes taking place in mental health services globally.
- The role of the mental health nurse continues to evolve in response to changing societal needs and priorities for health and social care.
- Mental health nurses are key contributors to mental health policy and in defining the vision for the future mental health of the population.
- The role of mental health nurses has to be positioned within the wider context of nursing, particularly the overall vision and strategy, professional standards of practice and behaviour changes in nurse education, and the developing evidence base of nursing.
- People who use mental health services can expect to receive skilled, compassionate care and support from competent and capable mental health nurses.
- There are a number of internal and external influences that will affect the future development of mental health nursing, including social and economic determinants and advances in the evidence base for the care and treatment of people with mental health problems.

INTRODUCTION

This chapter provides a broad overview of mental health nursing as it is currently practised in England. Since nurses are the largest group of professionals providing mental health care in most countries, the chapter will have wider value beyond England. It will also be of relevance to the many countries which have little or no information on their nursing workforce for mental health and limited knowledge of their impact on health outcomes. The chapter highlights some of the major government policies relating to mental health and their impact on mental health nursing. Worldwide many countries require a radical change in the delivery of mental health care, and some are yet to prevent abuses of human rights and discrimination against people with mental health problems. According to the World Health Organization, only 36 per cent of people living in low-income countries are covered by mental health legislation compared with 92 per cent in high-income countries.[1] Nevertheless, in some countries mental health care has undergone major changes and it is clear that governments are committed to improving services. Nurses have a central role to play in implementing these developments and initiatives. Mental health nursing is examined in the context of nursing more widely and the competencies, skills and capabilities required are described. The chapter concludes with a look at future trends and drivers which will affect the profession, including an emphasis on health promotion and the prevention of mental health problems, demographic changes and advances in digital technology.

MENTAL HEALTH NURSING TODAY

The role of the mental health nurse continues to evolve in response to changing societal needs and priorities for health and social care. Mental health nurses play a key role in delivering mental health services in many countries around the world. They work with people with mental health problems, their families and carers, across the life course. They work in a diverse range of settings, including acute admission wards, community teams, emergency departments, the independent and voluntary sectors, the criminal justice system and education. Globally, nurses represent the most prevalent professional group working in mental health services. The median rate of nurses in this sector (5.8 per 100,000 population) is greater than the rate of all other human resources groups combined. Being the largest professional group working in mental health services, mental health nurses have huge potential and opportunities to influence health and social care, and people's health outcomes. There are 95,913 nurses registered with the Nursing and Midwifery Council (NMC) with a mental health qualification in the UK. Out of these, 37,930 mental health nurses work in the NHS. The number of mental health nurses working in social care and in the voluntary and independent sectors is not known but is estimated at several thousand.

Worldwide there is a substantial gap between the burden caused by mental health problems and the resources available to prevent and treat them. It is estimated that 4 out of 5 people with serious mental disorders living in low- and middle-income countries do not receive the mental health services that they need. Depression alone accounts for 4.3 per cent of the global burden of disease and is among the greatest single causes of disability worldwide. It is estimated that the cumulative global impact of mental health problems in terms of lost economic output will amount to US$16.3 trillion between 2011 and 2030.[1]

Mental health problems are responsible for the largest burden of disease in England, 23 per cent of the total burden compared to 16 per cent for cancer and 16 per cent for heart disease. Mental disorder affects more than 1 in 4 of the population at any one time and costs the English economy £105 billion a year.[2] With increasing needs and expanding services, there is a pressure on workforce supply. It is vital that we invest in the current and future nursing workforce to have the capacity and capability to deliver services that provide a good experience and improved health outcomes for people with mental health problems. Health Education England (HEE) is responsible for overseeing and where necessary building the workforce. In 2015/16 HEE increased the number of mental health student nurse commissions by 3.2 per cent, which equals 3,243 student mental health nursing places altogether for England.

Following a number of high-profile national reports, such as the report of the Mid Staffordshire inquiry,[3] HEE invited Lord Willis to be the independent chair of the 'Shape of Caring' review to determine the future education and training of registered nurses and care assistants. The report published in March 2015 includes 34 recommendations under 8 broad themes. The recommendations and the implications for mental health nursing are discussed in more detail in chapter 73.

Developments in mental health services over the last decade have provided many opportunities for mental health nurses to expand their role, develop new skills and acquire more autonomy and responsibility. Many mental health nurses are specialists who prescribe medications and treatments and make referrals to other services. Some mental health nurses lead their own services and run their own clinics, assessing and caring for people who self-refer or are directly referred from others. Working in partnership with service users and carers, many have developed new services and models of care: for example, providing 24-hour crisis care; street triage – working with police officers as a first-line response for people with mental health problems; providing school-based early interventions and targeted mental health support for vulnerable children and their families; and assessing and supporting refugees and asylum seekers. The many varied new roles taken on by mental health nurses include nurse consultants, modern matrons and advanced nurse practitioners. It is clear from all these developments that mental health nursing is increasing in complexity and diversity. Mental health nurses seldom work on their own. Generally, mental health nurses work as part of a multidisciplinary team with psychiatrists, general practitioners, psychologists and social workers. The complexities of multidisciplinary team working are increasing as nurses take on new roles in integrated services such as the criminal justice system. Changes in mental health law have also enabled mental health nurses to take on roles previously held by other professionals, such as the 'approved' mental health practitioner. The development of these new roles is seen as important in strengthening the capacity of the profession, improving its image and making mental health nursing an attractive career option, enhancing clinical career structures and providing fulfilling jobs and opportunities.

UNDERSTANDING THE NATURE OF MENTAL HEALTH NURSING

The primary purpose of mental health nursing is to promote mental health and quality of life, and to deliver compassionate care and support to people with mental health problems, their families and carers. As with all professional groups, mental health nurses are encouraged to continuously reflect upon their role and on how they deliver care, and seek to improve the way they function and develop in response to changing needs and a rapidly transforming health and social environment. Through reflection and supervision it is important that mental health nurses explore the emotional impact of their work on self, and on their personal and professional values and beliefs. See Chapters 10 and 11 for further information on clinical supervision and critical reflection respectively.

The professional values base for mental health nurses is the key element underpinning practice (Box 1.1). Nurses continue to build on these as they aspire to provide the most humane care possible and strengthen the profession.

BOX 1.1: THE VALUES BASE FOR MENTAL HEALTH NURSING

Mental health nursing is based on clear values that include person-centred, compassionate and holistic care using a recovery-orientated approach which requires the formation of a therapeutic relationship between the nurse and the service user. It includes working collaboratively with family and carers. Central to this are the following underpinning principles that guide mental health nursing practice.

Human rights
Respect and uphold people's human rights, regardless of status. Promote awareness of human rights and challenge oppression.

Personalization
Support the individual's choice and control over their own life and services through care, support and empowerment.

Recognizing diversity
Recognize diversity including values, needs and circumstances of individuals, including their age, disability, gender, marital status, race, religion, sexual orientation, culture and individual choice.

Challenging inequality
Challenge discrimination, stigma and prejudice, and practise non-discrimination and equality.

Social inclusion
Promote social inclusion and enable people and communities to fully participate in society and contribute to community life.

Parity of esteem
Mental health should have the same value as physical health and people with mental health problems should have the same access and opportunities as anyone else.

Person-centred
Provide care tailored to each individual based on needs and goals that are significant to the person.

Strengths-based
Work collaboratively with service users to meet the needs of the individual and help people to make informed decisions about their care.

Respect
Value the whole person and the diversity of people who support and sustain him or her. Appreciate the contribution of families and carers and, where possible, enhance the contribution of others.

Partnership working and integrated care
Ensure care is integrated around the service user to enhance their quality of life and enable them to regain independence.

POLICY DIRECTION AND MENTAL HEALTH NURSING

Mental health policy defines the vision for the future mental health of the population, specifying the framework which will be put in place to manage and prevent priority mental problems. Mental health policy can coordinate essential services and activities to ensure that treatment and care are delivered to those in need, while at the same time preventing fragmentation and inefficiencies in the health system.

From a national policy perspective in England, the last few years have seen a transformation of mental health services across the country. The principle of parity of esteem (that mental health and physical health are regarded and valued equally) has been enshrined in legislation via the Health and Social Care Act 2012,[4] and the priorities for change and high quality care set out in *Closing the gap*[5] and *Achieving better access to mental health services by 2020*[6] have been delivered. Mental health nurses have played their part in making these improvements a reality at local level. It is important to acknowledge the considerable progress made, but we must build on this to deliver benefits for all service users and their carers. As a profession, we need to be clear about our contribution not only to the current delivery of effective services but also to the future. Mental health nurses are central to developing and providing services that are innovative and responsive, and which are organized around the needs of service users. The government's strategy, set out in *No health without mental health* (2011),[2] adopts a new approach whereby change is to be achieved by adopting more localized control, a focus on mental health outcomes, early intervention, prevention and promotion of health. The strategy set out six shared high-level health objectives, outlined in Box 1.2.

A significant amount of progress has already been achieved, including the introduction of the first access and waiting time standards in mental health. There has been a national roll-out of Improving Access to Psychological Therapies (IAPT). Significant achievements have been made in crisis care driven by the Crisis Care Concordat,[7] with a reduction of 55 per cent in the use of police cells as places of safety (from 8,000 to less than 4,000 cases) over 3 years. *Positive and proactive care: reducing the need for restrictive interventions*[8] has resulted in mental health services introducing restrictive interventions reduction programmes. Time to Change, the country's largest anti-stigma and discrimination campaign, has seen a 6 per cent improvement (representing more than 2.5 million people) in public attitudes to people with mental health problems in 3 years.

In 2016 the Independent Mental Health Taskforce to the NHS in England published the *Five year forward view for mental health* (see 'Relevant web pages').

BOX 1.2: THE SIX MENTAL HEALTH OBJECTIVES

More people will have good mental health
More people of all ages and backgrounds will have better wellbeing and good mental health.

Fewer people will develop mental health problems – by starting well, developing well, working well, living well and ageing well.

More people with mental health problems will recover
More people who develop mental health problems will have a good quality of life – greater ability to manage their own lives, stronger social relationships, a greater sense of purpose, the skills they need for living and working, improved chances in education, better employment rates and a suitable and stable place to live.

More people with mental health problems will have good physical health
Fewer people with mental health problems will die prematurely, and more people with physical ill health will have better mental health.

More people will have a positive experience of care and support
Care and support, wherever it takes place, should offer access to timely, evidence-based interventions and approaches that give people the greatest choice and control over their own lives, in the least restrictive environment, and should ensure that people's human rights are protected.

Fewer people will suffer avoidable harm
People receiving care and support should have confidence that the services they use are of the highest quality and at least as safe as any other public service.

Fewer people will experience stigma and discrimination
Public understanding of mental health will improve and, as a result, negative attitudes and behaviours to people with mental health problems will decrease.

Source: Department of Health, *No health without mental health: a cross-government mental health outcomes strategy for people of all ages.* London: COI: 2011: 6.

From a public consultation involving over 20,000 people, the report sets out the start of a 10-year journey to further transform mental health service based on the priorities of prevention, access, integration, quality and a positive experience of care. Mental health nurses will be crucial in bringing about the changes identified in the report and to drive forward these improvements.

THE WIDER NURSING CONTEXT

Before considering the competencies, capabilities and skills of mental health nurses, we must be mindful that mental health nursing is only one field of nursing, and, like all registered nurses, mental health nurses are expected to meet the essential mental and physical health needs of people of all ages and conditions. Current policy for mental health care in England and the role of mental health nurses in its delivery has to be positioned within the wider context of nursing, particularly the overall vision and strategy, our professional standards of practice and behaviour, changes in nursing education, and the developing evidence base for nursing. *Compassion in practice: nursing, midwifery and care staff - our vision and strategy* (2013)[9] identifies six qualities (6 Cs) that are required of all nurses, midwives and care staff (see Figure 1.1). The next section examines the applicability of the 6 Cs for mental health nursing.

Care based on choice and inclusion

In common with nurses working in other fields of practice, mental health nurses provide person-centred care and treatment to meet people's physical, psychological, social, mental and spiritual care needs. This includes providing support and involves families, carers and friends who play a significant role in people's lives in a way that supports their recovery. Providing person-centred care is a leading value of mental health nursing. There are a number of definitions of person-centred care. In general it is taken to mean seeing the person as a unique individual, taking into account their expectations and preferences and responding in a flexible manner through engagement built on empathy and trust which forms the basis of the nurse–patient therapeutic relationship.

In 2011 the National Institute for Health and Care Excellence (NICE) issued guidance and best practice advice on improving the experience of people who use adult NHS mental health services. The guidance aims to promote person-centred care that takes into account service users'

needs, preferences and strengths. People who use mental health services should have the opportunity to make informed decisions about their care and treatment, in partnership with their health and social care practitioners.[10] If service users do not have the capacity to make decisions, health care professionals should follow the Department of Health's advice on consent and the code of practice that accompanies the Mental Capacity Act 2005.[11] The Mental Capacity Act[12] aims to protect people who lack mental capacity but need to be deprived of liberty in order to receive appropriate care and treatment in hospitals and care homes.

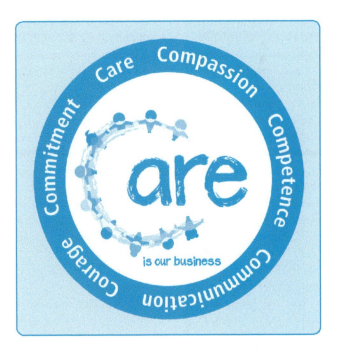

Figure 1.1 The '6 Cs' vision for nurses, midwives and care staff in England. (Source: Department of Health. *Compassion in practice: nursing, midwifery and care staff - our vision and strategy.* London: DH, 2013: 28.)

If the service user consents, families and carers should have the opportunity to be involved in decisions about treatment and care. The Triangle of Care[13] is a good example of carers and staff working together to improve carer engagement in mental health services, and provides examples of partnership working between service users, their carers and staff.

Mental health nursing is distinctive because at its core is the professional therapeutic relationships nurses form with the people they care for. See Chapter 3 for more information on developing and maintaining therapeutic relationships. It is about mental health nurses' ability to deliver care in a way that focuses on the therapeutic use of self, and using this dynamic process to facilitate improvement in the health and well-being of others.

Mental health nurses use a range of relationship-building and communication skills to work in partnership with people to support them in their recovery. These include an ability to offer specific interventions, such as psychological therapies, family therapies, and other relationship and communication-based group and individual interventions.

Compassion, communication and therapeutic relationships

Compassion is how care is given through relationships based on empathy, respect and dignity. Developing a therapeutic relationship between the mental health nurse and the service user is the essence of mental health nursing and is critical to the success of any nursing intervention. The nurse's skills in developing, maintaining and ending a therapeutic relationship are crucial to promoting recovery and improving health outcomes. These skills include self-awareness, therapeutic communication involving verbal and non-verbal communication, attentive listening, setting clinical boundaries and the therapeutic use of self.

Therapeutic use of self involves nurses applying their own personality factors, perceptions, judgements and insights in an intentional way. Mental health nurses need to empathize with the people they care for and show warmth and respect for them. The values and qualities that service users repeatedly state they find helpful in mental health nurses, and which they find aid their recovery, include being friendly and approachable, being consistent and honest, and having integrity. Taken together, this is what good mental health nursing should look like.

The code: professional standards of practice and behaviour for nurses and midwives[14] articulates clearly that nurses should put the interests of people using or needing nursing first. Nurses must make sure that the care and safety of people using the service is their main concern, preserving their dignity, treating them with respect and upholding their rights. They must challenge any discriminatory attitudes and behaviours towards those receiving care.

Courage – evolving responsibilities, safety and protection

Courage enables us to do the right thing for the people we care for, to speak up when we have concerns and to have the personal strength and vision to innovate and to embrace new ways of working. People with mental health problems are often very vulnerable, not least due to the stigma and discrimination they experience. Mental health nurses are well aware of the vulnerability of the people in their care, but improving patient safety in mental health is a significant challenge. Recent developments have increased the nurse's role in improving safety. Mental health nurses are expected to speak out against poor practice and discriminatory attitudes, including those situations which oppose the freedom of choice of the individual. Failure to do so damages the trust which is the basis of the therapeutic relationship, and could contravene the human rights of the individual.

The Equality Act 2010[15] replaces all previous anti-discrimination legislation and requires public bodies to have due regard to the need to eliminate discrimination and to advance equality of opportunity and foster good relations between people who share certain protected characteristics and those who do not. The protected characteristics are age, disability, gender reassignment, pregnancy and maternity, race, religion or belief, sex and sexual orientation. The Act provides an important legal framework which should improve the experience of all mental health service users, particularly those from black and minority ethnic communities.

The NMC Code (2015)[16] is clear that nurses must raise concerns immediately if they believe a person is vulnerable or at risk and needs extra support and protection. Nurses must be aware of and conform to the relevant laws and policies relating to protecting and caring for vulnerable people, including the Mental Capacity Act (MCA).[11] In particular nurses need to be familiar with the principles and main provision of the MCA to understand when a person may lack the capacity to take particular decisions for themselves and to know when decisions should be taken in their best interests. The Deprivation of Liberty Safeguards were introduced in 2009 and are part of the Mental Capacity Act 2005.[11] The safeguards are used to protect the rights of people who lack the ability to make certain decisions for themselves and make sure that their freedom is not inappropriately restricted. They do this by empowering people to make their own decisions wherever possible and, when necessary, making sure that decisions made on their behalf are in their best interests.

Safeguarding describes the function of protecting adults and children from abuse and neglect, and it is central to mental health nursing due to the vulnerability of those whom nurses care for. It involves protecting the most vulnerable individuals and communities, as well as promoting the safety, health and well-being of all. Abuse is a violation of an individual's human and civil rights by another person(s). It is about the misuse of power and control that one person has over another. Where there is dependency, there is a possibility of abuse or neglect unless adequate safeguards are in place.

The rights and procedures for NHS staff to raise concerns about safety, malpractice and wrongdoing in clinical practice are popularly known as whistleblowing. Nurses are supported to speak out about concerns in care through the national whistleblowing policy for the NHS. The NMC provides guidance and toolkits for nursing staff.[16] The Care Quality Commission (CQC) has also published guidance for NHS staff about whistleblowing and how to raise concerns with the CQC if they do not feel able to report their concerns internally.[17]

Commitment to promoting recovery

A commitment to service users and to society is a cornerstone of what mental health nurses do. We need to build on our commitment to improve care and the experience of service users. There are many areas in mental health care that require commitment, but two particular examples where much progress has occurred (though more still needs to be done) are promoting recovery and parity of esteem.

[Recovery is] … a way of living a satisfying hopeful and contributing life, even with limitations caused by illness. Recovery involves the development of new meaning and purpose in one's life as one grows beyond the catastrophic effects …[18] (p.15)

In recent years there has been a clear expectation from service users and carers to have choice in the services they receive, to have information and support to manage their own mental health, and for services to be based on the principles of recovery. High quality mental health services are seen as recovery-focused. Services that use recovery as the guiding vision provide care that is focused around the needs of the service user, and extend beyond care and treatment to helping people rebuild their lives and do the things that are important to them, helping them take control and responsibility and live the life they choose. This approach has changed the way we think about the role of mental health nurses. Recovery-focused approaches mean that mental health nurses must be able to work alongside people in a way that supports them to live meaningful and satisfying lives, as defined by them, in the presence or absence of symptoms.

The experience of mental health problems and recovery is a deeply personal process that is unique to the person. For mental health nurses this means they need to work in a way that shifts the emphasis from being seen as 'experts' towards working in a way that recognizes and maximizes the person's own expertise and strengths. Recovery means new ways of working, including new skills and values that enable people's self-direction and social inclusion. The recovery approach helps and focuses us on providing person-centred care, with a shared responsibility for positive risk taking. Chapters 35 and 36 provide a fuller explanation of the recovery approach.

Mental health nurses often have to care and provide treatment for people who are detained under the Mental Health Act without those people's consent. In such an event it is important that the guiding principle of the Act's Code of Practice are applied. Nurses taking action without a person's consent must attempt to keep the restrictions they impose on the person's liberty to a minimum, having regard to the purpose for which the restrictions are imposed. Mental health nurses have to deal with difficult and sometimes threatening situations.[8,19] Workplace violence is often associated with mental health services, and figures reported for physical assaults on NHS staff would support this view, with 47,181 total physical assaults reported in 2013/14.[20] Mental health nurses are trained in the special skills required to identify a build-up of tension and to be able to defuse it by preventing escalation to more violent behaviour. A more detailed account of nursing the person who is extremely distressed and disturbed is provided in chapter 25.

Commitment to parity of esteem

Parity of esteem means mental health having the same value as physical health. Unfortunately, service users still complain that their physical health needs are often ignored by staff. They frequently complain that the side effects of their antipsychotic medication have not been monitored or managed. Evidence clearly shows that people with mental illness have poorer physical health than the general population. They also have difficulties accessing and using general health services. Whereas previously mental health nurses tended to see physical health and mental health separately, generally this is no longer the case. The NMC *Standards for competence for registered nurses* (2014)[21] clearly state that all registered nurses are expected to meet the essential mental and physical needs of people of all ages and conditions. Following on from the White Paper *Choosing health*,[22] recommendation 7 of the Chief Nursing Officer's (CNO's) 2006 review of mental health nursing[23] proposed that mental health nurses will have the skills and opportunities to improve the physical well-being of people with mental health problems.

Mental Health Act 1983: Code of Practice

Promoting good physical health is a requirement of the *Mental Health Act 1983: Code of Practice*.[24] The Code requires commissioners and providers to ensure that patients living with a mental problem receive physical health care that is equivalent to that received by people who are not living with a mental problem. Commissioners should ensure that long-term physical health conditions are diagnosed and treated, and that patients receive regular oral health and sensory assessments and, as required, are referred to appropriate specialists. Physical health and health promotion are covered in more detail in chapters 69 and 70 respectively.

The Code highlights that patients detained under the Act are at particular risk of comorbidities. It emphasizes that commissioners should build into their procurement outcomes the requirement for physical health checks, and physical health care planning. Reporting arrangements should include evidence that physical health issues have been routinely considered for every individual patient for whom they have commissioned services.

MENTAL HEALTH NURSES – COMPETENT AND CAPABLE

Definitions

Competence is what 'individuals know or are able to do in terms of knowledge, skills and attitudes'[25] (p.799).

Capability is the 'extent to which an individual can apply, adapt and synthesise new knowledge from experience and so continue to improve their performance'[25] (p.799).

A 'competency framework' is a structure that sets out and defines each individual competency (such as problem solving or people management) required by individuals working in an organization or part of it.

The terms 'competency' and 'competencies' focus on the personal attributes or inputs of an individual. They can be defined as the behaviours (and technical attributes, where appropriate) that individuals must have, or must acquire, to perform effectively at work. 'Competence' and 'competences' are broader concepts that encompass demonstrable performance outputs as well as behaviour inputs, and may relate to a system or set of minimum standards required for effective performance at work.

To deliver mental health care and improve people's mental health, nurses require a mix of behaviour, attitude and action that results in the highest quality care, which is both safe and effective. This requires having the right numbers of nurses with the right values and having mental health nurses with the right competencies and capabilities to meet service users' needs now and in the future. In mental health, considerable time and effort has gone into identifying core competencies and capabilities for mental health nurses, particularly at the point of registration.

The ten essential shared capabilities: a framework for the whole of the mental health workforce

Following the publication of the National Service Framework for Mental Health (NSF)[26] and the NHS Plan (NHSP),[27] the Capable Practitioner Framework (CPF) was developed and a mapping exercise of mental health education and training in England took place.

The CPF described the capabilities that all staff should have and what would be expected by some specialists. Nationally the CPF was well received and was used to influence curriculum development, training needs analysis and personal development planning.

The outcome of the national mapping exercise showed that there were significant gaps in the pre- and post-qualification training of all professional staff working in mental health in their ability to deliver the NSF and the NHSP. Significant omissions included service user and carer involvement, mental health promotion, values and evidence-based practice, working with families, multidisciplinary working and working with diversity.

The results of this work led to the development of the Essential Shared Capabilities (ESC).[28] These were developed in a wide consultation with service users, carers and health care staff. The ESCs are the top capabilities required to achieve best practice for education and training for all staff who work in mental health services (see Box 1.3).

The ESCs make explicit what should be included as core in the curricula of all pre- and post-qualification training for professional affiliated staff, as well as being embedded in induction and continuing professional/practitioner development (CPD) programmes. The ESCs were not intended to replace the CPF, the National Occupational Standards or the NHS Knowledge and Skills Framework (KSF), but were complementary to these frameworks and provided the mental health specific context and achievements for education, training and CPD at pre-registration/qualification stage.

Best practice competencies and capabilities for pre-registration mental health nurses[29]

The best practice competencies and capabilities for pre-registration for mental health nursing were developed to complement the CNO's review of mental health nursing.[23] The CNO review was established following a number of structural changes and development of mental health services and to provide a future focus for the profession. Both the review and the guidelines involved a wide consultation exercise including practising mental health nurses, mental health nursing academics, service users, carers and service managers. The competencies and capabilities reflect the main areas of the CNO's review of mental health nursing. They are mapped against previous work by the NMC in setting learning outcomes for pre-registration nursing programmes, the ESCs for mental health practice, the National Occupational Standards for Mental Health, and Skills for Health competencies for mental health practice. In order to be fit to practise as a registered nurse, students need to have the best competencies and capabilities. These include developing and promoting positive attitudes to people with mental health problems; engaging with service users, carers and families through the therapeutic use of self; and understanding the central role of interpersonal relationships and empathy in mental health nursing (see Box 1.4).

BOX 1.3: THE TEN ESSENTIAL SHARED CAPABILITIES FOR MENTAL HEALTH PRACTICE

1. *Working in partnership.* Developing and maintaining constructive working relationships with service users, carers, families, colleagues, lay people and wider community networks. Working positively with any tensions created by conflicts of interest or aspiration that may arise between the partners in care.

2. *Respecting diversity.* Working in partnership with service users, carers, families and colleagues to provide care and interventions that not only make a positive difference but also do so in ways that respect and value diversity, including age, race, culture, disability, gender, spirituality and sexuality.

3. *Practising ethically.* Recognising the rights and aspirations of service users and their families, acknowledging power differentials and minimising them whenever possible. Providing treatment and care that is accountable to service users and carers within the boundaries prescribed by national (professional), legal and local codes of ethical practice.

4. *Challenging inequality.* Addressing the causes and consequences of stigma, discrimination, social inequality and exclusion on service users, carers and mental health services. Creating, developing or maintaining valued social roles for people in the communities they come from.

5. *Promoting recovery.* Working in partnership to provide care and treatment that enables service users and carers to tackle mental health problems with hope and optimism and to work towards a valued lifestyle within and beyond the limits of any mental health problem.

6. *Identifying people's needs and strengths.* Working in partnership to gather information to agree health and social care needs in the context of the preferred lifestyle and aspirations of service users, their families, carers and friends.

7. *Providing service user-centred care.* Negotiating achievable and meaningful goals, primarily from the perspective of service users and their families. Influencing and seeking the means to achieve these goals and clarifying the responsibilities of the people who will provide any help that is needed, including systematically evaluating outcomes and achievements.

8. *Making a difference.* Facilitating access to and delivering the best quality evidence-based, values-based health and social care interventions to meet the needs and aspirations of service users and their families and carers.

9. *Promoting safety and positive risk taking.* Empowering the person to decide the level of risk they are prepared to take with their health and safety. This includes working with the tension between promoting safety and positive risk taking, including assessing and dealing with possible risks for service users, carers, family members and the wider public.

10. *Personal development and learning.* Keeping up-to-date with changes in practice and participating in life-long learning, personal and professional development for one's self and colleagues through supervision, appraisal and reflective practice.

Source: Department of Health. *The ten essential shared capabilities: a framework for the whole of the mental health workforce.* London: DH, 2004: 3.

REFLECTION

- What does caring mean to you as a mental health nurse?

- What skills are required for mental health nurses to work in partnership with service users?

- What do you understand by compassion and its relevance for mental health nursing?

- Compare the principles underpinning the recovery approach with a service in which you have experienced working or training. Can you identify ways the service could develop its approach to focus more on recovery?

- How much is your own practice based on the recovery approach?

- What do you understand by parity of esteem? Do you think mental health nurses should be trained to carry out physical health assessments?

BOX 1.4: BEST PRACTICE COMPETENCIES AND CAPABILITIES FOR PRE-REGISTRATION MENTAL HEALTH NURSES

- Promote a culture that values and respects the diversity of individuals, and enables their recovery
- Use a range of communication skills to establish, maintain and manage relationships with individuals who have mental health problems, their carers and key people involved in their care
- Promote physical health and well-being for people with mental health problems
- Promote mental health and well-being, enabling people to recover from debilitating mental health experiences and/or achieve their full potential, supporting them to develop and maintain social networks and relationships

- Work with individuals with mental health needs in order to maintain health, safety and well-being
- Work collaboratively with other disciplines and agencies to support individuals to develop and maintain social networks and relationships
- Demonstrate a commitment to the need for continuing professional development and personal supervision activities, in order to enhance the knowledge, skills, values and attitudes needed for safe and effective nursing practice

Source: Department of Health. *From values to action: the Chief Nursing Officer's Review of Mental Health Nursing.* London: DH, 2006: 5.

THE CRAFT OF CARING

Being a competent and capable mental health nurse means providing care effectively. It means nurses being able to use their skills and knowledge in responding to the service user's needs and becoming fully engaged with them, using a person-centred approach. This involves combining those aspects that make up the art and science of nursing and is often referred to as the craft of caring. As society becomes more dependent on technology, it is often easier to identify and give prominence to the scientific aspects, which nurses need to know – for example, the functioning of the central nervous system, cognitive development, administering medicines and monitoring their side effects. These are all important to mental health nursing.

On the other hand, the art of nursing is more than just knowing; it is relationship-based and includes the way nurses use the caring relationship to listen to someone who is depressed, and what they say to someone who is distressed because they are hearing voices. The art is in the way the nurse provides information and uses every contact in a meaningful way. It is the application of all the knowledge and skills of the nurse to provide excellence in carrying out nursing.

These actions require nurses to practise to become confident in how best to engage with service users and meet their needs. The craft of caring requires using every opportunity for nurses to grow in their ability, constantly improving and polishing their approach, gaining mastery over their craft.

The proper focus of nursing is said to be the craft of caring and the value of care is defined by those who receive it.[30] The next section examines whether mental health nurses satisfy the needs and expectations of service users.

THE VIEWS OF PEOPLE WITH LIVED EXPERIENCE: SERVICE USERS AND CARERS

The views of and expectations of mental health nurses held by people with a lived experience, service users and carers, are essential to understanding the contribution the profession makes to their care, treatment, health and well-being. Such feedback identifies areas for improvement and future development. Mental health nurses are highly valued by people with mental health problems, and their families and carers. People want nurses to treat them with compassion and dignity; they want them to recognize and respect their diverse needs, and to consider their views and feelings.

A systematic review by Bee et al.[31] relating to service users' views of mental health nurses identified that a large number of studies reported on the range of skills, qualities and responsibilities that service users thought essential to effective mental health nursing. Service users' views of the key factors that make up the service user and mental health nurse relationship were of central importance. Service users like continuity of care and familiar staff. They do not like high staff turnover, high levels of staff sickness and the increasing use of temporary bank/agency staff. Similar findings have been reported more recently suggesting that suicidal patients may be put at risk by a reliance on inexperienced and agency nurses.[32] The importance of service users spending more time with mental health nurses has been a constant theme throughout a number of studies and reports. One-to-one time is seen as an opportunity for service users to express how they are feeling, to discuss worries and problems and to explore possible solutions. Bee et al.[31] concluded that there is a consistently identified core set of views among service users that involve an expectation that mental health nurses will fulfil a multi-faceted role that combines practical and social support alongside the more formal psychological interventions. Services users expect mental health nurses to possess and exhibit both specific clinical skills and more generic skills and attributes related to effective interpersonal communication. The importance of spending individual time with service users has been acknowledged with the introduction of the 'protected time' initiative. However, evaluation studies of the use of protected time in mental health services shows there is still much variation in practice.[33]

Feedback from service users, carers and families has become formalized with the introduction of the Friends and Family Test (FFT). It asks people if they would recommend the services they have used. When combined with supplementary follow-up questions, the FFT provides a mechanism to highlight both good and poor patient experience. This kind of feedback is vital in transforming NHS services and supporting patient choice.

NATIONAL REVIEWS OF MENTAL HEALTH NURSING – LESSONS LEARNT

National reviews of mental health nursing usefully serve two functions. First, they provide us with a snapshot of the state of mental health nursing during a particular historical period, and second they help drive improvements and help us prepare for the future.

Psychiatric nursing – today and tomorrow (1968)[34]

This review took place in 1968. The report focused particularly on inpatient psychiatric nursing at a time when there were approximately 130,000 inpatients, mostly contained in old Victorian asylums. The role of the mental health nurse has changed radically since this review, particularly with the process of de-institutionalization, whereby many service users are treated and cared for in the community.

Working in partnership: a collaborative approach to care (1994)[35]

About 25 years later, a further comprehensive review of mental health nursing took place with the aim 'To identify the future requirements for skilled nursing care in the light of developments in the provision of services for people with mental illness'[35] (p.vi). The review clearly identified that the work of mental health nurses rests on their relationship with people who use mental health services and that the relationship should have value to both partners.

The review followed the significant changes which had occurred in service provision, in professional roles, in education and in the development of research. However, the important major change was working in partnership with service users. Service users expect to be treated equally and to work in partnership with nurses, and the review clearly articulated that the principle of user and carer choice needed to be firmly established as a basis for the practice of mental health nursing.

From values to action: the Chief Nursing Officer's review of mental health nursing (2006)[29]

In 2005 the CNO for England set up a review of mental health nursing to address the question 'How can mental health nursing best contribute to the care of service users in the future?' The review, published in 2006, set out a vision for mental health nursing for the next 10 years. The vision articulated the values that should inform every aspect of mental health practice, including the requirement that mental health nurses should incorporate the principles of the recovery approach into every aspect of their practice. In addition, the vision called for all mental health nurses to reduce health inequalities and ensure all groups in society receive an equal service.

The review aimed to improve the outcomes and experience for service users and carers. In order to do so, mental health nurses were to be equipped with the skills to develop and sustain positive therapeutic relationships, which should form the basis of all care. They were to provide person-centred and holistic care, taking into account physical, psychological, social and spiritual needs. Nurses were expected to promote good health as well as treat ill-health. It also set out the following aims:

- Inpatient care should be improved.
- Mental health nurses need to be well trained in risk assessment and management.
- They should work closely with service users and others to develop realistic individual care plans.

The following features should characterize a positive, modern, profession:

- Mental health nurses should focus on working directly with people with high levels of need and supporting other workers to meet less complex needs.

- Pre-registration training courses should be reviewed to ensure that essential competencies are gained.
- Career structures should be reviewed according to local needs and a range of new nursing roles should be developed.
- The recruitment and retention of mental health nurses needs to be improved.

Evaluation of the Chief Nursing Officer's review of mental health nursing in England (2009)

The impact of the CNO's 2006 review on mental health trusts (MHTs) and higher education institutes (HEIs) was systematically evaluated. The results show that, while the review was accepted in MHTs, implementation varied considerably and it was difficult to demonstrate that any changes or improvements were directly attributable to the review. Poor implementation of the recommendations seems to be associated with a lack of an implementation plan at both national and local level, and competing Trust priorities. Many MHTs reported making progress towards implementation; however, detailed case studies of selected

Trusts did not support this assertion. In contrast, in HEIs there were many examples of the review guiding revision of mental health nursing education curricula. There was a clear shift towards recovery approaches and working in partnership with service users, carers and stakeholders.

> ### REFLECTION
>
> - What are the mental health nurse's responsibilities in combatting discrimination and advancing equality?
> - Can you describe the principles of the Mental Capacity Act 2005 and the statutory framework for assessing decision-making capacity and determining someone's best interests?
> - Do you think mental health nurses promote health improvement by using every contact they have with service users as an opportunity to encourage people to adopt health-promoting behaviours, such as stopping smoking?

THE FUTURE OF MENTAL HEALTH NURSING

Section 6 examines the development of mental health nursing in the twenty-first century. However, there is a need to end this chapter by highlighting some recent developments and levers for change, which will have major implications for mental health nursing. First are the findings from the Mental Health Taskforce and the *Five year forward view for mental health*. Mental health nurses must articulate their contribution to the future and find new solutions and different ways of working to tackle the challenges identified.

Second, HEE is holding engagement events across the country on the recommendations of the Lord Willis Report, which will inform the HEE Board on which recommendations to take forward, and how these might be implemented. Third, the CNO is about to publish a new nursing strategy which will have implications for all nurses.

In addition to developments in national policy, there are a number of internal and external influences that will affect the future development of mental health nursing. These include the advances in the evidence base for the care and treatment of people with mental health problems, and social and economic determinants. Three areas of particular note are described in this final section. These are, first, the importance of mental health promotion and the prevention of mental health problems; second, the changing demographic picture; and third, technological advances.

Mental health promotion and the prevention of mental health problems

It is well established that, among other factors, poor childhood experiences, inadequate housing and unemployment increase the likelihood that people may experience mental health problems and that the course of any subsequent recovery will be affected. As life expectancy increases, it is critical that healthy life expectancy increases, including mental health. Our knowledge base about which interventions and factors work to improve well-being and prevent problems developing is steadily increasing. All mental health nurses will need to maximize their role in promoting health and well-being by providing advice and support on the preventable aspects of mental health problems. They will be expected to work across all levels of practice, at individual, community and population level. There is an increasing policy drive to develop services and interventions that support population health.

Demographic changes

The biggest challenge facing every health and care system in the world is the fact that people are living longer and many have increasingly complicated health and care needs. There are 4.4 million people aged over 75 in England, and by 2026 it is estimated there will be 6.3 million over 75s. By 2018, 3 million people will have three or more long-term conditions, including dementia (the current economic impact of dementia in the UK is £26.3 billion). The need to improve dementia care has been highlighted in a number of policy documents, including the *Prime Minister's challenge on dementia* (2015).[36]

Mental health nursing needs to develop to meet the changes in population demographics and health demands, for example at the very start of life. Improving the health and well-being of children has the biggest impact on their future health in adulthood. A good start in life and positive parenting are fundamental to lifelong resilience to adversity. This is particularly important because half of lifetime mental health problems have already developed by the age of 14.

As outlined in the government's mandate to HEE, there is an expectation that training programmes will be developed that will enable health and care employers to ensure all staff have an awareness of mental health problems and how they affect their patients. The mental health and well-being of children and young people is a core theme of both the Health Visiting implementation plan and the national school nurse development programme.

Mental health nurses and technological innovations

The societal explosion in the use of digital information and communication technology (ICT) is mirrored in mental health nursing, and nurses are becoming increasingly familiar and engaged with its use. Social media, including Facebook and Twitter, have enabled communities of mental health nursing practice to develop and cut across hierarchical and organizational boundaries. For example, @WeMHnurses connects mental health nurses, enabling them to talk and share ideas and information, while #mhnursechat has grown as a voluntary social-media-based discussion and networking forum. Communication technology is helping to make care more collaborative; multidisciplinary teams can share records between professional groups and settings. Community mental health nurses have remote access to records on tablet computers during home visits, enabling them to immediately record assessments and conversations with service users and carers.

No health without mental health[2] recommends the increased use of ICT to improve care and access to services. Eight National Institute for Health Research (NIHR) Healthcare Technology Co-operatives have been established to work collaboratively with industry to develop concepts of new medical devices, health care technologies and technology-dependent interventions that improve treatment and quality of life for patients. MindTech is one of eight

NIHR Healthcare Technology Co-operatives in England, with the aim of identifying unmet clinical needs in mental health and dementia, collaborating on developing and testing a range of new technologies, and providing advice and knowledge exchange to help increase their adoption.

NICE has approved the use of computerized cognitive behavioural therapy (CCBT) for the treatment of depression, generalized anxiety disorder and panic disorder. CCBT is the name used for delivering CBT via computers, tablets and phones, usually online. Research suggests it can be just as effective as having face-to-face therapy with a therapist if people are also supported by a remote therapist.

As well as CCBT there are a range of other online mental health services available to support people with their mental health. There are a number of advantages of using online mental health services, including their 24-hour availability and easy access. Service users have greater engagement in their care and this can allow earlier detection of problems, more timely adjustment of treatment and shared decision making. Online mental health services have shorter waiting times for NHS referrals, and service users do not need to travel to clinics and outpatient departments.

Despite the clear potential of digital technology to connect people and health data in new ways, the Chief Medical Officer (CMO) offers a word of caution in terms of major issues that need to be addressed, including patient safety, confidentiality, security, and ensuring that patients and their needs remain at the centre of technology development and implementation. Regulatory guidance on m-health apps was published by the Medicines and Healthcare Products Regulatory Agency (MHRA) in March 2014, and work is underway to develop a regulatory framework.

In future the use of digital technology may no longer be an option for mental health nurses, but a requirement, as its uptake becomes more standardized. Mental health nurses will be in a prime position to test new technologies for their usability, safety and clinical effectiveness. (Further information on health care technology and mental health nursing can be found in chapter 72.) They can ensure that the use of technology empowers service users and that both they and their needs remain at the centre of its development and implementation. Mental health nurses can make the most of these opportunities to improve aspects of care and coordination, they can develop and add to the emerging evidence base for the effectiveness of digital technology, and they can ensure that the opportunity provided by data sharing between service users, carers and clinicians does not threaten privacy but is used to improve safety and quality.

CONCLUSION

This chapter has provided a broad overview of mental health nursing as it is currently practised. It has highlighted some of the major policy developments and new ways of delivering services, and how these influence the profession. It is clear that the government is committed to pushing forward with further improvements in mental health services. Together with the changing demographics, and pharmaceutical and technological advances, the future sets a challenging agenda for mental health nurses to meet the increasing health needs of the population. Such development cannot be achieved without paying attention to the skills and capabilities of the workforce. Mental health nursing will continue to develop and adapt, using new technology, and will be at the forefront of reforming services, making a difference to people's lives across the life course.

SERVICE USER COMMENTARY

Sarah Markham

This chapter provides a truly comprehensive overview of both the role of the mental health nurse and mental health nursing, both as they are now and how they might develop as the twenty-first century progresses. The author should be commended for his ability to capture and highlight the most pertinent aspects of the diverse nature of the profession.

The chapter begins by noting the demand for mental health nurses (the largest group of professionals working in mental health services) and the wide range of settings in which they perform their role. Having justified the need for mental health nurses in terms of the high incidence of mental disorders in the population, the author goes on to outline both the innovative and expansive nature of mental health nursing in terms of partnership working and co-facilitation, in relation to both service development and service user involvement.

Changes in mental health law have also enabled mental health nurses to take on roles previously held by other professionals and the implications of this for the profession are explored, together with the part mental health nurses have played in implementing national policies and initiatives such as Improved Access to Psychological Therapies (IAPT). The author also reminds the reader of the wider context of mental health nursing as but one nursing speciality, and the commonalities of ethos and motivation in all areas of nursing practice. Providing person-centred care is a leading value of mental health nursing and this is explored in all its aspects.

I am glad to see that due weight is placed on the quality and dynamic nature of the professional therapeutic relationships formed by nurses with the people they care for, and the multi-dimensional nature of this interactive interface. The therapeutic use of self, i.e. the integration of a nurse's personality into the interpretation and implementation of his/her role, with a view to improving therapeutic outcomes, is also explained, giving an indication of the depth and sophistication involved in good nursing.

With a reference to the Equality Act 2010, the importance of the role of the mental health nurse as an advocate for patients who may be quite vulnerable and the (potential) victims of mental health stigma is outlined, together with the responsibilities of safeguarding and patient safety. The potential (contentious) imbalance of power between mental health nurses and their patients, especially in the context of detention under the Mental Health Act, is mentioned without perhaps sufficient attention to the distress this may cause service users. This is followed by a more detailed exploration of the nature of mental health nursing competency and the Ten Essential Shared Capabilities for Mental Health Practice.

Last, but definitely not least, is coverage of the increasing value placed on gathering patient (and carer) experience with a view to influencing and improving mental health services. The chapter finishes with an exposition of the future of mental health nursing in the wake of the findings from the Mental Health Taskforce and various initiatives currently in implementation. (See chapter 73 for more detail on mental health nursing in the twenty-first century.)

For mental health nursing students, this chapter provides an excellent introduction to the profession which will definitely impress upon the reader the importance and multi-dimensional nature of the role. In fact, any interested party – professional, public or patient – would find this chapter interesting and informative.

Sarah Markham, BA (Hons), MA (Cantab), PhD, is a Visiting Researcher at King's Clinical Trials Unit, IoPPN, King's College London, UK.

References

1. WHO (World Health Organization). *Mental health action plan 2013–2020*. Geneva: WHO, 2013. Available from: http://www.who.int/mental_health/publications/action_plan/en/ [Accessed 8th June 2016].

2. UK Government. *No health without mental health: a cross-government mental health outcomes strategy for people of all ages*. 2011. https://www.gov.uk/government/uploads/system/uploads/attachment_data/file/213761/dh_124058.pdf [Accessed 8th June 2016].

3. Francis QC, R. *Report of the Mid Staffordshire NHS Foundation Trust Public Inquiry*. London: TSO, 2013.

4. The Stationery Office. *Health and Social Care Act*. London: TSO, 2012.

5. UK Government. *Closing the gap: priorities for essential change in mental health*. 2014. Available from: https://www.gov.uk/government/uploads/system/uploads/attachment_data/file/281250/Closing_the_gap_V2_-_17_Feb_2014.pdf [Accessed 8th June 2016].

6. UK Government. 2014. *Achieving better access to mental health services by 2020*. https://www.gov.uk/government/uploads/system/uploads/attachment_data/file/361648/mental-health-access.pdf [Accessed 8th June 2016].

7. Department of Health. *Transforming care: a national response to Winterbourne View Hospital, Department of Health Final Report*. London: DH, 2012.

8. Department of Health. *Positive and proactive care: reducing the need for restrictive interventions*. London: DH, 2014.

9. Department of Health. *Compassion in practice: nursing, midwifery and care staff - our vision and strategy*. London: DH, 2013.

10. NICE (National Institute for Health and Care Excellence). *Service user experience in adult mental health: improving the experience of care for people using adult NHS mental health services [CG135]*. London: NICE, 2011.

11. The Stationery Office. *Code of Practice to the Mental Capacity Act 2005*. London: TSO, 2007.

12. Her Majesty's Stationery Office. *The Mental Capacity Act 2005* (Eng.). London: TSO, 2005.

13. Carerstrust. *The Triangle of Care*. London: Carerstrust, 2012.

14. NMC (Nursing and Midwifery Council). *The code: professional standards of practice and behaviour for nurses and midwives*. London: NMC, 2015.

15. Her Majesty's Stationery Office. *Equality Act 2010* (Eng.). London: HMSO, 2010.

16. NMC (Nursing and Midwifery Council). *Raising concerns: guidance for nurses and midwives*. London: NMC, 2015.

17. CQC (Care Quality Commission). *Raising a concern with CQC: a quick guide for health and social care staff about whistleblowing*. London: CQC, 2014.

18. Anthony W. Recovery from mental illness: the guiding vision of the mental health service systems in the 1990s. *Psychosocial Rehabilitation Journal* 1993; **16**(4): 11–23.

19. MIND. *Mental health crisis care: physical restraint in crisis. A report on physical restraint in hospital settings*. London: MIND, 2013.

20. NHS Business Services Authority, NHS Protect. Reported physical assaults on NHS staff in 2014/15. 2015. Available from: http://www.nhsbsa.nhs.uk/Documents/SecurityManagement/Reported_Physical_Assaults_2014-15_-_FINAL_Published_Figures(1).pdf [Accessed 23rd August 2016].

21. NMC (Nursing and Midwifery Council). *Standards for competence for registered nurses*. London: NMC, 2014.

22. Department of Health. *Choosing health: making healthy choices easier*. London: DH, 2004.

23. Department of Health. *Best practice competencies and capabilities for pre-registration mental health nurses in England: the Chief Nursing Officer's Review of Mental Health Nursing*. London: DH, 2006b.

24. The Stationery Office. *Mental Health Act 1983: Code of Practice*. London: TSO, 2015.

25. Fraser SW, Greenhaigh T. Coping with complexity: educating for capability. *British Medical Journal* 2001; **323**: 799.

26. Department of Health. *National Service Framework for Mental Health (NSF)*. London: DH, 1999.

27. Her Majesty's Stationery Office. *The NHS Plan: a plan for investment: a plan for reform*. Norwich: HMSO, 2000.

28. Department of Health. *The ten essential shared capabilities: a framework for the whole of the mental health workforce*. London: DH, 2004.

29. Department of Health. *From values to action: the Chief Nursing Officer's Review of Mental Health Nursing*. London: DH, 2006a.

30. Barker P (ed.). *Psychiatric and mental health nursing: the craft of caring*, 2nd edn. Boca Raton, FL: CRC Press, 2008.

31. Bee P, Playle J, Lovell K, Barnes P, Gray R, Keeley P. Service users' views and expectations of UK-registered mental health nurses: a systematic review of empirical research. *International Journal of Nursing Studies* 2001; **45**(3): 442–57.

32. University of Manchester. *National Confidential Inquiry into Suicides and Homicides by People with Mental Illness Annual Report 2015*. England, Northern Ireland, Scotland and Wales: University of Manchester, 2015.

33. Edwards K, Dhoopnarain J, Fellow J, Griffith M, Ferguson D, Moyo L, Adamson N, Chaurura A. Evaluating protected time in mental health care. *Nursing Times* 2008; **104**(36): 28–9.

34. Central Health Services Council. *Psychiatric nursing: today and tomorrow*. London: Report of the Standing Mental Health and the Standing Nursing Advisory Committee, HMSO, 1968.

35. Department of Health. *Working in partnership: a collaborative approach to care. Report of the Mental Health Review Team*. London: HMSO, 1994.

36. Department of Health. *Prime Minister's challenge on dementia 2020*. London: DH, 2015.

Further reading

Baggott R. *Understanding health policy, 2nd edn*. Bristol: Policy Press, 2015.

Callaghan P, Repper J, Lovell K, Playle J, Baker J, Clifton A, Shaw T, Stacey G, Nelson P, Minshull S, Swarbrick C, Schneider J, Watkins M. *Evaluation of the Chief Nursing Officer's review of mental health nursing in England: Report to the Department of Health Policy Research Programme*. Nottingham: University of Nottingham, 2009.

Department of Health. *Annual report of the Chief Medical Officer, public mental health priorities: investing in the evidence*. London: DH, 2013.

Glasby J, Trew J. *Mental health policy and practice*, 3rd edn. London: Palgrave Macmillan, 2015.

Hall A, Wren M, Kirby SD. *Care planning in mental: promoting recovery*, 2nd edn. Chichester: John Wiley and Sons Ltd, 2015.

Halpern D. *Inside the nudge unit: how small changes can make a big difference*. London: WH Allen, 2015.

Health and Social Care Information Centre. *Mental health bulletin. Annual report from MHMDS returns 2014–15*. 2015. Available from: http://www.hscic.gov.uk/catalogue/PUB18808 [Accessed 8th June 2016].

Health Education England 2015. *Raising the Bar Shape of Caring: A Review of the Future Education and Training of Registered Nurses and Care Assistants*. 2015. Available from: https://www.hee.nhs.uk/our-work/developing-our-workforce/nursing/shape-caring-review [Accessed 8th June 2016].

NHS Business Services Authority. Reported physical assaults on NHS staff figures. Available from: http://www.nhsbsa.nhs.uk/3645.aspx [Accessed 8th June 2016].

NHS England. *Commissioning for quality and innovation (CQUIN): 2014/14 guidance*. London: NHS England, 2014.

NHS England. *The Friends and Family Test: a short guide for patients*. 2014. Available from: http://www.nhs.uk/friendsandfamily [Accessed 8th June 2016].

NMC (Nursing and Midwifery Council). *Standards for competence for registered nurses*. London: NMC, 2014.

Royal College of Psychiatrists. *Report of the second round of the National Audit of Schizophrenia (NAS2)*. London: HQIP and the Royal College of Psychiatrists, 2014.

Sainsbury Centre for Mental Health. *The capable practitioner: a framework and list of the practitioner capabilities required to implement the National Service Framework in Mental Health*. London: Sainsbury Centre for Mental Health, 2001.

WHO (World Health Organization). *Mental health atlas*. Geneva: WHO, 2014. Available from: http://www.who.int/mental_health/evidence/atlas/mental_health_atlas_2014/en/ [Accessed 8th June 2016].

WHO (World Health Organization). *mHealth. New horizons for health through mobile technologies*. 2013. Available from: http://www.who.int/goe/publications/goe_mhealth_web.pdf [Accessed 8th June 2016].

Relevant web pages

Making Every Contact Count. http://www.makingeverycontactcount. co.uk/

Mental Health Foundation. https://www.mentalhealth.org.uk/

MIND. http://www.mind.org.uk

NHS England. Compassion in practice. https://www.england.nhs. uk/nursingvision/compassion/

NHS England. Five year forward view. https://www.england.nhs. uk/ourwork/futurenhs/nhs-five-year-forward-view-web-version/5yfv-exec-sum/

NICE (National Institute for Health and Care Excellence). Guidance and advice list. https://www.nice.org.uk/guidance/published

Rethink Mental Health. E-learning platform. http://rethinkelearning.clcmoodle.org/local/sites/rethinkelearning/customlogin/

Rethink Mental Health. Physical health check flyer with basic facts about physical health checks. https://www.rethink.org/media/813628/Rethink%20Mental%20Illness%20Physical%20Health%20Check%20Flyer.pdf

Skills for Care. http://www.skillsforcare.org.uk/Home.aspx

Social Care Institute for Excellence. e-Learning. http://www.scie. org.uk/publications/elearning/sexualhealth/index.asp
This is a sexual, reproductive and mental health resource developed for the busy mental health professional, as an easy-to-use guide to key aspects of sexual and reproductive health in the context of mental illness.

YoungMinds. http://www.youngminds.org.uk

2 Ethics and mental health nursing

VINCE J. MITCHELL

LEARNING OUTCOMES

- To recognize the ethical dimensions of mental health nursing practice.
- To be able to evaluate some key ethical theories and frameworks.
- To know how to apply ethical concepts to practice situations.
- To be aware of the implications of different approaches for the service user in mental health care.
- To be able to reflect on your ethical responses in professional practice.

SUMMARY OF KEY POINTS

- Mental health nurses make ethical decisions in everyday practice.
- There needs to be an awareness of the background of unequal power and potential coercion in mental health practice.
- Key ethical concepts such as autonomy, dignity and compassion need to be critically examined.
- Ethical frameworks such as the four principles approach can help the nurse understand competing demands when making a decision.
- Character and emotion have a central role to play in making a wise decision.

INTRODUCTION

The idea that nursing is fundamentally a moral pursuit is not new.[1,2] This chapter aims to demonstrate how nursing ethics is part of everyday practice, and is not just reserved for unusual case studies. It will consider ethical ideas that are important for aspiring mental health nurses and suggest how these ideas can be drawn on to help resolve some of the more difficult situations that may be faced in practice.

Mental health nursing can be a challenging undertaking, and asking people to think about ethics may seem to be adding yet further complexity to the endeavour. However, nursing is not merely about doing what is effective; it also involves being a good nurse and doing right by those in your care. This can be challenging due to the nature of mental health nursing, which is often practised in the context of an imbalance of power between those providing care and the people who are receiving it. This context inevitably affects the relationships nurses form with those in their care, and the ethical implications of this will be explored.

MAKING ETHICAL DECISIONS IN DISPUTED TERRITORY

As discussed in chapter 4, caring for people with mental distress raises a number of controversial issues. Not least is the fact that treatment for mental illness can be administered against the will of service users. Philosophical debates abound as to whether mental distress is something that can be effectively treated as an *illness*, or whether it is better understood *socially* as a metaphor constructed by society to control unusual thoughts and behaviour.[3] Whatever position is held in these debates, the reality of the potential use of force affects relationships, even when force is not involved. When a nurse has a conversation with a service user about the benefits of being 'concordant' with psychiatric medication, this choice may well be made with the knowledge of both parties that long-term refusal could result in some form of compulsory treatment.

Nonetheless, Gray[4] argues that persuading service users to take medication is a valuable part of the caring role. In his view, accepting a refusal of treatment at face value, even from a person with full mental capacity, is 'misplaced progressive liberalism' (p.150), which wrongly assumes that the person has reflected on the consequences of his or her choice. Gray promotes the use of adherence therapy to promote medication concordance and is also willing to consider cash incentives to help persuade people.

For Gray, the *effectiveness* of the intervention is paramount and the right to refuse should not be overly emphasized, as service users tend to underestimate their risk of relapse. Yet should the central concern be with *effective* treatment or with building a collaborative therapeutic relationship with those in our care, even when the latter means accepting a service user's wish to refuse the treatment prescribed? Other fields of practice respect someone's right to refuse treatment, even when their refusal is considered unwise. If mental health nursing is going to be different in this regard, then a case needs to be made as to why.[5] (For further discussion of freedom and consent, see chapter 18.)

Seemingly, an impasse looms between those who wish to prioritize what is considered to be in a service user's best interests and those who wish to give more weight to a service user's claim to self-determination. It can perhaps be agreed that nurses need to be judicious with their professional power and exercise it only for the good of nursing those in their care. Nonetheless, establishing how to be a good nurse in this context is not straightforward.

> ### REFLECTION
>
> Consider the ways in which the use of professional power might affect the therapeutic relationship. What are the ethical issues that this raises?

ENGAGING WITH ETHICAL ISSUES

Nurses make ethical choices not only as citizens but also as professionals who are accountable for the care that they give. This may involve a certain amount of negotiation between personal morality and what is expected in their professional role. There may be times when nurses feel that they have not acted ethically, personally and/or professionally. This may be due to external constraints such as law, policy, work hierarchy or a lack of resources. Alternatively, it may be due to internal constraints such as lacking assertiveness or competence, or having a fear such as losing one's job.[6] Feeling constrained from doing the right thing in these ways is said to cause the nurse *moral distress*.

It has been argued by Johnstone and Hutchinson[7] that the term moral distress is misleading, both because of its underlying assumption that nurses' thwarted moral judgements are the right ones, and by casting doubt on whether the nurse is genuinely powerlessness to act. Nonetheless, empirical studies suggest that this distress exists for mental health nurses.[8,9] Though unpleasant, having sensitivity to ethical issues provides the nurse at least with the opportunity to try to improve the situation for those in their care.

Professionally, nurses are expected to behave with good conduct and character at all times. As such, individual nurses need to navigate ethically through complex scenarios in a way that meets professional obligations. Professional codes offer a minimum standard below which nurses should not fall. For example, the Nursing and Midwifery Code of Practice in the UK[10] expects practitioners to care for people with *respect*, *dignity* and *compassion* at all times. However, in order to ensure that these requirements are responded to in a way that is meaningful, and not seen merely as clichés, it is necessary to explore the meaning behind the concepts.

Furthermore, there are times when particular dilemmas arise. In order to aim for the right course of action, the nurse may wish to draw on a decision-making framework. A well-known example is the medical ethics framework of Beauchamp and Childress.[11] This seeks to draw on commonly held moral norms in the form of four equally significant principles: autonomy, beneficence, non-maleficence and justice. These can be briefly summarized as:

- *autonomy*: respecting and supporting decisions made with autonomy;
- *beneficence*: relieving, lessening or preventing harm and providing benefits balanced against risk and cost;
- *non-maleficence*: avoiding causing harm;
- *justice*: fairly distributing benefits, risks and costs.

The first three principles will be considered in some depth below. The fourth refers primarily to justice at a policy level and allocating resources in a way that is fair and non-discriminatory. Though relevant, this aspect will not be focused on here. (For a discussion of policy issues, see chapter 68.)

The four principles are recognized as a sound starting point for ethical practice, though further ethical exploration is required to solve disagreements about how the principles should be balanced.[12] A number of common dilemmas in mental health nursing will be analysed using this basic structure, before moving on to a discussion of dignity and the place of virtues such as compassion in being a good nurse.

ETHICAL CONCEPTS RELEVANT TO MENTAL HEALTH NURSING

Autonomy, beneficence and non-maleficence

As suggested above, the mental health nurse can be in a pivotal position in deciding how to proceed when the wishes of someone in their care differ from what is believed to be in their best interests by the mental health team. This can be understood in terms of a possible tension between *autonomy*, the right of people to think and decide for themselves, and *beneficence*, which entails an obligation to promote good outcomes.[11]

It is not only treatment that raises this tension. Consider case study 1.

CASE STUDY 1

Bill is recovering from a recent psychotic episode and is an inpatient in a mental health unit. He wishes to go out for a walk. He continues to believe that people are after him but these ideas are less intense than before. In the past going out has made his paranoia worse and sometimes he can be at risk from the environment due to being distracted by hearing voices. The nurse thinks it might be better for Bill's welfare to stay on the unit; however, he is insistent that he has a right to go out. Bill is not detained under mental health legislation but the nurse knows that it is within her power to use a legal holding power if she feels that is justified.

The nurse may feel empowered to exercise a professional judgement that Bill's mental health is not good enough for him to go out. However, Bill states that he has a 'right' to go out. (For further discussion of legal and human rights considerations, see chapter 67.)

REFLECTION

Does Bill have a point? What are the relevant *ethical* factors for the nurse in this situation?

By saying he has a right to go out, Bill is asserting his autonomy to make decisions about his own life. Usually, persons have the right to make choices, even if these are seen as unwise. Many of us choose to drink too much, smoke, get into debt, do extreme sports and so on. People may say phrases such as 'well it's his choice', thus putting the responsibility on the person making the decision. In these cases, the decision is being respected, though autonomy is being supported only in a *negative* sense in that there is no interference with the choice being made.

Yet, the context cannot be ignored here. Bill is a mental health service user, which means that people have a professional duty to care for him, and as such non-interference may be seen as negligence. *Beneficence* requires that harm is lessened and that any benefit promoted needs to be balanced against risk. In some ways it may benefit Bill therapeutically to go out, but the risk may outweigh this, and so it would not be beneficent to allow Bill to go out, and to promote it may be seen as against the principle of *non-maleficence*.

Nonetheless, this does not mean that Bill's freedom can be restricted without good reason. For example, if the nurse was simply more comfortable with the idea of Bill remaining on the unit, that would not be sufficient justification. In this case the nurse may not have Bill's welfare at the centre of her decision and as such the action is not beneficent. She is merely being *cautious* in order to prevent her own discomfort. In this situation, Bill could probably legitimately complain that his right to autonomy has been overridden. Furthermore, it can be seen as causing harm to Bill by preventing him from realizing his wishes. As such it would also be in opposition to a principle of non-maleficence, which states that harm should be avoided.

However, let us assume that the nurse genuinely believes that Bill is making an unwise choice that is going to put him at enough risk that he should not go out. Should Bill's choice be overridden to protect his welfare? One way to justify this is to state that Bill does not have sufficient cognition or awareness to exercise autonomy and so cannot take responsibility for his welfare. This would mean that the principle of respecting autonomy is no longer able to balance the other principles, thus tipping the decision in favour of beneficence. However, in order to make the assertion that exercising autonomy is not possible, it is necessary to consider the concept in more depth.

Deeper views of autonomy

Autonomy is generally understood to be a capability for self-governance, but the elements required to have this capability are not generally agreed upon.[13] Often, autonomy requires not only the ability to have preferences but to reflect on those preferences and be able to assess their validity.[13,14] Virtually all views agree that merely making a free choice is not sufficient. A decision made with autonomy needs to meet certain conditions, and often this means making a choice that is aligned with the overall values held by the person concerned.

Some deeper views of the concept state that a choice is not made with autonomy unless it has a moral element. Autonomy in this sense is about making choices that are not only free but *justifiable*.[15] Others, in the tradition of the ethics of care, argue that autonomy needs to be understood as being based in *relationships*. This is known as *relational autonomy*. It states that people rely on the support of others such as friends and family, and as a result make choices in an interdependent rather than independent way.[16]

It may be that Bill is able to exercise autonomy in some of these senses but not others. If Bill is able to exercise autonomy only in a more limited sense or only to a limited degree, then his wishes are more likely to be outweighed by other ethical considerations. Nonetheless, it is important to ensure that some of these deeper considerations are not lost in pursuit of a quick and easy solution.

It is worth noting that these deeper views of autonomy cut both ways. The nurse must also be able to reflect on *her* decision and whether it is justifiable. Taking on a relational view, choices ideally should be made collaboratively within a therapeutic relationship with the service user, which is reciprocal and trusting. Furthermore, the nurse needs to reflect on her influence in the situation and whether it is being misused. (For more discussion on developing and maintaining therapeutic relationships, see chapter 3.)

Paternalism, coercion and power

When the pursuit of beneficence involves overriding a person's wishes or actions in order to promote their own welfare, this is known as *paternalism*.[11,14] As outlined, such acts of beneficence can be justified when it is believed that the individual no longer has the capability to take responsibility for his/her own welfare. This is controversial, as those making judgements about someone's competence do so from a position of *power*. This can lead to the concern that service users are (in reality) only considered to be competent to exercise autonomy when they are in agreement with mental health professionals.[17]

Furthermore, there is a tendency for nurses in psychiatric care to use *coercion*,[1,17,18] even in voluntary admission.[19] O'Brien and Golding[17] define coercion as 'any use of authority to override the choices of another' (p.168). They argue that, though coercive practices can have a paternalistic justification, this is overused. They also suggest that mental health nurses can believe that coercive practices are allowed, due to their belief that service users cannot make acceptable decisions for themselves.

Consider case study 2.

Initially, it seems that similar questions need to be asked about this scenario as for the one involving Bill above.

CASE STUDY 2

Edna is a heavy smoker and has chronic obstructive pulmonary disease. She is also an inpatient on a psychiatric unit and has a diagnosis of schizophrenia. Edna appears to understand that smoking is bad for her and that it may shorten her life. Nonetheless, it has been decided that, in the interests of her health, Edna's cigarettes are kept in the nurse's office and that she only has one an hour. Otherwise, Edna chain smokes, which exacerbates her condition and requires her to have an increase of her treatment with Salbutamol. Edna passively adheres to this arrangement, though there are times when she wants more cigarettes than she is 'allowed'.

Is Edna able to exercise autonomy about her choice to smoke? If the answer to this is yes, it might be imagined that no further discussion is needed. Yet, even if Edna is able to make an autonomous choice, do the nurses still have a responsibility to preserve Edna's health because she is an inpatient?

The nurses might decide that, even though Edna appears to understand that smoking is not good for her health, they cannot allow her to harm herself in this way while she is in their care. In the previous scenario with Bill, there was only a *risk* of harm, whereas in this case Edna is actually harming her health. Nurses may feel that their own autonomy is being unreasonably restricted if they are unable to fulfil their duty of care by at least restricting the amount Edna smokes.

REFLECTION

Should the nursing team act paternalistically in order to prevent Edna harming herself with smoking? As this is a team decision, what might you do as an individual nurse if you disagree with the decision that has been made?

Now consider the following.

CASE STUDY 2 (continued)

One day Edna manages to get hold of some extra cigarettes and is seen smoking them. Edna likes to have a daily trip out but it is decided by the nurses on duty that Edna should not go out today as she has failed to stick to the 'boundaries' regarding her cigarettes. The staff defend this as it will 'encourage' Edna in the future to stick to her smoking restriction in the interests of her health.

Seemingly, a further line has now been crossed. Edna is now being *punished* with the hope that a positive outcome will be brought about. This action is more clearly coercive. It involves the use of authority to deprive Edna of her leave, along with the aim that she will make a different choice in the future due to the threat of her leave being restricted again.

As well as being coercive, it can also be criticized as *infantilizing*, meaning that Edna is being treated in a child-like way. Justification could be sought by the argument that there is no moral difference between this and occasions when society seeks punishment for adults who break the law. However, this argument would probably be misapplied, as no law has been broken and the sanction here is only intended to prevent Edna from harming herself, a choice that many would believe is Edna's own.

Finally, let us consider that Edna decides after a few months of this arrangement that she should stop smoking for her health. The staff are pleased that Edna has reached the 'right decision'. However, this decision is being made in a context. Relational views of autonomy suggest that no one really makes a free decision because we are influenced by those around us. Better decisions can be made by having *supportive* relationships with those we trust to help guide us. On the other hand, they can be influenced negatively by *oppressive* relationships.

If a relational view of autonomy is taken, then the problem moves to determining whether the relationship Edna has with the nurses is a supportive or oppressive one. The reality that nurses are in a position of power is obvious. It also appears that Edna has been somewhat infantilized by the relationship. When Edna has attempted to exercise self-determination, this has been punished and the threat of further punishment is used to coerce Edna to agree to the arrangement in the interest of her health. Yet the nurses might see their role as supportive if they believe that Edna responds to these clear boundaries.

Ultimately, it is up to the nurses, and probably the wider multidisciplinary team, to *judge* whether the balance between autonomy and paternalism has been weighed appropriately. Nonetheless, it is worth noting that, even if substantial weight is given to Edna's autonomy, it is still the staff who have the power to decide the balance, not Edna herself.

REFLECTION

Consider the source of power in the nurse–client relationship. How free should service users be to make choices about their care and treatment? When might coercion be justified?

Dignity

Dignity is a concept which is familiar to many, but, as with autonomy, there are a variety of ways to understand it. It is fair to say that most people are able to get a sense of the difference between a dignifying and an undignifying situation for a human being. Shotton and Seedhouse[20] suggest that anyone who has found themselves in a 'degrading situation' knows what dignity is (p.246). In everyday life we make efforts to do things such as protecting the privacy of our bodies, behaving in a polite way, or attempting to appear knowledgeable to others or calm under pressure. There is a sense that we already know what dignity is for ourselves and this can be generalized to help honour it for others.

The link is commonly made between dignity and autonomy. This stems from the classical philosophical idea that the source of our dignity as human persons is found in our ability to act with autonomy.[21] If this argument is accepted, then failing to respect someone's autonomy *also means* that we are not respecting their dignity as a person. It may suggest to some that dignity is therefore simply a matter of upholding someone's wishes. However, as case study 3 shows, this may not be the case:

CASE STUDY 3

Eric spent many years homeless. He developed a long-term psychosis and is now a resident of a home for people recovering from long-term mental health problems. Due to his many years on the road, Eric has a preference to eat separately from the other residents, crouching down using a plate he puts on the floor. Eric says he does not feel comfortable eating with others at the table and his choice is respected. One day, a visitor comes to the home. She is horrified to see Eric eating in such an 'undignified' way. She complains, saying there are certain things that just should not be allowed.

The visitor is making a judgement about what is dignified, perhaps based on what she feels would be dignified for herself based on her preferences. However, Eric's preferences are different. As such it may not be fair for the visitor to make this judgement as Eric is merely exercising his own preferences.

On the other hand, it is possible that an *objective* view of dignity is being taken, which means that it is being seen as existing independently of someone's individual (subjective) experience.[22] The argument could be put forward that there are indeed certain things that human beings should not be encouraged or allowed to do. In other words, there are certain standards which apply for human beings in general. So, the argument could proceed that, because we are intelligent cultured beings, we need to eat in a way that reflects this. A similar argument could be put forward to justify a decision to dissuade someone from wearing clothes that are unclean or considered inappropriate. However, on closer examination, it appears that at least some of these decisions are still based on *cultural* expectations. In some parts of the world eating crouched down with your hands off a plate on the floor is considered acceptable. A study by Edlund et al.[23] found that dignity indeed has a *relative* component which is highly changeable depending on culture in a society and all the norms and rules that it involves.

This suggests that calls to dignity need to be carefully employed. Some forms of dignity are linked to autonomy, but nurses have to exercise caution when acting to uphold dignity in a way that conflicts with autonomy. This is because the justification for enforcing social norms is more controversial, and again brings the discussion back to the disputed issue of whether enforcing such norms is the proper focus of mental health nursing.

> ## REFLECTION
>
> What does dignity mean to you? How might you uphold the dignity of those in your care? Should this be your primary concern, or are other factors equally or more important?

Contrasting consequentialist and deontological ethics

Rather than judging an action as right or wrong based on whether it respects the autonomy or dignity of those involved, another approach, *consequentialism*, evaluates goodness solely on the *outcome* produced.[24] Importantly, this outcome needs to have a greater good *overall*; it cannot maximize a desired value just for *particular* individuals if that is achieved at the expense of the overall good. It is necessary, therefore, to decide how a good outcome is to be measured. In utilitarianism, a state of affairs is judged as good depending on the amount of happiness that is produced. The downside, at least in classical act-utilitarianism, is that this means that it is allowable for the rights of individuals to be disregarded by an action, as long as overall happiness is maximized as a result.

Consider case study 4.

From a consequentialist point of view, the action of lying in this situation is justified as long as the act of lying brings more good into the world than telling the truth. At face value, this seems to be the right thing to do.

BEING A GOOD NURSE

Wisdom and courage

The four principles approach has been used above to provide a framework that can help lead the nurse to an ethical solution. A process of *weighing and balancing* the four

> ## CASE STUDY 4
>
> A woman with dementia keeps forgetting that her husband has died. She used to ask the nursing staff when he was coming to visit. When the woman was told that her husband had died, she became very distressed, affecting the happiness of both her and those around her. About an hour later, she would forget but then after some time she would ask again. Each time she was retold, it was like hearing the news for the first time. The nurses therefore decide to tell a therapeutic lie that her husband is away on a business trip and will see her when he gets back. She accepts this and is much happier as a result.

Furthermore, there is evidence that therapeutic lying is indeed prevalent in the field of dementia care, though there is reluctance to endorse the practice officially.[25,26]

The dilemma arises because lying is seen in *deontological* (duty-based) views of ethics as being wrong. This is because it is disrespectful to lie to people as it affects their ability to exercise their autonomy. It may also be seen as undignifying, as to believe a lie can make people appear foolish to others. Many people would expect to be told the truth by a medical or nursing professional, and, arguably, *trust* is founded on the existence of a mutual respect of autonomy.[15]

However, there are two factors that appear to make it justifiable in the example above. Firstly, there is a large amount of distress caused by telling the truth and there seems to be no distress resulting from the lie being told apart from (perhaps) the distress felt by the person telling the lie. Secondly, due to the woman having dementia, some pressure can be put on the notion that she has the same right to be told the truth as somebody with normal mental capacity. She seems unable to retain or reflect on the information, which makes her ability to respond to the truth in an autonomous way more questionable.

It is worth noting at this point that the principle of beneficence, described above, can also be used to justify telling a lie in this and other situations. Consequentialism can be aligned with this principle in that both aim to maximize benefits and minimize harm. Nonetheless, the extent to which we have obligations to maximize these benefits in a *general* sense, such as helping people with whom we have no personal connection, is debatable.

principles is required, and this involves using deliberation and judgement. This suggests that applying the four principles or any other ethical framework to guide *conduct* is only part of the picture; the capability to make a good judgement requires good moral *character*.[11]

The development of good character is the fundamental concern of *virtue ethics*. Such an approach requires the nurse not merely to ask what he/she ought to do in a particular situation, but to examine how she can be a good nurse. When making decisions, the nurse can call upon *professional wisdom*. This involves firstly being able to appreciate the ethical components in a given situation. Secondly, it involves exercising moral imagination in order to see a challenging situation in a different light and therefore respond in a more reflective way.[27] (For further discussion on critical reflection, see chapter 11.)

Along with wisdom, another core virtue for a good nurse is *courage*.[28–30] Mental health nurses may find themselves in situations where they feel physically or psychologically threatened. In such situations the easy course of action may be tempting even if it is not the right course of action. A courageous nurse acts in a way that he/she sees as right, and can also be seen as someone to emulate by other nurses.

To illustrate, let us return to the example of Bill above. Here the nurse believes it would be better for Bill's welfare to stay on the unit. It was argued above that the nurse should not make the decision that is merely the most comfortable for her. She may have known Bill for years and feel compassion for his situation. She may nonetheless believe that in this situation he needs to be kept safe. The nurse may feel fear in this situation if Bill becomes angry. The nurse may also experience self-doubt if other colleagues question her decision and she will need to judge whether their views are wise. Due to all these factors, courage is required to see the decision through, and take the course of action that a good nurse would choose.

The same would apply if the nurse made the opposite judgement and allowed Bill to leave. Initially this might seem the easier choice, to acquiesce to Bill's request. However, the nurse then has to have the courage to carry the anxiety of taking both a personal and professional risk. If Bill comes to harm, she may well feel personal guilt and fear that she has not been professionally wise. However, if she genuinely believes that this is the right course of action, then again she needs to have the courage of her convictions. In a similar vein, the good nurse will often have to show courage in order to speak out against unacceptable practice.

Compassion and the ethics of care

Along with wisdom and courage, a good nurse also shows *compassion* for those in her care. Calling attention to the importance of compassion in everyday practice is increasingly being seen as a central concern in both nursing and medical ethics.[31,32] Compassion and the related virtue of *receptivity*[33] are highly dependent on the nurse engaging with her emotions and feeling empathy for those in her care.

This approach is in tune with an *ethics of care* which also focuses on emotions, responsiveness and relationships as a priority in the moral life, rather than abstract rules and reasoning. The ethics of care focuses primarily on the claims made on us by particular people with whom we form a caring relationship.[34] In this way it often stands in opposition to consequentialism discussed above.

Let us reconsider the example already described of the woman with dementia who has forgotten that her husband has died. The nurse could approach this problem in a purely *cognitive* way. She could weigh up the pros and cons of telling or not telling a lie. She could consider the rights of the service user and of those around her before carrying out her action. This could be done in an effective manner and a decision reached. Yet, if she feels nothing, then both virtue ethics and an ethics of care would suggest that something vital has been lost. Telling the truth in a matter-of-fact way, even if the nurse believes this is the most respectful thing to do, could be seen as cold by other receptive individuals. Instead the nurse should connect compassionately with this situation.[35] Whether the care provider tells the truth or a white lie, the key ingredient is the compassionate motivation originating from good character.

Mentors

It is beyond the scope of this chapter to give a full account of all the virtues that may be relevant to nurses in this and other situations. Along with compassion and courage, other virtues that have been highlighted as important for nurses are a sense of honesty, justice, tolerance and open-mindedness.[28,29] There are times when these virtues might conflict but, as with the four principles, the virtuous individual is expected to be able to employ each virtue in a measured manner with wise judgement.

All virtues need a positive moral climate in which to flourish.[30] This can be cultivated by having mentors in practice,[36] a familiar notion for nursing students. Virtues are learned by modelling character and behaviour on those of virtuous exemplars.[37] This may seem initially a somewhat highfaluting notion, but it draws from the idea that nursing students may find that they admire one or more professionals in particular, and want to be a good nurse like those individuals. From a virtue ethics perspective, approaches such as consequentialism and deontology fall short, as they demote the importance of character in virtues such as kindness.[38] Put simply, it is not enough just to *act* with kindness; the nurse should *be* kind, and this requires emotional involvement.

> ### REFLECTION
>
> What sort of character qualities does a good nurse have? Can you think of a nurse in your experience who has these qualities? How might you cultivate such qualities in your own character?

Evaluating the role of virtue ethics

The usefulness and reliability of virtue ethics as a sole theory for making ethical decisions in professional life is open to challenge. Holland[39] argues that though virtue ethics makes a valuable contribution to *personal* ethics in terms of how to live a good life as a human being, it is not appropriate for the professional sphere. Holland argues that professional ethics needs to be kept separate from professional ethics, as there is no 'nursing nature' towards which virtue ethics can aim. However, as argued by Putnam:[38] 'Virtue ethicists assume that a human life is a whole and that the virtuous individual manifests his or her character traits to different situations, personal as well as "professional"' (p.143).

So virtue ethics downplays the distinction between personal and professional ethics. As pointed out by Putnam, it hardly seems appropriate for someone to be kind, courageous, honest, and so forth at work, but then not at home. Virtue ethics is about having the *character* to be a good nurse. It seems fair to state that good character is not something which can be switched on or off, though different qualities may be required at different times.

A second criticism of virtue ethics is that the approach is circular.[40] How is it possible to know who a good nurse is, when a good nurse is defined based on the actions that a good nurse would choose? One answer to this (at least from a virtue ethics perspective) is that certain character traits are seen as good by bringing positive 'warm' feelings to those who are similarly receptive.[33] In other words, developing empathy can help us with identifying other good people and modelling their actions. Nonetheless, this may be seen as overly *subjective*, thus casting doubt on the ability of virtue ethics to guide action fairly.

As such, an approach that combines virtue ethics with the use of commonly agreed moral principles may be more easily defended. Another alternative is to combine the four principles framework discussed above with the ethics of care. Here the principles are 'infused' with care to take more account of relationships and emotion in the care encounter.[41]

CONCLUSION

Mental health nurses work in disputed territory. Coercion is a real possibility for many receiving mental health care, and the potential use of force by mental health professionals inevitably affects the nature of the therapeutic relationship. A good nurse needs to behave virtuously and make sound ethical decisions while being mindful of this imbalance of power. Decision-making frameworks such as the four principles approach can help the nurse to understand the competing moral elements in the decision-making process. However, ultimately, the character of the nurse comes to fore. Good nurses are receptive to the thoughts and feelings of those in their care and aspire to be compassionate, courageous and wise in their responses.

SERVICE USER COMMENTARY

Sarah Markham

The author demonstrates a firm grasp of the tension that can exist in the relationship between mental health nurse and patient due to the (at times significant) imbalance in power between the two, and the difficulties and moral dilemmas that may arise as a consequence. He quotes Gray without more than a superficial questioning of assumptions such that adherence to prescribed medication is always the best choice. However, as the nurse may not necessarily be an expert in pharmacology/prescribing practice, he is right not to delve too deeply into this area. Prescribing is in virtually every case and to varying degrees a question of trial and error; the responsible clinician/psychiatrist is the best judge and therefore his/her expertise should be respected and adherence advocated, unless it emerges that the patient is suffering undue distress.

The author makes good use of reflective questions throughout the chapter which focus on various ethical considerations pertinent to those in the nursing role.

The author shows a sensitive understanding of the moral distress nurses might experience because of external and internal constraints on their practice and the very human question: 'Did I do my best?'

The author draws the (nursing) reader's attention to the medical ethics framework of Beauchamp and Childress as a resource to draw upon when the minimum standard demanded by professional codes of practice provide insufficient guidance, and he gives a realistic example of how to use it in practice. He also presents a balanced view of the use of coercion, and again illustrates it via a case study and a perceptive use of a variety of perspectives.

A similar practical approach is used to examine the deployment of key ethical theories, such as contrasting consequentialist and deontological ethics.

Overall the chapter is informative and appropriately provocative and capable of immersing the (nursing) reader in the challenging and at times perplexing world of professional ethics.

Sarah Markham, BA (Hons), MA (Cantab), PhD, is a Visiting Researcher at King's Clinical Trials Unit, IoPPN, King's College London, UK.

References

1. Olsen DP. Influence and coercion: relational and rights-based ethical approaches to forced psychiatric treatment *Journal of Psychiatric and Mental Health Nursing* 2003; **10**: 705–12.

2. Gastmans C, Dierckx de Castele B, Schotsmans P. Nursing considered as moral practice: a philosophical-ethical interpretation of nursing. *Kennedy Institute of Ethics Journal* 1998; **8**: 43–69.

3. Szasz TS. *The myth of mental illness – foundations of a theory of personal conduct*. New York: Harper & Row, 1974.

4. Gray R. Cash, choice, antipsychotic medication and the mental health nurse. *Journal of Psychiatric and Mental Health Nursing* 2015; **22**: 149–53.

5. Barker P, Buchanan-Barker P. First, do no harm: confronting the myths of psychiatric drugs. *Nursing Ethics* 2012; **19**: 451–63.

6. McCarthy J, Gastmans C. Moral distress: a review of the argument-based nursing ethics literature. *Nursing Ethics* 2015; **22**: 131–52.

7. Johnstone M-J, Hutchinson A. 'Moral distress' – time to abandon a flawed nursing construct? *Nursing Ethics* 2015; **22**: 5–14.

8. Lűtzén K, Scheiber R. Moral survival in a nontherapeutic environment. *Issues in Mental Health Nursing* 1998; **19**: 303–15.

9. Austin W, Bergum V, Goldberg L. Unable to answer the call of our patients: mental health nurses' experience of moral distress. *Nursing Inquiry* 2003; **10**: 177–83.

10. NMC (Nursing & Midwifery Council). *The Code: professional standards of practice and behaviour for nurses and midwives*. London: NMC, 2015.

11. Beauchamp TL, Childress JF. *Principles of biomedical ethics*, 7th edn. New York: Oxford University Press, 2013.

12. Gillon R. Defending the four principles approach as a good basis for good medical practice and therefore for good medical ethics. *Journal of Medical Ethics* 2015; **41**: 111–16.

13. Christman J. Autonomy in moral and political philosophy. In: Zalta EN (ed.). *The Stanford encyclopedia of philosophy*, Spring 2015 edn. Available from: http://plato.stanford.edu/archives/spr2015/entries/autonomy-moral/ [Accessed 5th June 2016].

14. Dworkin G. *The theory and practice of autonomy*. Cambridge: Cambridge University Press, 1988.

15. O'Neill O. *Autonomy and trust in bioethics*. Cambridge: Cambridge University Press, 2002.

16. Mackenzie C, Stoljar N. Introduction: autonomy refigured. In: Mackenzie C, Stoljar N (eds). *Relational autonomy*. New York: Oxford University Press, 2000: 3–31.

17. O'Brien AJ, Golding CG. Coercion in mental healthcare: the principle of least coercive care. *Journal of Psychiatric and Mental Health Nursing* 2003; **10**: 167–73.

18. Duxbury, J. Editorial: minimizing the use of coercive practices in mental health: the perfect storm. *Journal of Psychiatric and Mental Health Nursing* 2015; **22**: 89–91.

19. O'Donoghue B, Roche E, Shannon S, Lyne J, Madigan K, Feeney L. Perceived coercion involuntary hospital admission *Psychiatry Research* 2014; **215**: 120–6.

20. Shotton L, Seedhouse D. Practical dignity in caring. *Nursing Ethics* 1998; **5**: 46–255.

21. Kant I. Groundwork of the metaphysics of morals. In: Kant I. *Practical philosophy*. Trans. Gregor M. Cambridge: Cambridge University Press, 1996 [originally published 1785]: 37–108.

22. Gallagher A. Dignity and respect for dignity – two key health professional values: implications for nursing practice. *Nursing Ethics* 2004; **11**: 587–99.

23. Edlund M, Lindwall L, von Post I, Lindström UÅ. Conceptual determination of human dignity. *Nursing Ethics* 2013; **20**: 851–60.

24. Darwall S. Introduction. In: Darwall S (ed.). *Consequentialism*. Malden, MA: Blackwell, 2003: 1–7.

25. James IA, Wood-Mitchell AJ, Waterworth AM, Mackenzie LE, Cunningham J. Lying to people with dementia: developing ethical guidelines for care settings. *International Journal of Geriatric Psychiatry* 2006; **21**: 800–1.

26. Culley H, Barber R, Hope A. Therapeutic lying in dementia care. *Nursing Standard* 2013; **28**: 35–9.

27. Banks S, Gallagher A. *Ethics in professional life: virtues for health and social care*. Basingstoke: Palgrave MacMillan, 2009.

28. Armstrong AE. Towards a strong virtue ethics for nursing practice. *Nursing Philosophy* 2006; **7**: 110–24.

29. Sellman D. *What makes a good nurse: why the virtues are important for nurses*. London: Jessica Kingsley, 2011.

30. McKie A, Swinton J. Community, culture and character: the place of the virtues in psychiatric nursing practice. *Journal of Psychiatric and Mental Health Nursing* 2000; **7**: 35–42.

31. Dewar B, Adamson A, Smith S, Surfleet J, King L. Clarifying misconceptions about compassionate care. *Journal of Advanced Nursing* 2014; **70**: 1738–47.

32. Zulueta PC. Suffering, compassion and 'doing good medical ethics'. *Journal of Medical Ethics* 2015; **41**: 87–90.

33. Slote M. *From enlightenment to receptivity: rethinking our values*. New York: Oxford University Press, 2013.

34. Held V. *The ethics of care: personal, political and global*. New York: Oxford University Press, 2005.

35. Tuckett AG. The experience of lying in dementia care: a qualitative study. *Nursing Ethics* 2012; **19**: 7–20.

36. Woods M. Nursing ethics education: are we really delivering the good(s)? *Nursing Ethics* 2005; **12**: 5–18.

37. Begley AM. Practising virtue: a challenge to the view that a virtue centred approach to ethics lacks practical content. *Nursing Ethics* 2005; **12**(6): 622–37.

38. Putnam DA. A reply to 'Scepticism about the virtue ethics approach to nursing ethics' by Stephen Holland: the relevance of virtue in nursing ethics. *Nursing Philosophy* 2012; **13**: 142–5.

39. Holland S. Scepticism about the virtue ethics approach to nursing ethics. *Nursing Philosophy* 2010; **11**: 151–8.

40. Holland S. Furthering the sceptical case against virtue ethics in nursing ethics. *Nursing Philosophy* 2012; **13**: 266–75.

41. Edwards SD. *Nursing ethics: a principle-based approach*, 2nd edn. London: Palgrave Macmillan, 2009.

Further reading

Banks D, Gallagher A. *Ethics in professional life: virtues for health and social care*. Basingstoke: Palgrave Macmillan, 2009.

Barker P. *Mental health ethics: the human context*. London: Routledge, 2011.

Beauchamp TL, Childress JF. *Principles of biomedical ethics*, 7th edn. New York: Oxford University Press, 2013.

Edwards SD. *Nursing ethics: a principle-based approach*, 2nd edn. London: Palgrave Macmillan, 2009.

Johnstone M-J. *Bioethics: a nursing perspective*, 5th edn. Sydney: Churchill Livingstone, 2009.

Sellman D. *What makes a good nurse: why the virtues are important for nurses*. London: Jessica Kingsley, 2011.

Relevant web pages

Values based practice
http://www2.warwick.ac.uk/fac/med/study/research/vbp/

3 Developing and maintaining therapeutic relationships

ROSIE STENHOUSE AND CHRYS MUIRHEAD

LEARNING OUTCOMES

- To be able to identify the key features of therapeutic relationships.
- To be able to discuss the role of therapeutic relationships in mental health nursing.
- To understand the impact of the context on the therapeutic relationship.
- To be able to describe the processes you would engage with to develop and maintain therapeutic relationships.

SUMMARY OF KEY POINTS

- Therapeutic relationships involve working in partnership with patients. Nurses should work alongside patients, focusing on a definition of their needs.
- People make sense of and express their experiences using stories. Listening to and engaging with patients' stories is key to developing an understanding of their perspective, developing and demonstrating empathy, and valuing them as a person.
- Therapeutic relationships occur in a context in which power is a key component. Nurses need to recognize how the structures and values of the mental health system impact on their relationships with patients.
- Rogers' core conditions of empathy, congruence and unconditional positive regard, as well as the concept of therapeutic alliances, are central to the development and maintenance of therapeutic relationships.

INTRODUCTION

This chapter represents a collaborative effort to examine and discuss those things that we think are important for the development and maintenance of therapeutic relationships. As a collaborative act, the writing of this chapter required us to negotiate how best to present our positions – derived from different experiences, training and knowledge bases – whilst avoiding replicating the power dynamics so often experienced between patient and nurse. Fundamentally we agree on a great many things with regard to what constitutes a useful therapeutic relationship. However, our voices are different, they speak from different places drawing on different experiences and positions within mental health care, and it was important to us that this chapter presented these voices as having equal authority rather than allowing the academic or professional voice to dominate.

It is for this reason that we have chosen to write in a style that breaks some of the norms of academic writing in order to usurp the authority that this style of writing gives the professional voice.[1,2] This chapter is therefore written in a manner that clearly identifies our different voices, whilst also drawing together the learning from each.

The collaboration involved in writing this chapter, with its sensitivity to issues of power in the writing relationship, also symbolizes our understanding that therapeutic relationships are inscribed with power. We therefore briefly explore power as one of the contextual factors that impacts therapeutic relationships.

Chrys

At times the discussion that follows might seem disjointed. This is sometimes how the nurse–patient relationship feels, and it has been a conscious decision to retain this feature rather than develop a smooth, singular narrative.

A NOTE ABOUT LANGUAGE

Chrys

I identify as a survivor of mental illness and psychiatric treatment, and do not accept the biological nature of psychiatry. Therefore I will be using alternative terms for medical language, for example drugs not medication, labels not diagnoses, etc. In so doing I am recognizing the power of language and my ability to take back the power, to deconstruct the psychiatric notes and reconstruct my story in a way that is acceptable, to me.

Rosie and Chrys

We will use 'he' and 'she' randomly when referring to the nurse rather than 'he/she'. Throughout, we use the word 'patient' to refer to the person who is relating with the nurse in the context of mental health care. We are aware of the choice of other terms that could have been used – service user, survivor, consumer – however, like the term 'patient', each of these terms signifies different experiences of power within the relationship. We understand that people who use mental health services will define their position in relation to these services differently, and ask that readers are equally aware.

DEFINING THE THERAPEUTIC RELATIONSHIP

Rosie

Within the literature, the therapeutic relationship is generally regarded as a key facet of mental health nursing.[3-6] Research has identified that the therapeutic relationship may be the means through which healing occurs regardless of the psychological therapy used.[7,8] It is a particular form of nurse–patient relationship; purposeful and intentional. The purpose of the relationship is to support the person to expand their capacity to deal with life. Interactions are oriented towards a particular outcome; supporting the person's existing capacity to develop and make change. To this end, the therapeutic relationship is an intentional activity which the nurse should devote time and energy to developing and maintaining.

The focus of the relationship should remain on the needs of the patient, and the nurse's actions are guided by this.[5,9-11] Barker and Whitehill[11] align this aspect of mental health nursing with the concept of craft where, unlike in art or science, the object is assigned meaning by the recipient. The power to define the meaning of the situation therefore sits with the patient rather than the nurse. It follows, then, that to act therapeutically, the nurse needs to elicit and work with the patient's understanding of the situation, developing a partnership. This requires two-way communication, and the development of a relationship based on trust and respect in which different views and options can be discussed.

Research has identified that, when asked, nurses and patients identify similar ideas about therapeutic relationships.[12] However, despite this, patients describe occasions when they did not experience relationships with nurses as therapeutic.[13-15] The literature points to a number of contextual reasons that may lead to this experience.[16-18] We will examine some of these contextual issues later.

Chrys

I believe a therapeutic relationship or helping alliance in psychiatric settings is very similar to friendships made over the years, with people of like minds. Therefore in the mental health setting it should be no different from the 'real world' and should be grounded in equality, reciprocity and level playing fields. It should be about getting alongside a person rather than doing things to or for a person. It should also be about sharing experiences, as if nurse and patient were on the same side of the fence. The challenge in the psychiatric setting is that personal stories are usually only shared by patient or carer and then written down in the notes. This is not to advocate mental health nurses revealing their whole life story, issues and problems, but to demonstrate vulnerability and being human, allowing the person/patient to be the expert of their own experience.

As a community development worker since 1980 I have engaged in an empowering way with people, where the aim has been to enable, to inform and to create spaces where people can learn, grow and become independent, emancipated members of their community. It has meant that from the beginning the end was in sight. You might describe this as having an exit strategy from the entrance door. I see this as being therapeutic and in the best interests of the 'other'. I would like mental health nurses to empower patients and, in so doing, be empowered themselves. The challenge, as ever, will be in the dynamics of the nurse/patient/psychiatrist triangle.

The following quotations capture the power of human-to-human interaction, and taking the side of the 'other' and the possible need to negotiate difficult dynamics to facilitate change:

The more radical the person is, the more fully he or she enters into reality so that, knowing it better, he or she can transform it. This individual is not afraid to confront, to listen, to see the world unveiled. This person is not afraid to meet the people or to enter into a dialogue with them. This person does not consider himself or herself the proprietor of history or of all people, or the liberator of the oppressed; but he or she does commit himself or herself, within history, to fight at their side.[19] (p.39)

Change means movement. Movement means friction. Only in the frictionless vacuum of a nonexistent abstract world can movement or change occur without that abrasive friction of conflict.[20] (p.21)

Rosie

Your focus on the human connection as a key element of the therapeutic relationship resonates with findings of Welch's[21] small qualitative study of experienced mental health nurses' perceptions of what makes a difference in the therapeutic relationship. In this study, empathy, authenticity and congruence were identified as the main qualities or attributes of effective interpersonal nursing.

The human element of the therapeutic relationship is also evident in patients' accounts of what they are expecting from mental health nurses. Service user participants in the study by Barker et al.[22] reported a desire for closer, more reciprocal relationships, and in Moyles'[15] study they expected a nurturing relationship which they only experienced briefly at the point of admission. As in the study by Stenhouse,[13] patients in Moyles'[15] study expected that the nurses would actively seek to create therapeutic relationships with them as a means of therapy and were disappointed when this did not happen.

Chrys

I appear to be different from the patients mentioned in your study and Barker et al.,[22] in that I wasn't looking for therapeutic support from nurses. As a psychiatric inpatient on three separate occasions (1978, 1984, 2002), for up to 4 weeks at a time, I formed therapeutic relationships with my peers, other psychiatric inpatients, and found the peer support to be both a survival mechanism and a way of

being in solidarity with others in a similar situation. The main reason I didn't form helpful alliances with nurses in psychiatric settings was because of being resistant to treatment and therefore subject to coercive drug treatment.

The earlier two inpatient stays were as a result of painful childbirths and diagnoses of puerperal psychosis. The treatment consisted of antipsychotics and separation from my babies, a painful course of action which further alienated me from the staff, although I wouldn't have wanted my baby sons to be in a psychiatric hospital. I made a full recovery after a year by tapering the drug and getting back on with my life.

In 2002, after 17 years of good mental health, I experienced another altered mind state when I was 50 and menopausal. Again I entered a psychiatric ward voluntarily, but was detained for 72 hours when I was resistant to remaining a patient, on seeing what the ward was like. Again I formed therapeutic relationships with fellow patients, who showed me the ropes. Risperidone was given to me in pill form, which I swallowed. As usual, the antipsychotic depressed me, and after discharge I was prescribed venlafaxine and then lithium as my flatness of mood continued. I found that psychiatric drugs for me weren't therapeutic.

It was at this point that I eventually experienced a therapeutic relationship and alliance with a community psychiatric nurse, a woman about my age who visited me in my own home and shared personal experiences of her home life and circumstances. I felt that we were more like friends than nurse and patient. She helped signpost me to different activities, listened to my concerns, and was a confidence builder and stepping stone to volunteering opportunities. She took early retirement and discussed this with me at the time. Her trust in me meant that I felt valued, and it was reciprocated. It made all the difference to my recovery.

Rosie and Chrys

So what we are identifying are some key features of the therapeutic relationship as an intentional activity which is orientated towards the needs of the patient, but in which the nurse develops a relationship that is reciprocal and human. It is these latter features of the relationship which Chrys identifies that highlight the need for the nurse to be able to work between the personal and professional self. This requires self-awareness and conscious use of personal experience as the basis for interaction, while ensuring that the boundaries of such interaction do not lead to the nurse using the relationship to satisfy her own needs.

Listening to stories

Rosie

We have just identified how the therapeutic relationship is a dialogical relationship through which nurses and patients come to know each other, and work towards mutually agreed goals for the benefit of the patient. But how can we come to know the experience of another person? This is a problem identified by Laing,[23] who recognized that experience is individual, and invisible, except through its expression:

> *'I cannot experience your experience. You cannot experience my experience. We are both invisible men. All men are invisible to one another. Experience used to be called The Soul. Experience as invisibility from man to man is at the same time more evident than anything'* (p.16).

It is generally understood that experience is expressed through the stories we tell ourselves and each other about events.[24-26] As we tell stories we make sense of our experiences as well as express them for others to hear. Stories therefore form a vital element of the therapeutic relationship. Through listening to patients' stories we can find out how they perceive the world, how they understand their problems as having come about, their values and their goals. Listening to people's stories enables us not only to get a sense of 'what' is happening but also 'how' they make sense of it. Understanding how a person makes sense of what is happening to them is important, as it allows us to shape our interactions in a way that conveys empathy. By taking the time to listen to the patient's story, engaging with it and asking questions arising from it, we also demonstrate that we are valuing the patient as a person.[27]

Taking time to listen to a person's story enables the person to develop their story in line with what is important to them using their own language. Allowing a person to develop their story requires the nurse to focus on what is being set out in front of them, allowing questions to arise from what they are hearing so that they are probing for greater detail.

Through active engagement with the patient's story, the nurse can demonstrate a desire to understand the patient's perspective, demonstrating empathy and placing importance on the individuality of the patient. Valuing the person's individuality enables the nurse to understand how they have constructed their identity and their relation to the context of their lives. This is important not only because these factors drive behaviour, but also because the problems which bring patients into contact with mental health services are experienced in the context of their lives, and therefore need to be understood in that context.

Stories also offer an opportunity to explore new ways of understanding the world, because they are the means by which people make sense of what happens. As a person tells their story they are encouraged to take different perspectives by the response of the listener. This new learning is applied to the story as we re-tell it, allowing us to see alternatives to our original understanding of events. In this way storytelling can also facilitate problem solving as part of the work of the therapeutic relationship.[27,28]

Chrys

I have found when reading the psychiatric notes of family members that what is written can tell a different story from our experiences of the events that happened. I describe this as a 'work of fiction'. It has often seemed that notes are written up to justify an action or a reaction to a person's behaviour. I'm thinking of both patient and carer. 'Difficult and demanding mother' was a phrase used to describe an occasion when I questioned what was going on in the ward, why certain things were or were not happening. My response as a mother and writer has been to blog about it or to write emails to people in positions of power so that my side of the story can be told and listened to. You might describe this as taking back the power.[29]

I have advocated for family members and others so that their story and voice are listened to. I think it's about bringing balance to a situation, or redressing the balance, so that the being 'done to' becomes doing or being with.[30]

REFLECTION

How can the nursing notes be written so that they accurately reflect the person's story and not the nurse's interpretation of events or experiences? How can the person be involved in writing their own notes?

Rosie

Chrys, what are your thoughts about stories and being listened to? Do nurses take time to listen to your story? If they don't listen to your story, how does that feel/what is the impact on your relationship with them? I know that in my research[13,16] a couple of the participants pointed out that the nurses couldn't possibly understand what was happening to them as they never came and asked them.

Chrys

In my experiences of psychiatric inpatient care it always felt like a 'them and us' scenario, both in the earlier inpatient stays and the latter one which was in a different health board area. Having entered a psychiatric ward with a psychosis or altered mind state meant a disconnect from the beginning, and the coercive drug treatment only increased the gap and the mistrust. Of my three sons who have like me experienced psychoses and inpatient treatment, only one of them formed therapeutic alliances with nurses both in hospital and out in the community. He prefers being in a relationship with a nurse to one with a fellow patient. I think that he would say the nurses understand him and he sees them as both equals and colleagues. I should add that he lives in a different health board area to the one where the rest of us accessed psychiatric treatment. He trusts the nursing staff and I have found them also to be respectful of me as a carer and mother. This wasn't the case for my other two sons.

THE CONTEXT OF THERAPEUTIC RELATIONSHIPS

Rosie and Chrys

What we have just talked about is the definition, or the ideal, of the therapeutic relationship. We also identified that the patient experience might not match the nurses' intentions. Some of the reasons for this mismatch can be identified when considering the context of therapeutic relationships. Relationships develop in a particular socio-political and historical context which, through the development of norms, is often experienced as the taken-for-granted backdrop to mental health care. Across history it is possible to see how prevailing social attitudes towards mental illness have led to the development of particular treatments and services.[31–33]

At present, the prevailing ideology which underpins policy and practice is recovery (see chapter 35). Therapeutic relationships within the context of recovery are underpinned by the concepts of hope, collaboration, relationships, strengths and finding a purpose or meaning.[34] As Barker and Buchanan-Barker[35] write: 'We believe that the key to "recovery" is to be found in "story telling". By "bearing witness", or "telling my story", people discover the "personal truth" of their own life - as opposed to the artificial, theoretical "truths" offered by different psychiatric professionals'.

However, this occurs within a mental health care system which exerts its power through systems of diagnosis and application of mental health legislation.[36] As a representative of this system, the position of the nurse in relation to the patient is always associated with power, and such power impacts on the development of therapeutic relationships.

Chrys

I think the psychiatrist is the invisible third person in every relationship between a nurse and patient. The psychiatrist makes decisions on diagnoses, treatment and drug prescribing. The nurse carries out these decisions, some of which he may not be in agreement with. Therefore the nurse may see himself as being disempowered in the relationship with the psychiatrist and at the same time being an advocate for the patient at clinical meetings.

REFLECTION

Think of ways in which the disempowerment of a nurse's relationship with a psychiatrist may be of benefit in the therapeutic relationship with a patient. How might this power imbalance help in the alliances formed with patients and increase understanding of the patient perspective and their feelings of powerlessness?

One of the big issues relating to power is the use of the Mental Health Act. Mary O'Hagan[37] writes that:

The four cornerstones of a recovery approach are hope and belief in people's potential, self-determination over their lives, the choice of a broad range of services, and equal participation in their communities. Legal coercion, through mental health legislation, empowers selected mental health professionals with support from the police and the judiciary to detain people in hospital, treat them without their consent, place them in solitary confinement (seclusion), and in many jurisdictions to compel people to take treatment in the community. Legal coercion erodes all the cornerstones of the recovery philosophy, yet it remains a core response in our mental health systems.

Rosie

Morgan and Felton[38] also identify tension between the ideology of recovery and mental health legislation. They cite the increasing use of community treatment orders (CTOs) as a threat to these cornerstones of recovery, rendering it a rhetorical exercise. In situations where the patient is being treated under a section of the mental health legislation, the problem of power can interfere with the development of the therapeutic relationship. However, even in situations of voluntary treatment, patients are aware of the potential power of the Mental Health Act.[39,16] (For detailed discussion of the related issues of freedom and consent, see chapter 18.)

Chrys

As a psychiatric inpatient the voluntary act of putting myself into a psychiatric ward for respite and care, after experiencing an altered mind state, led to my being detained and made to swallow antipsychotic drugs. This meant my relationships with the mental health nurses felt unequal from the offset and I distrusted their actions.

REFLECTION

How can you help to build an equal relationship when trust may have been eroded and/or agency (the capacity of individuals to act independently and to make their own free choices) denied?

Rosie

As well as issues of power, research from the patient and nurse perspective has identified features of the care context that impact on the therapeutic relationship. Much of this work has been carried out in hospital wards. However there are many issues regarding the context that are transferable to the community context. Particular issues are the experiences that patients identify of the nurses not being accessible, often because they are undertaking other, non-patient-centred tasks, such as admin and ward management.[13,17] A lack of time being offered or, even when there is time, interruptions can lead to a lack of interaction.[18] While these issues may seem to be particular to the inpatient environment, it is possible for the pressure on nurses in the community to impede the time offered to the therapeutic relationship, and distractions within the home environment – television, other family members, animals – can impact on the quality of relating.

Previous experience of developing close relationships in inpatient settings has been found in one study to correlate with the ease with which patients developed therapeutic relationships in an outpatient setting.[40] In Chrys's stories above, the impact of her previous experience of relationships in inpatient care on her relationships with the nurses during subsequent admissions is clearly demonstrated.

THE THERAPEUTIC RELATIONSHIP AS A JOURNEY

Rosie

In her writing in the 1950s, Peplau identified that the nurse–patient relationship proceeded through three overlapping phases of orientation, working and resolution.[4] Subsequent authors have identified other models of three phases arising out of work with patients[14] and nurses.[41] While the phases derived from the work of these authors are labelled differently, the utility in conceptualizing the nurse–patient relationship as a journey with different phases lies in the understanding that it flows through a process of getting to know one another, setting goals and working together to reach a final phase of negotiating disengagement as patients develop their capacity to cope.

KEY FEATURES OF THE THERAPEUTIC RELATIONSHIP

Within the research literature, regardless of how the journey of the relationship is conceptualized or whether the focus is on the nurse or patient perspective, there are a number of key features of nurse–patient interaction that are identified as contributing to the development of therapeutic relationships. These are empathy, authenticity, trust, openness, genuineness, congruence, partnership/mutuality, dignity, respect[41–43] and being listened to/nurses giving time.

These were also identified above in Chrys's discussion of the therapeutic relationship. We will therefore discuss Rodgers's core conditions – empathy, congruence and unconditional positive regard – and collaboration or alliance as the means through which all of these features might be addressed within the relationship.

Empathy

Chrys

Mercer and Reynolds[44] identify that 'Clinical empathy involves an ability to: (a) understand the patient's situation, perspective, and feelings (and their attached meanings); (b) to communicate that understanding and check its accuracy; and (c) to act on that understanding with the patient in a helpful (therapeutic) way' (p.S9).

Rosie

The definition above highlights some important aspects of empathy. In particular, it is notable that the authors view empathy as more than simply understanding how another person feels, and that it involves actively engaging with the patient to test interpretations, and then using this information as the basis for action. A range of communication skills are used to demonstrate empathy, including active listening and reflective statements. The ability to empathize guides the nurse's interactions with the patient, enabling them to collaborate and work towards jointly identified goals.[45]

Chrys

I have found as an activist and campaigner in mental health matters that sharing stories of lived experience is a powerful way of eliciting empathy and understanding in the hearer and listener, and can influence positive change. However, in the psychiatric or mental health setting, stories become symptoms and behaviours that result in diagnoses and treatment being written up in the notes.

Here is the dilemma of the nurse as an interface between the psychiatrist and patient, and the challenge of being empathic and congruent to the patient while having to report at clinical meetings on how the patient is 'presenting' or behaving. As a carer advocating at clinical meetings for family members I am aware of the power imbalances for both nurses and patients. I wonder if this might be an opportunity for a more therapeutic alliance between nurse and patient that may lead to more collaborative stories of people who are patients receive top billing rather than being an afterthought or postscript.

Congruence

Rosie

Congruence, or genuineness, relates to the fit of the nurse's inner experience with his outer expression and is sometimes termed *authenticity*. This condition requires the nurse to be self-aware, and to give something of himself. It brings to the fore issues of boundaries between the personal and professional self. While the judicious use of self-disclosure might enhance the therapeutic potential of the relationship, this should only ever be carried out in the best interests of the patient. The ability to make judgements about what and when to disclose comes with experience and through reflection on practice.

Achieving such authenticity in therapeutic relationships may be challenging. The professional status of the nurse requires that he does not allow his emotional state to reduce the quality of care provided, and impact negatively on the therapeutic relationship. Nurses must therefore undertake emotional labour[46] as they manage their emotional responses to patients. Emotional labour aims to induce a positive emotional response and the feeling of being cared for in others[46–48] through the nurse's suppression or induction of emotion in herself, in line with the feeling rules of a particular care context.

Smith[48] identified emotional labour as central to the nurse–patient relationship, and the experience of care. This is supported by Gray's[47] conclusion in a small qualitative study of nurses', GPs', student nurses' and lecturers' understanding and experience of emotional labour. He states that 'emotional labour informs interpersonal relationships and sustains the quality of nurse–patient care. Emotional labour is potentially of great therapeutic value'[47] (p.173).

While emotional labour might be a feature of quality nurse–patient relationships, it is also effortful. If not attended to it may lead to stress and 'burn out' in nurses. Clinical supervision (see chapter 10) provides the opportunity to discuss the emotion-related issues that arise through caring for patients.

Unconditional positive regard

Rosie

Unconditional positive regard is often discussed in terms of being non-judgemental. That is, the nurse interacts with the patient in a way that conveys acceptance of who they are. In order to practise in a manner that conveys unconditional positive regard and makes patients feel valued, it is necessary for nurses to recognize their own value systems and how these may conflict with those of others, creating judgement.

REFLECTION

Our interpersonal interactions are influenced by both our personal and professional value systems. These value systems develop through experience and education over the course of our lives, and for most of us form the taken-for-granted norms of our everyday world. We are often unaware of the values that guide our interactions and only become aware of them when something conflicts with our taken-for-granted view of the world. Take five minutes to identify some of your personal and professional values? How do these values impact on your interactions with patients?

Chrys

'As a qualified community education worker, the core conditions', according to Carl Rogers 'were taught and learned, and underpinned our practice.' These underpinned my practice. In addition, reflection-in-action[49] was a key part of being an effective, empowering communicator.

A practitioner's reflection can serve as a corrective to over-learning. Through reflection, he can surface and criticize the tacit understandings that have grown up around the repetitive experiences of a specialized practice, and can make new sense of the situations of uncertainty or uniqueness which he may allow himself to experience.[49] (p.61)

I think that mental health nurses working in inpatient settings may find it more challenging than their community-based counterparts to foster and maintain empathy, congruence and openness in their relationships with patients. They will on occasion be faced with mentally distressed people who test their patience to the limits, and ward conditions that may be less than favourable, for example lack of privacy, mixed gender wards, limited resources, reduced staff numbers or temporary staff. Nurses are only human and should have the space to develop their authenticity, improving their practice. The key to this will be good management and relationships between nurses on the ground and in the offices.

When I have raised issues in nursing practice, from the carer perspective, it resulted in more note-writing training sessions. I found this puzzling and would have preferred a focus on relational interactions, reflecting on practice and involving people with lived experience in staff training workshops. Face-to-face working with people in mental distress has to be the most challenging of interactions, and learning or training in this area could be of real benefit in these interactions, helping to foster more therapeutic relationships.

Therapeutic alliances

Chrys

In everyday life situations, connections with fellow human beings are often what make sense of it all – the feeling that we are not alone on this planet, that another person understands us and has really listened to our story. If it can happen with a stranger on a bus or park bench, then there is no reason why it shouldn't be happening between a mental health nurse and their patient. I think the challenge is to see the person and not the label,[50] and this begins in the psychiatric setting.

Rosie

In her definition of the therapeutic relationship at the beginning of this chapter, Chrys equated a good relationship to an alliance. Alliance or collaboration also underpins the concept of recovery. In their study of nurses' and patients' experience of collaboration, McCloughen et al.[12] found that patients found it difficult to collaborate with nurses, felt devalued, and often ended up simply going along with the nurses' desires.

Interestingly, this conflicts with the nurses' perceptions that they were working collaboratively with patients. The patients identified that improved communication, listening to their stories, and the nurses having the authority to make decisions about the issues they raised would improve their experience.

CONCLUSION

Rosie and Chrys

In this chapter we have examined a number of factors that contribute to the development of the therapeutic relationship. These include intrapersonal factors such as value systems, and personal attributes, as well as consideration of the context of mental health nursing practice. The literature indicates that it is possible to develop and nurture therapeutic relationships in which nurses actively seek to engage with patients, focus on their needs, and attend to their story to collaboratively identify their needs within the context of their lives.

The evidence from the patient experience literature highlights the need for nurses to make time for patients. Initially, at least, this will involve actively seeking out the person and engaging with them. Such engagement may take the form of a verbal interaction if the person is amenable to this. However, where a person's mental distress has resulted in withdrawal from social interaction, the simple process of being with, and present for, the person, in a way that enables them to feel that their distress and current emotional state has been acknowledged, may be what is required.

Whatever the form of the interaction, it is necessary for the person to feel that the nurse is present for them in that relationship. Presence involves focusing one's being on what is happening in the interaction without allowing external demands to intrude. Interacting with people in a

way that involves presence, even if it is only a brief encounter, promotes the sense of being valued and respected.

Where developing a relationship ends and maintaining it begins is not clear-cut, and the ways of interacting at the beginning are not necessarily changed at the point of maintaining the relationship. What might demarcate the two is the change in power relations as the relationship progresses. At the beginning of the relationship, particularly if the person is beginning contact with mental health services, the nurse may need to develop a much more structured relationship with the person. At this point the balance of power sits with the nurse, who sets boundaries and guides the structure of the interactions. As the relationship develops, a collaboration can occur, enabling shared goal setting, and the role of the nurse changes in relation to the patient.

Finally, let's return to the concept of craft developed by Barker and Whitehill,[11] introduced at the beginning of this chapter. We would like to reiterate that, if caring is conceptualized as a craft, then it is the *recipients*, not the providers, of that care who must validate the activities of the nurse as *caring*. It follows that, if one of the keys to caring is the development and maintenance of therapeutic relationships, it is imperative that mental health nurses have the skills, attributes and knowledge to develop high quality relationships that are experienced by the patient/person as *caring*.

References

1. Bertram V. Theorising the personal: using autobiography in academic writing. In: Jackson J, Jones J (eds). *Contemporary feminist theories*. Edinburgh: Edinburgh University Press, 1998: 232–46.
2. Lather P. *Getting smart: feminist research and pedagogy with/in the postmodern*. New York: Routledge, 1991.
3. Buchanan-Barker P, Barker P. Observation: the original sin of mental health nursing? *Journal of Psychiatric and Mental Health Nursing* 2005; **12**: 541–9.
4. Peplau HE. *Interpersonal relations in nursing*. Basingstoke: Macmillan Education, 1998.
5. Altschul A. A personal view of psychiatric nursing. In: Tilley S (ed.). *The mental health nurse: views of practice and education*. Oxford: Blackwell Science, 1997: 1–14.
6. Munro S, Baker J. Surveying the attitudes of acute mental health nurses. *Journal of Psychiatric and Mental Health Nursing* 2007; **14**: 196–202.
7. Hewitt J, Coffey M. Therapeutic working relationships with people with schizophrenia: literature review. *Journal of Advanced Nursing* 2005; **52**(5): 561–70.
8. Cahill J, Paley G, Hardy G. What do patients find helpful in psychotherapy? Implications for the therapeutic relationship in mental health nursing. *Journal of Psychiatric and Mental Health Nursing* 2013; **20**: 782–91.
9. Reynolds W, Cormack D. *Psychiatric and mental health nursing: theory and practice*. London: Chapman and Hall, 1990.
10. Barker PJ, Reynolds W, Ward T. The proper focus of nursing: a critique of the 'caring' ideology. *International Journal of Nursing Studies* 1995; **32**(4): 386–97.
11. Barker P, Whitehill I. The craft of care: towards collaborative caring in psychiatric nursing. In: Tilley S (ed.). *The mental health nurse: views of practice and education*. Oxford: Blackwell Science, 1997: 15–27.
12. McCloughen A, Gillies D, O'Brien L. Collaboration between mental health consumers and nurses: shared understandings, dissimilar experiences. *International Journal of Mental Health Nursing* 2011; **20**: 47–55.
13. Stenhouse R. 'They all said you could come and speak to us': patients' expectations and experiences of help on an acute psychiatric inpatient ward. *Journal of Psychiatric and Mental Health Nursing* 2011; **18**: 74–80.

14. Coatsworth-Puspoky R, Forchuk C, Ward-Griffin C. Nurse–client processes in mental health: recipients' perspectives. *Journal of Psychiatric and Mental Health Nursing* 2006; **13**: 347–55.

15. Moyles W. Nurse–patient relationship: a dichotomy of expectations. *International Journal of Mental Health Nursing* 2003; **12**: 103–9.

16. Stenhouse R. *Unfulfilled expectations: individuals' experiences of being a patient on an acute psychiatric inpatient ward.* Saarbrucken, Germany: Lambert Academic Publishing, 2013.

17. Clarke L, Flannagan T. *Institutional breakdown: exploring mental health nursing practice in acute inpatient settings.* Salisbury: APS Publishing, 2003.

18. Cleary M, Edwards C. 'Something always comes up': nurse–patient interaction in an acute psychiatric setting. *Journal of Psychiatric and Mental Health Nursing* 1999; **6**: 469–77.

19. Friere P. *Pedagogy of the oppressed: 30th anniversary edition.* New York: Continuum, 2006.

20. Alinsky S. *Rules for radicals.* New York: Random House, 1971.

21. Welch M. Pivotal moments in the therapeutic relationship. *International Journal of Mental Health Nursing* 2005; **14**: 161–5.

22. Barker P, Jackson S, Stevenson, C. What are psychiatric nurses needed for? Developing a theory of essential nursing practice. *Journal of Psychiatric and Mental Health Nursing* 1999; **6**: 273–82.

23. Laing RD. *The politics of experience and the bird of paradise.* London: Penguin, 1967.

24. Frank AW. *The wounded storyteller: body, illness, and ethics.* Chicago: University of Chicago Press, 1995.

25. Gee JP. The narrativization of experience in the oral style. *Journal of Education* 1985; **167**(1): 9–35.

26. Riessman CK. *Narrative analysis.* Oakland, CA: Sage, 1993.

27. McLeod J. *Narrative and psychotherapy.* London: Sage, 1997.

28. White M, Epston D. *Narrative means to therapeutic ends.* New York: W.W. Norton and Co., 1990.

29. Coleman R. *Recovery: an alien concept?* Gloucester: Handsell, 2000.

30. Hanson B, Taylor MF. Being-With, Doing-With: a model of the nurse–client relationship in mental health nursing. *Journal of Psychiatric and Mental Health Nursing* 2000; **7**(5): 417–23.

31. Pilgrim D, Rogers A. *A sociology of mental health and illness.* Buckingham: Open University Press, 2010.

32. Porter R. *Madness: a brief history.* Oxford: Oxford University Press, 2002.

33. Foucault M. *Madness and civilisation: a history of insanity in the age of reason.* New York: Vintage, 1988.

34. Repper J, Perkins R. *Social inclusion and recovery: a model for mental health practice.* London: Bailliere Tindall, 2003.

35. Barker P, Buchanan-Barker P. The Tidal Commitments: extending the value base of mental health recovery. *Journal of Psychiatric and Mental Health Nursing* 2008; **15**: 93–100.

36. Muirhead C. I would like to see a reframing of psychosis. *Mental Health Nursing* 2013; **33**(4): 7.

37. O'Hagan M. Legal coercion: the elephant in the recovery room. *Scottish Recovery Network.* Available from: http://www.scottishrecovery.net/resource/legal-coercion-the-elephant-in-the-recovery-room/ [Accessed 5th September 2016].

38. Morgan A, Felton A. From constructive engagement to coerced recovery. In: Coles S, Keenan S, Diamond B (eds). *Madness contested: power and practice.* Ross-on-Wye: PCCS Books, 2013: chapter 4.

39. Campbell P. Challenging loss of power. In Read J, Reynolds J (eds). *Speaking our minds: an anthology.* Basingstoke: Palgrave, 2000: 56–62.

40. Sosnowska M, Prot-Klinger K, Scattergood M, Paczkowska M, Smolicz A, Ochoka M. The therapeutic relationship and patients' experience of interpersonal bonds – research conducted in outpatient mental health care. *Archives in Psychiatry and Psychotherapy* 2013; **1**: 11–18.

41. Miner-Williams D. Connectedness in the nurse–patient relationship: a grounded theory study. *Issues in Mental Health Nursing* 2007; **28**: 1215–34.

42. Dziopa F, Ahern K. Three different ways mental health nurses develop quality therapeutic relationships. *Issues in Mental Health Nursing* 2009; **30**: 14–22.

43. Awty P, Welch A, Kuhn L. A naturalistic inquiry of registered nurses' perspectives and expectations of psychodynamic therapeutic care in acute psychiatric inpatient facilities. *Archives of Psychiatric Nursing* 2010; **24**(2): 104–13.

44. Mercer S, Reynolds W. Empathy and quality of care. *British Journal of General Practice* (Quality Supplement) 2002; **52**: S9–S13.

45. Perraud S, Delaney KR, Carlson-Sabelli L, Johnson ME, Shephard R, Paun O. Advanced practice psychiatric mental health nursing, finding our core: the therapeutic relationship in 21st century. *Perspectives in Psychiatric Care* 2006; **42**(4): 215–26.

46. Hochschild A. *The managed heart: commercialization of human feeling.* Berkeley, CA: University of California Press, 1983.

47. Gray B. The emotional labour of nursing: defining and managing emotions in nursing work. *Nurse Education Today* 2009; **29**: 168–75.

48. Smith P. *Emotion work: can nurses still care?* Basingstoke: Palgrave, 2012.

49. Schon D. *The reflective practitioner: how professionals think in action.* New York: Basic Books, 1983.

50. Scottish Government 'See Me' anti-stigma campaign. Available from: http://seemescotland.org.uk/ [Accessed 10th May 2014].

Further reading

Bach S, Grant A. *Communication and interpersonal skills for nursing.* Exeter: Learning Matters, 2009.

Collins S. Good communication helps to build a therapeutic relationship. *Nursing Times.net* 13 May 2015. Available from: http://www.nursingtimes.net/nursing-practice/specialisms/educators/good-communication-helps-to-build-a-therapeutic-relationship/5003004.article [Accessed 14th September 2016].

Combs G, Freedman J. Relationships, not boundaries. *Theoretical Medicine* 2002; **23**: 203–17.

Dziopa F, Ahern K. What makes a quality therapeutic relationship in psychiatric/mental health nursing: a review of the research literature. *Internet Journal of Advanced Nursing Practice* 2008; **10**(1).

Smith P. *Emotion work: can nurses still care?* Basingstoke: Palgrave, 2012.

Relevant web pages

Muirhead C. Chrys Muirhead writes. Weblog. ChrysMuirheadWrites.blogspot.co.uk

Rogers, Carl http://www.simplypsychology.org/client-centred-therapy.html

Narratives in mental health https://www.hindawi.com/journals/nrp/2011/293837/

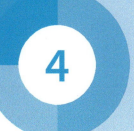

4 The politics, care and confinement of the mentally ill

LIAM CLARKE AND PHIL RUTHEN

LEARNING OUTCOMES

- To understand the history of psychiatric care and confinement.

- To have a fuller awareness of the interplay between confinement, therapy, politics and morality.

- To begin to understand the concept of community care as an extension of (psychological) confinement.

- To appreciate the roles of gender, class and economics in the political construction of institutional centres of care.

- To be able to integrate these outcomes with strategies of caring, formulating an approach that does not reject medically based perspectives but incorporates them into the craft of caring.

SUMMARY OF KEY POINTS

- The history of psychiatric care is grounded in ambivalence, both in its intent and in its practice.

- This ambivalence takes the form of a balance between therapeutics on the one hand and a perceived need for confinement and safety on the other.

- Although the structures and frameworks of delivering care alter and change, from asylum to hospital, to community and outreach programmes, it is argued that these two fundamental themes of coercion and benevolence are still sustained, albeit in more subtle forms.

- Increasingly, their forms are becoming less subtle. In the event of compliance with a treatment order, for instance, a patient can be recalled to custodial care.

- An important and continually neglected point is the denial, within British contexts, of the considerable political forces – typically played out in gender, class,

and economic terms – that impinge on many aspects of the delivery of care.

- Many nurses have had to struggle (with varying levels of success) against the limitations of institutional care and the ongoing social/political expectations of nurses.

- Current debates about nurse prescribing reflect the ambivalence about the role and identity of mental health nurses.

- Within strictures and sometimes against opposing forces, nurses have developed caring packages, and have developed the craft of caring in interpersonal terms.

- In a climate of tight fiscal management, prioritization of mental health has become a central issue, both for professionals and for society in general.

INTRODUCTION

In the beginning was Bedlam: initially called the Priory of St Mary of Bethlehem, this was later bowdlerized to Bethlem, or Bedlam. In the thirteenth century it was the only 'lunatic enclosure' in England and was probably privately owned. For an entrance fee, inmates could be viewed as though they were in a freak show, although at the time there were hardly more than a half-dozen patients.

Bedlam is important, because much of psychiatry's reputation would rest on how it was perceived over time. For example, the passage of time has canonized an image of affluent people paying to watch confined, brutalized, terrified lunatics. However, history contrasts this image with that of the 'liberating' activities of Philippe Pinel in Paris and the Tukes in England. Allderidge[1] notes that histories of Bedlam utilize few primary sources, resulting in widespread assumptions about its meagre provision and commercial proclivities. The brutality which endured until the eighteenth century is hardly denied but, as Allderidge shows, things are more complicated than that. By 1677, for instance, Bethlem's rules stated that: 'None of the Officers or Servants shall at any time beat or abuse any of the Lunatics in the said hospital, neither shall offer any force unto them but upon absolute necessity for the better government of the said Lunatics'.[2] In other words, whatever may have prevailed on the 'shop floor', force was not seen by the Bethlem authorities as ordinarily acceptable. Also, its provision of two wards for 'incurables' suggests that, for some (other) patients, recovery was a realistic aspiration. All these changes occurred within the political context of their times. In general terms, therefore, medicalized approaches to 'care' were gradually politically validated via governmental legislation. Treatments could either be brutal or weird in the extreme. Doctor Cox,[3] for instance, suspended patients from the ceiling in a contraption that rotated them 100 times per minute; unsurprisingly, many hastily reported a marked improvement in their condition.

The practice of paying to watch lunatics had become an established custom since the time patients were first incarcerated, and not just as a money-earner. In 1673, a new building, at Moorfields, replaced the old Bethlem and although – like the later Victorian asylums – its outward appearance was grand, on the inside it was anything but. Inmates were still put on display, this time along two galleries, one above the other. In addition, 'on each floor a corridor ran along a line of cells, with an iron gate in the middle to divide the males from the females'[4] (p.519).

BEYOND BEDLAM

After Bethlem, from the early eighteenth century, other asylums sprang up, mostly as a result of local initiatives, and these constituted the first wave of public asylums in England. The first, St Luke's, London, began under the guidance of William Battie, whose *Treatise on madness* had become very influential. Unsurprisingly, one of his initial actions was to ban asylum sightseers. St Luke's also broke with the past by accepting medical students. Although this suggests a newfound liberalism in English psychiatry, it was the arrival of 'moral therapy' at the York Retreat which heralded fundamental shifts in how lunacy was conceived and managed. Spearheaded by a Quaker family, the Tukes, its most significant innovation was a recognition that communities of carers and patients could be a force for good. Rather than using the established practices of trying to alter the lunatic's will, by medicine fair or foul, patients were now gently coerced, much as a kind parent would 'inculcate' good behaviour in a child. The intent, via praise as well as caution, was that inmates might recapture a measure of dignity and self-control. In her history of the Retreat, Ann Digby[5] notes that this liberalism was not new but rather was premised on received ideas of ethical and rational justice coupled with the growing abandonment of physical restraints. This matters, because it points towards the development of caring strategies that would ultimately evolve from the idea of treating people as individuals who are deserving of empathy and positive regard.

However, the Retreat had little direct influence on contemporary asylum practices *at the time*, perhaps unsurprisingly given the uniqueness of its religious disposition but, as well, the overriding dead hand of a generally conservative and cultural attitude towards how 'the mad' should be managed. True, there were some instances of liberal treatment in the early asylums, with some of them showing commendable tolerance of inmates' behaviour[6] (ch.10), but they could never fully ignore political pressure which forced their maintenance of a custodial role; furthermore, the sheer 'bricks and mortar' density of the asylums, of their presence, made liberalism extremely unlikely. For example, their perimeter walls could be as much as 15 feet high. Although this prevented the 'gaping at the lunatics' phenomenon, which, despite Battie's efforts, had continued into the early nineteenth century, their primary intention was to prevent escape. The devil, of course, is often in the detail, and Smith[7] reminds us that the fine grounds were restricted to fee-paying inmates, with the pauper lunatics taking their exercise in airing yards. The frightening conduction of sound (particularly at night), the poor diet, the bland hospital garb and the dead hand of unremitting routine bludgeoned individuality and, all told, endured into the second wave of Victorian asylums. Developing an ethos of care, in such conditions, must have been extraordinarily difficult. Even today, we take insufficient account of how intrusive organizations can be when developing person-centred methods of care.

For Roy Porter,[8] the story of English madness began in the late eighteenth century, and psychiatric institutionalization was the key to its history. From its beginnings, confinement has presented a fundamental challenge to practical psychiatry and care. Particularly difficult for nurses is the growing problem of reconciling custody and care.

Bethlem was hardly a prototype, but it influenced subsequent developments nationally. At Bethlem, the natural impetus had been to chain and punish, and although, even by the late sixteenth century, more enlightened treatments, coupled with some compassion, emerged,[8,9] the custodial impetus remained strong. The unleashing of restraints at Hanwell by John Connolly, in September 1839,[10] was a watershed, mainly on account of Hanwell's (large) size and Connolly's charismatic leadership. By the mid-nineteenth century, political dissatisfaction with custodialism and coercion was coalescing into a social push for change. In 1845, change came in spades with the passage of 'arguably the most significant mental health legislation of the century'[7] (p.275). This legislation required county magistrates to establish pauper lunatic asylums, with a remit that they follow Connolly's principles of unrestraint and care. By now, general standards of physical care had improved, but we must not suppose that the push for more civilized programmes came from within the existing mental institutions. Porter[8] has argued that what the nineteenth-century changes represented was an unprecedented public-spiritedness: Victorian England 'was, after all, a time of great men, of great vision, of great achievement'[11] (p.90), and with a political disposition to attack problems with verve and tenacity. The Victorians did not invent compassion for the plight of mad people, and their asylums lasted a mere century. Nevertheless, theirs was an extraordinary optimism, and achievement, all the same.

MORAL STRICTURES

To what extent did moral therapy (at the Retreat) reflect moral expectations generally? To what extent did moral therapy constitute, and camouflage, more subtle forms of restraint? Smith[7] observes that:

> *Moral treatment comprised more than a gentle, considerate approach. There were also aspects which sought to alter inappropriate behaviour. By 1800, the conception was widely accepted that the doctor had to gain ascendancy over the madman as a precursor to curative treatment. (p.191)*

This is important because even allegedly liberal psychiatric regimes can mask manipulative practices. For example, therapeutic communities[12] typically advocate principles of democratization, permissiveness, communalism and so on. However, these principles may cloak a deeper imperative such that, if the workings of the community break down, more traditional forms of management will re-emerge to put matters right. Lindsay,[13] a therapeutic community resident, noted that whenever matters became intolerable, conventional regimes surfaced to restore equilibrium.

These back-up systems imply a complicated overlap between public and institutional expectations, whereby institutions may display progressive practices such as unlocking doors, patients wearing their own clothes, participating in care plans and so on – features that represent development at one level, but whose apparent liberalism allows confinement and control when required.

Michel Foucault's[14] take on confinement is interesting. Confinement is the 'invention of a site of constraint, where morality castigates by means of administrative enforcement ... institutions of morality are established in which an astonishing synthesis of moral obligation and civil law is effected' (p.56). Although Foucault was primarily criticizing the York Retreat, with its abolition of physical constraints and instigation of a generally caring milieu, his criticisms just as easily apply to progressive movements generally. For Foucault, the Retreat substitutes the 'free terror' of madness with a stifling anguish of responsibility where, for the inmates, fear no longer waits outside the asylum gates but now resides within their newfound experience of conscience and normality.

Rather than punish guilt, the asylum now organizes it, and an illusion of (moral) therapy is created. Hand in hand with this, a slower development of asylum management occurs, largely giving way to an awareness of the need for rationality. An emergent medical professionalism slowly proceeds towards more open regimes of care: however, aided and abetted by the arrival of physical treatments, this has led to the objectification of patients, which can result in their experiences becoming separated from those of the general population. This causes concern about what is perceived as the dehumanizing of patients via a 'medical model' – a situation that psychiatric nurses strive to ameliorate.

Insightful obeisance

Much of Foucault's work is premised on the idea of patients as unwilling or ignorant participants in their treatment when, actually, patients can be complicit in their treatment or even detention. For instance, the first patients at the York Retreat were themselves Quakers and thus probably did not experience its 'moral management' as irksome or unwarranted.

However, a libertarian agenda drives much of Foucault's writing and one suspects that his conclusions do not always reflect available evidence. Contrary to Foucault, Digby's account[5] of the York Retreat is consistent with the high praise generally warranted by its humanitarianism. A measure of its openness, for example, was the fact that less than 5 per cent of inmates were restrained at any time and then only if violent or suicidal. Many of its inmates mixed freely with visitors; they dressed ordinarily, took tea with the governors and even, now and then, ventured outside the Retreat's walls.

However, Digby does support Foucault's assertion about moral control by highlighting the Retreat's implicit threat of restraint, as well as its religious training and work regimes. The problem with Foucault's perspective is that restraint does not preclude good therapeutic intentions. The basic aim of the Retreat was to allow people to recollect their senses by appealing to their unaffected faculties. In this, they were influenced by John Locke's assertion that insanity is a disturbance of the association of ideas, not of the spirit, nor of morality. If what they desired was improvement in moral probity, this may have been the true purpose of their regime.

Separation

One of Foucault's themes is that in the seventeenth century a grand confinement of society's rejects and misfits took place, eventually culminating in the building of the Victorian asylums. However, seventeenth-century confinement schemes were parochial in nature: much of the management of madness was in (often lucrative) private houses or in families (the latter classically realized in Bronte's *Jane Eyre*), and it was not until the early nineteenth century that a widespread separation of the mad was attempted.

Separation meant new rules: distancing patients from everyday life now implied human inferiority and a risk to society. However, the conventional view is that 'asylum colonization' was a positive outcome of Victorian political altruism coupled with an acceptance of medicine's growing confidence in managing the insane. Commenting on this, Andrew Scull[15] stated:

> *The very language that is used reflects the implicit assumptions which for many years marked most historians' treatment of the subject – a naive Whiggish view of history as progress, and a failure to see key elements of the reform process as sociologically highly problematic. (p.2)*

Foucault's view of pre-nineteenth-century society is that it is at ease with madness: in a sense, the village fool is indeed a fool, 'but he's our fool': he possesses consensual worth because, as yet, no epistemology exists by which to debar him. In this, Foucault attacks psychiatric science, which, he alleges, objectifies patients and thus marginalizes them. He has a point, since the close of the eighteenth century saw the advent of philosophical and scientific rationalism – with their offspring, sociology and psychology – a time when religious thought was superseded by humanist (scientific) discourse. Thus, psychiatry invents a concept of madness in which unreason is no longer considered virtuous. Thus Foucault's 'madman' – combined roughly of two parts noble savage and village buffoon – moves from his primitive but socially viable status, to that of mental defective where, in effect, medical expertise thwarts his moral status.

Many, of course, disagreed with this perspective. According to Edward Shorter,[16] prior to the building of asylums, people 'were treated with a savage lack of feeling … there was no golden era, no idyllic refuge from the values of capitalism. To maintain otherwise is a fantasy' (p.4).

In the context of a belief in 'golden eras' when the 'village idiot' was accorded a social status, however meagre, Shorter's point is well taken. However, Foucault's notion is not about how people treated one another – life was nasty, brutish and short for everyone – but that 'the mad' were now confined on grounds of disease, and were now conceptually excluded by scientific norms.

THE PRINCIPAL ISSUE

It is important to consider whether asylums were a product of Victorian paternalism, or a result of increasing medical power, part of whose agenda was to protect society from the criminal and/or eugenic propensities of the mentally ill. Edward Shorter crisply sets out the debate:[16]

> *To an extent unimaginable for other areas of the history of medicine, zealot-researchers have seized the history of psychiatry to illustrate how their pet bugaboos – be they capitalism, patriarchy, or psychiatry itself – have converted protest into illness, locking into asylums those who otherwise would be challenging the established order. (p.viii)*

On the other hand, Andrew Scull notes that:[15]

> *The direction taken by lunacy reform in the nineteenth century is thus presented as inevitable and basically benign – both in intent and in consequences – and the whole process crudely reduced to a simplistic equation: humanitarianism + science + government inspection = the success of what David Roberts calls the great nineteenth-century movement for a more humane and intelligent treatment of the insane. (pp.2–3)*

The issue is the extent to which elements from one or other of these strands holds true. Nietzsche states that, ultimately, all argument represents 'a desire of the heart', and this topic certainly feeds conflicting prejudices towards psychiatric practice.

The interpretations of anti-institutionalists were written up in a more creative and radical style than traditional accounts. That said, their argument that nineteenth-century reforms operated not as an outcome of Victorian benevolence, but as an attempt to corral troublesome citizens, is now seen as overly simplistic, as well as perhaps being aligned with radical political philosophies that were prevalent in the 1960s.

For example, while acknowledging the use of asylum patients as cheap labour, as well as the recurring violence and abuse of rights, Kathleen Jones[17] nevertheless states that asylums could be humane and intelligent. She asserts that much that has been written about asylums is biased, and that we should set aside our own prejudices and look at asylums in their contemporary context. What this might mean, for instance, is that, given the conditions of nineteenth-century working-class life, both in the workhouses and generally, asylum admission may well have been a blessing. For Jones, removing mentally ill people to rural hospital outposts protected them from unsanitary urban living conditions. Extraordinarily, Peter Ackroyd[4] records that Bethlem had a fresh water supply from an artesian well, which indeed conferred a lifetime's freedom from cholera. The location of asylums in rural areas was probably more to do with finance, the imperative being to purchase building land in cheap, non-urban settings. But it also of course flags up the endemic relationship between social class and psychiatry, the difficulties of separating out the two, as well as the difficulties of setting up communication systems between staff and patients. Embryonic forms of relationship-building depended upon language skills, and the comparative differences of these among different class groups may have been problematic.

So why were the Victorian asylums built?

Certainly 'social control' cannot be discounted at a time of political concern about public disorder. The asylums satisfied Victorian altruistic inclinations towards lunatics; however, the secondary purpose, to make the streets safe, cannot have been far from their minds. That said, the therapeutic ambitions of interested parties cannot be set aside lightly. In Walton's view,[18] the promise of 'cure' may have partly forced the development of asylum psychiatry. Undoubtedly, some anticipation of psychiatric cure prevailed for at least some mental states. As such, the new 'mad doctors' (as they were first called) needed a medical arena in which to work, and, with the new public asylums, they got it.

Also, asylums became places for working-class people to send relatives whose behaviour rendered them unsuitable for family living, at a time when market economics was leading to a separation of home and workplace. At a time when many people worked at home in 'cottage industries', the insane might be looked after at home. By the 1890s, however, asylums were populated by 'the impossible, the inconvenient and the inept'[15] (p.370). Whereas the old madhouses had accommodated obvious cases of madness, the clientele of the Victorian asylums was much broader. Scull[15] notes that in 1891 there were 15,853 institutionalized pauper lunatics in London but that this had increased to 26,293 by 1909. Since this sudden increase in numbers hardly reflected an increased incidence in mental illness, the implication is that some form of 'social cleansing' was at play. The governing principle seems to be that power elites restrict hapless, unproductive people; and if this interpretation is unpalatable, you may prefer the establishment view that Victorian altruists sought to help mentally unwell people through benevolence. Of course, both views can cohere: there are examples of magistrates and doctors incarcerating people so as to maintain social order but, equally, many of the relatives of these people appealed for this action to be taken, presumably in the 'best interests' of their relatives.

REFLECTION

In what ways can confinement be utilized as a liberating force, with regard to someone's personal psychology?

The nature of the beast

Although the nineteenth-century asylums housed many people who would today be diagnosed as 'schizophrenic', the variation in cases was remarkable. Walton[18] describes the case of Emma Blackburn, who, after spending 5 months in the Haslington workhouse, was admitted to an asylum in 1871. She was said to be suffering from 'political excitement'. According to the notes on her case, she looked healthy and robust, but after being admitted to the asylum, occasionally shouted and cried, was sometimes argumentative and at other times unresponsive, and had difficulty sleeping. Partly as a result of being given morphine but also, I imagine, the sheer horror of her predicament, she deteriorated, and after 2 years she died. Such cases were hardly rare, and although beliefs about women and madness varied across political and social dimensions, Elaine Showalter[19] states that:

The prevailing view amongst Victorian psychiatrists as that … women were more vulnerable to insanity because the instability of their reproductive systems interfered with their sexual, emotional, and rational control. (pp.55–6)

Skultans[20] agrees, saying that women were viewed at being at risk of insanity if they engaged in intellectual activity, from which their reproductive role precluded them.

REFLECTION

- Several issues can be weighed up at this point before moving into the 1950s and what can be called the modern era. For example, note the emphasis on female anatomy and vulnerability and how this increased in inverse ratio to women's demands for education – as well as growing assertiveness about their changing social roles. We universalize this point when we argue that psychiatric practice rarely fails to conform to prevalent social attitudes and mores.

- Also note how we have graduated from the asylum as a building, into its subsequent designation as hospital, and on to its fragmentation into 'services in the community'. It is at this point that we might ask whether change is necessarily superficial and designed to camouflage that which remains fundamentally the same. For instance, does the apparent sophistication (and rationales) of forensic systems ensure their continuance as forms of custodialism?

- Look especially at how different historians 'read into' events sometimes widely differing interpretations. To what extent do such interpretations influence contemporary perceptions of the profession and its varying activities? What kind of history does a profession require to further and underpin its ongoing designs and ambitions?

- The craft of caring can be traced throughout this history but mainly by implication. In some cases – such as the creation of therapeutic communities – we can gauge the theories behind change, but in many other cases we may suppose at best that human nature expressed its better aspects in those caring for people, be they called inmates, patients or just persons.

- Consider the present-day issue of nurse prescribing. Which historical accounts and rationales would be favoured by prescribers, as opposed to non-prescribers?

- Remember that history – as opposed to 'the past' – happens now: there are axes to grind and stories to tell. Bear this in mind as you continue to read on to where we are now and beyond.

THE 1950s ONWARDS

From the 1950s, psychiatry painstakingly got its medical act together: concepts of pauper lunatics were long gone and therapeutic zeal mushroomed. The eagerness to cure proceeded along two different fronts. One was social in nature and composed of two strands, namely the therapeutic community 'proper' (typified by the work of Maxwell Jones at the Henderson Hospital), and a therapeutic community 'approach' reflected in less radical activities such as unlocking doors and minimizing regimentation.[21] Nurses in the main favoured the approach followed by Maxwell Jones, probably because it fostered a more social domain, which would allow them – the nurses – to develop interventions that made sense within the larger therapeutic milieu. Jones actually required a multidisciplinary approach since by definition it complied with his group methods. Therefore nurses were able to formulate caring packages that now had the backing of well-founded theories, as well as support from sister agencies. See chapter 57 for further discussion on therapeutic communities.

A second front was a single-minded dedication to applying physical treatments that would halt mental illness once and for all. These two fronts could be linked in complex ways.

For example, William Sargant – doyen of physical treatment methods – insisted that phenothiazine drugs sounded the death knell of the asylums, since they allowed previously troublesome, withdrawn or disturbed patients to return home. Thus begins the mythical 'phenothiazine revolution', the supposed 'real' reason behind the unlocking of hospital doors and other liberal progressions. In addition, this false dawn detracted from psychiatric nurses' education, playing down more humanistic actions on their part. Indeed, many were lulled into a belief that, given the 'breakthrough' nature of these new drugs, more social or psychotherapeutic-based responses to people's distress would diminish. In fact, the post-war period was more intricate than this, with changing hospital practices stemming mainly from changing attitudes towards mental illness and its causation. The sobering spectacle of soldiers going to war in apparently good mental health, and returning psychologically wrecked, suggested that mental illness need no longer be seen, necessarily, as a pathology of the nervous system. That mental illness could come about, or at least be mediated by, social events severely dented the traditional regard for mental distress as 'inborn and irredeemable'.

The shortfalls of benevolence

By the mid-twentieth century, the Victorian mental hospitals were becoming subject to criticism and review. David Clark (personal communication), medical superintendent at Fulbourn Hospital, has usefully separated them into three groups:

- The first, influenced by therapeutic community principles, achieved a good level of care for their patients.
- The second, much larger, group remained institutionalized but with a paternal/maternal approach and minimal punitiveness.
- The third group were 'the bins': large hospitals situated near cities and operating at a low point of restrictive and punitive care.

Martin's *Hospitals in trouble*[22] chronicles the failures of this last group, as well as the abuses inflicted on patients. Writing in the 1950s, Johnson and Dodds[23] reported that hospitals viewed their patients as undeserving nuisances (cited in Porter[6]).

The problem was partly the hospitals themselves. As Gittins[24] observes, 'class, gender and categorizing illness were literally built into the hospital infrastructure' (p.5). Their architecture was closely linked to their function, so that no matter how hard an enlightened staff might try to encourage good care, the institutions themselves hobbled all that occurred within them (see chapter 8 in Scull[15]). And, of course, we can add the abysmal overcrowding and a demoralized nursing staff saddled with the thankless task of trying to contain it all while attempting to sustain programmes of care and rehabilitation. It says a lot about human will that, amidst sometimes harsh regimentation, there are innumerable instances of companionship between nurses and patients. Confinement had always meant separating the sexes: eugenic fears of the mentally ill reproducing with abandon were always strong. At first sight, therefore, the instigation of sexually integrated psychiatric wards always looked like progress. But it merely showed (again) how patients become a means of accomplishing (ostensibly liberal) professional ends. Notwithstanding the serial humiliations of older people now exposed to 'integration', this 1970s 'reform' went ahead anyway. These changes were well meant but, regrettably, the idea of asking patients what they might want was still some way off. That some of these old people, with attitudes rooted in an earlier age, might object to being nursed among the opposite sex, being too polite, too circumspect, was left to mental health nurses to deal with as best they could. One of the advantages of developing person-centred plans is that individual schedules of help can cut across official regimes, because they are geared to individual people. In this way, caring techniques could provide help not just to clients but, in the case of ward integration, to relatives who also needed reassurance.

REFLECTION

How might you feel about being confined in a place of care, against your wishes?

Into the community

If, over the years, mental hospitals had weathered a growing liberal condemnation, it was, at least, criticism that stemmed from professional and ethical concerns. By the 1970s, however, liberalism had become fair game for politicized economics and the closure of expensive hospitals in favour of community care. The precipitous implementation of community care, however, could only mean a shortfall of actual or efficient care; in fact, the 'plight' of the mentally ill under 'care in the community' became a sorry conclusion to a century that had started with such high hopes. Cataloguing community psychiatric grief is beyond the scope of this chapter, so I will focus on one or two aspects only.

Smith's outline[25] of assertive outreach shows how its initial intentions quickly coalesced around primary concerns with medication and the professional difficulty of 'non-compliance' by whatever name. Chapter 56 concentrates on assertive outreach. In Smith's view there has been:

a reemergence of old institutionally based ideas of biomedical illnesses requiring control, containment and, in particular, pharmacological treatments – the very issues that led to 'learned helplessness' for so many people in asylums.

In effect, a spreading therapeutic bureaucracy ensnares patients, so that their continued monitoring by professionals – their continued membership of the community – becomes contingent on complying with medication.
(pp.7–8)

Hemming et al.,[26] concerned that the restrictive functions of assertive outreach might take hold in the public imagination, tried to provide a definitive (warmer) account of it but which, in its detail, matches the findings of Smith. All told, Hemming et al. describe a world where patients who typically fail to comply with their treatments are deemed in need of clinical supervision, especially in relation to risk assessment. Associating the mentally ill with concepts of risk is about fixing them within a community so as to maintain a policing role over them.[27] Views such as these gave way to concerns about psychiatric patients' civil rights, which is a debate that continues apace under the guise of ethics and patients' demands. Italian psychiatry had taken a radical libertarian shift, which had proved influential to some British psychiatric thinkers. However, the 'Italian Experience', as it came to be known, was not all it seemed. The debate that followed revived much of the rhetoric and discourse of the past concerning the moral worth of psychiatry as a medical speciality. Professor Jones visited various centres in Italy and her reports contradicted those that had praised the Italian changes as revolutionary and widespread. In fact, Jones stated, the successful closure of mental hospitals had only happened in Trieste, with other centres only partially implementing community programmes because they were hindered by an ongoing lack of resources. In some ways, Jones's account calls into question what had become accepted at face value, and pointed out that what actually was happening in Italy was more piecemeal and problematic. But Jones's account was more than this. Stung by the criticism that she favoured mental hospitals, but, more so, dismayed that Italian psychiatry exulted in its hospital closures, Professor Jones went on to reiterate her lifelong contention that the quality of care is what is really important, rather than where patients are housed. This, of course, partly misses the point, because it does matter where psychiatry is practised: the architectural environment of patients does encourage deterioration and development of stereotypical beliefs and behaviours. At the same time, though not unaffected by their surroundings, codes of conduct, in respect of caring for patients, had usually resulted in nursing care premised upon regard for and acceptance of patients' behaviour.

Trieste was the natural home of the Italian reform and Jones praised it as a fascinating experiment in human relationships. She describes a carnival atmosphere combined with a refreshing rejection of professionalism, with everybody on first name terms and everyday life being replicated as far as possible. However, the problem, she believed, was that, by and large, the Trieste experiment was not replicated elsewhere, other than in a half-hearted fashion. Also, some categories of patients, for example those with dementia, were excluded. However, these reservations hardly detract from the idea of professionals engaging in human relationships in a positively crafted humanistic way.

In the long run, the ideas that propelled Italian radicalism are what matter, because a central criticism of psychiatry is its unacknowledged political intent. The role of

psychiatric dissidence is to critique psychiatry's rationale as much as the vagaries and mishaps of its practice. This is why criticism is viewed as intolerable by the psychiatric establishment. So Jones ends her commentary on Trieste with references to 'frolic radicalism' as well as its appeal to the non-rational aspect of the human mind. There is a stern warning that the Italians are not above confusing politics with psychiatry, added to which is the admonition that symbols and dogma are still powerful in a country with such a strong attachment to Catholicism. The implication here is that a dogma-free Britain – unencumbered by symbols – is not the ideal place for radical applications of psychiatric care. Granted, British practitioners would hardly align themselves with political parties or even claim that their work was directly political. Yet few would deny that mental illnesses are managed within conventional norms of what counts as acceptable social behaviour.

Psychiatric practices probably do not travel well – as current difficulties with ethnic minority mental health demonstrates – and what works in Trieste might not go down well in Tunbridge Wells. Nevertheless, the 'Italian Experience' reminded us that psychiatry can still be perceived as a malevolent force, particularly when it ignores the political and economic dimensions of mental distress. According to Phil Barker[28] (p.738), contesting this situation requires psychiatric nurses to answer the following questions:

- What challenges does caring present to you?
- How do you deal with such challenges?
- Who do you turn to when you run out of solutions?
- How has your idea of caring changed since you first decided to become a nurse?

REFLECTION

Are we, as professionals, sufficiently conscious of how momentous it is to take someone's freedom away?

ACCOMMODATING LOSS

As we accommodate to the loss of mental hospitals, combinations of legal restrictions and concerns with 'non-compliance' echo older desires to confine 'the mad', whether for their own or for society's good. The Victorians believed that their lunacy mansions were a solution; we came to dislike their form while continuing to harbour respect for their function. In effect, the repressive elements of the hospitals carried over into the development of less obtrusive ways of managing insanity, systems containing the power to treat if required and even if objected to by patients, such objections being transformed to a symptomology. To attribute

legitimacy to such objections is seen (by medicalists) as heartless; heartless, that is, not to treat the symptoms even when this requires preliminary confinement. Such confinement will henceforth depend more on community-processed restrictions, such as 'at risk registers', 'assertive outreach programmes' and 'community treatment orders'. As psychiatry becomes ever more convinced of the rightness of biotechnology, its self-assurance may become less susceptible to the influence of non-medical thinking.

Yet the insistence (and optimism) of psychiatric nurses for working therapeutically with patients is undiminished.

This insistence is not misguided, nor is it cynical. It is an aspiration that finds expression in innumerable encounters between nurses and patients daily. Regrettably, personal expressions of humanity now operate within a collective commitment which errs on the side of confinement, even if, in many cases, this is seen as a prerequisite to providing care. Even if, as has been argued,[27] a policing role is endemic to psychiatric nursing, it is the regrettable and objectionable necessity of that role that should govern its expression. In psychiatry, confining some patients may be immoral: indeed, the effect of psychiatric diagnoses can be to collapse ethical concerns about removing people's rights.

Is it really the case that nurses can make choices as to how to act in someone's interest? The politics of care depend heavily upon politics per se. In the contemporary world of psychiatric care and administration, few, if any, professionals can escape governmental diktat. Indeed, it is a frequent complaint that dissenting voices are silenced and innovation of any kind is played down.

Confinement under the rubric of 'forensic services' continues, and even if one concedes that confinement is a necessary prerequisite to caring for recalcitrant patients, is it not doubly necessary, therefore, to be wary of actions which, although intentionally benign, nevertheless marginalize people? It may be that significant numbers of nurses being all too willing to take up the mantle of 'nurse prescribing' diminishes the 'humanizing functions' of nurses. Whatever the efficacy of drugs, nurse prescribing alters the relationship between nurse and patient inasmuch as it circumscribes how he/she might react to a patient's reluctance to actually take that medication. To whom will patients now turn where there are differences of opinion between them and the prescriber? Who now will give that support and information necessary for them to come to terms with how they are medicated and treated? How do nurses now craft procedures of care and therapy in conjunction with their prescribing of drugs? It might entail complexities of responses whereby patients can recognize the wide context of empathy in which such prescriptions take place.

SERVICE USER COMMENTARY

Phil Ruthen

Liam Clarke's chapter is important as much for its inclusion as its content. That Clarke's chapter presents much of its subject matter to be taken as read is, I think, a positive measure of where the 'canon' of accepted ideas and history is now situated. Like other authors, he values the insights but increasingly recognizes the limitations of Foucault for contemporary ranges of enquiry. The socio-political debate, coupled with a questioning of the underpinning of imperatives of care,[29] offers opportunities to prevent the mental health system from being confined to deterrents.

This approach has implications for mental health service construction and practice, the basis on which it is formulated, and for whom. Where multidisciplinary teams respond to mental health requests, society's and psychiatry's delegation to team members of therapies, prescribing, and law enforcement can become a performative act between care, empathy, social support, intervention and obligations to systemic and management structures. Clarke's words are apt: 'even allegedly liberal psychiatric regimes can mask manipulative practices'.

Today, economic and legislative imperatives to intervene in certain pre-defined circumstances, coupled with moral mandates 'to care' – to create 'better people' – work within a system that is already uncertain of how to value an individual subject in distress (and the fact that it is still often described as a 'system' is telling in itself). A value or 'need' judgement implicitly enters triage and referral protocols. Here, 'best interest' can indeed struggle to be a positive agency for the prevention of unnecessary confinement.

Opposition can arise when the means and content of mental health promotion and health services, in their construction, codification and delivery, are not informed and structured from inclusive service user/survivor perspectives (for example, Sweeney et al.[30]). Selection and extrapolation of peer-reviewed 'survivor' research offering alternate perspectives remains an ethical goal for achieving equality in evidence promotion, and increasing awareness of people's difference. Also, trauma-informed research methodologies (for example, Mead;[31] Mead et al.;[32] and, for a discussion of ethics and empathy in the mental health context, see Estroff[33]) and social discourse theory methods re-position the subject, whom medical research often treats as an experimental repository of data, rather than as an individual person. Chapter 2 focuses on ethics and mental health nursing.

Yes, the examination of physical places of confinement matters; in south London appalling ward conditions exist side by side with high-tech research facilities. However, social anxieties exist – external, internalized; as does the internalizing of mental health 'labels', law and regulation, alongside contradictions in continuing policies such as community treatment orders, or a Care Plan Approach morphed into a recovery or well-being plan that struggles to break free from previous risk-averse, confining templates. Yet a vibrant, if small and variable in influence, anti-psychiatry movement exists; confinement is, as it always was, an imperfect method of maintenance and control. Mary O'Hagan stated: 'compulsory treatment sets out to control who you are, whereas compulsory detention merely controls where you are'[34] (p.4). Pilgrim and Rogers pertinently summarize objections to the *raison d'être* of the psychiatric discipline, and associated professional interventions: 'although patients complain about waiting lists, professional attitudes, and poor communication, few would question the enterprise of medicine itself. By contrast, psychiatry has always been thus challenged'[35] (pp.120–1) (see also the peer-led national online archive of mental health and survivors' movements[36]).

To Clarke's summary can be added the former asylums' eugenic history of racial segregation, genetic theories and experimentation. Additionally, the 2003 independent inquiry following the death by restraint in hospital of David Bennett produced recommendations for systemic improvements in mental health care, highlighting the need to pursue the question of care construct origins. In reporting evidence of institutional racism in mental health services, it intended to inform all relevant agencies and processes to further progressive policy making, and cultural sensitivity developments.[37] How far nursing and mental health systemic cultures are able to integrate social and personal responsibility with 'a more caring, less medic-based grasp' is open to question; but they retain the potential to do so.

The history of psychiatric care is weighted heavily by the dichotomy – to the extent that there is one – between custodialism and the delivery of therapy. There are two aspects to this: the first is the actual dichotomy itself, but more important is the issue of the extent and/or depth of its discussion by nurses. To confine someone – particularly when against their will – is to impose a fundamental shift in their status as (free) persons. Crucially we have done this, almost arbitrarily, by drawing on medical knowledge, relying for example on a diagnosis of schizophrenia, in some cases, as grounds for such confinement. Whatever the truth or otherwise of

medical diagnoses, one of its major effects has been, and is, to kill discussion. The State buys into psychiatry on this – as it does in no other sectors of human rights – and although psychiatry has been curtailed by some legal processes, its diagnostic decisions have generally held sway. We have noted that economic strictures have curtailed the sweep of medical jurisdiction in other disciplines now assuming decision-making responsibility within overall health provision. However, the issue is less the dissemination of professional responsibilities as much as the degree to which other, once secondary, professionals adhere to medical-diagnostic thinking in their decision making: so far, this is what they have done. As noted, the fact that nurses are now prescribing medicines is surely evidence of their acquiescence to medical thought.

That there has failed to materialize, within forensic services, any clear, alternative voice grounded in ethics, or even a view stemming from some consciousness of how a nursing 'voice' could differ, is worrying. To be empathic within a confined milieu, with a person who wants to leave, and in which one has been instrumental in that confinement, is a hard call.

Nurses do have a noble history but, as well, a troubling one with respect to detaining people involuntarily. It may be that the best avenue open to nurses is at least to retain an awareness of the negativity of confinement, and especially of how it is legitimated via diagnostic identities. It is also important to fight against those voices that deplore such concerns as these as outmoded, romanticized rhetoric. Actually, as I gaze up at the 18-foot iron fence surrounding my local forensic unit, I am persuaded that we have never had a greater need for vigilance on this matter.

References

1. Allderidge P. Bedlam: fact or fantasy. In: Bynum WF, Porter R, Shepherd M (eds). *The anatomy of madness: essays in the history of psychiatry*, Vol. II. London: Tavistock Publications, 1985: 17–33.
2. Minutes of the court of governors of Bridewell and Bethlem, 30 March 1677.
3. Cox JM. *Practical observations on insanity in which some suggestions are offered towards an improved mode of treating diseases of the mind to which are subjoined remarks on medical jurisprudence as connected with diseased intellect*, 2nd edn. London: Baldwin and Murray, 1896.
4. Ackroyd P. *London: the biography*. London: Chatto and Windus, 2000.
5. Digby A. *Moral treatment at the Retreat 1796–1846*. In: Bynum WF, Porter R, Shepherd M (eds). *The anatomy of madness: essays in the history of psychiatry*, Vol. II. London: Tavistock Publications, 1985: 52–72.
6. Porter R (ed.). *The Faber book of madness*. London: Faber & Faber, 1991.
7. Smith LD. *Cure comfort and safe custody*. London: Leicester University Press, 1999.
8. Porter R. *Mind-forg'd manacles*. Harmondsworth: Penguin Books, 1990.
9. Andrews J, Briggs A, Porter R. *The history of Bethlem*. London: Routledge, 1997.
10. Jones WL. *Ministering to minds diseased: a history of psychiatric treatment*. London: William Heinemann Medical Books, 1983.
11. Winchester S. *The surgeon of Crowthorne: a tale of murder, madness and the Oxford English Dictionary*. London: Penguin Books, 1999.
12. Jones M. *The therapeutic community: a new treatment method in psychiatry*. New York: Basic Books, 1953.
13. Lindsay M. A critical view of the validity of the therapeutic community. *Nursing Times (Occasional Papers)* 1982; **78**: 105–7.
14. Foucault M. *Madness and civilisation: a history of insanity in an age of reason* (trans. R. Howard). London: Tavistock Publications, 1967.
15. Scull A. *The most solitary of afflictions: madness and society in Britain, 1790–1990*. London: Yale University Press, 1993.
16. Shorter E. *A history of psychiatry: from the era of the asylum to the age of Prozac*. Chichester: John Wiley, 1997.
17. Jones K. The culture of the mental hospital. In: Berrios GE, Freeman H (eds). *150 years of British psychiatry 1841–1991*. London: Gaskell, 1991: 17–28.
18. Walton JK. Casting out and bringing back in Victorian England: pauper lunatics, 1840–70. In: Bynum WF, Porter R, Shepherd M (eds). *The anatomy of madness: essays in the history of psychiatry*, Vol. II. London: Tavistock, 1985: 132–46.
19. Showalter E. *The female malady: women, madness and English culture, 1830–1980*. London: Virago Press, 1987.

20. Skultans V. *English madness: ideas on insanity 1580–1890.* London: Routledge and Kegan Paul, 1979.

21. Clark D. *Administrative therapy.* London: Tavistock, 1964.

22. Martin JP. *Hospitals in trouble.* Oxford: Blackwell Science, 1984.

23. Johnson D, Dodds N. *The plea for the silent.* London: Christopher Johnston, 1957.

24. Gittins D. *Madness in its place: narratives of Severalls hospital, 1913–1997.* London: Routledge, 1998.

25. Smith M. Assertive outreach: a step backwards. *Nursing Times* 1999; **95**: 6–7.

26. Hemming M, Morgan S, O'Halloran P. Assertive outreach: implications for the development of the model in the United Kingdom. *Journal of Mental Health* 1999; **8**: 141–7.

27. Morrall P. *Mental health nursing and social control.* London: Whurr, 1998.

28. Barker P (ed.). *Psychiatric and mental health nursing: the craft of caring,* 2nd edn. Boca Raton: Taylor & Francis, 2008.

29. Foucault M. *Society must be defended.* New York: Picador, 2003: chapter 11.

30. Sweeney A, Beresford P, Faulkner A, Nettle M, Rose D (eds). *This is survivor research.* Ross-on Wye: PCC Books, 2009.

31. Mead S. Rights, research, liberation. Shery Mead Consulting, 2001. Available from: www.walsh.org.nz/file/jigsaw/PDFs/4-rightsresearchandliberation.pdf [Accessed 2nd August 2016].

32. Mead S, Hilton D, Curtis L. Peer support: a theoretical perspective. *Psychiatric Rehabilitation Journal* 2001; **25**(2): 134–41.

33. Estroff SE. Subject/subjectivities in dispute: the poetics, politics, and performance of first-person narratives of people with schizophrenia. In: Jenkins JH, Barrett RJ (eds). *Schizophrenia, culture, and subjectivity.* Cambridge: Cambridge University Press, 2004: 282–302.

34. O'Hagan M. Force in mental health services: international user/survivor perspectives. Keynote address, Australian and New Zealand College of Mental Health Nurses 29th International Conference, Rotorua, September 2003.

35. Pilgrim D, Rogers A. *A sociology of mental health and illness,* 2nd edn. Buckingham: Open University Press, 1999.

36. Mental health and survivors' movements and context. Available from: http://www.studymore.org.uk/mpu.htm [Accessed 27th June 2016].

37. Report of the independent inquiry into the death of David Bennett, presented to the Secretary of State for Health and the Norfolk, Suffolk and Cambridgeshire Strategic Health Authority, Wednesday 17 December 2003 (set up under SHG (94)27) having limited powers.

Further reading

Buchanon A. *Care of the mentally disordered offender in the community.* Oxford: Oxford University Press, 2002.

Eastman N. *Forensic psychiatry.* Oxford: Oxford University Press, 2012.

Jones A. *Nurse prescribing in mental health.* Chichester: Wiley, 2009.

Kettles A. *Forensic mental health nurses in acute settings.* London: Quay, 2007.

McGanley G, Bartlett A. *Forensic mental health care: concepts, systems, and practice.* Oxford: Oxford University Press, 2010.

Trenoweth S, Lynch JE. *Contemporary issues in mental health nursing.* Chichester: Wiley, 2008.

Relevant web pages

Flexible Assertive Community Treatment Model. https://www.eaof.org
Rethink. www.rethink.org.uk
Mental Health Care. www.mentalhealthcare.org.uk
Mind. www.mind.org.uk

Generating nursing knowledge

TIM THORNTON, DAVID CREPAZ-KEAY,
SEBASTIAN BIRCH AND JAN VERHAEGH

LEARNING OUTCOMES

- To be able to list some fundamental distinctions between kinds of knowledge: understanding versus explanation, tacit versus explicit, facts versus values.

- To be able to articulate some of the key properties of knowledge in general.

- To know how to differentiate between explanation and understanding.

- To be able to compare different views of the subjectivity or objectivity of value judgements.

- To be aware of examples of tacit knowledge.

- To be able to outline the advantages of and challenges to the co-production of knowledge.

SUMMARY OF KEY POINTS

- Nurses need knowledge because nursing is a practical discipline: the craft of caring.

- Nursing knowledge involves both explaining events scientifically, and understanding people by making rational sense of them.

- Care requires knowledge both of facts and of values, and these have different sources and methods.

- Nursing craft involves tacit practical know-how as well as explicit theoretical knowledge.

- Nursing practice draws on a potentially unlimited set of other disciplines to inform patient care. This places a heavy burden on knowledge-based practice.

- The co-production of knowledge suggests a more equal role for patients and service users, providing a richer source of knowledge, but also some challenges.

- Because nursing care has to select from a body of general knowledge to match a particular patient's needs, it is an art or craft as well as a science.

INTRODUCTION

What kind of knowledge underpins good nursing practice, the craft of caring? Is it a unified field? And if not, what are the appropriate methods for arriving at new knowledge?

In this chapter, we will consider three important distinctions which divide up forms of knowledge and argue that, in each case, nursing knowledge is found on both sides of the divide. Nurses must be able to *understand* their patients/service users as well as *explain* the course of their illnesses. They must know about *facts* and about *values*. Also, since nursing is a craft, they must have the *tacit* knowledge as well as the *explicit* knowledge of their profession.

This suggests that nursing knowledge is not a single unified field but rather draws on a range of different disciplines. Given the nature of knowledge itself, a range of quite different approaches is necessary to generate new knowledge. The challenges are increased in mental health care in particular, by the aim of co-producing knowledge with patients or service users. Finally, we will suggest that, because nursing has to draw on a range of different disciplines, the skill of identifying the right pieces of knowledge appropriate for each particular patient or service user lies at the heart of nursing. Although underpinned by scientific knowledge, this ability to judge what is relevant can helpfully be interpreted as an art or a craft.

This chapter concerns some deep philosophical questions about the kind of knowledge nurses need to have. Our contention is that knowledge of a variety of different kinds lies at the heart of good nursing care. Acquiring, combining and applying expertise across a range of disciplines with the goal of patient care is *the* key practical and philosophical challenge of modern nursing.

THE VALUE OF KNOWLEDGE

> ### REFLECTION
>
> Why should nurses aim to have knowledge of their subject? What is the value of knowledge? Think about this question before reading on. One clue might be to think about possible opposites to knowledge. If nursing practices were not based on knowledge, on what might they be based? Write down some ideas.

Defining the value of knowledge is difficult. We will approach it via a preliminary question: what is knowledge, or what does 'knowledge' mean? Now there might *not* be a very helpful or informative answer or definition. However, some general features of knowledge can be learnt from particular examples. Suppose that staff nurse Robin knows that, because it is 5pm, service user/patient Terry is due for medication. If so, Robin must take it to be true that it is time for his medication. That is, she must at least *believe* it. ('At least' because we often use the word 'believe' when we are *not* sure we do *know* something. 'Do you *know* that?' 'Well I *believe* it'.) Second, if Robin does know that Terry is due for medication, then Terry must *really* be due for medication. *If* Robin has knowledge, what she believes *must* be true.

Third, Robin's belief cannot merely be accidentally true. Neither a reckless guess nor an ungrounded hunch can support knowledge, even if they turn out to be true. They might, too easily, not have been true. But knowledge can be undermined, even when one does one's best. Suppose Robin believes that it is time for Terry's medication because she knows that he takes medication every day at 5pm and she believes, by looking at the ward clock, that it is now 5pm. But suppose that the normally reliable ward clock had, in fact, stopped the day before. By lucky chance, however, it is now nearly 5pm. If so, although Robin has a true belief that it is time for Terry's medication, she does not *know* it. If she had looked at the clock an hour earlier, she would have formed the *false* belief that it was 5pm and thus time for his medication then.

These constraints on knowledge have motivated a definition which dates back 2,000 years to the Greek philosopher Plato: knowledge is *justified, true belief*. The idea is that needing a justification for a belief (for it to count as knowledge) should rule out merely lucky true beliefs. But this prompts a question: in the example of Robin and the stopped ward clock, does that work?

> ### REFLECTION
>
> Does the traditional analysis give the correct account of Robin? Here is a clue: ask whether Robin has a justification for thinking the time is 5pm and also ask whether her true belief is lucky. If the answer to both is 'yes', then the traditional account does not address the problem of luck. If it does not, could some modification be made to the definition?

We will return to this question shortly.

As well as trying to rule out merely lucky true beliefs, justification also plays a second role which is helpful for thinking about the challenge of generating nursing knowledge. It provides a way, or a method, or a route, to aim at true beliefs. It is one thing to worry that one's beliefs about the latest medication for mental illness may not be right, but quite another to work out *how* to avoid being wrong.

Suppose a hospital authority issued an instruction that *all nursing staff should replace any false beliefs they hold with true beliefs*. On the face of it, this seems a good aim. But would the instruction help? The problem is that 'from the inside' true beliefs and false beliefs seem the same. To hold a belief is to hold it to be true. To believe that something is not true is precisely not to believe it. Thus beliefs which are, in fact, false are not transparently so to someone who holds them. So the instruction is not helpful.

By contrast, the following instruction would help: *replace any beliefs that one holds without justification with beliefs that do have justifications or grounds*. One can tell whether one believes something for a reason, or with a justification. Further, by aiming at having only justified beliefs, one should in general succeed in reaching true beliefs since justification is, in general, conducive to truth. Any 'justification' which did not increase the chances of a belief being true would not be a justification for it after all. This approach lies at the heart of evidence-based medicine, but applies more broadly.

Although justification can play this second, helpful role of providing a concrete way of aiming at true beliefs, it is not so successful in the first role mentioned above: ruling out being merely true by luck. As the example of Robin and the stopped clock illustrates, Robin *does* have a justification for believing that it is 5pm: she can point to the clock. Nevertheless, her belief is only true by luck because, as the narrator of the film *Withnail and I* says, even a stopped clock gives the right time twice a day. So she has a justification for a belief and the belief is true, but no one would say that she *knows* the time.

Although the definition that knowledge is justified, true belief dominated philosophy for 2,000 years after Plato, the problem that one might have a justified, true belief but still not have knowledge was first pointed out in the 1960s by the philosopher Edmund Gettier using an example like this one.[1] What do such examples tell us about the nature of knowledge in general and how, in practice, to acquire it?

It may seem that, as a definition of knowledge, 'justified, true belief' must fail (because Robin has justified, true belief but she still does not have knowledge). But a better response is to argue that the example really shows that Robin does not really have a *proper* justification, a good enough justification for knowledge in the context. Knowledge can still be correctly understood as justified, true belief, but not everything that one might think of as a justification (in the example, looking at the ward clock) really is a justification (because the clock has stopped). Knowledge and justification are a pair of concepts that one learns at the same time. The definition highlights the essential connection between them. The route to knowledge that underpins nursing practice will be, as suggested above, through suitable justification.

We will end this section by returning to the question we first raised. Why should nurses aim to have *knowledge* of their subject? What is the *value* of knowledge? Part of the answer is this: because knowledge, unlike, say, mere rumour or public opinion on which nursing might otherwise be based, is by definition true, aiming at knowledge is aiming at truth.

Now it may seem obvious that in a purely theoretical or contemplative discipline one should aim at truth for its own sake. Cosmologists, for example, want to understand how the universe works just for the sake of understanding it. But there is a further reason for nurses to aim at truth. This is because nursing is a *practical* discipline, a *craft* of caring. It aims not just to understand health and illness but to make a difference, to change people's states of illness to health. And in general, actions – such as medical interventions – based on true beliefs are more likely to succeed than those based on false ones. So nurses should aim at having true beliefs in order that their practical interventions in the lives of their patients are more likely to be successful. But because there are no intrinsic signs or symptoms of true beliefs that mark them out from false beliefs, the route to this is via a suitable justification which forms part of the conceptually rich idea of knowledge.

In this section, we have raised a fundamental question: why should nurses aim at knowledge? By 'unpacking' the concept of knowledge, we have suggested answers which connect to the value of truth, the role of justification as a way of aiming at truth and the practical ambitions of nursing to intervene in patients' lives.

But although we have talked about nursing knowledge, there are reasons to think that the diversity of forms of knowledge that nurses need to know makes the phrase 'nursing knowledge' potentially misleading. Towards the end of the chapter we will provocatively suggest that there is no such thing as 'nursing knowledge' and show how this connects to the idea that nursing is as much an art or a craft as it is a science. But in the next three sections, we will discuss some broad divisions of kinds of knowledge, and suggest that nursing straddles each divide. Hence, in each case, the generation of new knowledge to underpin practice has to draw on distinct methods and approaches, which adds to the challenge of being a modern nurse.

EXPLANATION AND UNDERSTANDING

In the first section we asked what knowledge was and considered the definition: 'justified, true belief'. The question, and the discussion which followed, may suggest that knowledge is a single, unified sort of state. In fact, however, what is called 'knowledge' can be further subdivided.

One way to divide up knowledge is to divide it very finely by subject matter. For example, knowledge of human physiology subdivides into knowledge of the

skeletal system, the muscular system, the immune system, the renal system and so on. Knowledge of the skeletal system subdivides into the ribs, vertebrae, cranium and so on. But while the facts concerning the skeletal system differ from those of muscular system, there is no reason to think that the *form* of knowledge differs in these cases. *What* one knows differs, but the *nature* of knowledge itself does not.

Some divisions, however, do seem to concern not just *what* is known – the facts – but the *way* it is known. Consider these two examples of patient history.

- Mr Smith is a 65-year-old man who visits his GP because recently he needs to pass urine more frequently but is having difficulty. With his permission, his GP performs a digital rectal examination of Mr Smith's prostate. He also requests an oncology appointment for a prostate-specific antigen test whose levels are raised if there are cancerous cells in the prostate, as well as to run an ultrasound in order to determine its size. From these diagnostic tests, the stage and grade of any cancer in Mr Smith's prostate can be determined, and the progress of the disease monitored and treatment adjusted accordingly.
- Miss Singh is a 23-year-old who has been referred to a community mental health team by her GP because she has recently had very strong feelings and ideas to end her life. With her consent, a nurse asks Miss Singh some questions and hears that she has been finding it hard to fall asleep, that she struggles to get out of bed and her appetite has dropped considerably in the past few months. She cannot plan for or see any happiness in her future. The nurse thinks that these could be some symptoms of depression and asks about Miss Singh's past. Miss Singh's mother passed away a few years ago and this event left her depressed. After some further questions, the nurse discovers that it is approaching the anniversary of Miss Singh's mother's death.

REFLECTION

What are the typical indicators that one is on the right track for grasping the biological course of a disease? And what are the typical indicators that one is on the right track for understanding the development of a patient or service user's attitude to their diagnosis? Are they the same?

In both cases, GPs and nurses aim at knowledge: a truthful reasoned account. In one case, the justification flows from a process of looking at medical records and diagnostic tests, and in the other from a process of asking questions and having a conversation. Despite sharing the aim of knowledge, these two accounts appear to have different structures. One accords with a structure of biological processes described by physiological laws of nature. The other has a psychological structure of thinking, feeling and acting for reasons.

The idea that there is a difference of kind between these forms of knowledge dates back to debates about psychology in the late nineteenth century called, in German, the *Methodenstreit*. The philosopher and psychiatrist Karl Jaspers is of particular relevance to mental health nursing. Like now, psychiatry at the start of the *twentieth* century was

dominated by neuroscience and the assumption that mental illnesses were really brain illnesses. Jaspers thought that biological psychiatry had been taken too far, and stressed the need for *understanding* in addition to *explanation*. While explanation tracked objective measurable symptoms, understanding was necessary to grasp subjective symptoms. Taking empathy to be a key aspect of understanding he said:

Objective symptoms can all be directly and convincingly demonstrated to anyone capable of sense-perception and logical thought; but subjective symptoms, if they are to be understood, must be referred to some process which, in contrast to sense perception and logical thought, is usually described by the same term 'subjective'. Subjective symptoms cannot be perceived by the sense-organs, but have to be grasped by transferring oneself, so to say, into the other individual's psyche; that is, by empathy. They can only become an inner reality for the observer by his participating in the other person's experiences, not by any intellectual effort.[2] (p.1313)

The distinction between explanation and understanding can be thought of as the difference between deriving events from general scientific natural laws concerning what typically happens, versus fitting them into patterns of *good* reasons, what *should* happen, what makes shared sense.

The distinction has an echo in the balance in contemporary mental health care between evidence-based medicine (EBM) on the one hand, and person-centred care on the other. While EBM emphasizes the importance of generalities by privileging evidence derived from large-scale randomized controlled trials (RCTs), person-centred care stresses the importance of a focus on individual patients. For detail on evidence-based medicine see chapter 6.

To practise a craft of caring, nurses need knowledge that spans both sides of this distinction. They need to grasp the laws that govern the workings of human physiology and which describe the course of illnesses, including mental illnesses. But they also need to be able to *understand* mental health service users or patients: their hopes, fears, beliefs, desires and experiences. This is knowledge of central importance for health care.

How then is it possible to generate new nursing knowledge on both sides of this conceptual divide? New *explanatory* knowledge – that is, knowledge based on natural scientific laws – is the focus of EBM, whose main approach is the RCT or, even better, the meta-analysis of RCTs. Such knowledge is underpinned by research that seeks out larger and larger study groups in order to avoid the potential biases introduced by small populations and particular researchers.

New knowledge from the other side, the understanding rather than explanation side, of the distinction calls for a different approach: to continue to listen to the changing beliefs, wishes and feelings of patients, recognizing that listening is a skill that can be practised and developed. By contrast with the ever more general perspective of explanation, looking away from the individual to the general population-based research of EBM, the key focus for *understanding* is away from the general and towards the individual patient.

KNOWLEDGE OF FACTS AND VALUES

In the previous section, we outlined the importance of a distinction between explanation based on general laws, and understanding individuals in a distinctive way by trying to interpret their utterances, experiences and actions in ways that make shared sense. In their influential book *Evidence-based medicine: how to practise and teach EBM*, David Sackett and colleagues define EBM as follows. 'Evidence-based medicine is the integration of best research evidence with clinical expertise and patient values'[3]. This is a surprising definition. Normally the focus of EBM is on the first element of that three-part division: research evidence. But Sackett et al. widen their definition to include two further aspects: expertise and values. They give a further brief preliminary sketch of each as follows.

> *By best research evidence we mean clinically relevant research …*
>
> *By clinical expertise we mean the ability to use our clinical skills and past experience to rapidly identify each patient's unique health state and diagnosis, their individual risks and benefits of potential interventions, and their personal values and expectations.*
>
> *By patient values we mean the unique preferences, concerns and expectations each patient brings to a clinical encounter and which must be integrated into clinical decisions if they are to serve the patient.[3] (p.3)*

This broad definition suggests a further important distinction for the craft of caring: that between facts and values.

Nurses need to know about research evidence concerning the workings of the brain and mind – the biomedical facts – but also about values: those of their patients and service users, and also their own, and those of broader society. They need to know not just about evidence-based but also about values-based practice. This prompts the following question: is knowledge of values a kind of knowledge distinct from knowledge of facts?

Let us take an example. Mrs Jones is a 29-year-old mother of one. She has a diagnosis of bipolar affective disorder, which is successfully managed by sodium valproate. She and her partner are planning to try for another child. This poses two risks: first, the risk of neural tube damage in the potential child, birth defects and developmental delay; and second, the risk of Mrs Jones developing post-partum psychosis. She has some choices. She may well wish to continue taking sodium valproate, with a full understanding of the risks to her child. Perhaps she has been on other mood-stabilizing medication in the past and has found the side effects unbearable. A further issue could be that Mr and Mrs Jones express a desire that, if Mrs Jones were to become psychotic after childbirth, she be treated at home rather than in a mother and child unit. This again contravenes best practice. But there could be reasons why Mr and Mrs Jones would wish for treatment at home.

As we stressed at the start, nursing is a practical discipline. It aims to change the world as well as understand it. So a case like this prompts the question: what is the right course of action? An informed answer will include the best medical evidence for the likely prognoses of interventions. But knowledge of the biomedical facts is only part of the story. Another part might be relevant economic facts concerning treatments permitted by the National Institute for Health and Care Excellence (NICE). But another will concern the *values* relevant to a decision. These will include those values encapsulated in mental health law concerning capacity. They will include a range of ethical factors, some of which will command wide agreement while others will be contentious. Yet others concern the wishes, hopes and fears of, primarily, the patient or service user.

Outlining the nature of values-based practice is beyond the scope of this chapter. But it is obvious that knowledge of facts and values can be very different. There is no equivalent of RCTs to decide how we ought to act. The closest equivalent, in the case of medical ethical values, might be knowledge of ethical principles, such as the 'four principles' approach of respect for beneficence, non-maleficence, autonomy and justice.[4] But whereas physical forces, for example, can be added together using the mathematics of vector addition, there is no general mathematics for saying when, for example, the principle of autonomy should trump beneficence and when the other way round. Further, ethical values are merely one subset of the values, preferences and traditions that need to be taken into consideration in values-based practice, and thus the prospects for codifying all the value judgements relevant for clinical decisions are unpromising.

Some proponents of values-based practice argue for an even more dramatic difference in the nature of knowledge of facts and values. The psychiatrist and philosopher Bill Fulford, for example, thinks that values are subjective. They lie merely in the eyes of the beholder. Fulford thus argues that successful values-based practice in mental health care does not aim at a correct judgement but at following a good process.[5] It is a matter of following the appropriate deliberative process, exercising good communication skills, and seeing what view emerges, rather than aiming to get the values in a particular situation objectively right.

Others argue that, even though there is no algorithm for forming a view of what to do in a particular situation, that does not rule out the idea that value judgements aim at truth, that value judgements are objective.[6] On this latter view, while knowledge of values is not reducible to, or codified in, general principles, it is still a form of knowledge of the values inherent in the clinical situation.

But whatever the best view of values-based practice, there is no doubt that values-based practice and evidence-based practice call on different kinds of expertise based on a sensitivity to different features of the world: the biomedical facts and patients' and others' values. Nurses need both, however.

Is it possible to generate new knowledge of values relevant for nursing practice? (We considered new knowledge of explanatory facts relevant for nursing practice in the previous section.)

> ### REFLECTION
>
> Think for a moment about the kind of skills that might be involved in values-based practice. Do they depend on knowledge of values? If so, how does one acquire such knowledge?

This is a difficult question for which there is no clear-cut answer. To begin, it depends on the view of values one takes. If one thinks that value judgements are subjective, then there are no new truths about values to be discovered, because there are no truths about values, merely new truths about what people, as a matter of fact, like or dislike. But, even so, there may be new approaches to values-based practice in the way that Fulford's or the 'four principles' approaches were both new developments in their day.

If, on the other hand, one thinks that values are real or objective features of the world, then the possibility of new general knowledge of values will hang on the possibility of a kind of moral – and other value – progress. On this view, the present-day rejection of the historical claim that plantation slaves who had a compulsion to run away suffered a form of mental illness, 'drapetomania', is a piece of moral progress and hence new knowledge of the values that underpin mental health and illness. It is a piece of *knowledge*, on this view, because reasons can be given to justify the claim that there was something wrong with thinking of such behaviour as pathological. Exploration of such reasons is as much the development of a kind of sensitivity to other people as it is learning general rules.

TACIT AND EXPLICIT KNOWLEDGE

The characterization of EBM by Sackett and colleagues discussed above also highlights a further distinction of kind within nursing knowledge. Sackett defines expertise as the 'ability to use our clinical skills and past experience to rapidly identify each patient's unique health state and diagnosis, their individual risks and benefits of potential interventions, and their personal values and expectations'[3] (p.3).

This characterization contains two elements already mentioned in the previous distinctions. Clinical expertise is directed towards individuals and their unique states and circumstances, picking up the understanding side of the first distinction (explanation versus understanding). It is also directed at their values and expectations, picking up the values side of the second distinction (knowledge of facts versus values). But it also suggests a practical recognitional skill is in play, and that suggests a third important distinction: between explicit and tacit knowledge. This also reflects the idea that nursing is a craft of caring.

The idea of tacit knowledge was first promoted by Michael Polanyi. In his book *The tacit dimension*,[7] he says:

> *I shall reconsider human knowledge by starting from the fact that we can know more than we can tell … Take an example. We know a person's face, and can recognize it among a thousand,*

> *indeed among a million. Yet we usually cannot tell how we recognize a face we know. So most of this knowledge cannot be put into words.[7] (p.4)*

Tacit knowledge is *tacit* because it is 'more than we can tell'. We cannot *tell how* we know things that we know tacitly. But why not? Surely to be a form of knowledge, there must be something – some *content* – known? On the standard model of knowledge, this content is a belief (for example, *that Terry is due for medication*). But if so, why can this not be put into words?

> ### REFLECTION
>
> What kind of thing could be known but could not be put into words? Do we use the word 'knowledge' about anything other than knowing facts, knowing *that* something?

Polanyi himself suggests a clue to this riddle:

> *I may ride a bicycle and say nothing, or pick out my macintosh among twenty others and say nothing. Though I cannot say clearly how I ride a bicycle nor how I recognise my macintosh*

(for I don't know it clearly), yet this will not prevent me from saying that I know how to ride a bicycle and how to recognise my macintosh.[8] (p.88)

Polanyi suggests that we use 'tacit' for knowledge of how to do something: practical knowledge. When one knows *how* to do something, one knows *something* but typically one cannot put it fully into words. Nursing, being a practical discipline or a craft of caring, contains much practical, tacit knowledge. This includes knowledge of how to do things: basic clinical skills, but also the recognitional skills mentioned by Sackett et al.[3]

That recognitional skills are tacit is important to mental health care. For the last 50 years, both of the main diagnostic manuals for mental illness (the World Health Organization's *International classification of diseases* (ICD) and the American Psychiatric Association's *Diagnostic and statistical manual* (DSM)) have adopted an 'operationalist' approach. Syndromes are described by lists of observable or expressible symptoms. Presented with an individual, the diagnosis of a specific syndrome is justified because he or she has enough of the relevant symptoms which can be, as closely as possible, 'read off' from their presentation. Such an approach to diagnosis emphasizes explicit knowledge.

Nevertheless, there remains a key role for tacit knowledge because there is always a gap between even a very thorough *description* of a symptom and its *expression* by a particular patient or service user at a particular time.[9] The skilled practitioner learns to see that the words set out on the page apply to the lived experience before them. This skill is not itself a matter for explicit knowledge since, sooner or later, whatever is written down in general terms has to be applied on the ward. It is a practical skill in recognition.

We suggested in the first section that knowledge cannot rest merely on luck and still count as knowledge. Although Robin had a true belief that it was time for Terry's medication, she did *not* know it.

REFLECTION

Does the incompatibility of knowledge and luck – for example, the fact that one cannot gain knowledge by forming a belief which is true only because of a piece of good luck – also apply to tacit knowledge? Stop reading and think what might be the equivalent for practical or tacit knowledge of justification for explicit knowledge. How does practical or tacit knowledge avoid resting on mere luck?

The clue is in the idea that tacit knowledge is a form of practical knowledge or craft, and that practical knowledge is a skill. So the equivalent of justification for tacit knowledge is having developed a general ability through practice, repetition and criticism. This suggests the route to new practical or tacit knowledge for nurses: the arduous work of moving through the hierarchy connecting novice to expert practitioner.[10,11]

IS THERE SUCH A THING AS NURSING KNOWLEDGE?

In the previous three sections, we have examined three distinctions that apply to the knowledge that underpins nursing care. Knowledge can concern explanation (using laws of nature) or understanding (making sense through reasons); it can concern facts or values; and it can be explicit or tacit. In each case, we have argued that nursing practice should be based on knowledge from both sides. This suggests that the way to learn and to generate new knowledge, both individually and as a discipline, varies.

In this section we wish to raise a more provocative question: is there such a thing as 'nursing knowledge'? This is not the same as asking whether nursing should be based on knowledge and whether nurses should keep up to date with new developments and findings. Of course it, and they, should. But is there a characteristic unified field of knowledge that could helpfully be called 'nursing knowledge' and can it help to define nursing itself? In an article called 'Defining nursing knowledge', Angela Hall suggests that the answer to both is 'yes'. She says: '"What is nursing knowledge?" is a complex question, the answer to which helps define nurses as a profession'[12] (p.34). We think that the answer to both questions is 'no', and that this places a particular burden or duty on nurses.

We have argued that the knowledge nurses need to have lies on both sides of a range of significant distinctions. This suggests that 'nursing knowledge' is not a simple unified kind at all, but instead comprises different kinds or sorts, all of which are necessary for the practice of nursing.

To reject the idea that there is a unified underlying concept of 'nursing knowledge' is not to reject the idea that the different aspects highlighted in this chapter are all important and all are kinds of knowledge. They are – but they are gathered together to underpin the nature and role of the profession of nursing: the skilled craft of caring for patients and health service users. Nursing knowledge is *whatever knowledge is needed for that craft*.

This places a heavy burden on nursing as a profession and on individual nurses in maintaining their knowledge base. It is impossible to put limits in advance on the areas of human inquiry which might provide knowledge relevant for improving patient care. Even now, nursing education draws on the biological sciences and chemistry, psychology, communication, management science and moral philosophy. The duty for the future is to keep an open mind to developments from any other discipline that might have a bearing.

CAN NURSING KNOWLEDGE BE *CO-PRODUCED*?

Much of the discussion of nursing knowledge focuses on the *nurse* as acquiring and having knowledge. But it is also important to consider the role of the patient or service user and in particular to consider their role as co-producer of knowledge.

Historically, the role of the patient has been a passive one. The patient was thought of as the 'problem' needing to be solved. That patients may themselves have knowledge has been regarded as a mixed blessing, with the role of nurses and clinical professionals being to extract the 'wheat' of knowledge from the 'chaff' of patients' descriptions of their experience. This process is rendered more difficult in mental health nursing, where there may be a concern that the patient lacks insight and that their testimony may therefore be unreliable. As well as making the generation of knowledge more difficult, this observer/object relationship can lead to therapeutic conflicts.

Modern nursing has seen the development of service user/patient involvement, expert patients, self-management and peer support. These developments have changed the role of the patient from passive recipient of nursing to active player in a partnership. The term 'co-production' is applied to these and other partnerships. Chapter 35 looks in more detail at partnerships and the recovery approach and chapter 50 considers collaborative care planning. Co-production typically involves both professionals and service users (and often informal carers) bringing their skills and experience to a joint process that creates something new. This collaborative approach can be applied to the process of generating knowledge, both at the individual case level, and at a more widespread level in developing research and practice.

> ### REFLECTION
>
> Consider the idea of nurses and patients co-producing knowledge. What are the challenges? What are the benefits?

Some of the challenges involved in this co-production will depend on the nature of knowledge. If, for example, we consider the definition 'justified, true belief', then we need to consider whether both 'justification' and 'truth' can have common meaning to nurse and patient. Nurses are trained to assess information in a particular way; patients are not. Patients are living the condition, and living with the consequences of the condition; nurses are not. We also need to consider the power differences that exist as a result of the respective roles of nurse and patient, including the legal powers that may affect the relationship. See chapter 3 for more detail on developing and maintaining therapeutic relationships.

While these may be challenges, the differences in perspective, experience and even perception also offer potential benefits. This chapter has highlighted the diversity of forms of knowledge needed for nursing care. If we ensure that knowledge is co-produced, this broadens the experience and values that contribute to knowledge.

THE ART OR CRAFT OF NURSING CARE

We began this chapter by asking the very general question: why should nurses aim to have *knowledge* of their subject? What is the *value* of knowledge? One way to address that is to consider the nature of knowledge itself. On a traditional view dating back to Plato, knowledge is a state that fuses belief, truth and justification. This highlights the intimate connections between these concepts. Given this, nurses should aim at knowledge because, among other things, knowledge supports successful action and nursing is a practical discipline or craft.

Despite the *general* argument for the importance of knowledge for nursing, subsequent sections have highlighted the different kinds of knowledge that underpin nursing care, calling for quite different ways of acquiring new knowledge. Thus it seems that there is not a single unified field that nurses should aim to know. This suggests a central task for nurses as experts in diverse forms of knowledge.

In the presence of a particular individual, nurses have to select the knowledge appropriate to 'each patient's unique health state and diagnosis, their individual risks and benefits of potential interventions, and their personal values and expectations', in Sackett's words.

This task fits a distinction between what the philosopher Immanuel Kant calls 'determinate' and 'reflective' judgement in his *Critique of judgment*:[13] 'If the universal (the rule, principle, law) is given, then judgment, which subsumes the particular under it, is determinate … But if only the particular is given and judgment has to find the universal for it, then this power is merely reflective'[13] (p.18). In a *determinate* judgement, one already knows the general concept that is relevant to a particular instance, and deduces from it something that follows from that. For example, if one knows that Mrs Jones is suffering from mild depression and one knows that those who are mildly depressed are likely to respond well to CBT, then one knows that Mrs Jones is likely to respond well to CBT. CBT is discussed in more detail in chapter 40.

The case of a *reflective* judgement is different. It corresponds to the case of meeting a particular individual and seeking out the general concepts that fit him or her; for example, that he or she is suffering from depression. Kant argues that this is an essentially *imaginative* task involving a 'subjective harmony of the imagination with the understanding'. But he also thinks that this harmony is the source of pleasure in understanding art.

Because nursing has to draw on an open-ended list of other disciplines to match knowledge to the particular needs of individuals, it requires the exercise of what Kant calls reflective judgement. But further, if Kant is right, then the *knowledge* at the heart of nursing, the *knowledge* to select the right subsidiary scientific and other knowledge called for by particular patients in particular situations, is an art. As much as it involves science, nursing care is a practical art or a craft.

CONCLUSION

Nursing, the craft of caring, should rest on knowledge because it aims to intervene in people's lives, and interventions based on truth are more likely to succeed. Aiming at knowledge, a fusion of justified or grounded true beliefs, suggests a route to this end. But the knowledge that underpins good caring practice lies on both sides of three fundamental divides (understanding versus explanation; facts versus values; tacit versus explicit) and so 'nursing knowledge' is not an intrinsically unified field. Rather, it is unified by the needs of the craft of caring. This fact, in turn, suggests that the key intellectual skill nurses need is the art, or craft, or know-how, to select from the full range of human knowledge what is relevant to a particular individual, in a particular context, with his or her needs.

SERVICE USER COMMENTARY

Jan Verhaegh

Health problems are always problems of the whole person. This means that they have a biological, psychological and social dimension. In the Netherlands we have physicians who treat mainly the physical dimension, psychotherapists who treat mainly the psychological dimensions and nurses who take care of both the physical and psychological dimensions. In some institutions nurses, who have the greatest contact with patients, are called 'socio-therapists' because of their focus on the social dimension. They have the knowledge and skills necessary to teach their patients how to cope with challenging social situations through practice and role play, as well as teaching broader interpersonal skills in order that their patients are empowered to cope better with life in the community. But they also need wider knowledge of their patients' social worlds, such as what it means to live in a patriarchal unequal world that can lead to violence, abuse, mistreatment and so on, and thus in turn to mental and physical health problems.

For example, recent research links the intelligence of people with Asperger's syndrome to the experience of social stress because of bullying, social conflicts and exclusion, which can in turn lead to psychosis.[14] The most intelligent young people suffering from Asperger's syndrome are 18 times more likely to develop psychosis than a neurotypical child. To take care of such people, nurses need knowledge of the biological, psychological and social dimensions of health and illness.

References

1. Gettier E. Is justified true belief knowledge? *Analysis* 1963; **23**: 121–3.
2. Jaspers K. The phenomenological approach in psychopathology [1912]. *British Journal of Psychiatry* 1968; **114**: 1313–23.
3. Sackett DL, Straus SE, Richardson WS, Rosenberg W, Haynes RB. *Evidence-based medicine: how to practise and teach EBM.* Edinburgh: Churchill Livingstone, 2000.
4. Beauchamp TL, Childress JF. *Principles of biomedical ethics.* Oxford: Oxford University Press, 2001.
5. Fulford KWM. Ten principles of values-based medicine. In: Radden J. (ed.). *The philosophy of psychiatry: a companion.* New York: Oxford University Press, 2004: 205–34.
6. Thornton T. Radical liberal values based practice. *Journal of Evaluation in Clinical Practice* 2011; **17**: 988–91.
7. Polanyi M. *The tacit dimension.* Chicago: University of Chicago Press, 1967.
8. Polanyi M. *Personal knowledge.* Chicago: University of Chicago Press, 1962.
9. Sims A. *Symptoms in the mind: an introduction to descriptive psychopathology.* London: Baillière Tindall, 1988.
10. Benner P. Using the Dreyfus model of skill acquisition to describe and interpret skill acquisition and clinical judgment in nursing practice and education. *Bulletin of Science, Technology & Society* 2004; **24**: 188–99.
11. Dreyfus H, Dreyfus S. *Mind over machine: the power of human intuition and expertise in the era of the computer.* New York: Free Press, 1986.
12. Hall A. Defining nursing knowledge. *Nursing Times* 2005; **101**: 34–7.
13. Kant I. *Critique of judgment.* Indianapolis: Hackett, 1987.
14. Selten JP, Lundberg M, Rai D, Magnusson C. Risks for nonaffective psychotic disorder and bipolar disorder in young people with autism spectrum disorder: a population-based study. *JAMA Psychiatry* 2015; doi: 10.1001/jamapsychiatry.2014.3059.

Further reading

Armstrong A. *Nursing ethics: a virtue-based approach*. London: Palgrave, 2010.
This book gives an account of nursing ethics.

Benner P. Using the Dreyfus model of skill acquisition to describe and interpret skill acquisition and clinical judgment in nursing practice and education. *Bulletin of Science, Technology & Society* 2004; **24**: 188–99.
This article provides a discussion of Dreyfus's hierarchy of skills applied to nursing.

Gascoigne N, Thornton T. *Tacit knowledge.* Durham: Acumen, 2013.
This book provides a wide-ranging discussion of tacit knowledge.

Loughlin M (ed.). *Debates in values-based practice: arguments for and against*. Cambridge: Cambridge University Press, 2014.
This book provides a discussion of the subjectivity or objectivity of values-based practice.

Pritchard D. *What is this thing called knowledge?* London: Routledge, 2006.
This book provides an introduction to philosophical accounts of knowledge in general.

Reed J, Ground I. *Philosophy for nursing*. Boca Raton: CRC Press, 1996.
This is a general book on philosophy for nursing.

Relevant web pages

The analysis of knowledge. *Stanford Encyclopaedia for Philosophy*. http://plato.stanford.edu/entries/knowledge-analysis/
This entry contains a substantial bibliography for the philosophy of knowledge.

Collaborating Centre for Values-Based Practice. http://valuesbased-practice.org/
The Collaborating Centre for Values-Based Practice promotes discussion of knowledge of values in health care.

International Network for Philosophy & Psychiatry. http://inpponline.com/
The International Network for Philosophy & Psychiatry promotes research on the philosophy of mental health care more broadly.

Polanyi Society. http://www.polanyisociety.org/
This society is dedicated to promoting Polanyi's views of tacit knowledge.

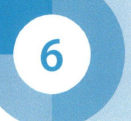

6 Evidence-based practice in mental health care

HUGH McKENNA

LEARNING OUTCOMES

- To be able to define evidence-based practice.
- To be aware of the issues around terminology in this field.
- To gain an insight into the politics and ethics of evidence-based practice.
- To know when it is legitimate not to use what appears to be best evidence.
- To know the barriers to using evidence-based practice.

SUMMARY OF KEY POINTS

- The involvement of service users in identifying and assessing what is and what is not good evidence is crucial.
- The plethora of terms to describe evidence-based practice is confusing and, in some cases, contradictory.
- There is a relationship between the different types of evidence and the different research methods.
- Research-based practice is not the same as evidence-based practice.
- When there is solid evidence to show that a specific intervention works, political pressure and financial stringencies have often led to it being rationed.

- There are key differences between the craft of nursing and the science of nursing, and how they are linked to evidence.
- Nursing interventions can be influenced by the concepts of certainty and agreement with existing practices.
- Four types of evidence – empiric, ethical, aesthetic and personal – are used interchangeably by practising nurses and are often traded off against each other.
- On occasion, clinicians, managers and researchers can inadvertently ignore the best available evidence.

INTRODUCTION

I had the pleasure of writing the chapter on evidence-based practice in mental health in the last two editions of this textbook. As readers would expect, over this time there have been considerable changes in how evidence is perceived and applied. More books and papers have been written on the subject, and I will refer to those that I believe are pertinent.

To an extent I have become cynical about fads and fashions in nursing. I am old enough to remember primary nursing, the nursing process, nursing standards, nursing models and the named nurse. All of these were laudable initiatives, driven and applied by people who wanted to improve the care of service users, their families and communities. I am also a little sceptical about the term 'evidence-based practice' because it erroneously gives the impression that all of practice should be grounded in the existing evidence. There are two things wrong with this; first, evidence does not exist and may never exist for all nursing interventions, and second, nursing practice should be informed by evidence but not slavishly based on evidence. Therefore, I suppose the right terminology is evidence-informed practice rather than evidence-based practice. However, everyone appears to use the latter term and so I too will reluctantly use it in this chapter.

REFLECTION

Consider the terms 'evidence-based practice', 'practice-based evidence' and 'evidence-informed practice'. Which do you prefer and why?

I propose to set you some challenges in this chapter and to be controversial in order to make you test your own assumptions. I will revisit the issue of terminology in a little more detail and try to get underneath the origin of evidence-based practice. Because of its large size and hence its costs, nursing as a profession cannot escape the attention of politicians. Even the production and use of evidence to underpin practice have political implications; I will explore this later. Finally, as I suggested above, evidence should not be swallowed whole; rather, experienced clinical staff should select the best available evidence to inform their practice. Nurses have been taught to be critical and selective in their acceptance of research studies. They should be equally critical and selective in their acceptance of available evidence. Later I will outline occasions when it is acceptable to accept the best available evidence and where one can reasonably reject such evidence.

EVIDENCE-BASED PRACTICE – ITS ORIGINS

It is generally agreed that, as a movement, evidence-based practice was 'kick-started' by a lecture given by Archie Cochrane in 1972. He was a physician and epidemiologist who aroused a lot of interest by pointing out that many decisions about health care are made without up-to-date evidence. However, his 1972 Rock Carling Lecture, entitled *Effectiveness and efficiency,* was a culmination of concerns he had expressed over many years. He argued that: 'Health services should be evaluated on the basis of scientific evidence rather than on clinical impression, anecdotal experience, "expert" opinion or tradition'[1] (p.317).

The lecture was stimulated by his experiences as a prisoner of war during the Second World War, when he noted that people were dying because of the medical attention they received, rather than the lack of it. Reflecting on this, Cochrane stated:[2]

> I would gladly have sacrificed my freedom for a little knowledge. I had never heard then of 'Randomised Controlled Trials', but I knew there was no real evidence that anything we had to offer had any effect … and I was afraid that I shortened the lives of some of my friends by unnecessary intervention. (p.82)

Around a hundred years previously, Florence Nightingale noted that medical care during the Crimean War did not have much effect on morbidity and mortality. Borrowing from Dante's *Inferno,* she asserted that due to the hazardous nature of care and treatment in the Barrack Hospital at Scutari, the words 'Abandon hope all ye who enter here' should be written over the entrance[3] (p.127).

In the twenty-first century, health care is still hazardous. In London in 2003, Don Berwick compared the lives lost each year with the number of encounters needed for each lost life.[4] Compared to ultra-safe activities like scheduled airline trips or train trips, the number of deaths from health-related interventions puts it in the dangerous category of deaths per 1,000 encounters. This makes the incidence of health care-related deaths much higher than road traffic deaths. This is a disaster, and to help reduce this death toll evidence-based practice has been promoted within government policy in the UK, Europe, the USA and Australia. More recently, nurses came under severe criticism for the poor quality and safety of care in the Mid Staffordshire Trust.[5] Therefore, it is not surprising that there is a call for practice to be informed by the best evidence available.

THE PROBLEMS WITH TERMINOLOGY: A MOVEABLE FEAST

Fifteen years ago a Canadian physician called David Sackett wrote and spoke about 'evidence-based medicine' (EBM)[6] (p.19). Soon after this, some nurses took up the baton and wrote about 'evidence-based nursing'.[7] Shortly after, the term 'evidence-based health' emerged, as did 'evidence-based management' and 'evidence-based policy'[8] (p.62). It seemed that the mere act of putting the words 'evidence-based' in front of something added to its credibility and made it seem more serious and scientific.

Over the years the service user movement has gathered pace. If they so choose, it is now commonplace for service users to be involved in decision making about their care.[9] A more recent manifestation of this phenomenon is the involvement of service users in the research process itself.[10] Traditionally, patients and members of the public played quite a passive role in nursing research. They were mainly subjects, participants or respondents who supplied the researchers with the necessary data. This has been described as the 'theft' or 'piracy' of people's lived experience by researchers.[11] Occasionally, the researchers established 'research advisory groups' and asked patients or members of the public to be members. Such groups met every few months and, in some cases, this was tokenism, a ploy to show the grant-awarding body that the researchers were taking cognisance of the views of service users and the public. It is now expected that service users will be involved as partners in the research process from design to dissemination.

Service users should also be partners in the planning and delivery of care. However, there is a danger that this could also be seen as tokenism, or a remnant of the age-old view that the doctor and the nurse know best. I think readers would agree that, if service users are to participate much more fully in their treatment and care, they must be provided with adequate information to do so – thus leading to what has been termed 'evidence-informed service user choice'.[12] It is important to realize that such user involvement may bring about a new way of perceiving what evidence is.[9] In addition, what in the past were viewed as anecdotal stories have gained some validity because they are now seen as valuable human testimony.

REFLECTION

Give three reasons why it is important to involve service users and/or their families in health care decision making.

I hope that you have not been confused too much by the variety of terminology. To simplify it for you, I can state with a degree of certainty that what they all have in common is that they call for practice or decisions or policy or management to be grounded in the best *available* evidence.[13]

You will note here that the word 'available' is emphasized. This is because for some practices the best available evidence may be very old, or indeed there may be no evidence available at all! In the past, some mental health interventions and decisions were based on routine and ritual, passed down from one generation of nurses to the next, often without rhyme or reason. Perhaps such behaviours did not do the service users any harm, but there again they may not have done them any good either.

I want to share with you some early definitions of evidence-based practice. One reason for doing this is that they stand the test of time. They also illustrate perfectly the confusion that exists about what exactly 'evidence' is! Of the many available definitions, here are just two. Appleby[14] stated that evidence-based practice was 'A shift in the culture of health care provision away from basing decisions on opinion, past practice and precedent toward making more use of research evidence to guide clinical decision making'. McKibbon[15] put forward a less rigid definition of evidence-based practice: 'An approach to health care that promotes the collection, interpretation and integration of valid, important and applicable service user-reported, clinician-observed and research-derived evidence' (p.A10).

Look at these definitions carefully; notice that neither of them refers specifically to service user outcomes – a familiar pattern in most definitions of evidence-based practice. Rather, each concentrates on the 'thinking and doing' aspects of care, suggesting that the term 'evidence-based practice' relates specifically to the processes (or doing) of care and treatment. The fact that these processes should lead to positive outcomes is not a matter for explicit consideration by any of these authors. Therefore, clinical nurses may indeed be basing their clinical and managerial decisions on the best evidence available and they would be employing evidence-based practice as defined here. But this evidence could be having no impact or even a negative impact on service user outcomes. So, to use evidence to underpin practice and not evaluate its effectiveness is short-sighted.

Another thing to notice about these definitions is that what McKibbon would identify as evidence would not be perceived as such by Appleby. From Appleby's perspective, evidence is reliant solely on the existence of relevant research findings. In contrast, McKibbon stated that clinical expertise and service user preferences are also sources of evidence. This apparent contradiction may be explained by what the United States Preventive Services Taskforce referred to as 'Grades of Evidence' or what Muir Gray[16] called the 'Hierarchy of Evidence' (see Table 6.1).

You will note that the top four levels relate to quantitative research methods. In essence, it is really about counting, and this predilection with quantification has its roots as far back as the Middle Ages. For instance, Galileo[17] wrote: 'Count what is countable, measure what is measurable and what is not

Table 6.1 The hierarchy of evidence

Level I	Meta-analysis of a series of randomized controlled trials (RCTs)
Level II	At least one well-designed randomized controlled trial
Level III	At least one controlled study without randomization
Level IV	Well-designed non-experimental studies
Level V	Case reports, clinical examples, opinion of experts

Table 6.2 A reconfiguration of the evidence hierarchy

Level I	Opinion and views of experts
Level II	Service user preferences and narrative accounts
Level III	Clinicians' experiences
Level IV	Results of qualitative studies and quality improvement/audit activities
Level V	Results of quantitative research

measurable – make measurable' (p.104). But many of the issues of importance to mental health care and to service users defy quantification: how do you calibrate compassion? How do you quantify a presence? How do you measure empathy?

It is not unusual to hear the mantra that randomized controlled trials (RCTs) are the gold standard, the most highly prized source of evidence. This is a faulty assumption, as it depends on what the research question is. If I wanted to study the effects of a new drug on schizophrenia, then yes, the RCT may well be the gold standard. However, if I wanted to study people's experience of the effect of schizophrenia on them and their families, then the gold standard may be a qualitative phenomenological approach. It really depends on the question posed.

According to Muir Gray's hierarchy, narratives from service users specifically and word of mouth generally are not regarded as sound evidence. This is not the case in all professions. In the legal profession such evidence is highly valued,

and word of mouth is sufficient to put a person in prison for a long time, or in some countries to have a person executed.[18] In contrast, such sources are denigrated in most textbooks and articles about evidence in health care. Perhaps it might be more useful for a new hierarchy to be proposed (see Table 6.2).

As with the previous hierarchy, this one also has inherent problems. How can you decide whether a service user's account comes above or below the experience of clinicians? Obviously, it depends on circumstances; hierarchies belong to the world of quantification and we should question whether the quality of evidence should be tied to the quality of a research design!

You can see that the above definition by McKibbon[14] is the most comprehensive, and includes as evidence the comments of service users and the observations of clinicians as well as research findings. This fits well with what I alluded to when I referred to the involvement of service users in clinical decision making. You will not be surprised to note that not everyone would sign up to McKibbon's definition, and the political and practical reasons for this will be made clear later in the chapter.

RESEARCH-BASED PRACTICE OR EVIDENCE-BASED PRACTICE?

In most instances when people refer to evidence-based practice they are implying that the evidence was derived from research.[19] When you read chapter 7 on building practice from research, you will see that this is the most desirable option. However, for a discipline like mental health nursing, this can be problematic. For example, suppose the government issued an instruction stressing that mental health nurses should not undertake any procedures with service users unless they are based on up-to-date research evidence. The result would be that most nursing interventions would cease. This would not be unique to nursing; research studies have shown that many interventions undertaken by doctors are not underpinned by evidence.[20]

The American Psychological Association[21] defined evidence-based practice as 'the integration of the best available research with clinical expertise in the context of service user characteristics, culture and preferences' (p.273). This echoes the words of McKibbon,[14] but uncovers new definitional problems. For instance, what characteristics, culture and preferences are taken into account and how are these defined?

> **REFLECTION**
>
> Outline how culture could be taken into account as evidence.

Let us return for a moment to Archie Cochrane,[2] who could be called the father of the RCT. He also realized that research could not answer everything. He noted the importance of service user characteristics and preferences. He understood that sometimes other approaches were needed for human problems:

The Germans dumped a young Soviet prisoner in my ward late one night. The ward was full, so I put him in my room as he was moribund and screaming and I did not want to wake the ward … He had obvious gross bilateral cavitation and a severe pleural rub. I thought the latter was the cause of the pain and the screaming. I had no morphia, just aspirin, which had no effect … I felt desperate … I finally instinctively sat down on the bed and took him in my arms, and the screaming stopped almost at once. He died peacefully in my arms a few hours later. It was not the pleurisy that caused the screaming but loneliness. It was a wonderful education about the care of the dying. I was ashamed of my misdiagnosis and kept the story secret. (p.82)

So over time Archie Cochrane had other views about what may or may not be an effective intervention, and the importance of such psychosocial interventions will not be lost on mental health nurses.

Another important point to bring to the discussion is the eroding of evidence by time. What was good evidence last year may not be good evidence next year. At one time, and based on the best evidence available, boring holes in people's skulls (trepanation), spinning mentally unwell service users in a special chair (rotational therapy) and frontal lobotomies were perceived as good ways of controlling some symptoms.[22] Today, such interventions are rightly perceived as barbaric. I have no doubt that, in 50 years' time, interventions currently used as best evidence will be denigrated by society. No crystal ball gazing, but I doubt if current practices such as electroconvulsive therapy, major tranquilizers or service user care for weeks or months in acute admission wards will exist.

> ## REFLECTION
>
> Identify another clinical intervention that is currently based on research that you think will not be acceptable in 50 years' time. Why do we use that intervention now?

THE POLITICS AND ETHICS OF EVIDENCE-BASED PRACTICE

It has been maintained that there is a clash between evidence-based practice and how it is implemented in the health service.[23] Some intimate that it is often used to control costs. Readers should rightly enquire as to how service users' preferences and values fit with this approach to implementing 'best' evidence.

In essence, evidence-based practice has become a powerful political tool. One of the main reasons for this is that health care is becoming increasingly expensive. Therefore, if cash-strapped health service managers fund practices or expensive technologies that have not been proven to be effective, not only would this be a waste of scarce funds, but they could also make service users' conditions worse.

When there is sound evidence to prove the effectiveness of an intervention, it is not unheard of to find that some of these are rationed for economic reasons. Recent UK cases included surgeons refusing to carry out costly heart operations on people who smoke or liver transplants on people who continue to drink alcohol.[24] In the USA, there are many stories of service users being refused treatment because they are on Medicaid.[25] The obvious question is: will people who have a diagnosis of schizophrenia be refused expensive medical and surgical treatment because their future contribution to the economy might be perceived as negligible?

The ethical implications of this are obvious, and I fear such rationing will not go away. For instance, Jamie Horder in the *Guardian* reviewed several studies on the rates of mental illness.[26] He did this because he was intrigued by so many organizations in the UK asserting that one in four people will have a mental illness. He was unable to find a great deal of 'evidence' for this figure. However, he noted that a survey in 2009 came up with this figure when it asked people whether they had suffered symptoms in the past week (for most disorders).[27] He did come across a major survey in the US that found an estimated lifetime mental illness rate of no less than 50.8 per cent! He uncovered another study, this time in Dunedin, New Zealand,[28] which found that more than 50 per cent of the people surveyed had suffered from mental illness at least once by the age of 32. We may take it for granted that, if a family member has a mental illness, there is a good chance that other family members will be affected negatively through experiencing worry, stress or anxiety. In addition, many people who have serious physical problems will also have emotional problems. Therefore, in a population the size of the UK, there will never be enough therapists or mental health professionals to cope with the demand for therapy. In such cases, evidence-based, but costly and prolonged, interventions will continue to be rationed.

CATEGORIES OF EVIDENCE

Two distinct types of knowledge have been described by Rhyl.[29] These are 'know how knowledge' and 'know that knowledge'. The former is skills-based and involves knowing the mechanics of how to do something. For instance, you may know how to use a microwave or how to drive a car, but you may not know how the computer in a microwave is programmed or the mechanical theory of the internal combustion engine. In nursing, much of 'know how knowledge' is perceived as our craft. A craft can be defined as work that is undertaken with a skill that has been perfected over a number of years through observation, reflection and practice. It is not usually synonymous with a research-based activity. It could be argued by some that much of nursing is a craft developed over years of observation, reflection and practice. In contrast, 'know that knowledge' has its basis in empirical research and theory and is often perceived as our 'science'. It is reasonable to replace 'know how knowledge' and 'know that knowledge' with 'know how evidence' and 'know that evidence'.

Pierce identified seven ways of knowing.[30] Here, too, you can justifiably replace the word 'knowing' with the word 'evidence':

- knowing (evidence) based on the word of an authority figure;
- knowing (evidence) based on unverified hearsay;
- knowing (evidence) based on trial and error;
- knowing (evidence) based on past experiences (history);
- knowing (evidence) based on unverified belief;
- knowing (evidence) based on spiritual/divine understanding; and
- knowing (evidence) based on intuition.

More recently, Kerlinger[31] asserted that the way to verifiable knowledge is through rigorous research. Here 'hard' evidence is required in order to be certain that something is or is not true. But Kerlinger also identified what he thought were 'less respectable ways of knowing'. These are 'tenacity', 'authority' and *a priori*.

To illustrate Kerlinger's approach, we could take the example of the knowledge that using 'mindfulness' relieves anxiety in individuals that have obsessive compulsive disorders.[32] Nurses may take this as evidence for practice because such interventions 'have always been done this way' (tenacity) or the clinical nurse manager told them so (authority) or that it is reasonable to assume that if a person gets such support they will be less anxious (*a priori*). We could also have identified Kerlinger's preferred source of evidence – research; nurses provide service users who have obsessive compulsive disorder with 'mindfulness' therapy because this practice was proven effective through the collection and analysis of empirical data.

> ### REFLECTION
>
> Identify another nursing intervention that reflects Kerlinger's types of knowing. Which of the types do you believe is the most valid and why?

Like Muir Gray[16] (see Table 6.1 above), physical scientists like Pierce[30] and Kerlinger[31] feel comfortable building categories and hierarchies of evidence. In Kerlinger's scheme the empirical research method is supreme and intuitive knowledge occupies a lowly position. But for a practice discipline like mental health nursing, this may be an inappropriate way of viewing evidence. I remember working as a student on an acute psychiatric admission ward. The ward sister was an experienced clinician. One afternoon she asked me to keep a close eye on a particular patient. I did so and shortly afterwards he had a massive epileptic seizure, which was followed by another and another. Thankfully he recovered, but when I later asked the sister how she knew this was going to happen, she replied that she did not know how she knew – she just did! This type of intuitive evidence is very important and is a skill that many experienced mental health nurses possess. Polanyi has called it 'tacit knowledge'.[33] Not surprisingly, Muir Gray, Kerlinger and Pierce would not place much faith in it.

CERTAINTY AND AGREEMENT IN EVIDENCE-BASED PRACTICE

The world of mental health care, like life in general, is full of uncertainties, and we reach out continually for the 'will o' the wisp' that is certainty. There is an interesting link between certainty and agreement in health care leadership.[34] I believe this can be applied to evidence-based practice.

In Table 6.3, Quadrant 1 contains those interventions that have high levels of agreement but evidence of their effectiveness is far from certain. They tend to be practices that have been routinized. Most of these interventions do no real harm but they also do no real good – a waste of valuable and scarce resources. An example would be the use of unnecessary medications or unnecessary service user observations.

In Quadrant 2 are those interventions that have high levels of agreement and certainty. They represent the best available evidence. Here, undoubtedly, the interventions do more good than harm. One example would be cognitive behavioural therapy to improve functioning in acutely psychotic inpatients.

In Quadrant 3 are those interventions that have low levels of agreement and evidence of their effectiveness is far from certain. These interventions do no real harm but it is uncertain whether they do any good. One example is the use of nursing models where there is no consensus among clinicians as to the most appropriate ones to use or their effectiveness.

Finally, in Quadrant 4 are those interventions that have low levels of agreement but evidence of their effectiveness has been shown to be certain. Examples include the use of

Table 6.3 Certainty–agreement grid

	Far from certainty	Close to certainty
Close to agreement	1	2
Far from agreement	3	4

exercise for mental well-being. Here we know that these interventions do more good than harm but they are not universally incorporated into our practice or lifestyle.

> ## REFLECTION
>
> Identify another clinical procedure, intervention or practice in each of the four quadrants in Table 6.3.

The situation we should be aiming for is to eradicate interventions in Quadrants 1 and 3, increase the number of interventions in Quadrant 2 and continue to evaluate their effectiveness, and bring the interventions in Quadrant 4 into mainstream practice.

LEGITIMATE REASONS FOR REJECTING WHAT IS APPARENTLY BEST EVIDENCE

If I asked you whether you should use the best available evidence to underpin practice, you would probably say yes. Who could possibly be opposed to this? But I would argue that there are many reasons why best evidence should be ignored.

In 1978, Barbara Carper identified four types of knowing in nursing.[35] These were: *empirics*, the science of knowing; *aesthetics*, the art of knowing; *ethics*, moral knowing; and *personal knowing*. For the purpose of this chapter, I will replace the word 'knowing' with the word 'evidence'.

Empiric evidence

'Empirics' represents evidence that is obtained by rigorous observation or measurement. It is verifiable, objective, factual and research-based. This is the type of quantifiable and objective evidence seen in levels I to IV of Muir Gray's hierarchy[16] (see Table 6.1) and coincides with Kerlinger's empirical knowledge[31] and Rhyl's 'know that knowledge'.[29] I will argue that on occasions we can legitimately ignore this type of evidence because it is superseded or contradicted by one or more of the other three types.

Ethical evidence

'Ethics' represents evidence about what is right and wrong and what is good and bad, desirable and undesirable. It is expressed through moral codes and ethical decision making. In everyday practice, clinicians often have to make choices between competing interventions. These choices and judgements may have an ethical dimension, and selection of the most appropriate position or action requires careful deliberation. For example, some mental health nurses may decide not to participate in a particular treatment because of ethical concerns, even though the results from empirical research show that it is effective for some conditions. Take the example of electroconvulsive therapy; there is strong evidence that it does have a positive effect with some psychiatric conditions. However, ethically, some nurses may decide that they do not wish to participate in this intervention. The same applies to the early discharge of service users to a non-supportive environment because community care is perceived as preferable. Ethical

evidence may also be used to make decisions about the rationing of treatment, as described above.

Aesthetic evidence

'Aesthetics' gives us the evidence that focuses on the craft or art of nursing. It enables us to go beyond that which is explained by existing laws and theories and accept that there are phenomena that cannot be quantified. It reflects the 'craft of nursing' and Rhyl's 'know how knowledge'.[29] Therefore, intuition, interpretation, understanding and valuing make up the central components of *aesthetic* evidence. Polanyi's tacit knowledge, referred to above, would be a good example of this type of evidence.[33] I argue that, because of having *aesthetic evidence*, we can ignore *empiric evidence*. For instance, many research-based scales are used to assess and predict service users' risk of suicide. Nonetheless, the clinical judgement based on experience and intuition of an experienced clinician could overrule what the scales indicate. Similarly, research evidence may provide guidance on when service users can be discharged from treatment, but the intuitive expertise of the clinical nurse regarding the service user's discharge capability may justifiably override this.

Personal evidence

'Personal evidence' focuses on our own unique history, self-consciousness, personal awareness and empathy. It is possible that clinicians may reject empirical evidence because of what their personal evidence tells them. If, as various theorists argue, the craft of caring is an interpersonal process[36] in which interactions and transactions between people are central, then we must know our own strengths and weaknesses in order to be expert practising nurses. Invariably, what mental health nurses have in their therapeutic arsenal is themselves, and they use themselves therapeutically to make a positive difference to service users. Nurses often learn as much from a caring relationship as service users do, and a good caring relationship will depend on the nurse's own self-regard. So, personal knowing requires self-consciousness and active empathic participation on the part of the nurse.[37] This may on occasions override more empirically based evidence.

Experienced mental health nurses often use these four types of evidence interchangeably. For instance, they will be aware of the research and theoretical basis for providing medication by injection (empirics) and they have the skills and intuition to ensure the service user understands the treatment and is as comfortable as possible while receiving it (aesthetics). However, the issue of withholding medication because of the severe side effects and sometimes poor results is a moral decision to be made with the service user (ethics). Finally, knowing themselves and their inner resources is important in the construction of an inter personal therapeutic relationship with the service user, so as to establish trust and confidence and discuss openly the pros and cons of medications (personal evidence).

> **REFLECTION**
>
> Think of another clinical intervention that has empirical, ethical, aesthetic and personal evidence.

ILLEGITIMATE REASONS FOR REJECTING WHAT IS APPARENTLY BEST EVIDENCE

Over the years, I have been fortunate to lead research teams on a number of studies dealing with barriers to evidence-based practice.[38–40] One focused on community nurses and GPs, and the other on mental health nurses and their managers. Based on some of the findings from this work, I will deal briefly with what I see as the illegitimate barriers to evidence-based practice, erected by practising nurses, nurse managers, nurse educators and nurse researchers.

Practising nurses

Findings from one of these studies identified the entrenched attitudes of practising nurses as being the single most significant barrier to their use of evidence. Why should this be so? Well, let's face it, nurses are no different from anyone else and research evidence is not a sufficient reason to change practice. We know there is research evidence on the dangers of smoking or eating fatty foods or not taking enough exercise, but how many people change their behaviour because of such evidence? There is some research to suggest that this is caused by lack of confidence with regard to their practice.[41]

Nurse managers

Modern nurse managers are interested in evidence-based practice because they are interested in good clinical governance. But lack of management commitment may be one of the greatest barriers to nurses using research evidence. Often senior health managers have other commitments and do not perceive evidence as a core element in the provision of nursing services. It is not surprising that, in a setting with competing demands, no one is really going to believe that evidence-based practice is truly important unless the boss makes it important.

Researchers at the London Business School published a paper called 'Reclaim your job'.[42] In essence, they stated that managers' claims of lack of time and competing commitments are little more than excuses and mask their lack of purposeful engagement in supporting improved effectiveness. From studies undertaken over a period of several years, the researchers noted that 30 per cent of managers had low focus and low energy, causing them to procrastinate on making decisions. Forty per cent had high energy but low focus, distracting them from the task in hand. Twenty per cent had low energy but high focus, causing them to be disengaged. The best managers had high energy and high focus and as a result were purposeful in ensuring continuous improvement. They knew what mattered about their organization. This research has obvious implications for managers' support of evidence-based practice.

Nurse educators

Contrary to expectations, nurse educators do not always keep up to date with the latest evidence-based practice, and this can affect students' views on using evidence. At the best schools of nursing, student nurses are encouraged to ask questions and learn in a culture of critical enquiry. Much is written about the theory–practice gap. This writing tends to address the gap between what students learn in university and what is practised clinically. However, I believe there is another theory–practice gap. It is the gap between the latest research evidence and the curricular content that lecturers teach. It is my belief that nurses are best able to appreciate and use evidence when they have been learning from the beginning in an environment where knowledge is generated, challenged and tested as well as being taught,[43] but how many nursing schools or clinical settings could be described in this way?

Nurse researchers

Researchers may also inadvertently be a barrier to evidence-based practice. For example, think about the inability of clinical nurses to understand statistical techniques, the confusion that arises through conflicting research results or the use of too much research jargon. There is also the overwhelming number of published research papers available to clinical nurses. This latter issue is not new and is illustrated wonderfully by a building metaphor used almost 50 years ago by Raulin.[44] Let's suppose that the 'builders' (practising nurses) depend upon 'brickmakers' (nurse researchers) to produce usable bricks (research papers) so that they can make edifices (evidence-based interventions). Raulin described this as follows:

> And so it happened that the land became flooded with bricks. It became necessary to organise more and more storage places, called journals ... in all of this the brick makers retained their pride and skill and the bricks were of the very best quality. But production was ahead of demand and ... it became difficult for builders to find the proper bricks for a task because one had to hunt among so many ... It became difficult to complete a useful edifice because, as soon as the foundations were discernible, they were buried under an avalanche of random bricks. And, saddest of all, sometimes no effort was made to maintain the distinction between a pile of bricks and a true edifice.[44] (p.348)

Therefore, if we are not careful, practice can be choked with evidence-based guidelines, protocols and research reports. This has the potential to alienate practising nurses from research-based evidence.

There is a tendency for practising nurses to criticize nurse researchers for making their research complex and publishing it in journals that are not accessed by clinicians. There is also the possibility that nurse managers criticize clinical nurses for not wishing to change practice, while practising nurses criticize managers for not giving them the support or resources to implement evidence-based practice. This tendency to blame others for not supporting an evidence-based culture might be explained by the Japanese terms 'taseki', meaning 'your burden', and 'jiseki', meaning 'my burden'[45] (p.57). Shifting the burden (taseki) for not using best evidence is comforting. In contrast, accepting the burden (jiseki) is uncomfortable for the following reasons:

- limited slack in the workload for innovation;
- limited time to update;
- guilty feelings of your practice being outdated;
- fear of failure and unsafe practice;
- exposure to 'attacks' from outside;
- exposure to 'attacks' from inside;
- limited confidence;
- shifting the blame to others reduces anxiety.

Therefore when it comes to identifying the success of implementing evidence-based practice, taseki is much easier to adopt than jiseki.

CONCLUSION

Service users in need of health care deserve an intervention that has been proven to be effective.[46] As core members of the multidisciplinary team, mental health nurses strive to achieve this, and none of them would deny that sound evidence should be an integral part of clinical decision making. In over 30 years in nursing I have never known any nurse who comes to work to do a bad job.

The demand for up-to-date information to inform care and treatment highlights the importance of collaboration between policy makers, managers, researchers and practitioners. But the mere existence of evidence cannot alter the care of service users; it has to be used and its outcome evaluated.

A note of caution, though: nurses should not apply evidence in an unquestioning manner. The thoughtless use of weak evidence may do a great deal of harm and may become just as much a routine as the habitual acceptance of hand-me-down rituals.

Nurses are individually accountable to the public for the delivery of high quality care and for seeking ways to improve that care through evidence-based practice. Therefore, to look favourably on the use of evidence is to look favourably on quality of care. This means the willingness to accept that our favourite views and practices may on occasion be wrong. There are no reasons left why nurses should not be informing their decisions and interventions with the best available evidence – only excuses.

SERVICE USER COMMENTARY

From a service user perspective, the importance of high quality evidence-based practice in the care of individuals with mental health conditions is a crucial aspect of a positive engagement with professionals during the ongoing treatment that often characterizes the mental health experience. As a service user myself, who has experienced some very acute mental episodes, and as an individual who educates health care professionals to care for people with mental health issues that require interventions, I cannot overemphasize the importance of evidence-based practice. Evidence-based practice should have a central place in the care of people with mental health conditions in all contexts. Furthermore, the importance of evidence-based practice for service users has increased due to an exponential growth in evidence being available to all through the internet. This means that a service user can be as up to date with the latest evidence as the mental health professional who is treating them.

A good example of the importance of best evidence-based practice in addressing the needs of service users with mental health conditions became very apparent to me when I developed full-blown Stevens–Johnson syndrome as a side effect of being prescribed a commonly utilized drug in the treatment of bipolar disorder. If I had simply been told, 'If you get a rash when you have taken this medication, seek immediate medical help', this could have saved me and many others from experiencing the severe side effect of Stevens–Johnson syndrome which, if left untreated or not captured in time, can be fatal. This is an extreme but salutary example, for if it were not for the diligent observation of a nursing intern student I had been teaching who noticed the rash and then encouraged me to seek immediate medical treatment, it is possible that I would not have survived to write this piece advocating the importance of evidence-based practice. Put simply, the nursing intern was aware of the evidence relating to the medication and its contraindications and acted upon her knowledge of the evidence.

The poet Rudyard Kipling probably offers all health and social care professionals who work in the arena of mental health practice the simplest, yet most effective means by which to practise everyday evidence-based care in their interactions with people experiencing mental health conditions requiring professional interventions. In a verse of a poem from his publication *The elephant's child*, the poet advocates how, with a little reflection, evidence-based practice can be best achieved:

I keep six honest serving men
(They taught me all I knew),
Their names are What and Why and When,
And How and Where and Who.
I send them over land and sea,
I send them East and West,
But after they have worked for me,
I give them all a rest.

Rudyard Kipling

Kipling offers professionals working in mental health practice the notion that they should endeavour to seek out what the evidence says about a particular intervention, while also challenging them to consider what the evidence says about why a particular intervention should be chosen over another. What does the evidence tell professionals about the best environment to carry out an intervention? Does the evidence have something to say about when the best time to engage with a person with mental health issues might be, or indeed what does the evidence say about who might best assist a person with mental health difficulties during a crisis? Engagement in evidence-based mental health care can only be augmented using Kipling's six wise men: what, why, who, where, when and how. Such an evidence-based approach could lead to professionals becoming mindful, reflective and contemplative in their caring interactions with people with mental difficulties.

References

1. Dickersin K, Manheimer E. The Cochrane Collaboration: evaluation of health care and services using systematic reviews of the results of randomised controlled trials. *Clinical Obstetrics and Gynecology* 1998; **41**: 315–31.
2. Cochrane A. *One man's medicine*. London: BMJ (Memoir Club), 1989.
3. Nightingale F. *Notes on nursing: what it is and what it is not*. Edinburgh: Churchill Livingstone, 1859/1980.
4. Berwick DM. Improvement, trust, and the healthcare workforce. *Quality and Safety in Health Care* 2003; **12**: 448–52.
5. Francis R. *The investigation into Mid Staffordshire NHS Foundation Trust* (Francis Report 2013). Available from: http://www.kingsfund.org.uk/projects/francis-inquiry-report [Accessed 21st May 2016].
6. Sackett DL, Straus SE, Richardson WS, Rosenberg W, Haynes B. *Evidence-based medicine: how to practice and teach EBM*. Edinburgh: Churchill Livingstone, 2000.
7. Ingersoll G. Evidence-based nursing: what it is and isn't. *Nursing Outlook* 2000; **48**: 151–2.
8. Ellis P. *Evidence based practice in nursing: transforming nursing practice*. London: Learning Matters Ltd, 2010.
9. Tait L, Lester H. Encouraging user involvement in mental health services. *Advances in Psychiatric Treatment* 2005; **11**: 168–75.
10. Morrow E, Boaz A, Brearley S, Ross FM. *Handbook of service user involvement in nursing and healthcare research*. Chichester: Wiley-Blackwell, 2011.
11. Weinstein J (ed.). *Mental health, service user involvement and recovery*. London: Jessica Kingsley, 2010.
12. Entwhistle VA, Sheldon TA, Sowden A, Watt IS. Evidence-informed service user choice: practical issues of involving service users in decisions about health care technologies. *International Journal Technology Assessment in Health Care* (1998); **14**(2): 212–25.
13. Barker J. *Evidence based practice for nurses*. London: Sage, 2013.
14. Appleby J, Walshe K, Ham C. *Acting on the evidence*. Research Report. London: NAHAT, 1995.
15. McKibbon KA. Evidence based practice. *Bulletin of Medical Library Association* 1998; **86**(3): A10.
16. Muir Gray JA. *Evidence-based healthcare: how to make health policy and management decisions*. New York: Churchill Livingstone, 1997.
17. Whitehouse D. *Renaissance genius: Galileo Galilei & his legacy to modern science*. London: Sterling Publishing Company, 2009.
18. THE JUSTICE PROJECT, *Eyewitness identification: a policy review*. Washington: The Justice Project, 2009. www.TheJusticeProject.org.
19. Davies J. *Nursing and health: evidence based practice survival guide*. London: Pearson, 2012.
20. Brownlee S. *Overtreated: why too much medicine is making us sicker and poorer*. New York: Bloomsbury, 2007.
21. APA (American Psychological Association). *Report of the 2005 Presidential Task Force on Evidence-Based Practice*. New York: APA, 2005.
22. Greenberg D. 10 mind-boggling psychiatric treatments, *Mental Floss* 2012. Available from: http://mentalfloss.com/article/31489/10-mind-boggling-psychiatric-treatments [Accessed 21st May 2016].
23. Drisko J, Grady M. *Evidence-based practice in clinical social work*. New York: Springer-Verlag, 2012.
24. Jones J. Doctors stand by refusal to treat smokers: soapbox medicine or scientific medicine? *Independent* 30 May 2014. Available from:

http://www.independent.co.uk/news/doctors-stand-by-refusal-to-treat-smokers-soapbox-medicine-or-scientific-medicine-judy-jones-reports-on-a-divided-profession-1461741.html [Accessed 21st May 2016].

25. Ubel PA. *Physicians, thou shalt ration: the necessary role of bedside rationing in controlling healthcare costs*. Healthcare Papers: Longwoods, CA, 2002.

26. Horder J. One in four will get a mental illness. *Guardian* 24 April 2010.

27. HSCIC (Health & Social Care Information Centre). *Adult psychiatric morbidity in England – 2007, results of a household survey*. London: HSCIC, 2009. Available from: http://www.hscic.gov.uk/pubs/psychiatricmorbidity07 [Accessed 21st May 2016].

28. Moffitt T, Caspi A, Taylor A, Kokaua J, Milne B, Polanczyk G, Poulton R. How common are common mental disorders? Evidence that lifetime prevalence rates are doubled by prospective versus retrospective ascertainment. *Psychological Medicine* 2010; **40**(6): 899–909.

29. Rhyl G. *The concept of the mind*. London: Penguin, 1963.

30. Pierce CS. *Essays in the philosophy of science*. Indianapolis: Bobbs-Merrill, 1957.

31. Kerlinger FNB. *Foundations of behavioural research*, 3rd edn. New York: Holt, Rinehart & Winston, 1986.

32. Williams WG. *Mindfulness: a practical guide to pace in a frantic world*. London: Williams, 2011.

33. Polanyi M. *The tacit dimension*. London: Routledge and Kegan Paul, 1967.

34. Zimmerman B, Lindberg C, Plsek, P. *Insights from complexity science for health care leaders*. Irving, TX: VHA Inc., 1998.

35. Carper BA. Fundamental patterns of knowing in nursing. *Advances in Nursing Science* 1978; **1**(1): 13–23.

36. Peplau HE. Interpersonal relations: a theoretical framework for application in nursing practice. *Nursing Science Quarterly* 1992; **5**: 13–18.

37. Carper BA. Philosophical inquiry in nursing: an application. In: Kikuchi JF, Simmons H (eds). *Philosophic inquiry in nursing*. Newbury Park: Sage, 1992: 71–80.

38. McKenna HP, Ashton S, Keeney SR. Barriers to evidence based practice. *Journal of Advanced Nursing* 2004; **45**(2): 178–89.

39. Sinclair M, Hasson F, Richey R, Keeney SR, Poulton BC, McKenna HP. Innovative midwifery practice: a case study. *Evidence Based Midwifery* 2005; **3**(2): 56–63.

40. McKenna HP, Ashton S, Keeney S. Evidence based practice in primary care: a review of the literature. *International Journal of Nursing Studies* 2004; **41**(4): 369–78.

41. Taylor S, Allen D. Visions of evidence-based nursing practice. *Nurse Researcher* 2007; **15**(1): 78–83.

42. Ghoshal J, Bruch P. Reclaim your job. *Harvard Business Review* 2004; **82**(3): 41–5, 125.

43. Salmond S. Advancing evidence-based practice: a primer. *Orthopaedic Nursing* 2007; **26**(2): 114–23.

44. Bashford L, Slevin O. *Theory and practice of nursing: an integrated approach to caring practice*, 2nd edn. Cheltenham: Campion Press, 2003.

45. Shore D. *The trust crisis in healthcare, causes, consequences and cures*. Oxford: Oxford University Press, 2007.

46. Melnyk BM. *Evidence-based practice in nursing & healthcare: a guide to best practice*. Philadelphia, PA: Lippincott Williams & Wilkins, 2011.

Further reading

Bateman AW, Krawitz R. *Borderline personality disorder: an evidence-based guide for generalist mental health professionals*. Oxford: Oxford University Press, 2013.

Beautler LE, Norcross JC, Levant RF. *Evidence-based practices in mental health: debate and dialogue on the fundamental questions*. Washington: American Psychological Association, 2013.

Cohen A. *Delivering mental health in primary care: an evidence-based approach*. London: Royal College of General Practitioners, 2008.

Drake RE, Lynde DW, Merrens MR. *Evidence-based mental health practice: a textbook*. London: Norton Professional Books, 2005.

Milne DL. *Evidence-based clinical supervision: principles and practice*. Oxford: Blackwell, 2009.

Newell R, Gournay K. *Mental health nursing: an evidence based approach*. Edinburgh: Churchill Livingstone, 2009.

Priebe S, Slade M, Clare A. *Evidence in mental health care*. New York: Taylor and Francis, 2005.

Pryjmachuk S. *Mental health nursing: an evidence based introduction*. Los Angeles: Sage, 2012.

Sullivan P. Developing evidence-based care in mental health nursing. *Nursing Standard* 1998; **12**(31): 35–8.

Varcarolis EM. *Essentials of psychiatric mental health nursing: a communication approach to evidence-based care*. St Louis: Saunders Elsevier, 2009.

Webber M. *Evidence-based policy and practice in mental health social work (post-qualifying social work practice series)*. London: Learning Matters, 2011.

Relevant web pages

Bandolier. http://www.bandolier.org.uk/

British Medical Journal. Evidence-based nursing. http://ebn.bmj.com/

Nursing Research. Evidence-based nursing. http://nursingplanet.com/research/evidence_based_nursing.html

http://www.graziano-raulin.com/supplements/theoryimport.htm

Strategies for Nurse Managers. Evidence-based practice resource center. http://www.strategiesfornursemanagers.com/ebp_resource_center.cfm

7 Building practice from research

JOANNE McDONNELL

LEARNING OUTCOMES

- To have a broader understanding of issues faced when trying to build clinical practice on research findings and evidence.
- To have an increased awareness of varying perspectives on the application of research in practice.
- To have an increased awareness of barriers impacting on implementation of research into practice.
- To develop insights into ways to support more effective implementation of research in practice.

SUMMARY OF KEY POINTS

- An array of previous literature has shown that there are significant difficulties in applying research findings to mental health nursing clinical practice.
- There are some key barriers that need to be overcome if nurses are to be expected to use research findings successfully.
- Research findings must be used alongside a nurse's knowledge, skill and intuition and must be balanced with what the patient deems to be a positive outcome and experience.
- Individual patients may have their own unique ways of managing a mental health issue that may not be in line with research findings.
- Organizations need to do more to ensure their research strategies are robust and are explicit about the expectations of the role of the nurse.

INTRODUCTION

A close family member has helped me to develop this chapter by sharing her experiences of being an inpatient in a psychiatric unit a couple of years ago. She was an informal patient there and, when I visited, she would often have a long list of questions for me about why certain decisions were made. She did not even know what the term 'informal' meant and thought she had been sectioned.

When a diagnosis of 'adjustment disorder' was given, we all doubted how accurate it was and whether it was in fact the actual source of the problem, but the doctor knew best apparently. Having spent a total of approximately 30 minutes with her during her three-week-long stay, the doctor knew that this was her problem and that she needed antidepressants. Did the doctor know this intuitively, via experience, or come to this decision on a scientific basis? What my relative and her family thought she needed was a course of some type of psychological therapy to help her understand why she reacted so badly to certain stimuli or incidents in her life. She also needed to learn alternative ways of managing her feelings, other than using illicit substances and alcohol. We were not convinced that a course of antidepressants was going to achieve that. Prior to admission, when she was found threatening to jump from a bridge, it was not a genuine attempt at suicide, according to the nursing staff on the ward, who then shared this view with the doctor. On what basis was this view formed? Was an evidence-based tool used to ascertain her suicidal risk? Even if an evidence-based tool was used, how would we know if she would answer the questions honestly? Was this decision based on the fact that she had telephoned me asking for help rather than actually jumping? Or was it based on the fact that she had been drinking? Welsh and Lyons in 2001[1] discussed the complexities and factors of individuals' reactions to alcohol and how their desire to commit suicide may differ greatly. They asserted that excessive alcohol consumption might remove one person's volition to harm themselves but for another the opposite may be true. Had any scientific analysis gone into the decision-making processes surrounding my family member's care, or was this simply the opinion of staff? If it was based on the opinion of staff, how did they form this view? What goes into the decisions *you* make about patients in your care? Despite my professional background, we as a family were really struggling to see any clear, robust evidence to inform and support some of the decisions that were being reached.

For us as a family, the clinical decision that my relative was not actively suicidal raised many questions regarding how clinical decisions are made in practice and consequent treatment given, in addition to ensuring opportunities to prevent future recurrences were not missed. There is a whole array of research regarding management of low mood, suicide risk and prevention of suicide. As a family we were not at all confident that this was considered when decisions were made about our loved one's care. I must say that, as a registered mental health nurse myself, as well as a distressed relative, I was not confident that the staff were even aware of any research findings and that their views on her level of risk of suicide were in fact robust enough. An Australian study by Fisher in 2014[2] explored the use of psychological therapies by mental health nurses and concluded that mental health nursing was too focused on medical treatment and risk management, and that practice was dominated by the administration of medication, excessive documentation and patient observation. Could this be a factor in why psychological therapies were not even considered for my relative?

This chapter will focus on some of the difficulties faced when implementing research findings in practice, and it will explore varying perspectives on how nurses can get the balance right between the 'scientific' approach of the application of research in practice, and a clinician's intuition, experience and knowledge.

RESEARCH IN PRACTICE

> ### REFLECTION
>
> Consider the last time you read a research paper related to your daily practice. If you do not read them regularly, consider the reasons why not.

First of all, let us turn to the subject of research itself. I think we would all agree that it is really important that our practice is based on the most up-to-date research. Bryman[3] in his glossary of terms kindly provides us with definitions of key terms such as hermeneutics, epistemology, constructivism, univariate analysis, correlational statistics, phenomenology, grounded theory, to name a few. Shall I continue? There is a lot more to excite us all and encourage us to read on. As far back as 1995, McKenna[4] warned of the dangers of research reports being overloaded with jargon. Even though I myself have a Master of Research in Health Science, with Distinction, I still manage to switch off a few lines into a research study that spends more time talking about how the study was conducted than about the impact on a patient's life it could have as a result. Mental health academics do sterling work researching new and existing approaches in mental health. There is, however, still a commonly accepted gap between academics and clinicians on the front line. Many researchers have already written about it. Bowers et al.[5] expressed a view that they as academics may be missing out on ways to communicate effectively with practising nurses and may not be getting through to managers who are responsible for driving change in today's health service. They suggested that researchers needed to change their language, work with managerial and policy initiatives, and package and present their findings in ways that are attractive and understandable to clinicians. Cleary and Freeman[6] cited Gerrish and Clayton,[7] who suggested that nurses were more likely to develop their knowledge from local policy and procedure than from reading journals. McKenna[4] highlighted that psychiatric nurse researchers tend to publish in academic journals read mostly by other academics, and that their findings are reported mostly at conferences attended by other researchers. As I have always had a keen interest in research, I am one of those nurses who did attend such conferences and must say that from my experience I was definitely in the minority and did appear to be surrounded by academics primarily. It did help that I understood much of the terminology due to the education I had received via my Master's degree, but I still chose to attend the sessions that focused more on what the research had found and what it meant in practice than those that spent 75 per cent of the time justifying the methods they used to carry out the research and which featured words I still had to look up in the dictionary. Clearly, the methods used in research must be robust and transparent so that we can make informed decisions about whether or not the study will stand up to scrutiny, but I have always wondered if there is a better way. Bowers et al.[5] stressed that research findings that are presented as potentially generating quick and reliable improvements in outcomes are more likely to get drawn into practice and used.

THE APPLICATION OF RESEARCH TO POLICY

REFLECTION

Choose one of your local policies and procedures that focuses on a clinical intervention, such as management of self-harm. Review the evidence and the research it uses to inform the content, and consider how your practice compares. Consider visiting other areas both within and external to your organization and compare your practices to those as well.

I was a Head of Nursing in a large mental health trust when I was asked to write the policy on the management of self-harm. On reflection, it was not a topic to which I had overtly given lots of thought, except for my preconceived long-term notion that we had to keep people safe and stop them self-harming at all costs. In 2004, Zauszniewski and Suresky[8] described psychiatry and mental health nursing practice as being strongly influenced by tradition, unsystematic trial and error and authority. This is a view supported by many other researchers. Bartholomew and Collier[9] supported the view of Rodgers[10] who in 1994 suggested that there was a degree of fear in applying new knowledge because it challenged traditional and ritualistic practices. Wynaden et al.[11] supported this view and cited lots of work that supported a finding that a considerable part of nursing practice continued to be based on tradition rather than scientific evidence.[12–14] Zauszniewski and Suresky[8] also highlighted that, for practising nurses, it is challenging to break away from the routines and practices with which they are familiar and comfortable, and that 'old wives' tales' were still retold. When I was taught about self-harming, it was on an acute mixed ward in 1988. My job was to observe the patient and to stop her self-harming during my shift. At that time, I accepted this unquestioningly, and this appeared to be the view supported by many staff with whom I discussed it. It was only when I commenced the arduous task of writing the self-harm policy from scratch, and started to conduct a literature review on the subject, that I realized there were not just other options available, such as 'safe self-harming', but that there were different definitions and suggested causations and treatments for 'self-harm'. I had never been taught, nor actively considered, that there is a difference between the terms 'self-harm' and 'self-injury', and quickly realized that the suggested treatment options could be very different. While this had not directly impacted on my practice because I no longer worked on an acute ward, I did wonder why I had not heard much debate about such a controversial topic via the inpatient wards. I even discovered a very active group of people who considered themselves to be long-term 'self-harmers', who were adamant that they did not 'self-injure' in order to commit suicide or even to harm themselves. They were running an internet campaign to encourage organizations to recognize that, by stopping them self-injuring, nurses were in fact increasing the risk of propelling the need to self-harm to dangerously high levels. After a significant amount of research and after reviewing the National Institute for Health and Care Excellence (NICE) guidelines on the subject, my knowledge of and views on the management of self-harm had shifted significantly. I began to recognize that, for some people, self-injuring was their way of managing a variety of negative feelings, for a vast array of different reasons, and that many of them were adamant that this was not intended to harm themselves seriously or an active attempt at suicide. When this option was suddenly taken away from them, many of them genuinely believed that their risk of death became greater. On broaching the topic of safe self-harming being included in the trust policy with peers, however, I was almost universally ridiculed. I can absolutely understand the ethics surrounding this debate and also the essential discussion required that would promote the teaching of safer alternatives to self-harm based on each individual's unique reasons for self-harming, but I was quite surprised at how much resistance there was even to discussing it. I am renowned as quite a strong, tenacious and persistent character and yet I was increasingly frustrated by some of my peers' total disregard of the evidence with which I presented them. Holm and Severinsson[15] discussed how important it is for nurse leaders to have the skills required to make enlightened changes that meet the needs of both staff and patients. They quoted Jinks and Chalder[16] who in 2007 discussed evidence that the role of a consultant nurse requires a strong, forceful nature. Back in 1998, Gordon[17] recognized the difficulties faced by new nurses in being accepted into the professional team and yet still retaining the ability to critically evaluate practice advocated by more experienced, influential staff. This is a view supported by Bartholomew and Collier,[9] who suggested that nurses who trained a long time ago may have a lack of awareness of and not prioritize evidence-based practice. It is no surprise therefore that newly trained staff may have difficulties in constructively challenging existing practices and offering up new research findings that have the potential to change traditional approaches to caring.

> ### REFLECTION
>
> When you last noted the findings of a piece of research that had the potential to impact on your practice, did any factors get in the way of you changing the way you currently work based on the findings? List them.

Say, for example, you were a staff nurse on a long-stay older persons' ward in the late 1990s. You have several patients who require insulin and it has always been administered in the arm. How will you know when this recommendation changes, as it did, to the stomach? Has there been any further research on the best location on the body to give the injection or any new findings on absorption rate efficacy? Will you automatically be told via a change in organizational policy, or is it up to you as an accountable nurse to make sure your practice is up to date? The Nursing and Midwifery Council Code of Practice is clear when it tells nurses that we must always practise in line with the best available evidence.[18] Nurses need to be confident that they are ahead of the game when it comes to implementing research, as well as in the delivery of up-to-date practice in their clinical field. Lots of studies have been carried out to explore the reasons for the perception that nurses do not consistently apply the latest research findings to their practice in a timely manner. McKenna[4] claimed that mental health nurses have seldom been able to justify their actions by reference to research findings, and that their interventions, although carried out in good faith, are often the result of tradition and without empirical substance. He referred to his previous study of 1993,[19] in which 32 clinical nurse managers were asked what aspect of the practice being carried out in their clinical area was research-based. He found that none of the 32 could answer the question. It would be interesting to repeat this study to ascertain if anything has changed since then. McKenna also expressed a view that many of us would not argue with when he asserted that 'people with mental health disorders deserve a service which has been demonstrated through research to be the best that can be given'[4] (p.1257). Zauszniewski and Suresky[8] were also unequivocal when they claimed that nursing practice had been influenced by traditional wisdom passed down through generations by word of mouth and in published textbooks; they raised three crucial questions that seem as valid today as they were then:

1. Are psychiatric nurses aware of the efficacy of the treatments and interventions they provide?

2. Are they truly practicing evidence based psychiatric nursing?

3. Is there documentation of the nature and outcomes of the care they provide? (p. 130)[8]

An additional question might be: 'If there is evidence of the nature and outcomes they provide, do these outcomes match the desired outcome of the patient?'

There is also an array of studies that discuss why nurses should never rely purely on scientific evidence to guide their practice, and that 'tacit intuition' should never be ignored. Stickley and Phillips[20] cited Welsh and Lyons[1] who claimed that best practice should be based on intuition and tacit knowledge rather than the hierarchy of evidence offered. While research and evidence-based practice is clearly an essential component, Stickley and Phillips also questioned the validity of applying the hierarchies of evidence proposed by evidence-based medicine to mental health nursing theory and practice. Evidence-based practice is explored in chapter 6 of this book by Hugh McKenna, who discusses the differences between research-based practice and evidence-based practice, and the political and financial issues impacting on the implementation of specific interventions, despite there being solid evidence of their effectiveness.

In chapter 3, Rosie Stenhouse and Chrys Muirhead examine a number of factors that contribute to the development of the therapeutic relationship. They describe these factors as including intrapersonal factors, such as value systems, and personal attributes, as well as consideration of the context of mental health nursing practice.

Stickley and Phillips supported the views of Peplau,[21] who argued in 1952 that the quality of the therapeutic relationship is the very foundation of mental health nursing practice. Many of the studies that support this view discuss how factors such as compassion and nurses' intuition can be measured. Rasmussen et al.[22] found that experienced nurses were able to demonstrate a perceptual process of understanding a clinical situation through intuition, rather than the earlier stages where they relied more heavily on more experienced nurses. They also suggested that nurses need to recognize the value of individual human experience. This is an important point, which underlines that just because a piece of evidence or research dictates a finding, each of us as individuals may react very differently to having a mental health problem and that this will be largely based on each of us as a unique person, and our life experiences to date. Fisher and Happell[23] cited Whitley and Drake[24] who argued that translating findings from higher ranked research evidence may be scientifically sound, but that it fails to recognize the individual's experience of an illness and its treatment. This is a view supported by McAndrew,[25] who suggested that effective nursing relationships need to encompass an emotional human interaction where there is reciprocal involvement of the service user with the nurse. For example, in relation to an individual who may feel suicidal, studies may indicate that a high proportion of completed suicides are carried out by individuals under the influence of some sort of substance, as detailed in the 2014 National Confidential Inquiry.[26] Yet one nurse may know, either intuitively or via personal history, that a specific patient's risk is significantly increased only when he *abstains* from alcohol or drug abuse. Stickley and Phillips[20] cited the views of Margison[27] who argued that evidence-based practice as a model for planning individual care was deficient because of its generalizing nature; in other words, what works for the majority may not work for the individual. When I was a ward manager on two continuing care wards for people with dementia, reality orientation was a major part of what we were taught to do, alongside telling people with schizophrenia that the voices they heard were not real. One particular patient with chronic, late-stage dementia used to be convinced that we were all intruders in his house and he would randomly attack staff and patients, ordering them to get out. At that time, some staff used to go along with his view that it was his house and ask his permission for us to be there, and the situation would resolve quickly and without distress. Other staff felt that they had to religiously remind him that it was not his house and that he was in hospital because they needed to ensure he was being 'orientated to reality' as the theories suggested. This approach would almost always result in an aggressive incident, with staff trying to explain where he was to a man with very severe dementia who had little or no insight and was unlikely ever to regain it. This conflict often led the staff who 'went along with' his delusion to feel that they were somehow doing something wrong, and yet this course of action resulted in the most favourable outcome, both for this particular patient and for the staff. This may indeed make us wonder, when nurses apply what they are taught, either by more experienced nurses or in nursing school, what mechanisms they use that enable them to confidently challenge the 'way we do things'. Later research was no doubt carried out that may have disputed the efficacy of reality orientation for people with late-stage dementia, but at that time, on that ward, it either was not known about by the staff or had not been done yet. It would appear that this specific intervention had been the traditionally accepted approach for quite some time. A New Zealand study by Carlyle et al.[28] in 2012 suggested that the medical model of care constrained mental health nursing interventions, which potentially created tension between what nurses believe to be the most appropriate solutions to problems, and the actual options for responding that are available to them in their clinical setting. They proposed that mental health nurses often viewed their role as solely to support the work of the psychiatrist, and found it difficult to implement their own conceptual ideas in patient care. McKenna[4] also proposed that mental health nursing was underpinned by custodial and medical models and that traditional practice required obedience rather than enquiry. He referred to students who asked questions being perceived as troublemakers. It would be interesting to explore this view today and whether this perception remains. Stickley and Phillips[20] cited Allard,[29] who in 2002 recognized that, while evidence-based practice evolved through a reductionist scientific paradigm, human experience cannot easily be reduced. They also supported the view of Sackett et al.,[30] who argued in 1996 that the practice of evidence-based medicine meant the integration of individual clinical expertise with the best available external clinical evidence from systematic research. Fisher and Happell[23] also debated the importance of getting the balance right between the science and lived experience of patients when they argued that 'the need for the consumer voice and the importance of the lived experience of mental illness are not readily reconciled with a strong scientific paradigm that promotes detachment and objectivity' (p.179). Stickley and Phillips[20] concluded that, in their view, an approach was needed that focused on the lived experience of people, one that accepted that this lived experience constituted evidence in its broadest sense. A nurse may have a specific view on what works and what does not in practice, and who for example is genuinely suicidal and who is not, but it is important for the nurse to have a conscious awareness and understanding of how these decisions are being reached. Is it years of experience, detailed knowledge of an individual patient, tacit intuition, clear evidence of outcomes or just a personal opinion? In 2010, an Australian study by Cleary et al.[31] discussed the concept of 'facts versus proclaimed beliefs' and stressed how important it was for mental health nursing culture change in order to examine and challenge 'sacred beliefs' (p.47). Getting the correct balance between what mental health nurses know to be fact and what they believe to be fact is therefore crucial.

In 2009, Barker[32] expanded his concept of the 'craft of caring', describing the basis of good nursing practice as a combination of both art and science. He described the concept of the craft of caring as 'encouraging nurses to adopt a holistic approach to the practice of psychiatric and mental health nursing, rather than risk being trapped by technologically limiting approaches to treatment'.

It is also important to be aware of how personal attitudes may impact on practice. Happell[33] suggested that, once attitudes have been developed, they are not easily influenced and therefore tend to remain fairly constant in the absence of a strong reason to change them.

REFLECTION

Think about a nursing intervention that you carry out regularly. Is this intervention based on evidence, research or positive patient outcomes, or is it based on instruction and tradition?

BARRIERS TO THE IMPLEMENTATION OF RESEARCH IN PRACTICE

McKenna[4] believed that Hunt's[34] five reasons why practising nurses do not make use of research findings, published in 1981, were still valid:

1. They don't know about them.
2. They don't understand them.
3. They don't believe them.
4. They don't know how to apply them.
5. They are not allowed to use them.

The five points above may well be a starting point for nurses and organizations to review and evaluate, if they wish to improve their application of research in practice. An example I recall, which may demonstrate some of the difficulties faced by nurses when making a balanced decision regarding the application of research findings, was a debate regarding why the use of punch bags had been banned from all of the forensic wards in one organization. When challenged on why this decision had been made, a well-meaning manager advised that he had instructed his teams to remove all punch bags from wards because he had read an article in a weekly nursing journal that claimed they increased patient aggression rather than reduced it. Unfortunately, this article had only been an opinion piece, was only based on one ward and had not shown a full and balanced review of the available evidence, and the manager did not have the skills required to critically appraise it and make an informed decision on any implications for practice. McKenna[4] also warned of the dangers of mental health nurses using research unquestioningly, and argued that doing so is as bad as basing practice on tradition. He did, however, stress that the mere existence of research could not alter client care, and that one mental health nurse applying research findings in practice to improve care is of more value than dozens of nurses researching dichotomous topics that will never be disseminated. Bowers et al.[5] proclaimed that it would be a tragedy if research findings on how to prevent inpatient suicide, for example, remained stuck inside the pages of academic journals, never managing to reach a wider audience.

Nurses do sometimes also need to understand that not all research needs to involve a major, complex organizational change in order to be relevant. Even what may be considered as simple changes can have a big impact on patient care and experience. This could include starting up a peer support group focusing on a new initiative the nurse has discovered, or making sure all new patients admitted are offered the latest smoking cessation advice and access to services, or as basic as increasing awareness of particular side effects of food stuffs, such as the impact of caffeine on the bladder, and offering non-caffeinated alternatives. Small changes taken collectively can often have a big impact on patients' experiences of care. I still often see groups of nurses discussing the latest national award winners and hear them proclaiming to have 'already

been doing that for ages'. What is it that hinders practising nurses from publicizing their own good practice and writing about it? In 2007, Happell[35] suggested that there was a need to gain a greater understanding of the reluctance of nurses to publish. She recommended ways that nurses could develop their knowledge by disseminating research findings at conference presentations. Happell also suggested that, if nurses focused on presentations in the first instance, they may recognize that they have something interesting to say and be more likely to progress to a publication. She also highlighted how nurses may often choose to become involved in quality improvement projects rather than research-based ones, as this often removed some of the requirements, such as ethics approval. In 2002 Cleary and Horsfall[36] clearly advised that, whether or not the project is quality improvement or research, organizational approval is required, and this remains the case today. They described quality improvement projects as often involving investigation of problems at a local level for the purpose of improving clinical practice. In one of my previous roles, I was the organizational lead for two Trust-wide projects. One was the implementation of 'Essence of Care', a nursing back-to-basics-type benchmarking exercise, and the other 'Payment by Results', a new proposal for payment systems to Trusts. Both of these projects did in fact start off as quality improvement projects and ended up being presented at international research conferences, with the 'Essence of Care' work being published in two different nursing journals.[37,38] When I began work on both of these subjects, I had not anticipated either of them being in a position to be considered for publication or presentation at research conferences or events, and it was only on the advice of a lecturer colleague, who advised me on how to develop the robustness of the work, that I was able to even consider submitting them as abstracts to be presented on a broader scale. I did, however, fear the feedback from academic colleagues, as I had witnessed first-hand at events how publicly critical people could be over the perceived robustness of each other's work. While I understood that the method I had chosen to conduct the quality improvement project needed to be robust and transparent, as a nurse I did not particularly want to get into a debate about methodologies and flaws; I just wanted to concentrate on the difference that could be made to people's experiences of care by adopting some of the findings in practice. Happell[39] recognized that conference presentations are a good place for nurses to start, but also that many conferences tend to be dominated by academics and managers, which can leave clinicians feeing unprepared to present to such an audience. The role of research mentors may be an option for organizations to explore. Holm and Severinsson[15] also advocated the use of effective research mentors as a valuable way of helping nurses to develop research skills in the drive towards evidence-based practice. This could be developed in line with staff members who have recently completed studies and dissertations. Many large organizations continue to support staff to complete further education by way of time, access to data and financial support, but they may not be fully utilizing the findings from studies in their own organizations. When nursing staff complete work such as a dissertation, many of them may choose topics that are relevant to their own practice and organization, and use their own place of work to conduct the study. Yet many nurses complete their work and do not go on to disseminate it, either internally or externally, and there is often no organizational requirement for them to do so, nor clear processes for reviewing policies to take into account the findings.

> ### REFLECTION
>
> Attempt to establish how many nursing staff have completed further education studies supported by your organization in the past 3 years. Explore whether there is a system for approving such studies and sharing their findings and whether anything has changed as a result of them.

So it is quite clear that there is no quick win when it comes down to building your practice based on research. Lots of researchers have identified possible barriers to successful implementation and also suggestions for how they may be overcome. Bartholomew and Collier[9] cited MacGuire,[40] who in 1990 stated that the implementation of research-based practice is as much the responsibility of the organization as it is the individual. They also cited the work of Caine and Kendrick,[41] who found that, despite clinical managers having positive attitudes regarding the need for research-informed practice, they often became obstacles to implementation by not using their authority to the best effect and failed to take responsibility for the implementation of research initiatives. Fisher[2] suggested that nurses had identified the main barriers as bureaucratic practices, lack of time, insufficient staff or resources and a lack of peer support. Bowers et al.[5] suggested the following barriers to implementation:

- absence of clear advantage;
- lack of compatibility with perceived needs of staff;
- over complication;
- benefit not immediately visible;
- perceived irrelevance;
- not easily feasible;
- insufficient knowledge and skill;
- social networks interfering with dissemination;
- lack of adoption by opinion leaders in the team;
- lack of desire to change.

How does this list compare to your own views of why research is not implemented in practice? Bowers et al. did find that there was little guidance available on how to implement research in practice settings. Compare mental health nursing to acute nursing; is it acceptable not to use the latest research findings in a general physical health setting? If you believe there are differences in application, why is it acceptable in mental health?

> ### REFLECTION
>
> Think of ways in which you might help with research findings being built into practice in the area in which you work. What support might you need to make it work more effectively?

HOW TO IMPROVE THE IMPLEMENTATION OF RESEARCH IN PRACTICE

Bowers et al.[5] had many ideas for supporting more research being effectively embedded into practice. They suggested that job descriptions could be changed, nurses could be given clear research objectives and supervision, and improvement leads could be allocated for specific pieces of work that are regularly monitored and audited. They also suggested that academics should link their findings to systems that organizations are increasingly using to demonstrate measurement and effectiveness, such as score cards, dashboards, quality accounts and key performance indicators. In an Australian study in 2005, Cleary and Freeman[6] advocated the benefits of a beginner's guide to undertaking research. It detailed helpful, simple guides on helping nurses to understand the process of undertaking a research project, but did not address the implication for putting research into practice.

Another Australian study by Happell in 2004[39] detailed innovative approaches to enhancing clinical nursing research in the field by setting up a Centre for Psychiatric Nursing Research and Practice. One of the programmes on which this centre focused was the role of leadership and the application of research to psychiatric nursing practice. The programme developed a clinical research fellowship that was designed to support clinically based nurses to identify, appraise and utilize research that could serve as an evidence base for their practice. Participants were also asked to identify a policy, practice or procedure within their own work environment that was routine but did not have a known evidence base to support its efficacy. This study concluded that nurses in clinical practice, through participation in such programmes, were not only able to identify the potential relevance of research but also to play leading roles in establishing and carrying out a research agenda.

Back in 1995, Veeramah[42] summarized some suggestions from the literature that could be used to tackle some of the problems related to implementing research in practice that may well still be useful to consider today. These included staff being rostered to spend half a day each month exploring relevant research studies and disseminating findings to staff, developing research clubs[43] and reviewing research teaching in pre and post curricula.[44]

There are many very powerful and influential groups already in existence that may benefit from closer working relationships with each other. In the UK, for example, there is a very effective mental health nurse academics network and a very effective mental health nurse directors' forum. They may both mutually benefit from working more closely together on this subject. For example, the academics could provide high-level, plain English quarterly summary reports of latest research findings to directors of nursing who could in turn review their organization's performance against them and consequently influence the setting of organizational high-level objectives. Directors of nursing could then feed ideas for further research to academics and facilitate the use of their organizations for conducting some of the studies. Directors may wish to prioritize research that focuses on a clearly identified patient need that has the potential to change practice in their areas. This may help to narrow some of the gaps that have been previously identified between academics and practising clinicians.

It could be argued that all research is meaningless unless it can demonstrate a positive effect on patient care, experience or outcome. With this in mind, it is important always to consider that what may be deemed as important to nurses, doctors and academics may not be deemed as high a priority to patients. A study by Chambers et al. in 2013[45] cited a thematic data analysis by Strauss and Corbin[46] which found that patients' priorities included being treated with dignity and respect, involvement in decision-making processes, being given more information about their treatment, being offered access to more talking therapies and therapeutic engagement, access to daily activities and active listening by staff. Many of these issues remain topical and are still identified as areas requiring improvement in patient satisfaction survey results and regulatory body inspection findings today. There is also an existing array of published research studies related to the topics above that suggest clear recommendations for improvement. We should reflect on the reasons why these themes are often still as pertinent as they were nearly 20 years ago, despite the array of completed and published research.

Earlier on, you were asked to consider ways in which you might improve the application of research in practice. Table 7.1 aims to summarize some methods that various authors have suggested to improve success, in addition to some further suggestions from this chapter.

Table 7.1 Ways of improving the implementation of research in practice

Recommended action	Leads	Adapted from source where applicable
Quarterly summaries of completed research in a plain English, user-friendly format, reviewed by nurse directors and embedded within existing quality governance mechanisms.	Academic networks and nurse director networks	
All nurses having an objective within their job descriptions and appraisal systems to embed research into their practice and carry out a quality improvement project.	Nurses and organizations	5,39
Nurses to present improvement projects and/or research at conferences inside and outside the organization.	Nurses and organizations with support from academic institutions	35
Nurses to work towards publishing good practices in nursing journals.	Nurses and organizations	35,39
Develop robust organizational research strategies that: • identify organizational barriers that may impact on effective application of research in practice; • identify practical and planned approaches to overcoming some of the barriers to implementing research in practice; • include simple definitions of the differences between quality/service improvement, audit and research;	Organizations	34,5,6,31,35,39

(Continued)

Table 7.1 (*continued*)

Recommended action	Leads	Adapted from source where applicable
• use plain English and provide definitions of key terms; • simplify approval processes and systems; • agree simple pathways for conducting a piece of new service/quality improvement work; • have a clear and publicized process that supports all grades of staff to feel confident to make suggestions for improvements or changes in practice based on research findings; • are explicit about the expectations of certain roles within the organization, e.g. ward/team managers and trained nurses; • do not just focus on randomized controlled trials and ensure that the key role of nurses is explicit; • are clear how the results of research, including randomized controlled trials, are used and disseminated across your organization; • include detail that guides and assists staff to proactively seek out research relevant to their practice, develop their understanding of it, be able to critically evaluate it, understand how they can confidently use it and be supported from an organizational perspective to apply it to their practice with the support of the organization and leaders.		
Conduct a training needs analysis that is carried out in a transparent, structured way and is based on addressing perceived barriers to successful implementation of research in practice in your organization.	Organizations and teams	
Work with local academic institutions to review pre- and post-student nurse training curricula in a way that takes account of some of the barriers encountered to successful implementation.	Organizations and local academic institutions	42
Benchmark organization and teams to establish how much of current practice in clinical areas is based on research or an evidence base, versus traditionally accepted practices.	Organizations and nurses	4
Review current leadership and management commitment, views, skills and approaches to implementing research in practice in their areas.	Organizations with support from local academic institutions where required	
Be clear about the importance of the leadership role and have robust processes to assist with management of change factors.	Nurses and organizations	4,39
Agree quick-win actions such as teaching staff how to carry out an internet NHS Evidence search, hold annual clinician-focused best practice conferences that benchmark the best practice against available research, develop plain English research and good practice newsletters, promote the use of research mentors and dedicated intranet pages for informal publication and sharing.	Nurses and organizations	39
Review existing clinical policies, procedures and processes both locally and organization-wide to evaluate the robustness of the evidence base used to inform their content.	Nurses and organizations	39

(Continued)

Table 7.1 (*continued*)

Recommended action	Leads	Adapted from source where applicable
Develop a process for feeding back, sharing, analysing and using any findings or recommendations from pieces of quality improvement or research work conducted by organizational staff. This should include dissertations, publications and external conference presentations.	Nurses and organizations	
Make sure that quality accounts, dashboards, key performance indicators and patient/staff satisfaction and experience processes all include factors related to the use and application of evidence base and research.	Organizations	5
Consider building in dedicated time that is rostered which allows nurses to review the most recent research relevant to their field and present it to their colleagues.	Nurses and organizations	42
Develop research clubs, journal clubs, staff away days and support for writing for publication sessions.	Nurses and organizations	35,42
Review which NICE guidelines and standards are relevant to your organization and practice. Develop stricter enforcement of team, ward and organization's adherence to them. Ensure policies are based on NICE guidelines where applicable and are implemented and monitored in practice. Use commissioning levers and incentives to encourage the use of up-to-date research findings in clinical practice.	Nurses, organizations, regulatory and commissioning bodies	
Consider allocating senior nurses specific pieces of work on specific clinical topics to collate research evidence and then present their teams with summaries and recommendations for changing practice accordingly.	Nurses and organizations	5, 31

CONCLUSION

There are many factors that need to be considered when mental health nurses practise. Patients' individual experiences and outcomes; the strength of the therapeutic relationship; the nurse's skill, knowledge, intuition and experience; the robustness of evidence-based policies to support practice; and the application of measurable standards and research all have a part to play. This chapter has discussed many of the common barriers faced by mental health nurses that can hinder successful identification of relevant research and implementation of research in practice. I hope it has also shown that it is not just the application of research that is important, but how a nurse balances this with what the patient actually wants and what works for them. This is in addition to mental health nurses using their often extensive knowledge and experience to offer care that has taken into account a variety of factors. It is clear that the application of research in caring practice is far from easy, but it is most definitely a 'craft', and we all owe it to ourselves, our organizations, our patients and their families to do our very best to try to overcome the barriers to doing something that we all really know should be part of routine practice.

References

1. Welsh I, Lyons CM. Evidence-based care and the case for intuition and tacit knowledge in clinical assessment and decision making in mental health nursing practice: an empirical contribution to the debate. *Journal of Psychiatric and Mental Health Nursing* 2001; **8**(4): 299–305.

2. Fisher JE. The use of psychological therapies by mental health nurses in Australia. *Journal of Psychiatric and Mental Health Nursing* 2014; **21**(3): 264–70.

3. Bryman A. *Social research methods.* Oxford: Oxford University Press, 2004.

4. McKenna H. Dissemination and application of mental health nursing research. *British Journal of Nursing* 1995; **4**(21): 1257–62.

5. Bowers L, Pithouse A, Hooton S. How to establish evidence-based change in acute care settings. *Mental Health Practice* 2012; **16**(4): 22–5.

6. Cleary M, Freeman A. Facilitating research within clinical settings: the development of a beginners guide. *International Journal of Mental Health Nursing* 2005; **14**(3): 202–8.

7. Gerrish K, Clayton J. Promoting evidence based practice: an organizational approach. *Journal of Nursing Management* 2004; **12**: 114–23.

8. Zauszniewski JA, Suresky J. Evidence for psychiatric nursing practice: an analysis of three years of published research. *Online Journal of Issues in Nursing* 2004; **9**(1): 125–35.

9. Bartholomew D, Collier E. Research-based care on an acute inpatient psychiatric unit. *British Journal of Nursing* 2002; **11**: 876–84.

10. Rodgers, S. An exploratory study of research utilization by nurses in general medical and surgical wards. *Journal of Advanced Nursing* 1994; **20**: 904–11.

11. Wynaden D, Heslop K, Al Omari O, Nelson D, Osmond B, Taylor M, Gee T. Identifying mental health nursing research priorities: a Delphi study. *Contemporary Nurse* 2014; **47**: 16–26.

12. DiCenso A. Research: evidence based practice: how to get there from here. *Nursing Leadership* 2003; **16**: 20–6.

13. Parahoo K. Barriers to, and facilitators of, research utilization among nurses in Northern Ireland. *Journal of Advanced Nursing* 2000; **31**: 89–98.

14. Wynaden D, Landsborough I, Chapman R, McGowan S, Lapsley J, Finn N. Establishing best practice guidelines for the administration of intramuscular injections in the adult: a systematic review of the literature. *Contemporary Nurse* 2005; **20**: 267–77.

15. Holm AL, Severinsson E. The role of the mental health nursing leadership. *Journal of Nursing Management* 2010; **18**: 463–71.

16. Jinks M, Chalder G. Consensus and diversity: an action research study designed to analyse the role of a group of mental health consultant nurses. *Journal of Clinical Nursing* 2007; **67**: 1323–32.

17. Gordon NS. Influencing mental health nursing practice through the teaching of research and theory: a personal critical review. *Journal of Psychiatric and Mental Health Nursing* 1998; **5**: 119–28.

18. NMC (Nursing and Midwifery Council). Professional standards of practice and behaviour for nurses and midwives. 2015. Available from: https://www.nmc.org.uk/standards/code/read-the-code-online/ [Accessed 4th October 2016].

19. McKenna HP. Appraisal of clinical areas for mental health student placement. Unpublished report. University of Ulster, 1993.

20. Stickley T, Phillips C. Single case study and evidence-based practice. *Journal of Psychiatric and Mental Health Nursing* 2005; **12**: 728–32.

21. Peplau HE. *Interpersonal relations in nursing.* New York: G Putnam's Sons, 1952.

22. Rasmussen P, Henderson A, Muir-Cochrane E. Conceptualizing the clinical and professional development of child and adolescent mental health nurses. *International Journal of Mental Health Nursing* 2014; **23**: 265–72.

23. Fisher JE, Happell B. Implications of evidence-based practice for mental health nursing. *International Journal of Mental Health Nursing* 2009; **18**: 179–85.

24. Whitley R, Drake R. How do clients obtain mental health information? Commentary on consumer perspectives on information and other inputs to decision-making. Implications for evidence-based practice. *Community Mental Health Journal* 2008; **44**: 457–8.

25. McAndrew S. Broadening our horizons: seeing beyond the six 'C's to capture the depth of mental health nursing. *International Journal of Mental Health Nursing* 2013; **22**: 375–6.

26. National Confidential Inquiry into Suicide and Homicide by People with Mental Illness. *Annual report.* 2014. Available from: http://research.bmh.manchester.ac.uk/cmhs/research/centreforsuicide-prevention/nci/reports/ [Accessed 4th October 2016].

27. Margison F. Evidence-based medicine in the psychological treatment of schizophrenia. *Journal of the American Academy of Psychoanalysis and Dynamic Psychiatry* 2003; **31**: 177–90.

28. Carlyle D, Crowe M, Deering D. Models of care delivery in mental health nursing practice: a mixed method study. *Journal of Psychiatric and Mental Health Nursing* 2012; **19**: 221–30.

29. Allard S. A user/survivor perspective: what's beyond the evidence? In: Priebe S, Slade M (eds). *Evidence in mental health care.* Hove: Brunner-Routledge, 2002: 207–14.

30. Sackett DL, Rosenburg WMC, Gray JAM, Haynes RB, Richardson WS. Evidence-based medicine: what it is and what it isn't. *British Medical Journal* 1996; **312**: 71–2.

31. Cleary M, Horsfall J, Happell B. Developing practice in mental health settings. *International Journal of Mental Health Nursing* 2010; **19**: 45–52.

32. Barker P. *Psychiatric and mental health nursing: the craft of caring,* 2nd edn. London: Hodder Arnold, 2009.

33. Happell B. Influencing undergraduate nursing students' attitudes toward mental health nursing: acknowledging the role of theory. *Issues in Mental Health Nursing* 2009; **30**: 39–46.

34. Hunt J. Indicators for nursing practice. *Journal of Advanced Nursing* 1981; **16**: 89–114.

35. Happell B. Conference presentations: developing nursing knowledge by disseminating research findings. *Nurse Researcher* 2007; **15**: 70–7.

36. Cleary M, Horsfall J. Quality improvement projects: finding a pathway through policies. *International Journal of Mental Health Nursing* 2002; **11**: 121–7.

37. McDonnell J, Jones C. Benchmarking best practice in mental health care services. *Nursing Management* 2010; **16**(10): 20–4.

38. McDonnell J, Jones C. Overcoming the difficulties of benchmarking in mental health. *Mental Health Practice* 2010; **13**(6): 24–8.

39. Happell B. The Centre for Psychiatric Nursing Research and Practice: an innovative approach to enhancing clinical nursing research in the psychiatric/mental health field. *Issues in Mental Health Nursing* 2004; **25**: 47–60.

40. MacGuire JM. Putting nursing research findings into practice: research utilization as an aspect of the management of change. *Journal of Advanced Nursing* 1990; **15**: 614–20.

41. Caine C, Kendrick M. The role of clinical directorate managers in facilitating evidence-based practice: a report of an exploratory study. *Journal of Nursing Management* 1997; **5**: 157–65.

42. Veeramah V. A study to identify the attitudes and needs of qualified staff concerning the use of research findings in clinical practice within mental health care settings. *Journal of Advanced Nursing* 1995; **22**: 855–61.

43. Luckenbill-Brett JL. Use of nursing practice research findings. *Nursing Research* 1987; **36**: 344–9.

44. Closs SJ, Cheater FM. Utilization of nursing research culture, interest and support. *Journal of Advanced Nursing* 1994; **19**: 762–73.

45. Chambers M, Gillard S, Turner K, Borschmann R. Evaluation of an educational practice development programme for staff working in mental health inpatient environments. *Journal of Psychiatric and Mental Health Nursing* 2013; **20**: 362–73.

46. Strauss A, Corbin J. *Basics of qualitative research: grounded theory procedures and technique,* 2nd edn. London: Sage, 1998.

Further reading

Bryman A. *Social research methods*. Oxford: Oxford University Press, 2004.

De Vaus D. *Research design in social research*. London: Sage, 2008.

Department of Health. Statistical update on suicide. February 2015. Available from: https://www.gov.uk/government/uploads/system/uploads/attachment_data/file/405411/Statistical_update_on_suicide_acc.pdf [Accessed 19th November 2016].

Grix J. *The foundations of research*. Basingstoke: Palgrave MacMillan, 2004.

HM Government. Preventing suicide in England: two years on. Second annual report on the cross-government outcomes strategy to save lives. 2015. Available from: https://www.gov.uk/government/uploads/system/uploads/attachment_data/file/405407/Annual_Report_acc.pdf [Accessed 5th September 2016].

NICE (National Institute for Health and Care Excellence). Self-harm: the short-term physical and psychological management and secondary prevention of intentional self-harm in primary and secondary care. Available from: https://www.nice.org. uk/guidance/cg16/evidence/cg16-selfharm-full-guideline-2 [Accessed 5th September 2016].

NICE (National Institute for Health and Care Excellence). Self-harm in over 8s: long-term management. 2011. Available from: https://www.nice.org.uk/guidance/cg133 [Accessed 5th September 2016].

Polit DF, Beck CT. *Nursing research: principles and methods*. New York: Lippincott, Williams and Wilkins, 2004.

RCP (Royal College of Psychiatrists). Self-harm, suicide and risk: helping people who self-harm. 2010. Available from: http://www.rcpsych.ac.uk/files/pdfversion/cr158.pdf [Accessed 5th September 2016].

Robson C. *Real world research*. Oxford: Blackwell, 1993.

Samaritans. Suicide statistics report 2015. Available from: http://www.samaritans.org/sites/default/files/kcfinder/branches/branch-96/files/Suicide_statistics_report_2015.pdf [Accessed 5th September 2016].

Relevant web pages

CALM. Suicide stats and research. https://www.thecalmzone.net/about-calm/suicide-research-stats/

CQC (Care Quality Commission). http://www.cqc.org.uk

Department of Health. Research and innovation in health and social care. https://www.gov.uk/government/policies/research-and-innovation-in-health-and-social-care

Medical Research Council. http://www.mrc.ac.uk

The Mental Elf. http://www.nationalelfservice.net/mental-health/

Mental Health Foundation. Suicide. http://www.mentalhealth.org.uk/help-information/mental-health-a-z/s/suicide/

Mental Health Foundation. The truth about self-harm. http://www.mentalhealth.org.uk/publications/truth-about-self-harm

MHLDNDL (Mental Health & Learning Disability Nurse Directors' and Leads' National Forum). http://mentalhealthforum.org.uk

MIND. Self-harm. http://mind.org.uk/information-support/types-of-mental-health-problems/self-harm/

NHS Benchmarking Network. http://www.nhsbenchmarking.nhs.uk/index.php

NHS Choices. Clinical trials. http://www.nhs.uk/conditions/Clinical-trials/Pages/Introduction.aspx

NHS Choices. Quality accounts. http://www.nhs.uk/aboutNHSChoices/professionals/healthandcareprofessionals/quality-accounts/Pages/about-quality-accounts.aspx

NHS Choices. Self-harm. http://www.nhs.uk/conditions/Self-injury/Pages/Introduction.aspx

NHS Health Research Authority. Determine which review body approvals are required. http://www.hra.nhs.uk/research-community/before-you-apply/determine-which-review-body-approvals-are-required/

NHS Networks. https://www.networks.nhs.uk

NIHR (National Institute for Health Research). http://www.nihr.ac.uk/research/

NIHR (National Institute for Health Research) Clinical Research Network. Mental health. https://www.crn.nihr.ac.uk/mentalhealth/

NSHN (National Self-Harm Network) Forum. http://www.nshn.co.uk

RCN (Royal College of Nursing). Network for Psychiatric Nursing Research. http://www2.rcn.org.uk/development/nursing_communities/rcn_forums/mental_health/npnr

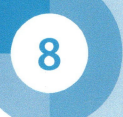

8 Nursing classification and care planning

KAY JANSEN, AMY COENEN AND NICHOLAS R. HARDIKER

LEARNING OUTCOMES

- To be able to discuss how using an electronic health record can facilitate care planning.

- To understand how using a personal health record can promote care coordination between nurses and service users.

- To know how to define interoperability and why this is important to health care providers and service users.

- To understand why standardized nursing terminologies are needed for interoperability of health data and information.

- To be able to provide examples of how to implement standardized terminology in a care plan.

SUMMARY OF KEY POINTS

- Despite the ubiquitous nature of information and communication technology, health care has proved to be something of an exception and remains relatively untouched by the 'digital revolution'
- The electronic health record has the potential to support mental health nurses through a number of means, including care planning that facilitates:
  - interdisciplinary care;
  - evidence-based practice;
  - care coordination;
  - service user participation, health literacy and self-management.
- In addition to identifying service user problems and nursing interventions, it is also important to identify service users' assets and strengths and to set goals or expected outcomes of care.
- The use of standardized terminology in the electronic health record can support nursing care planning.

INTRODUCTION

Information and communication technology (ICT) is an umbrella term that covers a broad range of communication devices such as computers and telephones and their supporting infrastructure such as software and networks. ICT makes possible the delivery of applications and services that we now take very much for granted; for example, email, online messaging, video and conferencing. ICT has become an important part of our lives – its use has very rapidly become the norm – and it is difficult to imagine how we managed just a few years ago without these tools and devices.

Despite the ubiquitous nature of ICT, health care has proved to be something of an exception and remains relatively untouched by the 'digital revolution'. There have been some notable successes, such as the widespread digitization of radiography. However, the uptake of ICT in health care has been at best patchy, and confined primarily to the hospital-based care of individuals with physical health issues (see chapter 69).

The reasons for the comparatively slow pace of progress of ICT in health care do not include a lack of desire. Many scores of individuals have been actively engaged in this agenda for many years. Conferences, some of which have been running for several decades, attract audiences in the thousands or tens of thousands, and the investment made over this period runs into billions or even trillions.

Nurses too have played their part, with active engagement stretching back at least to the time of the first computers, over half a century ago (some scholars would pre-date this by a further century, citing Florence Nightingale as one of our first health informaticians).

Despite this considerable effort, however, we are yet to see systems in routine use of ICT supporting nursing practice and enhancing health. This is even more evident in the area of mental health. The science is sound. The systems work. We have the necessary skills. What may be lacking is the knowledge or awareness about what is possible in supporting the craft of caring.

In this chapter we explore the potential benefits that ICT can bring to mental health nursing. However, we go beyond the usual expectations management (or mismanagement) approach, with its tendency towards over-promising and under-delivering. Instead, we seek to expand your thinking by providing realistic scenarios and describing in detail practical approaches to addressing, through the creative application of ICT and a focus on care planning, some of the issues that might arise.

While we acknowledge that a wide range of contemporary technologies will bring benefits to people and professionals alike, we make no apologies for avoiding the glitz and glamour of gizmos. Instead, we go back to basics and focus on the main currency of good nursing care – information.

ELECTRONIC AND PERSONAL HEALTH RECORDS TO SUPPORT CARE PLANNING

Advances in technology, such as the introduction of ICT, present potential opportunities to support nurses in delivering care using all components of the nursing process through electronic assessments and care planning. Care planning is a dynamic activity and the service user's care plan is a major component of the health record.

Health information systems, such as the electronic health record (EHR), are now the norm in many health care settings, for use by health care professionals, service users and family members. Nurses can maximize the potential of the EHR to improve service user outcomes. There is not one universally agreed upon definition of the EHR. For the purpose of this chapter, however, the EHR is defined by the World Health Organization[1] as a longitudinal electronic record of a person's health encounters across all types of health care settings. Ideally it should reflect the entire health history of an individual across his or her lifetime, including data from multiple providers from a variety of health care settings. An EHR is not simply the replacement of the paper record. It is intended to provide more functionality, such as decision support, to both health care providers and service users.

Specific examples of using the EHR are discussed here in regard to how it can improve care planning and support mental health nurses in (a) interdisciplinary care, (b) evidence-based practice, (c) care coordination across health care settings, and (d) promoting service users' and family members' participation in health. Examples of care planning in mental health care are also provided.

Supporting interdisciplinary care

The EHR has the potential to support mental health nurses through a number of means, including care planning. Developing a person-centred plan of care is an *interdisciplinary* activity that includes the service user and family. EHRs can provide a platform to enable all health professionals involved to communicate with each other to ensure a shared plan of care.

Nurses can use the care plan to contribute to the multidisciplinary problem list and identify specific nursing interventions and goals for each problem identified. In addition to identifying service user problems and nursing interventions, it also is important to identify service users' assets and strengths and to set goals or expected outcomes of care.

Mental health services have a long history of interdisciplinary approaches to care in many countries – more than 30 years ago the Department of Health in Ireland[2] recommended the establishment of multidisciplinary teams to adequately meet the needs of those with mental illnesses. Teams that represent different approaches to treatment and that involve the participation of people from a number of professional disciplines, such as those found in the Care Programme Approach (described in chapter 37), can provide truly holistic care to service users and their families across the boundaries of primary, secondary and tertiary care. Within an interdisciplinary team, each professional must be responsible for the quality of their care planning; including development of the initial care plan, evaluation of progress against the plan of care, and updating the care plan based on service user progress or decline.

An EHR can provide decision support for best practice in interdisciplinary care planning. Some basic components or functionality of the EHR can support the use, timeliness and coordination of interdisciplinary care planning. For example, interventions or treatments that are identified in a care plan can be used to guide ongoing documentation of care, confirming that specific interventions planned were indeed delivered or carried out. Another function of the EHR is to ensure that all professionals are notified when the plan has been updated or modified. Due dates for review of care plans can trigger alerts to those professionals involved.

Supporting evidence-based practice

Evidence-based practice for mental health nursing practice provides assurance that care is based on the best available research evidence, the nurse's expertise and experience, and the service user's preferences.[3] Some EHRs provide decision support tools for nurses. These tools might include alerts, drop-down menus or standard care paths to assist the nurses in documentation and decision making. (More information on evidence-based practice in mental health care can be found in chapter 6.)

More sophisticated EHRs provide links to the scientific evidence or published research to assist nurses in decision making. For example, when a nurse documents the nursing problem 'suicidal ideation' in the care plan, the EHR may provide an alert. This alert will guide the nurse in documenting a complete suicide assessment in the EHR. Based on the assessment data, decision support tools will trigger a list of interventions for the nurse to consider in planning care. (See chapter 46 for further details on crisis assessment and resolution.) The EHR can also provide access to evidence-based guidelines for planning care for service users who are suicidal.

Decision support tools, based on research, do not replace the nurse's clinical judgement. Rather, evidence-based decision making by the nurse includes applying not only the research knowledge but also the nurse's expertise based on experience and the service user's preference. In all cases, the nurse is responsible for clinical decisions made and for assuring the safety and best care for each service user.

REFLECTION

Do you use an EHR in your practice? How might an EHR support interdisciplinary, coordinated care across the many settings where mental health services are provided?

Care coordination

In many cases, a service user with mental health needs does not receive all of their health care services from one professional. Rather, service users tend to move through the health care system to access and receive care across health care providers as needed. *Care coordination* is an important aspect of the nurse's role in mental health. To assure holistic care, the nurse must have an understanding not just of the psychological aspects of health but also of the service user's physical, social and spiritual dimensions of health. The ability for all health care providers, with the permission of the service user, to access and share data across health care services is essential for coordination of care. Care coordination can improve quality and lower costs.[4] For example, laboratory or test results can be more readily shared via an EHR to improve care planning and reduce the ordering of redundant tests.

A role in some health settings is that of the nurse care coordinator. This role has been expanded in the care of persons with long-term illnesses, including those with mental illness. Nurses in these roles play an important part in ensuring that service users with mental illness have coordinated care across the continuum of services. Again, the EHR can support this nursing role by sharing data and information to ensure a more holistic perspective in care planning.

Supporting service user participation, health literacy and self-management

Care planning activities should involve the service user as much as possible. Service users should be present for care planning conferences or have the opportunity to review their care plan with a health professional. When the nurse meets with a service user, they can review the care plan together. The nurse can use this meeting as an opportunity for evaluating progress, lending encouragement and providing education. *Service user participation* in their health care decision has been demonstrated to improve health outcomes.[5]

A number of important concepts are related to service user participation, including health literacy and self-management. *Health literacy* has many definitions. It is more than the ability to read or access health information. Health literacy is the ability to use or apply health information in personal situations to improve health. Nursing interventions to promote health literacy include more than teaching about health conditions and treatments such as medication. In order to facilitate a service user's health literacy to enable them to participate in health decisions, nurses must have the cultural competency to assess all potential barriers.

With the introduction of the internet, access to health information has expanded dramatically. Nurses can encourage service users and family members to evaluate the quality of information available on the internet. Nurses can assist service users in accessing reliable resources on the internet and encourage discussion of information from these resources. Supporting health literacy is an important intervention to consider when planning care for service users and families with mental illness.

Health literacy is one aspect of self-management of disease or illness. *Self-management* is defined as the ability to actively manage one's own illness. There are many models of self-management but all include the individual's participation in health care. In addition to the web portals for service users to access data and information in their EHR, other ICT tools to promote service user participation are gaining popularity among health care consumers. These include applications for mobile telephones or other

mobile devices. Mobile applications can be used as alerts for medication reminders and to track symptoms or health behaviours. Evaluating when to use or not use ICT devices is an important part of individualized care planning.

> ## REFLECTION
>
> - Is health literacy a concept you are familiar with and something you attend to in your nursing practice?
> - Why is health literacy important to your service users?

NURSING CLASSIFICATIONS AND TERMINOLOGY STANDARDS

The success of ICT resources such as the EHR depends on *interoperability*. Interoperability is the ability for health information systems to share and use data across health providers and settings. If a service user visits the mental health clinic and notifies the nurse that s/he visited the emergency department (ED) last week and wants the nurse to review what occurred, the clinic and ED information systems must be interoperable to be able to share records.

An essential building block for interoperability of health information systems is terminology standards. Standards are needed for interoperability among information systems. In addition to sharing data, standards support the collection and storage of nursing data, within and across health information systems. If data are standardized, they can be collected once by the nurses in practice and reused many times. When standardized nursing data are saved, these data can be examined to describe nursing practice, including identifying nurses' contributions to health outcomes. Nurse researchers can study what nursing interventions for specific nursing diagnoses result in best outcomes.

Standardized data collected routinely in documentation of nursing care in the EHR can be reused to evaluate nursing care and inform nurses and administrators how to improve service user outcomes. These standardized data can be used for quality improvement, results reporting and targeted analyses. For example, if a mental health hospital wanted

to examine the use of a particular drug, the data warehouse for the EHR could be queried to extract all the coded data elements related to that drug. Combining drug use data elements with other data elements for analysis, such as time of day or age of service users, could provide meaningful information to a specific unit, hospital or region.

Efforts to advance terminology standards in nursing began many decades ago with the Nursing Minimum Data Set (NMDS).[6] The NMDS identified the need to standardize concepts to represent nursing diagnoses, nursing interventions and service user outcomes. Since 1988, a number of nursing classifications and terminologies have been developed and used to represent nursing practice in the health record. Some examples of nursing terminologies include NANDA,[7] which represents nursing diagnoses; and the Omaha System,[8] Clinical Care Classification (CCC)[9] and the International Classification for Nursing Practice (ICNP),[10] which represent all three NMDS concepts, i.e. nursing diagnoses, interventions and outcomes.

In the following section, examples of the nursing components of a service user care plan are provided using the ICNP. The ICNP is an international standard which is owned and maintained by the International Council of Nurses and is used to represent nursing diagnoses, nursing interventions and service user outcomes or goals.

CASE STUDY AND CARE PLAN USING STANDARD NURSING TERMINOLOGY

In this section a case study is presented to provide an example of a nursing care plan across time and various care settings (see case study 1). The standardized terminology used in this example is ICNP. The code for each concept is added in the care plan to display that each ICNP concept has a unique code. These codes can be stored in a relational database in the EHR data warehouse for future uses, such as evaluation of the quality of care.

Initial electronic care plan: diabetes clinic

After completing a comprehensive physical examination, history and laboratory tests, the collaborative care plan shown in Table 8.1 was developed with Mr Stevens and entered into the EHR to be used as the basis for future nursing documentation. For example, at the end of the first visit an alert was triggered by entering the nursing diagnosis

CASE STUDY 1: INITIAL ASSESSMENT IN A DIABETES CLINIC

Background information

Robert Stevens is a 58-year-old divorced male who was diagnosed 6 months ago with type 2 diabetes. He sees a nurse practitioner in a diabetes clinic every 2 weeks for ongoing diabetes management, including education and laboratory tests. Mr Stevens says he 'sometimes' does not administer his midday dose of insulin at work. He also does not do blood glucose testing before lunch and reports that 'it's too hard to do at work. I just can't do it there.' Mr Stevens understands his medical diagnoses and treatment and realizes that this behaviour impacts disease management. His haemoglobin A1C results ranged from 8 to 11 per cent over the last 6 months. Weight 99.31 kg; Height 180 cm; BMI 30.6; BP 146/90.

Current medical diagnoses

- Uncontrolled hypertension
- Type 2 diabetes mellitus
- Obesity

Past health history

Mr Stevens had an episode of major depressive disorder in his early 20s. He refused medication and therapy at that time. He has had 'several bouts' of depression over the last 30 years but never received treatment. He attributes his current episode of depression to the divorce. He has no history of hospitalization or surgery.

Medication history and allergies

Prescribed: pre-mixed insulin, t.i.d. before meals and antihypertensives, one tablet daily. Admits to forgetting to take antihypertensive medication 'sometimes'.

Over the counter medications: multivitamin 1 tablet daily; pain medication for headache less than one time per month.

- Herbal remedies: none.
- Side effects or problems with medication: none.
- Allergies: none known.

Social history

Mr Stevens has a full-time position as an accountant for a small printing company where he has been employed for 25 years. He was married for 30 years prior to his divorce 2 years ago. He has three married children and six young grandchildren who live within 20 miles of his home. He reports being 'very involved' with his family and reports that they are very supportive. Hobbies include fishing and bowling with friends and spending time with family. He has no religious affiliation. Never used tobacco; drinks 'occasionally' with friends – 1–2 beers per week. Mr Stevens has two brothers he rarely sees because they live 'far away'. His parents are both living and reside with one of his brothers.

Family history

Hypertension – both brothers and father; mother has major depression and takes an antidepressant medication; family history otherwise unremarkable.

'Risk for depressed mood' and the nursing intervention 'Screen for depressed mood' in the electronic care plan. This alert prompted the nurse to complete and document the result of the WHO (Five) Well-being Index for depression screening in primary care[11] during Mr Stevens' second visit. Periodic assessment of well-being, including mood and diabetes distress, is one of the Psychological Care recommendations in the International Diabetes Federation clinical guidelines.[12]

Each ICNP nursing diagnosis, intervention and outcome in the care plan has a unique identifier or code. The codes would not be shown with the concepts in the electronic care plan, but they are connected to the concepts and would be used to store data in the data warehouse for the EHR.

REFLECTION

- How does the electronic care plan in this case study demonstrate or exemplify collaborative care planning (see chapter 50)?

- What would improve the collaborative nature of this care plan?

Change in condition

The nurse and nurse practitioner have noted changes in Mr Stevens' behaviour, affect and appearance in the last 2 weeks. He is less verbal and social during visits; exhibits

Table 8.1 Electronic care plan for Mr Stevens

ICNP code	Nursing diagnoses	ICNP code	Nursing interventions	ICNP code	Expected outcomes
10027550	Hyperglycaemia	10040586	Assess preferences (diet and exercise)	10033685	Blood glucose within normal limits
		10044481	Assess adherence to diet		
		10024214	Assess obstructions to adherence		
		10024116	Teach about disease		
		10038051	Promote medication adherence		
		10041628	Promote adherence to exercise regime		
		10032034	Monitor blood glucose		
		10035286	Manage hyperglycaemia		
10022954	Altered blood pressure	10032052	Monitor blood pressure	10027647	Blood pressure within normal limits
		10044148	Teach about measuring blood pressure		
		10032121	Monitor weight		
		10021703	Promote medication adherence using a pillbox		
10021956	Knowledge of disease	10022537	Reinforce self-efficacy	10021956	Knowledge of disease
		10040501	Facilitate ability to participate in care planning		
10045702	Positive family support	10035927	Facilitate family ability to participate in care planning	10045702	Positive family support
10032329	Risk for depressed mood	10040636	Assess attitude toward health status	10038430	Positive psychological status
		10045022	Screen for depressed mood		

slowed movements; has depressed affect and is easily distracted; wears wrinkled clothes; and comes to appointments unshaven. When asked about these changes during a recent visit, Mr Stevens reports feeling 'sad' and 'tired all the time'. He also states, 'I know I've gained weight because I stopped taking my daily walk.' 'Maybe it's the depression again.' He denies suicidal ideation.

Upon further assessment, the nurse learns that Mr Stevens has not missed work but finds it very difficult to get out of bed in the morning. He has been experiencing problems falling and staying asleep during the last 2 weeks. His concentration is decreased and he is 'impatient with the grandkids'. He also reports that his children have noted that he doesn't seem to enjoy anything any more. His appetite is decreased and he does not have the energy to cook, so eats 'junk food' when he has an appetite.

Based on the recommendation from the International Diabetes Federation clinical guideline,[12] the nurse repeats the WHO (Five) Well-being Index. His score 6 months ago was 80 per cent and his current score is 8 per cent. The nurse knows that a score below 52 per cent indicates poor well-being, and a change in scores greater than 10 per cent indicates the need to test for depression.[11]

Additional data obtained during this visit include: weight: 97 kg (decrease of 2.31 kg in 6 weeks). Fasting blood glucose 150 mg/dL. The urinalysis and additional blood work are within normal limits.

When the nursing diagnosis 'Depressed mood' is entered in the electronic care plan, the following recommendation from the International Diabetes Federation clinical guideline[12] appears on the computer screen: 'Refer to a mental health-care professional with a knowledge of diabetes when indicated. Indications may include: severe coping problems, signs of major depression, anxiety disorder, personality disorder, addiction and cognitive decline'(p.27).

The nurse makes a referral to the psychiatrist who is affiliated with the diabetes clinic. Mr Stevens agrees to keep the appointment. The original care plan is updated with the nursing diagnoses, interventions and outcomes shown in Table 8.2.

Mental health intervention

The following day, Mr Stevens sees the psychiatrist. Based on past health history, physical examination, laboratory tests and a thorough psychological evaluation, the diagnosis of major depressive disorder is confirmed. The psychiatrist prescribes an antidepressant that does not cause weight gain and asks Mr Stevens' permission to include his family in a conference to discuss treatment recommendations. The family conference is attended by two of Mr Stevens' three children who accompanied him to the appointment. With family encouragement and support, Mr Stevens agrees to take the antidepressant medication and to allow one of his sons to stay with him as he adjusts to the medication (see Table 8.3).

Diabetic clinic follow-up

One week later, during his diabetic clinic visit, Mr Stevens reports nausea, loss of appetite and suicidal ideation. His fasting blood glucose is 300 mg/dL. Mr Stevens is taken by his son to the psychiatrist and subsequently admitted to an inpatient mental health facility.

> **REFLECTION**
>
> - In your work with service users, have you had access to care plans across the continuum of care?
> - How might sharing care plans across settings benefit service users, nurses and other health care providers?

Table 8.2 Updated electronic care plan 1

ICNP code	Nursing diagnoses	ICNP code	Nursing interventions	ICNP code	Expected outcomes
10022402	Depressed mood	10030734	Assess psychological status	10027901	Decreased depressed mood
			Provide emotional support	10027051	
		10032567	Refer to health care provider (for mental health assessment)		
		10036078	Promote family support		
10027226	Impaired sleep	10036764	Assess sleep	10030279	Adequate sleep
		10040380	Teach about sleep (sleep hygiene)		
10033399	Lack of appetite	10036614 10024618	Monitor food intake Teach about nutrition	10040333	Positive appetite

Table 8.3 Updated electronic care plan 2

ICNP code	Nursing diagnoses	ICNP code	Nursing interventions	ICNP code	Expected outcomes
10015356	Risk for suicide	10036336	Implement suicide precautions	10027938	Decreased suicide risk
10022626	Medication side effect	10043884	Monitor medication side effect	10040282	No medication side effect
		10021837	Manage medication side effect		
		10044614	Teach about medication side effect		

Inpatient mental health facility and summary

Mr Stevens participated in intensive cognitive behavioural therapy, group therapy and one family therapy session. He also received medication management and support in a safe environment. Nurses in the inpatient mental health facility continued to use the electronic care plan to guide interventions and documentation. As part of the routine assessment of service users admitted to the inpatient mental health facility, a physical risk assessment tool called the Serious Mental Illness Physical Health Improvement Profile[13] was administered by the mental health nurse (see chapter 69). Three health needs were identified from the 28 health parameters included in this risk assessment tool. The needs, which were consistent with those identified previously in his care plan, included blood pressure, glucose and sleep. No additional nursing diagnoses or interventions needed to be added to the plan of care. By the fifth hospital day, Mr Stevens no longer had suicidal thoughts, his sleep and appetite had improved markedly, medication side effects were reduced, and blood pressure and glucose were within normal limits. He was discharged and returned home with his daughter to recover further.

A Care Programme Approach (CPA) (discussed in chapter 37) was implemented when Mr Stevens returned to his own home 2 weeks after hospital discharge. Through this approach to care, he received home visits and phone calls from a community mental health nurse care coordinator who collaborated with the general practitioner and all of the health care providers in the diabetic clinic. Three months later, Mr Stevens no longer experienced any signs or symptoms of depression. He was able to return to work and to self-manage his diabetes and hypertension successfully with minimal support from the nurse practitioner at the diabetic clinic.

CONCLUSION

Care plans must be built on evidence and updated regularly to ensure effective, efficient, safe, quality care. The EHR can ensure that the nursing care plan is integrated with the interdisciplinary plan of care and available across care delivery settings. The use of standardized terminology in the EHR can support nursing care planning and the craft of caring.

SERVICE USER COMMENTARY

Writing as a service user with complex health issues, it is my view that any move to provide continuity of care through a common, systematic and effective approach of care planning has to be welcomed. While perhaps slow to embrace ICT in health care, examples of best practice can be found in intensive care units where essential minute-by-minute observations and changes in physical condition are effectively documented using ICT. In other areas, including mental health, my experience has indeed been 'at best patchy'. However, it is impossible to divorce physical and mental health issues in a patient, and the 'truly holistic care to service users and their families' approach is an ideal which should be striven for.

Care planning using EHRs has been of little benefit in my experience, and ways to 'improve service user outcomes' must be explicit and measureable to justify the time required to complete EHRs. Even in simple, let alone complex, cases, the ideal of including 'data from multiple providers' is a communication nightmare, in spite of a proposed vehicle which could enable such a vision. All health care providers would need to sign up to an all-embracing system, feel enabled and take ownership of the responsibilities and expectations placed upon them. To implement and achieve this approach, staff may not have 'all the necessary skills' for many reasons – age, interest, access to training and software, time to master updated technologies, aptitude and simply time. What can be achieved must be realistic for nurses to deliver, given time pressures, and must be of practical use for patients.

The care plan is interdisciplinary, but the issues involved in complex physical and mental health conditions require detailed understanding at a level which can provide challenges even for specialist nurses in specialized hospital departments, and may be too intricate to expect all nurses to be sufficiently knowledgeable to provide specialist interventions and goals. The input will inevitably vary from one nurse to another. Active involvement in my care plan is empowering if the result is effective. This can only happen if all are committed to the EHR and if sufficient time, funding and ongoing training are made available.

To enable such a system to operate effectively requires a commitment to the system, with diligent updating of information and responses to alerts. The false assumption that information has been communicated, understood and reacted to as appropriate has been a fundamental flaw in my experience of EHR use in mental health nursing. Crucial details have not always been communicated and/or noted, resulting in serious consequences through reliance on ICT as the communication tool.

All too often, certainly in mental health care, both ongoing and in crisis, the service user is asked and expected to know what they want, need, should do and so on. Frequently it is not possible for service users to know or articulate what would benefit them, and support tools to trigger interventions to consider could be valuable to include on care plans. 'Health literacy' requires input from reliable sources, extracted from the plethora of information available. Dedicated staff must be responsible for this as it is easy for the service user to become confused, led (worryingly) astray or struggle to access information intellectually or practically, depending on circumstances. The EHR could contribute to enabling patients to 'actively manage one's own illness' but only as part of the bigger picture. Service users will have access to varied ICT facilities, so it is important to realize the system may never be wholly inclusive for all, although that should continue to be its aim.

Interoperability has issues for practical implementation, including costing of resources, regular research, support to troubleshoot problems, cost of upgrades in software and hardware, and ongoing training, for which provision needs to be made in budgets locally and nationally. Clearly, the uniformity of standards is a crucial issue when using EHRs, and national agreement on the classification standards to be adopted could be difficult to achieve. Consideration will need to be given to training at undergraduate and postgraduate levels for continuing professional development in

this respect. Standardized data may also not always allow for the idiosyncrasies of service users – one size never fits all – and this must always be borne in mind, together with unexpected deviations from the norm. The option of a free text facility would be a positive move.

The case study clearly demonstrates how the EHR could be used comprehensively and collaboratively to provide excellent nursing care and support, and the alerts and drop-down menus provide prompts to optimize treatment and more focused/targeted plans and ideas for meetings with care coordinators and at CPA reviews. The specialized nursing interventions and expected outcomes could positively increase nurses' understanding of particular diagnoses which may be outside their regular training in complex and more obscure physical conditions. This could improve patient care and lead to more successful outcomes. However, the essential 'craft of caring' and clinical observation of the nurse can never be replaced by ICT alone; balance is required and traditional nursing skills must never be downgraded in favour of over- or total reliance on ICT and data to create care. It is important that the EHR should support but not subsume other aspects of care, as the primary role of any nurse is not that of an ICT worker.

References

1. WHO (World Health Organization). *Electronic health records: manual for developing countries*. Geneva: WHO, 2006.
2. Department of Health (Ireland). *Planning for the future*. Dublin: Stationery Office, 1984.
3. Melnyk BM. *Evidence-based practice in nursing & healthcare: a guide to best practice*. Philadelphia, PA: Lippincott Williams & Wilkins, 2011.
4. American Nurses Association. The value of nursing care coordination 2012. Available from: http://www.nursingworld.org/carecoordinationwhitepaper [Accessed 19th November 2016].
5. Street RL, Makoul G, Arora NK, Epstein RM. How does communication heal? Pathways linking clinician–patient communication to health outcomes. *Patient Education and Counseling* 2009; **74**: 295–301.
6. Werley HH, Lang NM (eds). *Identification of the nursing minimum data set*. New York: Springer Publishing Company, 1998.
7. NANDA International. *Nursing diagnoses 2015–17: definitions and classification*. Hoboken, NJ: Wiley Blackwell, 2014.
8. Martin KS. *The Omaha System: a key to practice, documentation, and information management*, 2nd edn. Omaha, NE: Health Connections Press, 2004.
9. Saba VK. *Clinical Care Classification (CCC) System. Version 2.5 (2nd ed). User's guide*. New York: Spring Publishing, 2012.
10. International Council of Nurses. *International Classification for Nursing Practice (ICNP)*. Geneva: International Council of Nurses, 2013.
11. Psychiatric Research Unit, World Health Organization Collaborating Centre in Mental Health. *WHO (Five) well-being index*. Geneva: World Health Organization, 1998.
12. International Diabetes Federation. Global guideline for type 2 diabetes 2012. Available from: http://www.idf.org/global-guideline-type-2-diabetes-2012 [Accessed 19th November 2016].
13. White J, Gray R, Jones M. The development of the serious mental illness physical Health Improvement Profile. *Journal of Psychiatric and Mental Health Nursing* 2009; **16**: 493–8.

Further reading

Anthony P, Crawford P. Service user involvement in care planning: the mental health nurse's perspective. *Journal of Psychiatric and Mental Health Nursing* 2000; **7**: 425–34.

Instefjord MH, Aasekjær K, Espehaug B, Graverholt B. Assessment of quality in psychiatric documentation: a clinical audit. *BMC Nursing* 2014; **13**: 32.

Mental Health Network, NHS Confederation. *The future's digital: mental health and technology*. London: NHS Confederation, 2014.

Truman C, Raine P. Experience and meaning of user involvement: some explorations from a community mental health project. *Health & Social Care in the Community* 2002; **10**(3): 136–43.

Tunmore R, Thomas B. Nursing care plans in acute mental health nursing. *Mental Health Practice* 2000; **4**(3): 32–7.

Relevant web pages

International Council of Nurses. eHealth 2015. http://www.icn.ch/what-we-do/ehealth/

International Council of Nurses. ICNP browser 2016. http://www.icn.ch/ICNP-Browser-NEW.html

International Council of Nurses. International Classification for Nursing Practice (ICNP) 2015. http://www.icn.ch/what-we-do/international-classification-for-nursing-practice-icnpr/

Spirituality, nursing and mental health

JOHN SWINTON AND SARAH GIBSON

LEARNING OUTCOMES

- To be able to define spirituality and religion.
- To recognize their differences, similarities and benefits for people living with mental health problems.
- To understand the relationships between spirituality, religion and mental health.
- To understand the nature of spiritual care.
- To identify practical ways in which they can be incorporated into recovery-oriented practice.

SUMMARY OF KEY POINTS

- Spirituality is something that is important for all service users.
- Spirituality manifests itself in a variety of different forms, not simply religion.
- Spirituality draws our attention to issues of meaning and purpose and away from issues of pathology.
- Spirituality forms a central dimension of the recovery model.

INTRODUCTION

In this chapter we examine the role of spirituality and religion in the experiences of people living with mental health problems. Through a combination of theoretical reflection and the sharing of our own personal experience, we offer insights into spirituality and spiritual care which we hope will enable mental health nurses to attend well to the spiritual dimension of lives.

SPIRITUALITY AND RELIGION

For the purposes of this chapter we will consider spirituality and religion as two separate things, while recognizing their deep interconnectivity at certain levels. *Spirituality* is a universal human experience, within which people seek to (re)gain, construct or maintain a sense of meaning, purpose, hope and value. This may not include a sense of God or the divine, though for some people it does, even if they have no formal connection to a religion. One of the authors of this chapter, John Swinton, has described spirituality in this way:

> *Spirituality is a subjective experience that exists both within and outside traditional religious systems. It relates to the way in which people understand and live out their lives in view of their ultimate meaning and value and includes the need to find satisfactory answers to ultimate questions about the meaning of life, illness and death. Importantly, spirituality provides a context in which people can make sense of their lives, explain and cope with illness experiences and find and maintain a sense of hope, inner harmony and peace in the midst of the existential challenges of serious mental health problems.*[1]

Religion is perceived as a formal system of beliefs held by groups of people who share certain perspectives on the nature of the world and that which they consider to be divine. These perspectives are communicated through shared narratives, practices, beliefs and rituals which, taken together, create particular world views. A world view has to do with the ways in which people see and interpret the world around them and make sense of their experiences within the world. It relates to the structures of belief and systems of practice that form any given religion. Religions therefore shape and form the ways in which those who participate in them see and respond to the world. A person's religion is thus seen to be a powerful force for shaping their understanding of their mental health problems. Religion can be intrinsic or extrinsic. Intrinsic religion is when a person perceives their faith as central to who they are and how they function in the world. Extrinsic religion is where the belief and practice is like a veneer, which people can strip off at any point if they lose interest. Importantly, the beliefs of a religious person form part of their world view, i.e. the way that they see and interpret the world and everything within it, including their mental health problems. It is important to notice that religion is not simply a legalistic adherence to a set of rules. Central to religion is the experience of *faith*, i.e. a deep and certain belief that the world has meaning and purpose and that God is in control. Extrinsic religion can be the simple holding to a set of rules; intrinsic religion requires faith and that faith shapes everything that a person experiences. For the purposes of this chapter, when we talk about religion we will be talking about intrinsic religion, which is marked by faith.

While both religion and spirituality differ in significant ways, they each strive to answer these four fundamental questions:

- Who am I?
- Where do I come from?
- Where am I going to?
- Why?

These are precisely the types of questions we encounter when we experience mental illness. Helping people to find satisfactory answers to such questions is central to spiritual care.

REFLECTION

Spirituality is not only something for religious people; it relates to all people. What might this mean for you?

ARE RELIGION AND SPIRITUALITY GOOD FOR YOUR MENTAL HEALTH?

The relationship between spirituality and mental health and ill-health has traditionally been somewhat fraught. Freud's thesis that religion is in fact a form of neurosis, which requires psychotherapeutic intervention to 'free' people from such an illusion,[2] set an unfortunate and in our opinion misleading precedent for suspicion around issues of the role of spirituality and religion in mental health and ill-health. However, recent empirical research has cast some considerable doubt on the suggestion that spirituality and religion are inevitably bad for people's mental health. There is a growing evidence base that supports the assertion that a person's spiritual belief system can have a profound effect on their physical and mental health. Religion and spirituality have been shown to be beneficial on a number of levels and in relation to a wide variety of conditions. The health benefits of religion include:

- extended life expectancy;
- lower blood pressure;
- lower rates of death from coronary artery disease;
- reduction in myocardial infarction;
- increased success in heart transplants;
- reduced serum cholesterol levels;
- reduced levels of pain in cancer sufferers;
- reduced mortality among those who attend church and worship services;
- increased longevity among the elderly;
- reduced mortality after cardiac surgery.[3]

Spirituality has been positively correlated with improving/enhancing a person's:

- sense of self;
- ability to form relationships with others;
- feelings about themselves, including the impacts of the physiological changes of ageing;
- level of self-esteem;
- self-image and self-perception.

There is also a growing body of evidence to suggest that religion and spirituality are beneficial for mental health. We are discovering that a healthy spirituality makes us happier, protects us from depression, makes us more secure, provides us with a stronger sense of self and, if our spirituality is manifested via religion, roots us firmly within a supportive community, which in turn has significant health benefits.[4–6] Such communities offer a 'meaning of life context' into which people can locate their own experiences, develop a sense of identity, find opportunities to acknowledge guilt and seek forgiveness, find assurance of ultimate justice and healing, discover helpful rites of passage and develop practices such as prayer, meditation and worship. Communities such as this act as a container for anxieties and longings, conscious and unconscious processes.[5]

People writing out of the lived experience of mental distress cite many examples of the ways in which their faith and spirituality have supported their path through and life with mental health problems,[7–11] bringing clarity,[12] meaning, community, forgiveness, contentment, self-esteem and self-awareness,[13] miraculous healing,[14] acknowledgement of pain and suffering and a way to frame difficult questions.[15]

CHALLENGES OF SPIRITUALITY, FAITH AND RELIGION

However, while there is a good deal of evidence for the positive effects of spirituality and religion, the literature also describes times when spiritual experiences and encounters with faith communities can be distressing, disturbing and difficult for people. Religion, control, obligation and rule keeping can all be negative for people with mental health problems, especially if a spiritual belief system is accompanied by punitive consequences for people who do not meet expectations of behaviour, holiness or goodness/perfection through their own efforts. Some religious perspectives on healing can put unhealthy pressure on people to 'get well', receive healing or work to get clean or holy. Likewise, if people do not meet such demands, issues of blame and shame can emerge. Importantly, while spirituality and spiritual practices can be good for people's mental health, the losses incurred in not being able to engage with spiritual practices in the same way when mentally unwell as one could when one was well (difficulties reading, comprehending, managing social or group situations/meetings, visiting, caring for others, undertaking roles within one's own community) can be deeply troubling. Finally, belief systems and communities which do not have space for doubt, fear, anger and confusion (the whole of human experience) can put people in situations that are anxiety-provoking and ultimately very unhelpful.

REFLECTION

- There is a solid evidence base to suggest that spirituality can be beneficial for health care in general and mental health care in particular.

- What difference might it make that spirituality is in fact an aspect of evidence-based practice?

Nevertheless, the fact that spirituality and religion can be problematic does not rule out spirituality and religion as important and useful. (The fact that medication can have side effects does not mean we do not use it.) It simply emphasizes the need to try to understand the ways in which a person's spirituality functions and manifests itself in times of illness and wellness and to use that knowledge effectively. This knowledge and understanding can then form an important component of collaborative care planning with service users and carers (see chapter 50).

WHAT DO SPIRITUALITY AND SPIRITUAL CARE LOOK LIKE?

With these initial thoughts in mind, we can now begin to seek an understanding of what spiritualty and spiritual care actually look like. If we were trying to teach the reader about the physical action of a medication, simply imparting facts and information within some theoretical frameworks might suffice. But spirituality is more complicated. Spirituality is not like penicillin! It is much more subjective and embodied. By definition, spirituality is not something that we can see or touch. It is a deep human experience that is best captured within the stories that we tell about our lives and the meaning and experience of that which we choose to refer to as 'spiritual'. Likewise, mental health problems are in essence stories. Mental health problems are meaningful human experiences, before and after the symptom labels and diagnostic language with which they become entangled. This is a very important point. It is easy to get caught up in the issue of diagnostic criteria and categories. Naming mental health problems in this way may be helpful insofar as it enables us to get some understanding of the technical details of the person's experience. However, there is a temptation to forget that diagnoses are maps of the territory and not the territory itself. If you are investigating a place that is not familiar to you, you need a map. A map will give you basic guidelines as to what the terrain looks like, what you should look out for and a basic idea of where you are going. But it is not until you get down onto the ground that you can really understand what the place you are visiting is like. Only then can you feel, touch and live with the intricacies of the landscape and the strangeness of the places that you visit. Diagnoses may be useful in enabling us to negotiate the basic terrain of mental health problems, but they do not tell us about the small things, the meaningful important details of the experience of madness and the powerful and important personal narratives that people share about their lived experience. When we come close and listen, we begin to see the importance of the spiritual.

That being so, the best way for us to take the reader into the heart of the issues that are the focus of this chapter is through narrative. We choose to tease out these issues by offering the reader our own stories. The following section will focus on our stories of spirituality and spiritual care, which are central to the craft of caring. In listening to these two stories it will be possible for the reader to gain important insights into the nature of mental health and the role of spirituality in facilitating healing and well-being.

JOHN'S STORY

I worked for many years as a mental health nurse and latterly as a community mental health chaplain. However, during my years of training, I never once had a lecture on spirituality or delivering spiritual care. It simply wasn't on the agenda in 1976, at least not in the way that it is today. So, I found myself as a well-educated charge nurse, with responsibility for the holistic care of many vulnerable people with no training or awareness of the role of spirituality in the practices of nursing. Looking back in the light of recent developments which have brought the issue of spirituality to the fore, such a lack of awareness of things spiritual seems more than a little odd. Of course, the basic principles of spiritual care in some ways always underpinned my practice. I respected people, valued their dignity, understood that their lives were meaningful and so forth. However, when it came to really understanding people's religious and spiritual experience, I must have inevitably been at a disadvantage.

Having nursed for 16 years, I made a move first into hospital chaplaincy and then into academia. But it is my time as a hospital chaplain that relates best to this chapter. I was employed as a community mental health chaplain to work specifically with people moving from long-term institutional care into the community. My task was to work alongside people with serious mental health problems to help them to have their spiritual needs met and, for some, to find a place within a faith community. In that situation spirituality was presumed to be a general concept that related to those things that offer people's lives meaning, purpose, hope, value and dignity. We worked with the idea that spirituality relates to the ways in which all of us try to answer the four key questions we highlighted previously: Who am I? Where do I come from? Where am I going to? Why?

These are the questions that all of the major religious traditions, in different ways, try to answer. But in a culture wherein not all people are religious, people use different ways to seek answers to these core questions. For some people their spirituality related to God and they were engaged, formally or informally, in a religious system. However, for others it had to do with different things. Some of the folks I walked with found their spirituality in things such as gardening, family, finding open spaces where they could feel in touch with nature, encountering places where they felt connected (clubs, community activities, football matches) and so forth. The key was to help people to recognize that life has meaning and that their stories were both valuable and purposeful.

This broad understanding of spirituality opened up some interesting possibilities for care and support. For example, one young man I worked alongside, George, was diagnosed with schizophrenia when he was 12. I first met with him when he was 26. He was quite upbeat and he had good reason to be so. He told me that he had a new friend. A couple who had volunteered on a befriending scheme had been visiting George for several weeks and their relationship seemed to be developing well. He told me something that was quite startling: 'You know John, I am 26 years old and this is the first time I have had a friend who is not paid to be my friend.' I found this quite profound and carry that with me even now. If spirituality is connectedness and if people often find it very difficult to find connections, then spiritual care in this broad sense is deeply important. Friendship is one mode in which spirituality finds embodiment. The questions: Who am I? Where do I come from? Where am I going to? Why? all find answers within one's network of friends. If that is the case, then creating spaces where friendships might become possible is surely a vital dimension of spiritual care. There is of course nothing wrong with having paid friends. It's just not what most of us want. Creating spaces where social networks can have the opportunity to develop is a basic human need and a spiritual task that belongs to all of us.

What I discovered in my work as a nurse and as a chaplain is that spiritual care hasn't so much to do with developing new competencies or fresh techniques. Spiritual care has to do with noticing the importance of relationships and meaning for the lives of all people and using that awareness as a focus for developing genuinely person-centred and spiritually aware practices and policies that take seriously the *whole* of our experiences and so embody the craft of caring. In my case I was working with an understanding of spirituality that included religion but was not defined by it. However, the support of religious faith itself can be a vital dimension of spiritual care, as Sarah's story makes very clear.

REFLECTION

- Spiritual care has to do with finding those things that bring meaning and purpose to someone's life, even in the midst of their struggle.

- What brings meaning and purpose to your life?

SARAH'S STORY

I have chosen to share these parts of my story with you to illustrate the value of a holistic approach to care, the misapprehension that people of faith experience in health care, and the foundation, strength and hope that faith and faith communities can offer people with long-term mental health problems. Whilst I understand that God may be viewed in different ways according to an individual's belief systems, I offer my experience from a Christian perspective: it all started for me when I was at university. Two terms into my degree course the cracks had begun to show. I started experiencing times of high anxiety, confusion and distress. So, since God promises to hear and answer our prayers for healing and protection, I met with some supportive Christian friends to talk, pray and send away the evil spiritual powers around me. After we prayed, I experienced God's love and felt assured of angels protecting me, enabling me to sleep. One morning, soon afterwards, two of my friends were praying separately when they each heard God the Holy Spirit prompting them to give me the same Bible verse: Zephaniah 3:17, 'The LORD your God is with you. He is mighty to save. He takes great delight in you. He quiets you with His love. He rejoices over you with singing.' My long mental health journey since then has been undergirded by this truth, and my experience of God's presence, love and most importantly His grace – His delight in me, His unmerited favour – not based on my performance, goodness, recovery or self-management skills but instead on Jesus Christ's perfectly lived life and death as redemption for all my mistakes and imperfections. My faith in Jesus Christ and His promise of life to the full gives me hope for ongoing healing.

Then, I had a lot going for me and a great boyfriend, now my husband of 20 years. I was from an evangelical charismatic Christian family and I knew I belonged to God. I headed off on an overseas orchestral tour for the short vacation after my exams but, by the end of this, my whole fragile world appeared to be tumbling down. I could barely eat for anxiety, I was continually shaking, needing to carry water for my dry mouth and unable to make simple daily life choices or keep track of my possessions. My friends and hosts overseas (whom I trusted because I recognized the Christian fiction on their shelves which included descriptions of the spiritual battles I was experiencing) supported and prayed with and advised me as best they could. I understood this as a spiritual battle (a fight against evil spiritual forces attacking me), and I was mentally, physically and emotionally exhausted. I was experiencing debilitating mental health problems for the first time. Yet even then, I knew God was with me. Even when everything else fell away, He was there. He knew. He was present by His Spirit and through His people, asking me to look them in the eye and see His love and care. I attempted to return to university but the anxiety immobilized and imprisoned me, leaving me unable to look after myself or communicate my distress. I could see that the psychiatrist who saw me then didn't understand my description of the spiritual battle I was engaged in and my strategies to pray, read my Bible and fight lies with truth. I still remember the way he stopped writing and looked enquiringly at me. I think, in his eyes, this just gave me more 'psychotic features'. I scrambled for the words to patch up my case for comparative sanity and defensively tried to explain the theological basis for my views and allay his fears. This experience taught me to discuss spiritual things in only vaguest terms within the mental health system for fear of being misunderstood and pathologized. Looking back, this was a narrow escape. This psychiatrist chose to send me home with my Dad rather than admitting me as an inpatient in my university town. As I left my bare student room in defeat, a concerned friend took me aside. 'You're not losing your faith, are you?' she asked. God remained the rock on which I stood when everything else was shifting at my feet. Respite at the home of my church youth leaders brought a gentle victory in that first battle. I started to learn the spiritual strategies of:

- allowing love to chase away paralysing fear and anxiety (1 John 4:16–19);
- receiving supernatural peace through thankful prayer (Philippians 4:6–7);
- replacing confusing lies with the Truth that sets us free (John 8:30–2, 36);
- finding hope for the future in my faith that God created us for a purpose (Ephesians 2:10).

These have served me well as I have learned to navigate complex terrains. Though stopped in my tracks on numerous occasions since by serious mental health problems, my life has gone on.

I was enabled to return to my studies with the support of my amazing moral tutor (my personal tutor responsible for pastoral care and arranging students' tutorial studies). I started to use my lived experience of mental health problems in my studies and to offer peer support and prayer to friends and see others gain freedom. Later, when finishing my degree, the disabling anxiety returned again. I made use of my supportive church community and the spiritual strategies above, which brought me a measure of peace, but I cried to God for real healing of the ongoing problems I was experiencing.

Often when I encounter God I see pictures in my mind. Then, I saw a table with a deep scratch on it and heard God say that He wasn't being slow in bringing my healing but rather taking care like a French polisher would gently restore that table. Looking back,

decades on, I can see that this long journey to healing has formed a deep peace and strength in me, as I have discovered my identity, value and courage to keep going by the grace of God.

At this time I had a community psychiatric nurse. This person took my mental health concerns seriously but also normalized my experiences, listened to how I was coping and arranged regular meetings. This offer of time, validation of my feelings and strategies for living through the anxious state I was in fitted alongside church-based pastoral care, prayer ministry and other mental health sources of support whilst I tried to learn how to take care of myself.

More explicitly holistic care came when I was in a later crisis and I needed help. After attempting to engage with NHS psychotherapy, I needed to find a place where I felt safe, where my physical, emotional *and* spiritual needs could be cared for. My GP supported a private out-of-area referral to Burrswood Christian Hospital so that I could go and get the help I needed. What I encountered in my weeks at Burrswood was amazing. God's presence was tangible. I had time to talk and pray with a chaplain and receive support from the nursing staff in the middle of the nights when I struggled to sleep. And all of this support was rooted in a shared faith in God who miraculously heals through relationship as well as through physical and emotional care. My main need in that time was to make sense of my psychological and emotional state and my life as a whole. (Who am I? How did I get here? Where am I going? Why?) I found this through spiritual experience, through insights from nature, through prayerful conversation with God. In a shocking vision, whilst I was in prayer in the Church of Christ the Healer, which is part of the hospital, God revealed a deep root of some my problems. I was able to take this and other questions and insights directly to therapy, back to God and to the chaplain, and to take time to piece together my own understanding whilst keeping in touch with a few family members. People walked gently alongside me in defined roles.

My counsellor, the chaplains, the nursing and medical staff and my husband were each available for me to bring different types of questions and insights and offer different approaches to enabling me to answer and understand these, whether with medical facts, practical advice on sleep and rest, accompaniment on my spiritual walk or providing safe space for questions and emotions in therapy. This combination of physical, psychotherapeutic and spiritual care and connection to people who seek to know and love me has been pivotal to my journey, and should be available to all people experiencing mental health crises. Burrswood became my place of safety for the coming years and the counsellor I met there still remains part of my three-sided self-care approach. As a Christian, I know she understands the spiritual insights that I have into my condition and works with me as I seek out more explicitly spiritual support through prayer or pastoral care at my church. She is also able to support me as I have to make decisions about choosing to explore care from primary or secondary mental health services, take time off sick from work or navigate the medical world of psychiatric diagnoses and medication as an adjunct to my usual preference for unmedicated self-management. But the bottom line is my faith in God. He is always with me. He never leaves me. He always understands and never gives up, even in my darkest times. He is kind and full of compassion, fiercely protective and just, yet forgiving. I have the privilege to know Him and to experience Him and His healing power directly and indirectly through the people He has put alongside me in my life – caring people who in some ways are like Him, looking me in the eye with love and helping me to see myself like He sees me – people who care more about my life and freedom than I do sometimes and who put up with my failings and weaknesses with compassion whilst wanting the best for me. I appreciate these people and hope that I can be like Him and like them alongside others.

REFLECTION

- Faith can be a source of hope and new possibilities. We must pay attention to it. It requires the gift of time.

- What needs to change for you to be able to listen to the spiritual dimensions of people's experiences?

SPIRITUAL CARE AND RECOVERY

These two narratives, which outline both a generic approach to spirituality and one rooted in religious faith, begin to highlight some important aspects of what spirituality is and how it might work itself out in the lives of people encountering mental health problems.

Having laid out a narrative perspective alongside reflections on the literature, we will now explore how the spiritual perspective that we are developing feeds into current ideas of mental health and in particular to the idea of *recovery*. The concept of recovery from mental distress as rooted in the 'survivor movement' emphasizes personal existential processes such as re-engaging with personally meaningful and purposeful activities that give hope, meaning and purpose[16] rather than medical measures of success (e.g. reduction of symptoms or inpatient admissions). UK mental health services are in the challenging process of being redesigned to be more 'recovery oriented'.[17] Chapters 35 and 36 provide further information on recovery. This should give greater priority to supporting people holistically in taking control of their own recovery processes (see chapter 50 on collaborative care planning with service users and carers). Such an understanding of recovery converges with recent accounts of spirituality, personalism and existentialism, while diverging from the dominant medical model with its stress on biological psychiatry.

Personal recovery has been defined by Anthony[18] as:

a deeply personal, unique process of changing one's attitudes, values, feelings, goals, skills, and/or roles. It is a way of living a satisfying, hopeful, and contributing life even within the limitations caused by illness. Recovery involves the development of new meaning and purpose in one's life as one grows beyond the catastrophic effects of mental illness. (p.12)

This contrasts with clinical ideas about recovery, which involve getting rid of symptoms and 'getting back to normal'. Some would argue that services should focus on both.[19] In practice, recovery means different things to different people. Its description and definition varies with people's diverse experiences of life, distress, diagnosis and services.[20–22] Kahlathil et al.,[23] for example, demonstrated the importance of culture, ethnicity, community and spirituality in their research on recovery narratives in setting out socio-cultural, personal and familial and biomedical contexts of distress, recovery and resilience for the Black women participating in their study. Spiritual components were significant both in descriptions of distress (e.g. loss of faith, spiritual crisis, feeling connected to the sufferings of others) and what helps (e.g. spiritual development of self, finding spiritual grounding).

Since recovery is self-defined, it is neither an endpoint or cure nor a simple linear process or journey. However, some have suggested components that it may include, such as hope, identity, meaning and control,[24] or domains it may encompass, including spirituality as just one of these.[25] Bird et al.[26] settle on 'Connectedness', 'Hope and optimism', 'Identity', 'Meaning and purpose' and 'Empowerment' (CHIME) as categories, while acknowledging difference in areas such as 'diagnosis and medication' and finding 'scepticism about recovery' itself.

With the obvious overlap in conceptual understandings of recovery and spirituality, orientation towards recovery should open up important personal and community spaces for spirituality and spiritual care. Spiritual care is not a mode of curing. Spiritual care (paying attention to issues of meaning, purpose, hope, value, connection to faith and God) is in essence a way of accompanying someone in their recovery, redefinition and perhaps spiritual *discovery* of the life they want, alongside, through and beyond experiences of mental health problems. Recovery has to do with *living well* with mental health problems (*meaningful* goals being personally determined rather than externally imposed and measured), regaining power and *control* over one's life (i.e. choosing how one wants to live, how and when to use different kinds of support and strategies), redefining or reaffirming one's *identity*, re-engaging in wanted roles, one's place in the family, the workplace, the faith community and wider community engagement. It means holding out *hope* and having hope and living again with hope. It means feeling able to take desired steps towards *purposeful* opportunities on offer. As Deegan[27] puts it: 'The goal of recovery is not to become normal. The goal is to embrace the human vocation of becoming more deeply, more fully human' (p.92).

Viewed in this way, spirituality (and, for some, faith or religion) is central to recovery.

The big questions we have highlighted thus far become central to the process of recovery:

- Who am I? ((re)discovering/defining identity and roles)
- How did I get here? (exploring control and context)

IMPLICATIONS FOR PRACTICE

Spiritual care is underpinned by the building and honouring of therapeutic relationships (see chapter 3) and should be considered an intrinsic part of collaborative care planning with all service users and carers (see chapter 50). With that in mind, we wish to offer the following recommendations for practice:

- Spiritual care is not a set of techniques or competencies. Rather it has to do with the enabling of carers to

- Where am I going? (hope defining purpose or life beyond)
- Why? (finding meaning)

Big Roy[28] describes this relationship between recovery, spirituality and the search for meaning:

I am going to talk about what recovery means for me. When people say there is no God, they want to suffer mental illness – either you'll want God or you'll find one. If people experienced what I feel, they would hope there is a God to save them. Communing with nature – when you sit alone – no matter how bad you feel you can see a meaning to it … What I see as God is not someone sitting on a cloud with a big stick – it is all that is out there – nature.[28] (p.39)

There is a good deal of evidence to support the suggestion that spirituality and recovery are deeply connected.[29] A review of the literature on spirituality and mental health[30] reported that hope, meaning and comfort are found in spiritual beliefs and practices and concurs that 'religion can play a central role in the process of reconstructing sense of self and recovery'[31] (p.369). Spirituality has long been acknowledged as part of many people's recovery narratives.[32] If spirituality supports recovery then, as Ashcraft et al.[33] argue from the US context, it is inevitably central to the business of 'holistic culturally competent recovery oriented' service provision (p.8). Mental health commissioners in England are also advised similarly that 'Spiritual care teams in mainstream services can also enable staff to recognise culture and belief as legitimate contexts in which to better understand mental health and emotional issues arising in all communities, and faith as a means for reflection and resilience and a protective factor'[34] (p.17).

So, spirituality and spiritual care, as we have outlined and illustrated them in this chapter, certainly live and breathe alongside explorations of recovery, and that being so, the concept and the practices must not be alien to nurses, since they are central to good person-centred holistic care and are 'the shared responsibility of all who work in the NHS'[35] (p.206).

do what they do already, but to *look* differently at those to whom they seek to offer care, to *listen* to the meanings of their experiences and to *see beyond* that which is expected.

- *Listen* to what makes sense to that individual person in front of you, rather than imposing external frameworks of meaning on experiences and difficulties.
- *Do not pathologize* spiritual ideas as just part of an illness, even if unusual or confused. They may be an

essential part of a person's solution to making sense of their experiences or finding meaning in their internal suffering. Do not see understandings of spirituality as *the problem* but rather as offering potential insights into parts of a person's particular solutions.

- *Recognize* spiritual needs and resources as part of holistic assessment and care planning.
- Be willing to *accompany* people on their journey as they seek to find answers to their big questions.
- *Respect* loss of hope, identity, meaning, purpose and control not as symptoms to treat but valid human experiences to walk through.

- *Have faith* in people's capacity to regain these essentials to life; *hold out hope* that losses can be regained.
- *Create space* for people with mental health problems to choose and engage with spiritual self-care strategies (e.g. creative and reflective processes, writing, singing, engaging with nature, forms of prayer worship and meditation, reading, giving) and recognize these as important to recovery/well-being.
- *Be willing* to support people with mental health problems to access and explain their experiences to members of their faith and wider cultural communities and help them to express felt needs for support and care.

CONCLUSION

In conclusion, there is no better way to sum up the things we have been trying to express in this chapter than by listening to and taking inspiration from these reflections of a mental health peer worker, rooted in their own lived experience of mental health problems:

I had been thinking about all the people who were sitting on locked wards, because they had, perhaps, gotten overwhelmed and confused about God or the devil or some combination thereof … about ghosts and the television … spirits in the pictures … telepathy with some big machine … a lifeforce relaying messages. How might their stories have been different if they'd had someone to talk with, someone to listen to

them, to support them in figuring out what their thoughts and feelings meant to them in relation to what was in their hearts?

Part of my current spiritual practice is hoping that the people who are confined by chemical and court order because they stumbled into feelings and ideas that they did not have a context for will find some light in their day, that the fire in their hearts will not go out, and that they will feel somehow that they are loved … and that they will believe it.[36]

Spiritual care is the beginning point for the renewal of our humanness.

References

1. Swinton J. Why psychiatry needs spirituality. *Royal College of Psychiatrists Newsletter* 2005; 1. Available from: http://www.rcpsych.ac.uk/pdf/ATT89153.ATT.pdf [Accessed 23rd August 2016].
2. Freud S. *The standard edition of the complete psychological works of Sigmund Freud*, Vol. 23, *The future of an illusion* (1927). Trans. Strachey J. London: Hogarth Press, 1968.
3. Larson DB, Swyers JP, McCullough M. *Scientific research on spirituality and health: a consensus report.* National Institute for Healthcare Research, 1997.
4. Koenig HG, Larson DB, McCullough ME. *Handbook of religion and health.* New York: Oxford University Press, 2001.
5. MacKenna C. Why mental health practitioners need to understand spiritual matters. In: Coyte M, Gilbert P, Nicholls V (eds). *Spirituality, values and mental health. Jewels for the journey.* London: Jessica Kingsley, 2007: 246–55.
6. Swinton J. *Spirituality in mental health care: rediscovering a 'forgotten' dimension.* London: Jessica Kingsley, 2001.
7. Mental Health Foundation. *The courage to bare our souls: a collection of pieces written out of mental distress.* London: Mental Health Foundation, 1999.
8. Coyte ME, Gilbert P, Nicholls V (eds). *Spirituality, values and mental health. Jewels for the journey.* London: Jessica Kingsley, 2007.
9. Chard Intentional Peer Support Group. *Turn towards the light. Stories of our journeys through mental health.* Chard Intentional Peer Support Group, 2010.
10. Webb D. *Thinking about suicide; contemplating and comprehending the urge to die.* Ross-on-Wye: PCCS Books, 2010.

11. Barlow S, Waite D. *Stepping through my nightmares. A true story of fear and hope set against the backdrop of the Gulf War.* Herford: Eagle, 2002.
12. Somers E. The journey. In: Mental Health Foundation. *The courage to bare our souls.* London: Mental Health Foundation, 1999: 25–6.
13. Were M. In: Mental Health Foundation. *The courage to bare our souls.* London: Mental Health Foundation, 1999: 27–8.
14. Stanbridge V. A religious experience. In: Mental Health Foundation. *The courage to bare our souls.* London: Mental Health Foundation, 1999: 19–20.
15. Harding E. Recovery – adventures in being. In: Chandler R and Hayward M (eds). *Voicing psychotic experiences: a reconsideration of recovery and diversity.* London: Pavilion, 2009: 85–100.
16. Deegan PE. Recovery as a self-directed process of healing and transformation. In: Brown C (ed.). *Recovery and wellness: models of hope and empowerment for people with mental illness.* New York: Haworth Press, 2001: 5–21.
17. ImROC (*Implementing Recovery through Organisational Change*). http://www.imroc.org [Accessed 5th June 2016].
18. Anthony WA. Recovery from mental illness: the guiding vision of the mental health system in the 1990s. *Psychosocial Rehabilitation Journal* 1993; **16**(4): 11–23.
19. Unger R. Moving beyond clinical recovery and personal recovery: reclaiming the possibility of full recovery. 2010. Available from: http://recoveryfromschizophrenia.org/2010/04/moving-beyond-clinical-recovery-and-personal-recovery-reclaiming-the-possibility-of-full-recovery/ [Accessed 5th June 2016].

20. Kalathil J, Collier B, Bhakta R, Daniel O, Joseph D, Trivedi P. *Recovery and resilience: lessons in healing from black women's stories*. London: Mental Health Foundation, 2011.
21. Turton P, Demetriou A, Boland W, Gillard S, Kavuma M, Mezey G, Mountford V, Turner K, White S, Zadeh E, Wright C. One size fits all – or horses for courses? Recovery-based care in specialist mental health services. *Social Psychiatry & Psychiatric Epidemiology* 2011; **46**: 127–36.
22. Turner K, Lovell K, Brooker A. '… And they all lived happily ever after': 'recovery' or discovery of the self in personality disorder? *Psychodynamic Practice: Individuals, Groups and Organisations* 2011; **17**(3): 341–6.
23. Kalathil J, Collier B, Bhakta R, Daniel O, Joseph D, Trivedi P. *Recovery and resilience: African, African Caribbean and South Asian women's narratives of recovering from mental distress*. London: Health Foundation, 2011.
24. Andresen R, Oades L, Caputi P. The experience of recovery from schizophrenia: towards an empirically validated stage model. *Australian and New Zealand Journal of Psychiatry* 2003; **37**: 586–94.
25. Working Together for Recovery. Spirituality. Available from: http://www.workingtogetherforrecovery.co.uk/spirituality.htm [Accessed 5th June 2016].
26. Bird, V, Leamy M, Twe J, Le Boutillier C, Williams J, Slade M. Fit for purpose? Validation of a conceptual framework for personal recovery with mental health consumers. *Australian and New Zealand Journal of Psychiatry* 2014; **48**(7): 644–53.
27. Deegan P. Recovery as a journey of the heart. *Psychiatric Rehabilitation Journal* 1996; **19**(3): 91–7.
28. Big Roy. Thank God for the trees. In: Chandler R, Hayward M (eds). *Voicing psychotic experiences: a reconsideration of recovery and diversity*. London: Pavilion, 2009.
29. Lukoff D. Spirituality in the recovery from persistent mental disorders. *Southern Medical Journal. Special Section: Spirituality/Medicine Interface Project* 2007: **100**(6): 642–6.
30. Mental Health Foundation. *The impact of spirituality of mental health: a review of the literature*. 1996. Available from: https://www.mentalhealth.org.uk/sites/default/files/impact-spirituality.pdf [Accessed 24th August 2016].
31. Mohr S, Huguelet P. The relationship between schizophrenia and religion and its implications for care. *Swiss Medical Weekly* 2004; **134**(25–6): 369–76.
32. Fallot D. Spiritual and religious dimensions of mental illness recovery narratives. *New Directions for Mental Health Services* 2007; **80**: 35–44.
33. Ashcraft L, Anthony W, Mancuso L. Is spirituality essential for recovery? *Behavioral Healthcare* 2010; **30**(7): 7–8.
34. Joint Commissioning Panel for Mental Health. *Guidance for commissioners of mental health services for people from Black and Minority Ethnic Communities*. 2014: 17.
35. Eagger S, Richmond P, Gilbert P. Spiritual care in the NHS. In: Cook C, Powell A, Sims A (eds). *Spirituality and psychiatry*. London: Royal College of Psychiatrists, 2009: 190–211.
36. MIA Correspondent. Spirituality & recovery, faith & mental illness. *Madinamerica.com*. 29 March 2013. Available from: http://www.madinamerica.com/2013/03/spirituality-and-recoveryfaith-and-mental-illness/ [Accessed 5th June 2016].

Further reading

Cook C, Powell A, Sims A (eds). *Spirituality and psychiatry*. London: Royal College of Psychiatrists, 2009.

Coyte ME, Gilbert P, Nicholls V (eds). *Spirituality, values and mental health: jewels for the journey*. London: Jessica Kingsley, 2007.

Gilbert P (ed.). *Spirituality and mental health*. Brighton: Pavilion, 2011.

Swinton J. *Spirituality and mental health care: rediscovering a 'forgotten' dimension*. London: Jessica Kingsley, 2001.

Relevant web pages

Mental Health Matters. http://www.mentalhealthmatters-cofe.org

Mental Health Project. http://www.mentalhealthproject.co.uk/resources.html

Mind & Soul. http://www.mindandsoul.info

Royal College of Psychiatrists. Publications archive: Spirituality and Psychiatry Special Interest Group. http://www.rcpsych. ac.uk/workinpsychiatry/specialinterestgroups/spirituality/publicationsarchive.aspx

Spiritual Crisis Network. http://spiritualcrisisnetwork.uk/about-us/

Spirituality Forum. http://www.spiritualitymentalhealth.org.uk/index.html

Clinical supervision

JOHN R. CUTCLIFFE AND KATHERINE OWEN

LEARNING OUTCOMES

- To be better able to identify the nature, rudiments and principal features of clinical supervision (CS), and in so doing be able to articulate what clinical supervision is and what it is not.

- To be able to discuss why CS is useful, if not necessary, for effective psychiatric/mental health nursing.

- To be better able to identify how engaging in effective CS can improve outcomes for clients, for nurses themselves and for the health care organization more broadly.

SUMMARY OF KEY POINTS

- There is no one singular, best way to operationalize CS; no 'one size fits all' model; no idealized, homogenized version of CS that all nurses should embrace. However, in order to be legitimately classified as CS, certain features, elements or principles need to be present.

- CS needs to involve at least two people meeting (including 'virtual' meetings) together for the purpose of engaging in CS.

- CS requires some engagement in reflection upon clinical practice (in its broadest sense).

- CS sessions and meetings have some degree of structure and have a specific over-arching focus – the development of therapeutic proficiency.

- CS must be a supportive, emancipatory process.

- CS involves a monitoring process: a self-driven, self-exploratory process of review of one's own accountability, practice, ethics and knowledge.

- CS must be concerned with growth and development and must thus be a learning process.

INTRODUCTION

Nursing is an interpersonal endeavour. Regardless of the particular setting, context, specialism or age group of the client(s), nursing inevitably involves interpersonal interaction. Moreover, the specialism of psychiatric and/or mental health (P/MH)* embraces the interpersonal nature of nursing[1-3] and sees this as *de rigueur* for effective psychiatric and mental health nursing care. Psychiatric and mental health nurses are now expected to provide care, in the occidental world, that is situated within a broader practice context epitomized by lifelong learning[4,5] and evidence-based practice.[6] Care often occurs in complex, highly challenging and emotionally charged situations and conditions. Not surprisingly, contemporary P/MH nursing literature is now replete with references to the demands on the nurse as a result of operating in these vagary-filled circumstances.[7,8]

---

* While being mindful of the existing debate and associated literature which highlights the significant problems in attempting to conflate 'psychiatric' with 'mental health' nursing (see Cutcliffe, Stevenson and Lakeman,[3] for instance), given the pre-determined title of this textbook and in the interests of consistency, the author has adopted the term P/MH nursing for this chapter.

One 'mechanism' or process that was introduced as a means to assist nurses to survive and thrive in challenging care environments and circumstances is clinical supervision (CS). From the 1920s/1930s in the USA,[9–13] CS was conceptualized as a democratic process concerned with professional growth and was to occur in a wholesome atmosphere of partnership, permissiveness and support. Similar supportive and developmentally driven approaches to CS have been advanced in Australia, New Zealand, Scandinavian countries, the UK and, to a lesser extent, Canada. Despite such developments, CS is still bedevilled by misunderstandings, misrepresentations and unwarranted encroachments and transgressions by those who would amalgamate CS with administrative/managerial supervision. Similarly, while there is evidence which points to a higher uptake of CS in P/MH nursing,[14] it cannot be said with any degree of empirical confidence that CS has become a key aspect of the culture and practice of *all* P/MH nurses, let alone nurses more broadly. Accordingly, this chapter will explore what CS is and what it is not and, in so doing, remind ourselves of the original and contemporary principles and components of CS. Following this, the chapter will focus in more detail on each of the six underlying principles.

WHAT IT IS AND WHAT IT IS NOT: THE ORIGINAL AND CONTEMPORARY PRINCIPLES AND COMPONENTS OF CLINICAL SUPERVISION

Together with esteemed colleagues and pioneers of CS in nursing,[15,16] I have written previously that there is no one singular, best way to operationalize CS; no 'one size fits all' model; no idealized, homogenized version of CS that all nurses should embrace. Given the wide and rich variety of settings, contexts, professional groups, client types, etc., with which nurses work, I regard this as axiomatic. That said, acknowledging the documented variation concerning certain aspects of CS in no way indicates that 'anything goes'; that any practice can accurately be termed and deemed to be CS. In order to be legitimately classified as CS. As with other systems of classification (see any biological taxonomy, e.g. Folkins and Bleile,[17] or mathematical taxonomy, e.g. Dunn and Everitt[18]), certain features, elements or principles need to be present. CS has a number of required principles, listed at the beginning of this chapter in the 'Summary of key points', and discussed in detail in this section.

Importantly, the last three principles – that CS must be a supportive, emancipatory process; involves a monitoring process; and that it must be a learning process – have been enshrined in the most popular model of CS. The most most complete and contemporary description and explanation of this model is provided by the original author herself.[19,20] These three components of CS are commonly referred to as: restorative (support), formative (development) and normative (standard setting). Even a cursory review of the relevant theoretical, empirical and discursive literature will show that multiple, often repetitive and sometimes contradictory definitions of CS exist. A number capture or allude to some (or all) of these principles, while others do not. Some of these discrepancies and contradictions can be attributed or traced to misunderstandings of original conceptualizations of CS and/or the encroachment of competing agendas into the domain of CS;* As a result of appropriate evolution and development of the theory and practice of CS this has given rise to multiple, 'spin-off', progeny and idiosyncratic versions of CS.

I have no interest in wishing to further 'muddy the conceptual waters' by offering yet another definition. Indeed, I will draw on the epistemology of theory and model construction (see for instance, Jaccard and Jacoby[21]) which argues that: (a) the world we experience (including CS) is complex and mostly hidden from view; and (b) people place concepts into relationships with other concepts and use these conceptual systems as guides to organizing and explaining the world they experience. Accordingly, this approach requires the scholar (researcher, nurse) to look 'beneath' the conceptual system of CS, consider the concepts and their relationships and, in so doing, identify and postulate the underlying assumptions of CS. As a result, such an examination shows that CS is necessarily:

- supportive;
- safe, because of clear, negotiated agreements by all parties with regard to the extent and limits of confidentiality;
- centred on developing best practice for service users;
- brave, because practitioners are encouraged to talk about the realities of their practice;
- a chance to talk about difficult areas of work in an environment where the person attempts to understand;
- an opportunity to ventilate emotion without comeback;
- an opportunity to deal with material and issues that practitioners may have been carrying for many years (the chance to talk about issues which cannot easily be talked about elsewhere and which may have been previously unexplored);
- not to be confused with or amalgamated with managerial supervision;
- not to be confused with or amalgamated with personal therapy/counselling;
- regular;
- protected time;

---

* For instance, the all too often encountered example of crude and misplaced attempts to conflate CS with administrative/managerial supervision.

- offered equally to all practitioners;
- a committed relationship (from both parties);
- separate and distinct from preceptorship or mentorship;
- a facilitative relationship;
- challenging;
- an invitation to be self-monitoring and self-accountable;
- at times hard work and at others enjoyable;
- learning to be reflective and becoming a reflective practitioner;
- an activity that continues throughout one's working life.

(adapted from Cutcliffe, Butterworth and Proctor,[15] and Cutcliffe, Fowler and Hyrkas[16])

Ultimately, CS has to be concerned with benefiting service users as well as health care practitioners. As each of us, to a greater or lesser extent, has 'paid for' health care services, and given that we are all either historically, currently, or perhaps will be some time in the future, recipients of health care, each of us has a personal, vested interest in receiving the very best care possible. In addition to our self-interests, our moral duty as P/MH nurses (and humanists) seems to require us to advocate that all our fellow humans and denizens/co-constructors of the 'Just City' should be provided with the best care possible. It has been argued that this 'best care possible' can only be delivered by the front line staff, who are sufficiently competent and healthy.[16] Effective CS, provided by a competent and well-prepared supervisor, can help practitioners become and remain sufficiently competent and healthy to provide the best care possible. Unless CS ultimately does have an influence on the care provided, it ceases to be what it was designed to be and becomes something of a rather narcissistic, self-absorbed activity for staff or yet another (unwanted) managerial monitoring tool.[16]

> **REFLECTION**
>
> Consider your own experiences of CS. What underlying assumptions can you detect?

We now move on to examine each of these principles in more detail.

CS needs to involve at least two people meeting (including 'virtual' meetings) together for the purpose of engaging in CS

It is perhaps tautological to point out that CS requires practitioners to meet together. CS involves at least two participants; there is the provider of the supervision (a.k.a. the supervisor) and the recipient(s) of the supervision (a.k.a. the supervisee(s)). Whether the CS

is operationalized in dyads (pairs) or a larger group (literature seems to suggest a maximum group size of 8), whether this occurs in a traditional, face-to-face setting or via a distance-learning medium (e.g. Skype, video conferencing), there is still a requirement for a meeting to occur. Spontaneous, occasional (sometimes referred to as informal) supervision can and does occur, but this should not be confused with actual or formal CS. CS then needs to be acknowledged as a deliberate rather than an accidental occurrence and, as such, needs to be a practice that occurs in 'protected time'. In other words, the time dedicated to CS sessions needs to be protected and not encroached upon. Furthermore, the meetings (or sessions) have a specific purpose(s); to provide staff with a forum or 'place' that is protected by confidentiality, and feels safe and supportive, in order to engage in critical reflection on professional practice. Furthermore, the purpose is to provide a space and opportunity to help practitioners become more self-aware, 'own' their practice and become more self-responsible. CS then is a purposeful act, and one that occurs within the boundaries of a negotiated working agreement (i.e. a contract). There is a deliberate attempt to co-create the conditions (e.g. responsibilities, roles, boundaries, etc.) necessary for effective supervision.

> **REFLECTION**
>
> Consider how formal CS differs from so-called informal CS. What implications arise from these differences?

CS requires some engagement in reflection upon clinical practice (in its broadest sense)

For many authors who have contributed to the extant literature in this area, reflection underpins much of the practice of CS (see, for instance, Fowler,[22] Gilbert,[23] Johns and Freshwater,[24] and Fowler and Cutcliffe[25]). It is difficult to see how any retrospective examination of either oneself (i.e. thoughts, feelings and actions), or *ex post facto* review of any clinical practice experience (for example, why did this client interaction result in an aggressive/violent incident?), or any retroactive consideration of how the broader environmental, milieu or policy context impacted your practice (or specific incidents), can even occur in the absence of reflection. Further, it is epistemologically more reasonable to accept the axiomatic relationship between CS and reflection once one has a robust understanding of the nature of reflection and how it is harmonious with the purpose and practices of CS. The origins of reflection and, with that, reflective learning and reflection on (or in) action, can be traced back to Dewey's work during the early part of the twentieth century.[26,27] For Dewey, reflective thought consisted of 'active, persistent, and careful consideration of any belief or supposed form of knowledge in the light of the grounds that support it and the further conclusions to which it tends'[27] (p.118).

Reflection, then, is a cognitive process; and as a process of, or approach to, learning, it clearly requires that the person making use of reflection (i.e. student, nurse, supervisee) engages in critical thinking. Participation in reflective thinking (and reflective learning) requires the learner to eschew 'received wisdom' and authoritative knowledge; to challenge taken-for-granted 'truths'. In some sense, then, reflective learning is a solipsistic endeavour or an attempt to 'temet nosce', wherein to 'know thyself' is a warning to pay no attention to the opinion of the multitude. These ideas can be found in the seminal work on different patterns (for some – forms) of knowledge in nursing; for instance, Barbara Carper's[28] work. While there may be aspects of critical thinking and solipsism in Carper's *personal* pattern (or form) of knowledge, it is her pattern (or form) termed *aesthetic* knowledge that is predominantly concerned with attempting to examine and understand oneself; particularly gaining a deeper understanding and insight into oneself within the 'framework' of one's clinical practice. However, it is worth pointing out that engaging in serious self-examination can be a daunting task. Atkins and Murphy[29] argue that effective reflection requires that the individual put aside any sense of defensiveness, attempt to remain open and transparent, and thus be willing to 'expose the self' – an exercise that many people find difficult to accomplish without guidance from a skilled person.[25]

According to Todd and Freshwater:[30] 'Reflective practice is a multidimensional process that seeks to problematize a broad range of professional situations encountered by the practitioner in order that they can become potential learning situations. This enables a continuation of learning, development and growth, both cognitively and emotionally, in and through their practice' (p.1384). Accordingly, while a perfunctory analysis of one's practice, attitudes or issues may enable confirmatory bias to occur (i.e. the common tendency that people have to search for or interpret information in a way that confirms their preconceptions), the critical thinking and problematizing of such phenomena seems to create developmental and growth opportunities for the reflective practitioner. See chapter 11 for further information on critical reflection.

While it may sound paradoxical, the problematizing of one's everyday practice and subjecting this to critical examination is entirely in keeping with the movement to becoming a more questioning discipline;[25] a discipline increasingly concerned with evidence-based practice rather than slavish adherence to ritual, authoritarian knowledge or established customs and practice. Chapter 6 looks in more detail at evidence-based practice in mental health care.

CS sessions and meetings have some degree of structure and have a specific over-arching focus – the development of therapeutic proficiency

CS sessions invariably have structure – they are not a 'free for all'. While the degree of structure can and does vary between different organizations, policies and practitioners, certain common (and some would say necessary) elements are included. As a result, some or all of the following are commonly considered:

- the creation of a collaborative CS working agreement at the start of a series of CS sessions. Referred to as a 'contract', 'working alliance' or 'working agreement', this agreement is discussed and negotiated (rather than imposed) and helps inform the remainder of the structure. Subsequent sessions may also include some form of review of this agreement;
- the frequency and duration of the CS sessions themselves;
- the different roles and responsibilities of both the supervisor and the supervisee;
- what type of learning styles the supervisee has, and how these can/should be woven into CS sessions;
- how CS can provide a forum for the celebration and deconstruction of 'effective' (or 'good') practices in addition to highlighting limitations, problems, gaps in awareness and exploring resolutions of clinical problems;
- how and when the CS experience and process is to be evaluated, and who has responsibility for initiating this evaluation;
- how supervisees can follow through by putting into practice those changes emerging from discussions during CS;
- how resistance, defensiveness and denial are to be considered if/when they occur in the CS;
- how parties can gain the most value from CS, and how it can be experienced as effective and valuable;
- issues related to documentation;
- confidentiality (this topic should be covered early on in discussions about structure);

- what is a legitimate topic or issue to discuss in CS and what is not;
- the boundaries and limits of CS (for instance, CS is not to be confused with personal therapy or individual performance plans, and should not become a 'gripe' session);
- ethical aspects of practice;
- whether there is to be a focus on problem resolution;
- whether or not the practice of 'homework' will be used;
- CS frameworks (CS frameworks guided by psychotherapy models seem to have potential utility);
- the practice of reflection and how reflection can/does occur;
- whether there are skills, attitudes and knowledge that might be transferred from the clinical context into supervision;
- whether or not 'best practice' guidelines and recommendations and/or latest research findings will be included as a legitimate aspect of CS discussions.

REFLECTION

What structural elements have you found to be helpful and less helpful when engaging in your own CS? What structural elements would you want in place?

CS must be a supportive, emancipatory process

Numerous scholars, clinicians and commentators have pointed out fundamental changes that have occurred to health care systems during recent decades. In the UK, for instance, the 1970s saw a major shift in care organization and delivery, from 'task orientated' to individualized, planned care (and the introduction of the nursing process seems to be bound up with these developments[25]). Rather than care being decided and delegated by a ward sister/charge nurse, and carried out by junior nurses, this shift required nurses to become more responsible for their own practice. Similarly, accountability began to move from the hierarchical structures embodied or personified by the ward sister and medical consultant to the individual nurse. Then, in 1992, this shift to personal accountability for nurses was codified in the development and publication of the UK of the Code of Professional Conduct[31] which made individual nurses accountable for their own actions.[25] Increased attention to individual accountability was further fuelled by tragic and major misdemeanours by individual nurses, the most notable example perhaps being the conduct of Beverly Allitt and the subsequent Allitt inquiry.

Developments and advancements in practice, alongside the growing agenda of cost-cutting and efficiency drives, resulted in nurses doing more – often with fewer nurses – with 'sicker' (more challenging) clients/patients. Fowler and Cutcliffe[25] summarized these changes and their effects on the support needs of nurses as follows:

The effects of these social, political, health and professional developments in the mid-1970's through to the late 1980's resulted in the gradual erosion of well-established support and supervision structures coupled with the increase in the severity of patients' conditions and volume and intensity of work. Additionally accountability at an individual level became established within the profession. By the late 1980's senior nurses were recognising the role of the nurse had changed and was continuing to change. However, the traditional support and supervision structures were no longer in existence or appropriate for the developing role. Thus a formalised structure of support and supervision which gave assurance of customer protection began to appear as a clinical need on the agenda of a number of senior nurses in the profession. (p.11)

It perhaps comes as no surprise, given the demise of traditional support systems, and the corresponding increase in accountability, responsibility and required proficiency, that nurses found themselves in need of support. As a result, together with my esteemed colleagues, we commenced our list of the essential elements of CS (see above) with the notion that it must be supportive; this was a deliberate, purposeful positioning. Similarly, consider Proctor's[20] stated position on this matter: 'Clinical supervision will be a major opportunity for professional and, hopefully, personal refreshment *so the restorative task in these stressful times should, I think, be placed first. If supervision is not experienced as restorative, the other tasks will not be well done*' (emphasis added) (p.25).

The need for support for nurses has been advanced and developed by a number of other authors. Aycock and Boyle[32], for instance, argue that there are few systematic supports in place to help nurses deal with their emotional responses to witnessing and working with tragedies, trauma, sadness, grief and loss. Coupled with this lack of support is the qualitatively and quantitatively different relationship that nurses have (or aspire to have) with clients. From a quantitative standpoint, it has been well documented that nurses spend more time in direct contact with clients than those in other disciplines.[33] They are, as Bush[8] highlights, 'sustained responders' who are thus expected to provide continuing (vs. time-limited, episodic) contact, presence and support to all patients. Further quantitative evidence of nurses' particular need for support resides in the frequency with which nurses encounter, witness and (vicariously) experience trauma. According to Showalter[34] and Yoder,[35] nurses not only encounter such trauma on a regular basis but moreover, when compared to first responders (e.g. emergency ambulance responders, firefighters, etc.) interactions and (often close) interpersonal relationships with clients (and their families) are maintained over time. Such a situation leads Bush[8] to argue that it is both the extended nature of the relationship with traumatized clients and the situating of the nurse in the middle of the care scenario that gives rise to a unique need for support.

From a qualitative point of view, P/MH nurses (at least those who practise from a humanistic perspective) seek to empathize with the client's experiences; they seek to establish close, trusting and, in some ways, intimate relationships with clients. They do not seek to distance themselves from the client and his/her pain, trauma or suffering; they do not avoid these difficult, painful subjects – on the contrary, they are willing to have a presence with the client as he/she tells his/her story. Chapter 3 considers developing and maintaining therapeutic relationships in more detail. This emotional closeness and willingness to empathize does not occur without cost, a cost which has been couched in terms such as 'compassion fatigue',[8,34,35] counter-transference, emotional burnout and vicarious traumatization. Such compassion fatigue occurs as a result of the accumulation of unresolved (unprocessed) stress, repeated exposure to emotionally charged and challenging situations, and/or repeated and continual immersion in the suffering experiences of the clients.[36] While there is no apparent consensus on which term(s) should be used to capture or depict the effects on and costs for nurses that result from empathic engagement with clients, there is little or no debate in the extant literature to suggest that this type of practice does *not* result in some cost to the nurse.

Accordingly, the literature in this area is clear in documenting the burden or cost that nurses incur as a result of engaging empathically and therapeutically with clients. This body of work also highlights how nurses have quantitatively and qualitatively different relationships with clients (when compared to other health care disciplines), and it further reports the demise (or at least diminution) of previous and traditional support systems. The case is clear: nurses need support, and thus the hegemonic position that support (the restorative component) needs to be central to the practice of CS is well founded.

> ## REFLECTION
>
> Has your own experience of CS been characterized and typified by an atmosphere of support? If not, what are the implications?

CS involves a monitoring process: a self-driven, self-exploratory process of review of one's own accountability, practice, ethics and knowledge

The second of these three domains, nominally referred to as the 'normative' component, is by far the most misunderstood and misapplied of the Proctor's[19,20] tripartite model.[13,37,38] Search the relevant literature on CS and you will invariably find that some authors have metamorphosed this domain from one concerned with *self-monitoring and self-evaluation* into the oversight of one's practice by managers, administrators or/and by those occupying some form of hierarchical position over the supervisee. This could not be more inappropriate, nor more damaging. The whole purpose of the normative domain can be captured by considering the phrases 'self-monitoring and self-evaluation'. Supervisees are required to reflect on their practice and consider the professional regulatory and accountability aspects of their conduct; there will inevitably be references to professional codes of conduct, codes of ethics, best practice guidelines, local or institutional policies and so-called standards of care. For some it could be described as (one way of) considering the quality control aspects of one's practice. However – and this cannot be over-stressed – it is the supervisees' (not the supervisor's) responsibility to engage in the juxtaposition of their practice, attitudes and knowledge with the relevant bodies of work pertaining to ethics, professional accountability and standards, best practice guidelines and so on. The purpose of the normative domain is to help the supervisees develop and refine their own self-monitoring practices – not in any way to subject themselves to some third-party evaluation.

It is perhaps worth stressing this point given the ongoing conflations of CS with administrative/managerial supervision (A/MS). In addition to the original conceptualizations and founding rudiments of CS (see above), numerous authors and agencies have highlighted how CS must be separate from A/MS. According to Paunonen and Hyrkas,[39] the Scandinavian countries deliberately eschewed having line managers acting as clinical supervisors due to the possible role conflict that could arise. The Nursing Midwifery Council (NMC; formerly the United Kingdom Central Council, UKCC)[40] was similarly unequivocal in avoiding the conflation of CS with A/MS.

While there are links between and complementary aspects of CS and A/MS – for instance, managers should be involved with implementing, supporting and evaluating CS. Amalgamating CS with A/MS invariably diminishes, if not eradicates, the more democratic, emancipatory, supportive and developmental aspects of CS.[13,37,41,42] In describing some of the problems arising from this amalgamation, Cutcliffe[43] highlighted that:

> *there is a tendency for those in senior roles to focus on performance and action rather than exploring the subtleties of process; there is the potential for material offered during supervision to be used in a disciplinary manner; there is the tendency to focus on management (normative) issues as the major agenda; and there is a confusion caused by the duality of supervisory and managerial roles. (p.140)*

The importance of maintaining CS and A/MS as distinct but complementary practices is further underscored when one acknowledges that there are already sufficient mechanisms and processes for surveillance and professional accountability in nursing. Yet, as highlighted earlier in this chapter, given the demise of 'traditional' and pre-existing support systems, what are lacking now more than ever are opportunities for personal/practice development in an entirely safe, yet challenging, and supportive, yet stimulating, interpersonal environment.

REFLECTION

Think about your own experiences of CS. Was there any evidence or experience of 'slipping' into administrative/managerial supervision? How did this impact on the experience?

CS must be concerned with growth and development and must thus be a learning process

The last of Proctor's[19,20] tripartite model components is termed 'formative' and this is concerned with the supervisee's learning, development and growth. From the original conceptualizations of CS (see above) to innumerable useful contributions to the extant literature in this area, to contemporary conceptualizations such as the position statement advanced by the UKCC/NMC,[40] descriptions and definitions of CS have invariably included the crucial element(s) of learning, growth and development of the supervisee. Indeed, I know of no published work which advances the view that CS is not, at least in part, concerned with the practitioner's (supervisee's) learning, growth and/or development. Accordingly, given the self-evident truth that CS is inherently concerned with learning, growth and/or development, the next logical step is to explore what form(s) of learning are incorporated by CS.

It may be of interest to note that, despite the (relatively) recent arguments for competency-based learning and competency-filled curricula,[44–47] such behaviouralist and competency-driven views of education are at odds with original conceptualizations of CS, which saw experiential learning as fundamental to effective CS. While clinical supervisors themselves appear to need certain competencies in order to be proficient (see Cutcliffe and Sloan[14]), learning for the supervisee is not competency-driven – it is experience-driven and thus concerned with experiential learning.

As stated previously in this chapter, Dewey's[26,27] significant and pioneering work on experiential learning is founded, at least in part, on the integrated concepts of experience and reflection; for Dewey reflecting on experience equals learning.[48] However, for Dewey there are some important caveats; in particular, the point that *not* all experience has the potential for learning – it is the particular 'quality' of an experience that provides a measure of its educational significance.[48] Accordingly, the experience needs to be internalized and positioned in relation to existing knowledge and earlier experiences. Subsequent important contributions to this body of work[49–51] draw attention to a further key element in experiential learning that separates it from other pedagogical approaches – namely that of where the 'locus of control' resides. Fowler[48] draws attention to the relevance of this phenomenon to the practice of CS:

> *For when the locus of control of what is learnt, lies with the individual or as in clinical supervision, the supervisee, then the potential for the challenge of social norms becomes a reality; a 'bottom up' rather than a 'top down' change agent. Thus in clinical supervision if the locus of control remains with the supervisee, then the potential for such 'bottom up' change and all its implications becomes a reality, and the phrase which is not an uncommon expression in some people's experiences of clinical supervision, of it being a 'life changing' experience, is better understood. (p.55)*

For Kolb,[52] another seminal contributor in this area, one of the three principal characteristics of experiential learning and development is that learning is best conceived as a process and ought not to be thought of in terms of behavioural outcomes. Indeed, for Kolb, it is the emphasis on process rather than behavioural outcomes that distinguishes experiential learning from traditional (behaviouralist) approaches to learning. Kolb reinforces his position by highlighting that the theory of experiential learning rests on a different philosophical and epistemological basis from behaviouralist (and thus competency-focused) education.

Learning, growth and development within (or via) CS are also premised on the notion of lifelong learning, and such a position is now clearly enshrined in the relevant nursing literature; particularly in the literature pertaining to 'fitness for practice', 'continuing professional education and development' and thus matters pertaining to ongoing nurse registration. Lifelong learning is now seen as necessary for continuing professional competence. This position has an intuitive logic to it, given the increasing pace of new health-care-related discoveries, practice development and evolution, and the sheer width and depth of relevant information that now exists. Recognizing that mental health practice does not remain static, notwithstanding the fact that changes to practice can be progressive or regressive,* any change to practice creates the need for reflection. The 'quality' experiences that ensue in a climate of practice evolution, for some, require, if not demand, that the practitioner reflect on these 'novel' situations. The case for experiential learning and reflection in CS as a principal source of growth and development is further underscored when one acknowledges the reality that contemporary mental health care now exists within the epoch of evidence-informed practice. Reflection on our practice and experiential learning within CS provides the tools by which each practitioner can examine his/her practice and consider decisions made and actions taken (or not taken) within the context of evidence. And lastly in this section, while it may be an uncomfortable truth for some, we are all 'works in progress'; we are all imperfect beings and imperfect practitioners – we will all make mistakes from time to time. The philosophy and practice of experiential learning seems to encompass the idea that mistakes are seen as almost inevitable and, moreover, are regarded as developmental, learning opportunities. Examination of errors or mistakes, within the safe atmosphere or environment of CS, can then serve as one mechanism for improving practice and reducing iatrogenic harm. As opposed to 'living in fear' of errors and exercising the fantasy of a mistake-free health care system, experiential learning and reflection allow each practitioner to embrace their imperfection(s) and use these as a springboard for improvement, growth and development. As Stephen Hawking puts it, 'One of the basic rules of the universe is that nothing is perfect. Perfection simply doesn't exist. So the next time someone tells you that you have made a mistake, you should simply say that maybe that's a good thing because without imperfection, neither you nor I would exist'.[53]

REFLECTION

Think about your own experiences of CS. In what ways were you encouraged to reflect on your practice? How did you find the experience of exploring and ultimately learning from any of your mistakes or errors?

CONCLUSION

In many contemporary health care settings, P/MH nurses have a pronounced need to engage in supportive, emancipatory CS, particularly given the demise of traditional support systems, the emotionally challenging demands of mental health care and their increased accountability and responsibility. While there is no one singular form of CS that is ideal for all, CS is not a 'free for all' and thus needs to have evidence of the underpinning rudiments and principles presented in this chapter.

SERVICE USER COMMENTARY

Katherine Owen

I have worked in mental health services in a variety of roles for over 25 years and have been a service user myself for the last 10. It has felt like a long, slow journey of realization that in order to provide the best care to other people I first need to look after myself. I consider CS very much as one strand of the support I need for myself in my clinical work with clients. I have experienced a variety of different forms of CS over the years, with several supervisors in various organizations, in groups, one to one, in person and via Skype, but all have offered me a safe place to reflect and learn and grow.

This chapter is a helpful exploration of what CS is and what it is not. It is usefully specific about the difference between clinical supervision and managerial supervision, and makes it clear that it is possible to get support that is really about restoration, development and learning, rather than managerial supervision, which can be more associated with other people's agendas, targets and definitions of what doing a job well means. Similarly, it clarifies the self-monitoring process in CS and importantly emphasizes that it is directed by the supervisee themselves as a means of growing self-responsibility, rather than a dynamic of being brought up short by someone in a position of power over you. I especially appreciated the discussion of experiential learning in the chapter. For me it has certainly been life-changing to discover that learning is a process, one in which mistakes are to be expected, and which redresses the balance between knowledge 'out there' with a growing sense of my own intuition and trust in myself.

---

* For instance, the relatively recent increases in the coercive nature of much of mental health practice for some is seen as a retrograde step.

CASE STUDY 1

Note: In the interests of maintaining confidentiality, while this case is based on a real CS encounter, all names, identifying features and details have been altered.

Margo was a mental health clinician specializing in counselling. She sought out Clinical Supervision from an experienced mental health practitioner. After negotiating and establishing contractual boundaries, and subsequent to several 'early' Clinical Supervision sessions, Margo wanted to discuss the challenging situation that she had encountered with one of the clients she was working with. Margo described situations where the client would engage in flattery of her; indeed such was the extent that Margo felt the client was flirting with her. However, days after the flirting episodes, the client was sharing with his co-residents that he and Margo were 'a thing' and that they had a 'special connection'. The supervisor asked Margo to say how it made her feel when she received these compliments, Margo admitted that it was 'nice to receive a compliment', though she was angered and upset as a result of the client sharing untruths with his fellow residents. The supervisor began by offering supportive statements, empathizing with the feeling of being deceived and let down by the client and by engaging in some appropriate self-disclosure; the supervisor stated that he had encountered similar situations in his past clinical work.

The supervisor encouraged Margo to consider what motivation(s) the client may have had for engaging in this behaviour, to make room for possible explanations other than the flirting actually being about Margo; could there be something else going on (under the surface, so to speak)? Margo began to recount that the client had a long history of failed interpersonal relationships with the opposite gender. His relationships tended to follow a pattern where, at first, he was charming and overly attentive, and ingratiated himself with women. This was inevitably followed by the bragging or boasting to his colleagues about his latest relationship and how he was such a success with the opposite gender.

In so doing, Margo was able to consider the client's behaviour towards her in the broader (and very important) context of his behaviour towards women per se. Margo began to see the behaviour more as a possible 'means to an end', rather than being about her specifically. Together with the supervisor, she began to explore some possible ways of responding to any future flattery. She began to explore the value of reiterating professional boundaries and reminding the client of the professional nature of the relationship. She was also able to reflect the attempt at flattery back to the client the next time he tried this. This led to the next few sessions with the client being the most constructive, exploratory and rewarding, where the client was able to begin to explore the motivations for his behaviour and how this was impacting on his relationships per se.

I agree that bravery is a necessary asset to have in order to engage with the process of reflection and self-evaluation. It can be uncomfortable to come face to face with your imperfections, blind spots and limitations. For me CS has been an invaluable support. I have been skilfully supported to see the opportunity for learning in difficult situations, which, left to my own thinking alone, could have led me to be overly critical of myself. I have been advised when I have flown close to the flame of wanting to 'fix' other people and their problems, and I have been gently shown my habits of relating which are not in my own awareness.

This chapter has helped remind me that my CS takes priority, along with a work–life balance, walks in nature, saying 'no' to over-committing myself and realistically pacing myself. All are equally important ways to look after myself and my own needs, so that I can then be more available to the needs of others.

References

1. Peplau HE. *Interpersonal relations in nursing: a conceptual frame of reference for psychodynamic nursing*, 2nd edn. New York: Putnam, 1988.
2. Barker P. *The philosophy and practice of psychiatric nursing.* Edinburgh: Churchill Livingstone, 1999.
3. Cutcliffe JR, Stevenson C, Lakeman R. Oxymoronic or synergistic: deconstructing the psychiatric and/or mental health nurse. *International Journal of Mental Health Nursing* 2013; **22**: 125–34.
4. Barnard AG, Nash RE, O'Brien M. Information literacy: developing life-long skills through nursing education. *Journal of Nursing Education* 2005; **44**(11): 505–10.
5. NMC (Nursing Midwifery Council). *Standards to support learning and assessment in practice: NMC standards for mentors, practice teachers and teachers.* London: NMC, 2008.
6. Trinder L, Reynolds S. *Evidence-based practice: a critical appraisal.* London: Blackwell Science, 2000.

7. Edwards D, Burnard P, Hannigan B, Cooper L, Adams J, Juggessur T, Fothergil A, Coyle D. Clinical supervision and burnout: the influence of clinical supervision for community mental health nurses. *Journal of Clinical Nursing* 2006; **15**(8): 1007–15.

8. Bush NJ. Compassion fatigue: are you at risk? *Oncology Nursing Forum* 2009; **36**(1): 24–8.

9. Day GA. Changing competencies of supervision. *Modern Hospital* 1925; **24**(5): 469–70.

10. Schmidt E. Principles and practices of supervision. *American Journal of Nursing* 1926; **27**(2): 119–20.

11. Wolf L. Development of floor nursing and supervision. *Hospital* 1941; March: 53–6.

12. Freeman R. Supervision in the improvement of nursing services. *Public Health Nursing* 1952; **44**(7): 370–3.

13. Yegdich T. Clinical supervision and managerial supervision: some historical and conceptual considerations. *Journal of Advanced Nursing* 1999; **30**(5): 1195–204.

14. Cutcliffe JR, Sloan G. Towards a consensus of a competency framework for Clinical Supervision in nursing: knowledge, attitudes and skills. *Clinical Supervisor* 2014; **33**(2): 182–203.

15. Cutcliffe R, Butterworth T, Proctor B (eds). *Fundamental themes in clinical supervision.* London: Routledge, 2001.

16. Cutcliffe JR, Fowler J, Hyrkas K (eds). *Routledge handbook of clinical supervision: global perspectives on fundamental themes.* London: Routledge, 2011.

17. Folkins JW, Bleile KM. Taxonomies in biology, phonetics, phonology, and speech motor control. *Journal of Speech and Hearing Disorders* 1990; **55**: 596–611.

18. Dunn B, Everitt BS. *An introduction to mathematical taxonomies.* New York: Dover Publications, 2004.

19. Proctor B. Training for the supervision alliance: attitude, skills and intention. In: Cutcliffe JR, Butterworth T, Proctor B (eds). *Fundamental themes in clinical supervision.* London: Routledge, 2001: 23–34.

20. Proctor, B. Training for the supervision alliance: attitude, skills and intention. In: Cutcliffe JR, Fowler J, Hyrkas K (eds). *Routledge handbook of clinical supervision: global perspectives on fundamental themes.* London: Routledge, 2011: 23–34.

21. Jaccard J, Jacoby J. *Theory construction and model-building skills: methodology in the social sciences.* London: Guilford Press, 2009.

22. Fowler J. Evaluating the efficacy of reflective practice within the context of clinical supervision. *Journal of Advanced Nursing* 1998; **27**(2): 379–38.

23. Gilbert T. Reflective practice and clinical supervision: meticulous rituals of the confessional. *Journal of Advanced Nursing* 2001; **36**(2): 199–205.

24. Johns C, Freshwater D. *Transforming nursing through reflective practice*, 2nd edn. Oxford: Blackwell, 2005.

25. Fowler J, Cutcliffe JR. Clinical supervision: origins, overview and rudiments. In: Cutcliffe JR, Fowler J, Hyrkas K (eds). *Routledge handbook of clinical supervision: global perspectives on fundamental themes.* London: Routledge, 2011: 8–20.

26. Dewey J. *Democracy and education. An introduction to the philosophy of education.* New York: Free Press, 1966 [1916].

27. Dewey J. *How we think.* New York: DC Heath, 1933.

28. Carper B. Fundamental patterns of knowing in nursing. *Advances in Nursing Science* 1978; **1**(1): 13–24.

29. Atkins S, Murphy K. Reflection: a review of the literature. *Journal of Advanced Nursing* 1993; **18**(11): 88–1192.

30. Todd G, Freshwater D. Reflective practice and guided discovery: clinical supervision. *British Journal of Nursing* 1999; **8**(20): 1383–9.

31. UKCC (United Kingdom Central Council). *Code of professional conduct.* London: UKCC, 1992.

32. Aycock N, Boyle D. Interventions to manage compassion fatigue. *Clinical Journal of Oncology Nursing* 2009; **13**(2): 183–91.

33. Page A (ed.). *Keeping patients safe: transforming the work environment of nurses.* Washington, DC: National Academies Press, 2004.

34. Showalter SE. Compassion fatigue: what is it? Why does it matter? Recognizing the symptoms, acknowledging the impact, developing the tools to prevent compassion fatigue, and strengthen the professional already suffering from the effects. *American Journal of Hospice Palliative Care* 2009; **27**(4): 239–42.

35. Yoder EA. Compassion fatigue in nurses. *Applied Nursing Research* 2010; **23**: 191–7.

36. Figley CR. *Compassion fatigue: coping with secondary post traumatic disorder in those who treat the traumatised.* London: Brunner-Routledge, 1995.

37. Cutcliffe JR, Hyrkas K. Multidisciplinary attitudinal positions regarding clinical supervision: a cross-sectional study. *Journal of Nursing Management* 2006; **14**: 617–27.

38. Bishop V. Clinical supervision and clinical governance. In: Cutcliffe JR, Fowler J, Hyrkas K (eds). *Routledge handbook of clinical supervision: global perspectives on fundamental themes.* London: Routledge, 2011: 113–24.

39. Paunonen M, Hyrkas K. Clinical supervision in Finland: history, education, research and theory. In: Cutcliffe JR, Butterworth T, Proctor B (eds). *Fundamental themes in clinical supervision.* London: Routledge, 2001: 284–300.

40. UKCC (United Kingdom Central Council). *Position statement on clinical supervision for nursing and health visiting.* London: UKCC, 2014.

41. Kelly B, Long A, McKenna HP. A survey of community mental health nurses' perceptions of clinical supervision in Northern Ireland. *Journal of Psychiatric/Mental Health Nursing* 2001; **8**: 33–44.

42. Epling M. Cassedy P. Visions from the classroom. In: Cutcliffe JR, Butterworth T, Proctor B (eds). *Fundamental themes in clinical supervision.* London: Routledge, 2001: 64–883.

43. Cutcliffe JR. Clinical supervision and reflective practice: symbient and integral aspects of the role of community psychiatric nurses. In: Hannigan B, Coffey M, Burnard P (eds). *A handbook of community mental health nursing.* London: Routledge, 2003: 132–44.

44. Lenburg CB. The framework, concepts and methods of the Competency Outcomes and Performance Assessment (COPA) Model. *Online Journal of Issues in Nursing* 1999; **4**(2).

45. JCAHO (Joint Commission on Accreditation of Healthcare Organizations). *Meeting the competency challenge in behavioral healthcare: the resource tool for behavioral healthcare human resource professionals who must meet the rigorous requirements of JCAHO.* Washington, DC: C&R Publications, Inc., 2000.

46. Calhoun JG, Dollett L, Sinioirs ME, Wainio JA, Butler P, Griffith JR, Warden GL. Development of an interprofessional competency model for healthcare leadership. *Journal of Healthcare Management* 2008; **53**(6): 375–89.

47. Yarbrough LA, Stowe M, Haefner J. Competency assessment and development among healthcare leaders: results of a cross-sectional survey. *Health Service Management Research* 2012; **25**(2): 78–86.

48. Fowler J. Experiential learning: an underpinning theoretical perspective for clinical supervision. In: Cutcliffe JR, Fowler J, Hyrkas K (eds). *Routledge handbook of clinical supervision: global perspectives on fundamental themes.* London: Routledge, 2011: 51–62.

49. Freire P. *Pedagogy of the oppressed.* London: Harmondsworth Penguin, 1972.

50. Illich I. *Deschooling society.* London: Calser and Buyars, 1971.

51. Rogers CR. *Freedom to learn.* Columbus, OH: Charles Merrill Publishing Co., 1969.

52. Kolb DA. *Experiential learning: experience as the source of learning and development.* Englewood Cliffs, NJ: Prentice Hall, 1984.

53. Hawking S. Stephen Hawking quote. Available from: http://www.goodreads.com/quotes/363982 [Accessed 6th June 2016].

Further reading

Cookson J, Sloan G, Dafters R, Jahoda A. Provision of clinical supervision for staff working in mental health services. *Mental Health Practice* 2014; **17**(7): 29–34.

Cutcliffe JR, Hyrkas K, Fowler J (eds), (2011). *Routledge handbook of clinical supervision: global perspectives on fundamental themes*, 2nd edn of *Fundamental themes in clinical supervision*. London: Routledge, 2011.

Cutcliffe JR, Sloan G. Towards a consensus of a competency framework for clinical supervision in nursing: knowledge, attitudes and skills. *Clinical Supervisor* 2014; **33**(2): 182–203.

Gonge H, Buus N. Is it possible to strengthen psychiatric nursing staff's clinical supervision? RCT of a meta-supervision intervention. *Journal of Advanced Nursing* 2015; **71**(4): 909–21.

Relevant web pages

Steven Power. Supervision resources. http://counsellingsupervision.blogspot.com/p/resources.html

Yale Program on Supervision. http://www.supervision.yale.edu/index.aspx

11 Critical reflection

JAN FOOK, JANE ROYES AND ANTHONY WHITE

LEARNING OUTCOMES

- To understand the basic meaning of critical reflection.
- To be aware of why critical reflection is important and some possible benefits of using it.
- To appreciate how critical reflection might be used in practical terms.

SUMMARY OF KEY POINTS

- Critical reflection is important to professional judgement and caring in the current environment.
- Critical reflection basically refers to 'learning from experience' using a framework of understanding about how power dynamics operate. This enables an ability to transform thinking and behaviour.
- There are many ways to critically reflect. The method covered in this chapter involves presenting critical incidents (examples of experience) and dialoguing about them in small groups.
- There are many benefits of critical reflection. They include personal and emotional gains, as well as professional improvement.

INTRODUCTION

Long ago Socrates called for reflection which involved 'the examined life' for ethical and compassionate engagement with the world and its moral dilemmas.[1] Dewey[2] wrote influentially about reflection as 'learning from experience' in the 1930s. So, why the current interest?

Contemporary contexts of uncertainty call for new ways to ensure that practice and care continue to be responsive to changing conditions. In a context of continual policy reviews and increasing austerity measures, it is difficult to build on existing knowledge and to know what works with any certainty.

The 'new professionalism'[3] also demands that decisions and actions must be justified in order to maintain client and patient satisfaction. These trends support better service delivery. However, when taken to extremes, they can also reduce definitions of good practice to measurable criteria only. When taken as the sole standards of professionalism, they disallow a holistic response to human need, and the ethical bases which underpin, and sometimes provide the rationale for, the care that professionals provide. The call for professionals to be reflective and exercise judgement in complex situations[4] is associated with a desire to honour the integrity which for many professionals lies at the heart of what and how they practise, and which many believe to be threatened by current workplace trends. Indeed, it might be argued that the 'craft of caring' itself is associated with 'relational wisdom'[5] or compassion – how relationships of empathy, respect and dignity are central to caregiving[6] (see chapter 3 for further information on developing and maintaining relationships). Recent calls for compassion in nursing[7] sound an alarm about how technocratic approaches to professional practice might fly in the face of what many of us believe – that the craft of caring should essentially define our professionalism.

In these circumstances critical reflection is highly relevant. It can help deal with uncertainty and complexity; make our practice more responsive to change; keep us more honest and accountable; and provide an ongoing way of evaluating what we do – all in conditions that are becoming more difficult for professionals to control. More fundamentally, it might also be used as a method of ensuring that the basic values that are inherent to our 'craft of caring' are upheld.

WHAT IS CRITICAL REFLECTION?

Critical reflection is understood in many different ways, and, being complex, it is difficult to pin down in concrete practice. Briefly, reflection is 'learning from experience'.[2,8] In straightforward terms, learning from experience simply involves re-examining past personally experienced events in order to make new meaning of them in the light of other (subsequent or current) experiences and contexts. The 'learning' should involve turning the thinking involved from that early event into a broader principle or guideline (by perceiving patterns or commonalities with other experiences or events). The learning, however, should enable more expansive and flexible ways of thinking and acting, rather than more rigid or restrictive thinking. For instance, if, as a service user, I have an annoying encounter with a health professional, I could decide to avoid health professionals in the future, or to take up a defensive stance before I meet the next one. On the other hand, I can try to work out what made the encounter annoying, and develop some guidelines for how I would like to set up the next encounter (for example, what questions can I ask and how?). The latter way of responding is clearly more flexible, and allows a greater range of actions. This is the type of learning from experience that is encouraged through reflection. This presumably also fits with Socrates' understanding of reflection which allows for more ethical and compassionate engagement.

What makes reflection 'critical'? There are two simple answers. First, the level of learning should be deep; that is, it should extend to being able to formulate guiding principles which touch on some fundamental values about yourself and other people, and your understanding of your own place socially and professionally. For instance, with the above example, the learning would be considered fundamental if you were able to create some understanding of why you (what was it about who you are, your situation?) found the encounter with the health professional annoying and what this says about you (and other similar situations) more generally. How can this learning inform the way you work more generally with other types of people?

The second aspect of 'critical' involves an understanding of power dynamics. So, for instance, if you appreciate that your own sense of yourself as powerless (as a service user) contributed to your annoyance, you would be beginning to delve into the more critical aspects of reflection. This understanding of power of course automatically creates a possible vision for how power inequalities might be better managed, and therefore how social encounters might be *transformed*.

In summary, then, critical reflection is a way of learning from or making deeper meaning of experience. It involves re-examining past experiences and turning the learning from these into more generalizable principles or guidelines. When an understanding of power and how it operates is included, the reflection can be critical in a *transformative* sense.

METHODS FOR CRITICAL REFLECTION

There are many different ways to critically reflect. The approach that I work with uses Schon's[9] reflective practice approach as a practical starting point (hunting for assumptions) within a broader framework of learning from experience (outlined above).

I have developed a structured model for critical reflection.[10] The practitioners participating in the critical reflection process bring an example of their own practice experience to reflect upon. Often these are 'critical incidents' or events that they feel are significant to their learning. They are encouraged to write this down beforehand, describing what happened in terms that are as 'raw' as possible. The reflection on this incident then involves two stages: a first stage where deep assumptions are unearthed, and a second stage where the impact of the awareness of these is reworked to give new guidelines for action. It is usually used in a small group setting, in an ethical learning climate.

The learning climate provides a clear space for practitioners to examine their work in a non-threating way, so that they feel safe enough to challenge their own work.[11] The learning climate focuses on how to help practitioners reflect for themselves – it enables people to *learn* how to reflect, rather than having other people's reflections imposed. People must be able to learn how to unearth their own underlying assumptions for themselves. The group creates an inquisitive (not judgemental) atmosphere by asking questions which help the person reflect by becoming aware of their hidden thinking. The questions, for example, may attempt to explore the origins of the thinking (for example. personal, cultural, social) – 'where does that come from?'; or the kinds of assumptions the person is making about others – 'I wonder what that person's perspective might be?' The first stage simply aims to uncover the person's assumptions so that they have an opportunity to examine them (and perhaps make assessments of their relevance in their own way) with further reflection.

In the second stage, the person is encouraged to reflect further on the hidden ideas that emerged in the first stage, perhaps noting whether they think that any further fundamental thinking has surfaced. They are then encouraged to think about what they want to change (thinking and actions) as a result of the new awareness. Ultimately they are encouraged to label this new approach to practice, using their own words. This constitutes an attempt to remake the meaning of their experience and new guidelines for action.

This model may be adapted in many different ways. Besides being used in small groups, it can also be used for self-reflection (that is, asking yourself the critical reflection questions) or in one-to-one supervision (chapter 10). It can also be used as a framework for written reflections in diaries, or for written reflective assignments.

BENEFITS AND OUTCOMES OF CRITICAL REFLECTION

Claims about the benefits of critical reflection range from more personal or emotional benefits, to those which contribute to better workplaces and practice improvement.[10] For example, practitioners often report feeling supported and able to overcome emotional blocks through reflecting on a difficult experience. Others consider themselves better able to work with colleagues whom they perceive as difficult, which makes for better teamwork. Some are able to find new ways of understanding, particularly the service user's perspective, which in turn assists them to find new strategies. As we have noted earlier, critical reflection may contribute to a better understanding of ourselves and others, and therefore enable a better 'craft of caring'.

In the following section we include examples of reflection from a social services setting. Although these are not mental health nursing examples, they are examples from different professions. All of us have conducted critical reflection with a number of different professionals, and we find that the process works in a similar way for all. Thus the process is clearly transferable. In fact, we find that professional differences fade away, simply because it is very fundamental assumptions, which are emerging. This is because, although we might have different training and backgrounds, ultimately we all share a similar basic set of assumptions about fundamental things such as what power is, or what change is.

> ### REFLECTION
>
> In order to make the examples below more relevant to yourself as a mental health nurse, you might like to think about experiences you have had which are similar.

PUTTING CRITICAL REFLECTION INTO PRACTICE: ANTHONY'S EXPERIENCE

I am an advanced practitioner based in a frontline children's safeguarding team within an inner London local authority. I support newly qualified social workers, as well as experienced staff, with the overall aim to improve practice standards. Facilitating critically reflective practice is key. I do this in groups as well as one-to-one. I have been involved in developing critical reflective groups in two major frontline services as well as within a children's centre and a complex needs team. All teams work with children and families.

The use of critical reflective practice is imperative for any practitioner's basic survival within the workplace. This is my own personal theory. Working in any challenging and demanding environment where the interactions between practitioners and family, patient, child and communities can be fraught will naturally cause some level of emotional discomfort.

I have found that this model of critical reflection can guide workers in understanding the transition from their own experience (something that happened in practice) to understanding how and more importantly why this is affecting them. This results in a change in their beliefs and practices.

Some challenges

While the social workers I worked with initially welcomed group-based critical reflective practice, this later became a challenge. Staff felt that protected time was needed, away from their desks, to participate in critical reflection, but making that commitment on the day of the group meetings has proved difficult. There is a prevailing culture in which staff feel that workload demands take priority. Therefore people need to be encouraged to make critical reflection a priority and not schedule other appointments when they know groups are running. It can also help to hold groups in the morning, or at a venue outside the office.

It is ironic that staff actually need critical reflection more at times of higher pressure but are less able to find the time in those crucial periods. It is therefore important that prior planning takes place, such as block booking group sessions and ensuring that a number of people are prepared to share incidents.

While we wanted groups to run and in doing so we wanted (and needed) people to attend, we had to be cautious about people just attending for the *sake* of it, as opposed to genuinely wanting to learn and support colleagues. I believe the former situation can be destructive. If the presenter shares their experience and sincerely wants to learn from it, and group members are quiet, evasive or non-engaged, this can have a negative impact on the presenter, leaving them feeling vulnerable and unsupported.

The model therefore appears to work best with colleagues who genuinely want to learn and support others even when they are not presenting their own incident. People do comment that they learn from listening to descriptions of other people's incidents. They notice similarities between the presenter's incident and their own experience. It is a far more productive session when those who attend a group are committed to critical reflection.

There needs to be some careful thought about the membership of each group. We consulted with staff about who they felt most comfortable with: the more comfortable they are, the more likely they are to share a critical incident and to explore the deeper meaning of this. For this reason also, groups which are made up of peers are more likely to be successful than those where a manager might be present.

An example of critical reflection

A critical incident was presented by a social worker, Ann, in a family assessment centre. It involved a mother (with two young children under 5) diagnosed with depression, and concerns about alcohol and cannabis use. Ann had been working with the family for around 6 months. The initial engagement was around family support; however, due to increasing concerns with the family, Ann was now asked to undertake a parenting assessment.

The critical incident occurred after a home visit that Ann undertook with her manager. The mother had been argumentative and challenging during the visit. Ann had noted a change in the mother's behaviour towards her over the last few weeks. The critical incident for Ann was when, after leaving the home visit, she told her manager that she did not wish to continue working with this family or the parenting assessment. The visit had occurred 3 days ago. Ann felt this was perhaps said out of frustration, as she was feeling tired and deflated in her work with the mother.

When presenting to the group, Ann said she wished to focus on why she felt so reactionary after the visit.

She wanted to explore, after many years of experience in working with challenging families, why she felt so frustrated about this particular family.

Stage one of the critically reflective process began by exploring Ann's feelings in the incident. She mentioned feeling tired and exhausted. She said the mother was bombarding accusations that she [Ann] was going to have her children removed. The group explored Ann's assumptions about the mother. Ann had assumed that this mother would participate well in the assessment. She described the mother as intelligent and insightful. The group aimed to explore what Ann's assumption of 'well' was and how she felt this reflected the past. Questions asked were:

- When you said 'participating well', can you tell us a bit more about that and what 'well' means for you?
- What do you expect from families you work with?
- What do you want for this family and this mother?

Ann shared her thoughts on change and stated that she hopes that all families she works with are able to change. The group asked about where she felt this mother was with change (in terms of her mental health, ability to care for the children) and Ann struggled with this. She felt that, in spite of the support she [Ann] offered and her capacities, she may not now be able to change. The group looked at what this felt like for Ann (in doing the assessment) and making the recommendation. She described a sudden sense of responsibility. The discussions involved some good questions about power, perceptions of power, who 'should' hold power, etc. Ann initially felt that the mother held the power as she was the driver for the assessment, but during the group discussion she began to feel that she [Ann] did. Ann felt the incident demonstrated the mother's understanding of where the power sat, and perhaps her own recognition that she cannot change or manage things in the way Ann may want.

Ann then thought that perhaps the incident was critical for her, as this was the point when she realized that *the mother could not make these changes and that this a real disappointment for her*. She had not anticipated this, and being there with her manager (that is, with her manager seeing this at first hand) made it all very real for Ann.

Ann spoke about feeling let down by her beliefs about change and felt she should 'be used to this'. Open questions about why she may then not be 'used to it' proved useful. Again it reflected how her beliefs about social work and organizational expectations perhaps differed from her own expectations of herself.

The second stage highlighted the main learning points for Ann. She felt that, during the process of stage one, she gained more insight about why she reacted in the way she did (not wanting to work with the case anymore). She felt that understanding more about the power dynamics was an important element, as was thinking about her acceptance of families not being able to change. Ann thought more deeply about why she wanted change so much for this family and wanted to take this point away to consider it further. In terms of changes she wanted to make, Ann felt more insightful about power and how this changes between social worker and service user. There was a sense of breakthrough in Ann accepting (or beginning to accept) that working with service users and families that do not or cannot change is both challenging and difficult. She almost felt that saying and owning this was a big step, since it is not perhaps something that is considered in her organization.

Overall, critical reflective practice has worked well within my organization. While it has been difficult to implement such a large change in the whole organizational culture, individual practitioners feel they have benefited from this. Although from an outsider's perspective, the learning may seem small-scale, the practitioners involved view this very differently. Staff share how positively conscious they have become about their learning experiences in their practice and they talk about ways they have, over time, thought about implementing change which is driven by their learning from critical reflective practice.

REFLECTION

Think about an experience of your own that you felt was significant, or critical to your own professional learning. What made it 'critical' for you?

PUTTING CRITICAL REFLECTION INTO PRACTICE: JANE'S EXPERIENCE

I am a qualified social worker and work as an educator in the Learning and Organizational Development Team for three inner-city London local authorities. Critical reflective practice has recently been introduced to the organization and is emerging as an important approach for learning and development for staff across the organization. The following section provides an overview of how it was introduced in the organization and has been used to enable practice development.

When I was a new manager in a social work team, a fatal fire in a client's home was a significant event that changed my professional career. Looking back, the incident was critical for me because I thought that I should have prevented the client from dying in the fire. I felt guilty and embarrassed about what had happened. Without using any framework to analyse my practice experience, I began to see myself as a 'bad manager'. I quickly lost my confidence. An investigation into the case concluded that the death of the elderly woman who died in the fire was accidental and the case was closed shortly thereafter. The incident, however, continued to resurface for me and I thought about it a lot. In an attempt to understand what had happened and whether it could have been prevented or I could have done something differently, I re-read the old case notes relating to the incident to see if there was any detail or procedure that I might have missed. I tried to discuss what had happened with a few trusted colleagues. 'You did everything you could,' they would say. I know this was to try and reassure me, but their advice never did feel quite right or help me understand why this experience had had such an impact on me; nor did it help me think through what I could learn as a result of what had happened. I also tried to discuss the case with the social worker whom I had supervised while she was working on the case. Our discussions usually broke down and finally we stopped talking about it. It was as though we blamed each other for what had happened.

Shortly after this incident, I left my management role and moved into social work education. I learnt more about the process of critical reflection and how it is used as a process to enable learning from critical incidents. With the support of a critical reflective practice group, I was able to analyse my critical incident and this has helped me understand my thinking and how I constructed my experience. It also provided new perspectives. The group helped me unearth my assumptions about being a 'bad' manager. My perception was that a 'good manager' knew all of the procedures. This view came from what I had observed of other managers. I explored my understanding of this through analysing the organizational context, and the high value that the organization places on completing the right forms and risk assessments.

I began to realize that I had seen the use of procedures and forms as a way of controlling the situation. I understand now that my over-reliance on procedures does not protect a client or me. This new awareness helped me to understand more about defensive practice and how this can contribute to a culture of fear and blame among professionals. It can take the focus away from the client and good practice. When things do go wrong on cases, I could see why anxieties were so heightened.

I also analysed my understanding of my manager role. I realized that in my transition from social worker to manager I needed to consider how my relationship to clients had changed – although I was indirectly involved in the case, my responsibility had changed to a supervisory role. I realized that I had not considered the perspective of the social worker who was working directly on the case and the support she may have needed before and following the client's death.

If professionals experience significant incidents, and these continue to resurface throughout their careers, what happens if they do not have an opportunity to understand them properly? If they are not able to reflect on their practice in depth, how do they move forward to practise with new awareness, changed thinking and confidence? My role in the training team allowed me a sphere of influence to explore these questions further. My new role was an opportunity to introduce critical reflection as a pathway for social workers to learn, develop and help change the culture of learning. This was an important part of practice development where learning from critical incidents could be utilized to help change both the practice of individuals and of the organization.

Setting up critical reflection in my organization

I set up the first critical reflective practice group with the support of Jan Fook after she had done some work with newly qualified social workers.

In the first group, I aimed to introduce the model and then, over time, support the group to learn how to facilitate sessions which they could then run within their own teams. This was the first time that social workers had been encouraged to learn about critical reflection and given space to practise it.

I ran these sessions with a group of approximately 25 people. The dynamics of the group provided some challenges for the learning environment. The group included a mix of managers and frontline staff – some people felt uncomfortable with this mix because sharing experiences was viewed by some as exposing their own weaknesses. This was threatening. Others found the process of experiential learning a challenge – this was particularly difficult for those more familiar with the didactic training approaches used by the organization. The busy nature of people's workplaces also meant that it was hard to take time out for slowing down and thinking and reflecting. One person openly admitted that he 'didn't have the patience to listen to other people's problems'. This also indicated a certain mindset among some practitioners about what constituted learning and useful forms of support for practitioners. Some of the more experienced workers struggled with a process which did not allow them to offer advice or affirmation. Others found the experience beneficial – most people had the chance to share their critical incident and were open to learning more about themselves and their practice.

It was through the people who attended the first critical reflective practice group that I was then able to make inroads into the organization and introduce critical reflection to other teams. The following section gives a brief overview of the different settings and groups that have since gone on to use critical reflection, and provides some highlights of what I have learnt so far.

Learning for a manager

A manager from a busy hospital social work team invited me to run critical reflective practice sessions with her team.

She scheduled four sessions over 4 months. I worked with a co-facilitator in the sessions. We introduced the model to the group and at each session one of the workers presented their critical incident. We supported each of them to use both stages of the model. The structured approach helped the group to focus on using the style of questioning that is needed to unearth fundamental assumptions. A key to the success of each session was the enthusiastic manager who had allowed the time and space for her team to meet. She conveyed that she wanted her practitioners to critically reflect to help them to deal with some of the challenges of their work and to use the model to think and talk about their practice. She believed that it was a supportive part of being a manager. At the end of one particular session the manager shared with the group what she had learnt and how she would change her management style to be more supportive.

A model for practice educators working with students

A practice educator workshop is run every month in my organization for social workers who supervise and assess social work students on placement. The workshops use a peer support model to share best practice and promote ways of working with students to help them learn. I had observed a tendency for these sessions to turn into 'moaning' about problems they were having rather than looking for solutions or sharing best practice. I introduced the model of critical reflective practice to the group to empower them to look at the problems that were presented differently. I felt that supporting them to critically reflect would also support them to assist their students' learning. What I found was that the process of critical reflection was new to the entire group and they needed to be trained in how to use the model and practise this at each session. All of them had critical incidents that they wanted to look at. This process of working with practice educators not only provided an insight into how the organization is supporting the next generation of social workers but also how we sometimes overlook what some of our most experienced professionals need for their own learning and development.

Occupational therapists and interprofessional working

A group of occupational therapists in the organization asked me to run a critical reflective practice session. When I first met with this group, they already had a supervision group in place and the critical learning climate had been established.

At one of the sessions, Freda presented an incident that involved her experience of managing a case with a client who had physical needs and was in a family with complex dynamics. Freda spoke openly about her concern for the person's social and emotional needs. She had not previously mentioned this in supervision, because she saw her role as confined to clients' physical concerns. As the session progressed, she became aware of the strong values she had about the importance of family. Rather than seeing the limitations of her practice and feeling unable to meet the person's social and emotional needs, she considered the perspectives of other professionals and whether indeed the family issues that she had identified for the client could be further supported by another professional such as a social worker. This then led her to consider the importance of working more closely with her professional colleagues. Freda moved on from seeing the limitations of her practice and the frustrations of this to now being able to meet the social and emotional needs of her client. This learning changed her planned approach to her work and her relationship with other professionals.

A framework for supervision groups

A supervision group for social workers that was already established was looking for a model that they could use at each session. I ran a number of sessions with the group but also invited one of the group members to co-facilitate, so that over time the group would be able to run their own sessions. The group's initial reactions to the model when it was taught were very positive, and comments were made such as 'this is what we should be doing' and 'this is how practitioners need to think and learn'. The facilitator role was important for the group because I observed that the group fell easily into old habits – it was easy to use the session as a case discussion rather than an opportunity to reflect deeply on the ideas inherent to their approach. The facilitator therefore had to work hard to enable the discussion to focus on the person and their experience of their incident, rather than analysis of the case. There was also a tendency for the group participants to offer advice. When this occurred, the facilitator needed to help the participants to change and adapt their statements into questions. Some interesting critical incidents were presented. For example, during one of the sessions the worker who was presenting openly spoke about how she 'was frustrated because the person wouldn't do what [she] thought was right for him'. By the end of the critical reflective session she talked about how she realized that she 'couldn't control everything in a client's life' and discussed changing her practice to reflect the need to respect the rights and views of the client. She also showed

insight into her understanding of power. What was remarkable about this group was how open and honest they were in talking about their personal values and how this influences their practice.

Concluding remarks

Regardless of whether practitioners feel ashamed, or proud, of something they have done, critical reflection can help them stand back and use a logical and systematic approach to learn more from it. For some, this may be uncomfortable, for others it is liberating, and for some it is both. Space and time to think are essential components for critical reflection to work at its best. Commitment is also needed from the group, to help create an environment of trust and positive regard. With the support of a facilitator and the group, practitioners can question where their thoughts come from and how this influences what they see and how they practise. Critical reflection can help a person shift their focus, and discover a new way of thinking and ways of doing things differently. It is a process of empowerment and transformation.

Critical reflection is a necessary part of how I now continue to develop and work. At the start of this section I referred to my critical incident of the fatal fire, and how through the process of critical reflection I was enabled to examine and learn from my experience. It was a process that helped me to move forward but more importantly to rebuild my confidence to practise. What I never envisaged, however, was how the change that I experienced then enabled me to help other social workers across the organization to learn and develop their practice. My new level of awareness about the benefits of critical reflection motivated me to influence and potentially change the culture of learning across the whole organization. What I have learnt from this whole experience is that an organization without critical reflection is an organization that may be missing out on learning.

> ### REFLECTION
>
> What assumptions do you think you make about the role of managers and what being a manager involves? How do you think these ideas have influenced the way you do your own work?

CONCLUSION

Can critical reflection help restore the craft of caring, and if so, how might it best be implemented as part of a programme of systematic learning for busy professionals in complex workplaces? We have attempted to shed some light on these two questions, through introducing a clear model for practising reflection; discussing

the perceived benefits of carrying out critical reflection in this way; and posing some practical issues for how it might work better.

Indeed, being able to practise the craft of caring is not the sole responsibility of individual nurses, nor of the organizations in which they work. It is surely a joint responsibility.

We hope this chapter has illustrated how being critically reflective, either in groups, in supervision, or even in one's own practice, can help to reconnect us with the fundamental values which underpin why we work in the people professions. This might carve a path for professionals and organizations to work together in practising, and creating an environment for, the craft of caring.

> ## REFLECTION
>
> How do you think you might integrate critical reflection into your own practice? What might be some of the difficulties involved in doing this?

References

1. Nussbaum M. *Cultivating humanity: a classical defence of reform in liberal education.* Cambridge, MA: Harvard University Press, 1997.
2. Dewey J. *How we think: a restatement of the relation of reflective thinking to the educative process.* Boston: Heath, 1933.
3. Leicht KT, Walter T, Saisanhea I, Davies S. New public management and new professionalism across nations and contexts. *Current Sociology* 2009; **57**(4): 581–605.
4. Polkinghorne D. *Practice and the human sciences: the case for a judgement-based ethics of care.* New York: State University of New York Press, 2004.
5. Swinton J. The wisdom of L'Arche and the practices of care: disability, professional wisdom and encounter-in-community. In: Bondi L, Carr D, Clark C, Clegg C (eds). *Towards professional wisdom: practical deliberation in the people professions.* Farnham: Ashgate, 2011: 153–68.
6. Department of Health. *Compassion in practice: nursing, midwifery and care staff: our vision and strategy.* London: The Stationery Office, 2012.
7. Department of Health. *Department of Health's response to the Francis Inquiry: Hard truths: the journey to putting patients first.* London: The Stationery Office, 2013.
8. Boud D, Keogh R, Walker D (eds). *Reflection: turning experience into learning.* London: Kogan Page, 1984.
9. Schon D. *The reflective practitioner: how professionals think in action.* New York: Basic Books, 1983.
10. Fook J, Gardner F. *Practising critical reflection: a resource handbook.* Maidenhead: Open University Press, 2007.
11. Fook J. Challenges of creating critically reflective groups. *Social Work with Groups* 2012; **35**(3): 218–34.

Further reading

Gardner F. Using critical reflection to research practice in a mental health setting. In: Fook J, Gardner F (eds). *Critical reflection in context.* London and New York: Routledge, 2013: 68–80.

Johns C. *Becoming a reflective practitioner*, 4th edn. Chichester: Wiley-Blackwell, 2013.

Tiberius V. The reflective life: character and the values we live with. 2005. Available from: http://www.scotsphil.org.uk/documents/TiberiusReflectiveLifeCh1-Introduction.pdf [Accessed 2nd September 2016].

Relevant web pages

Learning through reflection. www.nwlink.com/~donclark/hrd/development/reflection.html

Stanford Encyclopaedia of Philosophy. Reflective equilibrium. plato.stanford.edu/entries/reflective-equilibrium

Section 2

The foundations of mental health nursing

Classification of mental illness

DAVID KINGDON, SHANAYA RATHOD AND CAROLYN ASHER

LEARNING OUTCOMES

- To understand the importance of diagnosis for evidence-based practice and empowering and facilitating self-management.
- To understand the complementary importance of diagnosis, formulation and narrative.
- To be aware of the relationship of stigma to diagnosis.
- To have a broad overview of diagnostic categories.

SUMMARY OF KEY POINTS

- Classification and diagnoses in mental health are controversial and can be misused, but they are necessary for communication.
- Systems should be as reliable, valid, culturally appropriate and useful in clinical practice as possible.
- The key system used internationally is described in the Mental and Behavioural Disorders Chapter (V) of the *International classification of diseases* (10th edition).
- Broad diagnostic categories are used in treatment guidelines and these, rather than narrower categories, are most useful in clinical practice.

INTRODUCTION

Diagnosis and classification systems of mental disorders have raised controversy over many years. They have been extensively criticized as being:

- reductionist: i.e. simplistic, not providing a holistic view of the individual, reducing the person to merely a 'label';
- unreliable: i.e. not being repeatable from one psychiatrist (or anyone else making a diagnosis) to another; in other words, producing different diagnoses between different observers and also the same observer at different times in the person's episode of illness;

- invalid: i.e. not describing real entities in the world which are meaningful in terms of service user experience or needs, or indicating interventions to assist them.

Diagnosis has certainly been misused to categorize and depersonalize individuals with dismissal of their complex unique individual histories. This is not unique to psychiatry but is also a feature of other areas of medicine. This has discredited psychiatry in the view of many professionals and service users. The value of the individualized formulation has been highlighted as an alternative way of communicating in a meaningful and acceptable manner.

However, it is very difficult to get away from the inevitable tendency that we have to group and name phenomena, experiences and objects. This helps us make sense of the world which can otherwise seem chaotic and every new experience requires a completely new response. Classifications therefore have been developed for flowers, animals, furniture, diseases and music (rock, folk, hip-hop), to give just a few examples, but acceptance is needed of the limitations of such processes. See chapter 8 for a discussion on nursing classification and care planning. The advantages are that they ease communication and define groups which can be investigated. They also allow research into groups to be conducted, they allow treatments to be developed and prescribed, and they allow the individual to find out more about specific issues, such as depression or eating disorders.

Classification can occur at various levels. 'Mental health' and 'mental disorder' are broad descriptive terms and it is worth considering what they mean. The World Health Organization (WHO) says:

Mental health is defined as a state of well-being in which every individual realizes his or her own potential, can cope with the normal stresses of life, can work productively and fruitfully, and is able to make a contribution to her or his community.[1]

Mental disorder is the opposite – a state where mental health is impaired, causing distress or disability. However, people can often maintain good functioning and may not even be distressed by what to others may seem to be a mental disorder. For example, some people hear voices and value the experience. 'Normal' stresses, such as bereavements, can cause distress and there have been persisting arguments about whether these should be defined as disorders. However, to exclude anything that has an understandable cause would mean that many people with distress and disability from the consequences of life experiences might not receive the help from which they could benefit. The concept of 'mental illness' is helpful as it describes a situation where health is affected by a mental disorder (however caused), and a response by society is appropriate.

A core problem is the confusion about how mental disorder relates to mental illness. The *Diagnostic and statistical manual* (DSM)[2] in particular has struggled with this, and it seems to be attempting to define illness rather than disorder. Defining who is ill is really society's job, based on – but not the same as – a classification of disorders. The concept of illness is used to describe situations where support for individuals is appropriate. This is where their human experiences have caused and may continue to cause distress to them or otherwise interfere with their lives. They are consequently excused from some or all of their responsibilities (such as going to work

or washing the dishes), while they receive help to cure or cope with their problems – their illness. It can therefore relate to physical but also to mental functioning. Society, in a range of ways, often involving health professionals, determines receipt of the 'sick role'. Mental health professionals may guide this, but do not determine it. On that basis, it would be reasonable to say that bereavement may cause distress (mental disorder) but may not be an illness as most people accept and work through it. In some circumstances, the reaction to bereavement is so distressing and disabling that support is given – time off work and perhaps psychological help until recovery occurs. Refer to chapter 61 for a further discussion on bereavement and grief counselling.

Classification systems describe groups which resemble each other in ways that are meaningful: most such systems, such as those for flora and fauna, do not judge whether, for example, a flower is a weed or not (i.e. disordered or not), but simply whether it exists and whether it should be part of one group or another. So there is also a case for having a classification system of mental states or conditions rather than disorders. It would then be perfectly appropriate to provide evidence for the conditions, with relevant inclusion and exclusion criteria, for which there are effective treatments.

A further issue is whether mental disorders are appropriately classified, and the controversy over the DSM suggests that doubts about this remain. Despite this, practitioners, psychiatrists and therapists have grouped individuals together for the purpose of research and teaching, and broad categories such as those used in treatment guidelines (e.g. from the UK National Institute for Health and Care Excellence (NICE), and the US Schizophrenia Patient Outcomes Research Team (PORT)) have been widely accepted.

There remain some concerns about the terminology that is used, and 'schizophrenia'[3] and 'personality disorder'[4] have been particularly criticized in this context as stigmatizing or even, in the case of the latter, rather insulting. Alternatives that seem more acceptable to clients include 'psychosis' and 'emotional dysregulation/difficulties' or trauma-related terms.

While most people therefore agree with the benefits of having a classification system, the creation of classification systems in mental disorders has been fraught with challenges. There has been a lack of agreement among psychiatrists and other health professionals regarding the concepts upon which classification should be based: diagnoses can rarely be verified objectively in biological terms, and the same or similar conditions are described under a confusing variety of names, particularly in the schizophrenia group of disorders. Classifications of mental illnesses are snapshots of knowledge at a given point in time, and they evolve and change as our understanding of illness changes. Despite the challenges, it is widely acknowledged that there is a need for a universal language that can help professionals to communicate with each other and with patients. There are other reasons why we need classification systems. A diagnosis helps clinicians to plan management, prescribe treatments and acquire funding for certain treatments in the NHS such as clozapine and psychological treatment, and in the private sector through insurance. It can aid discussions on prognosis. Diagnosis is a prerequisite to research; for example, for understanding epidemiology and interventions and hence planning and costing services. Traditionally, mental health services have been commissioned through block contracts. Future payment in mental health is likely to be determined by diagnosis and care packages linked to the same. Therefore it is important to have robust and widely agreed systems of diagnosis.

However, there are particular disadvantages of classification systems and diagnosis that are specific to mental health. The stigma of mental illness continues to be a problem in society, and this is specifically linked to diagnosis. Classification systems are notorious for creating an illusion of discrete entities, whereas many mental disorders exist on a spectrum and are variants, often at the extreme, of individual lifestyles, beliefs and behaviours.

Homosexuality provided the most controversial representation of this, as it was defined by the DSM as a mental disorder until a vote of the American Psychiatric Association (APA) in 1973 overturned this decision. Culture also influences the way in which people attribute symptoms to mental illness, engage with services and choose treatments.

REFLECTION

- What problems have you found with using diagnoses?

- What problems have you found when you have tried to avoid using them?

- Are there particular times when diagnosis can be misunderstood?

- How would people find out about their conditions if they did not use names? Would looking up information on symptoms be sufficient?

WHAT CONSTITUTES A GOOD CLASSIFICATION SYSTEM?

Jablensky and Kendell[5] defined the criteria for assessing a classification system in psychiatry as:

1. *Reliability:* Reliability shows how far errors of measurement have been excluded from assessment. Diagnostic reliability can be improved by operational diagnostic criteria and by using structured interview schedules. Reliability establishes a ceiling for validity. Lower reliability means lower validity, but the converse does not hold true.

2. *Validity:* Validity establishes how far a test actually measures what it is supposed to measure, meaning 'the nature of reality'.

3. *Utility:* Utility is a graded concept and is partially context-dependent. The clinical utility of a classificatory system can be assessed empirically by taking into account its impact on three domains: its use in practice and in the decision-making process and its relationship to clinical outcome.

4. *Ease of use:* A classification system will only be used if it is convenient and relevant to clinical staff.

5. *Applicability across settings and cultures:* As we have mentioned, psychopathology and diagnosis can be influenced by culture, and generalizability is important.

6. *Meeting the needs of various users:* If a classification system is a language for communication, it should meet the needs of clinicians, researchers and users of mental health services.

THE MAIN CLASSIFICATION SYSTEMS

There are currently two widely established classification systems for mental disorders – Chapter V of the *International classification of diseases*,[1,6,7] and the *Diagnostic and statistical manual of mental disorders*[2] by the APA. There are other national classification systems, such as the Chinese and French systems, as well, but these are not used as widely.

The origins of the DSM date back to 1940, when the government wanted to collect data on mental illness. DSM-I was published by the APA in 1952 and since then it has evolved significantly, culminating in the latest DSM-5 which was published in May 2013. Reliability tests have been used in the development of the DSM-5.

The ICD-10 was published in 1992 and involved the efforts of 700 psychiatrists from 52 countries and cooperation with the APA. It had its origins in Bertillon's Classification of Causes of Death, which evolved into the International List of Causes of Death. Following this, the WHO in 1948 published the *International statistical classification of diseases, injuries and causes of death*. ICD-11 is due for release in 2017. Although there is an aspiration to harmonize the two systems, there have been important differences between them in the past (such as the criteria for schizoaffective disorder), and there are likely to be others in the future. See Boxes 12.1 and 12.2.

BOX 12.1: ICD-10: MENTAL AND BEHAVIOURAL DISORDERS (F00–F99)

F00–F09: Organic, including symptomatic, mental disorders

F10–F19: Mental and behavioural disorders due to psychoactive substance use

F20–F29: Schizophrenia, schizotypal and delusional disorders

F30–F39: Mood [affective] disorders

F40–F48: Neurotic, stress-related and somatoform disorders

F50–F59: Behavioural syndromes associated with physiological disturbances and physical factors

F60–F69: Disorders of adult personality and behaviour

F70–F79: Mental retardation

F80–F89: Disorders of psychological development

F90–F98: Behavioural and emotional disorders with onset usually occurring in childhood and adolescence

F99: Unspecified mental disorder

Both the ICD-10 and DSM-5 systems can be defined as 'categorical classifications'. In addition to categorical diagnoses, a dimensional approach used in the DSM-5 allows clinicians to rate disorders along a continuum of severity that eliminates the need for 'not otherwise specified (NOS)' conditions, now termed 'not elsewhere defined (NED)' conditions. The dimensional diagnostic system also correlates better with treatment planning. A multiaxial system was used in the DSM-IV but was not successful in practice, and so the DSM-5 now comprises three sections:

- Section 1: An introduction on how to use the updated manual.
- Section 2: An outline of the categorical diagnoses according to a revised chapter organization.
- Section 3: Diagnostic categories that require further research and/or more time for clinicians to become acquainted with before being included in Section 2, as well as usable tools that should enhance diagnosis of the conditions listed in Section 2. The latter includes patient-rated and clinician-rated measures of symptoms that cut across all DSM diagnoses, measures of disability, information about how cultural context can influence the presentation of mental illnesses, and an alternative model for diagnosis of personality disorders.

BOX 12.2: DSM-5: DIAGNOSTIC CATEGORIES

1. Neurodevelopmental disorders
2. Schizophrenia spectrum and other psychotic disorders
3. Bipolar and related disorders
4. Depressive disorders
5. Anxiety disorders
6. Obsessive–compulsive and related disorders
7. Trauma and stressor related disorders
8. Dissociative disorders
9. Somatic symptoms and related disorders
10. Feeding and eating disorders
11. Sleep–wake disorders
12. Sexual dysfunction
13. Gender dysphoria
14. Disruptive, impulse control and conduct disorders
15. Substance related and addictive disorders
16. Neurocognitive disorders
17. Paraphilic disorders
18. Personality disorders

ICD-10 also uses a multiaxial approach, with three axes and, as with DSM-5, personality disorder is not separated from other mental state disorders. The ICD-10 system recommends that where multiple Axis I diagnoses coexist (i.e. there is comorbidity) all should be recorded, beginning with the most prominent. The axes in ICD-10 are:

- Axis I: Current mental state diagnosis including personality disorder.
- Axis II: Disabilities.
- Axis III: Contextual factors.

Both systems promote a hierarchy in selecting diagnoses, with certain categories tending to be more dominant; for example, if someone meets criteria for an organic disorder and psychosis or a common mental disorder, a diagnosis of the organic disorder is made. This generally makes sense in that, for example, in delirium or dementia, psychotic or depressive symptoms are common but treatment will focus on the organic disorder first. However, as this example illustrates, it is limited and has meant that secondary diagnoses, such as depression, have been ignored when they may be treatable in their own right.

Operational definitions in the ICD-10 are less rigid than in DSM, as it is more clinically orientated and favours general descriptions. This flexibility poses disadvantages when a classification system has to serve a multitude of users. The ICD-10 allows clinical judgement to inform diagnoses, but this freedom makes it unsuitable for research purposes, necessitating the development of separate research diagnostic criteria.[7] Thus, different versions of ICD-10 now exist and these include the clinical version,[6] a version with diagnostic criteria for research (which resembles DSM in its use of detailed operational criteria) and a version for use in primary care,[7] the latter consisting of definitions of 25 common conditions as well as a shorter version of six disorders for use by other primary care workers.

CLINICAL GUIDELINES

In the past, diagnosis has been considered a medical responsibility, but in modern services, where many patients are not seen by doctors, there is a need for a system of allocation to diagnoses to guide practice. The use of clinical guidelines, such as those produced by NICE, is now required by monitoring organizations such as the Care Quality Commission in the UK. The guidelines used in mental health have been developed to cover broad categories, and allocation to these categories is necessary to inform good practice. Where there are doubts about allocation, medical opinion can be sought from GPs or psychiatrists. The UK guidance on *New ways of working for psychiatrists*[8] was developed with this multidisciplinary context in mind, such that psychiatric time was freed to facilitate advice to practitioners on diagnosis, safety issues and clinical management. However, the guideline groupings are relatively self-evident and it is arguable whether the sub-categories in ICD-10 and DSM-5 add much to them that is useful.[9] Major ones are:

- psychosis and schizophrenia;
- psychosis with substance misuse;
- common mental disorders (with specific guidelines for anxiety, depression, obsessive compulsive disorder, and post-traumatic stress disorder);
- eating disorders;
- personality disorders (including 'borderline');
- bipolar disorder;
- substance misuse;
- learning disability.

DIFFERENTIATING BETWEEN CONDITIONS

Diagnosis is currently based on identifying patterns of signs and symptoms that service users experience. There are no biochemical, neuroimaging or genetic tests relevant for clinical practice. Although this may be seen as a disadvantage to diagnosis in other areas, as mental illness by its nature involves a disorder of mental functioning (as opposed to demonstrable brain malfunction), it is not unreasonable to expect diagnosis to depend on identification of psychological and behavioural phenomena. This may be seen as subjective, but reliability can be achieved with the use of training, prompted by appropriate instruments. Much is made of the differences between individuals making diagnoses, but in practice, agreement around broad categories guiding management is usually achieved, and any changes that are made are carried out through a process of reassessment of evidence. The major categories, though not exhaustive, are given below and will be further briefly discussed.

Psychosis and *schizophrenia* are increasingly used interchangeably, with the former being increasingly preferred by service users, especially when linked to social categories.[10] Psychosis is a condition where the boundary between what is real and what is imagined is breached – so people hear voices that others cannot hear (hallucinate) and have beliefs which do not seem to be supported by evidence (delusions) – for example, that people are conspiring against them or that they hold a very high position. They may also be very difficult to understand, jumping from topic to topic (thought disorder). However, these alone are not sufficient for a diagnosis, as there is very good evidence that hearing voices is common in society, and beliefs that do not hold up to scientific scrutiny are similarly widespread. There is a continuum between psychosis and normal thought, and it is only described and diagnosed as an illness where it is seriously interfering with functioning or causing distress (usually to the person themselves, but occasionally to others) and therefore intervention or treatment becomes relevant. Usually this is a cooperative process between mental health or primary care professionals but not always – where safety issues or effects on health become sufficient for intervention to occur. Traumatic events in childhood are common, including bullying, but also childhood abuse, and this may sometimes lead to symptoms of emotional dysregulation ('borderline personality disorder') within which the hearing of voices and paranoia develop.[11] Disputes as to whether the person has schizophrenia or 'personality disorder' can arise and are not helpful, as individuals can have both ('traumatic psychosis'). They then require help for both types of experience.

Later onset psychosis is also recognized ('delusional disorder') where a specific delusion presents in an individual who is otherwise socially competent, and this can elaborate into a system involving neighbours, work colleagues and so on, and lead to conflict with them.

Psychosis with substance misuse, sometimes called 'dual diagnosis', or residual psychosis after substance misuse, is common and important to diagnose. 'Dual diagnosis' can also be used to describe psychosis and learning disability, so it is not a helpful term. Psychosis can be directly caused by drug misuse and then remit after the drugs leave the person's system, but psychosis can also persist after the use of drugs has stopped, especially in the case of hallucinogenics and stimulants including cocaine, amphetamines and cannabis (especially in higher concentrations). This group of people with psychosis have been found to have higher levels of positive (voices, delusions and thought disorder) and lower negative symptoms, and they are more sociable, but can be involved more in safety/risk issues than others with psychosis.

Bipolar disorder is a usefully descriptive term which has replaced 'manic depression'. It describes someone who has had at least one manic episode at some time. Mania describes a state that usually involves persistent elation (though it can also involve irritability and overactivity) lasting for at least 7 days. Hypomania is a term used to describe a less intense or persistent state and alone is not sufficient for a diagnosis under ICD-10. However, this has been confused by the introduction of categories in DSM-IV which use terms such as bipolar 2 and spectrum disorder: generally, research into treatments has not included these categories and there is considerable overlap with 'borderline personality disorder' and substance use disorders. Most patients with bipolar disorder – though not all – become depressed at some stage, and depression may persist or they may become euthymic (normal mood) between episodes.

Common mental disorders is a term used to group together anxiety disorders, depression, obsessive–compulsive disorder and post-traumatic stress disorder. In some ways this grouping helps, as there is considerable overlap between these categories, and the medications used, especially 'antidepressants', do not tend to differentiate between them. Nevertheless, each has specific guidelines provided, and psychological treatments, especially cognitive behaviour therapies, tend to use common principles and practices in engagement, formulation and so on, even if there is a variety of techniques used. As with psychosis, these disorders exist on a continuum: we acknowledge that anxiety and depression are appropriate in response to threat and loss (for example, bereavement), and indeed help us respond to them. However, even when it is clear that there is a cause for the distress, it can become overwhelming, and help can become necessary and desired – in other words, it becomes appropriate to treat, or help cope with, an anxiety state or depressive illness. Obsessive–compulsive disorder, which manifests itself through rituals and ruminations, is also on a continuum with normal preoccupation and routines, but reaches levels where intervention is appropriate and a diagnosis should be made to facilitate coping and treatment of distress and interference with functioning. Physical symptoms not caused by physical illness (somatic symptoms disorder – inappropriately known more commonly as medically unexplained symptoms) are common in primary care and acute hospitals and are often explained by anxiety or depression – and frequently respond to psychological treatment.

Eating disorders is a term used to describe anorexia nervosa (the diagnosis depends on characteristic beliefs and low body mass index) and bulimia (binge eating and vomiting). Obesity tends not to be included in this classification group, though strictly an eating disorder.

Personality disorder, as discussed previously, is a very unhelpful and stigmatizing term which overgeneralizes behaviour, especially when referring to relationships with others. Classification systems include a range of terms, most of which are unhelpful, as people do not present to services with, for example, narcissistic personality. They will present with, for example, depression or anxiety. The way they respond to these emotions will be affected by, and cause effects on, their relationships. 'Borderline' personality disorder is probably a more useful grouping, which presents as an emotional disorder with extreme but often fluctuating distress in the context of negative childhood experiences. Antisocial personality disorder (or similar terms) is also recognized but not responsive (yet, perhaps) to psychological treatment. It is arguable whether it is helpful to describe it as a mental disorder and rarely, if ever, does describing it as a mental illness help the individual (at least in the long term) or society. 'Conduct disorder', a diagnosis used for children, is arguably a more descriptive term, and treatment is offered for this for immediate management and prevention of progression into adulthood.

Substance use disorders include substance abuse and misuse, which are simply terms to describe different degrees of disorder (DSM-5 now just uses the term 'substance use disorders'). Abuse could be described as exceeding the recommended levels of alcohol intake or using any illicit drug, but in clinical practice it tends to be reserved for higher levels of use, including binge drinking, which cause damage to the individual.

Learning disability is described as 'mental retardation' in most countries and in ICD-10. It is defined as 'a condition of arrested or incomplete development of the mind, which is especially characterized by impairment of skills manifested during the developmental period, skills which contribute to the overall level of intelligence, i.e. cognitive, language, motor, and social abilities'. It can be mild, moderate or severe, and qualified by a statement of no, or minimal, or significant impairment of behaviour. 'Mild' is described in ICD-10 as an IQ of 50 to 69 or a mental age from 9 to under 12, so is often described as 'borderline'. In clinical practice, emotional and social factors are very important in addition to IQ in deciding whether someone needs support for their learning disability. People with learning disability are more likely than most to have additional physical and mental health problems.

CULTURE AND CLASSIFICATION

The role of culture in diagnosis and classification systems has been acknowledged and an outline for cultural formulation was first introduced in DSM-IV, based on the recommendations of an independent National Institute of Mental Health (NIMH) workgroup on culture[12] but there was no method for collecting the required information. Subsequently, guidelines and practical approaches to develop a cultural formulation were proposed.[13] DSM-5 describes five aspects of culture that need to be taken into account in formulation of any case: cultural identity of the individual, cultural conceptualization of illness, psychosocial factors and cultural stressors, cultural features of the relationships between the individual and others, and overall cultural assessment.

CONCLUSION

The diagnosis and classification of mental disorders do create confusion and controversy and some of the terminology used is unnecessarily stigmatizing. But broad categories (such as depression and psychosis) are necessary to guide treatment and research and to empower service users to understand, learn about and thus engage fully in their recovery process. The two systems that exist, ICD-10 and DSM-5, have much in common. However, the former is the one that is used for clinical and statistical purposes in the UK and most countries outside the USA.

SERVICE USER COMMENTARY

Carolyn Asher

This chapter is an interesting look at the area of diagnosis and categorization which so often leads to stigma and discrimination. The chapter brings an understanding of the way in which an individual, culturally sensitive formulation can be a vast improvement on an ill-fitting diagnostic system. The chapter looks at the criticisms of the categorization systems that surround diagnosis, and it also looks at the way categorization can lead to an individual having a label. Ideally people shouldn't be given a label, especially those labels that bring stigma and discrimination. The issues surrounding diagnosis and its patriarchal power-heavy perspective mean that something needs to change within the structures of categorization to limit the stigma and discrimination that diagnostic categories bring. However, research, NHS payment and treatment standards need to use categories (diagnoses) that are easily communicated so that everyone knows what is being discussed. I am happy to see the idea that life experiences are considered rather than a diagnosis, and that mental states rather than disorders could be an alternative for categorizing mental illness. This individualized method is sure to improve, as we spread and create more knowledge through the effects of research. With this in mind, mental illness will be seen in a different light and treatments should become less troublesome as the specific causes of and issues surrounding mental illness are discovered.

References

1. WHO (World Health Organization). *International statistical classification of diseases and related health problems 10th revision (ICD-10) version for 2010.* Chapter V. Available from: http://apps.who.int/classifications/icd10/browse/2010/en#/V [Accessed 27th June 2016].
2. APA (American Psychiatric Association). *Diagnostic and statistical manual of mental disorders, fifth edition (DSM-5).* Washington DC: APA, 2013.
3. Kingdon D, Taylor L, Ma K, Kinoshita Y. Changing name: changing prospects for psychosis. *Epidemiology and Psychiatric Sciences* 2013; **22**: 297–301.
4. Kingdon D. DSPD or 'don't stigmatise people in distress'. *Advances in Psychiatric Treatment* 2007; **13**: 333–5.
5. Jablensky A, Kendell RE. Criteria for assessing a classification in psychiatry. In: Ma M, Gaebel W, López-Ibor J, Sartorius N (eds). *Psychiatric diagnosis and classification.* Chichester: John Wiley & Sons Ltd, 2002: 1–24.
6. WHO (World Health Organization). *The ICD-10 classification of mental and behavioural disorders. Diagnostic criteria for research.* Geneva: WHO, 1992. Available from: http://www.who.int/classifications/icd/en/GRNBOOK.pdf [Accessed 27th June 2016].

7. WHO (World Health Organization). *Diagnostic and management guidelines for mental disorders in primary care. ICD-10 chapter V primary care version.* Göttingen: WHO/Hogrefe and Huber, 1996. Available from: http://apps.who.int/iris/bitstream/10665/41852/1/0889371482_eng.pdf [Accessed 27th June 2016].

8. Department of Health. *New ways of working for psychiatrists: enhancing effective, person-centred services through new ways of working in multidisciplinary and multiagency contexts.* London: Department of Health, 2005.

9. Kingdon D, Afghan S, Arnold R, Faruqui R, Friedman T, Jones I, Jones P, Lloyd K, Nicholls D, O'Neill T, Qurashi I, Ramzan A, Series H, Staufenberg E, Brugha T. A diagnostic system using broad categories with clinically relevant specifiers: lessons for ICD-11. *International Journal of Social Psychiatry* 2010; **56**: 326–35.

10. Kingdon DG, Ashcroft K, Bhandari B, Gleeson S, Warikoo N, Symons M, Taylor L, Lucas E, Mahendra R, Ghosh S, Mason A, Badrakalimuthu R, Hepworth C, Read J, Mehta R. Schizophrenia and borderline personality disorder: similarities and differences in the experience of auditory hallucinations, paranoia, and childhood trauma. *Journal of Nervous and Mental Disease* 2010; **198**: 399–403.

11. Kingdon D, Gibson A, Kinoshita Y, Turkington D, Rathod S, Morrison A. Acceptable terminology and subgroups in schizophrenia: an exploratory study. *Social Psychiatry and Psychiatric Epidemiology* 2008; **43**: 239–43.

12. Mezzich JE, Kirmayer LJ, Kleinman A, Fabrega H Jr, Parron DL, Good BJ, Lin KM, Manson SM. The place of culture in DSM-IV. *Journal of Nervous and Mental Disease* 1999; **187**: 457–64.

13. Mezzich JE, Caracci G, Fabrega H, Kirmayer LJ. Cultural formulation guidelines. *Transcultural Psychiatry* 2009; **46**: 383–405.

Further reading

Frances A. *Saving normal: an insider's revolt against out-of-control psychiatric diagnosis.* New York: Morrow, 2013.

Johnstone L. *A straight talking introduction to psychiatric diagnosis.* Ross-on Wye: PCCS Books, 2014.

Katona C, Cooper C. *Psychiatry at a glance.* Chichester: John Wiley & Sons, 2015.

Relevant web pages

Emotional Well-Being. http://www.emotionalwellbeing.southcentral.nhs.uk/conditions/diagnosis

WHO (World Health Organization). *International classification of diseases (ICD).* http://www.who.int/classifications/icd/en/

13 Assessment: the key to effective practice

TONY WARNE, SUE McANDREW AND FIONA JONES

LEARNING OUTCOMES

- To understand the importance of assessment in promoting good mental health care.
- To be able to identify the different phases of the assessment process within the context of developing a therapeutic relationship.
- To understand the use of self within the assessment processes.
- To be able to demonstrate the acquisition of knowledge and skills that would facilitate an accurate collaborative assessment.

SUMMARY OF KEY POINTS

- Assessment is an ongoing dynamic process.
- As a process, it moves through a number of phases, requiring the nurse to engage in a variety of roles.
- The purpose of assessment is to gather knowledge – professional and personal knowledge and patient experience – to enhance our understanding of the person and the context of their distress.
- The most important and valuable assessment tool is that of self.

- It is only when we are able to facilitate the telling of the story and respond with respect, empathy and compassion that we will be able to offer attuned, sensitive mental health care.

This chapter draws upon a case study of a patient called Tess to help you work towards achieving these learning objectives. At different points in the chapter a number of questions are presented to guide your thinking and further reading.

INTRODUCTION

Our starting point in this chapter is the notion that assessment should form the fundamental basis of good mental health nursing practice. Chapter 14 explores the types of assessment that are often used in mental health care, and while we may touch upon some of these assessments and the reason for their use, this chapter deals with the relationship between assessment, care, recovery and an individual's life journey, and the way all of us assess and make judgements. For further information on family assessment see chapter 15.

We all engage in making assessments every day of our lives. Making assessments is how we make choices, take decisions and make judgements about a whole range of factors that are likely to impact upon our lives. Some of these assessments will require time, information, reflection and knowledge, while others are likely to be more superficial and in the moment. However, almost all assessments and the consequential actions will be influenced by previous lived experience.[1]

REFLECTION

As a starting point: think of four people you know, two of whom you like and two to whom you have taken a dislike. Write down their first names and under each name write down the reasons you like/dislike each of them. Consider the list under each name and how it relates to the time you have known the person, knowledge about the person and where that knowledge came from, and previous experiences that have direct or indirect links with that person. With regard to the latter, consider whether these have been direct experiences of the person, or experiences of another person who reminds you of the person identified. Reflect on each of your lists and consider what has influenced your opinion of each person and how this might have impacted on your relationship with them. Now consider why you have been asked to undertake this exercise and how it might relate to your everyday clinical practice.

Our lived experience results from the experiences we are exposed to from childhood through adulthood and older age. The education we receive, both formal and informal, the relationships we form and the aspirations we hold for our own achievements will all contribute to how we assess situations. Our lived experiences are shaped and tempered by our values and beliefs and the cultural contexts in which we live.

Anticipation, probability and predictability are also factors that mediate the processes of assessment. The degree of importance we attach to these various factors will also be dependent upon the particular assessment situation, our previous experience and, to some degree, our expectations of the desired outcome. For example, working on a medium secure unit can often be anxiety-provoking for those unfamiliar with this situation, as it is often considered an 'unpredictable' setting. The anticipation, on the part of inexperienced staff, regarding the possibility of a person becoming aggressive and/or violent can create a tension that may lead to an undesirable outcome – a self-fulfilling prophecy – the person does become aggressive and someone may get hurt. However, if we can consider an alternative ending, staying calm while speaking to the person about their current distress, we are more likely to successfully achieve the desired outcome of gaining insight into and understanding of their problems.

In undertaking an assessment as part of our practice as mental health nurses, we will draw upon the same range of factors as those we use in 'everyday life'. It is the desired outcomes that are likely to be different, if only in the degree of purposefulness and the structure used in any particular assessment. As you will see from chapter 14, there are a number of assessment tools that have been developed through research-based approaches to aid the assessment process. Barker[2] notes that, despite this apparently scientific-based approach to assessment, where people are concerned, assessment is more an art form than a scientific endeavour. An example of this notion is to be found in the *Diagnostic and statistical manual of mental disorders* (DSM), first published in 1952 and currently in its fifth edition. Published by the American Psychiatric Association, the DSM has been praised for its work in attempting to standardize the criteria used in agreeing diagnostic categories. However, the DSM has also been heavily criticized[3] for its lack of scientific evidence, with categorization often being based upon the subjective opinions of a relatively small number of psychiatrists, who are likely to have a medicalized view of the world and of human distress. Further discussion on the classification of mental illness can be found in chapter 12. While the medical view continues to pervade the domain of mental health/illness, it is well worth visiting some of the work associated with those who challenge the contemporary paradigm of psychiatry. These include a number of seminal texts: Thomas Szasz, *The myth of mental illness*; Ronnie Laing, *The divided self*; and Michael Foucault, *Madness and civilization*, the latter portraying psychiatry as based on repression and control.

Our criticism of the medical model[4] is based upon the notion that how an individual experiences an illness, whether it is a physical or mental health problem, is always going to be different from how it is experienced by others. It will be different even when following some kind of assessment protocol and when similar symptoms are apparent.

Thus, we have long argued[5,6] that mental health nurses need to acknowledge the value there is in the evidence represented by an individual's own experience – something we have described as 'exper(t)ience' knowledge.[6] So when mental health nurses undertake an assessment, recognizing what is being said, or not being said, in a person's account of their current distress is as important as recognition of various clinical and psychological signs and symptoms.

CRAFTING AN ASSESSMENT TO DELIVER APPROPRIATE, COMPASSIONATE CARE

With regard to the 'craft of caring', as with any craft, be it painting a picture, producing a piece of music or building a boat, we need to be able to envisage the end product in its entirety so that we can use the skills and expertise necessary for successful achievement. In applying these principles to mental health nursing, before we can embark on care planning and interventions, we need to hear the telling of the story, to ask questions so we can clarify the priority of problems and collaboratively consider how these might be best addressed to achieve a successful outcome. Such questions, of course, are best answered by the person who is looking to us to provide support and care in their time of distress. Often such people present us with complex problems that at first may seem vague, but nonetheless are impacting on their life to such an extent that they have, or someone close to them has, been prompted to seek help. It is important that a careful and accurate assessment of the person and their situation is made at the beginning of the interaction so that we do not risk adding to their distress.

Nursing, and in particular mental health nursing, is a social activity and, as such, requires that we get to know and understand people by asking questions. Listening to and hearing the person's story and asking appropriate questions will facilitate our understanding of what has happened to that person, their perception of events, how it has impacted on their life and in particular their health, and their thoughts and feelings in the here and now. All of this important information will help us to make sense of what is happening in the person's life and enable us to collaboratively plan what might need to be done to provide appropriate individualized care at a specific time.

CASE STUDY 1

Tess is a 58-year-old woman who has been admitted with depression and/or anxiety. On admission she appeared very anxious and expressed worries as to whether she had locked the doors at her home. Tess lives alone as her husband died nearly 2 years ago. They had no children and it was a friend who had prompted Tess to go to her GP. Over the last few months she had been neglecting herself, not eating and not going to bed at night and had complained of persistent headaches. On meeting Tess initially, she is tearful, looks at the ground and is difficult to engage in conversation.

REFLECTION

- What problems might have led to Tess neglecting herself?

- What skills would you need to use to encourage Tess to tell her story?

- Who might you seek information from in order to learn more about Tess?

In many cases an individual's problems might be multidimensional, with many different causes, each of which might impact upon their mental health and well-being in different ways. The Mental Health Foundation[7] estimated that 33 per cent of all people visiting GPs have mental health problems, and 35 per cent of GPs' time is taken up with dealing with these problems. Many of those presenting at their GPs or accessing other health services for conditions such as stroke, coronary heart disease and diabetes will also have a high risk of related mental health problems (for example, anxiety and/or depression). In primary care, one in five consultations are for somatic symptoms for which no specific cause can be found. Of these, 50 per cent are thought to be related to mental health problems. Likewise, social issues like homelessness, unemployment, loss and so on can have a short- and/or long-term impact upon an individual's mental health and well-being. Therefore mental health nurses need to be skilled in recognizing what, in the moment, and for that individual person, is the area to focus upon.

Assessment has been described as the 'bookends' of nursing care,[2] the initial preliminary assessment being carried out when we first meet the person and the final assessment mapping out the person's preferred way of disengaging with the service. Of course, while the initial exploratory assessment and the final assessment represent the beginning and ending of formal care, assessment is an ongoing process that requires the nurse, in collaboration with the person, to continually re-evaluate their story as they progress through the journey of care.

Throughout this journey it is the interpersonal relationship that will play a central role. When thinking about this, we must consider first impressions, as the way in which we present ourselves as a mental health nurse will influence how the person responds in terms of the telling of their story and how they answer our questions. It is at that first meeting that engagement is likely to occur, the person looking for someone to hold their distress, the nurse showing their receptiveness to provide this service. It is only when such a platform for care has been established that the relationship can move on to embracing collaborative engagement, which has the potential to facilitate mental health care that is satisfying to all parties.[8]

While the focus of this chapter is on assessment, we cannot overemphasize the importance of the interpersonal relationship that begins with the first handshake, hello, eye contact and/or smile, and will go on to act as the lynchpin in the ability to provide good nursing care. Assessment is reliant on such a relationship, as it is only through understanding the person within the given context of their life that we will be able to deliver empathic mental health care within the realities of their world.

THE STAGES OF ASSESSMENT: WALKING IN TANDEM WITH THERAPEUTIC RELATIONSHIPS

The work of Peplau,[9] and her model for mental health nursing, was based on psychoanalytic and humanistic teachings. This model, which is most pertinent to mental health nursing, seeks to explicate the development of a therapeutic relationship, which is the core component of mental health nursing (see chapter 3 for further discussion on developing and maintaining therapeutic relationships). For Peplau, the relationship can be explicated through four phases with which the nurse, along with the service user, has to engage, in order to gain insight into and understanding of the person's world and how, at the present time, it is impacting on their mental well-being. The four phases are listed in Box 13.1.

The orientation phase involves 'getting to know' each other, listening to the person's perceptions of their problems and giving consideration to what immediate help might be offered. The identification phase involves the acknowledging and prioritizing of problems and thinking about how these might best be addressed over a given period of time. The exploitation phase is the 'working' phase, which requires engagement in therapeutic activity, exploring the various issues that are impacting on the person's mental health and exploiting the resources available to address such issues. Finally, the resolution phase involves the termination of the relationship, the person becoming independent of the relationship. As we suggested earlier, assessment is an ongoing process and therefore each of these four phases may remain pertinent throughout the person's care journey.

> ## BOX 13.1: FOUR PHASES OF THE THERAPEUTIC RELATIONSHIP
>
> 1. Orientation
> 2. Identification
> 3. Exploitation
> 4. Resolution

According to Peplau,[9] these four phases were complemented by six roles (since the inception of Peplau's theoretical model, a number of people from a variety of disciplines have added to the roles) which a nurse takes on at any given time in the trajectory of the person's illness. These consist of: stranger, resource person, teacher, counsellor, surrogate and active leader. 'Stranger' is self-explanatory; it is our initial meeting/s with someone and provides the foundation on which the future relationship is built (consider the reflection that we asked you to carry out earlier in this chapter). 'Resource person' is concerned with the provision of what is needed to facilitate understanding and meaning. This could be information and/or the right environment for a person sharing their distress. 'Teacher' refers to imparting knowledge that is required by the person seeking help. The counselling role is one in which the nurse helps the person to understand and develop meaning for their current circumstances and provides encouragement for change to take place. When adopting the surrogate role, the nurse enables the person to clarify areas of dependence, interdependence and independence. This role may also encompass advocacy. Finally, the role of leader requires the nurse to work collaboratively with the person in order for them to assume maximum responsibility in meeting their treatment goals.

These roles do not follow a linear process, but are dynamic. They require the nurse to move in and out of them according to what is occurring in the here-and-now relationship. For example, when thinking about the initial assessment, the nurse may well have to adopt the roles of stranger, teacher and resource person all within the first few minutes of meeting the person: as a stranger, meeting and greeting the person; as a teacher, explaining where things are, such as the toilets; and as a resource person, ensuring they are able to access a quiet place where they cannot be overheard and/or will not be interrupted. While nursing models can at times seem overly theoretical, the phases and roles we have identified above from Peplau's work are, to an extent, natural ones that we readily adopt in our everyday lives.

THE PURPOSE OF ASSESSMENT: KNOWLEDGE, KNOWING AND NOT KNOWING

The purpose of assessment is to develop a meaningful baseline from which we can gain insight into and understanding of the disruptions in a person's life and how, through interventions, this can be resolved to the person's satisfaction. It is about knowledge, knowing and not knowing. *Knowledge* – professional, personal and patient experience knowledge – helps us to integrate new understandings, while *knowing* allows us to draw

on such knowledge, but within the context of the here and now. Knowing therefore forms part of our capacity to explore social and personal narratives, allowing us to make sense of our own and other people's mental state in terms of experiences, feelings, needs and motivations.[10] Increasingly, it is accepted that effective mental health nursing should be predicated upon a balanced understanding of knowledge and knowing, drawn from the theoretical and practical service user experience and awareness of self.[11] Knowledge and language are inherent in all social discourses and have the power to enable inclusion or exclusion.[12]

Knowledge, as an integral part of assessment, is a three-way process, involving the individual, others (family, friends, colleagues) and the mental health care professional. Ideally, assessment should be a collaborative process with as much information as possible being obtained directly from the person, through the narration of their personal story and/or other forms of self-report and observation. Peplau[9] noted that observation is a key focus of assessment, and observation can be transformed by interpretation into meaningful explanation.

REFLECTION

- Think about the problems you identified earlier and how you might review these in the light of this new information.

- What life events do you think might be contributing to Tess's current mental health and well-being?

- In terms of how Tess is behaving, what do you think might be going on for her intra-personally?

- How might you be able to draw upon your own experience in order to develop a therapeutic relationship with Tess?

CASE STUDY 1 (continued)

The GP's referral letter states that she cannot find evidence of any underlying physical condition that might be the cause of Tess's headaches.

From Tess's friend you have established that Tess has no known history of depression or anxiety, but for the past 15 months she has slowly withdrawn from her previously active social life. She also tells you that Tess appeared to cope well after the death of her husband, but has become more anxious about money and personal security. For example, the friend explains how Tess has to check all the windows and doors are locked as soon as it gets dark. Tess is also reluctant to answer the phone or open her door after it has become dark.

Tess herself is still withdrawn and does not mix with others on the ward. She does not participate in any of the ward's activities. Her non-participation has been commented on at the weekly case review meeting and is taken as a symptom of her depression.

Sometimes, when the person is unable or unwilling to engage in providing information, then those significant others, relatives, friends and other professionals, become more important to the mental health nurse in gaining insight into the person's distress. Information provided by others may be invaluable in adding to our knowledge and helping us to build the bigger picture. While at times the information given by others might corroborate the story narrated by the person, it might also be contradictory. The latter can be useful as it has the potential to illustrate the differing perspectives and/or provide insight into existing relationships.

Regardless of who provides the information, the process by which it is collected can be formal or informal and is likely to be a mix of both. On some occasions using formal means of assessment could make the person feel uncomfortable and uneasy about telling their story. At other times asking for information formally will be appropriate; for example, asking other professionals for specific information about medication, sleep patterns and previous history of suicide behaviour.

The purpose of assessment is to gather sufficient knowledge to allow us to know the person within the context of his/her own life story, so that through collaborative working with the person we can develop a plan of care that will ensure the person achieves a successful outcome.

SELF AS AN ASSESSMENT TOOL

So far in this chapter we have identified the core components of assessment, the fact that it is an ongoing process, the phases and roles the nurse may adopt within the process and the types of knowledge that will be required to ensure accurate understanding of what has taken place and is taking place within the person's life. We have also mentioned evidenced-based assessment tools (discussed further in chapter 14), but perhaps the most important and valuable assessment tool is that of self.

It is suggested that all that can be known about the world can only come from our own particular point of view or our experiencing of it.[13] This supports the view that, as human beings, we bring our 'self' into the assessment encounter, complete with all our preconceived ideas, values, beliefs and socio-cultural nuances. Bion[14] put forward the notion of freeing ourselves of pre-conceived ideas and bias, by abandoning memory and desires so that existing knowledge does not get in the way and cloud our view when we are with those in distress. However, it is not easy to accept and validate the experience of another individual whose distress may show in a way that we prefer not to recognize (for example, being aggressive), or when the person him-/herself finds it difficult to acknowledge what has happened or is happening; (for example, the death of someone close).[15] Indeed, Rogers[16] suggested that what it means to be a human being cannot be taught, but rather it is something that every person must discover for themselves.

Reluctance on the part of the nurse to work with emotional distress, such as that often encountered within mental health care, could be the result of their own internal psyche, and influenced by their own social, cultural and political identity. Such experiences can have a direct impact on their openness and willingness to explore distressing, intimate and often sensitive issues. When a nurse feels insecure in addressing such issues, he/she is likely to try to assert competence and control through use of his/her own defence mechanisms.[17] Such defence mechanisms often include professional detachment, denial of personal feelings, the use of rhetoric and/or the pathologizing of what we do not understand.[18] For example, 'diagnostic overshadowing', whereby a person's mental health detracts from a physical health issue being taken seriously, has been recognized as problematic in psychiatric care.[19] It is important that as mental health nurses we gain insight and a better understanding of our own unconscious defences if we are to avoid the perpetuation of negative feelings and poor treatment decisions for those for whom we are providing care.

Likewise, overcoming fear of incompetence and trusting in self and personal ability are also important, but not always easy to achieve. It is well established that our experiences can be influenced by others,[20] and while the power of the other can be influential, we are responsible for our own attitudes and how we present ourselves in terms of the acceptance of others.[21,22] Rogers[16] identified three core conditions; accurate empathy, unconditional positive regard and congruence, that need to be present in our interpersonal encounters with those whom we are trying to help. Empathy is being able to demonstrate a genuine appreciation and understanding of the person's perspective of what is happening in their life. Unconditional positive regard involves attentive listening without interruption, judgement or the giving of advice, while congruence refers to the nurse's ability to relate to the person as him-/herself without hiding behind a professional façade.

The use of self as an assessment tool and the ability to achieve the above is not easy and, just as those in our care are seeking help to unpick the problems affecting their mental well-being, we to have to disentangle our own attitudes, values and beliefs so we are free to better hear and understand others. A good example of what we mean by this can be found in Irving Yalom's book, *Love's executioner and other tales of psychotherapy*, whereby the author uses case studies to expose some of his own foibles when working with people in distress. The utilization of clinical supervision as a platform for challenging our own attitudes, values, beliefs and fears, brought to the fore during our interpersonal encounters, is crucial in achieving this.[23] The importance of effective and regular clinical supervision cannot be underestimated as it affords the mental health nurse the opportunity to bring conscious awareness to aspects of the self that are hidden, but nonetheless present in our encounters with those who are seeking our help for their distress.[24] Chapter 10 provides further information on clinical supervision.

HEARING THE STORY, CONTEXTUALIZING THE PROBLEM

The Mental Health Foundation[25] reported that people using mental health services need the following; somewhere to feel safe and accepted, a place where there is someone to talk to when distressed, help in managing feelings, and support from someone who is willing to listen. In particular, if mental health nurses are to better understand the lived experiences of people experiencing mental health problems, in order to provide sensitively attuned quality nursing care with positive outcomes, hearing the story is central to the provision of that care.[26,27] It is suggested that moving away from the illness as the main focus, and consequently shifting away from the medical model, so as not to miss or discount important aspects of the story, is essential to hearing the story.[28] The telling of stories is promoted through the demonstration of compassion by the listener, with their attitude and subsequent dialogue being the vehicle that facilitates human engagement and understanding of the other's experience.[29] The way in which the story is heard (by the nurse) will set the scene for the remainder of the interpersonal interactions. Care needs to be taken in the way in which the story is told. It might not always be reiterated in chronological order, but events may be identified in terms of their importance, perhaps indicating priorities for the person trying to make sense of their own story.

CASE STUDY 1 (continued)

Two weeks have passed since Tess was first admitted to the ward. She continues to present with what are described as symptoms of depression, but she has indicated that she misses her husband and finds it hard and frightening to live on her own. Although Tess has good social networks, she feels as if she is constantly being told what to do and what might be 'good for her'. However, what she has not been able to do is freely and safely express these feelings.

PREPARED TO RESPOND: KNOWLEDGE, ATTITUDE AND BELIEFS

Consistency, respect, affirmation, empathy and staying with and holding the emotional distress will provide an emotional platform conducive to nurturing trust.[30] However, this can sometimes be a difficult interpersonal place to occupy for many mental health nurses. Additionally, some nurses become so intent on utilizing their theoretical knowledge, perhaps in the use of a structured assessment process, that this becomes a hindrance to the processes of '*knowing*', in that it is easy to become distracted from what we are experiencing, from learning from what is occurring in the here and now.

However, responding to what is only available as theoretical knowledge can also provide a sanctuary for the mental health nurse who unconsciously wishes to distance themselves from the emotional zeitgeist of their patients and, in so doing, avoid the personal consequences implicit in the emotional burden of caring.[17] So in order to avoid becoming involved with an individual's emotional distress, some nurses will develop and maintain a '*professional distance*' in their nurse–patient relationships. However, in order to know the world of the person and subsequently understand the context of their distress, it is necessary to find out what their experience is at that particular time, and what sense and meaning they attach to that experience. With this in mind, the ongoing assessment can only be effectively performed with the person actively engaging with the process. There has to be a partnership, a coming together of the person seeking help and the nurse whose role is that of assessor, which promotes an interpersonal connection that will facilitate the development of a therapeutic relationship. It is this relational aspect of nursing that will lay the foundation for the all-important therapeutic relationship.[31]

We argue that the behaviour and thinking identified above reinforce the 'doing' and 'being' of mental health care. The doing of mental health care relies much more on the utilization of the 'professional self', which is concerned with reinforcing professional distance and boundaries. The being (of a mental health nurse) draws upon both the 'professional self' and the unconscious 'personal self' and the impact this 'self' has on the development of, and engagement with others in our everyday practice.

CONCLUSION

Within this chapter we have considered assessment and how, rather than it being a one-off occurrence, it is an ongoing process. It has a beginning, involving an orientation phase, and an ending, the resolution phase. What happens in between is the telling of an ongoing dynamic story, a personal narrative that will change as understanding and meaning mediate the distress that was initially experienced. While the story is pivotal to understanding the context of a person's mental distress, the development from day one of an interpersonal therapeutic relationship is central to the role of the mental health nurse. The accuracy of the assessment will act as a blueprint for the planning and delivery of care. To achieve the latter, the mental health nurse has to engage in various phases and roles, but most importantly he/she has to recognize 'self' as the main assessment tool. Taking on responsibility as the assessor, the nurse has to have an awareness of their own personal values, beliefs and prejudices, while simultaneously showing compassion through acceptance of and respect for the person who is seeking their help. Mental health nurses are in a privileged position as it is they who often get to carry out the assessment. It is in this early engagement process – the person looking for someone to hold their distress, the nurse showing their receptiveness to provide this service – that a platform for care can be established. The relationship will then move on, embracing collaborative engagement that is likely to promote mental health care that is satisfying to all parties.

References

1. Ariely D, Wertenbroch K. Procrastination, deadlines, and performance: self-control by precommitment. *Psychological Science* 2002; **13**: 219–24.
2. Barker P. *Psychiatric and mental health nursing: the craft of caring*, 2nd edn. London: Hodder Arnold, 2009.
3. National Institute for Mental Health. Transforming diagnosis. Available from: http://www.nimh.nih.gov/about/director/2013/transforming-diagnosis.shtml [Accessed 19th May 2016].
4. Warne T, McAndrew S. Bordering on insanity: Mis Nomer, reviewing the case of the condemned women. *Journal of Psychiatric and Mental Health Nursing* 2007; **14**: 155–62.
5. Warne T, McAndrew S (eds). *Using patient experience in nurse education*. London: Palgrave, 2004.
6. Warne T, McAndrew S (eds). *Creative approaches to health and social care education*. London: Palgrave, 2010.
7. Mental Health Foundation. *Starting today: the future of mental health services*. London: Mental Health Foundation, 2013.
8. McAndrew S, Chambers M, Nolan F, Thomas B, Watts P. Measuring the evidence: reviewing the literature of the measurement of therapeutic engagement in acute mental health inpatient wards. *International Journal of Mental Health Nursing* 2014; **23**: 212–20.
9. Peplau, H. *Interpersonal relations in nursing*. New York: Putnam, 1952.
10. Warne T, McAndrew S. Painting the landscape of emotionality: colouring in the emotional gaps between the theory and practice of mental health nursing. *International Journal of Mental Health Nursing* 2008; **17**(2): 108–15.
11. Warne T, McAndrew, S. Re-searching for therapy: the ethics of using what we are skilled in. *Journal of Psychiatric and Mental Health Nursing* 2010; **17**: 503–9.
12. Foucault M. *The archaeology of knowledge*, trans. AM Sheridan Smith. New York: Pantheon, 1970.
13. Merleau-Ponty M. *The visible and the invisible: followed by working notes*. Evanston, IL: Northwestern University Press, 1968.
14. Bion WR. *Learning from experience*. London: Heinemann, 1962.
15. Davidson B. What can be the relevance of the psychiatric nurse to the life of a person who is mentally ill? *Journal of Clinical Nursing* 1992; **1**(4): 199–205.
16. Rogers CR. *Client-centered therapy: its current practice, implications and theory*. London: Constable, 1951.
17. Warne T, McAndrew S. The shackles of abuse: unprepared to work at the edges of reason? *Journal of Psychiatric and Mental Health Nursing* 2005; **12**: 679–85.
18. Gallop R, O'Brien L. Re-establishing psychodynamic theory as foundational knowledge for psychiatric/mental health nursing. *Issues in Mental Health Nursing* 2003; **24**: 213–27.
19. Jones S, Howard L, Thornicroft G. 'Diagnostic overshadowing': worse physical health care for people with mental illness. *Acta Psychiatrica Scandinavica* 2008; **118**: 169–71.
20. Spinelli E. *Practising existential psychotherapy: the relational world*. London, Thousand Oaks, CA, New Delhi: Sage, 2007.
21. Sartre JP. *Hope now: the 1980 interviews*. Chicago: University of Chicago Press, 1996.
22. Frankl VE. *Man's search for meaning*. New York: Rider, 2004.
23. Lakeman R, McAndrew S, McGabghann L, Warne T. That was helpful, no one has talked to me about that before: valuing the therapeutics of research participation. *International Journal of Mental Health Nursing* 2013; **22**: 76–84.
24. Heath H, Freshwater D. Clinical supervision as an emancipatory process: avoiding inappropriate intent. *Journal of Advanced Nursing* 2000; **32**(5): 1298–306.
25. Mental Health Foundation. *Our own mind*. London: Mental Health Foundation, 1997.
26. Barker P, Buchanan-Barker P. Myth of mental health nursing and the challenge of recovery. *International Journal of Mental Health Nursing* 2011; **20**(5): 337–44.
27. Hewitt J, Coffey M. Therapeutic relationships with people with schizophrenia. *Journal of Advance Nursing* 2005; **52**(5): 1–10.
28. Kliewer S, Saultz JW. *Healthcare and spirituality*. Milton Keynes: Radcliffe, 2006.
29. Frie R. Compassion, dialogue, and context: on understanding the other. *International Journal of Psychoanalytic Self Psychology* 2010; **5**: 451–66.
30. Isay RA. *Commitment and healing: gay men and the need for romantic love*. Hoboken, NJ: Wiley, 2006.
31. Wright K, Jones F. Developing healthy working relationships for people with borderline personality disorder who self harm: re-adjusting perceptions, the service user's view. *Mental Health Practice* 2012; **16**(2): 31–5.

Further reading

APA (American Psychiatric Association). *Diagnostic and statistical manual of mental disorders, fifth edition (DSM-5)*. Washington DC: APA, 2013.
Foucault M. *Madness and civilization: a history of insanity in the age of reason*. London: Random House LLC, 1988.
Laing R. *The divided self: an existential study in sanity and madness*. London: Penguin, 2010.

Szasz TS. *The myth of mental illness: foundations of a theory of personal conduct*. New York: Harper Perennial, 1974.
Szasz TS. Mental illness is still a myth. *Society* 1994; **31**(4): 34–9.
Yalom ID. *Love's executioner: and other tales of psychotherapy*. New York: Basic Books, 2012.

Relevant web pages

Centre for Mental Health. http://www.centreformentalhealth.org.uk/
Deprivation of Liberty, Safeguarding and You. https://www.gov.uk/government/publications/deprivation-of-liberty-safeguards-forms-and-guidance
Mental Health Foundation. http://www.mentalhealth.org.uk/
Mental Health Nurses Association. http://www.unitetheunion.org/how-we-help/list-of-sectors/healthsector/healthsectoryourprofession/mhna/

MIND. http://www.mind.org.uk/
Movement for Global Mental Health. http://globalmentalhealth.org
Rethink Mental Illness. http://www.rethink.org/
Safewards. http://www.safewards.net/
World Association of Social Psychiatry. http://waspsocialpsychiatry.com

The nature and types of assessment

PAUL FALLON AND G~

LEARNING OUTCOMES

- To understand the need to choose the appropriate method of assessment to obtain accurate information to inform the care of the service user.
- To be able to describe the key components of an initial mental health assessment.
- To understand the difference between an assessment and a collaborative formulation.

SUMMARY OF KEY POINTS

- There are a number of different assessment types, and the choice of assessment will be influenced by a range of factors, including the purpose of the assessment, the type of information required and the amount of information required to complete the assessment.
- The best assessments are collaborative in nature.

- Assessments should guide the nurse on future care.
- Assessments can be experienced as intrusive by service users and nurses need to be sensitive to the feelings of the service user when exploring areas of their lives that they may be reticent about discussing.

INTRODUCTION

This chapter includes the reflections of a service user who wishes only to be known as 'G~'; G~ reflects on their experiences of being assessed by and building a therapeutic relationship with the other author of the chapter (myself). G~ reflects on how difficult it is to discuss their ongoing thoughts about how invasive and negative they find the world and how these thoughts lead them to often think about killing themselves. They then talk about how paradoxically the fact that I accept their right to hold such views and be able to express them makes them feel that they have a choice and that this means that 'being *able* to bow out persuades me to try and find meaning and beauty to carry on, live with worry, wait longer, give possibilities a chance'.

My contact with G~ includes a two-way process of communication and a two-way process of assessment. As in any human interaction, both parties assess each other, and nurses should always remember that what they say, how they say it and why they say it is constantly being thought about by their service users. For my part and in my role as a mental health professional, assessment includes an evaluation of G~'s social situation, including their mental health and the nature and degree of any risks. It is clear that they understand this, from their statement that they feel the need to be 'cagey' at times because they believe that 'nothing would precipitate that ending more abruptly than imminent restriction of choice to bow out if I'd had enough'. G~'s reflections offer valuable insights into the nature of the assessment process, as they highlight the differing agendas that each participant in the assessment process has and how they negotiate a shared space where they can be honest to a degree that allows understanding of each other's position.

In chapter 13 the authors discuss how assessment in mental health is key to effective practice. The information we gather via assessments helps us better understand our service users and this improves our ability to work with them in a therapeutic, recovery-focused manner. The assessment processes that mental health nurses engage in come in many forms. The changing nature of mental health nursing in the modern world has gradually expanded the scope of the aspects of a person's life that now come the under the auspices of mental health services. This is especially so in community settings, where health and social care staff often work closely together in integrated teams, working as care coordinators with an increasing amount of generic working. In these settings nurses perform not just traditional 'health' type assessments but also many assessments that were historically the remit of social care staff. In a broad sense the categories of the biological, social, psychological, cultural and spiritual domains remain the same; however, the specific aspects of a person's life that are now assessed by mental health nurses have expanded significantly. For example, as well as the expected domains of mental health such as mood, psychosis or risk, assessments are now also required for the commissioning of packages of care and finding and funding of appropriate accommodation placements.

As societies become more risk averse, governments place increasing responsibilities on health and social care organizations and their staff to manage the risks that people, including people with mental health difficulties, are exposed to or could pose to themselves or others. An example of this is pre-birth risk assessments that are now carried out on pregnant women under mental health services. In some parts of the world, it is not just the client who is subject to assessment; for example, in the UK, the Department of Health[1] lays out the responsibilities for statutory services to assess not only the needs of clients but also the needs of their carers. Chapter 15 discusses in detail the important role that carers often play in service users' lives and the different methods of assessment that services use to assess families and carers.

Though some assessments can be considered 'one-off' events, the majority of assessments are better perceived as part of an ongoing dynamic process, in which every meeting between staff and service users is an opportunity to assess the service user and, if necessary, to update assessment documentation. Therefore, when we discuss assessment tools, it is vital to remember that the completed tool is only wholly accurate at the moment it is completed and should be seen as a 'live' document, subject to revision whenever necessary. This is especially true of assessments pertaining to mental state and/or risk, where changes in environmental factors can have an immediate influence on the individual, leading to significant changes in their mental state. An example of this is where a person already low in mood subsequently experiences an adverse life event, such as a relationship breakdown; this can often lead to their mood lowering even further, which could then lead to an increase in the degree of risk that they pose to themselves or others.

ASSESSMENT METHODS: THE NEED TO BE SYSTEMATIC

The assessment method is how we collect information.[2] To collect information, we have to be systematic and scientific in our methods to ensure that what we gather is accurate, so that others can make the appropriate clinical decisions based on the information provided in the assessment. The method chosen for assessment should be that which is thought to be most likely to gather the required information about the particular aspect of the service user's life that the nurse is interested in finding out more about. Two questions must be asked of the method chosen. First, is it valid, i.e. will it assess what we want it to assess? Second, is it reliable, i.e. will it consistently generate the same information each time it is used?[3] Therefore well-established tools with proven validity and inter-rater reliability should be chosen where these exist. There is no point in re-inventing the wheel and trying to devise an assessment method if there is one that is already widely used in clinical practice. In many areas of clinical practice, the organization will already prescribe which tools clinicians use; this is especially the case with tools for risk assessment and assessment of mental state, as health organizations aim to standardize approaches to assessment to ensure a uniformity of assessment-driven care, as far as possible.

SOURCES OF INFORMATION

Where we collect information from can have a considerable influence on the quality of the assessment we produce. In general, collecting the information from the person concerned themselves provides us with primary data, which should theoretically be the most accurate we can gather.

However, other sources can be as important. For example, significant others, such as family and close friends, may have noticed a decline in the service user's mental health that they themselves have become too distracted to notice. Therefore they may be better able to describe the course of the illness and may even be able to point to a particular adverse life event that may have been significant in provoking the current episode of illness. Family and significant others are often the first people to alert services to concerns about an individual's mental health, especially if the individual themselves has lost sight of just how ill they have become.

Service users can sometimes be reticent or unable to disclose what they are actually experiencing psychologically; people can feel embarrassed or actually find it difficult to find the words to describe what is happening to them. This can be true of people experiencing psychotic symptoms such as auditory hallucinations or paranoid delusions, where the individual may no longer be certain of what is real and what is a symptom of their illness, and the confusion and anxiety associated with these experiences can profoundly influence what information the service user is able to give. Sometimes the person is uncomfortable discussing how they are feeling, especially if they fear that the consequence of opening up to mental health staff could lead to an enforced period of hospitalization. It could be that previous experience of admitting to thoughts of suicidality led to enforced hospitalization and they want to avoid losing control over their life choices (see G~'s reflections below). Therefore, though the service user should be the main focus for collecting information, other sources may provide collateral and in some cases vital information. These sources include family and significant others, clinical notes, other partner agencies such as the service user's general practitioner and also colleagues that may be involved with the service user or have significant knowledge of them from previously working with them.

THE FOUR MAIN METHODS OF ASSESSMENT

There are a number of methods that can be used to gather information, including observation; interviews; diaries, logs and personal records; and questionnaires and rating scales.[2] These four approaches are not mutually exclusive; for example, the nurse completing a side effects rating scale has to observe the service user closely to be able to accurately rate the nature and degree of the side effects present. Indeed, all assessments require good observational skills, as sometimes people tell us a different story with their body language than they do verbally. Therefore, though the nurse assessing for side effects is essentially completing a tick box rating scale, this requires close observation of a service user.

1. Observation

When we observe, we use all of our senses, our vision, our hearing, our sense of smell and sometimes even our sense of touch. The use of observation skills is practised across all the nursing disciplines. In the field of mental health we observe people's behaviour, including both their physical and verbal behaviour, to enable us to make inferences about their mental well-being. However, these observations tell us little unless they also take into account the context within which the person is acting.[3] This is especially true of people from different cultural backgrounds that may, for example, have a totally different way of expressing their distress or of explaining unusual sensory experiences such as auditory hallucinations. If we ignore or do not try to understand these differences when assessing their behaviour, we may make very poor judgements that may have very damaging consequences for the individual.[4]

Therefore an understanding of a host of factors concerning the service user, including their pre-existing social circumstances, usual way of behaving, social values, belief system and cultural factors, helps us to assess whether their current behaviours are indicative of a change in their mental well-being. This obviously means that it is easier to make more accurate assessments and inferences from behaviour for people of whom we have prior knowledge. In clinical practice, however, we often meet new service users, and that lack of contextual knowledge can lead clinicians to make assumptions that are erroneous. A famous example of this was the experiment carried out by David Rosenhan and others in 1973, in which he and a group of researchers feigned mental illness to gain admission to psychiatric hospitals in the USA, but, once admitted, stopped mentioning any psychotic symptoms and began behaving in their usual manner. Despite the fact that they were no longer exhibiting any symptoms, staff interpreted much of their behaviour as indicative of mental illness. For example, one nurse labelled the note-taking of one of the researchers as 'writing behaviour' and considered it pathological.[5] Given the dangers inherent in making assumptions about service users, nurses should try to be as objective as possible and record only observable facts on the basis of what they see and hear.[2]

2. Interview schedules

Interview schedules are a method of collecting information that is superior to questionnaires and rating scales, as they allow more flexibility on the part of the interviewer and therefore more exploration of the subject. This ensures that greater detail is gathered and therefore, hopefully, results in a better-informed assessment. They are by necessity still very structured tools for conducting assessments. In research terms they would be described as comprising a 'shopping list' of topics that the researcher wants to address.[6] The structure ensures that the tools are standardized so that all staff within an organization are conducting assessments in the same way and the same topics are covered. Though structured, most interview schedules are not so structured that they prescribe the actual questions to ask (see the example below of an initial mental health assessment tool which includes areas to be covered and then suggests some prompts and bullet points of possible questions). The more structured an assessment tool is, the more likely it is that the conversation will be stilted and rapport difficult to establish. One of the hardest parts of interviewing is getting the balance right between maintaining good eye contact when establishing rapport and trying to write down what is being said. Taking some brief notes is necessary to ensure that all the important information is recorded, so that the full assessment can be written up after the interview.

THE INTERVIEW PROCESS

In chapter 3, the inter- and intrapersonal aspects of building a relationship to help understand the service user's perspective were discussed. As part of the 'craft of caring', we have to consider the processes involved in interviewing and assessing service users. There are a number of key components that help to ensure that the interview is a productive experience for both the service user and the nurse. First, the nurse should introduce themselves and ensure that the interview takes place in a comfortable and quiet environment to try to put the service user at their ease and ensure confidentiality. Second, the nurse must explain the purpose of the meeting. If the assessment is part of an admission to a ward, for example, then this must be explained, as service users at the point of admission are often distressed or distracted due to their emotional and psychological state, and can find the process bewildering or unsettling.

In community settings, referrals to community mental health teams (CMHTs) come from agencies such as general practitioners (GPs), housing providers and inpatient units. In the case of GPs, often the purpose of these referrals is to request an assessment from mental health specialists so that advice on how best to support and treat their service users can be given. Therefore the nurse must explain that the purpose of the meeting is to conduct an assessment of their current circumstances and to arrive at a shared understanding of how these have impacted on their mental well-being, and that they will be providing advice to the referrer to help them care more effectively for them. However, people often think they are coming to the CMHT for treatment and/or therapy; this may be true for some, but the majority will have just one meeting where the assessment takes place and then they will be discharged with advice on management being sent to the referrer. Therefore, it should be explained what will happen as a consequence of the assessment. On a hospital ward it is usually obvious that the assessment is part of the admission process. In the community it needs to be explained that the likely outcome of the assessment is that advice will be provided

to the person who referred them and the assessment is probably a 'one-off' meeting. This enables the assessor to establish a boundary to the assessment process and set the agenda for the meeting.

When conducting an interview, the interviewer should attempt to make the experience approximate to a natural conversation as much as possible. This means that sometimes, if the service user wants to talk about issues in a different order from that laid out in the interview schedule, the interviewer should be confident enough to allow the assessment to move out of sequence. Good interviewers are very familiar with their assessment schedules and are able to allow the conversation to flow, encouraging the service user to open up, while at the same time guiding the interview back onto the areas of the assessment not yet discussed, ensuring that all the topics are covered.

REFLECTION

What factors do you have to consider when choosing which assessment tool is the most appropriate to use in any given situation?

CHALLENGES IN THE INTERVIEW PROCESS

It has already been highlighted that conducting an interview can be very challenging, as the interviewer has to make the process as close to a natural conversation as possible, to put the service user at ease. This increases the chances of the service user feeling able to open up to questioning during the assessment. Other challenges include maintaining eye contact while taking notes and allowing the conversation to divert at times from the order laid out in the schedule. There are other challenges too; for instance, on occasions the service user may only have attended the assessment because of pressure from friends or family and may be reticent about engaging meaningfully with the interviewer. Sometimes the service user may be reticent about disclosing information about traumatic life experiences to a stranger due to their feelings of guilt or shame. In these situations it is vital that the interviewer is sensitive to the feelings of the service user, and that they try to encourage them to engage in the process, while making clear that it is their choice how much they are willing to engage and how much they are willing to disclose. Giving the service user choice and a degree of control often makes them more at ease and hence more likely to engage in the assessment interview.

Another challenge that is becoming more common in mental health services is the need to use interpreters in assessments. In recent years and for various reasons there have been large migrations of people moving around the world. Some of these people may have pre-existing mental health problems; others have experienced significant trauma before or during their migration. A consequence of this is an increase in the number of people presenting to mental health services in countries where they do not speak the local language. This presents a number of challenges for the interviewer. First, it is rarely a good idea to use family or friends as the interpreter; for many reasons, especially confidentiality, service users are less likely to be forthcoming if they have to discuss issues through family members. Also, family members will have their own preconceived ideas about the service user, their capabilities and events in their life, and these can be at odds with the service user's perception of them, sometimes leading to arguments during the assessment. Their emotional attachment to the service user makes it difficult for them to remain detached enough to merely interpret and not engage in the interview themselves, further lengthening what would already be quite a long process.

Second, whether they are a family member or an interpreter hired from an agency, it should not be assumed that the interpreter has a good knowledge of mental health issues. It is always prudent to ask the interpreter before starting the interview what their experience of mental health is because this will affect how the interviewer asks the questions. For example, if the interviewer asks 'Do they hear voices?', this could easily be misinterpreted as 'Can you hear people's voices?' or variants of this if the interpreter knows little of psychotic symptoms. The question should be along the lines of 'Do they hear voices when there is no one else around and other potential sources such as the TV and radio are not turned on?' This approach of keeping the questions clear and unambiguous should be taken when working with interpreters to avoid the interpreter mistakenly asking incorrect questions. Third, though having an interpreter from the same cultural background can sometimes be reassuring for the service user, this cannot be taken for granted, and so it is best to check with both parties before commencing the assessment that there are not any potential cultural issues that would impede the assessment process.

BOX 14.1: EXAMPLE OF THE AREAS AN INITIAL MENTAL HEALTH ASSESSMENT TOOL SHOULD COVER IN A COMPREHENSIVE HOLISTIC ASSESSMENT

Presenting problem and history of presenting problem: Who has made the referral? What is the purpose of the referral? What does the service user perceive to be the main problem? Record verbatim. Consider the nature, onset, existing treatment, severity, alleviating/aggravating factors, duration, recent stressors.

Past mental health history: Chronological account of duration, nature and management of past mental ill-health, including dates, symptoms, diagnosis, treatments (including non-pharmacological), hospital admissions (including formal detention), outcomes. Did the service user seek help for previous episodes of mental ill health?

Physical health/medical history: History of medical illness, disease, conditions, surgery, diagnosis, symptoms, treatment, outcome. Are there links to psychiatric symptoms or psychiatrically linked health problems?

Personal and family history: Family history of mental health problems, parental occupation and sibling ages. Account of the service user's life from conception to the present, difficulties during birth, separation from mother, developmental milestones. Describe dynamics and workings of the family unit; positive relationships, parenting, who raised the service user. Consider school life, peer relationships, experimentation with substances, antisocial behaviour, academic abilities and qualifications, marital and sexual history, children, occupational history, support networks, aspirations. Consider need for carer's assessment. Check for predisposing, precipitating and maintaining factors for the presenting problem.

Medication: Current medication, include those for physical as well as mental health, dose and duration; side effects; compliance; drug allergies; previous medications.

Alcohol history: Current number of units per week, type of alcohol, length of use if problematic, dependence, seizures, previous use, impact on social circumstances.

Drug history: Type, quantity, method of administration, effect and reason for use, sharing of equipment, costs and financing, debt, impact on social circumstances. Include current and past use.

Forensic history: Chronology of previous offences, charges, convictions and sentences. Include those offences not brought to the attention of the police. Attitude toward offences and subsequent impact on service user's life. Cases pending.

Premorbid personality: Service user's personality and day-to-day functioning before onset. Characteristics of cognition, mood and behaviour.

BOX 14.2: MENTAL STATE EXAMINATION

Appearance and behaviour: Clothing, ethnic origin, gender, tattoos, piercings, scarring, make-up, alertness and movement, rapport, eye contact, interaction.

Speech: Rate, volume and quality, fluency and coherence.

Mood: Record subjective mood verbatim. Record objective assessment. Note changes during assessment. Diurnal variation, irritability, tearfulness.

Anxiety: Type, triggers, emotions, physiology, behaviours, coping strategies.

Sleep: Insomnia, disturbances to pattern and reasons for these, early morning waking.

Appetite: Appetite, dietary intake, nutrition, dieting, weight loss (intentional/unintentional), disordered patterns.

Motivation: Energy levels, fluctuations, changes in activity, libido, impact on activities of daily living, enjoyment and interests.

Cognitions: Alertness, cooperation, orientation, memory, concentration, attention, naming, repetition.

Thoughts: Formation of thoughts, thought disorder, delusions/overvalued ideas. Content: preoccupations, worries, recurrent thoughts, intrusions, suicidal thoughts.

Perceptions: Illusions, hallucinations (auditory, visual, tactile, gustatory, olfactory), dissociation, depersonalization, derealization.

Insight: Awareness and understanding of problem; attitudes, feelings and behaviour; need for treatment.

BOX 14.3: INITIAL RISK SCREENING

(A full risk assessment must be completed whenever screening indicates clear risks.)

Consider safeguarding of adults or children during the screening process.

Domains of risk: to self, to others, self-neglect, vulnerability/exploitation.

Capacity/deprivation of liberty safeguards.

Third party information: Who is providing the information? Is there permission to share?

Formulation.
Management plan.

(All actions need to include the person responsible for the action and a time frame. Include details of next review, if applicable. If a further review is not going to take place, be clear about this. Use numbered bullet points.)

BOX 14.4: FORMULATION

Near the end of the above assessment is the heading 'formulation'. Formulating is a process often used in cognitive therapy, and when used in a mental health assessment it improves the quality of the outcomes of the assessment process. A formulation is the process in which the assessor and service user work together to describe and then explain the issues highlighted in the assessment. In a broad sense it generates a hypothesis about the causes, precipitants and maintaining influences of a person's psychological problems.[7] The purpose of a formulation is to guide therapeutic interventions to relieve service user distress and build resilience.[8] In the process of collaboratively explaining how and why a service user arrived at the situation they are now in psychologically and materially, the formulation normalizes the presenting issues, validates the service user's experiences and can make complex issues seem more understandable. It also focuses on the service user's strengths and resilience, and therefore adds a positive aspect to the assessment process, which otherwise may have been primarily focused on current challenges and worsening mental health.

REFLECTION

Can you explain the difference between an assessment and a formulation?

SERVICE USER'S PERSPECTIVE: THE REFLECTIONS OF G~ ON BEING ASSESSED

Speak~ I remember Dr Fallon (Paul) does make notes sometimes as we speak. Wallpaper~ always above board, this becomes no more noticeable than wallpaper. Here~ under other circumstances I would be second-guessing and doubling back in damage-limitation, but not so here.

Lifeline?~ Rory Bremner's verbal tic on TV when impersonating MP Tony Benn: 'I'm not mad, you know', an apt disclaimer on disclosures like: my phone phobia challenged not by a dentist appointment but Jonathan Miller requesting my first call in 18 months, set up to fail … or contacting Martin Scorsese, for what, a lifeline?

Fantasy~ between the blanks where I can't tell the time on the clock and a potential that fell by the wayside, whatever former high-flown fancies of 'best writer in the …' leaving lightning traces of synapses across the page … instead of knotted anguish … eccentric to start with before things go wrong, still I believe sessions distinguish my reality and bleak observations from fantasy.

Morale~ I only censor darker observations on reality from human regard for Paul's spirits, as no good can come of bringing folk down to my low morale. Time~ a sane sign: sensitivity to my fellow man, not entirely wrapped in my own head as I am for much of the time.

Die~ I *can* express a darker inclination to die. Important~~ that's important. Action~ from the start, I sense what to disclose to defend my freedom of action. Cagey~ even writing now, I see I'm cagey. Enough~ nothing would precipitate that ending more abruptly than imminent restriction of choice to bow out if I'd had enough.

E)~ being *able* to bow out persuades me to try and find meaning and beauty to carry on, live with worry, wait longer, give possibilities a chance, bad luck to turn around, ensure I don't die wishing I'd tried c) or d) or e).

On~ sessions find middle-ground between respecting Paul's professional obligations and my need to be free, raising the subject only carefully. Echo~ so monitoring is a double echo. Feedback~ feedback.

Future~ Paul understands I find the future terminally hopeless and I understand Paul believes in the future. Compartment~ I understand Paul manages stress by compartmentalizing and Paul understands I hold off pressure by living inside my one compartment.

Sessions~ my visceral distress at an invading culture that fells trees everywhere like it fells hope and culls the vulnerable crashes my stability and pervades some sessions. Catastrophic~ so it could sound paranoiac when I called in panic because council chainsaws without notice had entered without consent to fell the spindly trees in my garden, which I found catastrophic. Home~ Paul's help hearing all that, taking time to see for himself, made the situation real and grounded all those alarms I sensed coming ever closer to home. Positive~ sometimes confirmation is more practical help than disclaiming catastrophes or being positive.

Bits~ all my time alone, retreating from society, keeps me from breaking to bits. Disintegrating~ shopping, under assault, head down heads off constant signs that my neighbourhood/society/country/world is disintegrating. Everybody's~ stranded in the present that abandoned the past, and abandoned by the past that had a better future than what it was traded for, my future long gone and so is everybody's.

Rough~ I'm atomized by it, something immeasurable slips between the lines, something missing turns to magical thinking as a first draft of a last resort against a mathematical certainty that can pinpoint pointlessness in the early hours where truth goes homeless and peace sleeps rough.

Outside~ a cable hangs loose halfway up the wall outside. Brain~ it led to an aerial I had taken off the roof that used to run poison through the wall and into my TV 100 different ways to feed into my brain. Improvement~ cutting off that signal was a key improvement. Cognitive-analysis?~ is this too cognitive for cognitive-analysis?

Exist~ to be able to try, to find mental space, to face a book, to string words that hold my identity together, and to let a squirrel's way of being displace mine – while government-driven psychology sets piledriving targets~goals~targets~goals~targets where we make up the numbers in fractions and remainders of ourselves, and every obsessive-compulsive result sets up another quantified worry and in all that cognition no space for meaning and no space for beauty to exist.

Number-crunching~ so I am grateful for the hand-crafted genuine space to make sense at C.H. free of number-crunching. Sense?~ does that make sense? Sure~ I'm not sure. Trying~ but the success of the space is typing this and still trying.

Squirrels~ my buffer: books/films/nostalgia/trees and feeding squirrels. Nostalgia~ books are my brickwork, films are a window on the world, and I find hope backwards in nostalgia.

Mind~ squirrels move much the same way, straight up, straight down, zigzag, as my mind.

Privacy~ my brittle peace-of-mind is this monastic privacy. Between~ what I must do and what Paul would do otherwise in my place is tacitly understood in the space between. Clinicians~ I never press for agreement because understanding is already more than I could expect of most clinicians.

Head~ it's a rare occasion to come out of the past for a moment and in that space hear my mind meeting someone outside my head. Sound-check~ like a sound-check. Extremes~ going home afterwards, these words recall part of who I was or am, and I piece together patterns of extremes.

Sampled~ that sounds a fanciful way to relate a session, but spend time alone like I do (voluntarily, not self-pity but self-preservation) then it's as rare a touchstone as I've just sampled.

3. Diaries, logs and personal records

Diaries can be useful tools to aid reflection on the part of the service user. They are commonly used by substance misuse services to help people log exactly how much of a particular substance they are abusing. They are also commonly used as therapeutic tools, for example, in the case of a mood diary in which a service user records their moods on a daily basis, as this helps identify changes to their mood and any possible triggers for this. Using a diary is a very straightforward, easy and cheap way of recording data. However, depending on how much data is recorded, the actual analysing of it can be more time-consuming.

The mood diary can also be used to track progress over time and, if progress has been made, can be an excellent source of positive reinforcement. Of course, a regular criticism of this approach[2] is that by focusing on an issue such as one's mood the person may develop an increased awareness of the problem and lose a sense of perspective on its actual importance. This could then lead to an increased emotional awareness of the issue, again possibly amplifying its emotional burden.

4. Questionnaires and rating scales

Questionnaires are a very common way of collecting information. They can be seen being used on most high streets and are freely available online. They are also the most common method of data collection in health research.[9] Most questionnaires that nurses administer are used for two main purposes: diagnostic and record-keeping.[9]

They explore, describe or assess a phenomenon, but do not necessarily measure it. There are a number of such tools used in mental health to measure a wide variety of aspects of the services user's experiences, from symptoms associated with depression or psychosis through to customer satisfaction surveys used to measure the satisfaction of the service user experience. Questionnaires contain questions that reflect the attributes of the concept under study and tend to use closed questions of the yes/no agree/disagree variety.

Rating scales differ from questionnaires in that they are made up of a list of items or statements that the respondent is invited to rate, each rated statement is given a score and the total score is given an interpretation.[9] In mental health, many rating scales are used to screen for the presence of a particular disorder, symptom or behaviour. Confusingly, some are described as questionnaires, such as the PHQ9 (Patient Health Questionnaire 9),[10] when in fact they are strictly speaking rating scales. Some rating scales follow the model of the Likert scale, which usually uses a five-point scale from 'strongly agree' at one end, to 'don't know' in the middle, to 'strongly disagree' at the other end. In nursing and health, however, most rating scales measure the presence of symptoms of a particular disorder such as depression and may have an item such as 'feeling good about myself' which is rated along a scale of 'never', 'rarely', 'some of the time', 'often' or 'all of the time'. Though both rating scales and questionnaires offer a quick and simple way of measuring standardized sets of phenomena across individuals, they are both subject to the same criticisms. First, as they are self-report scales, scores can be exaggerated or minimized by the person completing them. Second, given the limited amount of information they include in each question, some questions are open to interpretation and therefore may mean different things to different respondents. Third, as they are so highly structured, they lack flexibility both in the amount of detail the respondent can put into their answer and also more generally in the interaction between the nurse and the respondent.

> **REFLECTION**
>
> From your own experiences in practice, which types of assessment successfully engaged the service user in the assessment process, generated useful clinical information and appeared to be positive therapeutic experiences?

CONCLUSION

This chapter has highlighted the vast array of issues with which service users present to mental health services. These include their symptomatology, domains of risk, parenting skills, housing issues and need for packages of care, all of which require different types of assessment. Choosing the most appropriate assessment method is vital to ensure that the correct information is gathered to inform decision making and care planning. Assessment should be a collaborative process, and if it involves a formulation it can help the service user make sense of their current emotional and psychological state. Given the complex nature of service user presentations, conducting

assessments can be a challenging process that requires nurses to be well trained and fully conversant with the chosen tool.

As G~ so eloquently describes, service users are aware that the information that they give to nurses can have implications for themselves and therefore sometimes carefully decide how much they disclose to 'defend my freedom of action'. What G~ also makes clear is that service users value the time that staff spend with them while engaged in assessments, and nurses should not underestimate the powerful therapeutic effect that the feeling of being listened to and understood can have on them.

References

1. Department of Health. *The Care Act (2014)*. Available from: http://www.legislation.gov.uk/ukpga/2014/23/contents/enacted/data.htm [Accessed 22nd November 2016].
2. Barker PJ. Assessment methods in psychiatric and mental health nursing. In: Barker PJ (ed.). *The craft of caring*, 2nd edn. London: Hodder Arnold, 2009: 75–84.
3. Barker PJ. *Assessment in psychiatric and mental health nursing*. Cheltenham: Nelson Thornes, 2004.
4. Fernando SJM. *Mental health, race and culture*. London: Palgrave, 2002.
5. Rosenhan D. On being sane in insane places. *Science* 1973; **179**: 250–8.
6. Robson C. *Real world research*, 3rd edn. Chichester: John Wiley & Sons, 2011.
7. Wells A. *Cognitive therapy of anxiety disorders*. Chichester: John Wiley & Sons, 1997.
8. Kuyken W, Padesky CA, Dudley R. *Collaborative case conceptualisation*. New York: Guilford Press, 2009.
9. Parahoo K. *Nursing research, principles, process and issues*. London: Macmillan Press, 1997.
10. Spitzer RL, Kroenke K, Williams JB. Validation and utility of a self-report version of PRIME-MD: the PHQ primary care study. *Journal of the American Medical Association* 1999; **282**: 1737–44.

Further reading

Bateman AW, Krawitz R. *Borderline personality disorder: an evidence-based guide for generalist mental health professionals*. Oxford: Oxford University Press, 2013.
Cromby J, Harper D, Reavey P. *Psychology, mental health and distress*. Basingstoke: Palgrave Macmillan, 2013.
Heyman B (ed.). *Risk, health and health care: a qualitative approach*. London: Arnold, 1998.
Kelly BD. Globalisation and psychiatry. *Advances in Psychiatric Treatment* 2003; **9**: 464–74.
McEvoy P, Richards D. Gatekeeping access to community mental health teams: a qualitative study. *International Journal of Nursing Studies* 2007; **44**: 387–95.

Relevant web pages

Centre for Mental Health. www.centreformentalhealth.org.uk/
The Centre for Mental Health acts as a bridge between the worlds of research, policy and service provision by attempting to influence policy via high quality research.

Mental Health Foundation. www.mentalhealth.org.uk
This website provides an excellent range of research reports, campaigning material and educational guides.

Conducting a family assessment

CATHERINE GAMBLE, CHRISTINE LEWIS, JOHN BAKER AND RUTH ALLEN

LEARNING OUTCOMES

- To understand the purpose, benefits and challenges of undertaking family assessments.
- To be aware of the implementation of the Care Act 2014.
- To comprehend the impact mental illness can have on families.
- To be aware of information-sharing protocols.
- To be able to critique evidence-based assessment tools.
- To know how to incorporate assessment strategies into clinical practice.

SUMMARY OF KEY POINTS

- People with mental health problems do not recover in isolation; family and friends play an important role.
- Practitioners should consider families in assessment processes.
- Evidence-based tools support the development of support programmes for families.
- Sharing information and knowledge is valuable in supporting and engaging families.
- Communication and therapeutic interpersonal skills are key in enabling families to work in partnership with mental health services.

INTRODUCTION

There is a growing awareness that a person's recovery from mental illness is largely dependent upon the informal support they receive. Yet when people experience mental illness, most families, friends and carers are unaware of how to cope with it.[1] Consequently, this sense of powerlessness reduces coping strategies and increases social isolation, and has been found to cause depression and physical health problems.[2]

Family carers offer governments a low-cost way to support people with long-term health conditions. Public services could not function without the massive contribution they make. The input of carers saves the country approximately three times the UK's defence budget.[3] This figure has risen by almost 40 per cent since 2007, when the value of carers' input was put at £87 billion; this is a clear sign of the growing number of families who are taking on caring responsibilities. Government census data[4] released in December 2012 revealed that the greatest rise has been among those providing over 20 hours' care, the point at which caring starts to have a significant impact on the carer's health and well-being.

Over the last 50 years, health care delivery has changed significantly; people with mental health problems increasingly undergo treatment in their homes, with families and informal carers playing a pivotal role. For this reason, as mental health nurses are more likely to have day-to-day contact with families than any other professional group, an important part of the role is being able to assess what support systems people have, ascertain whether informal caregivers have the resources to provide care and to prevent serious health problems, and identify ways to support caregiver health and well-being.

BACKGROUND

Over the past 50 years psychiatric beds have been decommissioned and community care has been promoted. During this period, carers and family members have undertaken the majority of home care and support. There has been recognition of the value of this informal role, yet empirical research also identified that family factors influence people's relapse rates, illness course and outcome.[5] People living among families and informal carers involving high levels of criticism or emotional over-involvement tended to have poorer outcomes than those exposed to warm, appreciative attributes, positive interaction patterns and coping strategies.[6] Unfortunately, some professionals unwittingly used this evidence to promote negative attitudes towards families. In recent years, however, an attitudinal shift has occurred; studies have shown that family interventions reduce the number of relapse events and hospitalizations[7] and have encouraged more professionals to provide therapeutic interventions and work proactively with families to enhance their coping skills and increase their well-being.[8] Indeed, from their onset, some training programmes have promoted service users and carers as valuable members of curriculum development and teaching teams.[9]

However, away from the research and mental health teaching environments, mental illness remains outside one in four people's experience. When mental illness does occur, families can feel shocked, confused and isolated. The world they enter is frightening and the rules are unknown.

Families are often left to cope alone for long periods. The time of greatest need is the time when families have the least knowledge and information. Information and communication are often inadequate or hit and miss, and some families never get adequate support, do not recognize when they need it, or do not know they have needs and rights to support, information and involvement.

They used lots of terms I didn't understand. I couldn't keep asking what it meant because I felt stupid.

Jane, mother

When my Dad was terminally ill in general hospital I was treated with compassion. When my husband was admitted to a mental health ward I was turned away.

Dee, partner

It was critical for my own health to be able to access services. The information on what can be provided is really valuable; after 5 years of supporting my wife I have only just learnt I can apply for a carer's respite grant which has been wonderful.

Brian, husband

DEFINING WHAT A CARER IS

The definition of an informal 'carer' varies according to context. Carers' organizations and advocates usually use the term broadly to mean anyone providing unpaid care and support to a person with a disability, illness, frailty or other problems in coping with daily life. Since the Carers and Disabled Children Act 2000 was passed, carers have had a right to have their needs assessed, and professionals should support them in their caring role.[10] To be eligible for funded carers' support, according to current legislation (which guides local authority assessments of need and provision of services), carers generally are required to show that their relative is not receiving long-term care and demonstrate they provide 'substantial and regular' care. They need to request an assessment from a local authority (or an NHS Trust with delegated social care responsibilities) and then have their eligibility for funded services or other support assessed against local criteria.

The Care Act 2014 makes more provisions for carers and recognizes their needs more comprehensively.[11] This means three significant changes to the previous law on carers' assessments:

1. It removes the requirement for the carer to actively ask for an assessment (i.e. it should be offered as routine).
2. It removes the requirement for the carer to be providing substantial care on a regular basis. Instead, the only requirement is that the carer 'may have needs for support – whether currently or in the future'.
3. If both parties agree, the Care Act allows for joint assessments of service users' and carers' needs, enabling more sensible and personalized family- or couple-based support arrangements.

Carers are usually not charged for the services they receive, but local authorities can charge under the Care Act. If deemed eligible, carers can receive personal budgets and direct payments in their own right, just like service users. Carers can also be provided with support through additional services being provided to the person they care for.

Young carers (aged under 18) are eligible for support under children and families legislation, as are parent carers of disabled children. However, the Care Act now enables parents of people approaching the age of 18 to receive earlier assessments of their needs (and the needs of the young person) to improve their transition to adult services.

CHRISTINE'S REFLECTIONS

As a family carer, I support a relative and a friend who have schizophrenia. I am a volunteer and activist in mental health, focusing particularly on families' and carers' issues. In this role I help to facilitate a carers' support group and train mental health staff to engage with families and support them effectively.

Carers come from all walks of life, income groups and ages. The quotations I use from other family members in these reflective sections highlight this. They are parents, grandparents, step-parents, partners, siblings, sons, daughters and friends. The people they care for are some of the most vulnerable – the least able to speak up for themselves. Family members are sometimes reluctant to identify themselves as 'carers' as they see the role as part of their 'normal' family responsibilities. They may be slow to recognize that they have needs of their own which are distinct and separate from those of their relative.

'Carer' or 'family member'
We tend to think in terms of 'the service user' and 'the carer'. But severe mental illness affects the whole family. Family members often react in different ways to their relative's illness and the illness impacts in different ways. Everyone in the family has their own individual needs and strengths and is on their own path towards recovery, as well as supporting their relative. Understanding the nature of relationships and interactions is key to working supportively with them.

MEETING CARERS' NEEDS WITHIN THE NHS

NHS Trusts have a broad range of responsibilities towards carers, families and friends. NHS organizations and those who work in them are responsible for ensuring carers are involved optimally in service user assessments, care and crisis plans, reviews and risk management. NICE 2014 guidance[2] recommends that NHS Trusts provide psychosocial interventions to families, including the person using services, where appropriate, to support them to be able to live well together and to help reduce stressors and causes of tension or conflict. There are also specialist family therapy services available which may be able to support carers and family members alongside the service user. Trusts should also provide support, advice and guidance to individuals and to groups of carers, often in relation to specific conditions or needs groups. Where Trusts have delegated responsibility for social care functions, staff are tasked with identifying and providing assessments,

advice, information and services to carers – currently specifically 'substantial and regular' carers, but this is widened under the Care Act 2014.[11]

Overall, it is important to make a clear distinction between what is required by legislation (the Care Act), which is 'owned' primarily by social services, and a more generic appraisal which focuses on families' general need for information and support, and the level and amount of caring they are able to provide. Caregiving should be recognized as an activity with perceived benefits and burdens. Caregivers may be prone to depression, grief, fatigue, financial hardship and changes in social relationships. They may also experience physical health problems,[12] and perceived caregiver strain has been associated with premature institutionalization for care recipients, along with reports of unmet needs.[13] Such evidence further reinforces the need for services to assess carers' needs and support them.

CHRISTINE'S REFLECTIONS

The Care Act 2014 now gives carers a clear right to receive services, and places new duties on social services to identify and assess our needs. Consistent, national criteria for assessing carers' eligibility to receive services and support are very welcome. Mental health carers sometimes feel that generic carers' assessments are geared more towards those with physical conditions and personal care needs than to the specific needs of mental health carers. It will be important, and could be quite challenging, to ensure that mental health issues are adequately assessed, and that the new system does not unintentionally disadvantage mental health carers. I think carers' perception of the purpose of the carers assessment might change if it is regarded, or presented to them, much more as a test of eligibility than was formerly the case.

There may be a need to consider how to support carers and families in their caring role, irrespective of whether or not they are assessed as 'eligible' for social services support under the Care Act. There may be carers who are not assessed as eligible for services in their own right but still have considerable needs in their caring role.

FAMILY ASSESSMENT PROCESS

Caregiver assessment is a systematic process of gathering information about a caregiving situation to identify the specific problems, needs, strengths and resources of the family care giver, as well as the ability of the caregiver to contribute to the needs of the care recipient.[13] (p.225)

The purpose of family assessment is:

- to identify individual and carers' experience, expertise and knowledge in terms of stresses, concerns and coping styles;
- to determine what to offer and when;
- to develop shared understanding of needs, support plans and strengths to build on;
- to provide recognition, help and support for their caring role.

Prior to undertaking a family assessment it is important to do the following three things.

1. Consider the use of interpersonal skills

The concept of 'the craft of caring' dictates that the basis of good nursing practice is a combination of both art and science, encouraging nurses to take a holistic broad approach to engage both services users and their families. Family members really appreciate having their experiences and contributions to their relatives' care and their needs and strengths acknowledged, understood and valued. An important part of the process is an ability to take an emotionally intuitive appraisal of families' experiences, perspectives and needs. There are a variety of different 'art' (qualitative) and science (quantitative) methods to undertake this task. The first qualitative skill is to actively listen. The opportunity to 'share their narrative' is widely acknowledged to be of powerful benefit to families who may have struggled to access appropriate help. Indeed, although families' experiences have common themes, individual involvement in mental health services will be different. To avoid making judgements or painting everyone's experience with the same brush, it is important not only to use evidence-based tools but also to consider the skills and attributes required to assess and work with families. A small number of studies[14-16] have provided an overview of what competencies, qualitative personal qualities and interpersonal characteristics may be 'helpful', such as being able to create a calm atmosphere, being non-judgemental and being interested (see Box 15.1 for further skills required). Finding something likeable about the family really helps, and actively listening to identify family members' strengths, skills and abilities is the first step in achieving this.

2. Be supportive and non-judgemental, and have a clear rationale for your intention to collaborate and work together

Families are often vulnerable and can be at a very low ebb when initial contact is made, which can make them ambivalent and/or oversensitive to 'assessment' terminology. Assessment processes might be perceived as criticism, as all too often assessment of carers can feel like a tick-box exercise, which does not produce useful outcomes, and when this happens carers lose confidence in the process. In such instances, it is important to explain how working with families will help to address past engagement errors. Discussing the origins of such ambivalence can also provide a window of opportunity to introduce and highlight that, while families and service users go through mental health services, treatment delivery can be benchmarked against the six key Triangle of Care[19] standards to achieve better collaboration and partnership (see Box 15.2).

3. Be competent, and know what to offer and when

Appraising a family's needs and undertaking a carer's assessment is often perceived by professionals as difficult, because it is not within their competence, because it is in the domain of another profession or because the assessment process is too time-consuming and may expose a lack of ability to deliver. The challenge of offering assessments to families is further compounded by professionals not knowing what to offer and when.[20] Mohr et al.[21] postulate that this may be because families' experiences fluctuate; they are individuals on their own journey recovering from agonizing trauma. As they move through pre- and post-diagnosis events, such as being ignored when asking for help or dealing with difficult or strange behaviours, learning to cope with guilt, resentment and anger and becoming advocates, in many ways they become their own worst enemy. At the assessment stage, it may be evident that each member is recovering differently, going through different stages at different times, and there is no guarantee that they will get to the end of the journey together or in agreement that their management style worked. Indeed, during initial meetings most families will recall stories of muddling through, like being on a rollercoaster, and may use phrases like 'the blind leading the blind'. Caring for somebody with a serious mental illness (SMI) can become all-consuming. Family members can start to normalize some very odd behaviours, shut the door on friends and stop having a life of their own.

A failure to understand where family members are on this experience continuum also leaves practitioners unclear about how they can help[20] and researchers being disappointed by the difficulty of engaging carers in programmes that offer help.[22] Recent investigations into the support needs of siblings have also revealed a need to enhance siblings' knowledge about psychosis and their coping capacity, thus potentially improving their own mental well-being and promoting their contribution to service users' recovery.[23]

A triage approach to family inclusion[20] can provide a framework to ensure everyone in the family gets access to appropriate service provision and is appropriately targeted for support at a time when they need and require it (see Figure 15.1).

In seeking to implement family work into routine practice, Mottaghipour and Bickerton[24] used Maslow's Hierarchy of Needs principles to develop a conceptual 'Pyramid of Family Care' (see Figure 15.2). The base of the Pyramid addresses the families' basic need for assessment and information about SMI and mental health services, while the top of the Pyramid incorporates complex family circumstances through formal family therapy. The hierarchical model supports the assessment process as it outlines a minimum standard of care to guide practitioners and, like the triage model (see Figure 15.1), it assumes that a broad application of simple interventions can be delivered by mental health teams to address the majority of families' needs.

> ## BOX 15.1: INTERPERSONAL SKILLS AND ATTRIBUTES FOR WORKING WITH FAMILIES
>
> - Positive understanding attitude
> - Ability to use Rogerian principles[17]
> - Ability to engage and involve family members
> - Good communication skills
> - Experience of group work
> - Confidence in handling conflict
> - Knowledge and understanding of normal family systems and how they function
> - Skills in applying components of family work
> - Openness to reflect on own practice
> - Willingness to use supervision
> - Competence in co-working, problem solving and facilitation[18]

> ## BOX 15.2: TRIANGLE OF CARE STANDARDS
>
> 1. Carers and the essential role they play are identified at first contact or as soon as possible thereafter.
> 2. Staff are 'carer aware' and trained in carer engagement strategies.
> 3. Policy and practice protocols re: confidentiality and sharing information are in place.
> 4. Defined post(s) responsible for carers are in place.
> 5. A carer introduction to the service and staff is available, with a relevant range of information across the care pathway.
> 6. A range of carer support services is available.

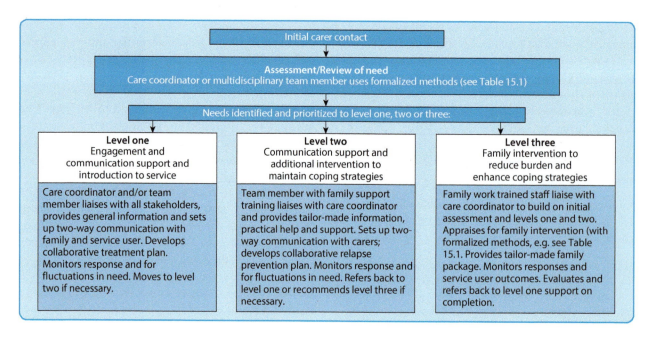

Figure 15.1   A triage approach to carer inclusion.

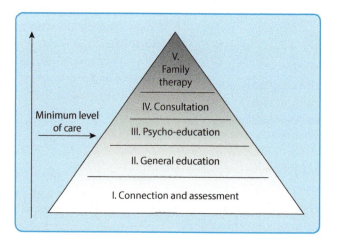

Figure 15.2   Pyramid of family care.

CHALLENGES OF IMPLEMENTING FAMILY ASSESSMENT

The uptake and successful implementation of family assessment is multifactorial. Potential recipients may be hindered by significant care burdens, and practical challenges such as travel and competing demands for time and energy are common.[25] Some may consider 'form filling' to be a barrier to engagement, especially if families' competence to care is felt to be under scrutiny, or if the tools used are lengthy or if they are perceived to have little value when the process results in little or no action. Sessions are also often scheduled when practitioners are available, and not when suitable for service users or their families. Additionally, families may not wish to identify themselves with psychiatric services; airing concerns in public when surrounded by the stigma of mental illness can be daunting. They may

have had negative past experiences with services, believe that nothing will help, or worry about losing confidential relationships with other family members or about losing autonomy.[6] Moreover, many service users lose close contact with their families – often, sadly, the illness itself has driven the family apart. Too often, mental health professionals just accept this as the norm. However, the assumption that carers will reject offers of help or feel bombarded by the process has to be reviewed. Mental health professionals need to do much more to encourage and support service users to stay in touch with their family, because there are such clear and obvious advantages for everyone if the family is involved. To achieve this, clinical experience suggests that practitioners need to adapt and be flexible.

METHODS OF ASSESSMENT

Most families want to talk about what has happened, and the assessment process can provide a platform to obtain a family history and facilitate a background discussion about familial relationships, and who is involved and supporting whom. A useful way to support this level of enquiry and promote dialogue is to compile a genogram,[26] as illustrated in Figure 15.3. From this it is possible to determine that Jane, the service user who has experienced a psychotic episode for the first time, has one sister (females are represented as circles), who is married with one daughter (Jane's niece). Jane's parents are still alive, her father (males are represented as squares) has two brothers and her mother has a sister. Her paternal grandmother has died (as the circle contains an X) and so has her maternal grandfather. Jane is separated from her husband (illustrated by the line through) and has no children. She had commenced divorce proceedings and family arguments about this decision meant Jane no longer felt welcome in her parents' home. The development of this genogram and the narrative that occurred during its construction provided an initial hypothesis regarding stress vulnerability and what may have exacerbated Jane's psychotic experience.

The assessment process can provide direction. After genogram discussion and development, the next step would be to facilitate a formal appraisal of family need. Outcome-orientated assessments encapsulate the extent to which interventions do what they are intended to do (for further guidance, see chapter 13). It can be very reassuring when sound, practical interviewing and rating procedures are therapeutically utilized, since this process demonstrates that assumptions are not being made, that accurate observations are sought and that systematic procedures to identify tailor-made interventions are being implemented. Overall, information obtained via systematic assessments on areas such as carer strain, and managing and understanding of mental illness at baseline and post-family work intervention, provides clear evidence that change can occur (see Table 15.1 for examples).

Overall, the family assessment process is valuable because:

- assessment tools can be selected to meet families' specific needs;
- being familiar with the tools enables practitioners to administer them sensitively and interpret them wisely;
- assumptions about how to intervene are less likely to be made.

SHARING INFORMATION AND CONFIDENTIALITY

The key is for mental health professionals to encourage good communication, while respecting everyone's need for privacy. The aim is inclusion and the greatest possible independence and self-management for the service user. For this reason, it is important to understand how to share information and overcome issues of confidentiality.

The beneficial effects of including family members in the planning and treatment of people with mental health

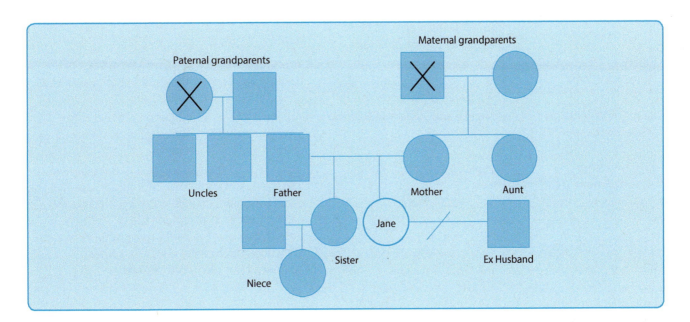

Figure 15.3 An example genogram.

Table 15.1 Assessment types and synopsis

Assessment name and reference	Assesses	Synopsis
Carer Strain Index (CSI)[27]	Caregiver strain among long-term family caregivers Self-report can be left with family for them to complete and return Originally developed for carers of older adults	Contains 13 questions that measure strain related to care provision: financial, physical, psychological, social and personal Can be used to assess individuals of any age who have assumed the caregiving role
Carers' Assessment of Difficulty Index (CADI)[28]	Difficult experiences and stressors Self-report can be left with family for them to complete and return	Contains 30 statements made by carers regarding the difficulties they experience and how stressful they find it
Carers' Assessment of Management Index (CAMI)[29]	Coping, stressors and management styles Originally developed for carers of those with dementia and learning disability	Contains 38 statements which carers have made about the coping strategies they use and how helpful they find them Builds on carer strengths and provides a baseline for engagement discussion
Experience of Caregiving Inventory (ECI)[30]	Difficulties, burden and coping Self-report can be left with family for them to complete and return	66 questions cover 10 domains; the first eight are described as negative (e.g. difficult behaviours; stigma; problems with services, etc.); the other two focus on positive areas such as personal experiences and relationships. Useful engagement discussion tool that provides a baseline to direct intervention
Carers' and Users' Expectations of Services: Carers' version (CUES-C)[31]	Service expectation Can be used as a supplement to others described or as a stand-alone, to facilitate discussion and as a baseline to direct intervention	Self-rated 13-item questionnaire, which addresses areas such as how to get help, information about care workers, information about the illness; involvement in planning of treatment, relationships; well-being; risk and safety
Knowledge about Schizophrenia Interview (KASI)[32]	Understanding of schizophrenia Can act as a follow up for RAI or as a stand-alone. Uses outdated terminology but helps to formulate development of psycho-education packages	Examines cause, prognosis, symptoms, medication and management
Relatives Assessment Interview (RAI)[32]	Global assessment Used to obtain information to help direct family intervention	Covers seven key areas, such as client's family background, contact time, current problems and effects of the illness on the carer
Family Problems Questionnaire (FPQ)[33]	Objective and subjective burden	Contains 29 items that focus on burden, and support received by professionals and from members of social networks
Family Coping Questionnaire (FCQ)[34]	Global assessment of coping styles	Self-administered 34-item questionnaire divided into sub-scales, including: information, positive communication, maintenance of social interest, patient's social involvement, use of drugs and alcohol, collusive reactions, non-compliance with prescribed treatments, search for spiritual guidance and talking with friends

problems are reinforced throughout this chapter. Despite this recognition, the carer's need for information has to be balanced with the service user's right to privacy.

Ethical dilemmas and confidentiality issues are frequently encountered in everyday practice, and it is therefore important to consider potential factors which may promote or hinder information-sharing processes. Despite knowing that families can play a significant role, many professionals remain uncertain about how to share information; hence many families report feeling undervalued and being left out of the communication loop.[35]

For those working within child and adolescent services or with older age groups, or for those who have experience of working with families, this dilemma is not as prevalent. In these service areas, family inclusion is more commonplace; because of capacity and consent issues, they are also more likely to be perceived as allies, so some sort of respectful contact is usually possible. Even if their family appears crucial in supporting an adult of working age, if service users withdraw their consent, breaching their rights to confidentiality is commonly mentioned as an engagement barrier by staff.[35]

Until recently there has been a lack of research in this area. To address concerns consistently raised by families, Slade et al.[36] assessed mental health sharing practices across the UK. Three groups informed the multiple method design: a core research group, an expert panel and a virtual electronic panel. All had service user, carer, professional, support worker and academic representation. Qualitative interviews of 24 participants were used to assess involvement in mental health, how confidentiality affected roles, where information sharing worked well and how information sharing could be improved. Data were also synthesized from policy reviews, surveys of current practice and qualitative interviews. The study identified 56 policies and 35 supporting documents, but only five provided any practical guidelines on how to share information. A review of these policies highlighted that those co-authored with carer groups advocated the use of advance statements to record preferences for who should be involved during relapse or times of crisis. The national survey of current practice included service users ($n = 91$), carers ($n = 329$) and professionals ($n = 175$). The majority of the carer sample reported they were well supported in terms of access to general information. However, when asked about the reasons why professionals did not share personal information, 47 (28 per cent) reported that confidentiality was given as the reason. The majority (57; 35 per cent) of carer respondents reported they had not been asked about it; 35 service users (21 per cent) did not provide consent, nine (5 per cent) were unable to give it, and 32 (19 per cent) were not asked to provide it. Reasons given by professionals included service users providing consent and then changing their mind, language barrier problems, and the carer not being next of kin. In contrast, more than half of service users ($n = 91$) stated that their families should have access to personal information and 47 (55 per cent) were comfortable with their carer being involved and 47 (55 per cent) stated that professionals should offer their families separate support.

Overall, Slade et al.'s findings[36] challenged the idea that service users were not willing for their families to be involved in their care, and highlighted the value of mental health professionals having a positive, inclusive attitude and taking a proactive role in engaging them. In this way they are more likely to be able to influence multidisciplinary decision making. To achieve this goal, Slade et al.[36] identified good practice principles for information sharing, listed in Table 15.2.

Table 15.2 Good practice principles for information sharing

	Carers	Service users	Professionals
Good practice principles	Knowing how to explain to service users about the carer's 'need to know' Seek information/support from another professional source	Consent must be obtained before information is shared	Collect consent Establish effective communication and maintain dialogue
	More consultation and improve professionals' attitudes	Identify information person feels comfortable sharing	Acknowledge distress and recognize the carer's role and their rights
	Attend care planning meetings	Use an advocate or support network	Share information on a general (hypothetical) basis
	Identify need through carer assessment process	Consider long-term relationships before deciding to share information	Talk to carers about confidentiality and professional codes of conduct

In cases of serious disagreement, carers, service users and professionals should use the framework for best clinical practice (see Figure 15.4).

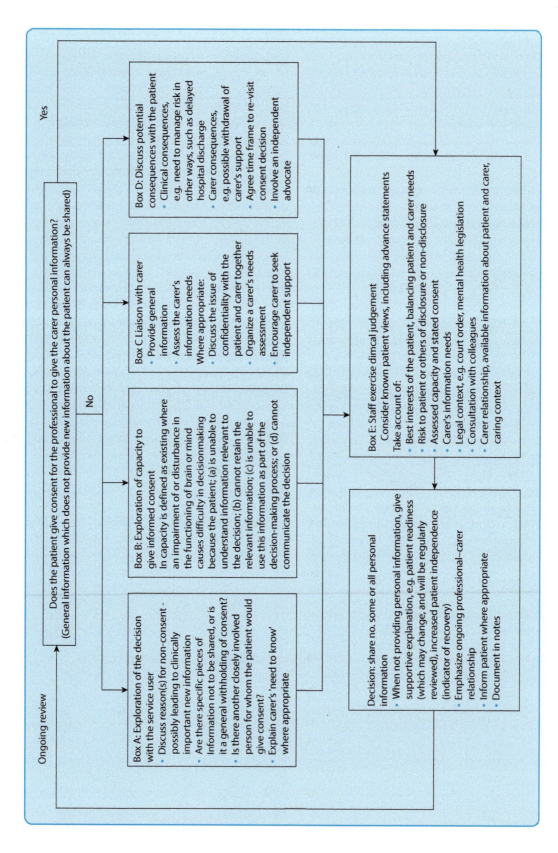

Figure 15.4   Framework for best clinical practice when consent is not given to share information.

Referring to the best clinical practice framework,[36] consider the following clinical examples through the following steps:

- exploration of the decision with the service user;
- exploration of capacity to give informed consent;
- liaison with carer;
- discuss potential consequences with the patient;
- staff exercise clinical judgement.

1. A family member rings the team to ask whether their relative, who they live with, has been admitted yet.
2. A brother questions his sister's capacity and tells staff he knows she isn't taking her medication.
3. A young carer (aged 15) visiting his mother asks the nurse what is wrong with Mummy.
4. A service user states he does not wish his parents to know his diagnosis.
5. A service user has not told his new bride that he was previously sectioned under the Mental Health Act and admitted to a forensic ward following a severe psychotic breakdown after stabbing his female neighbour in the foot.

Confidentiality would be breached if a diagnosis or personal information was shared without a person's consent. There are no 'right' or 'wrong' answers among the aforementioned examples, but they illustrate the value of the framework in supporting teams' decision-making processes in everyday clinical practice. Indeed, the framework has proved invaluable when teams need to articulate and give families a rationale for why particular decisions regarding information sharing have been made.

Confidentiality is generally not broken when practices are openly shared and inclusive and all parties know how decisions have been made. Indeed, there is a growing evidence base developed in Finland that demonstrates the value of routinely including families and people's social networks and taking an 'Open Dialogue' approach. In the 1980s psychiatric services in Western Lapland dealt with one of the highest incidences of schizophrenia in Europe. By using 'Open Dialogue' approaches, that is supporting people's networks of family and friends as well as respecting the decision making of the individual with psychosis, they now report significantly better outcomes. For example, around 75 per cent of those experiencing psychosis have returned to work or study within 2 years and only around 20 per cent still take antipsychotic medication at 2-year follow-up.[37] This Finnish alternative to traditional mental health services for people diagnosed with psychosis such as schizophrenia highlights that, with appropriate support, families and friends can bear extreme crisis situations and tolerate the uncertainty, so that in time shared meaning usually emerges, stigma reduces and thus a recovery paradigm is endorsed by those involved.

CHRISTINE'S REFLECTIONS

Carers are aware of the complex ethical dilemmas that can arise regarding confidentiality and information sharing. Getting it right makes a tremendous difference to the service user's recovery and their carers' and families' well-being and peace of mind. If handled badly, this can cause more distress and anguish than almost anything else.

For the family, it cuts both ways – we want to receive sufficient information about our relative's illness and treatment to help us support their recovery. We also want to give mental health professionals information about what we know about our relative and what we observe when they become unwell, so that we can help them, and at times, it is equally important that our rights to confidentiality are protected.

Service users often turn away from their carer or family when they become ill, just at the time when everyone could benefit most from sharing information – and this situation can seem difficult or impossible to resolve.

INVOLVING FAMILY AND FRIENDS IN MEDICINES MANAGEMENT

Like many others, Leroy's family (see case study 1) were integral to his treatment and recovery. Yet professionals often exclude families from discussion about pharmaceutical treatments and especially side effects. Medication conflict can feature prominently within families; many have conflicting beliefs about its value and purpose, and are ill-prepared to take on an administration role.[39] Unwittingly, family members can be perceived as agents of control, so requests to adhere to treatment are either ignored or provoke tension. However, families can offer a wealth of information about past treatment failures and successes, they often monitor an individual's treatment adherence and they are a reliable source of determining relapse. This knowledge can only be obtained when they are actively involved in an assessment process. However, it is widely known that carers feel excluded from services and receive limited education/information, particularly about medicines. For some families, developing the confidence and skills to take an active part in treatment decisions may take some time. Family intervention can support this competency development so that families can become more involved in care plan discussions around medicines and treatment.

CASE STUDY 1

Leroy, aged 27, has experienced three psychotic relapses, resulting in two admissions. He was severely bullied at college, smoked cannabis heavily and is now isolating himself from friends and family. His mother, Mel, who had never been included in Leroy's care or participated in a carer's assessment, contacted his mental health team to determine what could be done to address his social isolation. Follow-up contact was made through Leroy's care coordinator during a Care Programme Approach (CPA) review.[38] This CPA highlighted the need to recognize the importance of family support, but also to ensure that Leroy's experiences were contextualized and treated more effectively. Using the best clinical practice framework (see Figure 15.4), the care coordinator gained Leroy's consent to meet Mel and other members of his family to share understanding, collate experiences and assess their support needs.

This process involved meeting family members individually to gain their perspectives and understanding (see Figure 15.5). Leroy has a brother, his father works long hours and he describes his mother as playing a pivotal role in the family, but he acknowledged that he had other significant family members, such as his aunt and grandparents who had recently moved back to the Caribbean. While generating a genogram (see Figure 15.3 for an explanation), concerns were raised about how to find sufficient time to meet everyone. For this reason, a number of assessment strategies were chosen. Leroy's brother completed a CSI[27] and his father a CUES-C.[31] The care coordinator and his mother completed an RAI[32] together, at a mutually convenient time at home.

Having collated these baseline assessments, it was possible to summarize the family needs as wanting more information about:

- what services could provide, whom to contact and when;
- crisis planning and care plan management (see chapter 50);
- psychosis, treatment approaches and how to anticipate relapse and understand stress vulnerability;

- how to support Leroy to overcome his lack of motivation, social skills and concentration;
- how to cope as a family, stay on good terms, maintain personal activities and find employment.

Integrating family work into Leroy's routine care would:

1. increase his family's knowledge and understanding of psychosis and stress vulnerability, including raising their awareness of early warning signs of relapse and ways to proactively anticipate them;
2. promote communication between family members, including how to feel heard, make requests of each other and express concern;
3. re-establish relationships (especially with Leroy's friends and his brother) and enhance working alliances with professionals;
4. build on the family's strengths; signpost them to other carer support services and recovery college carer programmes; and increase everyone's problem-solving skills and coping strategies;
5. overcome obstacles preventing independence and life goals being achieved.

The results of these assessments were also drawn upon to describe the structure and flow of family meetings, as outlined in Figure 15.5. On sharing this draft structure, Leroy's care coordinator and another family work trained team member negotiated what should be prioritized, the duration of forthcoming meetings and who should be involved.

Leroy's recovery goals also included:

- individual problem solving to increase his motivation, activity levels and social and independent living skills;
- determining whether he was experiencing symptoms of post-traumatic stress syndrome following being bullied at college, as recommended by NICE schizophrenia guidance;[2]
- assessing side effects and examining Leroy's motivations to continue to take prescribed medication.

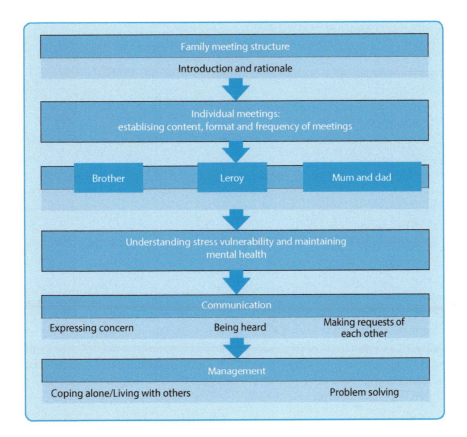

Figure 15.5 Family meeting structure and format.

Collaborative working is about being open and sharing information honestly, and ensuring full discussions on aspects that are important to the service user. Service users and carers should feel that they are active partners in treatment decisions and have influence regarding the frequency and format of treatment reviews.

SHARING AND GIVING INFORMATION ABOUT MEDICATION

Information sharing with service users and carers is notoriously poor. Carers have been asking for clear, unbiased information about medicines for some time. Information sheets provided with medicines are often inadequate or unclear. Without this information, families can on occasion attribute the side effects of medication to a person's illness. Key issues which can all be side effects that can cause tension within families include weight gain, sexual dysfunction and lack of motivation. Without proper knowledge, service users and their families can be powerless to modify behaviours, encourage alternatives or develop a healthier lifestyle.

Promoting knowledge and understanding about psychotropic medication and treatment influences with an individual (see chapter 48) and their family will mean they become a more active part in treatment decisions. As part of a family intervention package, it is useful to have meaningful discussions about diagnosis and pharmacological treatments. What are the families' views, knowledge and past experiences of psychotropic medicines, including dosage and circumstances? These views are often the most important factor of adherence. Indeed, without sensitivity, aspects of treatment and culture can exacerbate engagement barriers, particularly for those from black and ethnic minority families.[40]

> *Black and ethnic families are very distrusting of services. Having been in mental health for so long I can understand why. There is something about stigma. They are frightened to share information in case they are prejudged.*
>
> **Carer support worker 2**[40]

The UK African Caribbean population are diagnosed with schizophrenia more frequently than any other ethnic group and are more likely to access psychiatric services via the police and under compulsion. The Aetiology and Ethnicity in Schizophrenia and Other Psychoses (AESOP) study in three cities (London, Nottingham and Bristol) reported that it takes African Caribbean people longer to obtain a diagnosis, and when they do receive treatment, this usually involves higher doses of medication and limited or no access to psychological therapies, such as family therapy.[40]

Table 15.3 Family decision making around treatment

Family decision making around treatment	Meeting prescribers
Looking back – doing a timeline	Identify the objectives
Checking out familial beliefs about treatment	Rehearse the points you want to get across
Assessing and enhancing the person's ability to take medication, and the carer's ability to support medication taking	Write things down (take notes)
	List questions
Checking the pros and cons of medication	Share advance directive and crisis plan arrangement
Looking forward	
Working with beliefs about medication	
Evaluating the service user's and carer's experience of medication	
Addressing consent and planning for crisis	
Constructing advance directive	
Enabling carers to provide an intention of involvement at times of crisis or relapse	

The Culturally-adapted Family Intervention (CaFI) for African Caribbeans project is currently investigating the implementation and acceptability of family work for this community.[41] Their findings have yet to be published, but in the meantime Harris et al.[39] highlight some useful exercises to aid families' understanding and decision making around treatment and to help them when meeting prescribers (see Table 15.3).

Overall, the family can play an important role in monitoring side effects, particularly those which may influence the dynamics within a close relationship, such as sexual dysfunction or weight gain. The importance of the family in helping maintain good physical health cannot be underestimated.

Working with people and their families to derive maximum benefit from medicines takes skill and knowledge. Many medication management education programmes have been developed, incorporating supervision, and practitioners would be advised to access training for further knowledge.[39]

CONCLUSION

This chapter has sought to highlight the needs of families and how to assess their needs effectively. Practitioners are generally focused towards working with patients as individuals, but the techniques to promote family inclusion are clearly within mental health nurses' skill set and expertise. As a whole, mental health services would improve if early engagement and family inclusion principles were embraced in all aspects of care.[42]

I feel so much better. I have learnt how to talk to my daughter. I made a lot of mistakes and sometimes still do. Now I am more confident and relaxed and this is helping my daughter in her recovery.

Sunita, parent

CHRISTINE'S FINAL REFLECTIONS

After reading this chapter try to routinely:

- 'think family' and work supportively with carers – in this way everyone benefits, most of all the person with mental health problems;
- work collaboratively with families – building their capacity to support their relative makes *your* job easier as well as theirs;
- remember that, although families share broadly the same issues, every family's experience and everyone's story is different and individual. Their needs and, equally important, their strengths may not be immediately apparent;
- deliver sensitive assessment processes and follow these up with collaborative work which supports families' needs and plays to their strengths.

References

1. Shore L. Inside caring in mental health. In: Gamble C, Brennan G (eds). *Working with serious mental illness: a manual for clinical practice*, 2nd edn. London, Elsevier: 2006, 11–22.

2. NICE (National Institute for Health and Care Excellence). *Schizophrenia: psychosis and schizophrenia in adults: treatment and management*. NICE clinical guideline CG178, 2014. Available from: www.nice.org.uk/CG178 [Accessed 21st May 2016].

3. More than 2 million people give up work to care for relatives. *Guardian* 7 March 2013. Available from: http://www.guardian.co.uk/society/2013/mar/07/2-million-work-care-relatives [Accessed 21st May 2016].

4. Young H, Grundy E. *Who cares? Geographic variation in unpaid caregiving in England and Wales: evidence from the 2001 census*. Population Trends: Office of National Statistics, 2005. Available from: https://www.researchgate.net/publication/7718590 [Accessed 2nd October 2016].

5. Stern S, Doolan M, Staples E, Szmukler G, Eisler I. Disruption and reconstruction: narrative insights in to the experiences of family members caring for a relative diagnosed with serious mental illness. *Family Process* 1999; **38**(3): 353–69.

6. Kuipers E, Bebbington P. Research on burden and coping strategies in families of people with mental disorders: problems and perspectives. In: Sartorius N, Leff J, Lopez JJ (eds). *Families and mental disorder: from burden to empowerment*. Chichester: Wiley, 2005, 217–34.

7. Pharoah F, Mari J, Rathbone J, Wong W. Family intervention for schizophrenia. *Cochrane Database of Systematic Reviews* 2010; **12**: CD000088.

8. Kuipers E, Onwumere J, Bebbington P. Cognitive model of caregiving in psychosis. *British Journal of Psychiatry* 2010; **196**: 259–65.

9. Gamble C. The Thorn Nursing Programme: its past, present and future. *Mental Health Care* 1997; **1**(3): 95–7.

10. Department of Health. Carers and Disabled Children Act, 2000, Chapter 16. Available from: http://www.legislation.gov.uk/ukpga/2000/16/pdfs/ukpga_20000016_en.pdf [Accessed 21st May 2016].

11. Horne S, White J, Kirthi-Singha A. Consultation on funding formulae for implementation of the Care Act in 2015/16. Department of Health, Social Care Local Government and Care Partnerships Directorate Analytical Unit. Available from: http://consultations.dh.gov.uk/social-care-funding-1/allocations-for-2015-16/supporting_documents/scallocationscondoc.pdf [Accessed 21st May 2016].

12. Thornton M, Travis SS. Analysis of the reliability of the Modified Caregiver Strain Index. *Journals of Gerontology* 2003; **58B**(2); S127–S132.

13. Feinberg L, Houser A. *Assessing family caregiver need: policy and practice considerations*. Washington, DC: AARP Public Policy Institute, 2012.

14. James C, Cushway D, Fadden G. What works in engagement of families in behavioural family therapy? A positive model from the therapists' perspective. *Journal of Mental Health* 2006; **15**(3): 355–68.

15. Stanbridge RI, Burbach FR, Lucas AS, Carter K. A study of families' satisfaction with a family interventions in psychosis service in Somerset. *Journal of Family Therapy* 2003; **25**: 181–204.

16. Fadden G. Training and disseminating family interventions for schizophrenia: developing family intervention skills with multidisciplinary groups. *Journal of Family Therapy* 2006; **28**: 23–38.

17. Rogers CR. *Way of being*. Boston: Houghton Mifflin, 1980.

18. Gamble C, Sin J, Kelly M, Moone N. The development of a Family Intervention Competency Assessment and Reflection Scale (FICARS) for psychosis. *Journal of Psychiatric and Mental Health Nursing* 2013; **20**(8): 744–51.

19. Triangle of Care. 2013. https://professionals.carers.org/working-mental-health-carers/triangle-care-mental-health [Accessed 3rd October 2016].

20. Gamble C. Family intervention. *Psychiatry* 2007; **6**(9): 367–72.

21. Mohr W, Lafuze J, Mohr B. Three stages of caring opening car-egiver minds. *Archives of Psychiatric Nursing* 2000; **14**(5).

22. Szmukler G, Kuipers E, Joyce J, Harris T, Leese M, Maphosa W, Staples E. An exploratory randomised controlled trial of a support programme for carers of patients with a psychosis. *Social Psychiatry and Psychiatric Epidemiology* 2003; **38**: 411–18.

23. Sin J, Henderson C, Pinfold V, Norman I. The E Sibling Project – exploratory randomised controlled trial of an online multicomponent psychoeducational intervention for siblings of individuals with first episode psychosis. *BMC Psychiatry* 2013; **13**: 123.

24. Mottaghipour Y, Bickerton A. The Pyramid of Family Care: a framework for family involvement with adult mental health services. *Australian e-Journal for the Advancement of Mental Health (AeJAMH)* 2005; **4**(3).

25. Lobban F, Barrowclough C. *A casebook of family interventions for psychosis*. Chichester: John Wiley & Sons Ltd, 2009.

26. Rogers JC, Rohrbaugh M. The SAGE-PAGE trial: do family genograms make a difference? *Journal of the American Board of Family Practice* 1991; **4**(5): 319–26. In: *The Cochrane Central Register of Controlled Trials (CENTRAL)* 2016; **1**. Available from: http://onlinelibrary.wiley.com/o/cochrane/clcentral/articles/090/CN-00080090/frame.html [Accessed 21st May 2016].

27. Robinson BC. Validation of a carer giver strain index. *Journal of Gerontology* 1983; **38**: 344–8.

28. Charlesworth GM, Tzimoula XM, Newman SP. Carers Assessment of Difficulties Index (CADI): psychometric properties for use with carers of people with dementia. *Aging & Mental Health* 2007; **11**(2): 218–25.

29. Nolan M, Keady J, Grant G. CAMI a basis for assessment and support with family carers. *British Journal of Nursing Quarterly* 1995; **4**(14): 822–6.

30. Szmukler GI, Burgess P, Herman H, Benson A, Colusa S, Bloch S. Caring for relatives with serious mental illness – the development of the Experience of Caregiving Inventory. *Social Psychiatry and Psychiatric Epidemiology* 1996; **31**: 134–48.

31. Lelliot P, Beevor A, Hogman G, Hyslop J, Lathlean J, Ward M. Carers' and users' expectations of services – carer version: a new instrument to support the assessment of carers of people with a severe mental illness. *Journal of Mental Health* 2003; **12**(2): 143–52.

32. Barrowclough C, Tarrier N. *Families of schizophrenic patients: cognitive behavioural intervention*. London: Chapman and Hall, 1995.

33. Morosini PL, Roncone R, Veltro F, Palomba U, Casacchia M. Routine assessment pool in psychiatry: the questionnaire of family attitudes and burden. *Italian Journal of Psychiatry and Behavioural Sciences* 1991; **1**: 95–101.

34. Magliano L, Guarneri M, Marasco C, Tosini P, Morosini PL, Maj M. A new questionnaire assessing coping strategies in relatives of schizophrenia patients: development and factor analysis. *Acta Psychiatrica Scandinavica* 1996; **94**: 224–8.

35. Solomon P, Molinaro M, Mannion E, Cantwell K. Confidentiality policies and practices in regard to family involvement: does training make a difference? *American Journal of Psychiatric Rehabilitation* 2012; **15**(1): 97–115.

36. Slade M, Pinfold V, Rapaport J, Bellringer S, Banerjee S, Kuipers E, Huxley P. Best practice when service users do not consent to sharing information with carers. *British Journal of Psychiatry* 2007; **190**: 148–55.

37. Seikkulaa J, Alakareb B, Aaltonena J. The Comprehensive Open-Dialogue Approach in Western Lapland: II. Long-term stability of acute psychosis outcomes in advanced community care. *Psychosis: Psychological, Social and Integrative Approaches* 2011; **3**(3): 192–204.

38. Department of Health. Refocusing the care programme approach policy and positive practice guidance, 2008. Available from: http://webarchive.nationalarchives.gov. uk/20130107105354/http://www.dh.gov.uk/prod_consum_dh/ groups/dh_digitalassets/@dh/@en/documents/digitalasset/ dh_083649.pdf [Accessed on 21st May 2016].

39. Harris N, Baker J, Gray R (eds). *Medicines management and mental health care*. Oxford: Wiley-Blackwell, 2009.

40. Morgan C, Kirkbride J, Hutchinson G, Craig T, Morgan K, Dazzan P, Boydella J, Doody GA, Jones PB, Murray RM, Leff J, Fearon P. Cumulative social disadvantage, ethnicity and first-episode psychosis: a case-control study. *Psychological Medicine* 2008; **38**(12): 1701–15.

41. Edge D. HS&DR - 12/5001/62: Culturally-adapted Family Intervention (CaFI) for African Caribbeans with schizophrenia and their families: a feasibility study of implementation and acceptability. Available from: http://www.nets.nihr.ac.uk/projects/hsdr/12500162 [Accessed 21st May 2016].

42. Schizophrenia Commission. *The abandoned illness: a report from the Schizophrenia Commission*. London: Rethink Mental Illness, 2012.

Further reading

Cockburn P, Cockburn H. *Henry's demons: living with schizophrenia, a father and son's story*. London: Simon and Schuster, 2011.
Male family members rarely share their experiences of caring. The unique angle of this book is that the narrative is told from a father and his son's (service users) perspective. It provides insight into Henry's schizophrenia and his father's understanding of the illness and the impact it can have on familial relationships.

Lobban F, Barrowclough C. *A casebook of family interventions for psychosis*. Chichester: John Wiley & Sons Ltd, 2009.
This readable, user-friendly guide to family intervention discusses family needs and illustrates different intervention approaches. It outlines how to tailor family interventions to meet different needs, for example, working via an interpreter or working with families in which multiple members suffer mental health problems.

Smith G, Gregory K, Higgs A. *An integrated approach to family work for psychosis: a manual for family workers*. London: Jessica Kingsley, 2007.
This manual for working with families of people with severe mental illness discusses what constitutes family work, when it might be offered, and how and where it might be applied. The book addresses both theory and practice, and concentrates on the experience of mental illness for the service user and their family, providing a focus for intervention.

Relevant web pages

Meriden Family Programme. http://www.meridenfamilyprogramme.com/
On this site you will find useful information and resources if you are a person living with mental health issues, a carer, family member, friend, mental health professional or commissioner.

Open Dialogue. http://opendialogueapproach.co.uk/
This site introduces the principles of 'Open Dialogue' and resources. It also provides updates on training programmes and literature.

Rethink Mental Illness. http://www.rethink.org/
This site helps people living with conditions such as schizophrenia, bipolar disorder, personality disorders and others to recover a better quality of life.

Rethink Mental Illness. Siblings Network for brothers and sisters. http://www.rethink.org/carers-family-friends/brothers-and-sisters-siblings-network
This is an excellent resource to support siblings and introduce them to the Siblings Network.

16 Assessing risk of suicide and self-harm

KEITH WATERS AND ALYS COLE-KING

LEARNING OUTCOMES

- To understand how to assess risk in a reliable and consistent way, using evidenced-based and peer-reviewed clinical tools and frameworks to structure and record the assessment which will then help to inform the corresponding safety plans and treatment goals.

- To understand that every patient at risk of suicide needs a co-produced safety plan, and not just those patients deemed to be of higher risk.

- To be aware of the importance of asking and exploring for the presence of suicidal thoughts, and the importance of co-creating actions with the patient and carer to mitigate the risks identified.

- To understand the relationships among the risk factors relating to self-harm and suicide.

- To be aware of the importance of the craft of caring and its central role in guiding practice.

- To understand how national guidelines and policies help to inform the craft of caring for those at risk and those with suicidal thoughts.

- To recognize the strengths as well as the limitations of risk factor identification and assessment frameworks, tools and approaches.

SUMMARY OF KEY POINTS

- Suicide is preventable, and we need a new narrative, so that instead of focusing on 'characterizing, quantifying and managing risk' we talk about 'compassion, safeguarding and safety planning'.

- Self-harm and suicide are sometimes viewed as separate entities, and sometimes viewed as being 'on a continuum'.

- By believing we can make a difference, we will engage with confidence, compassion and competence with our patients.

- Suicidal people are extremely ambivalent, and their lives can be saved up until the final moment. Compassionate communication with people at risk of suicide can save lives, is essential to the quality of the

- information underpinning an assessment and can be the tipping point back to safety.
- A variety of theoretical models are described, to help understand suicide and self-harm.
- Suicide and self-harm assessments are described, along with training approaches and risk assessment tools.
- Suicide prevention is everyone's business and we are all part of the solution. The question we all should be asking is: 'What can be done to enable this person to not want to end their life today … this week … this month?'

- At the heart of the craft of caring is the process of working with an individual using clinical experience, a compassionate approach and the best available research and clinical evidence. This will support co-working, negotiation and participation and ways of working therapeutically with people who have suicidal thoughts and are at risk of suicide or self-harm.
- The evidence and guidance in this chapter apply to people of all ages. The chapter contains quotations from service users, derived from consultations, to emphasize specific points.

INTRODUCTION

Suicide and self-harm cause significant emotional distress, mortality and morbidity. Suicide is the 14th highest cause of death worldwide, responsible for 1.5 per cent of all mortality.[1] Suicide and harming one's body in various ways has been a feature of human behaviour throughout history and has evoked a wide range of human reactions. These include: heroic glorification, anger, sympathy, dismissal and moral or religious interpretations. During the fourth and fifth centuries, suicide was termed 'self-killing' and it was viewed as a mortal sin. Anyone who died by suicide was buried in unconsecrated ground. During the thirteenth century the legal term for suicide in the UK was 'self-murder' and the perpetrator was deemed to have committed a 'heinous crime'. In the early nineteenth century, a more pathological[2] understanding of suicide and suicidal behaviour started to emerge, according to which the individual was thought to be a victim of illness.[3] In the twentieth century people were thought to be victims of risk factors. This resulted in changes in the law. The UK Suicide Act 1961 stated that it was not a crime to take one's own life,[4] although it still remained a crime to assist someone in suicide. Today, suicide and suicidal behaviours are understood to be a manifestation of emotional distress,[5,6] rather than a primary disorder. For some, suicide is the end point of a complex history of risk factors and distressing events.[7]

Nurses, as frontline practitioners, are well positioned to detect and respond to those who are distressed and at risk of suicide or self-harm. The process of clearly identifying those who are significantly at risk remains a challenge that may be fraught with difficulties, but forms an important component of mental health nursing. There is a considerable amount of information available about self-harm and suicidal behaviours from a range of sources, including historical accounts, research, psychological autopsies, and accounts of people with lived experience who have attempted suicide, and their carers and relatives. There are also a variety of theoretical perspectives that assist in our understanding of self-harm and suicidal behaviours. These behaviours emerge from a complex interplay[8] of individually sensitive

markers for that person. When assessing for risk of suicide and self-harm, it is important to identify evidence-based risk factors. However, evidence-based risk factors do not necessarily assist in predicting individual risk at a given moment because they are based on predicting the risk of a population across its lifetime.

Individual suicides or acts of self-harm may be extremely difficult to predict. The existing risk assessment tools have poor predictive ability if they are only used to target care at those identified as high risk.[9–11] Mental health nurses can assess risk in a reliable, evidenced-based and consistent way using evidenced-based and peer-reviewed clinical tools to structure and record the assessment, which will then help to inform the corresponding safety plans and treatment goals. It is imperative that the craft of caring and clinical experience are part of the approach that informs the completion of the risk assessment tools.[12] The National Institute for Health and Care Excellence (NICE) guidelines state that everyone should receive a psychosocial assessment following self-harm.[13] The importance of a thorough assessment is also supported by findings from the National Confidential Inquiry,[14,15] which highlights the need for assessment and management of patients at risk of suicide. The presence of suicidal thoughts is not a feature of mental illness and could be considered to be a normal reaction and extreme response to distress, despair and difficulties in the human condition. Some illnesses have a higher incidence of suicide and self-harm.[9,10] However, suicide is not the inevitable outcome in psychiatric conditions. The risks of suicide and self-harm in depression, for example, although higher than in the general population, still mean that more people with depression do not take their lives than do.[1]

For instance, less than 5% of people admitted to hospital for treatment of an affective disorder die by suicide; most people with a psychiatric disorder will not die by suicide, nor will they experience suicidal behaviour. Thus, although the presence and accumulation of psychiatric disorders are risk factors for suicidal behaviour, they have little predictive power, and perhaps more importantly do not account for why people try to kill themselves. (p.28)

SERVICE USER'S PERSPECTIVE

A member of SH.SH. (Stop Hiding Self-Harm, a self-help group), with a long history of involvement with services and previous self-harm, says:

It's not the mental illness that makes me self-harm or feel suicidal, but the mental illness may make me more vulnerable to the other problems and difficulties that I'm facing.

REFLECTION

Based on your clinical experience so far, do you believe that mitigation of suicide risks can potentially help to save lives?

All suicidal thoughts require a response and safety plan because the prediction of suicide risk is fraught with difficulty and the level of accuracy is questionable.[6] The transition from mild and fleeting suicidal ideation to making an actual attempt at suicide is a highly complex issue and we still do not fully understand how suicidal thoughts progress. It is therefore proposed that the only safe response is to adopt a suicide mitigation approach.[6,16,17] Suicide mitigation starts from the assumption that suicidal thoughts need to be taken seriously and met with compassion and understanding on every occasion in order to engage positively with the person. A thorough structured assessment should be undertaken, using clinical tools to identify all risk factors and red flag warning signs, with an appropriate and proportionate action to mitigate each risk. The Classification of Suicidal Thoughts[6] provides a common language to describe the nature and intensity of suicidal thoughts. Use of common language to describe suicidal thoughts after undertaking a thorough assessment can help to improve the consistency, accuracy and appropriate prioritization of referrals.

New evidence suggests that there is more of an overlap between suicide and self-harm than previously thought, so self-harm should be taken seriously.[18,19]

REFLECTION

How do you feel about managing ambivalence and uncertainty arising from the fact that service users may be having conflicting feelings about wanting to live and wanting to die?

This chapter explores the issues raised in this introductory section, and provides guidance for understanding the risks and protective factors, which in turn will influence interventions and approaches.

SELF-HARM AND SUICIDE: A CONTINUUM OR SEPARATE ENTITIES?

In the UK the legal definition of suicide comes from verdicts given by a coroner following an inquest if it is determined that there was clear evidence showing beyond reasonable doubt that the person had intended to and acted to end their life.[20] A less stringent definition of suicide is used in clinical practice, which extends to include those deaths that occurred as a result of an act of self-harm.[14,15] This includes people who have undertaken an act with an intention to do harm to themselves, which resulted in their death. Studies on suicide will generally include this broader definition, which encompasses not only coroners' suicide verdicts but also includes other verdicts, such as open, narrative and accidental.

Although the function of self-harm may not be to end one's life, there is a link between self-harm (see chapter 22) and suicide. There is strong evidence to show that the risk of suicide among those who have self-harmed[21,22] is much greater than that of the general population, as is the risk of premature death.[23] The relationship between self-harm and suicide is conceptualized in Figure 16.1.

Many people who manage their distress using self-harm, especially self-cutting, report that their actions do not have suicidal intent.[24] Some report that their self-cutting is a way of preserving their life and ameliorating any suicidal thoughts, ideas or further actions. One view is that non-suicidal self-injury (NSSI)[24,25] should not be viewed on the continuum of self-harm and suicide. There are debates about whether people who carry out NSSI are a heterogeneous group and whether this is creating a false dichotomy.[19]

Self-harm can be categorized as behaviours that cause harm to the body, either directly with immediate tissue damage (direct self-harm), or indirectly, potentially leading to progressive long-term illness (see Box 16.1).

When considering direct and indirect self-harm, where does body art in the form of tattoos or body piercings fit? There are reports of these being used as coping mechanisms as well as having some potentially addictive-type properties.

For the purposes of this chapter, self-harm is defined as 'Any act of self-poisoning or self-injury carried out by an individual irrespective of motivation'[13] (p.6). For the nurse undertaking a risk assessment, it is important to gain an understanding of the function of the behaviour for the individual and the best way to support them to stay safe.

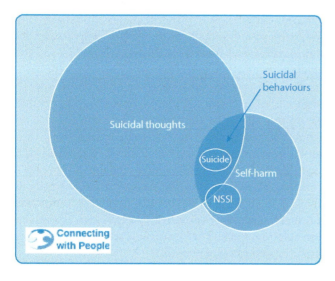

Figure 16.1 Relationship of self-harm to suicide. With kind permission from Connecting with People.

REFLECTION

Thinking about your clinical experience so far, do you feel able to provide a safe environment to ask service users about suicidal thoughts?

BOX 16.1: TYPES OF SELF-HARM

Direct self-harm
Cutting
Burning
Scalding
Picking
Head banging
Hair pulling (including eyelashes, eyebrows, etc.)
Excessive nail biting
Swallowing sharp objects or harmful substances
Inserting foreign bodies into skin or body cavities

Indirect harming behaviours
Driving too fast
Getting into fights
Self-denigration
Risky sexual practices and multiple sexual partners
Alcohol, especially binge drinking and other substance use (frequently associated with loss of control, increased recklessness and threat to life)
Involvement with crime
Putting oneself into dangerous situations
Remaining in unsatisfactory relationships/situations (not to be mistaken for situations of domestic abuse where the victim is unable to leave)
Isolation (often self-imposed)

Source: From Cole-King,[60] *Therapeutic assessment of patients following self-harm.* With kind permission of Sage Publications.

NATIONAL GUIDANCE, POLICIES AND EVIDENCE

National policies for suicide prevention have an established international history. They are informed by clinical, epidemiological and social research. It is important for nurses to be aware of these, as they are evidence-based and influence local policies and clinical guidelines.

Preventing suicide in England[7] sets out the strategic objective of reducing the suicide rate and providing better support for those bereaved or affected by suicide. The six key areas highlighted for action also inform the mental health nurse in relation to risk assessment and response – in particular, actions to reduce the risk of suicide in key high-risk groups, tailored approaches to improve mental health in specific groups and reducing access to means of suicide. Nurses need to be aware of the key high-risk groups that are prioritized for prevention (see Box 16.2) and the tailored approaches in Box 16.3.

Previous strategies in England have promoted useful instruments and guidance including *Preventing suicide: a toolkit for mental health services,*[26] which contains links to a range of useful resources.

The NICE guideline on the management of self-harm in primary and secondary care[13] provides guidance on the identification of needs for those who have presented to services within 48 hours of self-harm. It identifies the need to

BOX 16.2: HIGH-RISK GROUPS PRIORITIZED FOR ACTION

Young and middle-aged men
People in the care of mental health services, including inpatients
People with a history of self-harm
People in contact with the criminal justice system
Specific occupational groups, such as doctors, nurses, veterinary workers, farmers and agricultural workers

Source: Adapted from *Preventing suicides in England.*[7]

BOX 16.3: SPECIFIC GROUPS FOR WHOM APPROACHES SHOULD BE TAILORED TO IMPROVE MENTAL HEALTH

Children and young people, including those who are vulnerable such as looked-after children, care leavers and children and young people in the youth justice system
Survivors of abuse or violence, including sexual abuse
Veterans
People living with long-term physical health conditions
People with untreated depression
People who are especially vulnerable due to social and economic circumstances
People who misuse drugs or alcohol
Lesbian, gay, bisexual and transgender people
Black, Asian and minority ethnic groups and asylum seekers.

Source: Adapted from *Preventing suicides in England.*[7]

BOX 16.4: GUIDELINES FOR THOSE WORKING WITH PEOPLE WHO SELF-HARM

Aim to develop a trusting, supportive and engaging relationship with them.
Be aware of the stigma and discrimination sometimes associated with self-harm, both in wider society and in the health service, and adopt a non-judgemental approach.
Ensure that people are fully involved in decision making about their treatment and care.
Aim to foster people's autonomy and independence wherever possible.
Maintain continuity of therapeutic relationships wherever possible.
Ensure that information about episodes of self-harm is communicated sensitively to other team members.

Source: Adapted from *Self-harm: longer-term management,* NICE clinical guideline 133.[27]

BOX 16.5: FACTORS TO TAKE INTO ACCOUNT IN RISK ASSESSMENT

Methods and frequency of current and past self-harm
Current and past suicidal intent
Depressive symptoms and their relationship to self-harm
Any psychiatric illness and its relationship to self-harm
The personal and social context and any other specific factors preceding self-harm, such as specific unpleasant affective states or emotions and changes in relationships
Specific risk factors and protective factors (social, psychological, pharmacological and motivational) that may increase or decrease the risks associated with self-harm
Coping strategies that the person has used either to successfully limit or to avert self-harm or to contain the impact of personal, social or other factors preceding episodes of self-harm
Significant relationships that may either be supportive or represent a threat (such as abuse or neglect) and may lead to changes in the level of risk
Immediate and longer-term risks

Source: Adapted from *Self-harm: longer-term management,* NICE clinical guideline 133.[27]

reduce stigma, the need to promote understanding of those who have self-harmed and the need for a full physical and psychosocial assessment.

The NICE guideline on the longer-term management of self-harm[27] is concerned with the longer-term psychological treatment and management of both single and recurrent episodes of self-harm. It identifies the importance of person-centred care and presents key aims for those working with people who self-harm (see Box 16.4).

This guidance highlights the importance of working with the patient to identify the specific risks for them (see Box 16.5).

BOX 16.6: FACTORS THAT SHOULD BE TAKEN INTO ACCOUNT WHEN ASSESSING NEEDS

Skills, strengths and assets

Coping strategies

Mental health problems or disorders

Physical health problems or disorders

Social circumstances and problems

Psychosocial and occupational functioning, and vulnerabilities

Recent and current life difficulties, including personal and financial problems

The need for psychological intervention, social care and support, occupational rehabilitation, and also drug treatment for any associated conditions

The needs of any dependent children

Source: Adapted from *Self-harm: longer-term management,* NICE clinical guideline 133.[27]

All assessments following self-harm should follow a bio-psychosocial approach and should form part of a comprehensive clinical assessment. A needs-based assessment should identify factors outlined by NICE guidance (see Box 16.6) which will help identify both risk factors and protective factors for both self-harm and suicide.

In 2007 the Department of Health in the UK published guidance entitled *Best practice in managing risk,*[28] which promotes the adoption of a more systemic approach to risk assessment, risk management and regular training. The document sets out a framework of principles to underpin best practice, and also provides resources to guide and support risk assessment and management. It emphasizes that best practice involves making decisions based on: knowledge of the research evidence, knowledge of the individual patient, their social context, knowledge of the patient's own experience and the practitioner's clinical judgement. It states that risk tools are an aid to clinical decision making, and not a substitute for it. When risk tools are used, it is important that information from all other aspects of the patient's life and current situation is considered. Any risk management plan is only as good as the time and effort put into communicating the findings to others.

Risk factors can be classified as static or dynamic.[28–30] Static factors are unchangeable – such as previous histories, previous self-harm or suicide attempts. Dynamic factors can change over time – for example, someone's environment, attitudes and beliefs. The changeable nature of dynamic factors makes them potentially more amenable to management. Dynamic risks may reduce as care and

support are provided to address background difficulties, engage protective factors, increase hopefulness and reduce entrapment issues. However, other factors can play a part in increasing risk, such as re-exposure to distress, loss, crises, rejection, and mental illness features not improving or deteriorating. Substances the person may take also need to be considered, especially those that may be potentially disinhibiting or depressing to their actions. Alcohol is frequently involved in both self-harm and suicide,[31,32] and is often taken within hours of an act. So, while in the 'cool light of day' the ability to manage and resist difficult thoughts may be present, adding alcohol to the mix (and it does not need to be a lot) can significantly change the risk profile. Another dynamic factor to consider is the potential increase in risk in an improving or remission phase of depression or long-term mental illness, when the sufferer may now have more energy, awareness and insight to consider carrying through an act which may not previously have been the case.

REFLECTION

Consider your views on the role and value of risk screening and assessment tools.

Guidance from the Department of Health[28] describes three main ways to assess risk: clinical, actuarial and structured professional judgement. A clinical approach with information obtained during clinical assessment may be viewed as anecdotal, potentially unstructured and inconsistent, with no formulation. The actuarial approach relies on tools and information based on those factors that have been associated with increased risk in population samples. This approach should be used with caution, because it is the individual that is important. They can be used as part of the assessment of risk process, but should not be used in isolation. The use of structured professional judgement in assessing and managing risk is the recommended approach. It is interesting to note that this theme of caution in using tools to predict risk is highlighted in the NICE guidelines[27] on the long-term management of self-harm, which state: 'Do not use risk assessment tools and scales to predict future suicide or repetition of self-harm' (p.8). Again, it is important to acknowledge that various tools and approaches can be very helpful in informing the situation. It is, however, important that the risk formulation is developed using all the information available. Also important to remember is that risk factors affecting the person can change, sometimes rapidly.

National strategies and guidance are developed using detailed analysis of the available evidence and consultation. They are compiled by experts in the field, including those with lived experience and carers. It is vital that nurses are familiar with these to ensure best practice in the assessment of self-harm and suicide risk.

MODELS AND APPROACHES TO AID ASSESSMENT AND UNDERSTANDING

Assessment of a patient risk of suicide or self-harm is a complex process, requiring the collection and collation of both historical and current risk factors, alongside protective factors. These are needed in order to try to develop a formulation to understand what these factors might mean for each individual. Past behaviour will often give an insight into the ways in which someone is likely to respond. Simply put, nothing predicts behaviour better than previous behaviour, so in the area of suicide and self-harm risk, previous experiences of suicidal thoughts, plans and actions need to be considered should the patient face a similar set of circumstances in the future. Guidance given for the best practice in management of risk is that previous behaviour should not be considered in isolation;[28] however, it can help to inform the formulation.

From a global perspective,[33] most people who die by suicide are viewed as having psychiatric disorders, notably mood, substance-related, anxiety, psychotic and personality disorders, with comorbidity being common. However, psychiatric diagnoses on their own are not sufficiently sensitive to differentiate the smaller group who have mental disorders who do take their own lives from the majority who do not, which limits their ability to give further insights into the aetiology of self-harm and suicidal behaviour.[34,35]

Family history of suicidal behaviour is important, as are upbringing, exposure to suicidal behaviour by others, reporting of suicide in the media and availability of means. The presence of hopelessness has long been cited[36,37] as an important predictor of suicide, as has worthlessness. In a study of psychological process and repeat suicidal behaviour,[38] entrapment and frequency of previous suicide

attempts are two aspects that seem to be strong predictors of a future suicide attempt. Other known risk factors include impulsivity and aggression in the person's history and current presentation.[1,9]

The clinical-based risk factors may help inform the nurse conducting the assessment about those who are likely to develop self-harm and suicidal thoughts, but may be less robust predictors of those who would act on these thoughts. It is a combination of both art and science when assessing risk[12] that helps to guide the craft of caring.

A new approach is actively to mitigate those static risk factors that cannot be removed and are not amenable to reduction; for example, a recent bereavement or a family history of suicide. This approach ensures that the nurse, in collaboration with the patient, considers both an immediate and longer-term action to mitigate each identified risk.[6] The key to this approach is an emphasis on collaboration rather than direction. The patient should feel comfortable with their safety plan and agree to the interventions documented in the plan. This is particularly important with respect to provision of access to out-of-hours support when people are often at their most vulnerable. Note that the detail captured in an immediate safety plan will depend on the seriousness of a person's suicidal thoughts, their degree of planning, their ability to delay a possible suicidal act and the presence of protective factors. If their suicidal thoughts are classified as dangerous, or dangerous and imminent, when there is detailed planning, and there is a lack of protective factors, the nurse will need to take a more 'directive' approach rather than 'co-create' a safety plan to keep the patient safe.[6]

THEORETICAL APPROACHES

Suicide risk is determined by thoughts of death (suicidal ideation), hopelessness, the methods considered, development of a plan (and the degree and seriousness of that intent), risk factors and 'red flag'[6] warning signs. Open questions should be used initially, allowing for exploration in order to facilitate an honest answer. The follow-up questions should then be clear and direct, using closed questions for clarification, leaving no room for misunderstanding.

Having suicidal thoughts is not necessarily an uncommon experience when one is facing problems or distress, or experiencing a crisis. Suicidal thoughts usually start because people feel overwhelmed by their problems or their situation. They do not necessarily want their life to end; they just want to escape from intolerable distress. A number of psychological perspectives may make a person more prone to self-harm and suicide. Losses and abandonment[36] in relationships are common precipitants

in both self-harm and suicide. Defeat and entrapment are powerful concepts, particularly when the person sees no positive future and no way out of their current situation. Self-harm is associated with difficulties in problem solving,[38] especially linked to relationships. Social perfectionism[39] can also be a powerful influence. Those with strong social perfectionism traits are critical of themselves, and often believe that others are more critical of them than is actually the case.

Thomas Joiner[40] proposed the interpersonal-psychological theory of suicide. This is when an individual will not die by suicide unless both the desire to die by suicide and the ability to do so exist simultaneously. His theory asserts that desire for death occurs when people hold two specific psychological states in their minds simultaneously, and when they do so for long enough. These two states are perceived burdensomeness and a sense of low belongingness or social alienation. Joiner's theory suggests that nurses need to be alert to their patients' levels of belongingness, burdensomeness and acquired capability (especially previous suicide attempts), as this knowledge will support their assessment and response. Joiner suggests that having previously self-harmed confers a degree of capability, which is increased if there is access to potentially lethal means. Capability may also be increased if the person is more habituated to pain, injury or death. This model also helps, to some extent, to explain the longer-term risk of suicide in those who self-injure, even when the self-injury is not usually accompanied by suicidal intention.

A person who engages in self-injury is often managing intense negative emotions, while desiring them to change. Once someone has 'crossed a threshold' of being able to inflict violence on themselves and their behaviours become more habituated, their capability increases. For those who self-injure as a coping strategy, one of the dangers is in relation to what happens next time, if the self-injury does not produce the desired effects or if the usual method used for coping is no longer available. Having already crossed a threshold of harming and needing to use harm as a way of controlling emotions, the risk is that the next act may be one that is more dangerous and could be lethal.

David Klonsy[41,42] has further developed Joiner's approach to try to understand suicide in an 'ideation to action framework' of suicide theory and prevention. This framework proposes that there are two separate explanations for those who develop suicidal ideation as opposed to those who progress to attempts. More stressors, fewer reasons to live and less fear hasten the transition from ideation to attempts. In the development of suicidal ideation, Klonsy states that a combination of emotional pain and hopelessness must be present for the development of suicidal ideation. Ideation is more likely to become active if the pain increases and the connectedness to others declines, which increases the risk of suicide. If the investment in life is greater than the pain, that could be protective. The progression from ideation to an attempt occurs when the person is capable of attempting an act and the fear of attempting is less than the person's capability at that time. This is consistent with Joiner's theory.

Rory O'Connor's Integrated Motivational–Volitional Model of Suicidal Behaviour (IMV)[43] also relates to capability. It maps the relationship between background and trigger events and the importance of entrapment. The IMV model of suicidal behaviour may provide a useful framework on which risk assessment could be based.

O'Connor has also been involved in developing a pathway model which helps illustrate how self-harm and suicide can develop.[8,44] The model draws on a wide variety of research and evidence-based material. It shows a pathway from exposure to self-harm and suicidal thoughts through to acting on them. The model illustrates that the outcome of suicide is determined more by the person's access to methods that are likely to be lethal, while self-harm is the outcome when the method available and used is unlikely to result in death.

Figure 16.2 is a progressive model that can help a practitioner to gain an understanding of the areas that need to be explored in order to develop a comprehensive risk assessment. The model also embraces: epidemiological approaches, clinical perspectives, psychological and social context and psychological understanding. Each individual's picture emerging from this model will be different, helping to highlight the risk factors in the person's history and current situation, as well as potentially protective factors.

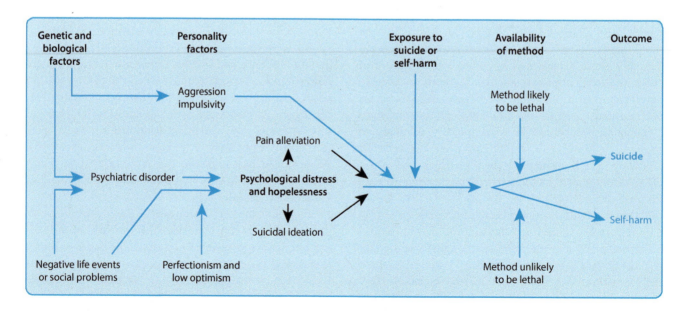

Figure 16.2 Suicide and Self-harm Pathway Model. (Source: From Hawton, Saunders and O'Connor.[8] Self-harm and suicide in adolescents. With kind permission of Elsevier.)

UK-DEVELOPED TRAINING

In the UK, two not-for-profit organizations have developed training programmes in self-harm and suicide awareness and responses using the latest clinical and research evidence. Both provide worksheets or tools that can be used by those who have received their training to augment any local systems, tools and processes. These resources assist in the assessment and response to risk of suicide or self-harm and the development of safety plans.

The training programmes share some common approaches and theoretical origins. Both identify the importance of suicidal thoughts and the importance of mitigation.[17] The programmes acknowledge that currently total prevention may not always be possible; however, active mitigation for those factors identified for the patient is important. Both programmes emphasize the importance of awareness, understanding and attitude.

There are also a number of both organizational and professional barriers to the identification and mitigation of suicide risk that are extremely important to identify and minimize.[6] The Connecting with People (CwP) training explicitly covers unconscious factors. It involves raising awareness and compassion, a robust governance framework and building emotional resilience and resourcefulness.

STORM[45] incorporates a micro-skills approach, and provides an opportunity to see filmed clinical assessments. Attendees are filmed while role-playing the micro-skills required.

Both training programmes provide a variety of tools and approaches that those trained are able to use. Both emphasize the importance of a common language. 'Low', 'medium' and 'high' risk are the terms used by STORM to categorize risk. CwP includes a number of practical clinical tools that produce a sophisticated risk assessment in the context of a robust governance framework. These include the Classification of Suicidal Thoughts, which provides a common language and consistency of approach. It introduces the descriptors of passive, active, dangerous, and dangerous and imminent suicidal thoughts. Using a standardized language permits greater clarity, accuracy and consistency of practice over time and across patient groups. Notably, CwP emphasizes that all patients need a co-produced safety plan and not just those judged to be at higher risk.

Suicidal thoughts can be extremely variable in nature. With a common language and terminology, alongside a uniform, structured approach to suicide mitigation, communication is improved between those people experiencing suicidal thoughts and those working to help them, such as health care professionals, their carers and the third (voluntary) sector.[6]

The tools and worksheets also offer a framework for documenting notes from assessment, including mental state examination. This information needs to be recorded consistently and in a structured way to provide robust evidence of assessment of risk. They also inform the completion of any other preferred risk assessment forms and approach, and thus do not require a redesign of the risk assessment documentation currently used within an organization. Safety plans are integral to working with the patient to create a positive therapeutic relationship. The training enables practitioners to support patients to co-produce a safety plan by instilling hope and helping them to identify their own reasons for living and ways to resist or manage suicidal and self-harm thoughts and feelings.

Both STORM and CwP resources not only help gain an understanding of the patient's experience but can also be used to help both the nurse and the patient monitor changes over time. Both training programmes advocate a person-centred approach,[46] a sensitive and compassionate communication style and co-creation of safety plans to help mitigate the risk of suicide or self-harm (chapter 3). The importance of the Triangle of Care, to include a patient's carers, friends[47] and relatives, is also a feature of both programmes.

ASSESSING A PATIENT AT RISK OF SUICIDE

Suicide is a complex phenomenon and so every nurse who assesses risk needs to adopt a multidimensional approach. While assessment tools may provide useful guidance, especially guarding against complacency and overconfidence, the fundamental basis of risk assessment must involve a thorough examination of the individual. This should include their risks, needs and protective factors and their interpersonal and social circumstances. Such an assessment by nurses needs to be carried out on a regular basis in the context of appropriate clinical supervision. Assessing the risk of suicide and self-harm should generally not be seen as a process that is separate from the clinical assessment and the ongoing assessment of the patient's needs, problems and strengths.

Using risk assessment scales to predict suicide risk is inaccurate and may in fact be dangerous,[48] however we know they are in current use and so we provide an overview with a warning that they should not be used to make care decisions based on the numerical score. Many risk assessment tools exist, and a selection will be reviewed briefly in this section. Most risk assessment tools include known risk factors from clinical and epidemiological research. They usually include demographic, social, historic, clinical and psychological risk factors. They also function to record findings, and as a communication aide to others. Such tools include the FACE Risk Profile,[28] the Sainsbury's Clinical Risk Management document,[49] the Nurses' Global Assessment of Suicide Risk (NGASR),[50] the Emergency Department Risk Assessment Matrix,[50] and locally derived tools that include known risk factors and personal, situational and historical factors. They also provide the opportunity for a narrative approach, including a formulation and an estimate of risk. Some, like the NGASR, attempt to score the level of risk, although no wide-scale, quantitative validation of the tool has been conducted.[50] With all risk assessments, caution is urged, as a patient may be at high risk of suicide even in the absence of membership of a high, risk group. Conversely, not all members of high-risk groups are equally at risk of suicide. Suicidal thoughts (and risk) can vary across a relatively short period.[6]

Following an act of self-harm, it is important to establish whether suicidal intent was a motivating factor for this act. If the answer is 'yes', interventions must be geared towards keeping the patient safe, and a full suicide risk assessment, plan of action and support appropriate to the risk are necessary.[13] Ambivalence is common in self-harm and suicide,[51] so trying to understand the degree to which the person wanted to live or die at the time of the act is helpful. Tools like the Beck[28] and Pierce[52] intent scales are helpful in determining suicide intent at the time of their act. It may be useful to differentiate between the suicide intent and medical lethality of self-harm.[6] Caution is needed in interpreting the scoring in isolation, as a low score could result from a patient being unaware that their self-harm was of such a medical lethality. Some patients may find their self-harm highly cathartic and an initial high intent may convert to a low-risk situation. Other tools that may help the nurse as part

of a comprehensive holistic assessment following self-harm include the Manchester Self-harm Rule & ReACT,[53,54] the Barratt Impulsivity Scale[55] and the SAD PERSONS Scale.[56]

> ## SERVICE USER'S PERSPECTIVE
>
> When I first went to my doctor, I wanted to be diagnosed with an illness to be treated and made better. Initially I was angry when this didn't happen. Now I see my self-harm differently and don't see it as an illness but as a way of coping with the other problems and difficulties I have.
>
> It's why I do what I do that is important for me and not what I do. Sometimes it is to feel something when feeling numb; other times it's to help me feel better.
>
> *A recent SH.SH. member*

Bolton and colleagues recommend considering suicidal thoughts and behaviour as an important therapeutic target.[11] The best 'low-level intervention' is a positive and compassionate clinical encounter, whereby nurses diligently identify and mitigate all risks, promote protective factors, instil hope and co-produce a safety plan with explicit reference to removal of means. It is not uncommon to hear nurses asking colleagues if they have 'done a risk assessment', where the understanding is that a tool or document has been completed. However, risk assessment as part of the craft of caring is far more complex and comprehensive than simply completing a tool and should never be viewed in this way.

TELLING THE STORY: A COMPASSIONATE APPROACH

The use of all available recorded information is an important aspect of the assessment of risk. It can help to validate or triangulate information obtained in the clinical interview and from carers.[48] The decision about when to review recorded information should be made on an individual basis. In some circumstances, it may be preferable to hear the patient's story first, followed by reviewing case notes. On other occasions it may be better to establish as much information as possible prior to the clinical assessment (see chapter 13).

Undertaking a suicide risk assessment is potentially lifesaving, but the clinical encounter is utterly dependent on what the patient chooses to reveal or keep hidden. In making a 'diagnosis' of suicide risk, we rely on our patient to trust us with often painful and difficult disclosure of their suicidal thoughts.[6] It is important to provide an environment where the patient feels safe to tell their story and able to share their history, thoughts and feelings. The nurse also needs to be able to generate a rapport[9] and trusting

relationship based on acceptance of the person and instilling hope for the future whenever possible (chapter 3). Developing an approach based on compassion can help to facilitate a relationship of openness and sharing with the patient.[47] It also provides ways that can help the patient and the nurse to cope with what at times may be difficult questions and difficult revelations.

Compassion is 'a deep awareness of the suffering of oneself and of other living things, coupled with the wish and effort to relieve it'[57] (p.xiii). The components of compassion can be subdivided into two basic psychologies. The first is the preparedness to pay attention to and turn towards suffering rather than try to avoid it and block it out. The second psychology is developing the skills and wisdom to be able to help alleviate and prevent suffering.

These two psychologies can be broken down further into a series of attributes and skills, as represented in the compassion circles shown in Figure 16.3. The inner circle represents the attributes of the first psychology of being

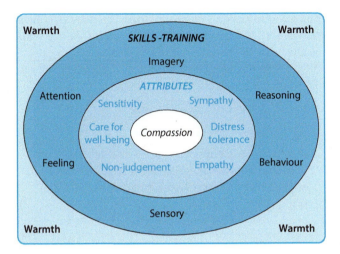

Figure 16.3 The compassion circle: key attributes of compassion (inner ring) and the skills needed to develop them (outer ring). (Source: From Gilbert,[57] *The compassionate mind*. With kind permission of Constable & Robinson.)

able to engage with and make sense of suffering. This can be broken down into six attributes. The first of these is caring for well-being by being motivated to engage with suffering. Here we can also explore our own motivations. Why do we want to engage with people's pain? How might this motivation help or hinder us? It is not uncommon for the distressed patient to be highly sensitized to the responses of others and they may have experienced rejection, abandonment and negative attitudes. It is important that the nurse tries to establish a caring and trusting interaction in the early stages of the contact (see chapter 3).

The second attribute is sensitivity. Developing sensitivity means being in touch, moment by moment, with the person, which makes one less likely to turn a blind eye or use denial or justification to avoid engaging with painful things.[58] Sympathy is the third attribute. As we attend to suffering, sympathy can help us to connect emotionally with another person. The fourth quality is capacity for tolerance of difficult emotions or distress. In suicidal patients this can stop many difficult emotions within the clinician, and the clinician's ability to tolerate their own anger or anxiety is important. The fifth quality is empathy, and this is more of a cognitive capacity to make sense of the patient. Whereas sympathy is an automatic emotional connection, empathy requires more effort. Imagine walking in the shoes of the patient. What must it be like to live the life they are living, and what has got them into the state where they want to harm themselves and their lives? Empathy, bridging into the experience of the patient, is not always easy and again this is where capacity to tolerate distress becomes particularly important. The final quality is being non-judgemental.

The second psychology is the capacity to require the wisdom to be able to alleviate and prevent suffering, which

also has a series of competencies. We begin with attention, which is the ability to bring to mind and pay attention to things that are likely to be helpful. It is important that we are able to reason in compassionate ways that are both wise and knowledgeable. Compassionate feelings are often about kindness, but not always. Sometimes emotions that facilitate compassion are more active. Compassion behaviour is often related to courage, and that is the ability to face frightening things. For example, the agoraphobic patient has to learn to go out and face anxiety and in that way move towards alleviating and preventing the difficulties.

When working with compassionate approaches in the context of suicide and self-harm, these qualities are important in the craft of caring when working with very distressed minds.

The aim of a psychosocial assessment following self-harm is to explore the factors that led up to the act, including the circumstances surrounding the self-harm, to undertake a risk assessment and to co-create a safety plan. There is a need to maintain a degree of flexibility of approach to match the patient's situation and enable them to tell their story. For the most part, the approach will require open questions and clarification of any ambiguities by reflecting back information in the form of a summary. However, there will be times when direct questioning, particularly in relation to self-harm and suicidal intentions, will be needed. The best approach to direct questioning is to develop a semi-structured conversational style. An approach described as 'stages of revelation'[12] provides a useful pathway. This approach allows the patient to start to feel at ease and more comfortable about discussing suicidal thoughts and ideas and acknowledge that we take their difficulties seriously.

The initial development of rapport will influence the assessment. Exploring the story in a chronological style early on in the assessment interview can help to encourage the patient to describe their childhood and upbringing. The focus can then shift to how they have coped with life events and milestones, their strengths and their connectedness. Within the semi-structured interview, the nurse will also need to look out for non-verbal communication.

The clinical assessment (see chapter 13) should clarify current problems, difficulties and strengths. It should contain a clear understanding of current and previous aspects of mental health, not only for the patient but also their family histories of mental illness, suicide and self-harm. It is important to facilitate a detailed exploration of current thoughts, plans and intent. Their previous history, childhood and development and family histories along with current social, financial and physical health aspects will need to be addressed. In considering the pathways to suicide model,[8,44] it is important that these areas are covered and supported by clinical tools. In assessing risk, all this information needs to be collated together, including information from other sources, in order to inform the risk assessment formulation. Wherever possible and safe to do so, sharing this with the patient and others involved in their care will aid understanding about the current situation and the importance of the safety plan.

> ## REFLECTION
>
> How will you ensure you care for yourself and your own emotional needs so that you are able to engage compassionately with patients who are suicidal?

CONCLUSION

Assessment of a patient at risk of suicide or self-harm is part of everyday practice for the nurse working in mental health. Suicide and self-harm cannot be accurately predicted[48] and so the process could be considered a combination of both art and science, highlighting the importance of the craft of caring. An initial assessment can itself be very therapeutic, particularly when it may be one of the few times the person has had the chance to tell their story, to be believed and to have the opportunity to gain some understanding. Generally speaking, the more areas that are covered and the more that is known, the better the formulation and understanding of risk should be. The more we can 'get alongside' our patient's experiences then the better able we are to respond fully to them in a compassionate way, to instil hope and to begin the process of recovery (see chapter 36).

However, we can never be assured that we have identified or understood all the risk factors for a patient, and also life is forever changing, not only day to day but sometimes minute to minute. So, in reality, a 'risk assessment' should not just be about 'doing a risk assessment' as part of a clinical assessment interview, but a process of constantly considering and reviewing risk in light of changes. The use

> ## SERVICE USER'S PERSPECTIVE
>
> Listen to me first; then together we may be able to start to put in place the building blocks for hope. Don't try to force this too quickly.
>
> *SH.SH. member*

of evidence-based and peer-reviewed clinical tools can significantly improve the quality and consistency of assessments and improve the risk assessment formulation.

The nurse should not feel that they are alone in completing an assessment and formulation of risk. The importance of sharing with colleagues and seeking their views is an essential part of the process. This helps to reduce the potential for emotional exhaustion and burnout.[59] A compassionate approach can provide better experiences for the nurse and the patient; alongside improving clinical outcomes,[60] sharing and supervision are vital, not just for the care of the patient but also for the care and emotional resilience of the nurse.

ACKNOWLEDGEMENTS

Thanks to Derbyshire Voice members, a user-led organization which plays an important part in working to improve mental health services across Derby City and Derbyshire. Thanks also to Claire Shortland and members of SH.SH. for their assistance in compiling this chapter, the opportunity to share their experiences and the provision of quotations to inform the text.

Thanks to Rory O'Connor and Paul Gilbert for their support, guidance and advice respectively on the 'Models and approaches' and 'Telling the story' sections; to Gavin Peak-Jones for help with the manuscript; and to many colleagues and contacts who have helped and supported this chapter's development.

References

1. O'Connor RC, Nock MK. Suicide 2: the psychology of suicidal behaviour. *The Lancet Psychiatry* 2014; Early Online Publication, 2 May: 27–39.
2. Marsh I. *Suicide: Foucault, history and truth*. Cambridge: Cambridge University Press: 2010.
3. Pritchard C. *Suicide – the ultimate rejection?: a psychosocial study*. Buckingham and Bristol, PA: Open University Press, 1995.
4. Suicide Act 1961. Available from: http://www.legislation.gov.uk/ukpga/Eliz2/9-10/60/section/1 [Accessed 31st August 2016].

5. Royal College of Psychiatrists. *Self-harm, suicide and risk: helping people who self-harm*. College Report CR158. London: Royal College of Psychiatrists, 2010.

6. Cole-King A, Green G, Gask L, Hines K, Platt S. Suicide mitigation: a compassionate approach to suicide prevention. *Advances in Psychiatric Treatment* 2013; **19**: 276–83.

7. Department of Health. *Preventing suicide in England: a cross-government outcomes strategy to save lives*. London: HMG/DH, 2012.

8. Hawton K, Saunders KEA, O'Connor RC. Self-harm and suicide in adolescents. *Lancet* 2012; **379**: 2373–82.

9. Morris R, Kapur K, Byng R. Assessing risk of suicide or self harm in adults. *British Medical Journal* 2013; **347**: f4572.

10. Cooper J, Kapur N. Assessing suicide risk. In: Duffy D, Ryan T (eds). *New approaches to preventing suicide: a manual for practitioners*. London: Jessica Kingsley, 2004: chapter 2.

11. Bolton JM, Gunnell D, Turecki G. Suicide risk assessment and intervention in people with mental illness. *British Medical Journal* 2015; **351**: h4978.

12. Anderson M, Waters K. Recognition and therapeutic management of self-harm and suicidal behaviours. In: Callaghan P, Playle J, Cooper L (eds). *Mental health nursing skills*. Oxford: Oxford University Press, 2009: chapter 17.

13. NICE (National Institute for Health and Care Excellence). *Self-harm: the short-term physical and psychological management and secondary prevention of self-harm in primary and secondary care. NICE clinical guideline 16*. London: NICE, 2004, with changes in 2011.

14. National Confidential Inquiry into Suicide and Homicide by People with Mental Illness. *Suicide in primary care in England: 2002–2011*. Manchester: University of Manchester, 2014.

15. National Confidential Inquiry into Suicide and Homicide by People with Mental Illness. *Annual report*. Manchester: University of Manchester, 2013.

16. Cole-King A, Green G, Wadman S, Peak-Jones G, Gask L. Therapeutic assessment of patients following self- harm. *Royal College of General Practitioners Journal for Associates in Training* 2011; **4**(5): 278–87.

17. Cole-King A, Lepping P. Suicide mitigation: time for a more realistic approach. *British Journal of General Practice* 2010; **60**: 3–4.

18. Klonsky DE, Alexis MA. Differentiating suicide attempters from suicide ideators: a critical frontier for suicidology research. *Suicide and Life-Threatening Behavior* 2013; DOI: 10.1111/sltb.12068.

19. Kapur N, Cooper J, O'Connor RC, Hawton K. Non-suicidal self-injury v. attempted suicide: new diagnosis or false dichotomy? *British Journal of Psychiatry* 2013; **202**(5): 326–8.

20. Gunnell D, Hawton K, Kapur N. Coroners' verdicts and suicide statistics in England and Wales. *British Medical Journal* 2011; 343: doi: 10.1136/bmj.d6030.

21. Hawton K, Bergen H, Kapur N, Cooper J, Steeg S, Ness J, Waters K. Repetition of self-harm and suicide following self-harm in children and adolescents: findings from the Multicentre Study of Self-harm in England. *Journal of Child Psychology and Psychiatry* 2012; doi:10.1111/j.1469-7610.2012.02559.x.

22. Murphy E, Kapur N, Webb R, Purandare N, Hawton K, Bergen H, Waters K, Cooper J. Risk factors for repetition and suicide following self-harm in older adults: multicentre cohort study. *British Journal of Psychiatry* 2012; **200**(5): 399–404.

23. Bergen H, Hawton K, Waters K, Ness J, Cooper J, Steeg S, Kapur N. Premature death after self-harm: a multicentre cohort study. *Lancet* 2012; **380**: 1568–74.

24. Butler AM, Malone K. Attempted suicide v. non-suicidal self-injury: behaviour, syndrome or diagnosis? *British Journal of Psychiatry* 2013; **202**: 324–5.

25. Hooley JM, St Germain SA. Should we expand the conceptualization of self-injurious behaviour? Rationale, review, and recommendations. In: Knock MK (ed). *The Oxford handbook of suicide and self-injury*. Oxford: Oxford University Press, 2014: 47–58.

26. National Patient Safety Agency. *Preventing suicide: a toolkit for mental health services*. London: National Reporting and Learning Services, 2009.

27. NICE (National Institute for Health and Care Excellence). *Self-harm: longer-term management*. NICE clinical guideline 133. London: NICE, 2011.

28. Department of Health, National Risk Management Programme. *Best practice in managing risk*. London: Department of Health, National Risk Management Programme, 2007.

29. Cole-King A, Parker V, Williams H, Platt S. Suicide prevention: are we doing enough? *Advances in Psychiatric Treatment* 2013; **19**: 284–91.

30. Kettles AM, Woods P. The theory of risk. In: Woods P, Kettles AM (eds). *Risk assessment and management in mental health nursing*. Oxford: Wiley-Blackwell, 2009: 49–75.

31. Haw C, Hawton K, Casey D, Bal E, Shepherd A. Alcohol dependence, excessive drinking and deliberate self-harm: trends and patterns in Oxford 1989–2002. *Social Psychiatry and Psychiatric Epidemiology* 2005; **40**(12): 964–71.

32. Bergen H, Hawton K, Kapur N, Cooper J, Steeg S, Ness J, Waters K. Shared characteristics of suicides and other unnatural deaths following non-fatal self-harm? A multicentre study of risk factors. *Psychological Medicine* 2011; DOI:10.1017/S0033291711001747.

33. Hawton K, Van Heeringen K. Suicide. *Lancet* 2009; **373**(9672): 1372–81.

34. Bostwick JM, Pankratz VS. Affective disorders and suicide risk: a reexamination. *American Journal of Psychiatry* 2000; **157**: 1925–32.

35. Adler PA, Adler P. The demedicalization of self-injury: from psychopathology to sociological deviance. *Journal of Contemporary Ethnography* 2007; **36**: 537–70.

36. Kolinsky DE, Kotov R, Bakst S, Rabinowitx J, Bromet EJ. Hopelessness as a predictor of attempted suicide among first admission patients with psychosis: a 10-year cohort study. *Suicide and Life Threatening Behaviour* 2012; **42**(1): 1–10.

37. O'Connor RC, Smyth R, Ferguson E, Ryan C, Williams JM. Psychological processes and repeat suicidal behavior: a four-year prospective study. *Journal of Consulting and Clinical Psychology* 2013; **81**(6): 1137–43.

38. Townsend E, Hawton K, Altman DG, Arensman E, Gunnell D, Hazel P, House A, Van Heeringen K. The efficacy of problem-solving treatments after deliberate self-harm: meta-analysis of randomized controlled trials with respect to depression, hopelessness and improvement in problems. *Psychological Medicine* 2001; **31**: 979–88.

39. O'Connor RC, Whyte MC, Fraser L, Masterton G, Miles J, MacHale S. Predicting short-term outcome in well-being following suicidal behaviour: the conjoint effects of social perfectionism and positive future thinking. *Behaviour Research and Therapy* 2007; **45**(7): 1543–55.

40. Joiner TE. *Why people die by suicide*. Cambridge, MA: Harvard University Press, 2007.

41. Klonsky ED, May AM. Differentiating suicide attempters from suicide ideators: a critical frontier for suicidology research. *Suicide and Life Threatening Behaviour* 2014; **44**(1): 1–5.

42. May AM, Klonsky ED. Assessing motivations for suicide attempts: development and psychometric properties of the inventory of motivations for suicide attempts. *Suicide and Life-Threatening Behaviour* 2013; **43**(5): 532–46.

43. O'Connor RC. The integrated motivational–volitional model of suicidal behaviour. *Crisis* 2011; **32**(6): 295–8.

44. Centre for Suicide Research, Department of Psychiatry, University of Oxford. Assessment of suicide risk in people with depression: clinical guide. 2013. Available from: http://cebmh.warne.ox.ac.uk/csr/clinicalguide/docs/Assessment-of-suicide-risk--clinical-guide.pdf [Accessed 10th September 2016].

45. Gask L, Lever-Green G, Hays R. Dissemination and implementation of suicide prevention training in one Scottish region. *BMC Health Services Research* 2008; **8**: 246.

46. Watkins P. A person-centred approach to assessment. In: *Mental health nursing. The art of compassionate care.* Oxford: Butterworth Heinemann, 2001: 45–55.

47. Worthington A, Lead PR. *The Triangle of Care – carers included: a guide to best practice in acute mental health care.* London: National Mental Health Development Unit, 2010.

48. Chan MKY, Bhatti H, Meader N, Stockton S, Evans J, O'Connor RC, Kapur N, Kendall T. Predicting suicide following self-harm: systematic review of risk factors and risk scales. *British Journal of Psychiatry* 2016; **209**(4): 277–83.

49. Morgan S. *Clinical risk management. A clinical tool and practitioner manual.* London: Sainsbury Centre for Mental Health, 2000.

50. Cutcliffe JR, Barker P. The Nurses' Global Assessment of Suicide Risk (NGASR): developing a tool for clinical practice. *Journal of Psychiatric and Mental Health Nursing* 2004; **11**(4): 393–400.

51. Hines K, Cole-King A, Blaustein M. Hey kid, are you OK? A story of suicide survived. *Advances in Psychiatric Treatment* 2013; **19**: 292–4.

52. Pierce DW. The predictive validation of a suicide intent scale: a five year follow-up. *British Journal of Psychiatry* 1981; **139**: 391–6.

53. Cooper J, Kapur N, Mackway-Jones K. A comparison between clinicians' assessment and the Manchester Self-Harm Rule: a cohort study. *Emergency Medicine Journal* 2007; **24**: 720–1.

54. Steeg S, Kapur N, Applegate E, Stewart SKL, Hawton K, Bergen H, Waters K, Cooper J. The development of a population-level clinical screening tool for self-harm repetition and suicide: the ReACT Self-Harm Rule. *Psychological Medicine* 2012; **42**: 2383–94.

55. Stanford MS, Mathias C, Dougherty DM, Lake S, Anderson NE, Patton JH. Fifty years of the Barratt Impulsiveness Scale: an update and review. *Personality and Individual Differences* 2009; **47**(5): 385–95.

56. Bolton JM, Spiwak R, Sareen J. Predicting suicide attempts with the SAD PERSONS scale: a longitudinal analysis. *Journal of Clinical Psychiatry* 2012; **73**(6): 735–41.

57. Gilbert P. *The compassionate mind.* London: Constable & Robinson, 2009.

58. All Party Parliamentary Group on Suicide and Self-Harm. *The future of local suicide prevention plans in England. A report by the All Party Parliamentary Group on Suicide and Self-Harm Prevention. Chair Madeleine Moon MP.* London: All Party Parliamentary Group on Suicide and Self-Harm, 2013.

59. Leineweber C, Westerlund H, Chungkham HS, Lindqvist R, Runesdotter S, Tishelman C. Nurses' practice environment and work-family conflict in relation to burn out: a multilevel modelling approach. *PLoS ONE* 2014; **9**(5): e96991, doi:10.1371/journal.pone.0096991.

60. Cole-King A, Gilbert P. Compassionate care: the theory and the reality. *Journal of Holistic Healthcare* 2011; **8**(3): 29–37.

Further reading

Baughan J, Smith A. *Compassion, caring and communication: skills for nursing practice.* Cambridge: Pearson, 2013.

Chambers C, Ryder R. *Compassion and caring in nursing.* Abingdon: Radcliffe Medical Press, 2009.

Department of Health. Compassion in practice. 2012. Available from: http://www.england.nhs.uk/wp-content/uploads/2012/12/compassion-in-practice.pdf [Accessed 31st August 2016].

Henden J. *Preventing suicide: the solution focused approach.* Chichester: John Wiley & Sons, 2008.

Neff K. *Self-compassion: stop beating yourself up and leave insecurity behind.* New York: Harper Collins, 2011.

O'Connor R, Platt S, Gordon J (eds). *International handbook of suicide prevention.* Chichester: Wiley-Blackwell, 2011.

Relevant web pages

Self-harm and suicide

Connecting with People. Staying safe if you're not sure life's worth living. http://www.connectingwithpeople.org/StayingSafe

Connecting with People. U can cope. http://www.connectingwithpeople.org/ucancope

MIND. Suicidal feelings. http://www.mind.org.uk/information-support/types-of-mental-health-problems/suicidal-feelings/#.V8btRzVmrLl

Samaritans. I want to kill myself. http://www.samaritans.org/how-we-can-help-you/what-speak-us-about/i-want-kill-myself

PAPYRUS. https://www.papyrus-uk.org/

Stamp Out Suicide. http://www.stampoutsuicide.org.uk/

Survivors of Bereavement by Suicide. http://uk-sobs.org.uk/

NICE (National Institute for Health and Care Excellence). https://www.nice.org.uk/

Centre for Mental Health and Safety. http://research.bmh.manchester.ac.uk/cmhs

WHO (World Health Organization). Suicide data. http://www.who.int/mental_health/prevention/suicide/suicideprevent/en/

National guidance, policies and evidence

Department of Health. Suicide prevention strategy for England. https://www.gov.uk/government/publications/suicide-prevention-strategy-for-england

Department of Health. Suicide prevention: second annual report. https://www.gov.uk/government/publications/suicide-prevention-second-annual-report

NICE (National Institute for Health and Care Excellence). Self-harm in over 8s: short-term management and prevention of recurrence. https://www.nice.org.uk/guidance/cg16

NICE (National Institute for Health and Care Excellence). Self-harm in over 8s: long-term management. https://www.nice.org.uk/guidance/cg133

NICE (National Institute for Health and Care Excellence). NICE pathways: self-harm overview. http://pathways.nice.org.uk/pathways/self-harm

Training and resources to support the process of assessing and responding to patients at risk of self-harm or suicide

ASIST (Applied Suicide Intervention Skills Training). https://www.livingworks.net/programs/asist/

Connecting with People. http://www.connectingwithpeople.org/

Glasgow Suicidal Behaviour Research Laboratory (SBRL). https://sites.google.com/site/suicidalbehaviourresearchlab/

Kevin Hines story. http://www.kevinhinesstory.com/

Oxford Centre for Suicide Research. http://cebmh.warne.ox.ac.uk/csr/profile.html

STORM. http://www.stormskillstraining.co.uk/

17 Engagement and observation of people at risk

FIONA NOLAN, CAREN WATSON AND MARY ELLEN KHOO

LEARNING OUTCOMES

- To understand methods used to manage risk in inpatient wards.
- To understand differences in levels of observation used in inpatient wards in the UK.
- To be able to critically evaluate the effectiveness and use of observations on acute wards.
- To understand the impact of observations on the patient, carers, staff and ward environment.
- To be able to evaluate the use of alternative means of engagement on wards.

SUMMARY OF KEY POINTS

- Observation is the principal tool for risk management in UK acute wards.
- If undertaken by unskilled staff, observation can have a negative impact.
- Intensity or levels of observation are determined by ongoing assessment of risk, which can be subjective and varied in implementation.
- Observation can provide opportunities for therapeutic engagement and activity.
- Safe ward environments can be promoted through use of additional interventions such as protected engagement time, Safewards and Star Wards, all of which place staff engagement with patients at the heart of ward activity.

INTRODUCTION

This chapter will explore some of the methods used in acute inpatient mental health wards to manage and minimize risk. While acute wards are the focus of our discussion, similar risks are frequently presented in other areas, such as long-stay rehabilitation wards, wards for older people and residential services, and in service users' homes. Clinical policies may differ between services, but the clinical skills required by staff to manage risk are transferable between settings and are at the heart of mental health nursing.

The aim of a hospital admission is to provide a safe and contained environment for people while they are acutely unwell. However, there are associated dangers, including risk of harm from others who are unwell, trauma from observing disturbed behaviour in others, institutionalization, harm caused by medication, being physically restrained by staff and the impact of being away from friends and family. There has been an increase in suicides of people under the care of mental health services in the UK since 2009, particularly in crisis resolution/home treatments teams,[1] which indicates the importance of a thorough risk assessment to guide professionals.

These assessments allow informed judgements to be made about the likelihood of a risk behaviour or event occurring. Ward staff should continually assess risk, as it can change frequently and will vary between patients. Past behaviour can be a helpful indicator of potential risk, and information should be gathered from patient records, the patient and both formal and informal carers. However, it is important to examine the context and circumstances of previous risk incidents in order to establish their current relevance. Changes in circumstance such as age, mental state, medication, ward environment and support from peers on the ward may all have an impact. Current risks should be identified in the person's care plan, with details of the steps that should be taken to minimize each risk. This plan should be written in collaboration with the patient, and all issues should be discussed with them to ascertain how they view their situation and what help they feel they need. Consideration should be made about any access to items that may be used to cause harm, such as ligatures, medication and sharp items. If items are removed from the possession of patients, the rationale should be explained in an empathetic manner, with staff giving reassurance and explanations and expressing awareness that the process may be distressing.

OBSERVATION

One of the main interventions used by ward nurses to maintain safety and minimize risk is observation. The term implies a distance and separation between the staff member and patient, but the intervention can have considerable therapeutic benefit if carried out in an empathetic and skilled manner.

Despite the widespread use of observation, there was no national policy in the UK to guide its implementation for many years. In 1999 the Standing Nursing and Midwifery Advisory Committee (SNMAC) published practice guidance in order to minimize the variance between observation practice and policies across the UK. This included a recommended classification of formal observation into four different levels: general, intermittent, within eyesight and at arm's length.[2] This guidance described observation as 'a minimally restrictive intervention of varying intensity in which a member of the healthcare staff observes and maintains contact with a service user to ensure the service user's safety and the safety of others'. The phrase 'maintains contact' was important here as it conveyed the essential ingredient of engagement and interaction. More recently, the National Institute for Health and Care Excellence (NICE) has revised its guidelines on the management of violence, which includes modified observation levels for inpatient mental health wards.[3] This guidance is applicable to England and Wales, and differs slightly from guidance in Scotland[4] and Northern Ireland.[5]

The observation classifications as defined by NICE[3] are as follows:

Low-level intermittent observation. This is the baseline level of observation on mental health wards. The frequency of observation is every 30 to 60 minutes, and is also known as general observations. The staff member carrying out these observations will also check each patient's whereabouts, what they are doing and who they are with. The staff member will also check for potential hazards, including those in the ward environment. These checks are often characterized by a staff member walking round with a clipboard making notes, but they provide the opportunity for regular interaction with each patient. A skilled nurse or healthcare assistant will use these observations as an opportunity for engagement, and will overcome the potential for the clipboard and checklist to function as a barrier between them and the patient.

High-level intermittent observation. This is used where there is an increased risk of harm occurring but that risk is not immediate. The frequency of observation is 15 to 30 minutes. Ideally, the intervals between these checks vary, to reduce their predictability. For example, a patient who has suicidal or self-harming intentions may be more likely to see a window of opportunity if they know nursing staff will next be checking them in exactly 15 minutes, as opposed to a random time between 5 and 20 minutes. Intermittent observations can be used to monitor for a range of risk behaviours and can be stopped and started at any time. These checks are often used with newly admitted patients until a more detailed risk assessment can be developed, and are also known as primary or intermittent observations.

Continuous observation. This is used when there is an immediate risk of harm occurring, and is also known as constant special observations, 'specialing', enhanced observations, close observations or 1:1 observations. It requires a designated member of staff being with a patient all the time, either within eyesight or at arm's length. The former involves accompanying the patient at all times to be aware of their whereabouts and behaviour, and to allow immediate intervention if necessary. The latter is more intrusive and should only be used when the patient is deemed to be of immediate danger to him-/herself or others and the staff need to be close enough to intervene as quickly as possible. This method of observation is particularly invasive and involves accompanying the patient to the toilet, to the shower/bath and when dressing, and it severely impinges on privacy.

Multi-professional continuous observation. This is used when a patient is at the highest risk of harming themselves or others. The patient is kept within eyesight of two or three staff members and at arm's length of at least one staff member. Once again this type of observation is very intrusive and, for that reason, as with continuous observation it should only be used as a last resort. Patients presenting with such levels of risk should be considered for referral to a psychiatric intensive care unit.

How is the observation level determined?

As mentioned, there is no standard method by which observations are either implemented or their level or intensity decided, and there is variation between hospitals and even individual wards.[6] A number of factors need to be considered when assessing the need for increased observation, including current mental state; a presence of suicidal ideation or command hallucinations which the patient is finding hard to resist; history of self-harm, suicide or harm to others; and history of absconding from care. General observations are now standard practice in acute wards, which may have reduced the use of continuous observations, although this is yet to be evidenced. It is important to note again that risk will fluctuate over time, and observation levels should be reviewed at least daily. Previous knowledge and relationships built between staff and patients can greatly assist in managing their risk when first admitted to a ward. A new or unknown patient will require a greater degree of caution from staff, and strategies to manage risk may be in place for somewhat longer than with patients with familiar or predictable needs and behaviour.

The responsibility and decision-making process for increasing or reducing observation levels have evolved through the years. Ideally, any decisions about observation levels should be made with participation from all professionals involved, from carers and from the patient themselves; however, in practice that is not always possible, particularly at evenings and weekends.[7] Nurses traditionally have been able to increase observation levels but not reduce them, but increasingly this is changing, with qualified nurses in some organizations being able to decrease the level of observations in accordance with a plan that has been agreed earlier with a doctor, provided that the rationale is fully documented.

Who carries out observations?

Ideally, observations should be performed by a staff member who knows the patient and is familiar with their risk assessment and care plan. Some organizations may require that the higher levels of observations are carried out by a qualified nurse. While the process of observation seems simple, in reality it is incredibly complex and its effectiveness will be dependent on staff skills, the constraints of the physical environment, and how the observation is interpreted within the system, by the patient and staff. Observation provides an opportunity for engagement and development of the therapeutic relationship (see chapter 3 for more detail on developing and maintaining therapeutic relationships). However, the numerous demands on the time of regular ward staff mean that observation is more likely to be delegated to more junior members or to temporary bank and agency staff who may not have an established therapeutic relationship with the patient. It is vital that full handovers are given to any staff conducting the observations and the patient should be involved in this process whenever possible. Local policies should have a maximum time limit during which a staff member should be with a patient as an 'observer', of between 1.5 and 2 hours, so staff should be rotated or regular breaks given.

Observation is a skilled activity, and training is recommended for all relevant staff.[2] However, there is no evidence to indicate that this training is provided in UK inpatient settings, particularly for temporary staff. Staff should have knowledge and understanding of the concept of risk assessment, how to talk to patients at risk, the therapeutic opportunities of observation, how to make the environment safe and how to record observations. This is in keeping with the craft of caring, which identifies many aspects of the competent and compassionate mental health professional.

DOCUMENTATION

As with all interventions, observation should be clearly documented. This is important for transferring information between colleagues on the ward, but the records may also be used for audit purposes and as evidence if a serious incident occurs. Recorded information for high-level intermittent and continuous observations should include the patient's whereabouts, their mental state, engagement and interaction and any observed risk behaviours. More creative uses of documentation could include a checklist handed over at each shift, containing potential tools for observations which are tailored to the needs and preference to assist staff in conducting observations of individual patients, such as exercise and interaction. The checklist should indicate which tools have been utilized, and to what effect.

IMPACT OF OBSERVATION ON PATIENTS

The impact of observation will vary greatly depending, among other factors, on how much the patient has been involved in the decision, who is carrying out the observation, individual attitudes and the environment. Potential positive effects include increased feelings of containment and safety and creating an opportunity to establish therapeutic engagement between staff and patients. However, before some patients find being under observation an intrusive, humiliating and degrading experience. Stewart et al.[6] found that aggression, particularly verbal, was more common during the observation period than before, which suggests that being constantly observed can be distressing and can increase the likelihood of aggressive outbursts. In a study by Bowles et al.[8] one woman describes how being under observation made her feel 'incarcerated': 'There is nothing more degrading than having to go to the toilet in front of a complete stranger. There is nothing more frustrating than trying to have a meal with someone watching you take each mouthful, and there is nothing more childish than having someone look over you while you sleep' (p.257).

Further negative connotations of this process were outlined by the SNMAC:[9] 'Unfortunately, users often perceive observation as a custodial and aversive procedure … Nurses may reinforce these views of observation … because they do not have skills and confidence to engage with the patient or clear guidelines as to the kind of nursing care that a person under observation should receive' (p.15, section 2.5.4).

Some organizations maintain observations without having additional staff to carry them out, thereby reducing the time available for other patients. Reducing risks for one patient through close monitoring and observation may therefore increase risk for others through reducing the staff time available for them.

Night checks, which form part of general or intermittent observations, can be particularly frustrating for patients as it can mean they are disturbed at regular intervals throughout the night. Nursing staff have a responsibility to check each patient, looking for evidence of breathing or movement, which might involve shining torches through the window or opening bedroom doors while patients are sleeping. It is important that nursing staff find the least intrusive methods possible to carry out these observations to minimize disturbance to patients. This should be done on an individual level with each patient through negotiation; it may involve moving the bed into the eyeline of a window, or leaving a bedroom door partially ajar, or there may be agreements with some patients that during the night time while they are in their room with the door closed staff should not disturb them. The level of risk needs to be balanced with the patient's right to privacy, dignity and a good night's sleep.

IMPACT OF OBSERVATION ON STAFF

The potential impact of observation on staff will be mitigated by factors including the role and experience of the staff member, the patient who is under observation, work pressures including the needs of the other patients and ward environmental factors. Positive effects on staff may include feeling reassured that the patient is safe, and feeling useful, as if they are 'doing something', providing opportunities for ongoing assessment and engagement[10] and reducing the likelihood of adverse events occurring.

Potential negative effects include a detrimental impact on the therapeutic alliance, feeling overly intrusive, boredom and, particularly if they have not been involved in the decision-making process about the implementation of observations, a lack of autonomy. It is unlikely that staff will derive job satisfaction from performing observations. At best they may have a sense of passive lethargy, of powerlessness; at worst they may feel degraded, helpless, and involved in an intervention that they feel is counter-therapeutic but that they have little power to change. The negative impact on morale is potentially great. Johnson et al.[11] found that a significant protective factor in maintaining job satisfaction is the level of autonomy staff have in their work. Both staff and patients can therefore be adversely affected if placed in a position whereby they are forced to engage in observations, and this is likely to be detrimental to their therapeutic relationship.

Buchanan-Barker and Barker[12] argue that observation is the 'original sin of mental health nursing', identifying it as an outdated intervention inherited from a less enlightened era. They highlight that observation in practice is something that is done 'to' rather than 'with' the patient and therefore has the potential to obstruct the development of genuine therapeutic relationships. They advocate that the relationship that is developed with patients should be meaningful for nurses and that there should be some recognition that conducting observations can be an intense period wherein good or bad relationships can be formed. The craft of caring advocates the use of time spent with patients for positive impact on the individuals (staff and patients) and on the therapeutic relationship. See chapter 3 for more discussion on developing and maintaining therapeutic relationships. Observations can be costly, in terms of both opportunity and finance. Nursing staff may feel frustrated if they have other tasks to complete and they juggle to balance the competing demands on their time in a pressured environment. Bowers and Park[13] demonstrated that observations can be a significant cost pressure, in one case accounting for up to 20 per cent of the nursing budget. A clear link between the number of continuous observations and hours of bank staff use has been demonstrated.[14] High-level intermittent observations were demonstrated to be significantly less costly in the City 128 study of 136 wards in England.[15]

IMPACT OF OBSERVATION ON CARERS

A potential impact on carers of the use of observation may be a feeling that their friend or relative is safe due to the constant proximity to staff. Conversely, they may feel that the intervention is intrusive. Carers should be involved in the decision to implement observations, but the authors feel that this rarely happens in practice. Confidentiality of patient care may be an impediment to carer involvement in some cases, but speed of access to the carer when decisions are made would be important in ensuring that they are informed and involved in the process. The use of advance decisions or crisis plans should be prioritized for patients who have been in hospital previously, as these plans identify what they and their carer would like to happen in a crisis and can include instructions about the use of observations.

There is evidence to suggest that involvement of families in mental health care can improve safety.[1] The National Confidential Inquiry into Suicide and Homicide by People with Mental Illness (2015) recommends improved communication between staff and families, with inclusion of carers at every step of an admission to hospital; from assessment to care planning to discharge planning.

> **REFLECTION**
>
> - What interventions or strategies could you put in place to reduce the need for observations with high-risk patients?
> - Which situations do you think justify higher levels of observation, and consequent infringement of privacy?

EFFECTIVENESS OF OBSERVATION

We have very little evidence on how effective observations are in preventing adverse events. Some of the difficulties in carrying out evaluations of the intervention include variation in how it is carried out in different organizations and a lack of consistent policy and clinical guidelines to direct practice. If a trial of the intervention were to be carried out, it would entail an ethical dilemma in carrying out research that involves withholding a potentially lifesaving intervention in order to test its effectiveness.[16]

Stewart et al.[6] found that continuous observations may be effective in reducing the risk of suicide for newly admitted patients. Further discussion on assessing risk of suicide and self-harm can be found in chapter 16. The City 128 study[15] reported that high-level intermittent observations may reduce the incidence of self-harm and was more acceptable to patients than continuous observations.

A systematic review of containment strategies used in mental health wards indicated that the lack of randomized controlled trials in this area means that no recommendations can be made about the benefits or harm of containment strategies, including the use of observations.[17]

> **REFLECTION**
>
> - What difficulties do you imagine would arise after observing a patient on a one-to-one basis? Would this influence the relationship with your patient?
> - How do you think observations impact on the therapeutic relationships between staff and patients?

ALTERNATIVES TO OBSERVATION

Despite its widespread use, it is clear that there is little empirical evidence to support the effectiveness of observation in managing risk, and its potential negative impact can outweigh its potential positive impact. Bowers[18] identifies observation as one of several containment strategies used by ward staff, and defines containment as 'any staff procedure directed at keeping patients safe' (p.178). He describes some of these strategies as coercive and some as therapeutic, and proposes that containment is divided into four categories:

1. *responsive containment*, which is an immediate short-term response to a harmful behaviour;
2. *preventative containment*, which is used in advance to stop a harmful event from occurring;
3. *blanket preventative containment*, which consists of procedures that are applied to all patients and are often policy-led;

4. *therapeutic preventative containment*, which maintains safety while having a beneficial effect on the patient's mental state.

Examples of other containment strategies include de-escalation techniques, time out (when patients spends time alone away from communal areas, often in a bedroom), locking ward doors, the use of physical restraint, the use of PRN medication and seclusion.

ENGAGEMENT

Therapeutic means of managing risk and collaboration with patients and carers have increased in importance and recognition over the past 10 years. NICE[19] recommends shared decision making between staff and patients when considering treatment options. Developing a sense of community and shared purpose on inpatient wards has the potential not yet evidenced to reduce the need for observations and other more restrictive containment techniques. This could be facilitated through empowering patients by informing them of all activity where possible – for example, having the staff duty rota available for patients to see. For some patients, hospital can provide relief and sanctuary from loneliness, abuse or relationship difficulties in the home. Establishing relationships with peers and staff members can be stabilizing and productive. Ward routine, and understanding the routine, can be important; every ward should have ward routine and activities clearly outlined – for example, on notice boards, on leaflets supplied on admission. It is important that a stable and predictable environment is provided for patients. Regular engagement with staff, and availability of staff to attend to patients needs as they arise, are important characteristics of ward practice.

There is some evidence that ward patients spend most of their time alone, with one study reporting that nurses spent less than half their time with them, and that this time decreased with increasing seniority.[20] This study found that the majority of patient interactions were with health care assistants, student nurses and domestic staff. The number of acute inpatient beds has been reduced over the past 16 years since home treatment teams were introduced in the UK, resulting in an increased proportion of detained patients in acute wards. There is limited evidence concerning levels of acuity in wards; however, use of the Mental Health Act can be a proxy indicator. Increased detentions under the Mental Health Act would imply increasingly risky patients, with higher levels of need, requiring an increasingly skilled staff group to provide the help they need. The ability of staff to engage in therapeutic relationships with patients presenting with risky behaviour in acute settings is therefore more necessary than ever.

There is a distinct lack of policy in the UK concerning staff and patient engagement, and what there is has little empirical backing. A number of theoretical models have been developed in recent years to try to address the question of engagement. The Tidal Model[21] promotes the use of engagement as a way of developing self-directed recovery through exploring a person's experiences. The model moves away from the traditional role of the professional as an 'expert' and instead emphasizes the importance of the person's 'voice' as an instrument of recovery.

Protected engagement time (PET) is a practical model that has developed in the last decade and is a way of managing staff time on inpatient wards in order to increase quantity and quality of interactions between staff and patients, and promote a safe environment. Although there are no national guidelines on how to implement PET, the concept involves ring-fencing a set period of time regularly (e.g. 1 hour per day) where staff do not engage in administrative or other duties and spend that time focused on patients. Despite its widespread use, its effectiveness has not been demonstrated, and a programme of evaluation is underway in England, funded by the National Institute of Health Research (NIHR), with results anticipated in early 2017.[22]

One model, Safewards, has been demonstrated to reduce conflict on acute inpatient wards.[23] This model consists of a complex framework to elucidate the factors that influence conflict and containment on mental health wards[24] and has led to the development of 10 interventions for ward staff. They are based on improved communication and understanding between staff and patients, with the use of positive language and a consistent approach. It is being increasingly adopted not only across the UK but in many other countries, including Australia, New Zealand, Denmark, Finland, Ireland and the USA.

Star Wards is another UK initiative, developed to help improve people's experiences on mental health wards.[25] It was established by Marion Janner following her admissions to an acute mental health ward in London, and is based on the sharing of ideas, best practice and benchmarking tools in order to improve patient quality of life and treatment outcomes.

SUGGESTIONS FOR RESEARCH

Trials of observation levels in inpatient wards have not been performed, due to ethical considerations of withholding the invention. However, there is potential for wards or hospitals to be randomized into an intervention consisting of specific training for staff in conducting observations, compared to a control group of wards or hospitals without that training. The potential for advance decisions to assist staff in deciding whether to place someone on high-level or continuous observations has not been investigated and is a further area for future research.

CONCLUSION

Managing risk is at the heart of mental health care in acute inpatient wards and requires effective therapeutic engagement between staff and patients. Approaches to risk management are varied, but in these settings in the UK the use of observation at increased levels has been standard practice for over 15 years. The potential positive effect on maintaining patient safety has to be weighed against the potential for intrusion to patients' privacy, the negative impact on the staff conducting the observations and the cost to the NHS.

Further research would be helpful to guide clinical services in the use of observation; to identify the staff training needed to enhance outcomes; and to understand the effect on patients, staff and carers.

ACKNOWLEDGEMENT

Our friend and colleague Caren Watson passed away on 3rd January 2017 after a 4 month illness. She is sorely missed but her dignity and kindness will always be remembered.

References

1. HQIP (Healthcare Quality Improvement Partnership). *National confidential inquiry into suicide and homicide by people with mental illness*. 2015. Available from: http://www.bbmh.manchester.ac.uk/cmhs/research/centreforsuicideprevention/nci/reports/NCISHReport2015bookmarked.pdf [Accessed 4th June 2016].
2. Standing Nursing and Midwifery Advisory Committee. *Practice guidance. Safe and supportive observation of patients at risk. Mental health nursing: addressing acute concerns*. London: Department of Health, 1999.
3. NICE (National Institute for Health and Care Excellence). Violence and aggression: short-term management in mental health, health and community settings. 2015. Available from: https://www.nice.org.uk/guidance/ng10 [Accessed 4th June 2016].
4. Scottish Government. Observation of people with mental health problems. 2002. http://www.gov.scot/Publications/2002/08/15296/10452 [Accessed 4th June 2016].
5. Northern Ireland Health and Social Care Board. Regional guideline on the use of observation and therapeutic engagement in adult psychiatric inpatient facilities in Northern Ireland. 2012. Available from: http://www.hscbusiness.hscni.net/pdf/ST_Special_Observations_Final_2012.pdf [Accessed 4th June 2016].
6. Stewart D, Bowers L, Ross J. Managing risk and conflict behaviours in acute psychiatry: the dual role of constant special observation. *Journal of Advanced Nursing* 2012; **68**(6): 1340–8.
7. Addo M, McKie A, Kettles, A, Gibb J, Gass J, Yule M. Are nurses empowered to make decisions about levels of patient observation in mental health? *Nursing Times* 2010; **106**(9): 26–8.
8. Bowles N, Dodds P, Hackney D, Sunderland C, Thomas P. Formal observations and engagement: a discussion paper. *Journal of Psychiatric and Mental Health Nursing* 2002; **9**: 255–60.
9. Standing Nursing and Midwifery Advisory Committee. *Mental health nursing: addressing acute concerns*. London: Department of Health, 1999.
10. Vrale GB, Steen E. The dynamics between structure and flexibility in constant observation of psychiatric inpatients with suicidal ideation. *Journal of Psychiatric and Mental Health Nursing* 2005; **12**: 513–18.
11. Johnson S, Osborn DP, Araya R, Wearn E, Paul M, Stafford M, Wellman N, Nolan F, Killaspy H, Lloyd-Evans B, Anderson E, Wood SJ. Morale in the English mental health workforce: questionnaire survey. *British Journal of Psychiatry* 2012; **201**(3): 239–46.
12. Buchanan-Barker P, Barker P. Observation: the original sin of mental health nursing? *Journal of Psychiatric and Mental Health Nursing* 2005; **12**: 541–9.
13. Bowers L, Park A. Special observations in the care of psychiatric inpatients: a literature review. *Issues in Mental Health Nursing* 2001; **12**: 769–86.
14. Kettles A, Addo M. Observation intervention: time for an overview. *Journal of Psychiatric and Mental Health Nursing* 2009; **16**: 813–21.
15. Bowers L, Whittington R, Nolan P, Parkin D, Curtis S, Bhui K, et al. *The City 128 study of observation and outcomes on acute psychiatric wards. Research report*. London: City University, 2007.
16. Manna M. Effectiveness of formal observation in inpatient psychiatry in preventing adverse outcomes: the state of the science. *Journal of Psychiatric and Mental Health Nursing* 2010; **17**: 268–73.
17. Muralidharan S, Fenton M. Containment strategies for people with serious mental illness. *Cochrane Database of Systematic Reviews* 2006; **3**: 1–10.
18. Bowers L. On conflict, containment and the relationship between them. *Nursing Inquiry* 2006; **13**(3): 172–80.
19. NICE (National Institute for Health and Care Excellence). *Service user experience in adult mental health: improving the experience of care for people using adult NHS mental health services*. 2011. Available from: https://www.nice.org.uk/guidance/cg136 [Accessed 4th June 2016].
20. Sharac J, McCrone P, Sabes-Figuera R, Csipke E, Wood A, Wykes T. Nurse and patient activities and interaction on psychiatric inpatients wards: a literature review. *International Journal of Nursing Studies* 2010; **47**: 909–17.

21. Barker P. The Tidal Model: developing an empowering, person-centred approach to recovery within psychiatric and mental health nursing. *Journal of Psychiatric and Mental Health Nursing* 2001; **8**: 233–40.

22. Nolan F, Fox C, Cheston R, Turner D, Clarke A, Dodd, E, Khoo ME, Gray R. A feasibility study comparing UK older adult mental health inpatient wards which use protected engagement time with other wards which do not: study protocol. *Pilot and Feasibility Studies* 2016; **2**(7).

23. Bowers L, James K, Quirk A, Simpson A, SUGAR, Stewart D, Hodsoll J. Reducing conflict and containment rates on acute psychiatric wards: the Safewards cluster randomised control trial. *International Journal of Nursing Studies* 2015; **52**(9): 1412–22.

24. Bowers L. Safewards: a new model of conflict and containment on psychiatric wards. *Journal of Psychiatric and Mental Health Nursing* 2014; **21**: 499–508.

25. Janner M. Starwards. *Healthcare, Counselling and Psychotherapy Journal* 2006; **6**(3): 32.

Further reading

Killaspy H, Johnson S, Pierce B, Bebbington P, Pilling S, Nolan F, King M. Successful engagement: a mixed methods study of the approaches of assertive community treatment and community mental health teams in the REACT trial. *Social Psychiatry & Psychiatric Epidemiology* 2009; **44**: 532–40.

Pereira S, Woollaston K. Therapeutic engagement in acute psychiatric inpatient services. *Journal of Psychiatric Intensive Care* 2007; **3**(1): 3–11.

Rooney C. The meaning of mental health nurses, experience of providing one-to-one observations: a phenomenological study. *Journal of Psychiatric and Mental Health Nursing* 2009; **16**: 76–86.

Relevant web pages

Safewards. www.safewards.net
Star Wards. www.starwards.org.uk
Tidal Model. www.tidal-model.com

Freedom and consent

HELEN LEIGH-PHIPPARD AND ALEC GRANT

LEARNING OUTCOMES

- To understand the rhetoric of empowerment in relation to freedom and consent for mental health service users.

- To able to reflect on risk as it relates to issues of freedom and consent.

- To be aware of how this field is impacted by the environmental and cultural contexts of practice, care and nurse education.

SUMMARY OF KEY POINTS

- The rhetoric of empowerment should be challenged.
- There is a marked absence of a mental health nurse presence on Twitter, in spite of the fact that this form of social media has proved empowering for service users.
- Being regarded as a source of risk can have a direct effect on service users' freedom, in a climate where

'risk management' may refer more to nurses avoiding blame than caring for people.

- Genuine empowerment of service users and carers involves regarding their lived experience as a valuable resource that should be integral to all nursing education.

INTRODUCTION

We hope in this chapter to challenge some conceptual sacred cows within mental health nursing. Drawing primarily on the British experience and literature, we aim to encourage readers to engage productively in relatively *unspoken* aspects of the area of freedom and consent. There is much that is good and useful practised in the name of psychiatric–mental health nursing. However, like Glenister,[1] we believe that it may, at worst, be characterized by institutional and professional denial around specific areas of user freedom. Although knowledge of mental health law is essential to nursing practice,[2–5] as both symptom of and defence against denial, nurses frequently displace disturbing aspects of users' freedom onto legal concerns such as capacity and risk, without even considering that the way in which, for example, 'risk'

is conceived, might in itself have consequences for service user freedoms (see also chapter 36 on the recovery approach and risk management).

We invite psychiatric–mental health nurses to begin to combat the above trend by seriously engaging in three related challenges.

First, the rhetoric of empowerment needs to be questioned. At worst, this rhetoric can seduce student nurses into imagining service users are genuinely situated at the centre of their care, with nurses free to co-facilitate this process.

Second, we need to consider how the conception/ construction of risk means that freedom and consent for mental health service users signifies something rather different to that which applies to the rest of the population.

Finally, nurses must engage with the problems endemic to the environmental and cultural conditions which 'set the scene' for the services that users receive and nurses deliver and, equally importantly, for the education of nurses in our higher education institutions.

Each segment of this chapter is composed of two parts: a discussion that sets out the theoretical issues and a subsequent dialogue conducted between the authors that is framed by this discussion. We are using dialogue as an autoethnographic practice here,[6] in a deliberate attempt to trouble current psychiatric–mental health nursing policy literature, and to allow for a more reflexive exploration of issues and contexts. Alec is a Reader in Narrative Mental Health at the University of Brighton with a professional background in mental health nursing and cognitive behavioural psychotherapy. He is also a mental health survivor.[7] Helen is a mental health service user (and a former academic) in the Carer and Service User Group (CUSER) at the University of Brighton.[8]

THE RHETORIC OF EMPOWERMENT

For service users to experience more freedom and equality in participating in their own care and treatment, they must harness their power positively. However, the concept of *empowerment* is problematic and needs to be considered across several contexts. The growth of the user movement, taken at face value, envisions an increasingly vocal collective, promoting the need for nurses and other mental health workers to listen *seriously and meaningfully* to users and engage with them in collaborative decision making;[9–11] to involve them in nursing educational programmes;[12] and to enable them to take more control than has hitherto been the case over their own care management.[13] (See also chapter 37 on the Care Programme Approach.) However, this rosy view needs to be balanced by an awareness of the institutionally endorsed order and control characteristic of inpatient and community settings,[1,7,9,11,14] and by what Morrall describes as a thinly disguised tokenism.[15]

What empowerment means in practice for nurses also hinges on them taking a position with regard to the supposed ethical demands of their role. This is by no means straightforward, as a range of possible future ethical and professional identities seduce nurses. They are invited to choose, for example, between the comforting certainties promised by so-called evidence-based practice;[16] a humanly 'ordinary and decent' view of their future role;[17] or a more esoteric view of psychiatric–mental health nursing as a uniquely and essentially spiritual form of engaging with the humanity of those in psychic distress.[18] However, nurses may discover that, in practice, their professional role socialization is shaped more by institutional[1] and organizational[19] factors than either they or psychiatric–mental health nursing luminaries would care to admit.

Alec

I think this is the problem of 'agency versus structure'. When user freedom and consent issues are violated, mental health nurses often seem to individualize responsibility and blame – the 'few bad apples' argument – rather than recognizing that the behaviour of nurses generally is shaped in large part by their work situations and wider socio-cultural (macro) organizational systems.

Helen

As a service user contributor to a mental health nursing programme, I often explore with students how they have been able to develop really positive 'human' therapeutic relationships with service users while on practice placements. But I am often saddened to hear them say that they have only been able to do this because they are students. Some even add: 'Of course, I won't be able to do this once I'm qualified because I simply won't have the time'. Even as students on placements they are 'learning' that they will not have time to listen to service users in a therapeutic relationship once they are fully qualified. How does that fit with what they are being taught in the classroom? Regardless of what they are taught about person-centred practice, they know absolutely that once they are employed their actual practice will be shaped by institutional and organizational demands.

REFLECTION

Is it possible for service users to be meaningfully empowered within the existing mental health system? If not, what would need to change, structurally and/or culturally, for this to become possible?

The rhetoric of empowerment: identity construction

The rhetoric of empowerment exists within a broader force field of *identity* and *relational politics* in mental health in twenty-first-century Britain.[20] A cacophony of voices declare the meaning of being a nurse or a service user. In addition to the demands upon nurses to work actively at ethical and professional identity construction, user needs articulated around issues of freedom and consent will vary as a function of ethnicity, cultural and religious diversity, gender, sexuality, resistance to representation, and the increased tendency for individual and corporate self-definition.

This picture of active identity shaping is in turn inseparable from the broader context of an information society saturated with ever-increasing forms of textual representation.

This has been taken a stage further by the public engagement of mental health services with social media.[21] Nurses and, increasingly, users enthusiastically engage in hyper-real dialogue, in which problems concerning user empowerment, freedom and consent are vigorously discussed – sometimes intelligently, sometimes defensively.

Notwithstanding institutional factors constraining development, in a postmodern vision of psychiatric–mental health nursing, possibilities thus exist for nurses to combine multiple approaches to, and skills in, developing their craft. The craft of caring may be regarded as each mental health nurse's individualized application of a blend of different types of useful knowledge in their work with users, in an attempt to work alongside them in a helpful way. What constitutes 'useful knowledge' in this context is likely to be a constantly changing blend of professional and broader cultural ways of knowing, applied in myriad different permutations.

This points to the existential angst that undoubtedly accompanies such a plethora of choices. It is not really surprising that mental health nurses displayed a tendency towards binary logic in the closing years of the twenty-first century with regard to what constitutes the proper focus of psychiatric–mental health nursing.[22–29] A constant – but now arguably anachronistic[30] – effect of this was to relegate the lived experiences and needs of service users around freedom and consent in favour of privileging the dominant agenda of any one particular camp.[31–33] However, the twenty-first century is perhaps witnessing a consolidating growth in the development of communities of mental health users and survivors who are challenging this agenda with increasing confidence and authority.[34]

Alec

As we have noted in our work,[11] new stories have emerged in the last 20 years or so which shift the balance of power more in the direction of user and carer lived experience as an alternative, but equally valid, knowledge base. This challenges the hegemony of professional and policy-driven knowledge.

Helen

A good example of some of the vexed issues related to the rhetoric of empowerment in the twentieth century lies in the use of social media. I find Twitter, in particular, a very useful source of social support, information and networking in mental health. Yet generally, when I say this to a mental health professional, it is met with a sharp intake of breath and a warning of 'the risks'. When I reply that I have been using Twitter for a number of years, I am well aware of the risks but believe that the benefits far outweigh them, I am quickly dismissed with a 'harrumph' of dismay.

There is a very robust and supportive mental health community on Twitter. I am rarely trolled (that is, harassed online), I use Twitter responsibly and I know when to leave a potentially inflammatory or triggering conversation. I have made many new friends and a number of 'virtual colleagues' there. Like other parts of the internet, Twitter can be a source of inaccurate and misleading information, but it can also be enormously helpful and empowering for service users, for whom information is a key source of power. The mental health community on Twitter is a huge resource which is freely available, a resource which includes a vast range of interested and interesting people with valuable skills and knowledge which they are willing to share. This is a community which includes lawyers, police officers, social workers, psychiatrists, journalists, psychologists, counsellors, campaigners, advocates, mindfulness practitioners, service users and carers – and from all around the world. Conversations on Twitter are not subject to traditional boundaries that govern access to information, such as education, class, wealth and geography; in the context of mental health this means that service users can, and do, converse as equals with mental health and other professionals.

Although NHS Mental Health Trusts, the Royal College of Nurses (RCN) and other nursing bodies have a presence on Twitter, their accounts are largely used for promotional and policy purposes. Mental health nurses are largely noticeable by their absence. A small number of individuals tweet in a personal capacity while declaring their professional status, and there are probably others who simply do not declare their professional status and are perhaps tweeting under pseudonyms, but their obvious numbers are few. I do not see why it is not possible to separate the personal from professional while nevertheless bringing professed nursing qualities – of compassion and caring – to the public debate, yet in the world of social media the divide between nurses and service users could not be wider.

I'm guessing more nurses don't contribute because of that idea of risk that seems to dominate mental health nursing, but there is an important conversation about mental health being had every day now on Twitter; if mental health nurses are not there, then they are not part of the conversation. Indeed in a #WeNurses chat on Twitter on 13 February 2014 at 8–9 pm about 'Student Nurses and Social Media' @DGFoord (David Foord, Director of Quality at Luton Clinical Commissioning Group) insisted in a tweet that Nursing and Midwifery Council (NMC) Code 61 implies a requirement to uphold the nursing profession's reputation by engaging with the public on social media:

'NMC Code '61 You must uphold profession's reputation at all times' This is not passive, we must actively do this including on SoMe [social media] #WeNurses – 13 Feb[35]

More positively, a small group of mental health nurses are now contributing to the #WeNurses community chats under the hashtag #WeMHnurses.

Do nurses have an obligation to participate in public 'conversations' about health care on social media in order to help the public understand the practice of their health care and to have the practice of their health care informed by the public?

The rhetoric of empowerment: freedom and consent

In terms of the capacity of nurses to engage meaningfully with user empowerment, a further and related problem with the rhetoric of empowerment is the continued *over-investment* in humanistic principles in psychiatric–mental health nursing curricula.[17,19,32,36]

Their uncritical acceptance serves to conceal or marginalize several problems related to user freedom and consent. First, in terms of the broader contemporary dialogue, the assumption that users are free to make informed choices about what they need or want when they may be lacking in sufficient control,[37] readiness to change,[38] self-esteem,[39] hope that change is possible,[40,41] or the belief in a successful outcome to such an intervention to make those choices in the first place,[41,42] may amount to unwitting abuse on the nurse's part.

There is a further contemporary difficulty with the modernist notion of the coherent 'growing person', from the social constructivist perspective.[43] This notion makes little sense within a postmodern interdisciplinary world view, which envisions and articulates the experiences of multiple, fractured and distributed selves, reflected in service users' perspective and related literature.[11,44–46]

The need for mental health nursing to challenge the cosy overemphasis on caring enshrined in person-centred curricular approaches is long overdue. More attention needs to be accorded to what nurses need to do to avoid fulfilling their future institutional capacity to engage in violence, coercion and control.[1,47] The notion of the self-actualizing user also seems fatuous in the light of environmental and organizational problems in inpatient[7,9,11] and community mental health care.[14] These serve to disadvantage users and will be addressed more specifically later.

Alec

For the last decade or more I have been bothered by the rhetoric of partnership, empowerment and related concepts in the mental health nursing professional and policy literature. The problem for me with potentially laudable slogans and approaches like 'the gift of time' and the Tidal Model is that they seem to sidestep the lived, psychosocial experiences of users and survivors of institutional psychiatry.

Helen

I remember the first several years I was in mental health services when I was 'stuck', not really getting the help I needed, before anyone was attempting to offer me any kind of proper recovery approach or help. All I was given was medication which just made things worse, I couldn't have therapy, and I remember the frustration of being asked time and again by mental health nurses what would help me, what my triggers were, what had made me so ill, why I felt the way I did, what I needed by way of support, why I felt so hopeless, why I had no self-esteem, why I didn't believe things could get better. The things I knew I wanted, the things I thought might actually help, I couldn't have, and by the time I knew the answers to the other questions I didn't need the mental health nurses any more.

As for service user involvement, I think the relationship between service providers and 'involved' or 'engaged' service users is a very complicated one. There is definitely an element of service providers finding ways of effectively 'choosing' the service users who might be involved in a particular project. My own experience is that, as a well-educated and articulate service user, I found that when I first became involved with a local participation project I was in high demand. However, as I gained confidence and my need for local services lessened, I became more outspoken and sometimes challenged the dominant NHS position in meetings. I quickly found that I wasn't in such high demand any more.

Have you ever been in a meeting that has had 'service user participation' in which one or more service users has challenged the dominant 'NHS' view of that meeting. What was the response to that challenge? Was it welcomed? Or were attempts made to sideline or silence the challenge? Did the challenge make people feel uncomfortable? How did it make you feel?

FREEDOM, CONSENT AND THE LANGUAGE OF RISK

At risk or risky?

Freedom and consent in mental health services are necessarily tied up with the concept, and the assessment, of risk.

How much freedom a mental health service user can have is dependent on the risk they are deemed to present. However, the language of risk is tied up with power: it is determined by practitioners and often does not reflect the concerns of service users and/or carers. Mental health service users often find themselves being perceived as a source of risk rather than 'at risk' and indeed the fact that they are seen as a source of risk by others can have a direct effect on their freedom: 'There is a clear connection between perceptions of risk and access to rights: the more risky you are seen to be by others, the fewer rights you have access to'[48] (p.3).

When risk is discussed in the context of mental health, it is usually with reference to the risk of potential harm someone poses either to themselves or to others, as expressed in the Mental Capacity Act 1983. The very term 'risk management' frames risk as something which is to be discussed in terms of who is to blame when things go wrong, rather than in terms of how to care for people who are 'at risk'.

In a survey of service users' experiences of risk management, Sheldon found that for mental health professionals risk management was a protection from possible accountability and recriminations.[49] Simpson, a community psychiatric–mental health nurse researcher, with clinical experience of assertive outreach work targeted at homeless mental health clients, sees this as a consequence of the introduction of the supervision register alongside the Care Programme Approach (CPA):

> *the soft police control role is experienced by many nurses as shifting the emphasis towards monitoring people – making sure you keep in contact with people … this results in a blame culture … organizational blame and avoiding risk. All emphasis is on maintaining contact and being seen to do that. If someone commits suicide or kills someone then the finger of blame points at the CPN (Community Psychiatric Nurse).[50]*

If service users are to be supported within a recovery-based approach, then there is a need for changes in the way risk is understood, managed and negotiated with people using mental health services, so that they are supported and enabled to take positive and exciting risks that promote independence and improve quality of life.

Without the opportunity to take risks, recovery can never take place (see also chapter 36, on the recovery approach and risk management).

Alec

Risk-averse cultures are infantilizing. Decisions are made for rather than with service users, in ways that inhibit growth and change. In my 26 years as a mental health nurse turned cognitive behavioural psychotherapist, I advocated therapeutic risk taking in my practice, with my students and in print.

Helen

When I was first ill, I often felt that I was given freedoms I didn't want, while not being given freedoms I did want. I was left for weeks at a time in a state of absolute crisis, very much at risk, with very little support and nowhere to go out of hours, while at the same time being given little choice about taking medication, no other treatment whatsoever and regularly threatened with the possibility of a section, and threatened with forced ECT (electroconvulsive therapy) under section, if I didn't comply. Even today, when I feel much more empowered, because I manage my mental health problems well and without medication, I still feel I don't have the freedom I should have because, when I am struggling and perhaps should be seeking support from services, I don't. I'm afraid that I may find myself having to explain again why I don't want to take medication, that I'll have to go back into defensive mode, that instead of getting help and support of the kind I want – person-centred help and support that recognizes that I don't want meds and values my own expertise in managing my symptoms – I'll get arguments, condescension and perhaps even threats. I know what kind of support I need, but I get by without it because I'm not sure I'll get it.

> ### REFLECTION
>
> How far should positive risk taking be encouraged in a recovery-oriented service?

ENVIRONMENTAL AND CULTURAL CONTEXTS OF PRACTICE

Inpatient services

> *… acute wards resemble jails and by extension, the nurses jailors.[51] (p.184)*

A reduction over the years in long-stay facilities, the failure to provide adequate community services, and the more recent demands that austerity has placed on public finances have led to increased pressure on the use of acute psychiatric services. More than 1,700 NHS mental health beds were closed between April 2011 and October 2013,[52] while the number of people subject to detention and/or treatment under the Mental Health Act has risen by 12 per cent in the past 5 years.[53] The general picture of acute inpatient wards in England is bleak: although costly, there is little evidence that inpatient stays are clinically effective[54] or cost-effective,[55] or that they provide much more than custodial care.[56]

Acute inpatient wards can become ridiculously overcrowded and a 'dumping ground for people whose community care has broken down'[57] (p.3); one London hospital was recently found to be using seclusion rooms as temporary bed spaces.[58] Not surprisingly, wards can be 'dangerous and chaotic, with staff always "fire-fighting", with violence common and absconding everyday occurrences'[57] (p.4).

Patients admitted on a voluntary basis often experience the admission as coercive, with many subsequently attempting to leave, only to be compulsorily admitted to prevent them from doing so: the Care Quality Commission (CQC) found in January 2014 that this was happening in 20 per cent of cases.[53] There seems to be a consensus across the user, carer and professional literature that acute inpatients often feel deprived of therapeutic activity and sufficient contact with nurses, and at times feel at risk of physical and sexual assault. The 2006/7 National Audit of Violence found that 43 per cent of working-age adults on acute inpatient wards had felt upset or distressed and 15 per cent reported being physically assaulted[59] (p.8). In the 2008 Healthcare Commission Review of Acute Inpatient Mental Health Services, 'one in every nine trusts was scored weak on the criteria for providing individualized care and for ensuring safety'[59] (p.24); it is worth noting that in this context 'weak' means 'the performance of this trust does not meet the minimum requirements and the reasonable expectations of patients and the public'[59] (p.20).

It is perhaps not surprising in this context that the CQC recently reported that 27 per cent of care plans for patients treated under the Mental Health Act showed no evidence of patient involvement[54] (p.3). The CQC also reported staff using 'subterfuge' or threats to induce patients to consent to informal admission to hospital, or to prevent them from leaving, and sometimes not knowing which patients had been admitted informally and which were detained. What this means is that treatment decisions are being made without valid consent, and that voluntary patients face the powers of the Mental Health Act without its protections.

In the *Guardian* newspaper in January 2014 Nathan Filer, a former mental health nurse, writes about the voluntary admission of his friend Byron Vincent to an acute psychiatric ward in Bristol's Southmead Hospital in 2011. The ward was very short-staffed and facing closure and, consequently, although Byron would sometimes be asked if he would like to go for an escorted walk and always said yes, these walks never actually happened. Whenever he suggested he might go for a walk alone, 'it was made clear to me in no uncertain terms that I'd be restrained until they could have me sectioned. I was only a voluntary patient in name'.[60] As Filer comments:

> *The kinds of 'holding powers' that Byron is referring to are in place as an emergency measure, not to dangle over a patient as a negotiation tool. For a person to remain 'voluntary' with the looming threat of detention should they try to leave, effectively incarcerates them – but without any of the rights ... that the Mental Health Act provides.[60]*

Mental health service users do not have the same rights as others because there is the possibility of taking away their freedom through the use of the Mental Health Act: they face the possibility of detention and treatment without consent (see also chapter 67 on Mental health, the law and human rights). Faulkner notes that this raises important issues about the circumstances in which a person's rights can be compromised by the risk they are believed to present, primarily to other people but also to themselves[48] (p.26). She concludes that this makes it all the more important to include people in the risk assessment made about them, as well as to ensure they are aware of their rights.

> *Each step in the process of developing a risk management plan should be based on discussions between the service user and those involved in their care. The service user should be offered the opportunity to take a lead role in identifying the risks from their point of view, drawing up plans for dealing with difficult situations, and indicating the sort of support that they would prefer: service users and carers are often in the best position to comment on the robustness and practicality of the plan.[61] (p.21)*

Alec

For meaningful, effective and truly therapeutic relationships between nurses and service users to be realized, nurses need to take critically reflexive steps to avoid being socialized into the control agenda of institutional psychiatry. We point out in our work together that users actually finding such relationships often seems more a matter of luck than a regular provision.[6,11]

Helen

The Healthcare Commission's Pathway to Recovery report talks about the importance of focusing on the individual, and recommends setting aside one-to-one time for staff to build up therapeutic relationships with service users[59] (p.29). None of this is rocket science. Endless reconfigurations of mental health services to 'improve' them miss the point: you are never going to make services work well unless you invest in people, because it is people and relationships, not structures, that make the most fundamental difference to service users.

It has always been people, particular individuals who have built a relationship with me and tried to make a difference to me and for me, that have helped me in my recovery. Some have done it better than others, but they have all cared about me as a human being, they have often tried to help me find ways round or through 'the system'; some have certainly helped in spite of it. There have also been people who have not helped, people who have most definitely not listened to me, whom I have fought against and with whom I most definitely did not have therapeutic relationships, but fundamentally my story is a story about people within a service structure, not a story about a service structure.

So I do think that having time for relationship building is an essential part of nursing: the Healthcare Commission is quite clear that 'protected therapeutic engagement time between mental health nurses and service users is recommended in national policy'[59] (p.27), and for me that should be the absolute centre of any acute inpatient service provision if that service is going to do anything other than confine people who are 'risky' until they aren't deemed risky any more.

> ## REFLECTION
>
> It is important that staff who work in inpatient services insist that the rights of their service users are upheld, because the service users themselves are often powerless. It is the responsibility of the staff in these services to work collaboratively and therapeutically with their service users. Given this, in what specific ways can you strengthen your advocacy and collaborative–therapeutic role in inpatient work?

Nursing education

If nurses and service users and carers are going to develop shared understandings of the meanings of freedom and consent, based on collaborative understanding and management of risk and relationship building, this has to begin at the beginning, with nursing education. Service user and carer involvement in nursing education has to be absolutely integral to design, delivery and assessment, and service users and carers need to be visible, tangible contributors to nursing degrees in person, in the same way as academic staff, and with similar status.

Involving service users and carers in nursing education from the outset (that is, from course design and admissions processes onwards) would have a number of potential benefits. It would remove any constructed barriers between them and us: such barriers are unnecessary anyway since we are all (nurses and academics included) potential service users. It would actively demonstrate partnership working between mental health professionals and service users. It would help to erode some preconceived stereotypes of mental health service users, for example, as incapable of work or reasoned argument. It would also help implicitly to shift power balances between mental health service users and professionals from the outset.

There is an underlying belief in academic institutions that knowledge gained primarily through lived experience is in some way inferior to and less valuable than that gained by academic study. But lived experience can teach nursing students to understand the real impact of their interventions (or the lack of them) and of the services within which they work on the service users they will meet, in a way that no amount of professional book learning will ever teach them.[7] Moreover, attending lessons taught by service users and carers, turning up on time for those classes, listening to those service users' stories, putting questions to them and responding to questions from them, are all experiences that are valuable first lessons in treating service users and carers with dignity and respect.

Alec

I'm left surprised and disappointed that the 'lived experience' paradigm has not found its way into the nursing/mental health nursing curricula to the degree that it should have by now.

Helen

I've read some of the literature on the 'difficulties' of service user involvement in nursing education. Often it's put down to the fact that service users can be unreliable because they are, after all, ill, or they struggle to commit, but when I read the literature I wonder if there are other reasons. I wonder if the service users are being properly supported, or if they are being treated as well as they might be. My own experience is that I am very well supported by a small group of brilliant mental health lecturers but we are still treated 'differently' – and, I would argue, like second-class citizens – by the wider university. We get paid a little less than visiting lecturers, because we are not 'professionals'. The mental health lecturers who support us have to fight very, very hard to protect us, and in particular to try to preserve funding for our essential support meetings. Our mental health lecturer colleagues work tirelessly to make us as integral to the mental health nursing degree as they possibly can, but it is always hard work to maintain our level of involvement in the degree whenever the curriculum changes, despite the consistently excellent feedback our classes receive from students. Our needs are not well understood within the university and we are often regarded as 'difficult' because we have special requirements which mean increased costs or timetable adjustments; for example, smaller classes because we are talking about difficult mental health experiences (hard to do in a large class of 40 students), late starts (because some of us are on psychiatric medications which make it very difficult to start at 9 am).

There are constant suggestions that service user narratives, which are a central part of our teaching, could be recorded on DVD and played to students, thus saving the cost of having actual service users in the classroom telling their stories in person. But I would argue that there would be human costs in doing this. Having a person in the room teaches the students something about a service user being a human being, about the importance of building a relationship with a person, and about freedom and consent. When I'm in a classroom telling my story,

I'm a human being choosing to tell that story, consenting to do so, building a relationship with those students by the telling of it, and when I answer their questions I'm consenting freely to do so. My story changes every time I tell it and I learn something from that, and every class of students hears something different as I restory it. If those students watch a DVD, there is no restorying; I'm not sure if there is even any consent, because although I might sign a consent form when the DVD is recorded, I would have no control over what happens to it afterwards – would I really want to consent to it being used in any way the university chose and for any audience? Perhaps more importantly, if the students have questions after watching the DVD, who speaks for me? Does the lecturer who is running the class? How can they? What would they say? How can they know what my answers would be? How can students learn from that?

REFLECTION

How important is it to listen to the experience of a real person in the classroom, rather than simply to read about their experience in a book or to watch a film or video? Does it make a difference to have a real person in the classroom, to be able to ask them questions and to have a conversation with them?

CONCLUSION

We began this chapter by challenging the rhetoric of empowerment. We questioned some of the dominant ideas about empowerment; in particular, that involving users both in their care and in wider organizational decision making is empowering, while in reality their choices are still defined by others. We also noted the marked absence (with a few exceptions) of nurses from the mental health community on Twitter, an arena which is proving empowering for service users, because, inter alia, it is not governed by organizational and institutional agendas.

We also looked at freedom, consent and the language of risk. We noted that being seen as a source of risk can have a direct effect on a service user's freedom. Risk management is discussed in terms of avoiding blame rather than in terms of caring for people 'at risk'. As a result of recent austerity measures in the UK, inpatient services have increasingly become about detaining and confining people, and the idea of building therapeutic relationships seems to have been lost. We concluded with the suggestion that, for genuine empowerment of service users and carers, and for a proper understanding of the ways in which freedom and consent can be undermined by their experience of mental health problems and services, lived experience should be integral to all nursing education.

References

1. Glenister D. Coercion, control and mental health nursing. In: Tilley S (ed.). *The mental health nurse: views of practice and education*. Bodmin, Cornwall: Blackwell Science, 1997: 43–57.
2. Department for Constitutional Affairs. *Mental Capacity Act 2005: code of practice*. London: Stationery Office, 2007.
3. Mind. *Mind guide to the Mental Health Act 1983*. London: Mind, 2012.
4. Mental Health Law Online. Available from: www.mentalhealth-law.co.uk [Accessed 20th October 2016].
5. Department of Health. *Reference guide to consent for examination or treatment*, 2nd edn. London: Department of Health, 2009.
6. Grant A, Leigh-Phippard H. Troubling the normative mental health recovery project: the silent resistance of a disappearing doctor. In: Zeeman L, Aranda K, Grant A (eds). *Queering health: critical challenges to normative health and healthcare*. Ross-on-Wye: PCCS Books, 2014: 100–15.
7. Grant A. Performing the room. In: Grant A, Biley F, Walker H (eds). *Our encounters with madness*. Ross-on-Wye: PCCS Books, 2011: 125–30.
8. Leigh-Phippard H. Surviving: from silence to speaking out. In: Grant A, Biley F, Walker H (eds). *Our encounters with madness*. Ross-on-Wye: PCCS Books, 2011: 103–9.
9. Campbell P. Listening to clients. In: Barker P, Davidson B (eds). *Psychiatric nursing: ethical strife*. London: Arnold, 1998.
10. Dunn C. *Ethical issues in mental illness*. Aldershot: Ashgate, 2000.
11. Grant A, Leigh-Phippard H, Short N. Re-storying narrative identity: a dialogical study of mental health recovery and survival. *Journal of Psychiatric and Mental Health Nursing* 2015; **22**: 278–86.
12. NMC (Nursing and Midwifery Council). *Standards for pre-registration nursing education (2010)*. London: NMC, 2010.
13. Rose D. *Users' voices: the perspectives of mental health service users on community and hospital care*. London: Sainsbury Centre for Mental Health, 2001.
14. Morrall P. *Mental health nursing and social control*. London: Whurr, 1999.
15. Morrall P. Clinical sociology and empowerment. In: Barker P, Davidson B (eds). *Psychiatric nursing: ethical strife*. London: Arnold, 1998: chapter 18.
16. Newell R, Gournay K (eds). *Mental health nursing: an evidence-based approach*. London: Churchill Livingstone, 2000.
17. Clarke L. *Challenging ideas in psychiatric nursing*. London: Routledge, 1999.
18. Barker P. *The philosophy and practice of psychiatric nursing*. London: Churchill Livingstone, 1999.
19. Grant A. Psychiatric nursing and organizational power: rescuing the hidden dynamic. *Journal of Psychiatric and Mental Health Nursing* 2001; **8**: 173–88.
20. Grant A. Knowing me knowing you: towards a new relational politics in 21st century mental health nursing. *Journal of Psychiatric and Mental Health Nursing* 2001; **8**: 269–75.
21. Mental Health Network/NHS Confederation. Joining in the conversation – social media and mental health services. Briefing 225. London: NHS Confederation, 2011.
22. Clarke L. Nursing in search of a science: the rise and rise of the new nurse brutalism. *Mental Health Care* 1999; **21**: 270–2.
23. Cannon B, Coulter E, Gamble C, Jackson A, Jones J, Sandford T, Sharkey S, Ward M, West L. Personality bashing. *Mental Health Care* 1999; **21**: 319.

24. Ritter S. Insulting distortion. *Mental Health Care* 1999; **21**: 319.

25. Rogers P. Arrested development. *Mental Health Care* 1999; **21**: 393.

26. Stevenson C. Power and control. *Mental Health Care* 1999; **21**: 393.

27. Duncan-Grant A. Misrepresentation, stereotyping, and acknowledging bias in science: responses to Liam Clarke. *Mental Health Care* 1999; **21**: 336–7.

28. Gournay K. What to do with nursing models. *Journal of Psychiatric and Mental Health Nursing* 1996; **2**: 325–7.

29. Barker P, Reynolds B. Rediscovering the proper focus of nursing: a critique of Gournay's position on nursing theory and models. *Journal of Psychiatric and Mental Health Nursing* 1995; **3**: 75–80.

30. Grant A, Biley F, Walker H, Leigh-Phippard H. The book, the stories, the people: an ongoing dialogic narrative inquiry study combining a practice development project. Part 1: the research context. *Journal of Psychiatric and Mental Health Nursing* 2012; **19**: 844–51.

31. Repper J. Adjusting the focus of mental health nursing: incorporating service users' experiences of recovery. *Journal of Mental Health* 2000; **9**: 575–87.

32. Dallard D. What does counselling do? A critical reexamination of Rogers' core conditions. *Mental Health Care* 1999; **21**: 383–5.

33. Rolfe G, Gardner L. The possibility of a genuine mental health nursing. In: Barker P (ed.). *Psychiatric and mental health nursing: the craft of caring*. London: Arnold, 2003: 552–8.

34. Grant A. Troubling 'lived experience': a post-structural critique of mental health nursing qualitative research assumptions. *Journal of Psychiatric and Mental Health Nursing* 2014; **21**: 544–9.

35. @DGFoord tweet, 8.20pm, 13 February 2014. The entire 13 February #WeNurses chat is available from: http://www.wecommunities.org/tweet-chats/old-chat-details/181 [Accessed 20th October 2016].

36. Grant A. Tales from the order of received wisdom (or some contemporary problems with mental health nurse education in Britain). *Journal of Psychiatric and Mental Health Nursing* 2002; **9**: 622–7.

37. Rotter JB. Generalized expectancies for internal versus external control of reinforcement. *Psychological Monographs* 1966: **80**(1): 1–28.

38. Diclemente CC, McCounnaughy EA, Norcross JC, Prochaska JO. Integrative dimensions for psychotherapy. *International Journal of Eclectic Psychotherapy* 1986; **5**: 256–73.

39. Fennell M. *Overcoming low self-esteem: a self-help guide using cognitive-behavioural techniques*. London: Robinson, 1999.

40. Snyder CR, Ilardi SS, Cheavens J, Michael S, Yamhure L, Sympson S. The role of hope in cognitive behaviour therapies. *Cognitive Therapy and Research* 2000; **24**: 747–62.

41. Grant A, Townend M, Mills J, Cockx A. *Assessment and case formulation in CBT*. London: Sage Publications, 2008.

42. Bandura A. *Social learning theory*. London: Prentice-Hall, 1977.

43. Rogers CR. *On becoming a person: a therapist's view of psychotherapy*. London: Constable, 1988.

44. Wetherell M, Maybin J. The distributed self: a social constructionist perspective. In: Stevens R (ed.). *Understanding the self*. London: Sage, in association with the Open University, 1997: 219–80.

45. Holstein JA, Gubrium, JF. *The self we live by. Narrative identity in a postmodern world*. New York: Oxford University Press, 2000.

46. Short N, Grant A, Clarke L. Living in the borderlands; writing in the margins: an autoethnographic tale. *Journal of Psychiatric and Mental Health Nursing* 2007; **14**: 771–82.

47. Zimbardo P. *The Lucifer effect: understanding how good people turn evil*. New York: Random House, 2007; see also www.lucifer-effect.com.

48. Faulkner A. *The right to take risks: service users' view of risk in adult social care*. York: Joseph Rowntree Foundation, 2012.

49. Sheldon K. Service users: experiences of risk and risk management. In: Whittington R, Logan C (eds). *Self-harm and violence: towards best practice in managing risk in mental health services*. London: Wiley-Blackwell, 2010: chapter 2.

50. Simpson A, personal communication with co-author, 2001.

51. Dodds P, Bowles N. Dismantling formal observation and refocusing activity in acute inpatient psychiatry: a case study. *Journal of Psychiatric and Mental Health Nursing* 2001; **8**: 183–8.

52. McNicoll A. Patients at risk as 'unsafe' mental health services reach crisis point. *CommunityCare*. 16 October 2013. Available from: http://www.communitycare.co.uk/2013/10/16/patients-at-risk-as-unsafe-mental-health-services-reach-crisis-point-2/ [Accessed 20th October 2016].

53. CQC (Care Quality Commission). *Care Quality Commission monitoring the Mental Health Act in 2012/13*. Newcastle upon Tyne: CQC, 2014.

54. Sainsbury Centre for Mental Health. *Acute problems: a survey of the quality of care in acute psychiatric wards*. London: Sainsbury Centre for Mental Health, 1998.

55. Minghella E, Ford R, Freeman T, Hoult J, McGlynn P, O'Halloran P. *Open all hours: 24-hour response for people with mental health emergencies*. London: Sainsbury Centre for Mental Health, 1998.

56. Mental Health Act Commission and Sainsbury Centre for Mental Health. *The National Visit: a one-day visit to 309 acute psychiatric admission wards by the MHAC in collaboration with the Sainsbury Centre for Mental Health*. London: Sainsbury Centre for Mental Health, 1997.

57. RCCPU (Royal College of Psychiatrists Policy Unit). *Acute mental health care: briefing note*. London: Royal College of Psychiatrists, 2009.

58. McNicoll A. Mental health patients admitted to seclusion rooms for up to five days due to lack of beds. *CommunityCare*. 16 January 2014. Available from: http://www.communitycare.co.uk/2014/01/16/mental-health-patients-admitted-seclusion-rooms-five-days-due-lack-beds/ [Accessed 20th October 2016].

59. Healthcare Commission. *The pathway to recovery: a review of NHS acute inpatient mental health services*. London: Commission for Healthcare Audit and Inspection, 2008.

60. Filer N. Mental health care: where did it all go so wrong? *Guardian*. 25 January 2014. Available from: http://www.theguardian.com/society/2014/jan/25/nathan-filer-mental-health-care-where-did-it-go-wrong [Accessed 20th October 2016].

61. Department of Health National Risk Management Risk Programme. *Best practice in managing risk: principles and evidence for best practice in the assessment and management of risk to self and others in mental health services*. London: Department of Health, 2007.

Relevant web pages

CQC (Care Quality Commission). http://www.cqc.org.uk

Mental Health Law Online. www.mentalhealthlaw.co.uk

#WeMHNurses Chat Archive. http://www.wecommunities.org/tweet-chats/chat-archive

#WeNurses. http://www.wecommunities.org

Archived #WeNurses chat on student nurses and social media. http://www.wecommunities.org/tweet-chats/old-chat-details/181

'I decided I wasn't going to be a diagnosis' – What does it mean to have a diagnosis of mental illness? The lived experience perspective

KATI TURNER

LEARNING OUTCOMES

- To learn about the experience and impact of receiving a mental health diagnosis from the lived experience perspective.

- To gain an awareness of the tensions between theoretical rhetoric and the lived experience of diagnosis, supported by references to the literature in the field.

- To link lived experience accounts with the practice of mental health nursing (the *craft of caring*).

SUMMARY OF KEY POINTS

- The experience of receiving a mental health diagnosis is often characterized by inconsistency and a lack of information.
- Significant levels of stigma and discrimination still surround a diagnosis of mental illness.
- The validity and place of a biomedical or clinical diagnosis in people's lives is being actively questioned by some.
- Issues around identity and self-stigmatization often follow a mental health diagnosis.

- Receiving a diagnosis is no guarantee of appropriate care: many experience poor or haphazard treatment.
- Current mainstream understandings of 'recovery' are sometimes at odds with the lived experience perspective.
- A humane and therapeutic relationship between nurse and service user is seen as an integral basis of mental health nursing.

19

'I decided I wasn't going to be a diagnosis' – What does it mean to have a diagnosis of mental illness?

INTRODUCTION

This chapter is written from the perspective of people with a lived experience of a mental health condition or illness. The aim of the chapter is to give voice to the person at the heart of a mental health diagnosis. The lived experience in mental health literature is frequently lost or overpowered by stronger or competing voices, and there is a dearth of literature concerning diagnosis from the service user perspective.[1] Yet it is often this voice of lived experience which can tell someone's story more powerfully than any traditionally accepted 'expert' clinical diagnosis or analysis.

In order to find out more about a range of experiences of mental health diagnoses, the author talked to a number of people over the age of 30, both individually and in groups. All the people who took part were recruited via a service user research reference group and were willing to talk in depth and reflect on their experiences. The quotations used in this chapter are taken from these discussions. Some of the recent literature relating to mental health diagnoses, stigma, treatment, care and recovery is also drawn upon, in an attempt to illustrate tensions between the theoretical rhetoric and the lived experience.

The men and women who took part in the discussions talked openly about their experiences of receiving a diagnosis, of living with their mental health condition and of the impact it had on their lives and those close to them. They also discussed the stigma which often surrounds mental illness and shared their personal stories of this. People talked about what had been helpful about receiving a diagnosis and what had not, and described their experiences of treatment received from various mental health services – within the community and in hospital. Finally, the discussions focused on the unique and vital role of mental health nurses in caring for those who receive treatment, and which skills, attributes and attitudes were most helpful for them to have.

A number of themes emerged from the discussions, many of them illustrating the challenges experienced by people coming into contact with a mental health system often perceived as harmful and in need of much improvement. Some of those key themes highlighted in this chapter are: the inconsistency and lack of information often accompanying a mental health diagnosis; the stigma and consequent discrimination which still surrounds mental illness, even in the eyes of some mental health professionals; the validity and place of a biomedical or clinical diagnosis in people's lives; self-stigma and identity following diagnosis; the often haphazard nature of treatment and care; the importance of developing internal coping mechanisms such as self-reliance and determination; and the humane and therapeutic relationship between nurse and service user, seen as an integral basis for the *craft of caring* of mental health nursing.[2]

RECEIVING A MENTAL HEALTH DIAGNOSIS

Diagnosis occupies a key position in the mental health system, as it is often the door that permits entry into that world and leads to far-reaching implications beyond it. The people who took part in the discussions had received a range of mental health diagnoses: paranoid schizophrenia; schizoaffective disorder; clinical depression; severe reactive depression; personality disorder; bipolar disorder; and anxiety disorder. They described the circumstances in which they had learnt about the diagnosis – usually from their GP (doctor) or a psychiatrist:

> I was diagnosed around 15 years ago ... finally came to this diagnosis after a few suicide attempts and hospital admissions ...
>
> I first went into hospital around the age of 20, I was sectioned and very afraid I wouldn't ever get out ... then in and out of hospital for the next 10 years ... I was in a ward round when given a diagnosis, lots of people were there, a psychiatrist, a social worker, a nurse, you are this, we all know best, they were all the authority figures.

These experiences echo the recent literature. Berk et al.[3] quote an average time of 10 years from onset to diagnosis for bipolar disorder, while Read et al.[4] draw attention in their study to the low percentage (7 to 34 per cent) of people with schizophrenia who are actually told their diagnosis.

Horn et al.[5] report that, for some, receiving a diagnosis comes as a relief, and this was reflected by some in the discussions:

> In a way it's a relief to have something to hold on to and know that there is actually something wrong with you, you're not just going a bit mad ... It helped in that it really answered the question, this is exactly how I feel so it fitted exactly how I felt.

But for others it had the opposite effect:

> I burst out in horror and said 'what is that?'
>
> First getting that bipolar diagnosis also felt very scary – like I have slipped into the severe and enduring box of mental health problems that are with you forever. I was worried about

What do people think and feel about having a mental health diagnosis?

19

the implications of this for all kinds of things, life insurance, driving, adoption, judgements of my suitability as a parent and worker.

A common experience reported by many people involved the manner and language in which a diagnosis was delivered. Rose[6] and Rose and Thornicroft[1] describe diagnosis as 'the formal status of psychiatric patient being conferred' (p.140) and refer to the inherent imbalance of power between those giving and those receiving a diagnosis. This was mirrored by many people's experiences:

The psychiatrist had no real interest in my story, what had led up to me having a breakdown. Everything was interpreted through the lens of ... diagnostic criteria. He was so busy asking me about my 'symptoms' that he forgot to talk to me, you know the person sitting right in front of him.

I have had diagnoses written in the letters or assessments ... these are often in different language or terms to the words used to me face to face in an appointment ... in my experience psychologists, counsellors and psychotherapists are much more careful and open with language.

People also referred to the less than acceptable level of information they were given about their condition:

I wasn't given any information about the illness: 'get on with it' was the impression I got.

I don't know what it is and to this day I have never been properly explained, all I was told

was vaguely, in layman's terms, you're a little bit schizophrenic and a little bit of a manic depressive, you have both of those attributes or both of those diseases and they affect you and you have to try and live with your illness and get on with it.

However, there is no doubt that receiving a diagnosis does not have to be a negative and fearful experience when care is taken to deliver it in a thoughtful and sensitive manner and the right level of information is given. Both Rose[6] and Thornicroft[7] refer to the possibility of diagnosis being a process of negotiation between service user and professional, and there are many examples in the literature of when receiving a diagnosis can lead to access to treatment and higher levels of self-management.[8–10] One member of the group discussions described a helpful approach:

The approach of the psychiatrist who gave me the diagnosis of 'Type II bipolar disorder rapid cycling' was really helpful ... It made sense to me and she described the experience of it very clearly. So that it fitted. I went away feeling that I had a new way of understanding what I was dealing with and could now make some steps to working out how to manage it.

REFLECTION

Put yourself in the place of someone who has just received a mental health diagnosis. How do you think you might react?

WHAT DO PEOPLE THINK AND FEEL ABOUT HAVING A MENTAL HEALTH DIAGNOSIS?

The manner in which a diagnosis is given can be instrumental in how people manage and make sense of their lives after receiving a diagnosis. A negative experience can often contribute to feelings of isolation and confusion, and people described periods following their diagnosis that were marked by fear, hopelessness and a sense of being controlled:

You go through the argument stage of asking why and is it just a way of controlling people ... you're going to be monitored for this amount of time, you're going to be medicated, you're going to be subdued – for a long time that's how I felt.

I feel like somehow before I was normal and then since 2000 I officially have depression and have to work my life around it and try and find medication or something that works for me.

People also expressed fears that a diagnosis could feel like a life sentence with no possibility of things being different, a prospect often reinforced by the rigidity of the diagnostic criteria and system:

No one's ever reassessed it, no one's ever turned round and told me you might have recovered from that.

I have said for years that I don't think I would any longer meet the diagnostic criteria for Type II Bipolar ... is this still my diagnosis? When I am most unwell I guess it is the type of label that I wonder if [it] might still fit. That makes me sad. I'd like to be completely free from that idea sometimes.

There is much in the literature concerning the links between identity and diagnosis. McCay and Seeman[11] refer to the concept of 'engulfment' – a process in which

19

'I decided I wasn't going to be a diagnosis' – What does it mean to have a diagnosis of mental illness?

individuals see themselves totally and solely in terms of their illness – and Korsbek[12] in her 2013 paper echoes this in relating her lived experience. This area was also keenly debated in the discussion groups, with people expressing a desire to live their lives in a way that was not defined by their diagnosis:

> *I've had a varied relationship with my mental health. When I am doing well I don't let it be my identity. I am me with many facets to my life story, many parts of me. Although I am a person who has had mental health problems, maybe a service user or survivor, it's very important above all to be a person … and to see my mental health lived experience (and experiences of diagnoses) as part of being Me.*
>
> *It's hard enough telling people you've got a mental health diagnosis, without telling them what the diagnosis is … it defines you as an individual … I just live my life … when I get home, I'm a husband, a father, a grandfather, I'm an individual … I'm so much more than a diagnosis.*

People also described their relationship with their 'illness' and the efforts they made to preserve a sense of self, rather than pathologize their lived experience:

> *I live with my difficulties like a troubled child. Some days she wants to get out of bed and do lots of things, some days she wants to hurt me, sometimes she's very creative. I have to look out for that part of myself now rather than ignore it. I still have ups and downs but I am so glad I don't pathologize my experience anymore.*

There was also discussion about who benefits from a mental health diagnosis and how much validity it has. Korsbek[12] makes a strong link between the recovery process and diagnosis, and suggests that it is equally valid for some people to actively resist or reject a diagnosis as it is for others to accept one. This perspective was reflected in the group discussion:

> *I think it just really helps them [mental health professionals], all it can do for us is maybe help us define ourselves a bit or find out some information about our so-called diseases.*
>
> *I would never be OK with being given a mental health diagnosis. Firstly I do not believe that the medicalization of my distress or my narrative has any scientific validity and secondly the word diagnosis or condition suggests that there is a medical solution to what I am struggling with.*

Some people also questioned the classification and wording around diagnosis:

> *I wish they would change the actual name of it [depression], then you could explain that this is an illness with extremes and a spectrum; it's not the same as saying 'I'm just a bit fed up today.'*

REFLECTION

Think about the different ways having a mental health diagnosis might impact on a person's life. How important do you think the manner in which a diagnosis is delivered is, and how might a person view themselves differently after receiving one?

EXPERIENCES OF STIGMA AND DISCRIMINATION

Despite recent campaign initiatives such as Time to Change (www.time-to-change.org.uk) and mental illness being acknowledged more openly by those in the media spotlight, stigma surrounding mental ill-health is still common. This is well illustrated in the literature,[13,5] with some diagnoses being singled out as carrying a particular stigma,[14,15] sometimes with the association of violence.[7] Jones and Hayward,[16] Hegner[17] and the Social Exclusion Unit[18] all refer to the public myths which surround mental illness, with Falk[19] calling it 'the ultimate stigma' (p.39). Many examples of this were cited by people in the discussion groups:

> *Anyone who knows about the media, the only time paranoid schizophrenics are ever mentioned is when they murder someone or they hold people up to ransom … so when*

> *I was told I'm paranoid schizophrenic that was quite, oh my god, what's going to happen … generally I don't tell people what my diagnosis is, I say I've got a mental health issue.*

However, it was generally agreed during the discussions that any mental health diagnosis or label carries a degree of stigma:

> *I don't know why there is such a stigma about it, I suppose people don't know how to deal with it, how to react and there are different levels … there's the whole idea of mental illness people find hard to deal with, they don't know if you're a bit mad or …*

Corrigan[20] discusses how a clinical diagnosis may exacerbate the perception among the general public of people with mental illness being essentially 'different'. These attitudes can often lead to instances of discrimination, and people in the group described feeling like 'social outcasts' and of being unfairly viewed as dangerous people:

[on becoming a social outcast] that's what happens once you get involved with the mental health system.

This discrimination can often extend into family and close relationships,[21–25] and there were many examples of this – and the subsequent effects – given in the group discussions:

I saw family members in a different light, I couldn't quite believe my siblings were my siblings, even they became unfriendly, then shunned me as well. It was as if having a mental illness, it rubs off, they also saw me as nothing.

For me, it's not something you want to go out and say to people … it's not got any easier telling people, for me it's like a real taboo subject … even my family it's like the unspoken thing, they'll never acknowledge it and that's quite hard.

People also expressed concern about possible future repercussions arising from the stigma surrounding mental health for their family members:

It's not like I can tell my children, even as they get older, it's becoming increasingly difficult to think: well how am I going to explain that, but it would be nice to think that the next generation might be a bit more accepting.

This [stigma] is present for me as a parent. 'People who know' may well already look at my husband with 'pity' since he takes a lot of responsibility for the things I can't or don't manage when I'm not doing so well. I'm not sure how I feel about my children looking back at their childhood through the lens of 'Mum being a bit mental at times'.

Experiences of stigma and subsequent discrimination – or the fear of it occurring – can lead to people 'self-stigmatizing', something which has been widely acknowledged in the literature.[26–32]

Corrigan[20] suggests that self-stigma can lead to feelings of shame and low self-esteem and, in a first-person account, Fox[33] describes her fear and subsequent isolation as a mother diagnosed with schizophrenia. Korsbek[12] states that 'depression, hopelessness, suicidal thought, internalized stigma and low self-esteem were all significant barriers

in my recovery process' (p.223). These experiences were mirrored in the group discussions:

It's more the fear of it … when I've been off sick in the past I'd come back to work … nobody would acknowledge that you'd been away … it was almost like nobody even dared even say anything, I find it really upsetting when people won't acknowledge it … to not say anything makes it so much worse because you just don't know what they're thinking.

I will generally avoid using specific diagnoses unless it is helpful to another service user for them to hear that I might have a similar experience. I fear that people who know my diagnosis may then be looking out for the signs and features and using this to understand me. I'm more comfortable with just me using it to understand myself. I don't want to be misunderstood, boxed or labelled or have some of my behaviour, ideas or approaches to things taken with a pinch of salt.

The consequent attempts that people made to hide their condition often added an additional strain:

That's part of the problem, not only are you dealing with an illness but you're having to cover it up and that in itself is very difficult and upsetting, I can't just say to someone, I've broken my leg, can you help me down the stairs or something … I can put on a front and … they would think nothing of it but it does take quite a lot of energy, putting on a front and pretending you're alright when you're not.

I have scars on my arms and legs and I have to be very careful about when I have them out. Sometimes I feel like I want to show the world that you can go right to the edge of death and come back stronger, but I know that the world is afraid. I don't want to frighten people who have never had to make that existential journey.

Perhaps one of the most concerning areas of stigma and discrimination around mental illness is that which is present within the medical profession itself. There are many examples in the literature,[34–37] and Corrigan[20] provides some disturbing examples of the subjective and judgemental language used by some mental health professionals to describe people diagnosed with personality disorder:[38,39]

People in the 'dramatic' cluster are rarely capable of empathy. They are often self-centred and prone to temper tantrums. They tend to be irresponsible, impulsive, and remarkably free of remorse.

19

'I decided I wasn't going to be a diagnosis' – What does it mean to have a diagnosis of mental illness?

Deceit, superficiality, and arrogance cloud all of their relationships …[39] (p.175)

They have great power to create confusion, disruption and violence in the workplace; their presence there is a stick of dynamite waiting for a match.[39] (p.222)

Some 15 years on, it seems that there are still examples of this attitude to be found, as related by some of the contributors to this chapter:

I went to a meeting recently where lots of psychoanalysts were and they were talking about personality disorder but they didn't say PD, they used the word 'psychopaths'. They kept saying it as if it was a perfectly OK way to describe another human being. Part of me wanted to pull an axe out and confirm their ridiculous beliefs, mainly it just made me want to cry because it feels like we still have so far to go.

We're all diagnosed with a particular mental health concern but it is generally based on one psychiatrist's opinion which is dangerous in itself. Because I could be seen by someone else and they diagnose me with something else … and on top of that, the nurse will just see on your file that diagnosis and it's their opinion and interpretation of that diagnosis … because

people will form opinions in their minds about a diagnosis.

Even where it appears that mental health professionals are well-intentioned, their unspoken acknowledgement of stigma and discrimination has not been experienced as helpful:

My GPs have often only referred to a diagnosis at the point that they are writing out a sick note. I have sometimes had to ask what the shorthand or letters mean since they appear to be using a code or trying to be kind by dumbing down the language used maybe to save me stigma or problems at work. This fuzzy approach can be unhelpful leaving me unsure what they think and whether I should be 'hiding something' in the way I talk too?

REFLECTION

Can you think of any instances of stigma and discrimination around mental health or ill-health that you have experienced or been witness to in your own life or work? Did this come from the media or people you know? What do you think are helpful ways to respond to attitudes like this?

EXPERIENCES OF CARE AND TREATMENT FOLLOWING DIAGNOSIS

It might be assumed that one positive outcome of making a clinical diagnosis is the ability to then identify treatment that is most likely to work for an individual.[40] Chapter 12 explains more on the classification of mental illness. However, many people described a lengthy process of different treatments – including medication, counselling, cognitive behaviour therapy (CBT), electroconvulsive therapy (ECT), primary and secondary health care and hospitalization – during the course of their lives, some of which had been helpful and some not:

It's not all been a bed of roses, I've stopped taking medication, I've got myself into fights, I've been hospitalized, sectioned under the MHA [Mental Health Act] a few times … I've had lots of different treatments … been through a wide gamut of different drugs … antidepressants, ECT.

It's not that treatable, it's not like I was diagnosed, given medication and that was that, I was better, nothing's ever really worked particularly well, it's a cyclical thing and I can be well on medication but I can also

be ill on medication … I feel like whatever help I have had hasn't really helped … ultimately it's something you have to get through yourself.

People also talked about some treatments only being effective at certain times of their illness or about hopes for some form of 'cure' or 'miracle' following a diagnosis:

And all the CBT, it is very good, it can only work at a certain point, I think if you're very depressed it doesn't work that well. I think if you're recovering … it can work quite well, I don't think it works very well for severe depression.

Ultimately I'm holding out for this miracle medication or cure … there's always this idea that until I was 28 or so I was alright so maybe's there's going to be a point when I'm suddenly OK again.

There were discussions about the levels of care received from different mental health professionals, with some being regarded as more beneficial than others. Negative experiences often seemed to follow instances where

Getting better/'recovery' from mental ill-health: an alternative approach?

19

communication was limited to diagnosis and a prescribed course of treatment:

> *The psychiatrist said to me 'you've got to get from a to b and you don't have a map'. And I sat there and thought I've come here to see you and that's what you say to me … I didn't appreciate it, I used to go there and come out in floods of tears, I thought I'll just go to my GP. I think the only person who did understand was the GP, even to this day.*
>
> *Psychiatrists and nurses couldn't ever see my viewpoint, it was always what my parents felt.*
>
> *I'd survived so much up until the point where I ended up in the psychiatric system. When I first saw a psychiatrist I imagined they would say something along the lines of 'Well done! You've managed to survive such a horrific ordeal so far, you've been so brave. We'll help you now and give you a bit of a break.' I couldn't have been more wrong.*

In the previous edition of this book, Barker et al.[2] discuss at length the 'craft of caring' of mental health nursing, placing the focus on the individual and advocating a humane and holistic approach which has as its basis the relationship between the nurse and the person in hospital. More on developing and maintaining therapeutic relationships are explored in chapter 3. This is echoed in the more positive experiences which people related:

> *The major support and help came from support and nursing staff … without their help and support I wouldn't be in the circumstances and situation I am in now, 15 years on from when I was diagnosed.*

> *My GP is very good but there's a limit to what she can do … she doesn't really know either, it's really up to me to decide whether to try a new medication or not … But it's really nice to know that she understands up to a point what it's like for me, she always tries to do something to help … just to have someone who understands and who is sympathetic, that helps a huge amount.*

However, there were concerns expressed about current mental health service provision, with fears that there would be less access to therapeutic services and more reliance on medication in the future. There was a feeling that the mental health system was becoming increasingly diagnosis-driven, where only a clinical diagnosis with a certain degree of severity could give a guarantee of treatment:

> *I don't demonstrate it in a way that's recognized … it's like what do I need to do? I know what I could do to get that help but I don't want to go down that road to get that help.*
>
> *The system is iatrogenic in the worst possible way. First my distress was labelled, either mad or bad. There was no enquiry, no attempt to understand my life, my story. The opposite of care. The most caring thing I could do for myself was to find a way to get help in spite of the system.*

REFLECTION

Do you think a diagnosis of a mental health condition or illness will always lead to the most helpful treatment and care? What obstacles might impede this?

GETTING BETTER/'RECOVERY' FROM MENTAL ILL-HEALTH: AN ALTERNATIVE APPROACH?

The voice of lived experience[41,42] has played an increasingly important role in helping to shape and develop current thinking about 'recovery' and mental ill-health. Korsbek[12] suggests a process which involves a 'transformation from patient to person' (p.222) and Beresford et al.[43] advocate a move away from the medical model to more socially orientated approaches. These sentiments were echoed in the group discussions:

> *Recovery is a strange word. It suggested there was a time when everything was rosy. I never felt OK and I never will. I am different, I think very deeply, I am sensitive and feel like I don't fit in. Accepting these things about myself has been*

immensely healing. I don't get the sense that I have anything to recover from. I haven't had the flu. I have had life. My life.

There is also an acknowledgment that the mental health system itself requires a transformation in order to be able to focus on an understanding of recovery 'as a personal and subjective experience'[44] (p.12) and that those working within it need to work more closely and collaboratively with service users and their families.[45,46] This would seem to suggest an inherent tension within a mental health system which is still fundamentally driven by clinical diagnosis. See chapters 35 and 36 for more detail on the recovery approach.

Regardless of how people in the discussion groups conceptualized or spoke about 'getting better', it was generally acknowledged that recovering from mental ill-health often does not follow a linear course, with some people describing periods of their life when they were either very well or unwell and unable to carry out the most basic of everyday tasks. However, even when people had been told they would not ever 'recover', they had gone on to lead fulfilling lives and described a process of coming to terms with and making sense of the diagnosis they had received:

I've been told I'll never make a recovery, that I'll be taking tablets for the rest of my life … After a while it opened my eyes … sent me on a challenge … I decided I wasn't going to be a diagnosis … I think it's perspective, how you see it, how you overcome it, the equation is, you have to deal with the anger, deal with the sense of loss and sense of regret that you might have … I'm now happily married, with a home I like, a loving wife, supportive family and friends that I know aren't going to judge me.

A key area which emerged in the group discussions was the development of personal attributes and skills – such as self-reliance and determination – which had helped people in their various journeys towards a better understanding of their mental health:

I had to become self-contained because I realized I cannot look to anybody to help me through, I have to look to me … sometimes I feel that if I don't do it it's not going to get done … Now I'm not really governed by anything, I'm my own person and that's keeping me safe and well.

I try not to look backwards, I deal with today, I look towards tomorrow and I try to make plans for a couple of months in advance … Meet new people, do different things, try and develop and progress, move on from being a diagnosis and not have someone pull me back or pull me down because of my diagnosis. I can be very determined … very fixed about what I want to achieve in my life.

These experiences are reflected in the literature, which describes a process of self-development and the change in identity from patient to person.[47–49] This move towards a social or relational sense of self, rather than the 'diagnosed' self, is also seen in the value people in the group placed upon 'peer support' – the understanding and support of others with similar experiences and the ability to empathize and offer support to others in return:

Me living through lots of different experiences of mental health has given me lots of ways I can empathize with others and that gives others strength and comfort. It's not all bad by any means!

I wish I had had someone with lived experience to explain to me what I know now.

The only positive signs in recent years is [sic] the development of the recovery college, the introduction of peer support workers and using the mentally ill on ward settings and in the communities.

REFLECTION

What do you think 'recovering' from a mental health condition or illness means? Can more socially orientated approaches work in tandem with traditional medical approaches, or do you think there is an inherent tension between the two?

ESSENTIAL SKILLS, ATTRIBUTES AND ATTITUDES FOR MENTAL HEALTH NURSES

The vital role that mental health nurses play in the care of people with a mental health diagnosis – both in inpatient settings and in the community – has long been acknowledged in the literature. Barker et al.[2] lay out their blueprint for the craft of caring, stressing the dynamic of working alongside and *caring with* people rather than *caring for* them. Many of these sentiments were echoed in the group discussions, which identified a number of key skills, attributes and attitudes that people agreed were vitally important for mental health nurses to have. One of these was an open, calm and caring attitude coupled with a holistic, non-judgemental approach which could see past the diagnostic label to the person within:

One additional person that you could be completely open with and you didn't have to talk in metaphors and pretend … whilst they may not understand exactly how you're feeling because they might not have experienced it, they accept what you're saying and [are] very sympathetic at the same time, can give you a bit of guidance … someone who can walk by your side a bit and help you.

… they [nurses] need to see themselves as that person and think what would I like if this was me? What if this was my daughter? They need to realize that we're all human.

Mental health nurses need to understand that people breakdown for all kinds of reasons. They shouldn't blame a person for their own distress. They certainly shouldn't interpret people's behaviour through their own, narrow medicalized perspective. People have been having breakdowns long before psychiatry came along. Mental health systems are the new things, people's sometimes troubled journeys through life are not.

The importance of establishing a therapeutic relationship between service user and nurse is prevalent in the literature (for example, Gilburt et al.,[50] Barker et al.[2]). Bray[51] talks about a 'healing relationship ... Offering help, that is, so that people can experience their distress and then see it both as the reasonable upshot of their life history and an opportunity for growth' (p.95). The importance of this healing relationship – regardless of diagnosis or treatment approach – was recognized by the chapter's contributors, with specific examples given of nurses needing to have a well-developed intuitive sense of someone's distress and being able and willing to listen:

An extra sensory perception – to be able to recognize that someone may be low before that person knows they're low ... and to know that that person is feeling low or stressed even if they can't express it, being able to just be there, be someone to talk to, bounce off of.

From my experience a good nurse is able to listen and pre-empt your conversation or jump in saying I know what you mean without you being able to express what you mean ... I've always found that to be a plus, the listening quality is really in place because that's what helps an individual to express yourself because you feel that the person is showing an interest ... body language and eye contact ... and if a nurse has those skills and is genuine ... you can pick it up and feel more comfortable in expressing themselves [sic] ... so it is a top priority.

Another key attribute discussed was the ability to encourage and help instil hope and self-reliance. Korsbek[12] refers to this 'message of hope' needing to start with the process of diagnosis, and Spandler and Stickley[52] suggest that hope and compassion are not just seen as an individual's attributes but are applied systemically as 'something which must be nurtured in context, through relationships, cultures and healing environments' (p.555). This was reflected in the group discussions:

They [mental health nurses] engendered hope more than anything ... I was at my worst, lowest ebb ... he came along and lifted me up.

They really need to give people hope ... instead of dishing out tablets. When they give you your diagnosis they need to be careful how they do it and they need to offer some hope – it's no good saying to somebody you're schizophrenic and you're going to be on tablets for the rest of your life ... they need to explain, there are ways we can help you, they need to be nice about it, to be kind, not to just [say], oh take these tablets and go away.

People also acknowledged some of the challenges that come with being a mental health nurse and drew attention to hierarchical relationships within the medical profession which they felt could have the potential to impinge upon the therapeutic relationship between nurse and service user:

I'm not a them, I'm not an us, I'm a me ... I would turn round and say to these nurses reading this book, you need to be able to stand up and be counted, if you have an opinion you need to be able to not worry about the authority figures and how influential they can be because your opinion can be just as influential.

The psychiatrist has the power over people's lives ... some nurses can be in awe of the doctors.

I think nursing is a very hard profession ... each service user does have different ways of wanting to be for want of a better word handled or spoken to – to get to grips with that, knowing your patient and to be able to help each and every one of them to the best of your ability would be straining on anybody, especially now with the turnover being so quick ... I'm not sure if the nursing profession is really being respected as it should be.

These opinions are echoed in the literature, which draws attention to inherent imbalances of power and systemic flaws which add to the challenges of mental health nursing.[53,54] Rose et al.[55] refer to both service users and nurses as 'two marginalised groups in the acute psychiatric care context' with the latter being 'bottom of the medical hierarchy' (p.94), and Crowe[56] recommends that 'mental health nursing practice needs to demonstrate an awareness of the power relations inherent in any diagnostic process and make attempts to redress these at both the individual and sociopolitical levels' (p.125). Elsewhere in the literature[57,58,2] lived experience and the service user perspective is regarded as a vital element in the journey to improve mental health services.

REFLECTION

Drawing on your experience, what other skills, attributes and attitudes do you think mental health nurses need to have?

19

'I decided I wasn't going to be a diagnosis' – What does it mean to have a diagnosis of mental illness?

CONCLUSION

We need to try to improve the system for future generations of mentally ill …

As seen from the contributions in this chapter, the lived experience of mental health problems is inherently painful, challenging and difficult. Added to this, the experience of being given a diagnosis of a mental health condition or illness can very often be a further blow to people who have already struggled for years either within or outwith the mental health system. We have seen how some people resist and reject their diagnosis as a result, while others continue to engage with the system despite their negative experiences as, in theory, diagnosis provides a pathway to the most appropriate treatment. When treatment is not successful or does not meet the expectations people have been given, this can compound negative experiences. Some people try, and succeed, in building a non-medicalized, social sense of self away from mental health services, and this is reflected to some extent in the co-opting of the recovery approach by mainstream mental health services. However, it must be acknowledged that very real tensions exist within a mental health system that is attempting to embrace social and humanistic models while ultimately being constrained and driven by a medical and diagnostically based system. It is all the more important, then, to emphasize the vital role that mental health nursing can play in people's mental well-being, in particular putting a caring and therapeutic relationship that is focused on hearing and understanding the lived experience at the heart of every interaction.

> ### REFLECTION
>
> How do lived experience accounts of receiving and living with a mental health diagnosis compare with others you have listened to or read about from other perspectives: for example, the perspectives of mental health professionals or academics?

References

1. Rose D, Thornicroft G. Service user perspectives on the impact of a mental illness diagnosis. *Epidemiologia e Psichiatria Sociale* 2010; **19**(2): 140–7.
2. Barker P (ed). *Psychiatric and mental health nursing; the craft of caring*, 2nd edn. Hodder Arnold: London, 2009.
3. Berk M, Dodd S, Callaly P, Berk L, Fitzgerald P, de Castella AR, Filia S, Filia K, Tahtalian S, Biffin F, Kelin K, Smith M, Montgomery W, Kulkarni J. History of illness prior to a diagnosis of bipolar disorder or schizoaffective disorder. *Journal of Affective Disorders* 2007; **103**: 181–6.
4. Read J, Haslam N, Sayce L, Davies E. Prejudice and schizophrenia: a review of the 'mental illness is an illness like any other' approach. *Acta Psychiatrica Scandinavica* 2006; **114**: 303–18.
5. Horn N, Johnstone L, Brooke S. Some service user perspectives on the diagnosis of personality disorder. *Journal of Mental Health* 2007; **16**: 255–69.
6. Rose D. *Users' voices, the perspectives of mental health service users on community and hospital care.* London: Sainsbury Centre, 2001.
7. Thornicroft G. *Shunned: discrimination against people with mental illness.* Oxford: Oxford University Press, 2006.
8. Mueser KT, Meyer PS, Penn DL, Clancy R, Clancy DM, Salyers MP. The Illness Management and Recovery program: rationale, development, and preliminary findings. *Schizophrenia Bulletin* 2006; **32**: Suppl. 1, S32–S43.
9. Salyers MP, Godfrey JL, Mueser KT, Labriola S. Measuring illness management outcomes: a psychometric study of clinician and consumer rating scales for illness self management and recovery. *Community Mental Health Journal* 2007 **43**: 459–80.
10. Mueser KT, Gingerich S. *Coping with schizophrenia: a guide for families.* New York: Guildford Press, 2005.
11. McCay EA, Seeman MV. A scale to measure the impact of a schizophrenic illness on an individual's self-concept. *Archives of Psychiatric Nursing* 1998; **12**: 41–9.
12. Korsbek L. Speaking out: illness insight and recovery: how important is illness insight in people's recovery process? *Psychiatric Rehabilitation Journal* 2013; **36**(3): 222–5.
13. Hamilton S, Lewis-Holmes E, Pinfold V, Henderson C, Rose D, Thornicroft G. Discrimination against people with a mental health diagnosis: qualitative analysis of reported experiences. *Journal of Mental Health* 2014; **23**(2): 88–93.
14. Crisp A. *Every family in the land: understanding prejudice and discrimination against people with mental illness.* London: Royal Society of Medicine Press, 2004.
15. Lequesne ER, Hersh RG. Disclosure of a diagnosis of borderline personality disorder. *Journal of Psychiatric Practice* 2004; **10**(3): 170–6.
16. Jones S, Hayward P. *Coping with schizophrenia: a guide for patients, families and carers.* Oxford: Oneworld Publications, 2004.
17. Hegner RE. Dispelling the myths and stigma of mental illness: the Surgeon General's report on mental health. *Issue Brief (George Washington University. National Health Policy Forum)* 2000; **754**: 1–7.
18. Social Exclusion Unit. *Mental health and social exclusion.* London: Office of the Deputy Prime Minister, 2004.
19. Falk G. *Stigma: how we treat outsiders.* New York: Prometheus Books, 2001.
20. Corrigan PW. How clinical diagnosis might exacerbate the stigma of mental illness. *Social Work* 2007; **52**(1): 31–9.
21. Corker E, Hamilton S, Henderson C, et al. Mental health service users' experiences of discrimination in England, 2008–2011. *British Journal of Psychiatry* 2013; **202**: s58–63.
22. Henderson C, Corker E, Lewis-Holmes E, et al. One year outcomes of England's time to change anti-stigma programme for service user-rated experiences of discrimination. *Psychiatric Services* 2012; **63**: 451–7.

23. Lasalvia A, Zoppei S, Van Bortel T, et al. Global pattern of experienced and anticipated discrimination reported by people with major depressive disorder: a cross-sectional survey. *The Lancet* 2012; **381**: 55–62.

24. Thornicroft G, Brohan E, Rose D, et al. Global pattern of experienced and anticipated discrimination against people with schizophrenia: a cross-sectional survey. *The Lancet* 2009; **373**: 408–15.

25. Thornicroft G, Kennedy R. Shunned. Discrimination against people with mental illness. *Journal of Occupational Psychology, Employment and Disability* 2009; **11**(56).

26. Rusch N, Corrigan PW, Todd AR, Bodenhausen GV. Implicit self-stigma in people with mental illness. *Journal of Nervous and Mental Disease* 2010; **198**(2): 150–3.

27. Biernat M, Dovidio J. Stigma and stereotypes. In: Heatherton TF, et al. (eds). *The Social Psychology of Stigma*. New York: Guilford Press, 2000: 88–125.

28. Dovidio J, Major B, Crocker J. Stigma: introduction and overview." In: Heatherton TF, et al. (eds). *The Social Psychology of Stigma*. New York: Guilford Press, 2000: 1–28.

29. Smart L, Wegner D. The hidden costs of hidden stigma. In: Heatherton TF, et al. (eds). *The Social Psychology of Stigma*. New York: Guilford Press, 2000: 220–42.

30. Smart L, Wegner D. Covering up what can't be seen: concealable stigma and mental control. *Journal of Personality and Social Psychology* 1999; **77**: 474–86.

31. Link BG, Phelan JC. Conceptualizing stigma. *Annual Review of Sociology* 2001; **27**: 363–85.

32. Ritsher JB, Otilingam PG, Grajales M. Internalized stigma of mental illness: psychometric properties of a new measure. *Psychiatry Research* 2003; **121**: 31–49.

33. Fox V. First person account: schizophrenia and motherhood. *Schizophrenia Bulletin* 2004; **30**(4): 763–5.

34. Lauber C, Nordt C, Braunschweig C, Rossler W. Do mental health professionals stigmatize their patients? *Acta Psychiatrica Scandinavica* 2006; **113**, Suppl. 429: 51–9.

35. Nordt C, Rossler W, Lauber C. Attitudes of mental health professionals toward people with schizophrenia and major depression. *Schizophrenia Bulletin* 2006; **32**: 709–14.

36. Peris TS, Teachman BA, Nosek BA. Implicit and explicit stigma of mental illness: links to clinical care. *Journal of Nervous and Mental Disease* 2008; **196**(10): 752–60.

37. Nehls N. Borderline personality disorder: gender stereotypes, stigma, and limited system of care. *Issues in Mental Health Nursing* 1998; **19**: 97–112.

38. Millon T. *Disorders of personality: DSM-III, Axis II*. New York: Wiley-Interscience, 1981.

39. Fischler GL, Booth N. *Vocational impact of psychiatric disorders: a guide for rehabilitation professionals*. Gaithersburg: Aspen Publishers, 1999.

40. Bentall R. *Doctoring the mind: who psychiatric treatments fail*. London: Penguin Books, 2009.

41. Gould D. *Service users' experiences of recovery under the 2008 Care Programme Approach: a research study*. London: Mental Health Foundation, National Survivor User Network, 2012.

42. Kalathil J. *Recovery and resilience: African, African-Caribbean and South Asian women's narratives of recovering from mental distress*. London: Mental Health Foundation, 2011.

43. Beresford P, Nettle M, Perring R. *Towards a social model of madness and distress? Exploring what service users say*. London: Joseph Rowntree Foundation, 2010.

44. Slade M, Amering M, Farkas M, Hamilton B, O'Hagan M, Panther G, Perkins R, Shepherd G, Samson T, Whitley R. Uses and abuses of recovery: implementing recovery-oriented practices in mental health systems. *World Psychiatry* 2014; **13**(1): 12–20.

45. South London and Maudsley NHS Foundation Trust and South West London and St George's Mental Health NHS Trust. *Recovery is for all. Hope, agency and opportunity in psychiatry. A position statement by consultant psychiatrists*. London: SLAM/SWLSTG, 2010.

46. Devon Recovery Research and Innovation Group (D-RRIG). *How can we use diagnosis to support people in their recovery? Guidance note no. 1*. Devon Partnership NHS Trust, 2013.

47. Davidson L, Strauss JS. Sense of self in recovery from severe mental illness. *British Journal of Medical Psychology* 1992; **65**: 131–45.

48. Roe D. Progressing from patienthood to personhood across the multidimensional outcomes in schizophrenia and related disorders. *Journal of Nervous and Mental Disease* 2001; **189**: 691–9.

49. Davidson L, Sells D, Sangster S, O'Connell M. Qualitative studies of recovery: what can we learn from the person? In: Ralph RO, Corrigan PW (eds). *Recovery in mental illness: broadening our understanding of wellness*. Washington, DC: American Psychological Association, 2005: 147–70.

50. Gilburt H, Rose D, Slade M. The importance of relationships in mental health care: a qualitative study of service users experiences of psychiatric hospital admission in the UK. *BMC Health Services Research* 2008; **8**(92).

51. Bray J. Psychiatric nursing and the myth of altruism. In: Barker P, Davidson B (eds). *Psychiatric nursing: ethical strife*. London: Arnold, 1998: 95–114.

52. Spandler H, Stickley T. No hope without compassion: the importance of compassion in recovery-focused mental health services. *Journal of Mental Health* 2011; **20**(6): 555–66.

53. Cleary M, Edwards C. 'Something always comes up': nurse–patient interaction in an acute psychiatric setting. *Journal of Psychiatric and Mental Health Nursing* 1999; **6**: 469–77.

54. Faulkner A. Institutional conflict: the state of play in adult acute psychiatric wards. *Journal of Adult Protection* 2005; **7**: 6–12.

55. Rose D, Evans J, Laker C, Wykes T. Life in acute mental health settings: experiences and perceptions of service users and nurses. *Epidemiology and Psychiatric Sciences* 2015; **24**(1): 90–6.

56. Crowe M. Psychiatric diagnosis: some implications for mental health nursing care. *Journal of Advanced Nursing* 2000; **31**: 583–9.

57. Walsh J, Boyle J. Improving acute psychiatric hospital services according to inpatient experiences. A user-led piece of research as a means to empowerment. *Issues in Mental Health Nursing* 2009; **30**: 31–8.

58. Rogers A, Pilgrim D, Lacey R, MIND. *Experiencing psychiatry: users' views of services*. Basingstoke: Macmillan Press in association with Mind, 1993.

Further reading

Flier N. *The shock of the fall*. London: Borough Press, 2014.

Gask L. *The other side of silence*. Chichester: Vie, 2015.

Greenberg J. *I never promised you a rose garden*. New York: St Martin's Press, 2009.

Jamison KR. *An unquiet mind: a memoir of moods and madness*. New York: Vintage, 1996.

Plath S. *The bell jar*. London: Faber & Faber, 2005.

Rogers A, Pilgrim D. *A sociology of mental health and illness*, 3rd edn. Maidenhead and New York: Open University Press, 2005.

Relevant web pages

HealthTalk. Mental health: ethnic minority experiences. http://www.healthtalk.org/peoples-experiences/mental-health/mental-health-ethnic-minority-experiences/getting-diagnosis

Here to Help. Dealing with a mental illness diagnosis. http://www.heretohelp.bc.ca/factsheet/dealing-with-a-mental-illness-diagnosis

MIND. Mental health problems: an introduction. http://www.mind.org.uk/information-support/types-of-mental-health-problems/

MindFreedom. Who we are. http://www.mindfreedom.org/who-we-are

Rethink Mental Illness. Diagnosis and treatment. http://www.rethink.org/diagnosis-treatment

Section 3

Caring for those experiencing mental health distress

The person who experiences anxiety

EIMEAR MUIR-COCHRANE, DEB O'KANE
AND KYLIE HARRISON

LEARNING OUTCOMES

- To be able to distinguish between tension, anxiety and anxiety disorders.
- To be able to describe the aetiology of anxiety.
- To be aware of the symptoms and relief behaviours of anxiety.
- To be aware of contemporary treatment options for anxiety disorders.
- To know how to develop self-management skills for your own anxiety in the nursing profession.

SUMMARY OF KEY POINTS

- Anxiety is a common condition and is very treatable.
- Symptoms of anxiety include physiological, psychological and behavioural elements.
- Individuals can learn to reduce their own anxiety through a number of strategies.

INTRODUCTION

Anxiety is one of the most common treatable mental disorders. Effective treatments include cognitive-behavioural therapy (CBT), relaxation techniques and occasionally medication. Anxiety disorders range from feelings of uneasiness most of the time to immobilizing bouts of terror. Here we shall discuss the most common anxiety disorders: generalized anxiety, phobias, obsessive–compulsive disorder and post-traumatic stress disorder. It is vital that nurses reflect upon their own experience of events that invoke anxiety and learn how to manage these feelings usefully, in order to be of use to those in their care.

KYLIE'S LIVED EXPERIENCE

As long as I can reality check that everything is OK, then I can get through my anxiety. Often something I did or said would cause me anxiety through constantly obsessing over it or concentrating on it, worrying about it and thinking I have done something wrong. Often I can't get it out of my head and it causes me to need to reality check with my colleagues, friends or family about the situation. As soon as I feel relief that the event was not as bad as I thought, I begin to relax.

Anxiety can be transferred interpersonally. For example, you arrive ready for an examination and find your fellow students extremely anxious. Interestingly, although you felt quite calm, now you find your anxiety levels increasing dramatically. Today, enough is known about anxiety to develop early intervention and prevention programmes. To that end, this chapter adopts a self-development approach so that nurses can develop their own anxiety management skills, and help service users facilitate their own anxiety management. Working with service users who are anxious is a craft of caring, one that can be taught and practised in powerful ways. Remember, if people in your care recognize your anxiety, this will elevate their own.

KYLIE'S LIVED EXPERIENCE

I have had anxiety practically my whole life. I suffered severe anxiety when I was 14 and nearly died. I suffered further anxiety to do with my bipolar disorder and the abuse of sexual assault that I endured during manic episodes where I would hitchhike and jump into strangers' cars. I have recently suffered anxiety because of a car accident.

THE NATURE OF ANXIETY

The experience of anxiety is a normal part of the human condition. Everyone experiences anxiety to varying degrees. Anxiety is usually a transitory response to threat or danger. Most people experience a knot in the stomach over mounting bills or just before a job interview at some point in their lives. Certain experiences and memories provoke anxious feelings in everyone, spurring us on, for example, to finish the essay that is due tomorrow. Nervousness in anticipation of an event is normal, yet the experience of anxiety can lead individuals to question the amount of choice and emotional control they have in their lives.[1] If people become preoccupied with unwarranted worries for longer than a short period of time or the feelings cause the person to avoid everyday activities, they may be described as suffering from an anxiety disorder.

KYLIE'S LIVED EXPERIENCE

Once I had a panic attack when I attempted to walk out on a wire 14 metres off the ground. People were on the ground encouraging me but I had to slow my breathing and basically get through my panic attack on my own. I managed to do this and I see this moment as a very empowering experience. Panic attacks on the ground didn't have the same power over me after that.

Think about what you have read of 'Kylie's lived experience' and consider the impact it is having on her life, both emotionally and physically. How would this anxiety impact on family and social life, such as relationships with a partner, a son or friends?

Anxiety disorders can have an underlying biological cause (e.g. thyrotoxicosis) and frequently run in families. Anxiety is also one of the most treatable mental disorders. It is characterized by a feeling of dread or uncomfortable anticipation, with physical, psychological, behavioural and cognitive features. Nurses are likely to come across people in their care exhibiting a variety of anxious responses to their situation. In general hospitals, many service users will be anxious about their medical condition, impending surgery or the experience of hospitalization itself. In mental health settings most people receiving care will demonstrate some anxiety, with a smaller number being so severely affected that they are unable to function normally in relation to work, family responsibilities and interpersonal relationships.[2] With such people, specific interventions, including medications, are usually required.

Prevalence of anxiety

Between 8 and 12 per cent of the population experience a pervasive level of anxiety that impedes their daily lives, with 2 to 4 per cent of the population believed to be experiencing an anxiety disorder at any one time. Baxter et al.[3] found a huge variation in prevalence across 44 countries (2.4 to 29.8 per cent), but this is thought to be due to methodological differences in the way studies were conducted. Anxiety is the most prevalent single psychiatric disorder of the modern era. People with anxiety disorders experience 7.4 per cent of all disability-adjusted life years (DALYS)[4] – that is, the times when they were unable to function fully as a result of a disorder. Loss of productivity from the paid and unpaid workforce has profound implications for the fiscal and social capital of a community and country.

The person who experiences anxiety

Research in the USA indicates that three of the five most productive things to invest in to reduce lost work productivity are migraine, anxiety and depression. Research in Australia has shown that women were more likely than men to have experienced anxiety disorders (12 per cent compared with 7 per cent).[5] Social anxiety disorder affects 13 per cent of the population; generalized anxiety disorder 3 to 5 per cent; and panic disorder 2 to 3 per cent of the population. Post-traumatic stress disorder (PTSD) occurs in reaction to a traumatic event, so incidence is dependent on the psychological impact of the trauma. Obsessive–compulsive disorders (OCD) affect 2 to 3 per cent of the population. Phobias and substance-induced anxiety disorders are less common. These Australian data are comparable with the incidence of anxiety globally. For more detail about the incidence of anxiety-related disorders, please see chapter 12.

KYLIE'S LIVED EXPERIENCE

My symptoms

I have had many panic attacks and these are more frequent when I am suffering severe anxiety due to early warning signs, and particularly moderate and severe signs of the mood swings of my bipolar disorder. I suffer from shortness of breath, rapid heart rate, feeling hot and feeling like I am going to die. I start catastrophizing small insignificant events where I think it's the end of the world.

How I cope with panic attacks

I take clozapine as my regular antipsychotic medication and I now take chlorpromazine for my anxiety as needed (PRN). I have a psychologist who takes me through CBT, and a psychiatrist who takes me through disassociation therapy. Recently when I had a car accident, I started having a panic attack. People who had witnessed the incident helped to slow my breathing and kept reassuring me that I was OK and safe. My breathing slowed down and very quickly my panic attack ended and I became calm. If no one had come to my aid, it might have been a different story.

My psychosis

Due to my first psychosis, I became convinced that I was in prison being interrogated. When I was being discharged from the city hospital to my country hospital, I began panicking that I was breaking out of prison and that my mum and myself would get into trouble. I had severe anxiety and was petrified. Once recovering at home with PTSD, I did not speak for 4 months. I stared at the white wall, not sleeping because I was anxious in the dark. I didn't want to sleep for fear of falling back into the blackness of the coma. I constantly thought about dying and would be in a catatonic state where I had constant anxiety and thought I was going to die.

My experiences when unwell

Another time I had been in a deep depression. My brother was having a big party for his 18th birthday. I forced myself to go there although I felt very uneasy. I had a massive panic attack in front of my brother's guests. My brother took me home but then I was too anxious to get out of the car.

Throughout my anxiety experiences there is lots of catastrophizing and 'what ifs' that come to my mind. During my manic episodes I would often end up alone with my psychosis, my thoughts and voices tormenting me as I waited in an emergency bed or seclusion room by myself. I would have panic attacks and plead for people to help me as I truly thought I was going to die. Often I would just need reassurance of my safety and to calm my breathing.

AETIOLOGY AND CONTEMPORARY TREATMENTS

Several theories purport to explain anxiety disorders. The biological view holds that anxiety disorders may have a genetic element, particularly OCD, and are associated with alterations in cerebral serotonin and dopamine. Learning theory supports the concept that anxiety is a conditioned response to specific environmental stimuli and has a biological survival value. The standard 'flight or fight' response, and the associated increase in heart rate and alertness, prepare the person for danger. Over time, how a person acts in response to a stressful event is often the result of learning. If too many stressors occur in a short period, the person may experience acute anxiety and exhibit maladaptive behaviour. An example of maladaptive behaviour may be an increase in alcohol consumption after the loss of a loved one through death or separation. Some theorists believe that social and cultural factors will determine how personality develops and how a person responds to stress. For example, a person with a negative self-image is more likely to have problems coping with an unexpected problem in their daily life than someone with a very positive self-image. CBT embraces a range of learning theories that view the way we feel, think and behave as inextricably linked. Thus a person with a poor self-image may have a disagreement with someone and conclude: 'That person does not like me', feeling anxious and sweaty and deciding to avoid social situations in future. CBT[6] is a relatively short-term treatment plan (6 to 8 weeks), which aims to teach a person how to relax, and how to recognize and cope with their anxious thoughts and feelings. CBT aims to help people become aware of their thinking style, replacing or reframing these with more positive ways of thinking, which can lead to an increase in self-confidence, problem-solving ability and reduced associated anxiety.

The assumption behind CBT is that dysfunctional behaviours are the presumed underlying problem.[7] CBT applies well-established learning principles to eliminate the unwanted behaviour and replace it with more constructive ways of thinking, feeling and acting. The major focus in CBT is to help the person examine and understand the world (their cognitions) and to experiment with new ways of responding (their behaviour). In this way the client can be helped to be future-focused and to behave more adaptively. Much has been learned in the past two decades about the treatment of anxiety disorders. Developments in neuro-imaging techniques have led to better understandings of the biology of OCD and the brain circuits that may be involved in the production of symptoms. The most effective treatment approach appears to be CBT,[7] consisting of exposure and response prevention and specific medications. Further information on CBT can be found in chapter 40.

Pharmacotherapy for anxiety is recommended, usually in combination with CBT, in the following circumstances:

- where there is comorbidity such as depression;
- when CBT is unsuccessful;
- when symptoms are severely disabling.

Benzodiazepines may be prescribed, but only for a couple of weeks as they are addictive. Refer to chapters 47 and 48 for further information on psychopharmacology.

Symptoms of anxiety

Use the material in Box 20.1 to explore the various dimensions of anxiety. In children, several other symptoms may

---

BOX 20.1: SYMPTOMS OF ANXIETY

Physiological
Shortness of breath
Dizziness
Choking sensation
Palpitations
Trembling
Sweating
Dry mouth
Decreased appetite
Nausea
Diarrhoea
Elevated blood pressure

Psychological
Affective (mood)
Fear
Terror
Dread
Sense of impending doom
Apprehension

Behavioural
Exaggerated startle reflex
Motor tension (foot tapping, restlessness)
Irritability
Nail biting
Altered sleep pattern (too much/too little/difficulty going to sleep or waking up)

---

be observable or reported by their parents, who may not recognize these behaviours as anxiety-related. Nurses are frequently in contact with adults and children who are either receiving care or who are family members of the sick person. Children often demonstrate anxiety symptoms as a response to the stress of what is happening around them. Symptoms include irritability, marked self-consciousness, excessive concern about the future and past events, a constant need for reassurance, unrealistic and excessive worry and distress on separation from parents. Children and adolescents with pervading anxiety require expert assistance through specialist intervention.

LIVED EXPERIENCE

'I would begin perspiring profusely, and once the nausea passed, I would be dripping with sweat. I felt faint, and I worried that I would pass out and vomit and aspirate and die.'[8]

Relief behaviours

Hildegard Peplau[9] identified a number of relief behaviours commonly occurring as an uncomfortable reaction to the experience of anxiety. These relief behaviours are often developed as a way for the person to reduce their anxiety by protecting themselves or escaping a threat. Such behaviours may include withdrawal, avoidance, risk taking, aggression and denial, to name but a few. They are often learned over time and are the physical manifestation of unconscious mechanisms to help the person cope with their feelings. Research has found that these relief behaviours, sometimes referred to as *safety behaviours*, prevent us from learning how to manage our emotions usefully and result in a reduced ability to learn new ways of coping. They can therefore become counterproductive rather than helpful in reducing a person's anxiety. Safety behaviour can be divided into preventative behaviour (behaviour that prevents future increased anxiety) or restorative behaviour (behaviour that delays the feelings associated with anxiety).[10] It is highly likely that these relief behaviours will manifest when people are under duress. Nurses need to be aware of their function to respond calmly and with compassion.

> ## REFLECTION
>
> Consider the behaviour of someone you may know who avoids a particular situation because it causes them anxiety. What are their observable behaviours? Do they appear to help in the short term? What about in the long term? In other words, do you think continuing with the behaviour will make the person more likely to engage in the anxiety-provoking situation in the future? What would you suggest to the person to help them find new ways of coping?

Health professionals should support the person with anxiety to consider constructive and functional ways of dealing with their anxiety, such as *realistic problem solving*. This refers to the individual exploring possibilities and potential solutions to their problem. For example, a person may learn to convert their anxiety into useful energies, such as exercising, to reduce their tension, thus resulting in the development of a useful coping skill.[3] See chapter 3 for more on how to engage and work with service users in their recovery journey.

The experience of anxiety

At a low to moderate level of anxiety, we experience a narrowing of perception. With increased muscle tension, our speech rate increases, with mixed feelings of challenge, confidence, optimism and fear. At a physiological level, anxiety activates the sympathetic nervous system, with an increase in blood pressure, heart rate and respiration, pupillary dilation and peripheral vascular constriction. Moderate levels of anxiety serve to improve performance, and even high levels of anxiety are often consistent with the demands of the situation. However, high anxiety can disable people to the extent that they find it difficult to perform everyday activities. It is normal to experience anxious thoughts, but it is the extent to which these thoughts render the individual able to carry out their normal activities that determines their disabling effect. Anxious thinking is often distorted thinking: anticipating that things are not going to turn out well and that you will not be able to cope (see 'Reflection'). This can increase anxiety and lead to depression if it persists. For example, if you see someone you know in the supermarket but they do not acknowledge you, an anxious thought may be, 'That person does not like me', but a more realistic thought may be, 'Oh, she has not seen me', or, 'She may be preoccupied'. CBT aims to help people understand their negative self-talk and to develop more positive and realistic patterns.

> ## REFLECTION
>
> Think about a time when you have felt extremely tense. Make some notes about your thoughts, feelings and sensations at the time. Then think about a time when you were extremely relaxed and make notes accordingly. What do you notice that is different?

ANXIETY DISORDERS

Anxiety can be disabling. The dysfunctional aspects are marked by three major components: behavioural avoidance, catastrophic cognition and autonomic hyperarousal.[11]

None of these components differentiates between normal and pathological anxiety. The only criterion is the level of interference in personal, occupational or social functioning. It is also incorrect to say that abnormal anxiety is just a matter of being too anxious at a time when others are not.

LIVED EXPERIENCE

'My hyper-alert nervous system produces palpitations, shaking, nausea, hot flushes, and feelings of impending doom. In this state, the feelings are so intense that I am utterly convinced that it will last forever; it is like being in hell.'[12]

Generalized anxiety

People suffering from a generalized anxiety disorder experience chronic exaggerated worry and tension that is more intense than the reality of the situation. A diagnosis is made if the person has spent at least 6 months worrying excessively about everyday problems.

CASE STUDY 1

An elderly woman is admitted to hospital after her daughter became increasingly concerned about her deteriorating physical activity and social isolation. The service user was bereaved 9 months ago. Since then she has become disinterested in activities she previously enjoyed. She says that she has gripping chest pains, that she often feels as if she cannot catch her breath and that her heart is pounding so loudly that other people can hear it. She is observed wringing her hands constantly and making multiple visits to the toilet.

Panic disorder

Panic disorder is characterized by a white-knuckled, heart-pounding terror that strikes with the force of a lightning bolt, without warning. Some people feel like they are going mad, being devoured by fear, or dying of a heart attack. Because they cannot predict these attacks, many experience persistent worry that another attack could overcome them at any time. Most panic attacks last only a few minutes but could last up to an hour in rare cases. With appropriate help, between 70 and 90 per cent of this group are helped within 6 to 8 weeks.[13]

Sometimes a combination of therapy and medication is the most effective approach to helping people manage their symptoms.

CASE STUDY 2

A 20-year-old student is admitted with a 6-month history of panic attacks. She has become unable to attend university regularly due to overwhelming and disabling feelings of choking, vomiting and difficulty in breathing. She failed her first year of study after she experienced 'blocks' during examinations. Since then her anxiety has worsened to the extent that she is extremely uncomfortable in public places, has difficulty swallowing and thinks she is losing her mind.

Phobias

Phobias are the most common form of anxiety disorder, affecting between 5 and 12 per cent of the adult population worldwide. Phobias occur in specific forms. A specific phobia is an unfounded fear of a particular object or situation, such as being afraid of dogs yet loving to ride horses, or avoiding flying on aeroplanes but being able to drive on busy highways. There is virtually an unlimited number of objects or situations that a person can be afraid of. Commonly people have phobias of snakes, spiders, open and/or closed spaces, dirt, blood, injuries and needles. Many of the physical symptoms that accompany panic attacks, such as sweating, racing heart and trembling, also occur with phobias.

Formal diagnosis is made when people experience extreme anxiety when exposed to a given situation or object and recognize that the fear is excessive or unreasonable, but are unable to change the feeling, with the result that normal routines, relationships and some activities are significantly disrupted. CBT has the best track record for helping people overcome phobic disorders. The goals of this therapy are to desensitize the person to feared situations and to teach the person to relax, and recognize and cope with anxious thoughts and feelings. Anti-anxiety agents or antidepressants may be also used to *minimize* symptoms in the short term. There are differing views about the combination of medication and CBT. Some would use a combination, but others advocate that the symptoms need to be treated, not suppressed by medications.

Obsessive–compulsive disorder

OCD affects almost 3 per cent of the world's population and is a major worldwide health problem. There are two main clinical aspects of this condition. An obsession is a persistent intrusive and unwanted thought or emotion that the person cannot ignore. A compulsion is a behavioural manifestation of the obsessive thought, resulting in the performance of a repetitious, uncontrollable, but seemingly purposeful act. For example, a person may have obsessive thoughts about cleanliness and the associated compulsive behaviour of repetitive hand washing, perhaps to the point of having excoriated skin on the hands from excessive washing. The compulsion becomes disabling when the person cannot carry on their normal daily activities due to the preoccupation with obsessive thoughts and compulsive acts.

CASE STUDY 3

A 35-year-old married man, Peter, who has two children aged under 5, is admitted with OCD. Two years ago he developed the obsessive thought that the chemical used to treat his roof was poisoning his children. He began washing his hands and clothes excessively to the extent that he was in danger of losing his job because of the time it took to repeatedly carry out these cleansing rituals. On admission, he was noted to be of low mood with an anxious presentation. He told the nurses that he was on the verge of going mad and was worried his wife would leave him. Peter was offered a mild antidepressant and a programme of CBT that involved exposing him gradually (systematic desensitization) to stimuli that triggered the anxiety, at the same time helping him to refrain voluntarily from hand washing.

Post-traumatic stress disorder

It has only recently been acknowledged that anyone who has experienced a traumatic event may experience *post-traumatic stress disorder* (PTSD), especially if the event was life-threatening. In the past, PTSD most commonly referred to victims of war who had experienced heavy combat. Common PTSD experiences include kidnapping, aeroplane crashes or other serious events, rape, natural disasters and war.[13] If the person is traumatized seriously by the event, the resulting psychological damage causes a significant impairment in the ability to maintain previous functioning, such as working or maintaining relationships. Symptoms can range from constantly reliving the event to a general emotional numbing. Persistent anxiety, exaggerated startle reflex, difficulty concentrating, nightmares and insomnia are common. Typically, people with PTSD avoid situations that remind them of the traumatic event, as this would trigger intense emotion and distress. For example, a person trapped on a road during a flood may deliberately avoid driving on that section of the road, even driving many kilometres to avoid the place of trauma. Research in this area has increased in recent decades, as individuals have developed PTSD after being involved in natural disasters, such as bushfires in Australia and floods in Europe. Depression is often experienced in PTSD, as is the use of prescription and non-prescription drugs and alcohol to dull emotional pain. Psychotherapy, CBT, medication such as antidepressants and anxiolytics, support from family and friends and relaxation techniques form the basis of treatment programmes with these service users.

NURSING STRATEGIES

Much of the work of nurses involved in the care of people with disabling levels of anxiety involves being with the service users, offering time for the service users to, as Barker[14] calls it, 'name their distress' (i.e. describe the meaning that they attribute to their experience). The loss of control service users feel due to their disabling anxiety is often an extremely important component of their distress, and therefore gaining control is a common goal. To that end the role of the nurse and structured programmes of therapy, such as CBT, involve creating a situation in which service users feels able to exercise choice about their future and how they think and feel about it. The relationship the nurse has with an anxious service user is extremely important if any interaction is to be meaningful. Carl Rogers[15] describes warmth, genuineness, empathy and unconditional positive regard as core dimensions of the nurse–service user relationship. If a nurse does not present a genuine demeanour or exhibits anxiety towards the service user, it is more difficult to be helpful. Nursing strategies can best be related to the level of anxiety a person is experiencing (mild, moderate or severe), rather than the diagnosis of the disorder

itself. See chapter 3 for more detail about the dynamics of the nurse–service user relationship and how nurses are required to exert emotional labour to alleviate distress for those for whom they care.

Box 20.2 provides advice on how to help someone who is experiencing a panic attack. The nurse should allow the service user to begin to ventilate and make sense of what is happening for them. From this starting point the nurse can begin to explore with the service users their coping resources by gentle inquiry into their perceptions of their social supports, economic circumstances, health status and cultural and spiritual beliefs. Particular attention also needs to be paid to the person's interpersonal resources, social skills and positive relationships with family and friends. Identifying a person's strengths and resources including positive motivation, drive, and personal and professional ambitions, value systems and self-esteem support a person on their road to recovery.[15] The way that people have coped with stress in the past is also a good indicator of their coping mechanisms. As has been previously discussed, people using relief behaviours over *time* generally

BOX 20.2: DOS AND DON'TS WHEN A PERSON IS HAVING A PANIC ATTACK

Do:

- Take some deep breaths yourself and remain calm and in an open posture.
- Encourage the person to take slow, deep breaths.
- Remind the person that the attack will pass and cannot harm them.
- Acknowledge their acute distress.
- Try and remove the person to a quiet place with some privacy.
- Stay with the person until they calm down.

Don't:

- Rush the person in any way.
- Express frustration.
- Tell the person that they are being ridiculous.
- Give orders.
- Tell the person to snap out of it or calm down (they can't).
- Encourage the person to face their fears (this is not the right time).

This checklist illustrates some simple strategies that might be employed if the person is in a state of high anxiety or panic. These emphasize the need for the nurse to remain with the service user and to present a calm demeanour. Working with anxious service users requires an initial assessment phase to gain a holistic picture of the person's situation and their potential and readiness to make positive changes. Gentle discussion of how the person makes sense of being in hospital or coming to community health services for assistance will provide useful contextual information. Asking 'What brought you here today?' can allow service users to begin to ventilate and make sense of what is happening.

find that they are not useful in adapting to expected or unexpected change and result in the person becoming cut off emotionally and often socially isolated. Effective coping skills include tackling the problem in a useful manner by seeking help or assistance. Searching for meaning, problem solving and evaluating how realistic personal expectations may be and readjusting some goals creates an opportunity to discover new strengths and resources. For each of the clinical cases cited, brainstorm nursing interventions that can assist these individuals while they undergo treatment.

ISSUES AND SOLUTIONS

It is not uncommon for people receiving treatment to develop a lowered mood, which prevents them from being able to undertake or complete aspects of their treatment, such as relaxation or CBT activities. The role of the nurse is vital in completing regular holistic assessments to recognize early warning signs of depression. If the person is depressed, treatment without medication is more difficult. Service users with OCD may initially find it very difficult to complete the suggested tasks and to practise relaxation methods they have been encouraged to use. They may complain of being too tense or develop further anxiety about the prospect of changing 'useless' behaviours, such as repetitive counting, checking and hand washing. If the person is admitted to hospital, it is not unusual for their compulsions to lessen dramatically in the first few days of hospitalization. However, once they have familiarized themselves with their new surroundings, the problematic behaviour re-emerges. Further, once the effects of treatment are manifest in a reduction in compulsive acts, different compulsions may emerge as the person's defence against anxiety. Understanding and support are vital to help service users deal with these eventualities.

LEARNING TO RELAX

It seems appropriate to approach the management of anxiety disorders by reflecting on our own anxiety and tension. If nurses can utilize basic self-relaxation techniques, it is likely that they will be more effective in helping people in their care to recognize tension and learn to relax and manage uncomfortable feelings and symptoms that interfere with their normal functioning.[1]

Relaxation training

Relaxation training involves the deliberate letting go of tension, whether *physical* (e.g. muscle tension or stomach cramps) or *psychological* (e.g. excessive worrying). When someone relaxes, the nerves in the muscles send messages to the brain that are distinctly different from those sent when anxious, tense or stressed. These different signals incur a general feeling of calmness in the person.[1]

Muscle relaxation has an effect on the nervous system, which manifests in physical and psychological ways, and is extremely useful in helping deal with feelings and experiences that disrupt everyday living. Relaxation training can help people who have been under stress for long periods, and who may have forgotten what it is like to relax and let go of their tension. Daily practice can help restore physical and psychological balance (equilibrium) and reduce tense feelings that include being jumpy, irritable and nervy, as well as physical manifestations of tension (such as stomach complaints, diarrhoea or constipation, and backache). Learning to relax can enable the control of uncomfortable levels of anxiety and tension in stressful situations.

To help people in your care learn to relax, it is vital that you examine and assess your own stress levels and anxiety (see Box 20.3). A small amount of stress is *necessary*, physically, to help us move about or exercise vigorously, and psychologically, to keep us alert to respond to a situation such as a job interview. However, a lot of the stress we feel is *unnecessary* and this can be determined by reflecting on the relationship between the level of tension and the activity involved, when the tension is not serving a useful function and where the level of tension remains high after the alerting situation has passed.

Progressive muscle relaxation

Like most things, relaxation training takes practice to be really effective. Encourage service users to persevere when they say, 'I'm too tense to relax', or, 'This is not for me, it's not doing me any good' (see Box 20.4). There are two core components to relaxation training: *recognizing tension* and *relaxing*. Progressive muscle relaxation training involves tensing and relaxing muscles in a repetitious fashion, moving from the hands to the shoulders, neck and head, and then down through the stomach, and back to the buttocks, legs and feet – tensing and relaxing alternately for about

BOX 20.3: ASSESS YOUR STRESS

Use the following questions to assess your own stress levels:

- Where do I feel tension? (e.g. in my chest, back, jaw, etc.)
- What are the characteristics of the tension? (e.g. fatigued muscles, soreness)
- What kinds of things lead to an increase in tension? (e.g. anger, loneliness, impatience, boredom)
- What external factors increase your tension? (e.g. loud noises, having to wait to be served, traffic, your relationships)

BOX 20.4: RELAXATION GUIDE

First of all, clear your mind of any worrying thoughts. Let your mind be calm. Practise breathing in, holding your breath for a few seconds and breathing out again. Try and control your breathing until it flows smoothly. Imagine that the tension in your body is flowing down and outwards, like water, every time you breathe out. Now it is time to relax your body, starting with your hands. For each muscle group, tense the muscles for 10 seconds, then let go and relax.

Hands: curl your hands into fists and relax.
Arms: tense the muscles in your arms and relax. Be aware of your biceps and the difference between tensing and relaxing them.
Shoulders and neck: shrug your shoulders up to your ears, hold for 10 seconds and relax.
Face: raise your eyebrows, hold and relax. Scrunch up your eyes, hold and relax.
Jaw: clench your teeth (not too tightly), hold and relax.
Chest: breathe in deeply, hold and relax.
Back: lean your head and back forward, hold and relax.
Bottom: tighten your buttock muscles, hold and relax.
Legs: push your feet firmly against the floor, hold and relax.
Lift your toes off the ground towards your shins, hold and relax.
Feet: gently curl your toes up, hold and relax.

Stay sitting quietly for a few minutes, enjoying the sensation of being relaxed. Take some slow deep breaths, and pay attention to your breathing. Try and practise every day; this will help your body to relearn how to relax and minimize tension building up.

10 seconds each time, usually over a 20- to 30-minute period. The best position is sitting comfortably with back straight, feet flat on the floor. It is generally advised not to lie down, as there is a good chance of falling asleep. So, sitting upright in a quiet warm place is a good option. Some people find other ways to achieve the same relaxation effect, through exercise, meditation, yoga or tai chi. All these provide an opportunity for self-reflection and letting go of the unnecessary stress we all carry, to varying degrees. If as nurses we can master the art of relaxation, we can model a relaxed and open demeanour to those around us. This, in turn, will increase the opportunity to build rapport and

trust with our service users, to explore how they view their concerns in a practical way and to reduce the amount of unnecessary and uncomfortable anxiety in daily life.

Being relaxed and having an open and compassionate demeanour are skills that have to be learned over time, and may not come easily, particularly for nurses who are naturally anxious. Witnessing relief behaviours such as acting out can be very stressful, and clinical supervision and opportunities to debrief, beyond the immediacy of the event, are important support strategies in the workplace.

Often, individuals experience more stress some time after experiencing some form of critical incident. Expressing personal judgement about a service user's problems is another potential sign that a nurse is under stress and could benefit from clinical supervision or mentoring. It is also common for health care staff, particularly nurses, to avoid people who are highly anxious. Recognizing the potential for such avoidance, and seeking the support of more experienced staff in working through such feelings, can facilitate and enhance personal and professional growth.

CONCLUSION

Gaining a personal and professional awareness of stress and anxiety is paramount when caring for people with anxiety disorders. Today, various interventions are helpful in the management of disabling anxiety. Being with anxious service users requires compassion and self-awareness, and understanding of the effect anxiety has on people's lives. By using different strategies, in a variety of health care settings, nurses can help people take control of their problems related to the experience of anxiety and manage them successfully.

References

1. Brown P. Anxiety, anxiety disorders and stress related illness. In Evans J, Brown P (eds). *Videbeck's mental health nursing*. Philadelphia, PA: Lippincott Williams & Wilkins, 2012: 230–1.
2. Dusek JA, Hibberd PL, Buczynski B, Chang BH, Dusek KC, Johnston JM, Wohlhueter AL, Benson H, Zusman RM. Stress management versus lifestyle modification on systolic hypertension and medication elimination: a randomized trial. *Journal of Alternative and Complementary Medicine* 2008; **14**(2): 129–38.
3. Baxter AJ, Scott KM, Vos T, Whiteford HA. Global prevalence of anxiety disorders: a systematic review and meta-regression. *Psychological Medicine* 2013; **43**(5): 897–910.
4. Whiteford HA, Degenhardt L, Rheim J, Baxter A, Ferrarie A, Erskine H, Charlson FJ, Norman RE, Flaxman AD, Johns N, Burstein R, Murray CJL, Vos T. Global burden of disease attributable to mental and substance use disorders: findings from the Global Burden of Disease Study 2010. *The Lancet* 2013; **382**: 1575–86.
5. Mental Illness Fellowship of Australia. Understanding anxiety. 2013. Available from: http://www.mifa.org.au/images/Documents/Wellways/164950%20Understanding%20Anxiety.pdf [Accessed 2nd July 2016].
6. Beyond Blue. Understanding anxiety. 2014. Available from: https://www.bspg.com.au/dam/bsg/product?client=BEYONDBLUE&prodid=BL/0384&type=file [Accessed 2nd July 2016].
7. Wells A. *Cognitive therapy: a practice manual and conceptual guide*. Chichester: John Wiley & Sons, 1997.
8. Stossel S. Surviving anxiety. *The Atlantic* 2014; Jan./Feb. Available from: http://www.theatlantic.com/magazine/archive/2014/01/surviving_anxiety/355741/2/ [Accessed 2nd July 2016].
9. Peplau HE. *Interpersonal relations in nursing*. New York: Putnam, 1952.
10. Helbig-Lang S, Petermann F. Tolerate or eliminate? A systematic review on the effects of safety behavior across anxiety disorders. *Clinical Psychology: Science and Practice* 2010; **17**: 218–33.
11. Slade M. *Personal recovery and mental illness: a guide for mental health professionals*. Cambridge: Cambridge University Press, 2009.
12. Time to Change. Anxiety disorder and what led me to write a book about mental health. 2014. Available from: http://www.time-to-change.org.uk/blog/anxiety-disorder-and-what-led-me-write-book-about-mental-health [Accessed 2nd July 2016].
13. Muir-Cochrane E, Barkway P, O'Kane D. *Mosby's pocket book of mental health*, 2nd edn. Chatswood: Elsevier Australia, 2014.
14. Barker P. *The philosophy and practice of psychiatric nursing*. London: Churchill Livingstone, 1999.
15. Rogers C. *Client-centred therapy*. Boston: Houghton and Mifflin, 1965.

Further reading

Burns D. *The feeling good handbook*. New York: First Plume Printing, 2001.
Forsyth J, Eifert G. *The mindfulness and acceptance workbook for anxiety: a guide to breaking free from anxiety, phobias, and worry using acceptance and commitment therapy*. Oakland, CA: New Harbinger, 2007.
Kennard J. *Overcoming worry and anxiety*. London: Sheldon Press, 2014.

Relevant web pages

Anxiety UK. https://www.anxietyuk.org.uk
This is a UK-based charity offering support to individuals and their families regarding all aspects of anxiety.
MIND. http://www.mind.org.uk
Anxiety. Moodjuice self-help guide. http://www.moodjuice.scot.nhs.uk/anxiety.asp
This website provides information and education about anxiety and how to manage it.

The person who experiences depression

IAN BEECH

LEARNING OUTCOMES

- To understand the nature of depression as experienced by the individual.
- To be able to identify and evaluate various theoretical explanations of the aetiology of depression.
- To be able to apply recovery-based approaches to helping a person who experiences depression.
- To understand various care and treatment approaches for depression.

SUMMARY OF KEY POINTS

- Depression is qualitatively different from merely feeling down.
- Nurses should adopt a pragmatic approach to helping those who are suffering.
- The over-arching concern when helping a person is not to cure the person's depression; it is to assist the person to find a way forward that enables meaningful everyday living.

INTRODUCTION

Until one has experienced a debilitating severe depression it is hard to understand the feelings of those who have it. Severe depression borders on being beyond description: it is not just feeling much lower than usual. It is quite a different state, a state that bears only a tangential resemblance to normal emotion. It deserves some new and special word of its own, a word that would somehow encapsulate both the pain and the conviction that no remedy will ever come.[1] (p.1)

The scientist and broadcaster Lewis Wolpert gives us one of the most important things to bear in mind when discussing depression: it is not merely feeling down or fed up, it is something very different from that. Wolpert[1] describes it as

being worse than anything else that he has ever experienced, including the death, from cancer, of his wife. This chapter provides some insights into the experience of depression for someone who suffers from it. The nurse, at least when working in an inpatient setting, in contrast to many mental health professionals, is the person who spends time with the person who suffers from depression rather than seeing the person on an organized sessional basis.

When student nurses begin their careers in mental health, there are a number of fears that it seems are common:

- 'What if something that I do or say makes things worse?'
- 'What if I give someone the idea of harming him- or herself?'
- 'What if I can't think of anything to say?'

When working with people who experience depression, all of these questions may arise, and nurses may deal with them in a number of ways. Some may retreat into a mind-set that believes that anything said or done by the nurse is incidental to a requirement to correct the person's brain chemistry by the administration of medication. Therefore all that is required is to manage risk and wait for the medication to work. Others may have undergone further training in a particular school of psychotherapy and may act as a 'nurse therapist' in a structured way. Most, however, will be somewhere in the middle, both administering medication and trying to engage with the person.

This chapter will focus on the craft of nursing people who experience depression. What follows will be considered from a broadly bio-psychosocial approach to providing nursing care. Therefore there will not be adherence to any single school of psychological thought.

WHAT IS MEANT BY THE TERM 'DEPRESSION'?

Most people understand what it is like to feel down or fed up. This can sometimes lead to responses such as the example given by the comedian Ruby Wax: 'a couple of phone calls telling me to perk up'. But, as she retorts: 'Perk up … Because I didn't think of that.'[2]

As the National Health Service information portal NHS Choices[3] tells us, depression is not simply a transient period of feeling down in the dumps or unhappy; it is something qualitatively and experientially different from that. A person experiencing depression will have some or all of these experiences for a prolonged period of time:[4]

- low mood that is largely unreactive to events occurring around the person;
- a mood that tends to be lowest when waking and may improve slightly as the day progresses but returns to being low the next day;
- tearfulness;
- social withdrawal;
- loss of energy;
- lack of ability to concentrate;
- loss of interest in relationships and sex;
- altered dietary pattern which might mean weight loss due to loss of appetite or weight gain due to comfort eating;
- feelings of guilt, worthlessness and self-loathing;
- recurring thoughts about death and dying, in some cases accompanied by a plan of how to commit suicide.

One of the problems for nurses in being with people suffering from depression is that the person often feels guilt, shame, hopelessness and worthlessness; the person may not be someone with whom it is stimulating to spend time. Compared with the person who is demonstrating manic behaviour or may be hearing voices, the person experiencing depression may even be boring and difficult to engage. The danger is that nurses may get distracted. The Mental Health Foundation gives figures of around 8 to 12 per cent of the population suffering from depression in any one year.[5] Given that suicide risk is significantly raised in those people who experience depression,[6] it is an important part of the psychiatric and mental health nurse's repertoire of skills to be able and willing to spend time in the company of people experiencing depression without becoming

MARTIN'S STORY

I worked as a residential social worker in the 1990s. To begin with I enjoyed my job and I liked working with the clients. After a while the organization changed and I was having to do things in my work that meant more writing and computer work.

I'm dyslexic and I've always struggled with that. The changes at work were really stressful for me. I kept falling behind with reports and other paperwork. My manager didn't seem to understand how difficult I found it and kept pushing and pushing.

I started to lose sleep. I was awake for hours every night thinking about what a failure I was. My wife got sick of me and we argued a lot. Thankfully she stuck by me and kept having a go at me to see my GP. She gave me antidepressants and signed me off on the sick.

I felt so bloody useless and I realized that everybody else – my wife, my kids, work – would all be better off with me gone.

I decided to kill myself and, funnily enough, once I'd decided that, I felt calmer and less anxious. I took an overdose of antidepressants but my wife found me and called an ambulance. They got me to A&E and from there I ended up in an acute mental health unit for about 3 months.

I haven't worked since. I finished work and went on benefits and I was in the doldrums for about 10 years.

distracted or bored. (See chapter 16 to learn more on assessing the risk of suicide and self-harm.)

REFLECTION

Think about your own experiences of being in the company of people suffering from depression. What feelings did you have? How easy was it to maintain focus on the person in the face of other distractions?

REASONS WHY A PERSON MIGHT EXPERIENCE DEPRESSION

At one time[7] nurses were taught a fairly simple explanation of how depression might come about:

- It could have a readily identifiable life event cause such as a bereavement, divorce or redundancy. This would be termed reactive or neurotic depression and was generally seen as the lesser of the two types.
- Alternatively, it could have no readily identifiable cause and so was deemed to emerge from within the person. This would be termed endogenous or psychotic depression and was seen as the more serious type of depression.

There are two obvious problems with such a classification. First, people's experiences do not conform to such narrow stereotypes. Some people might experience long-term, even life-threatening depression after a seemingly mundane life event, while others might experience a short-term depressive episode with no identifiable precursor. Second, both of these types of depression create potential problems for people diagnosed with depression. Someone seen as having a reactive depression could be seen, or see him-/herself, as weak, since others exposed to similar life events might overcome them without experiencing depression. Similarly, a person seen as having an endogenous depression can be seen, or see him-/herself, as having some fundamental flaw which predisposes the person to depression. In both cases such views encourage feelings of helplessness and self-blame.

Depression is classified according to two systems in modern mental health care. The American Psychiatric Association employs the *Diagnostic and statistical manual of mental disorders* (DSM), currently in its 5th edition (DSM-5).[8] As part of an integrated classification of health conditions, the World Health Organization (WHO) employs the *International classification of diseases and related health problems*, now in its 10th edition (ICD-10).[9] (See chapter 12 for further information on classification.)

There are now a number of explanations for why a person might experience depression.

Neurochemical explanation

This theory posits that a person experiences depression when there is an imbalance in the brain in certain chemicals that are responsible for neurotransmission. The imbalance may occur because a person is genetically predisposed to such imbalance, or s/he is subjected to such levels of stress that such an imbalance occurs, or in a metaphorical lottery ticket of depression a combination of genes and events is such that they combine to cause a chemical imbalance.

Scientists are not in agreement as to whether the same chemicals are implicated in all cases of depression. The usual suspects are serotonin and norepinephrine. Antidepressant therapy is predicated on the theory that the

MARTIN'S STORY

I had loads of different antidepressants over the years.

The worst one, I think, was amitriptyline.

It didn't half make me drowsy. I used to drop off in the middle of the day. Then one day I couldn't pee. I ended up in hospital and they put a catheter in. It seems my prostate had got bigger as I got older and this combined somehow with the drug to stop me from peeing.

Benign prostatic hyperplasia (BPH) is a common condition in men over the age of 50. In such cases care must be taken in giving amitriptyline as it has a common side effect of making the passing of urine difficult.

drug redresses the imbalance and so restores the brain of the individual to non-depressed function. Antidepressant drugs are inconsistent in their effectiveness. Different people respond to different antidepressants in different ways and some experience unpleasant side effects (see, for example, Martin's experience of amitriptyline[10]). Consequently, there is an element of trial and error in discovering the combination of drugs that might be effective for each individual. Some people find that, even after prolonged antidepressant therapy, they continue to experience depression. Chapter 47 contains more information on the use of drugs in the treatment of various mental health conditions.

The biological approach of relying on medication is somewhat problematic. It may be that different people have different chemical imbalances occurring in their brains that give rise to similar experiences and behaviour which society knows as depression. Equally it may be that the drugs in existence have the accuracy of a blunderbuss rather than a sniper rifle and are simply not refined enough to pinpoint the exact biochemical nature of people's depression.

Psychosocial explanations

There are a number of psychological and social explanations for depression. These include the psychodynamic theory[11] based on the principle that significant loss in childhood results in a distorted self-image based on a need for acceptance and approval by others. Interpersonal theory[12] suggests that depression is the result of negative interpersonal relationships and lack of positive reinforcement. Cognitive[13] explanations put forward the theory that depression is caused by negative thinking about self and the world. The social model considers social vulnerability to be the key to depression.[14]

NURSING APPROACHES

Crafting recovery

The nursing approach to working with a person who experiences depression is neither medicine nor psychotherapy. In working with people, nurses are in a position to promote recovery.

The notion of recovery from mental health problems is not new, but it is an idea that requires some understanding because the word 'recovery' can mean different things to different people. During historical research into Cardiff City Mental Hospital admissions in the early years of the twentieth century, it became apparent that people were often described as having 'recovered' from their condition and discharged home.[15] At the time this meant that the person was cured. They had recovered from their condition in the same way that we now consider a person to have recovered from a cold or influenza: they were returned to a state of health that they had prior to the condition. If the person was then readmitted at a later date, this was deemed to be a different illness.

When we talk of recovery today, we mean forward movement rather than returning back to some pre-condition state:[16] but forward movement from what starting point? Further information on recovery can be found in chapter 35.

Nora Jacobson[17] discusses a number of different ways in which people make sense of what is happening in their lives when they are described as having a mental illness. These include biological explanations, social explanations and environmental explanations. The point that Jacobson makes, which is important for nurses, is that if a person believes that what s/he is experiencing is the result of chemical imbalance in the brain it will lead to certain behaviour that is consistent with such a belief: taking medication willingly. If, however, the person believes firmly that what is happening is based in relationships or social circumstances, s/he may be less inclined to comply with a biomedical approach in the face of, for example, unpleasant side effects. The nurse needs to engage with the person who experiences depression at a mutually agreed start point, rather than trying to force the person into a belief system to which the person cannot relate.

The Tidal Model[18] is one approach that provides a framework in which a person's own story can be told by focusing on what is important for the person here and now. But how might the nurse work with a person who is uncommunicative, low in mood and withdrawn? Furthermore, if a person is intent on harming him-/herself, how might the nurse address the risk while being in a contrary position to that person? After all, the nurse wishes to keep the person alive while the person may wish to die.

Returning to some of the fears that students sometimes experience of not wishing to make things worse and not wishing to put the idea of suicide into someone's mind,

consider what we already know about depression. As we have seen, people experiencing depression lack hope, feel worthless and often ruminate on death.

Consider for a moment a person who is in an adult surgical ward awaiting an operation. How would that person feel if nurses avoid discussing the operation in spite of the fact that the person knows that an operation is imminent and the nurses know what the operation will be? In all likelihood that person would feel apprehensive, frightened and not a little confused.

Now consider a person experiencing depression. S/he knows that s/he feels depressed and suicidal. S/he knows that nurses know that s/he feels depressed and suicidal but no one will discuss it.

People experiencing depression can be thought of as existing on a continuum where ideas of suicide exist (see Figure 21.1).

> ### REFLECTION
>
> Consider your own thoughts on being with a person who wishes to die. What are your worries about the situation? What can you say to help?

It is important for nurses to find out where a person might be on the continuum. The only way to achieve this is to talk to people, to listen to them and to give them the permission to talk about things that they may feel they should not disclose. If we approach people in a guarded way and give them the impression that certain things are not to be

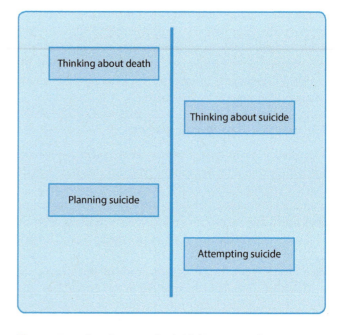

Figure 21.1 Continuum of suicidal intent and actions.

discussed, they will assume that we disapprove and will hide certain things from us.

The fear that we might put the idea of suicide into the mind of a person experiencing depression is, if we think about it, somewhat arrogant on the part of the nurse. How powerful do we think we are if we think we can convince someone to harm him-/herself by something we say? If we are indeed that powerful, why don't we simply tell people to get better?

The start of any piece of craft is the raw material: the block of wood or stone that becomes the figure, the oil paint and canvas that become the portrait. The craft of psychiatric and mental health nursing is no different. The raw material of working with people is the relationship. We need to approach people in such a way that they begin to feel that they can trust us. Chapter 3 addresses in more detail the concept of therapeutic relationships.

When we think about people we trust in our lives, one thing is fairly certain: those people did not make us trust them. Rather we trust people because they do not give us cause not to trust them. It is virtually impossible to make another person trust you, but very easy to give another person cause to not trust you. As nurses we therefore have to ensure that we do not give people cause to fail to trust us. There are a number of ways that we can inadvertently do this. These include giving people the impression that our time is too precious to be spent in their company, rushing them into complying with our agenda instead of paying attention to theirs, and letting them down by not following through on promises.

Egan[19] has described certain interpersonal skills that are helpful to mental health nurses in showing people attention and respect. He uses the mnemonic SOLER to assist in remembering it:

- S – Sitting squarely to the person
- O – Open posture with arms and legs uncrossed
- L – Leaning slightly forward
- E – Eye contact
- R – Relaxed posture

SOLER has been taught to many student nurses throughout their pre-registration nurse training for nearly 40 years since it was first introduced in the mid-1970s. It has more recently been criticized as somewhat stilted and formulaic, and as not taking into account human approaches such as touch. Theodore Stickley[20] proposes a new mnemonic, SURETY, as providing, perhaps, a better way of being with people in an effective helping way:

- S – Sit at an angle
- U – Uncross arms and legs
- R – Relax
- E – Eye contact
- T – Touch
- Y – Your intuition

For Stickley this approach is an improvement on Egan's, because it both allows for touch to be used as a means of providing comfort to the person and is less formulaic because it encourages nurses to use their intuition.

Coupled with learning to spend time with people in a way that portrays interest and concern, it is important to work at the person's own speed rather than trying to force the pace. Burnard[21] recommends the use of what he describes as phatic communication as a means of engaging with people, rather than launching straight into questions about symptoms. Phatic communication may be seen as small talk about the weather, sport, TV or anything that might help to break the ice. What this has the potential to achieve is that it demonstrates to the person who has low self-esteem and feels worthless that you are happy to spend time with them and that you value the person's company.

People experiencing depression can sometimes develop a hostile way of relating to others as a way of maintaining their own ideas of worthlessness, i.e. 'People have no time for me because I'm worthless so I won't have time for other people.' This can lead to nurses changing from what Watkins describes as being in a 'rescuer role' to a 'persecutor role'.[22] Rescuers see people as needing rescuing and expect those people to be grateful. Some nurses have a tendency to want to rescue people from their distress and to fix their problems. If the problem is not immediately fixable, the rescuer can become frustrated, and the rescuer turns into the persecutor, blaming the person for not wanting or trying to be fixed. Nurses can break this cycle by adopting a more neutral approach that does not take offence at the person failing to engage or being slow at getting mended.

> ### REFLECTION
>
> Consider your own expectations when you became a nurse. Did you want to help people? If so, did you enjoy it when people showed their gratitude? What about your feelings towards people who were less demonstrative of their gratitude?

When talking about her own experience of depression, Annie Altschul, the renowned nurse academic, once described how she needed the seemingly contradictory situation both of being able to have a nurse available to help her feel safe while also leaving her alone.[23] In other words, she wanted nurses to show her that they were comfortable in her presence without having an agenda of wishing to 'fix' her.

There is, of course, one situation where the relationship can wait. In order to form a relationship with a person, that person has to be safe and alive. Therefore in emergency situations the most important thing is to keep the person alive.

Barker and Buchanan-Barker term this psychiatric rescue.[18] To use their Tidal metaphor, you would not watch a person drown while sitting on the shore, stroking your chin and asking, 'How are you feeling?' You would throw a rope or a lifebuoy and pull the person out of the water and, after drying him/her off, then perhaps ask how s/he got in the water in the first place.

Once the person has been 'rescued', National Institute for Health and Care Excellence (NICE) guidelines recommend that people are involved in their own care decisions as much as possible.[24] Specialist therapeutic approaches recommended in the guidance include cognitive behavioural therapy (CBT) (see chapter 40), medication and sometimes electroconvulsive therapy (ECT). All of these require comprehensive assessment to assist in both the diagnosis of depression and identification of the nature and extent of the problems of living that the person experiences.

One tool that is available to nurses is the Beck Depression Inventory (BDI), which is a self-rating scale that looks at 21 areas of the person's life and gives each of these a score between 0 and 3. While the scores can be added and the total used as a diagnostic tool (0–13: minimal depression; 14–19: mild depression; 20–28: moderate depression; and 29–63: severe depression), a more comprehensive use is to focus on particular areas of the person's life that s/he identifies as important. It can be a useful adjunct for nurses to enable the person to tell his/her story as fully as possible.

In order to help the person to feel involved in his/her own care it is a useful approach to employ a Wellness Recovery Action Plan (WRAP).[25] This consists of three components: a daily maintenance plan, a crisis plan and a post-crisis plan. The daily maintenance plan helps the person to develop what works for him/her to maintain wellness on a daily basis. The crisis plan is an advanced plan whereby the person identifies what s/he would want to happen if things become critical. The post-crisis plan encourages the person to identify what has been learned from the crisis and what needs to change. More information on crisis assessment and resolution can be found in chapter 46.

A further helpful approach that nurses should incorporate into practice is to avoid concentrating solely on people's weaknesses. People who experience depression are only too aware of their weaknesses, but it is often forgotten how well they are managing in their lives. A person who is thinking constantly about suicide might be expected to carry out an attempt, and yet many people do not. It is helpful to know not just what may be making the person feel so down, but also why it is that the person is still alive; what is it that prevents the person from killing him-/herself? If we are able to discuss this with people, we can find some solid foundations to help craft recovery.

NICE guidelines recommend that a useful approach to helping people who experience depression is to help them to re-establish a good sleep pattern. Nurses can help this in a number of ways. Discussion of sleep hygiene measures with a person while putting together a daily maintenance plan may well be a useful intervention. Gega and Norman[26] describe sleep hygiene as having four components: behaviour, environment, diet and exercise. Suggestions that could be offered to someone include: altering his/her behaviour to try to establish a regular bedtime pattern; getting into a pre-bed routine by having a relaxing bath and limiting stimulation; not lying in bed trying to go to sleep, but getting up; having a cool, dark unstimulating bedroom; avoiding alcohol 3–4 hours prior to bedtime; avoiding caffeine in the late afternoon and evening; and trying to take exercise each day, if only going for a walk. People may have discovered other tips and techniques that they find work for them.

An important point to remember for nurses is that nothing works for everyone, but something works for each person. You should not become downhearted if you suggest something that you consider to be useful to someone and that person refuses to use it.

MARTIN'S STORY

I have to say that when I started to use a WRAP things improved loads. It helped me to sort out in my own mind the things that I used to do that were unhelpful and then I could try to make changes.

I think the biggest help for me is that instead of living in the past and worrying about how my job ended up, I've moved on now and don't think about it. I do all sorts of things now connected to teaching student nurses and I also interview them before they start their training.

One of the best things I've found to help me de-stress is I got an old JCB and I've slowly done it up over the last couple of years. I'm using it to landscape the land near my house. It's great. I just start it up and start digging and I can lose myself for a couple of hours.

REFLECTION

Consider what you think are sensible ways of helping you get a good night's sleep. How would you feel if you were to suggest these to someone else and that person was to reject them?

Medication

Nurses, with the exception of nurse prescribers, are not involved in deciding what medication a person should receive. Nevertheless, the majority of nurses are involved in the administration and monitoring of medication. Chapter 48 addresses issues of medication management. It is therefore incumbent on nurses to have an understanding of the medication employed in helping people who experience depression.

The drugs used in depression can be thought of in terms of groupings:

- drugs that inhibit the reuptake of serotonin into nerve cells;
- drugs that inhibit the reuptake of serotonin and norepinephrine into cells;
- tricyclic antidepressants;
- monoamine oxidase inhibitors (MAOIs);
- others.

All drugs are chemicals that have effects on the body. When the effect is desirable, we call it the therapeutic effect. When it is undesirable, we call it a side effect. In some cases, the side effect can become the therapeutic effect and vice versa depending on circumstances. For example, as we have seen in the case of Martin, the tricyclic antidepressant amitriptyline sometimes has a side effect of causing retention of urine, yet it is sometimes given to 'treat' difficulty in controlling the bladder at night (nocturnal enuresis). One of the balancing acts to be achieved with antidepressant medication is that of preparing people for the side effects, which can appear before the therapeutic effect. Each of the above groups has particular side effects. Comprehensive information on all of the drugs available cannot be provided here, so only pointers for good practice are suggested. As such, it is important for nurses to be up to date with the medication that is in common usage in terms of:

- recommended dosages;
- likely side effects;
- how long someone might need to take the drug before he or she can expect to experience any therapeutic effect;
- any special precautions or contraindications (when the medication might be inappropriate or dangerous);
- the answers to any common questions that someone prescribed the medication might ask.

More information about psychopharmacology can be found in chapter 47. However, it is important to remain up to date when looking at medication. New drugs come onto the market, while old ones fall out of favour or are removed from common usage. New precautions and instructions often appear after a drug has been in use for a while.

So, often, online resources are the most helpful. A good point of reference for both nurses and people prescribed antidepressant medication is the Norfolk and Suffolk NHS Foundation Trust Choice and Medication website (see 'Relevant web pages' below). This provides information about drugs in common usage in mental health, in readily accessible language.

If nurses are not transparent and honest with people about what to expect from medication, people will become suspicious of nurses' intentions. A person is far more likely to accept a side effect of a medication if s/he has been prepared for it than if it comes out of the blue.

Electroconvulsive therapy

Electroconvulsive therapy (ECT), in spite of the controversy that has surrounded it for a number of years,[27] remains a treatment for depression under NICE guidelines.[28] It is not the remit of this chapter to discuss the ethics of ECT. There are a number of constraints on its use and it is largely used as a treatment of last resort when other approaches have been deemed to be unsuccessful, or as a means of providing life-saving treatment. For nurses there are two aspects to the role of working with the person who is undergoing ECT. The first is that ECT is administered under general anaesthesia. This means that nurses need to be competent in the care of a person who is preparing for general anaesthesia and for the unconscious person directly after treatment. The second aspect is to help a person who has received ECT with the side effects that such treatment might bring about, such as headaches and memory loss, and to monitor the person's mood to evaluate whether the treatment might have had any effect.

Prior to treatment nurses should be aware of the required fasting times that local policy has in place for people undergoing general anaesthesia. The person should be encouraged to use the toilet prior to treatment and a checklist should be completed to ensure that dentures, prostheses, jewellery and nail varnish are removed. This is to ensure that nothing can injure the person while undergoing a seizure or, in the case of nail varnish, impede an accurate assessment of oxygenation in the unconscious person.[24]

Immediately after treatment the person will be unconscious for a short period of time. The nurse needs to ensure that the person's airway is clear and that oxygen, suction and monitoring equipment are in working order and the nurse knows how to use them. While unconscious, the person should not be left alone, and regular observations and recording of vital signs are necessary until s/he regains consciousness.

Once the person regains consciousness, s/he may feel nauseous, so a receptacle should be provided and possibly anti-emetic medication may be prescribed. As time progresses the person may feel soreness in the limbs and/or a headache. S/he should be encouraged to rest and possibly given mild analgesia.

Following ECT the person may experience short-term memory loss. The nurse should ensure that the person is not left to deal with this experience alone, as it can be frightening and disorientating. Further information can be found on the nursing role in ECT in chapter 62 of this book.

CONCLUSION

In summary, depression is something that should be taken very seriously by nurses. It is not merely a state of being 'down in the dumps'. There are significant risks associated with depression for the person who experiences it. People do die as a result of the suicidal ideation associated with depression. Notwithstanding this, nurses should neither adopt the attitude that there is nothing that can be done save to administer antidepressant medication, nor believe that they are helpless due to lack of expertise in psychotherapy.

Many years ago Hildegard Peplau described the role of the nurse as based on what she termed 'professional closeness'.[29] This is characterized as being different from physical closeness, which is simply doing physical things to people's bodies; from interpersonal intimacy, which is what happens between people who are intimate with one another; and from pseudo-closeness, which is an affected air of caring while remaining disinterested. Nursing as professional closeness, for Peplau, contained elements of personal closeness and of interpersonal intimacy, but there was no place for pseudo-closeness. This chapter has considered some of the skills that may go some way to crafting a helpful approach when caring for a person who experiences depression.

References

1. Wolpert L. *Malignant sadness: the anatomy of depression*. London: Faber & Faber, 2001.
2. Wax R. What's so funny about mental illness? 2012. Available from: http://www.ted.com/talks/ruby_wax_what_s_so_funny_about_mental_illness#t-96285 [Accessed 22nd June 2016].
3. NHS Choices. Clinical depression. 2012. Available from: http://www.nhs.uk/conditions/depression/Pages/Introduction.aspx [Accessed 22nd June 2016].
4. Royal College of Psychiatrists. Sample chapter from *Depression. The NICE Guideline on the Treatment and Management of Depression in Adults* (updated edition). London: Royal College of Psychiatrists, 2010. Available from: http://www.rcpsych.ac.uk/files/samplechapter/nicedepressionupedsc.pdf [Accessed 22nd June 2016].
5. Mental Health Foundation. The fundamental facts: the latest facts and figures on mental health. 2007. Available from: https://www.mentalhealth.org.uk/publications/fundamental-facts-about-mental-health-2015 [Accessed 25th July 2016].
6. Mental Health Foundation. Suicide and self-harm. 2000. Available from: http://www.mentalhealth.org.uk/publications/suicide-and-self-harm [Accessed 25th July 2016].
7. Ackner B. *Handbook for psychiatric nurses*, 9th edn. London: Baillière Tindall/Cassell, 1964.
8. American Psychiatric Association. *Diagnostic and statistical manual 5th edition*. Arlington, VA: American Psychiatric Association, 2013.
9. WHO (World Health Organization). *The international statistical classification of diseases and health related problems, ICD-10*. Geneva: WHO, 1994.
10. Howard R. Amitriptyline in BPH: increased risk of PVR and urinary retention. *Prescriber* 2008; 5 February: 42–5.
11. Hughes P, Riordan D. *Dynamic psychotherapy explained*. Oxford: Radcliffe Publishing, 2006.
12. Weissman M, Markowitz J, Klerman G. *Comprehensive guide to interpersonal psychotherapy*. New York: Basic Books, 2000.
13. Wills F, Sanders D. *Cognitive behavioural therapy: foundations for practice*. London: Sage, 2013.
14. Blazer D. *The age of melancholy: major depression and its social origins*. New York: Routledge, Taylor & Francis, 2005.
15. Beech I. The universal khaki: the impact of the Asylum War Hospitals Scheme on Cardiff City Mental Hospital 1915–1920. *Llafur: Journal of the Welsh People's History Society* 2005; **9**(2): 4–26.
16. Watkins P. *Recovery: a guide for mental health practitioners*. Edinburgh: Churchill Livingstone/Elsevier, 2007.
17. Jacobson N. Experiencing recovery: a dimensional analysis of recovery narratives. *Psychiatric Rehabilitation Journal* 2001; **24**(3): 248–56.
18. Barker P, Buchanan-Barker P. *The Tidal Model: a guide for mental health professionals*. Hove: Brunner-Routledge, 2005.
19. Egan G. *The skilled helper*, 9th edn. Pacific Grove: Brooks/Cole, 2010.
20. Stickley T. From SOLER to SURETY for effective non-verbal communication. *Nurse Education in Practice* 2011; **11**(6): 395–8.
21. Burnard P. Ordinary chat and therapeutic conversation: phatic communication and mental health nursing. *Journal of Psychiatric and Mental Health Nursing* 2003; **10**: 678–82.
22. Watkins P. *Mental health nursing: the art of compassionate care*. Oxford: Butterworth-Heinemann, 2001.
23. Altschul A. There won't be a next time. In: Rippere V, Williams R (eds). *Wounded healers: mental health workers' experiences of depression*. Chichester: John Wiley & Sons, 1985: 167–75.
24. NICE (National Institute for Health and Care Excellence). *CG90 Depression in Adults. NICE Guidance 2009*. Available from: https://www.nice.org.uk/guidance/cg90?unlid=4306996020163922547 [Accessed 25th July 2016].
25. Copeland M. *Wellness recovery action plan*. Dummerston, VT: Peach Press, 2000.
26. Gega L, Norman I. Cognitive behavioural techniques for mental health nursing practice. In: Norman I, Ryrie I (eds). *The art and science of mental health nursing: principles and practice*, 3rd edn. Maidenhead: Open University Press/McGraw-Hill, 2013: 317–45.
27. Breggin P. *Brain-disabling treatments in psychiatry: drugs, electroshock and the psychopharmaceutical complex*, 2nd edn. New York: Springer, 2008.
28. Nash M. *Physical health and well-being in mental health nursing: clinical skills for practice*. Maidenhead: Open University Press/McGraw Hill 2010.
29. Peplau H. *Interpersonal relations in nursing*. New York: Springer, 1991.

Further reading

Copeland ME. *Depression workbook*. Oakwood, CA: New Harbinger, 2001.

This is a useful resource to help people manage depression.

Milligan S, Clare A. *Depression and how to survive it*. London: Arrow, 1994.

Although a little dated now, the comedian Spike Milligan's collaboration with the psychiatrist Anthony Clare remains a useful insight into Milligan's periods of depression.

Plath S. *The bell jar*. London: Faber and Faber, 2005.

Sylvia Plath's classic novel draws heavily on Plath's own experiences of depression: a condition that would eventually take her life by suicide.

Relevant web pages

Bipolar UK. http://www.bipolaruk.org.uk

Bipolar UK supports people who suffer from bipolar disorder and associated problems including depression.

Depression Alliance. http://www.depressionalliance.org

The Depression Alliance provides a support network for people who experience depression and also a useful resource for those who endeavour to help them.

Norfolk and Suffolk NHS Foundation Trust. Choice and Medication. http://www.choiceandmedication.org/nsft

Time to Change. http://www.time-to-change.org.uk/category/blog/depression

Time to Change is a campaign to promote positive understanding about mental health problems and to reduce the associated stigma.

The person who self-harms

JANE BUNCLARK AND LOUISE STONE

LEARNING OUTCOMES

- To understand a definition of self-harm and its complexities.
- To understand why some individuals harm themselves, the associated factors and the methods used.
- To be aware of experience-based considerations in engaging and supporting this client group.
- To appreciate the key considerations of therapeutic interventions, in a multidisciplinary environment.
- To be aware of evidence-based guidance.
- To be familiar with service users' perspectives on interventions that are helpful or otherwise.

SUMMARY OF KEY POINTS

- Self-harm is complex to understand and define. Its motivation and purpose need to be understood.
- Self-harm arises from unmanageable emotions or memories and may be a means of coping.
- Factors associated with self-harm are broad, varied and individual, often with multiple causation.
- Self-harm is a symptom, not an illness, and is always symbolic.
- Understanding the function of self-harm guides nurses to support individuals in finding alternatives.
- Supervision and reflective practice help the worker to identify and address any re-enactments or other

difficulties that might arise in the relationship with someone who self-harms.
- Nurses take the lead in maintaining boundaries for consistency in therapeutic engagement.
- The nursing task is to support individuals in developing understanding and healthier coping mechanisms.
- Risk assessment is fundamental and needs to include the service user and carers.
- Risk assessment needs to sit alongside therapeutic risk taking.

INTRODUCTION

For most people, at both an individual and a societal level, self-harm is a complex and difficult phenomenon to understand – why someone inflicts pain, wounding or scarring when we try to avoid such damage. Self-harm is poorly understood and prompts ambivalent feeling in clinicians. However, nurses encounter individuals who self-harm in most settings. Often we are more sympathetic if someone states that they were attempting suicide rather than self-harming. Barker[1] frequently stresses that the focus of nursing is the craft of caring – that which helps bring together knowledge and aesthetics. For those who self-harm, the nurse's craft is to alleviate distress and to enable reparation, resolution and recovery.

Inflicting damage upon oneself is not a new phenomenon. Self-injury is an age-old and universal practice, and ceremonies involving blood, cutting and body modification appear in most cultures and religions. The use of pain and blood-loss often serve some social function at times of loss or bereavement. With a 3,000-year history, bloodletting, including through the use of leeches to cure physical and psychological conditions, has recently re-emerged, with research illustrating its usefulness in plastic surgery. Frequently blood, sacrifice and mutilation were found at the core of religion, for atonement of sin, spiritual advancement or purity. The Bible[2] documents rituals in which those who worshipped false gods slashed themselves with swords and spears; and self-cutting was associated with those possessed by demons.[3] Flagellation was a common practice in the thirteenth and fourteenth centuries among the fervently religious for penance and piety, and castration for religious purposes has been recorded over the centuries. The Hindu festival of Thaipusam involves sacrifice, including carrying *weighty* spikes inserted into the body or piercing with hooks and spears. Outside religious contexts, the history of punishment and torture is long and bloody, with mutilation and eventual death occurring throughout the centuries. Trephination, the ancient practice of making an opening in the skull to allow the escape or entrance of spirits, continues to be practised in parts of Africa, South America and Melanesia. At a more subtle level, the use of the skin as a tension reliever and a locus of healing takes many forms, including scratching and skin debridement.

The complexity of why individuals self-harm, and whether or not it is considered self-harm within their society, is confused by an array of terminology and lack of breadth in definition. Terminology includes self-injury, mutilation, para-suicide and deliberate self-harm. 'Self-harm' is currently most generally accepted, with the word 'deliberate' no longer preferred because many, including service users, considered it to be judgemental, ignoring the dilemmas that self-harm is not always 'deliberate' or 'intentional' – for example, if inflicted during dissociation. In terms of definition, the National Institute for Health and Care Excellence (NICE)[4] uses 'any act of self-poisoning or self-injury carried out by an individual irrespective of motivation' (p.5), which is somewhat more encompassing than their earlier[5] definition, with 'act' (p.21) amended to 'motivation'. This is a positive step, as 'act' is a poor determiner: many behaviours generally considered as 'suicidal' fall within the parameters of self-harm. A non-specific definition of motivation is helpful, as some experience interplay of both conscious and unconscious motivation. On the basis of my experience of nursing this group of individuals, I consider the NICE definition of self-poisoning or self-injury as still being too narrowly defined, as it excludes acts of omission of care (such as mismanagement of physical health), failure to protect oneself or gaining harm from others, and the interplay with eating disorders and substance misuse. I therefore suggest a more encompassing definition: 'an act to damage yourself without intending to die. This varies according to the situation and the individual carrying out the act and is a means of getting away from intolerable thoughts or feelings'[6] (p.7).

> ### SERVICE USER'S PERSPECTIVE
>
> I agree that having a broad, encompassing definition of self-harm is helpful, particularly in recovery. It is vital to remember when defining self-harm that self-harm is not the issue in itself – it is a behaviour used to express or serve some other need. As a behaviour that serves a purpose, more 'typical' self-harming behaviours, such as cutting, burning or overdosing, can be all too easily replaced by something else that is equally harmful to the individual. For me, what really helped in my recovery was being supported to be mindful around how I was behaving, and what purpose that behaviour was serving or what need it was meeting. At the time when I was unwell, staying up late and not eating properly were meeting a similar need for me as cutting, and being aware of that was important to my ultimately having a full recovery.

METHODS

A fundamental principle of understanding is having an *inclusive* definition of what might constitute self-harm.

In taking a longitudinal history, it may seem there were periods when a person abstained from cutting, etc., but

Table 22.1 Some methods of self-harm

Epithelial	Cutting
	Burning
	Scratching
	Abrasion
	Inserting objects under the skin
	Biting
	Hitting/punching self
	Pulling out hair
	Carving words on skin
Internal	Overdosing
	Substance misuse
	Ingestion of objects/caustic substances
Harm from others	Eliciting criticism or rejection
	Involvement in fights
	Contact sports
	Seeking attack, assault (physical, emotional, sexual)
	Abusive relationships
	Sex working
	Seeking physical restraint in hospital
	Refusing analgesia, including during suturing
Mind-altering methods	Bloodletting
	Overdosing
	Hanging
	Suffocation
	Substance misuse
	Purging
Omission	Failure to take prescribed physical medication
	Allowing wound infections
	Sleeping rough
	Poor hygiene/nutrition
	Deliberate recklessness

with inclusivity it could be revealed that in these periods the person was either at low weight or involved in unhealthy or abusive relationships. Thus the damage and maladaptive behaviours were constant.

Table 22.1 categorizes some methods of self-harm. However, there is some crossover between categories.

> **REFLECTION**
>
> Do you think you have missed ways in which your service users have damaged themselves?

PREVALENCE

Self-harm is common in young people, with recently rising rates,[7-10] and in college students.[11-13] The peak onset corresponds with pubescence[14] and about 10 per cent of adolescents report self-harm.[15,16] However, longitudinal studies indicate that 90 per cent of adolescents cease self-harm on entering adulthood.[17] The adult population reports approximately 4 per cent[18] engaged in self-harm; and it is more frequently found in women, and among lesbian, gay, bisexual, transgender groups,[19,20] those with socio-economic deprivation[21] and those identifying with 'Gothic/Emo' groups.[8,22] In the UK, Asian women are at higher risk compared to their white counterparts, but there are few studies comparing rates in other Black and Minority Ethnic groups.

Self-harm in the UK is one of the most common reasons for acute hospital admissions,[23] accounting for 200,000 hospital attendances annually,[24] with 40–50 per cent being repeat attendances,[25] the majority of which are due to overdoses.[26] Deaths worldwide in 2001 from self-inflicted injuries totalled approximately 800,000.[27] While being aware that self-harm is often not about committing suicide, clinicians need to recognize that these individuals are at greater risk of death, either intentionally or accidentally. However, a narrow definition does limit the accuracy of statistics.

WHAT MAKES PEOPLE SELF-HARM?

Individuals self-harm for many reasons; there is no single explanation that fits all, just as the initial trigger for the behavioural pattern is unique. Often someone may have an accidental injury and the relief they experience is such that, when distressed, they recall the relief and self-harm. The need to self-harm usually arises from emotions that are difficult to manage, with self-harm often being an outward demonstration of inner turmoil, trauma or crisis. Research and individual accounts show that many individuals struggle with intolerable distress or unbearable situations for some time before they self-harm.

SERVICE USER'S PERSPECTIVE

I started self-harming at a very young age and initially it was due to an accidental injury that I aggravated. For me, it wasn't a behaviour that was there all the time but something that became more prevalent during my teenage years. In actual fact, my most damaging self-harming behaviour began when I was admitted to an acute ward in a psychiatric hospital following an overdose (which I would consider a suicide attempt rather than self-harm). I think that this was due both to a pathologizing of the behaviour, rather than consideration of the underlying issues, and a lack of control, as staff struggled to manage my behaviour, rather than supporting me to manage it myself.

Pathologizing my behaviour, by which more than anything I probably mean giving me a label, is an interesting conundrum. At the time, I really wanted to be given a label – for someone to tell me that I had depression or something, because that would explain why I felt like this and why I needed to self-harm. I think that during my time in an acute setting, many professionals felt the need to give me a label, because if I had an illness then they could fix me, and 'fixing' me generally seemed to mean stopping me from self-harming,

not teaching me to tolerate and express the distressing emotions that I was managing through self-harm. The self-harm became the 'illness', and I think because of that it became part of my identity. At a time when I was struggling with low self-esteem and poor sense of self, I became defined by self-harming, which I think caused me to self-harm more.

Due to staff anxiety on the acute ward, many steps were taken to control me, and most of these were extremely unhelpful. Putting someone who self-harms on 1:1 observations around the clock might seem like a really logical idea – if you're watching them, then they can't self-harm. However, for me self-harm was a physical mechanism I used to control distressing emotions, so taking away that control wasn't helpful. It left me frustrated and constantly trying to work out how to get my control back in a constant battle with staff. This only left them and me frustrated, and the lengths that they would have to go to in order to keep me 'safe' would escalate to physical restraint and forced medication. I felt like the staff hated me. Ultimately giving me my control back – letting me take ownership of keeping myself safe – was far more useful.

(See chapter 17 for more information on the observation of people at risk.)

REFLECTION

What do you think of the service user's account? Can you think of occasions on which you have unknowingly entered a battle for control?

FACTORS ASSOCIATED WITH SELF-HARM

Abuse

Many individuals have experienced abuse in their early lives – physical, emotional or sexual. This can leave them feeling that they are 'to blame', guilty, in need of punishment or other unmanageable emotions.

Rape

The feelings described above might also arise from unwanted sexual experiences or rape. Some who experienced sexual abuse may believe that they deserve no better treatment and thus encounter further unwarranted sexual attacks.

Being bullied

Many individuals describe experiences of bullying at school, within social groups or at work. Often their experiences have been minimized or ignored by authority figures, leaving them unprotected and alone.

Difficult relationships within families

Some individuals come from divided, critical or violent environments, in which support for emotional development is absent. They might have lived in permanent fear, describing feeling as though they 'walk on eggshells'.

Parental separation

While parental separation is not necessarily harmful, the manner in which attention was given to young people's understanding of why this occurred and the impact on their attachments can hinder the development of a healthy sense of self. Young people may blame themselves, or think they need to 'side' with one parent over another. Similarly, parents' new partners and children may impact on the young person's place within the family, potentially leaving them feeling cast aside and powerless.

Bereavement

Bereavement is a period in which someone without inner coping resources may resort to self-harm. It is not only the loss that causes this reaction, but the lack of support or healthier coping skills to survive strong emotions.

Growing up

Adolescence is a time of turmoil for the healthiest of us; managing transitions, joining peer groups, emerging sexuality, and so on. However, for those without a supportive and enabling structure, it may be a time of isolation, self-doubt and confusion, and they may resort to self-harm.

Entering care

For some, entering care can be a relief from dysfunction or abusive families. For others, it may reinforce their belief that they are 'too hot to handle' and this may be cemented by multiple placements and associated broken attachments.

Problems with race, ethnicity, religion, sexuality, disability

As in the case of adolescence, individuals coping with and managing difference require supportive others. If these are absent, then self-harm may result.

High parental expectations

Some feel valued by their families only on the basis of their achievements, and as a mechanism for giving their family kudos. Perfectionist striving may leave them feeling that they are not good enough, as they are not accepted or loved for themselves.

Emotional neglect, lack of care or nurturing

Neglect, especially emotional/psychological, is hard to define and is frequently unseen or unacknowledged. However, growing up feeling unwanted or unloved, or that siblings are preferred, has profound effects. The belief that you are overlooked or unlovable is internalized leading to poor ego strength. This dilemma occurs for many who self-harm; they find it hard to understand why they feel 'different'.

SERVICE USER'S PERSPECTIVE

When my self-harming became severe, I started reading about it. What I can remember from that time is that much of the literature seemed to suggest that someone who self-harmed would have been sexually abused or have borderline personality disorder. For me, neither was the case. In fact, as I saw it, I didn't really have any dark issues in my past that would have caused me to end up in a psychiatric hospital. In some ways this made it more difficult – I felt like my 'stuff' wasn't good enough (or rather bad enough!) and for this reason I didn't really talk about it. It's really important to recognise that people self-harm for all kinds of reasons and the 'stuff' that has caused them to come on that particular journey can be wide and varied, but equally valid.

FUNCTIONS OF SELF-HARM

When nursing someone who self-harms, it is vital to explore the function their damage serves. Most individuals have a couple of 'preferred' methods, the choice of damage being dependent on what function or state of mind they are attempting to relieve. Self-harm is individual and personal, yet there are common themes expressed.

Destroying the body or making it less attractive

Scars, odours from burns, excessive obesity, and so on, can be used to make others 'back off' from unwanted sexual attraction, relationships or closeness, or communicate the disgust they feel for their physical self.

Regulation of distress/anxiety

Self-harm can be a 'knee jerk' reaction in which the body is used to release distress, anxiety or other unbearable emotions.

Distraction

Many who self-harm talk about how inflicting pain distracts them from their internal, unseen pain, almost as escapism, giving them a different locus of concentration.

Coping/survival

Many describe self-harm as a way of surviving unbearable memories or feelings, helping them cope with overpowering distress. It is thereby anti-suicidal.

Increased control

For some, self-harm provides a sense of control or mastery; of being in charge of one's life and what damage occurs. The damage is inflicted by them, not by others who may have inflicted damage before.

To feel real/ownership

Some individuals feel detached, like they are not 'living' in their bodies. This may previously have served some protective factor from traumatic experiences. Self-harm, pain or the sight of blood can act as a 'shock' into the here and now. Some speak of the reassurance gained from looking into lacerations and seeing bodily structures.

Testimony

Self-harm and scarification can offer a testament to what has been inflicted on bodies. Individuals speak of their scars showing something of their life story and struggles – almost as if their skin is a canvas, pointing to specific scars that relate to particular events.

Punishment of self or others

Early traumatic experiences can result in individuals feeling bad, contaminated or evil, and self-harm may be intended as either atonement or punishment. There is a perception of deserving punishment or a complex belief that they can punish others, often their abuser, through self-harm.

Cleansing

For some, self-harm serves the function of temporarily cleaning or purifying. Their sense of badness, evil, dirt, traumatic memories or unwanted feelings is evacuated through bloodletting. This is exemplified by those who eliminate their contamination into toilets, sinks, etc. For others, the use of bleaches and caustic substances hints at their sense of contamination.

To influence others

Some individuals have had repeated experiences of not being listen to or noticed, with protective figures perceived as 'turning a blind eye'. They might believe that communications via their body, if sufficiently severe, may elicit protection.

Communication

Self-harm is always a communication, either to self or to others, especially at times when people are unable to verbalize their emotions or their need for help. Self-harm could be viewed as a call for help, a hope that someone will notice and contain the emotions.

Re-enactment

While not universally acknowledged, self-harm can be seen as a replication of abusive experiences, with perhaps an unconscious hope that resolution or punishment will occur. The sense of breathlessness from ligature use or suffocation might be akin to a hand held over someone's face to quieten them. Re-enactment within self-harm might be represented in repeated attacks on particular parts of the body associated with particular memories of contamination; for example, insertion of blades vaginally.

Connection with inner world

However much damage an individual inflicts, it is only a glimpse of their internal damage. Attacks on their bodies can serve the function of making connections from their inner world to their physical self, showing others something of their damage.

Testing fate

Some individuals self-harm to test out whether they should live or die, almost as 'Russian roulette'. This is frequently seen in overdosing: at the point of ingesting the tablets, they want to die, but may subsequently alert others and receive treatment as their intent has altered.

Enacting the caregiver role

Paradoxically, self-harm may provide opportunities for individuals to self-care (or have nurses provide care) following injury. Many individuals have had difficult early attachment relationships with emotionally 'needy' parents, which may have involved lack of consistency in caregiving. Self-harm provides a mechanism for re-enacting and controlling the abuse/neglect and managing subsequent care and healing following injury.

SERVICE USER'S PERSPECTIVE

For me, understanding the functions of my self-harm was absolutely crucial to my recovery.

It was understanding what I was *really* doing when I self-harmed that gave me the insight to address the more difficult emotional and relational issues. For example, I came to realise that I often used self-harm as a way of communicating, and that this in turn would often have the result of influencing the behaviour of others. In these instances I was frequently using self-harm as a substitute for talking about the way I was feeling. By identifying this, I felt more empowered to speak and explore my feelings verbally. Similarly, I would use self-harm as an emotional outlet, giving me control over what felt like overwhelming and uncontrollable emotions. The realization of this gave me the courage to start to sit with my feelings and understand that difficult emotions don't last forever.

CHALLENGES OF NURSING INDIVIDUALS WHO SELF-HARM

Nurses have a key role in the care of individuals who self-harm, as they are uniquely placed by caring for the individual's bodily wounds as well as their minds, and will often have intense contact. Nurses are able to offer therapeutic relationships with patients, using the relationship for recovery and the hope of change (see chapters 3, 35 and 36). Nurses are able to model boundaries within relationships, and healthy ways of coping, while understanding the damage these individuals have encountered and replay upon their bodies – all within a compassionate and caring, yet challenging, encounter. Mental health nurses should be adept at balancing the dilemmas of risk management versus therapeutic risk taking. As discussed, the core concept in nursing this client group is that self-harm is a *symptom*, not the real problem. Just as individuals use their bodies as canvases for emotional management and expression, as nurses we can also be 'caught up' in providing interventions only at skin-level, thus ignoring the site of real damage – the individual's inner belief about themselves and their relationships.

In this work, anxiety will be ever present. Service users are frequently unable to manage their anxieties (intrusive thoughts or memories, overwhelming emotions, or 'split-off' parts of themselves experienced as critical, challenging voices), and these are communicated either overtly or subtly to nurses. Attention to containing anxiety is vital for the nurse to function, for the service user's containment and for the system to operate. For a nurse, engagement with someone who self-harms is difficult. Nurses may feel anxious, de-skilled, impotent, hopeless and responsible, perhaps similar to the way the service user feels. Winnicott[28] suggests that workers 'cannot avoid hating them and fearing them, the better he knows this the less will hate and fear be the motives determining what he does to his patients' (p.195).

This anxiety in clinicians manifests in various ways, sometimes in the involvement of multiple workers, each sharing part of the burden and thus making it harder to maintain a consistent, balanced approach. Nurses can be presented with the dilemma of being told secrets or receiving privileged information that is not to be shared with others; this is unhelpful to both colleagues and service users. Alternatively, the individual might be judged as challenging, manipulative or otherwise negatively, and discharged from services. Sometimes nurses are so distanced from involvement that they ignore the distress as 'just another crisis' in order to protect themselves. The relationship 'may be driven by the patients' and staff's wishes to deny feelings of pain, anxiety and despair about the level of pathology and disturbance'[29] (p.207). Service users find this neglectful and risk may escalate as they, perhaps unconsciously, battle to make nurses notice their distress through projection.[30] Organizations can become caught up in the same state of mind as service users, with nurses feeling criticized if someone self-harms or if self-harm is promoted as acceptable. 'Unless anxieties can be identified, addressed and contained within the system, it is likely that the system itself will produce defences that actively hinder rather than help therapeutic intervention'[31] (p.77).

In this work, nurses may encounter service users' desperate need for reparative relationships, driven by their lack of early parenting or containment. The nurse may find that relationships come to symbolize more than professional contact, due to the service user's need for reparation; this can result in it being impossible to fulfil their internal void, and thus whatever is offered is not good enough. Their desire for more time, more contact, and so on, will remain insatiable.

REFLECTION

Looking at the quotation below, do you think you may have 'slipped' into this dynamic?

'Nurses ... became either the punitive aggressors, who could not see her pain, or, if they could, blamed her for it, or the un-protective mothers who could be vigilant *only after* their child was hurt'.[32] (p.159)

NURSING APPROACHES TO WORKING THERAPEUTICALLY

Since, as already discussed, bodies are canvases of communication, nurses need to ensure that communication is at a verbal level. While service users repeat perverse damage on their bodies, practitioners should not repeat unhelpful, sadistic or ignoring responses. Instead they should offer supportive interventions, aimed at addressing the fundamental problem, rather than its outward manifestation. Nursing individuals who self-harm requires thoughtfulness, resilience, mindfulness (chapter 44) and maintenance of a therapeutic stance. Training, in whichever modality, supports nurses in conceptualizing dynamics, gaining knowledge and seeking meaning; without this, any understanding will be limited and symptom-focused, ignoring underlying difficulties and the healthier functions of service users. Nurses should be part of multi-professional teams, and should use collective thinking and reflective team discussions.

Regular, robust clinical supervision (chapter 10) is essential to examine the quality of relationships, to understand when re-enactments occur, to discuss anxieties, and to provide support for nurses hearing details of self-harm. Self-harm is always symbolic of other damage, and the more detail discussed, the less it will need to be enacted. Learning about repugnant details of what someone does with their blood, fat cells, and so on, will add to the risk assessment and will enable the individual to be understood at a deeper level. Supervision enables the dynamics around abuse to be addressed, as individuals who have experienced trauma may have learned to view life as offering only two roles – the abused or the abuser. This dynamic enters relationships, and nurses may be experienced as abusive or neglectful or feel abused or punished, through witnessing horrific wounds, rejections of help and crippling anxiety.

Consistent and standardized local protocols are necessary in all settings, with boundaries being set from the outset to manage expectations and provide safety for service users. This prevents the service user from being reconfirmed as 'special' or encountering a variety of anxiety-driven responses. 'The sufferer who frustrates a keen therapist, by failing to improve, is always in danger of meeting primitive human behaviour disguised as treatment'[33] (p.129). Protocols should be organizationally supported, such that nurses have a clear sense of their primary task, be it to support individuals to learn healthier coping techniques or to extinguish self-harm totally.

Risk assessment is fundamental, yet this service user group has additional complexities, and joint assessment by nurses and service users, including families/carers, is recommended. Joint risk discussions may enable the service user to consider their dangerousness, rather than being dismissive. It is important to note that risk is individual, that it cannot be totally eliminated and that assessment needs to sit alongside therapeutic risk taking. Nurses may wish to be helpful, but this distorts the responsibility boundary. The temptation to be risk-averse or overprotective, or not to allow service users to take responsibility for their behaviours and actions, must be resisted. (See chapter 16.)

REFLECTION

In supervisions and other reflective spaces, do you examine the quality of your relationship with service users and your valency[34] (i.e. your own capacity for patterns of behaviour in relationships) for particular roles?

BOUNDARIES – A FUNDAMENTAL CONCEPT IN CARING

Work with individuals who self-harm is based upon boundary maintenance. The transgression of boundaries in earlier life contributes to poor boundary recognition, such that fundamental boundaries of self/non-self are damaged and individuals have a desperate need to know

the limits within relationships. Individuals who self-harm attack not only the boundaries within relationships but also their primary boundary (their skin). The dilemma of re-enactment of boundary transgression is 'on offer' in contact, and the boundaries must be thoughtfully but not harshly maintained. The formation and maintenance of seamless boundaries and containing anxieties form the web that creates an environment that is sufficiently containing, such that engagement and difficulties can be addressed. Nurses are responsible for taking the lead in maintaining therapeutic relationships, neither offering friendship/ parenting nor being an inhuman, cold contact. Growth of the service user's insight and ability to hold responsibility occurs within boundaries, which need to be like skin: sufficiently flexible that cracks do not emerge, but with sufficient rigidity that therapeutic space is offered.

A multidisciplinary approach enables consistency for service users, ensures various disciplines are not 'split off', and precludes futile discussions about conceptual models or who holds more anxiety. Collectively the team can address dilemmas such as unwillingness to engage, criticism of care coordinators or responses to requests to change primary nurses. Negotiating team differences enables service users to witness the nurse tolerating and embracing difference and a consistent authority response. The team should not be thought of as knowing all the answers, but supporting service users to seek their own solutions. The most fundamental boundary is that of safety relating to self-harm – when to trust your service user to self-manage and when intervention is required – and therapeutic challenges test the permeability of this. Containment is 'The need for a vessel in terms of the community and the worker to be able to not

only hold onto the disturbance but digest and process it'[35] (p.145). Nurses are therefore tasked not only to manage self-harm, but to translate and share its meaning with service users to aid recovery – in essence, the craft of caring.

> ### SERVICE USER'S PERSPECTIVE
>
> My experience with many nurses was that they were very 'unboundaried' and I think that in the vast majority of cases this was with the very best of intentions, maybe because nurses simply didn't know what to do with me. What I needed more than anything at that point was for nurses to be clear and consistent in their responses to me, both individually and across the team. A lack of consistent boundaries across the team could result in patterns of behaviour emerging with different individual staff; for example, 'kicking off' when a particular nurse was on duty because I knew that her response was likely to be to have me physically restrained and injected rather than supporting me to find alternatives to regulate my emotions, or cutting when an especially sympathetic nurse was on duty because I knew that she would be more likely to spend time with me during her shift.

SUGGESTED INTERVENTION: 'SAFETY PLANNING'

Many individuals use self-harm to manage unbearable emotions due to a lack of opportunities to learn healthier coping strategies. Safety planning is a brief intervention to support individuals in searching for alternative coping strategies. The aims of safety planning are listed below.

1. Dispelling secrets

A dilemma in nursing this client group is the secretive nature of self-harm. Safety planning provides an opportunity to request help and involve others in an adult way, and it also supports the expectation that nurses (authority figures) will help protect. In practice, this may be that individuals inform nurses of their self-harm, such that risks and alternatives are considered.

2. Communication

Through safety planning, self-harm and underlying distress are moved from behavioural into verbal communication before self-harm occurs.

3. Reducing impulsiveness

Self-harm can be impulsive, a sudden reaction. Safety planning can break this pattern, providing a time delay from impulse to consideration of what they might 'do' to survive,

thereby acknowledging other possibilities, reducing impulsiveness and increasing healthy control.

4. Tolerating emotions

Safety planning can produce relief from difficulties of tolerating distress, by providing space before self-harm to identify and label emotions and support distress tolerance. This allows individuals to experience the shift and reduction of distressing feelings without the need to evacuate via self-harm.

5. Responsibility through self-direction

Ultimately, safety planning should become increasingly self-directed, with individuals using this technique without nurses' assistance.

6. Choice

Often the impulse to self-harm removes choice from the individual and the only answer is self-harm – almost as if self-harm has its own personality. The thinking space of safety planning provides opportunities for individuals to gain ownership of their actions, rather than automatically self-harming. Some speak of self-harm being their *only* choice, ever-present, under their control and a 'constant companion'. By verbally informing the nurse of the impulse to self-harm, the sometimes 'incestuous' relationship with self-harm is triangulated. The third person (the nurse) enters the dyadic relationship between the self-harm and the individual, to raise the notion of self-harm as a false solution. This poem by C (ex-service user) demonstrates the phenomenon:

Dear Self-harm,

Goodbye my lover, goodbye my friend, on you I no longer depend. You've comforted me

in my darkest hour; you've made me strong through your supposed power. I'll take some of you with me, your source and your marks, but I won't take the control you had over me – that I'm leaving behind. F** you, you b** you've robbed me of friends and hope. You were never truthful, never really helped, in fact you never really existed, I gave you power you didn't deserve.

SERVICE USER'S PERSPECTIVE

For me, safety planning was an incredibly helpful mechanism in reducing and subsequently eliminating my self-harming. Over the years, I have been exposed to a variety of efforts by professionals to stop me self-harming, including being on close observation, physical restraint, room searches and forcible medication. However, not one of these methods allowed me to stop *me* self-harming. Having the opportunity to choose to safety plan for 5 to 10 minutes allowed me a safe space to work through the methods I was going to use to avoid or delay self-harming. If I did self-harm after safety planning, there was no failure attached, on either my part or the part of the professional.

The physical treatment of self-harm is really important, and again I have experienced various versions of treatment. At one end of the spectrum, I would be given steri-strips and bandages and told to go and sort myself out; at the other end the practitioner would use that period of time when treating my injuries to try and talk to me about how I was feeling and why I had done it. For me, neither approach was helpful. The former approach has left me with some of the worst scars, mainly because trying to steri-strip your own arm is pretty impractical; the latter has both timing issues and huge potential for manipulation – learning that self-harming is going to result in an opportunity to talk after the event could encourage self-harm rather than talking about the feelings ahead of time. By far the most helpful response to my injuries was for a nurse to treat the wounds with care, calm and quietness – not asking why I had done it or whether it hurt, but simply and competently dealing with the injury at hand. I knew that I had the opportunity to talk prior to the injury (safety planning) and during my next 1:1 session.

REFLECTION

Are your conversations with service users only about why they self-harm, or also about the meaning for them?

WHAT TREATMENTS ARE KNOWN TO HELP?

While noting there are no proven effective treatments for recurrent self-harm, NICE,[36] states that the key aims and objectives of treatment should include the underlying principle of prompt, supportive assessment of psychological and physical difficulties, including pain management. There should be consideration of referral for further psychological, social and/or psychiatric assessment or treatment when necessary, which may include provision of 3 to 12 sessions of psychological intervention specifically structured for those who self-harm, aimed at self-harm reduction. A planned approach is recommended to include the service user, families and carers, with teams considering the issue of effective engagement, including discussion of harm-reduction strategies and the provision of information on long-term treatment, management and associated risks. For individuals with associated conditions, psychological, pharmacological and psychosocial interventions should be initiated.

Table 22.2 Psychological interventions for self-harm

Dialectical behaviour therapy (DBT)[37]	A multi-modal, psychological treatment, combining individual therapy, psycho-educational and skills group training. Includes a combination of cognitive-behavioural techniques for emotion regulation (distress tolerance, acceptance, and mindfulness) and is particularly effective for women with borderline personality disorder (BPD).
Mentalization-based treatment (MBT)	A complex psychological intervention (group/individual therapy) for individuals with BPD,[38] designed to increase individuals' ability to self-reflect. Based on the rationale that BPD is a developmental disorder of attachment, in which there is a failure to mentalize (ability to understand one's own and others' mental states).
Problem-solving therapy	There is supporting evidence that psychological treatments enhancing problem-solving skills may serve as a protective factor for individuals who repeatedly self-harm.[39]
Cognitive behaviour therapy (CBT)[40]	Structured, time-limited, individual therapy focused on problems concerning dysfunctional emotions, behaviours and cognitions. This has been adapted for recurrent self-harm.[36,41] A systematic review examining the effectiveness of CBT to reduce self-harm found some evidence of short-term reduction.

Psychological interventions

NICE recognizes that self-harm is driven by emotional difficulties and individuals' lack of skills to cope, and therefore interventions are aimed at reducing behaviours and enabling the individual to understand their unique contributing factors. The psychological interventions listed in Table 22.2 may be beneficial.

SERVICE USER'S PERSPECTIVE

In my personal journey, I found some of the therapeutic interventions mentioned in Table 22.2 extremely useful, particularly DBT. However, there were other experiences in a therapeutic setting which were equally valuable to me, including art therapy, creative writing, narrative telling and movement/dance therapy. All of these activities added a dimension beyond verbal expression or the use of bodily damage to communicate with others.

CO-PRODUCTION AND COLLABORATION

On reflection, this chapter symbolizes the essence of therapeutic engagement for nurses with those who self-harm. A nurse, asked to write about the issue, was tempted to be the 'knowing expert' based on clinical experience. Involving service users required renegotiating boundaries, and I was anxious about re-establishing contact as their lives have moved on to a journey of health, successful relationships, employment and 'normality'.

However, taking advice from colleagues (multidisciplinary engagement), I approached Louise and negotiated the boundaries of what we might say collectively – not without anxiety regarding contact, responsibility and level of familiarity. These concerns were echoed by Louise, but nevertheless negotiation occurred through expressing anxieties and re-setting boundaries. The resulting chapter is a co-production of working, thinking, insight and sharing. Neither the professional nor the recovered service user was the driver, for both parties brought insight, experience and wisdom. Our skills were different and the project moved from the professional being the leader, to the insights that Louise brought, the better writer and complete finisher leading our direction. In clinical settings, service users should also increasingly take the lead. I initially worried about whether Louise would be 'stirred up' by speaking about her experiences, but again I needed to remember to trust her self-management. In essence, the experience of writing about self-harm and the art of engagement was manifest in collaboratively presenting this chapter to you. We hope you enjoy the co-production, as we did.

CONCLUSION

Self-harm is complex to understand and define: anything can be turned into self-harm and no specific method should be viewed as only suicidal. It is not about the behaviour – rather about motivation and purpose (conscious and unconscious). Individuals self-harm because of unmanageable emotions or memories, and factors associated with self-harm are broad, varied and individual, often with multiple causation. It is important to understand that self-harm is not an illness and is always symbolic. Self-harm by omission needs to be recognized by nurses, in addition to more obvious methods. Many individuals have a 'preferred' method, and through unpicking the functions of each method, nurses will be guided to support individuals in finding alternatives.

This is not an easy group of individuals to nurse, and the process can leave nurses feeling anxious and disempowered, yet responsible. To address this, supervision and reflective practice are vital to prevent re-enactments or other harmful relationships from occurring.

Nurses are responsible for maintaining boundaries to support the individual in developing understanding and healthier coping mechanisms. Consistent, boundaried attachments are a vital element for therapeutic engagement. Holding secrets undermines your work, is detrimental to your colleagues and perverts relationships from being based on boundaried engagement. Risk assessment is fundamental, and it is vital to use the multidisciplinary team, the service user and families as integral in planning. Risk assessment needs to sit alongside therapeutic risk taking. The use of local protocols based on NICE guidelines is recommended.

References

1. Barker P (ed.). *Psychiatric and mental health nursing: the craft of caring*. London: Hodder Arnold, 2008.
2. Bible, First Kings 18:24–9.
3. Bible, Mark 5:2–5.
4. NICE (National Institute for Health and Care Excellence). *Self-harm: longer-term management*. National Clinical Guideline 133. London: NICE, 2011.
5. NICE (National Institute for Health and Care Excellence). *Self-harm: the short-term physical and psychological management and secondary prevention of self-harm in primary and secondary care*. Clinical Guideline. London: NICE, 2004.
6. HOTUSH (Helping others to understand self-harm) Crisis Recovery Unit, 2008 (unpublished).
7. Hawton K, Townsend E, Arensman E, Gunnell DJ, Hazell P, House A, et al. Psychosocial and pharmacological treatments for deliberate self harm. *Cochrane Database of Systematic Reviews* 1999; **4**: CD001764.
8. Young R, Sweeting H, West P. Prevalence of deliberate self harm and attempted suicide within contemporary Goth youth subculture: longitudinal cohort study. *British Medical Journal* 2006; **332**: 1058–61.
9. Plener PL, Libal G, Keller F, Fegert JM, Muehlenkamp JJ. An international comparison of adolescent nonsuicidal self-injury (NSSI) and suicide attempts: Germany and the USA. *Psychological Medicine* 2009; **39**: 1549–58.
10. Ross S, Heath N. A study of the frequency of self-mutilation in a community sample of adolescents. *Journal of Youth and Adolescence* 2002; **31**: 67–77.
11. Favazza AR, DeRosear L, Conterio K. Self-mutilation and eating disorders. *Suicide and Life-Threatening Behavior* 1989; **19**: 352–61.
12. Whitlock J, Eckenrode J, Silverman D. Self-injurious behaviors in a college population. *Pediatrics* 2006; **117**(6): 1939–48.
13. Gratz KL. Measurement of deliberate self-harm: preliminary data on the Deliberate Self-Harm Inventory. *Journal of Psychopathology and Behavioral Assessment* 2001; **23**(4): 253–63.
14. Patton G, Hemphill SA, Beyers JM, Bond L, Toumbourou JW, McMorris BJ, et al. Pubertal stage and deliberate self-harm in adolescents. *Journal of the American Academy of Child and Adolescent Psychiatry* 2007; **46**(4): 508–14.
15. Hawton K, Saunders KEA, O'Connor RC. Self-harm and suicide in adolescents. *Lancet* 2012; **379**: 2373–82.
16. Lloyd-Richardson EE, Perrine N, Dierker L, Kelley ML. Characteristics and functions of nonsuicidal self-injury in a community sample of adolescents. *Psychological Medicine* 2007; **37**: 1183–92.
17. Moran P, Coffey C, Romaniuk H, Olsson C, Borschmann R, Carlin JB, et al. The natural history of self-harm during adolescence and young adulthood: population-based cohort study. *Lancet* 2011; DOI:10.1016/S0140-6736(11)61141-0.
18. Briere J, Gil E. Self-mutilation in clinical and general population samples: prevalence, correlates, and functions. *American Journal of Orthopsychiatry* 1998; **68**: 609–20.
19. Skegg K. Self-harm. *Lancet* 2005; **366**: 1471–83.
20. Deliberto TL, Nock MK. An exploratory study of correlates, onset, and offset of non-suicidal self-injury. *Archives of Suicide Research* 2008; **12**(3): 219–31.
21. Hawton K, Harriss L, Hodder K, Simkin S, Gunnell D. The influence of the economic and social environment on deliberate self-harm and suicide: an ecological and person-based study. *Psychological Medicine* 2001; **31**: 827–36.
22. Moorey S. Managing the unmanageable: cognitive behaviour therapy for deliberate self-harm. *Psychoanalytic Psychotherapy* 2010; **24**(2): 135–49.
23. Evans MO, Morgan HG, Hayward A, Gunnell DJ. Crisis telephone consultation for deliberate self-harm patients: effects on repetition. *British Journal of Psychiatry* 1999; **175**: 23–7.
24. Hawton K, Bergen H, Casey P, Simkin S, Palmer B, Cooper J, et al. Self-harm in England: a tale of three cities. Multicentre study of self-harm. *Social Psychiatry and Psychiatric Epidemiology* 2007; **42**(7): 513–21.
25. Platt S, Hawton K, Kreitman N, Fagg J, Foster J. Recent clinical and epidemiological trends in parasuicide in Edinburgh and Oxford: a tale of two cities. *Psychological Medicine* 1988; **18**: 405–18.
26. O'Connor RC, Sheehy NP, O'Connor DB. Fifty cases of general hospital suicide. *British Journal of Health Psychology* 2000; **5**: 83–95.
27. WHO (World Health Organization). *Health-for-all targets. The health policy for Europe. Summary of the updated edition (EUR ICP HSC 013)*. Copenhagen: WHO, 1992.
28. Winnicott DW. Hate in the counter-transference. *International Journal of Psychoanalysis* 1949; **30**; 69–74.
29. Evans M. Problems in management of borderline patients. In: Jacob C, Adshead G (eds). *Personality disorders: the definitive reader*. London: Jessica Kingsley, 1998.
30. Klein M. Notes on some schizoid mechanisms. In: Money-Kyle R (ed.). *The writings of Melanie Klein*. Vol. 3, *Envy and gratitude*. London: Hogarth, 1946: 1–24.

31. Menzies Lyth I. The function of social systems as a defence against anxiety. In: *Selected essays, vol. 1*. London: Free Association Books, 1970.
32. Motz A. *The psychology of female violence: crimes against the body*. Abingdon: Taylor & Francis, 2008.
33. Main TF. The ailment. *British Journal of Medical Psychology* 1957; **30**(3): 129–45.
34. Bion WR. *Second thoughts: selected papers on psychoanalysis*. London: Heinemann, 1967.
35. Navarro T. Beyond keyworking. In: Foster A, Zagier Roberts V (eds). *Managing mental health in the community: chaos and containment*. London: Routledge, 1990: chapter 12.
36. NICE (National Institute for Health and Care Excellence). *Borderline personality disorder: treatment and management*. NICE Clinical Guideline 78. London: NICE, 2009.

37. Linehan MM, Armstrong HE, Suarez A, Allmon D, Heard HL. Cognitive-behavioral treatment of chronically parasuicidal borderline patients. *Archives of General Psychiatry* 1991; **48**: 1060–4.
38. Bateman A, Fonagy P. Mentalization-based treatment of BPD. *Journal of Personality Disorders* 2004; **18**(1): 36–51.
39. McLeavey BC, Daly RJ, Ludgate JW, Murray CM. Interpersonal problem solving skills training in the treatment of self-poisoning patients: a qualitative exploration of service-users' views. *BMC Public Health* 2007; **7**: 9–17.
40. Butler AC, Chapman JE, Forman EM, Beck AT. The empirical status of cognitive behavioral therapy: a review of meta-analyses. *Clinical Psychology Review* 2006; **26**(1):17–31.
41. Arntz A. Treatment of borderline personality disorder: a challenge for cognitive-behavioural therapy. *Behaviour Research and Therapy* 1994; **32**(4): 419–30.

Further reading

Babiker G, Arnold L. *The language of injury: comprehending self-mutilation*. Leicester: BPS Books, 1997.

Gardiner F. *Self-harm; a psychotherapeutic approach*. London: Brunner-Routledge, 2001.

Motz A. *The psychology of female violence: crimes against the body*. Philadelphia, PA: Brunner-Routledge, 2001.

Turp M. *Hidden self-harm: narratives from psychotherapy*. London: Jessica Kingsley, 2003.

Relevant web pages

http://www.behindthelabel.co.uk/

Mental Health Foundation. The truth about self-harm. https://www.mentalhealth.org.uk/publications/truth-about-self-harm

MIND. Self-harm. http://www.mind.org.uk/information-support/types-of-mental-health-problems/self-harm/

The Mix. Why do people self-harm? http://www.thesite.org/mental-health/self-harm/why-do-people-self-harm-5680.html

The Mix. Self-harm. http://www.getconnected.org.uk/get-help/harming-yourself/self-harm/

NSHN (National Self-Harm Network). http://www.nshn.co.uk/

Recover Your Life. http://www.recoveryourlife.com/

Royal College of Psychiatrists. Self-harm. http://www.rcpsych.ac.uk/mentalhealthinfoforall/problems/depression/self-harm.aspx

Self-Injury Support. http://www.selfinjurysupport.org.uk/home
This is a UK charity that offers support to people who self-harm, as well as resources and publications for professionals.

Time to Change. Blogs and †stories about self-harm. http://www.time-to-change.org.uk/category/blog/self-harm
This website contains blogs and stories from people with lived experience of self-harm.

YoungMinds. Self-harm. http://www.youngminds.org.uk/for_parents/whats_worrying_you_about_your_child/self-harm
This charity provides short films, publications and digital resource packs about self-harm.

Suicide

VANESSA GORDON, KAREN JAMES, MARION JANNER, KIRSTEN WINDFUHR AND ISABELLE M. HUNT

LEARNING OUTCOMES

- To understand what it can feel like to be suicidal.
- To be aware of the actions nurses can take to prevent suicide on their wards.
- To know how to conduct a good quality risk assessment.
- To be aware of strategies to reduce suicide outside of mental health services, such as in primary care.

SUMMARY OF KEY POINTS

- Mental health nurses play a crucial role in suicide prevention and in helping people to recover from a suicidal state of mind.
- A non-judgemental attitude and an in-depth understanding of the person you are supporting are essential components of effective risk assessment and suicide prevention.
- Key skills for the prevention of inpatient suicides include being observant and understanding the subtle cues that a person is in distress (being 'caringly vigilant and inquisitive').
- Implementation of the Care Programme Approach following discharge from hospital can save lives.
- Assessment of suicide risk should be ongoing and include a comprehensive formulation of risk that is tailored to the individual.

INTRODUCTION

Suicide is a major problem in the UK and its prevention is a priority worldwide. While there is no single or, in fact, simple way of preventing suicide, a wealth of progress has been made. The introduction of a more integrated approach, with the reduction of access to suicidal methods combined with a particular attention to high-risk groups, has helped to reduce the number of suicides. Furthermore, positive engagement with the media to ensure appropriate portrayals of suicide along with a continued drive to promote mental health and well-being is resulting in some encouraging outcomes.

What we do know is that suicide, its antecedents and the means by which people take their own lives are varied. Mental health nurses working within the paradox of suicide have a critical role to play. It is often the mental health nurse who is the last person to engage and build a meaningful relationship with these individuals, and who can provide a source of hope when all else appears to have ebbed away.

Such engagement in an often volatile, complex and highly emotive situation is one of the most important areas of care in which mental health nurses will deploy their skills, knowledge and experience. From my own perspective, this has to be one of the most demanding and rewarding aspects of the mental health nursing role.

This particular chapter focuses on the patient experience; the mindfulness, insight and intuition of the mental health nurse in practice; and the knowledge we have acquired from research.

SPEAKING FROM EXPERIENCE

To introduce myself – as an individual rather than just a suicide risk – I'm 54, Jewish, single, a co-parent of two learning disabled wonderful young men, blessed with loving, supportive and remarkably understanding family and friends, and I run the Star Wards mental health wards project.

It's important to state I'm in a secure position with my finances and home, without which I can't imagine still being around. My closest companion is my dog, Buddy – a gorgeous, super-docile, daft Tibetan Terrier who has been my support dog during the last 10 years of mental illness hell. Buddy is a familiar, and much loved, presence in the mental health hospital world. She even has a classroom named after her at South London and Maudsley's groovy Ortus learning centre! Luckily I'm relatively sane when not working and have enjoyed exquisite holidays in Cuba, Borneo and Madagascar during my illness.

The illness? The merciless, brutal borderline personality disorder (BPD), characterized by an inability to manage our feelings, intolerable emotional pain – and a compulsion to self-destruct both as a coping mechanism and as the ultimate, irreversible release from the torment. Before my BPD exploded 10 years ago, I was an unusually happy and dynamic little bunny, in a long-term relationship, the ending of which was the detonator to this very attachment-related illness.

The term 'suicidality' is unhelpfully broad, embracing everything from a fleeting thought to being right on the brink. For me, like many others, it's paradoxically not really about death – coffins, burial, others' bereavement, possibly an afterlife. Death is sort of 'collateral damage', a very reasonable price to pay for an unequivocal, permanent escape. I just want out. An exit from an intolerable existence.

The lowest-key, and therefore most manageable, manifestation of my suicidality is what feels like an involuntary or reflex observation. Sometimes it's more like a plea or a complaint. A protest. It's always the same comment: 'Want to die'. It's become my mantra, a brain-jerk reaction

to feeling anxious and, in particular, ashamed. Usually repeated several times till I notice what I'm saying to myself and try to stop it escalating into justification and then plans.

When things are particularly tough, the compulsion takes over. It feels like I've been on a quest the last 10 years for the one solution that will make life tolerable, by eliminating it and me. During those hours, I'm completely consumed by how to overcome the barriers to achieving this. There's the practical side: which method is the least ghastly for me and least traumatic for the person who finds me. I think I've cracked this but my enthusiasm for alternative options makes me highly receptive to new ideas. (I'm not going to be reading this book, for example, as additional options fuel my determination and distorted 'hope'.)

The automatic thoughts and the overwhelming compulsions are part of the madness. But I feel I have also developed a perfectly reasonable evaluation of the quality of my current and likely future life which confirm in a rational way that what is in my own interest is to call it a day. I'm immensely, unusually, lucky in having had a life rich in love, adventure, profoundly rewarding work and a large intake of Walnut Whips. Even if the future turns out to be OK, it isn't enticing enough to counteract the toughness of daily life.

So how come my quasi-actuarial calculation hasn't resulted in my self-liberation? There's a why and a how. The why is that being blessed with people who love me, especially my two lads, even my most imaginative rationalization of how they would be OK doesn't stack up. A few people would have their lives wrecked and others would suffer great pain. The how is a combination of what I can manage myself and having a small army of specialist professionals and services keeping me afloat.

Those times when I'm desperate to die, I experience a sort of 'inverse mindfulness' – I'm so utterly in the moment that I have no awareness of my surroundings (other than their lethal potential), time, even that my beloved Buddy is beside me. It's like being submerged in tar and darkness.

Usually I have to excavate each last gram of will-power to get through this, but when even that falters, I've been exceptionally fortunate to have had a psychiatrist/therapist who saw me weekly, on the NHS, for 7 years, and with a decreasing frequency determined by me over the last 2 years as I've become saner and more resilient. Anthony specializes in treating people with BPD, using a therapy created for people with BPD – mentalization-based treatment. Crucially for my survival, I have been able to phone or email Anthony between sessions if I'm really not coping.

Even this very unusual, deeply generous support hasn't been enough, and the charity I run found and paid for a crisis therapist. This (yet again very unusual!) arrangement is one that I feel should be a standard option for people at very high risk, enabling me to have specialist support from a therapist with whom I built a very trusting relationship. It meant that I could ring Patrick (who lives hundreds of miles away) any time in the evening or weekend and somehow he would always make himself available to get me through the crisis. For about 4 years I rang Patrick on average once or twice a week, in addition to a weekly 'check-in' call – i.e. therapy session.

Patrick is a genius therapist and mental health nurse, using a range of approaches, although the primary one was dialectical behavioural therapy, the most common specialist therapy for people with BPD (there were periods when I rang Patrick daily, our calls lasting anything from 1 to 3 hours).

Through this intensive support, I learnt how to weather the intolerable times – but for the first 8 years I was in such a state that I couldn't bring to mind what I needed to do, so Anthony and Patrick had to take me through the steps. I've been much more stable the last couple of years and have finally been able to implement coping strategies myself rather than relying on my therapists to walk me through them.

When I'm in my most suicidal state, I can only speak to people I know well, i.e. Anthony and Patrick. So paradoxically I don't ring the Samaritans when I'm particularly desperate to die. But I do contact them at other times and find it invaluable to talk through with a calm, non-judgemental, supportive, caring person what it's like coping with an overwhelming desire to be dead. They are a miracle organization.

There have been about six occasions when even Anthony and Patrick haven't been able to contain my suicidality, and I've ended up in hospital – only once on a section. Being in hospital is a good escape for me, although extremely trying for staff! I'm a nightmare patient because although the intensity of my yearning to be dead subsides in hospital (because inpatient care has done so well at making it very, very difficult to kill oneself in hospital), my compulsion to self-harm escalates. Like on most wards, self-harming is seen as totally dysfunctional, dangerous, shocking, etc. This might be the case, but the alternative of trying to resist the extreme frustration of not being able to use this coping mechanism ratchets up the compulsion. I admire (and promote!) the few hospitals where it's recognized that self-harming (which for most of us means cutting) has a valid function and patients are enabled to do this in as safe a way as possible.

The mid-way for me between killing myself and self-harming by cutting is taking overdoses. When life is so overwhelmingly complicated and excruciating, taking an overdose with the risk of dying and the capacity to reverse this at A&E is the one thing that gives me a sense of having some control over my situation. It's a mad Russian roulette of self-agency. I don't need, and rarely get, anyone telling me that this is a childish, selfish and expensive way of regaining my equilibrium. I know that. I really do get it. But the reality is that the (very traumatic and physically unpleasant) process does somehow reset my emotional thermostat and I can resume my (reluctant) life.

What else helps? Being treated with the same degree of understanding and empathy that Anthony and Patrick unfailingly show by other professionals. I'm always astonished and relieved how kind and non-judgemental ambulance staff are. Given how much of their time is spent with people who have completely involuntarily ended up on board, their humanity and ability to appreciate a very different type of crisis is one of the many wonders of our beleaguered NHS.

Most of my 'wish-list' for what the NHS could do to support people who are suicidal is pretty predictable – staff being trained by people with direct experience of suicidality, specialist services for people with BPD (which is still the relatively recent treatable kid on the block, having been regarded as hopeless till about 15 years ago), properly intensive support for those in crisis (not someone from the crisis team popping in for 10 minutes to ask if you've taken your medication) – in fact, everything contained in the recently published Crisis Care Concordat. The one useful contribution I can make is to strongly urge Trusts to introduce out-of-hours crisis therapists. However well we're supported in office hours, obviously our bad episodes don't conform to these times.

While writing this piece, I discovered what looks like a suicide note I wrote in 2006. I'd completely forgotten I'd written this. I've replaced people's names with an X.

You have all been so totally supportive. It's impossible to explain how I compartmentalise this but the best I can do is to say that when I'm feeling okay, and not suicidal, your love is incredibly sustaining and buoying. But when I feel like this, this is all there is. And all there is is the absence of X [my ex-partner]. And I want to be dead.

It's tempting to write something trite about 'try not to be too sad' but I know it will be devastating for some of you and intensely sad for others. It's said that suicide is a very selfish act and in this case it's true. It's something I want to do because it's the only viable way out of this pain and I'm blotting out what effect it will have on my much much loved family and friends.

I've appreciated so much what each of you have done, whether it's offering to come back from

anywhere in the world at any time (X), or greatly upping the frequency of meeting up with me (X, X, X, X) or being on top of my emotional state on almost a daily basis (X, X) or being able to tolerate and indeed solicit some of the more painful aspects of what I'm going through (X, X) or let me come and be part of the family every week (X) or be willing to do anything, including contacting me much less frequently than you'd like (X, X). Adding even a gram to X and X's pain feels indecent.

And the amazing X [my psychiatrist/therapist]. Will I be just chucking away a year of him having to put in an extra hour probably at home as a result of seeing me 8.30AM each week? And is there some awful suicide league table which I'll fuck up by my death? I'm so deeply grateful for his support, expertise and tolerance, and for him saying things like 'Fuck that for a game of soldiers'.

The note ends there, rather abruptly. Perhaps I felt a jolt of being supported by Anthony and this got me past this crisis. And I probably rang Patrick, my crisis therapist, at this point.

Marion Janner

REFLECTION

Read through Marion's narrative of her experiences. What role did mental health professionals play in her recovery? If you were Marion's mental health nurse, how might you have supported her?

Arguably one of the most important roles of inpatient mental health services is to provide support for people who are at an immediate risk of suicide. Within these services, it is mental health nurses who are the frontline carers for people who are suicidal. They must help people to recover a will to live,[1] as well as keep them safe from harm. This next section focuses on the actions nurses can take to prevent suicide on their wards.

The challenge of maintaining the therapeutic relationship and keeping a person who is feeling suicidal safe requires various skills of mental health nurses. (To find out more about therapeutic relationships, see chapter 3.)

Alongside the recognized skills of a caring, non-judgemental and understanding attitude toward the patient, bearing hope for recovery, and participating in a patient-centred relationship, mental health nurses must also maintain a constant awareness of the level of suicide risk.

Risk assessment is not a check-box exercise but draws on the instincts of the nurse and their knowledge and understanding of the patient. (Chapter 16 provides more detail on assessing risk of suicide and self-harm.)

People who are suicidal may resist protective efforts from clinicians and families. If someone is not able to make a decision about their care or is unable to develop an alliance with staff, then the risk for suicide is higher and the need to ensure safety is enhanced in situations of uncertainty. One of the most meaningful interventions for someone in distress is the presence of a caring nurse. 'Being with' a client who is in despair and mutually engaging in activities of his or her interest fosters a therapeutic relationship, and promotes participation in living. Even seemingly small and inconsequential activities can garner investment in life[2] and are the embodiment of the craft of caring.

The prediction and prevention of suicide within mental health services is difficult. Research studies have found just two predictors of suicidal behaviour; previous suicidal behaviour and depressive symptoms, both of which apply to large numbers of people under the care of inpatient services.[2] A major policy in England and Wales has focused on making the ward environment safer by removing potential ligature points and installing collapsible curtain and shower rails,[3] which has resulted in a reduction in the number of patient suicides.[4] Of course environmental policies will always play a part, but the ability to evidence the skills of the caring and compassionate mental nurse in suicide prevention has received less attention.

One study that has looked at this is that of Bowers et al.,[5] which examined the ways in which suicides were prevented on wards. In this study, researchers examined incident reports describing episodes of high-lethality self-harm (i.e. where there was a good chance that, if there had been no intervention, the person would have died) occurring during 1 year on inpatient psychiatric wards in England and Wales. Reports were collected from the UK's National Reporting and Learning database of reported patient safety incidents. The researchers looked at the circumstances of high-lethality self-harm, to discover how suicides were prevented on inpatient wards. The study found that over 70 per cent of suicides were prevented by the actions of nursing staff, illustrating the life-saving work that nursing staff do within these services every day.

Around 63 per cent of episodes of high-lethality self-harm took place in the private areas of the ward (bedrooms, bathrooms and toilets), and the highest number of incidents occurred in the evening. There was also an increase in high-lethality self-harm around midday and during evening nursing shift handovers.

A large number of these reports documented that suicides were prevented because staff were checking on patients regularly, either because they were placed under some form of intermittent observation, or as part of normal ward routine (e.g. during medication rounds, or mealtimes).

Understanding these potential risks and observing someone for signs of risks are critical. It is important that mental health nurses continuously observe and identify warning signs and should trust in their instincts to follow up whenever necessary. An observant nurse can respond to subtle patient cues and intervene at a time of increased distress. In the event of an actual attempt, the nurse can intervene immediately and provide emergency care to the patient who is frequently or constantly observed, and thereby diminish potential lethality.[6] (Chapter 17 provides further detail on engagement and observation of people at risk.)

These actions were described by Bowers at al. as being 'caringly vigilant and inquisitive'; a positive strategy for suicide prevention on inpatient wards. When the reports were examined in detail, the authors found a large number of people engaging in high-lethality self-harm were discovered because of staff being 'caringly vigilant and inquisitive'.

The concept of being caringly vigilant and inquisitive captures some key principles of good mental health nursing. These principles include having a sound knowledge of the patient as a person, and how they normally behave (so that you are able to notice when something is wrong), and constant attentiveness to their state of mind and whereabouts on the ward. Being caringly vigilant and inquisitive also means trusting your instincts, and having the confidence to act when you feel that something is not quite right.

'Caringly vigilant and inquisitive' encompasses seven different behaviours which are outlined below and are illustrated using examples taken from the incident reports studied by Bowers et al.:[5]

1. Noticing that a patient has been absent from communal areas for some time.
   'Staff became concerned when the patient was not in communal areas of ward. She was located in a toilet with a ligature tied tightly around her neck. She appeared to have lost consciousness, and was not breathing.'
2. Noticing that a patient appears physically ill.
   'A female patient came to the office and was observed to be dazed and pale in colour. The patient's bag was searched, there were empty packets of 32 tablets. She had taken the tablets as an overdose.'
3. Following a patient in distress.
   'The patient was in the garden and came up crying and ran into her bedroom. Staff were close behind and followed her in.'
4. Noticing that a patient is taking a long time in the toilet.
   'The patient went to the toilet and appeared to be taking a long time. Staff investigated & found she had formed a ligature from her bra.'
5. Noticing suspicious actions or behaviours.
   'The patient was lying on her bed, she turned on her front and staff saw her elbow moving slightly. Staff stood over the patient to see what she was doing and saw a strap wrapped around her neck.'
6. Listening carefully to safety calls.
   'The client was in the toilets. Staff called out to client but did not feel happy with the response. On opening the toilet door, client was found with a pyjama top wrapped around her head.'
7. Responding to an unusual noise.
   'I heard rustling from patient's bedspace, when I entered patient was lying on her bed with a plastic carrier bag over her head and attempting to tie it.'

This research has shown how being observant and vigilant has successfully prevented suicides on inpatient wards. Box 23.1 shows ways to incorporate being caringly vigilant and inquisitive (CVI) into your practice.

REFLECTION

Read through the examples from the incident reports listed above. What would you have done in these situations? Would you have picked up on the signs that something was not right? Would you have checked on the person? How might you incorporate being caringly vigilant and inquisitive into your practice?

BOX 23.1: BEING CARINGLY VIGILANT AND INQUISITIVE

- Talk about CVI with your colleagues, describe it and say when you are doing it.
- Identify, acknowledge and praise others when you see them doing it.
- Remind staff to be CVI during handover.
- Role model CVI, and request that those for whom you are responsible adopt this approach too.
- Include CVI in staff training or inductions.

PREVENTING SUICIDES DURING PERIODS OF TRANSITION

Periods of transition into and out of inpatient care remain a time of high suicide risk. Awareness of factors associated with high risk (e.g. self-harm; a short duration of mental illness), measures to reduce absconding or escaping from inpatient care, and enhanced support for patients in the early period of moving from inpatient to community care may help to reduce suicide.

Two recent case-control studies (studies which compared people who died by suicide with those who did not) examined factors associated with suicide among inpatients who died within the first week of admission, and patients who died within 2 weeks of leaving inpatient care (i.e. post-discharge).[7,8] Key risk factors for inpatient suicide were a history of self-harm, recent adverse life events, and short duration of illness (less than 12 months) – all of which increased risk more than three-fold. An important finding was the high percentage of patients (34 per cent) who died by suicide after leaving the ward without staff agreement or knowledge.[8] Within the 2-week period following discharge from inpatient care, 55 per cent of patients died within the first week of discharge, with 49 per cent dying before the first follow-up contact with mental health services.[7] Factors associated with increased suicide risk included recent adverse life events, a short (less than 1 week) last admission, older age, and comorbid psychiatric disorders. However, patients who had been receiving enhanced aftercare under the Care Programme Approach (CPA) were less likely to die by suicide. The successful implementation of the CPA requires ongoing evaluation and updating alongside the many tools or assessments that mental health nurses use. Any transition, whether leaving the ward or being discharged, may be distressing and fragmentation of the nursing experience once a person has been discharged needs to be redressed. (Further information on the Care Programme Approach can be found in chapter 37.)

There are now more suicides among patients under crisis resolution and home treatment (CRHT) services than among inpatients, reflecting the changing nature of how mental health services are provided (Figure 23.1).

MANAGING SUICIDE RISK

Although the factors associated with suicide risk are well known (e.g. self-harm), findings from the National Confidential Inquiry into Suicide and Homicide (NCISH) have shown that at the last contact clinicians often rate a person's suicide risk as low just before they take their own life (i.e. at the last point the clinician sees them). This is known

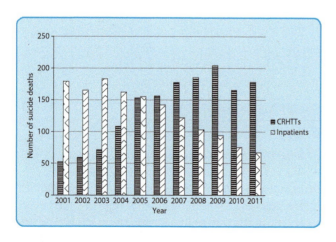

Figure 23.1 Number of suicides under crisis resolution and home treatment teams (CRHTTs) and in inpatient care in England, 2001–2011.

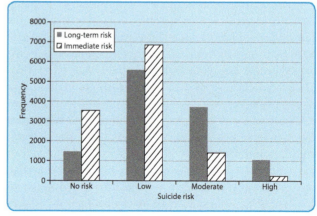

Figure 23.2 Number and percentage of clinicians' judgement of long-term and immediate suicide risk at last contact.

as the 'low risk paradox' (Figure 23.2).[9] There may be several reasons why clinicians underestimate the level of risk. The risk assessment process may have been satisfactory, but suicide risk might have changed between last contact with services and the suicide. Alternatively, it may be that the process of risk assessment itself was unsatisfactory. In June 2013, we reported on our study examining the process of risk assessment and management.[9] The aims were to develop an evaluation framework for assessing the quality of the risk assessment process, and to identify the quality of risk assessment and management prior to suicide.

The evaluation framework incorporated best practice guidance and relevant research, and included five domains against which quality was assessed:

- assessment of patient history;
- assessment of mental state and current circumstances;
- formulation of risk factors and disposal/management plans;
- communication of management plans;
- overall quality of the assessment.[9]

The inter-rater reliability of the quality of risk assessment between clinicians was good, indicating that the framework was a reliable means of assessing the process of risk assessment. In one-third of patient suicides (15; 36 per cent) the risk assessment process was judged to be unsatisfactory, particularly in the domains of risk formulation (i.e. an analysis of risks and risk factors) and management plans. The findings also showed that the patients' 'histories' were in some cases not sufficiently considered in the formulation of their suicide risk. In other cases, the management of the patients' risk did not follow on from the assessment of their risk. A good quality risk assessment and management plan should incorporate current mental state and past history. Importantly, assessment and management

of suicide risk should be tailored to the individual patient rather than relying on generic assessment and management tools, or 'tick-box' approaches to suicide risk.

> ## REFLECTION
>
> How might you construct an 'individualized' risk assessment? What kind of things would you need to consider to ensure you have tailored your risk assessment to the individual you are supporting?

The NCISH has for the first time shown a positive association between patient safety changes implemented by mental health services and a reduction in suicide rates. In our study, we reported a significant reduction in suicide rates in trusts that provided 24-hour crisis care, following recommendations made by the NCISH in '12 steps to a safer service'.[3,10] This was associated with a 19 per cent reduction in suicide rates. The implementation of dual diagnosis policies and multidisciplinary reviews following a patient suicide were associated with a 9 per cent and 10 per cent fall in suicide rates, respectively. Taken together, implementation of these recommendations was associated with 200 to 300 fewer patient suicide deaths. A UK-wide follow-up to the previous study suggests that a variety of service changes were associated with reduced suicide rates (e.g. assertive outreach; post-discharge follow-up).[11]

Key findings from the NCISH work are provided in a resource which has been developed for local audit and quality improvement. The freely available toolkit provides information on the recommendations, the data and source of information on which the recommendations are based, and a chart for trusts to note whether the recommendation has been implemented (see 'Further reading', NPSA, *Preventing suicide*).

SUICIDE IN OTHER HEALTH CARE SETTINGS

Approximately three-quarters of individuals are not in contact with mental health services in the year prior to suicide. Reducing suicide therefore requires a better understanding of suicide occurring in other health care settings, in particular primary care and emergency departments.

The majority of individuals are in contact with their GP prior to suicide, and an emphasis on prevention in this setting is important to reduce suicide.[12] Key messages for primary care services are to recognize markers of suicide risk such as frequent or increasing attendance, non-attendance, multiple drugs, and specific drug combinations (i.e. benzodiazepines and antidepressants). Incorporating mental health indicators in the annual health check may improve recognition of mental illness and encourage patients to attend their GP surgery. A 'flag' alert including these factors could also identify patients at risk of suicide.[12]

These measures may in part help to reduce suicide in individuals who usually do not attend, although suicide prevention in this group may be best addressed by voluntary or other agencies.[12] Our work also suggests that better liaison between primary and secondary services, including referrals, is an important factor in suicide prevention. For the emergency department setting, key suicide prevention measures include carrying out a psychosocial assessment in line with guidance from the National Institute for Health and Care Excellence (NICE).[13] Appropriate onward care (e.g. referral, treatment) may also be effective in reducing suicidal behaviour.[14] Finally, services should be aware that frequent attendance may be associated with increased suicide risk. This mirrors the finding of an association between increased attendance in primary care and suicide risk.[12]

CONCLUSION

As demonstrated in this chapter, there is clear evidence that the intuition and actions of mental health nurses save lives, and we hope the powerful insight into the service user experience provided here has illustrated the crucial role nurses can play in a person's recovery, as well as what it can feel like to be suicidal. Suicide prevention is difficult; however, we have learnt that there are a range of factors that commonly emerge as being part of the repertoire of suicidal thinking, such as low self-esteem, low self-worth and helplessness. Good risk assessment, effective communication and a high level of therapeutic intervention and engagement in person-centred delivery of care are essential components of suicide prevention.

Encompassing these different behaviours in nursing practice through the use of caringly vigilant and inquisitive clinical practice has shown to be life-saving. When delivering care, nurses should trust their instincts and follow this up if they feel a patient is at risk. Nurses should be observant and understand subtle cues of a patient's distress, an understanding which can only be developed by getting to know them and building the therapeutic relationship.

There has been a reduction in the numbers of people completing suicide on inpatient wards, but more needs to be done in other care settings. Most individuals who take their life by suicide are not known to mental health services and the challenge remains how to engage this section of the population.

References

1. Cutcliffe JR, Stevenson C, Jackson S, Smith P. Reconnecting the person with humanity. *Crisis: the Journal of Crisis Intervention and Suicide Prevention* 2007; **28**(4): 207–10.
2. Bowers L, Banda T, Nijman H. Suicide inside: a systematic review of inpatient suicides. *Journal of Nervous and Mental Disease* 2010; **198**(5): 315–28.
3. Department of Health. *Safety first. Five-year report of the National Confidential Inquiry into Suicide and Homicide by People with Mental Illness.* London: Department of Health, 2001.
4. National Confidential Inquiry into Suicide and Homicide by People with Mental Illness. *Annual report 2013: England, Northern Ireland, Scotland, Wales.* Manchester: University of Manchester, 2013. Available from: http://research.bmh.manchester.ac.uk/cmhs/research/centreforsuicideprevention/nci/reports/ [Accessed 20th September 2016].
5. Bowers L, Dack C, Gul N, Thomas B, James K. Learning from prevented suicide in psychiatric inpatient care: an analysis of data from the National Patient Safety Agency. *International Journal of Nursing Studies* 2011; **48**(12):1459–65.
6. Hawton K, van Heeringen K. Suicide. *Lancet* 2009; **373**: 1372–81.
7. Bickley H, Hunt IM, Windfuhr K, Shaw J, Appleby L, Kapur N. Suicide within two weeks of discharge from psychiatric inpatient care: a case-control study. *Psychiatric Services* 2013; **64**: 653–9.
8. Hunt IM, Bickley H, Windfuhr K, Shaw J, Appleby L, Kapur N. Suicide in recently admitted psychiatric in-patients: a case-control study. *Journal of Affective Disorders* 2013; **144**: 123–8.
9. National Confidential Inquiry into Suicide and Homicide by People with Mental Illness. *Quality of risk assessment report.* Manchester: University of Manchester, 2013. Available from: http://www.bbmh.manchester.ac.uk/cmhr/research/centreforsuicideprevention/nci/reports/RiskAssessmentfullreport2013.pdf [Accessed 23rd May 2016].
10. While D, Bickley H, Roscoe A, Windfuhr K, Rahman S, Shaw J, Appleby L, Kapur N. Implementation of mental health service recommendations in England and Wales and suicide rates, 1997–2006: a cross-sectional and before-and-after observational study. *Lancet* 2012; **379**(9820): 1005–12.
11. National Confidential Inquiry into Suicide and Homicide by People with Mental Illness (NCISH). *Patient suicide: the impact of service changes. A UK wide study.* Manchester: University of Manchester, 2013. Available from: http://www.bbmh.manchester.ac.uk/cmhr/research/centreforsuicideprevention/nci/reports/impact_of_service_changes.pdf [Accessed 20th September 2016].
12. National Confidential Inquiry into Suicide and Homicide by People with Mental Illness (NCISH). Suicide in primary care in England: 2002–2011. Manchester: University of Manchester, 2014. Available from: http://www.bbmh.manchester.ac.uk/cmhr/research/centreforsuicideprevention/nci/reports/SuicideinPrimaryCare2014.pdf [Accessed 23rd May 2016].
13. National Institute for Health and Care Excellence (NICE). *Self-harm: longer term management.* NICE clinical guideline (CG) 133. 2011. Available from: https://www.nice.org.uk/guidance/cg133 [Accessed 20th September 2016].
14. Da Cruz D, Pearson A, Saini P, Miles C, While D, Swinson N, Williams A, Shaw J, Appleby L, Kapur N. Emergency department contact prior to suicide in mental health patients. *Emergency Medicine Journal* 2011; **28**: 467–71.

Further reading

Department of Health. *Preventing suicide in England: a cross-government outcomes strategy to save lives.* London: Department of Health, 2012. Available from: https://www.gov.uk/government/uploads/system/uploads/attachment_data/file/216929/Final-assessment-of-impact-on-equalities.pdf [Accessed 26th November 2016]

NPSA (National Patient Safety Agency). *Preventing suicide: a toolkit for community mental health* (2011). Available from: http://www.nhsconfed.org/~/media/Confederation/Files/public%20access/Toolkit for community mental health.pdf [Accessed 26th November 2016]
This focuses on improving care pathways and follow-up for people who present at emergency departments following self-harm or suicidal behaviour and those who present at GP surgeries and are identified as at risk of self-harm or suicide.

Relevant web pages

National CAMHS Support Service. *Self-harm in children and young people handbook.* www.chimat.org.uk/resource/view.aspx?RID=105602

This provides basic information about self-harm in children and young people, with advice about ways staff in children's services can respond.

NHS Health and Wellbeing Improvement Framework. https://www.gov.uk/government/uploads/system/uploads/attachment_data/file/216380/dh_128813.pdf
Published in 2011, this is a tool for decision makers on boards, to support them in establishing a culture that promotes staff health and well-being.

National Confidential Inquiry into Suicide and Homicide by People with a Mental Illness. www.medicine.manchester.ac.uk/suicideprevention/nci
The National Confidential Inquiry into Suicide and Homicide by People with a Mental Illness provides regular reports on patient suicides and up-to-date statistical data. These reports highlight and make recommendations where clinical practice and service delivery can be improved to prevent suicide and reduce risk.

RCP (Royal College of Psychiatrists). Depression in older people. http://www.rcpsych.ac.uk/healthadvice/problemsdisorders/depressioninolderadults.aspx

Samaritans. Engaging the rail industry in suicide prevention and support. http://www.samaritans.org/for-business/rail-suicide-prevention/engaging-rail
Samaritans and Network Rail have established a joint, 5-year training, communications and outreach programme. Through joint working with partners including train operators and the British Transport Police, they aim to reduce suicides on the national rail network by 20 per cent. The project was launched in January 2010 and is initially focused on those stations most affected by suicide.

Support After Suicide Partnership (SASP). Help is at hand. http://www.supportaftersuicide.org.uk/help-is-at-hand
This is a resource to support people who have been bereaved or affected by suicide.

The person experiencing schizophrenia

JANET WOOD, NIALL McLAUGHLIN AND WARWICK OWEN

LEARNING OUTCOMES

- To be able to reflect on the service user's experience of psychosis to promote person-centred practice.
- To understand the impact of stress, trauma and implications for psychosocial intervention.
- To be aware of methods for engaging and working in creative ways with service users towards recovery to promote social inclusion.
- To be able to examine and practise strategies for service user self-management and building resilience.

SUMMARY OF KEY POINTS

- The craft of caring for the person experiencing schizophrenia involves joining them on a journey from illness to recovery – offering safety, validation, optimism and practical support.
- Joining them on that journey requires empathy, and

this can be located in the carer's own experiences and reactions to life events.

- Remaining strong enough to maintain empathy depends on the ability to use reflection and supervision skilfully.

INTRODUCTION

The defining characteristic of the craftsperson is that they work to the specification of the recipient of their work and the value of their work is primarily determined by that person.[1] However, the experience of schizophrenia can take people to a place where what they say they want, at their moment of greatest need, may differ greatly from what they would say was best for them if they were asked the question at a different time. So when we practise our craft as nurses with people experiencing a psychotic illness, how do we

know what they would have wanted and whether it is valid to progress on that basis?

Britain Thinks[2] represents the aspirations of Britain's 14- to 18-year-olds, and they reflect Maslow's hierarchy of needs in their prioritization of financial, emotional and domestic security. This survey also reveals a very pragmatic and realistic assessment by its subjects of the chances that mental illness will be a feature of their lives and that this will be an obstacle to attainment of their goals. Of those surveyed, 23 per cent believed that mental health problems were likely to be a feature of their lives and 65 per cent believed that these would pose a major obstacle to their attainment of personal aspirations. This may well reflect what they have already experienced in their own families – a parent, sibling, aunt or uncle whose independence, career progress or relationships have been stalled or disrupted by a 'breakdown'.

Nurses can be confident that in supporting service users to progress towards a feeling of security by the skilful deployment of time, optimism and compassion, across all practice contexts and diagnoses, that they will be perceived by beneficiaries of their craft as 'good nurses'.[3]

So, we have the concept of the 'good nurse' and we have the concept of youthful hope as vulnerable to catastrophic illness. Anyone who has suffered a cold or a stomach bug will recall that to wake up today with the same symptoms as yesterday is a demoralizing experience – even if we do not think that our futures are being taken away. Our young people may not themselves want fame and fortune, but currently there are celebrities who self-identify as being prone to depression or bipolar disorder, and this may offer some mitigation of their fears about these illnesses. There is little equivalent mitigating evidence to be found in the cultural representations of schizophrenia in the media that might challenge, rather than reinforce, catastrophic interpretations of this experience.

More work for the 'good nurse' to do, then. Thankfully we can be confident about what this nurse *is*, but what, specifically, when meeting a person experiencing psychosis or schizophrenia, are they to *do*?

Skilled practice of a craft involves creative use of tools which are refined by empirical evidence. If we can be confident that supporting people towards meeting baseline Maslowian needs is consistent with societal norms and expectations, and with patients' expectations of health care situations, then there need be no obstacle to using an evidence-based application to promote sustainable recovery. However, if we accept the proposition that a realistic appraisal of the difficulty of the recovery process is further compounded by personal experience, stigma and cultural representations, Lao Tzu's saying 'a journey of a thousand miles begins with a single step' becomes more of an omen than an inspiration. It would seem reasonable then that anyone who found even that first step challenging might prioritize other means of covering the distance. This is perhaps why a person overwhelmed by debt might buy a lottery ticket with their last pound rather than put it in a piggy bank. So the craft of the 'good nurse', in this context, is in synthesizing positive 'artistic' engagement orientated towards self-actualization with evidence-based (scientific) interventions that promote incremental and sustainable recovery. (See chapter 5 for more on recovery.)

If the craft of nursing combines the art of validating the dream of the thousand-mile journey and the science in enabling the first step, how better to inspire the traveller than to introduce them to someone who has already made the journey?

Peer-supported recovery is an ongoing process, but it is one that begins with a crisis which often triggers a profound reassessment by the service user of what an actualized self might be. This identity can only be expressed if we work in a person-centred way by understanding the service user's perspective on their situation. (See 'Further reading' for additional resources.)

SERVICE USERS' EXPERIENCES OF PSYCHOSIS AND SCHIZOPHRENIA

The concept of schizophrenia, with its roots in the medical model, is one that has been contested by psychologists,[4,5] sociologists[6,7] and service users. The person's experiences, such as voice hearing and unusual thoughts, frequently attributed to signs of schizophrenia, can in fact be interpreted from a range of perspectives by both professionals and the person themselves. For example, voice hearing may be explained as a sign of illness, telepathy, externalized thoughts or a religious experience. This range of perspectives can lead to confusion when people access mental health services and potentially creates barriers to engagement and development of the therapeutic alliance, considered crucial as a prerequisite to collaborative assessment and intervention. In this context, it can be seen that a broad-based approach is required that can encompass and acknowledge these perspectives.

> ### REFLECTION
>
> Think about someone you know or have worked with.
>
> - Do they have a definite diagnosis and, if so, how was it arrived at?
>
> - What terms are used by this person and others in relation to the diagnosis (such as 'schizophrenia/schizophrenic' or 'psychosis/psychotic')? Why might different words be used by different people for the same condition?

A specific diagnosis of, for instance, paranoid schizophrenia is often arrived at gradually. See chapter 12 for more on the classification of mental illness. First and early episodes are treated in accordance with the National Institute for Health and Care Excellence (NICE) 2014 guidelines[8] under the broader category of psychosis. It emerges from Warwick's story that he recognizes that he was given a diagnosis of paranoid schizophrenia, but he describes his experience as being of psychosis.

After my first breakdown at the age of 21, I was very compliant with what everyone told me to do. I was meeting my consultant regularly and checking out what I was allowed to do, but by the age of 25, inside I saw myself as being a young man who was able to be independent and manage my own life. So I stopped taking my medication and I eventually became more psychotic again.

Psychosis is unique to the individual. From my personal experiences of psychosis this can differ according to the trigger, mood or social situation.

1. *Trigger.* I may have managed my triggers for a long period of time; then a trigger, such as an old disagreement or misunderstanding, may cause me to get upset and then worry about the outcome.
2. *Mood.* A sensible active daily routine promotes good mental health. However, it's only human nature to want to escape this routine. In the case of psychosis this 'escape' may not be temporary and may suppress the previous good mood.
3. *Social situation.* There may be a disagreement, and if I am right, the other person may play on it and use my diagnosis as a method to convince others they are right. This may trigger/cause me to be embarrassed, which could have been otherwise avoided.

Psychosis occurs when I temporarily alter to a situation and feel out of character. When this repeatedly happens, it's time to seek help, as I am no longer my true self, as the ego has taken over.

REFLECTION

- How has the understanding of schizophrenia evolved historically as a phenomenon?
- Disclosure – what is it like to tell other people about your schizophrenia?
- Can the side effects of medication be worse than the symptoms of the illness?

Mental health nursing has traditionally taken a view of the whole person within the holistic model most commonly aspired to in practice.[9] In more recent years, mental health nursing has moved further towards psychosocial models, influenced by initiatives such as the Thorn Programme, and this has been a comfortable 'fit' with more traditional holistic approaches to practice. In addition to this, key psychosocial frameworks, such as that offered by the stress vulnerability model,[10] are sufficiently broad-based to take into account a range of perspectives on the person's experience of mental health problems, and importantly that of the person themselves.

WARWICK'S STORY: WHAT'S GOOD AND BAD ABOUT THE STRESS VULNERABILITY MODEL

I have had the opportunity to talk with other professionals, students and service users about the stress vulnerability model and how it relates to my personal narrative.

1. *Helpfulness.* The stress vulnerability model illustrates that the more stress someone is experiencing, the more vulnerable they become.
2. *Confidence.* Using the stress vulnerability model has given me the confidence to be open about the stress I experienced, when I was vulnerable to mental illness.
3. *Limitations.* As with any good model there are limitations. There is a lot of information to take in at once. However, for a service user who wants to learn about their personal psychosis, this provides plenty to discuss.

Warwick's story reveals that he was experiencing psychosis for the first time while his identity as a young person was being formed. Key moments in the emerging identity are expressed through the relationships that are formed within the institutional structures of services.

REFLECTION

Warwick's experience of psychosis, as described above, positions psychosis as a crisis of identity. What have been the key factors in the emergence of your identity – life events, rites of passage, family membership, social, professional or educational institutions?

The updated NICE guidelines[8] continue to support the use of psychosocial therapies, including cognitive behavioural therapy (CBT) and behavioural family therapy (BFT), for people experiencing psychosis and associated emotional problems. In addition to these, there is more emphasis on physical health monitoring, healthy eating and physical activity programmes, supported employment programmes, smoking cessation support, peer support and self-management. (See chapter 69 for more on physical health care.)

However, the issue of access to more specific psychological therapies such as CBT is a 'thorny' one, with the Schizophrenia Commission Report[11] finding that people experiencing psychosis either had not been offered this therapy or were faced with long waiting lists. A shortage of suitably trained CBT practitioners led the Commission to recommend that more health care workers such as nurses should be competent to offer psychosocial interventions to service users and their families. Despite the National Mental Health Strategy[12] promising increased access to psychological therapies for those with psychosis, this is unlikely to become a reality unless more specialist CBT practitioners are trained for working with this population, which seems to be a development that service users would welcome.[11] (See chapter 40 for more on CBT.)

WARWICK'S STORY: THE EXPERIENCE OF PSYCHOSIS

I enjoyed socializing with my friends. It is a big part of my life. I have a big social group and am close to a few of its members. Dad had recently passed away and we had moved to a smaller place nearer mum's work. When I say 'we', I mean mum, my younger brother Adam and myself. This move was convenient for me as I was nearer my friends.

There were a few girls I fancied, although I am currently single. I spend most of my time going to college, hanging out, or smoking cannabis. I know it's wrong but it makes me feel happy. Sometimes I want to stop smoking it, but there is always some about.

I am sure smoking cannabis gives me strange thoughts and feelings of grandeur. I also experience lows when I am not smoking it. I sometimes get quite angry and moody, especially with mum. She doesn't mind so much, but wishes I would talk to her about my problems.

Mum and I have always got on and are quite close. When dad passed away I felt guilty as I had not done that well in school and was still dependent on her. I knew she was upset about dad although we never spoke about it. Mum enjoyed her job; she is a manageress in a high street shop. Although the job is stressful, mum still finds time to look after me. The house is always tidy and dinner is always ready in the evenings. I do feel guilty as when mum's at work I don't get much college work done. I always attend college, but it's more to see my friends. I also feel guilty when I am smoking cannabis at college with my friends and mum is stuck at work.

Adam attends the same college as me, although he is attending a different course. As I did not do that well at school, I had limited choices and chose to take a science class. I want to be a lab technician when I leave college. Since I have been smoking cannabis I find it difficult to concentrate in class and never get any homework done.

I eventually finished college, although I did not have any certificates to prove this. Although I had attended the course and passed my exams, I had not produced a written portfolio of evidence. You were supposed to work on your portfolio in study time and at home. The idea was to add, little but often, to your portfolio, over the 3 years you were at college. At the end of the course the portfolio was supposed to count towards 60 per cent of my final grade.

I now had no prospects and a cannabis habit. This was depressing, and upsetting. I soon became withdrawn from my friends and began to experience psychosis. The stress of everyday life began to get to me. Although I still lived at home with mum, I had no money as I was not working. Mum said she would look after me but she would not pay for my social life. I had to find a job for that.

I became extremely vulnerable as I had no means of self-support or independence. I tried a few part-time jobs. None of them worked out, as the more money I had, the more cannabis I would buy. I would eventually continually be late for work or just not turn up. My addiction had got the better of me and my mental health was suffering.

Eventually mum asked me to go down the job centre and sign on. At least I had some income and the prospects of finding a job. I had to attend the job centre every 2 weeks to sign on. Having money was good but I was bored. All my friends now work for a living. I found this depressing, especially as some of them had quite good jobs. Adam is now working in London as a trainee stockbroker. Sam, my friend from college, does work in London, but his job pays well. He works in banking. I sometimes get depressed when I think about how they are enjoying their lifestyles and I am stuck at home in front of the telly.

I only blame myself and sometimes get psychotic. I never talk about it with mum but wish I could stop smoking cannabis, go back to college and turn my life around. I talked to Adam about this and he must have told mum as she arranged for me to meet a councillor. This was a help as I had someone to talk to.

PERSON-CENTRED CARE THROUGH PSYCHOSOCIAL INTERVENTIONS

According to NICE,[8] the aims of psychosocial interventions in psychosis are numerous, and include interventions to improve symptoms, but also to address vulnerability embedded in developmental processes. The aims therefore include: reduction of distress associated with psychosis experiences; promoting social and educational recovery; reducing depression and social anxiety; and preventing relapse. Interventions aimed at reducing vulnerability and promoting resilience are also likely to require a reduction in substance and alcohol misuse (for more information see chapter 31), promotion of social stability including family support, and dealing with the consequences of insecure attachment formation.

A bio-psychosocial approach is exemplified by the stress vulnerability model, but it is how this is used with service users that enables the person-centred approach in psychosocial interventions. The key skills of demonstrating active listening, empathic understanding, flexibility, collaboration and a Socratic questioning style enable the practitioner to work with psychosocial models and tools in a manner that is both respectful and curious about the person's 'story'. This includes the person's experiences, beliefs and understandings about their current and past circumstances. The use of a Timeline[13] to 'look back', alongside the stress vulnerability model, encourages the person to 'tell their story' in their own words from their perspective. This can promote engagement with the person and support information gathering (assessment) around current and past stressors, coping strategies used, early warning signs of mental health problems and strengths. Making use of the stress vulnerability model and Timeline in this manner can help to 'normalize' and 'de-catastrophize'[14] the experience of psychosis with the service user and their family, to reduce distress and address concerns generated by social stigma.[15–17]

WARWICK'S STORY: STARTING THE JOURNEY TO RECOVERY

I was referred on to a consultant psychiatrist as the counsellor recommended that I needed more therapy. I was diagnosed with paranoid schizophrenia, probably triggered by the life event of dad passing away, then progressed through regular use of cannabis.

My journey to recovery had started and I was now receiving professional help. I could see that mum was not so worried about me as she now also had someone to phone if I became psychotic. When I became psychotic, I would smash windows, slam doors until they broke or punch the walls.

Speaking to a professional helped me to put my life into perspective and review myself. My medication or the talking therapy must have worked, as it was now clear to me that one obstacle I had to overcome to get better was to give up the cannabis use. I began to cut it out until it was no longer a part of my personal life. My friends still enjoyed it but knew it was not for me.

Life is now good. I have a part-time job, the work is not glamorous as I stack bricks for a living. You know, I am so well at the moment that I don't think I need to take my medication. I will tell my consultant psychiatrist that I am still taking them and she will never know the difference.

Two months later, nobody had realized I was not taking medication. I thought: this is the ideal time to move on in my life. I began to think about what I could do with my spare time. I eventually packed my rucksack and headed off on the train to London. It's about an hour from where I live. I said goodbye to mum and left. She did not know I had one of her credit cards.

TRAUMA AND PSYCHOSIS

The impact of stress and trauma on the development of psychosis is an area of growing interest in the current literature[18] and is highlighted in the NICE guidelines.[8] It has been found that most individuals diagnosed with a psychotic episode also meet the criteria for post-traumatic stress disorder (PTSD). Despite this, trauma from both previous life events including physical or sexual assault,[19,20] the experiences of psychosis itself (distressing voices, beliefs and frightening treatment experiences) and PTSD symptoms are rarely recognized in services.[21,18,22,23] Additional types of trauma identified in people experiencing psychotic episodes can arise from current and past life experiences, such as military combat, experiences of serious accidents and disasters[21,18] and, more recently, cyber-bullying in young people.[24] Given this situation, it would be reasonable to assume that mental health practitioners including nurses would be equipped with the knowledge and skills to address this with clients and their families. However, the evidence suggests that there are barriers to mental health practitioners obtaining and following up on information about a client's trauma history, in terms of both skill and comfort levels.[25]

This issue is addressed by Putts,[25] who emphasizes the importance of establishing a 'rapport and a positive therapeutic alliance' (p.87) when conducting an effective clinical interview. More information on developing and maintaining therapeutic relationships can be found in chapter 3. This is so that ethical and safeguarding issues that may arise can be addressed with the client. In addition, it is so that specific types of information can be obtained, such as frequency of the startle response and nightmares; pre- and post-trauma functioning as a baseline for understanding the impact of trauma; client resiliency and coping methods; response to trauma; ongoing beliefs about the traumatic event (e.g. shame, responsibility, ongoing fear for safety); and social supports. An awareness of these specific types of information and the sort of questioning (Socratic) used to elicit it, in a sensitive and person-centred manner, can be integrated into the practitioner's work through use of the Timeline method, as previously discussed. As Putts points out, 'all clients should receive an assessment for trauma and PTSD following any psychotic episode, particularly with regard to the symptoms and treatment experiences of the psychosis itself'[25] (p.87). Indeed, despite another barrier to this work being cited as practitioners 'not believing the client', individuals appear to be accurate in reporting whether they have experienced a traumatic event and the impact of this.[26] Being open, curious and receptive to clients' experiences is a fundamental underpinning principle in psychosocial intervention work. This therapeutic style, used alongside the Timeline and stress vulnerability model, could be both engaging for the person and productive in trauma and PTSD assessment with those experiencing psychosis. Refer to chapters 13, 14 and 15 for further discussion on assessment.

As evidence that supports the association between traumatic life experience and psychotic states emerges, there have been questions about how these two phenomena are linked. Taking a psychological perspective, Morrison et al.[27] argue that both PTSD and psychosis are characterized by 'intrusions into awareness' (thoughts, images, impulses), and that the subsequent interpretation of these intrusions (flashbacks/hallucinations) leads to distress and avoidance. This highlights similarities between cognitive models of psychosis and PTSD. In a study testing this, Kilcommons and Morrison[28] found that negative appraisals (about the self) were associated with some psychotic experiences, especially hallucinations. These authors support the view that the beliefs people form as a result of trauma may lead to these individuals having an increased vulnerability to the development of psychosis. They tentatively conclude that findings support a view that trauma can lead to psychotic experiences, and that both PTSD and psychosis may be part of 'a spectrum of responses to a traumatic event' (p.357). The under-detection of PTSD in those with psychosis can mean it is untreated, and has a negative impact on the course of the psychosis – for example, by increasing the person's vulnerability to substance misuse. In addition, PTSD-related avoidance is likely to contribute to social isolation and loss of social support, thus increasing vulnerability to psychotic relapse. This association then between psychosis and PTSD is one that increases a person's vulnerability to both development and maintenance of psychosis if not detected. The authors recommend asking about post-trauma-related beliefs during the assessment process. NICE 2014 guidance cites some evidence for 'trauma re-processing therapy', a specific CBT-focused intervention. NICE recommends more research trials to look at these interventions and to target these towards those experiencing traumatic intrusions following a first episode of psychosis.

Specific screening tools can also be useful, but when PTSD is not the primary presenting problem, there is limited research to indicate which screening tools for PTSD symptoms could be used. The PCL-5, a self-report screening tool for PTSD,[29] has been used with psychosis, although some modifications have been made to this.[30,31] Using a screening tool alongside other methods of gathering information, such as the Timeline, could improve the recognition of PTSD in people presenting with psychosis.

While these psychological interventions require specific competencies and training as a CBT practitioner to implement them, it does open the way for thinking about the implications of this for other mental health practitioners working with people experiencing psychosis across a range of services.

In a literature review, key principles of trauma informed care are identified as:

Clients need to feel connected, feel valued, informed and hopeful of recovery; the connection between childhood trauma and adult psychopathology is known and understood by all staff; and staff work in mindful and empowering ways with individuals, family and friends, and other social services agencies to promote and protect the autonomy of that individual.[32] (p.52)

In this review, Walsh and Boyle indicate that many practices, such as ward rounds, search procedures, locked doors, mixed-sex populations and the use of seclusion and restraint, are re-traumatizing and are experienced by consumers as emotionally unsafe and disempowering (refer to chapter 25 for considerations of how to care for and support the person who is extremely distressed and disturbed).[33] To counter this, these authors see trauma-informed services as not just treating symptoms or syndromes related to trauma, but services where staff are aware of and sensitive to doing no further harm to survivors of trauma. They argue that 'the intent to do no further harm must drive a continued discourse for acute in-patient staff in trauma-informed care'[32] (p.58).

The DSM-5[34] distinguishes between schizophrenia and PTSD for the purposes of diagnosis thus: '[PTSD] may include flashbacks that have a hallucinatory quality and hypervigilance may reach paranoid proportions. But a [known] traumatic event of characteristic features relating to reliving or reacting to the event are required to make the diagnosis' (p.105). More detail on the classification of mental illness can be found in chapter 12.

REFLECTION

Devise your own timeline. Is there a key moment when your life could have taken a different course? Perhaps your subject choices at school? What might your life be like if you had chosen or acted differently? Were you able to make independent, informed choices or did you feel influenced by others?

WARWICK'S STORY: LEARNING FROM MY MISTAKES

London is fun, but mum's card isn't. I bought my train ticket, went out for dinner, got drunk and the money ran out. I only bought a single train ticket and cannot get home. I tried booking a room for the night but my card kept on getting declined. I felt extremely vulnerable and became psychotic. I did not want to phone mum. I instead slept rough in a park and decided to make it for myself in the morning.

When I woke up, I became delusional and believed I had some more money on mum's card. I headed off down to the nearest off-licence to buy some snacks for breakfast. I also fancied a drink. There was some money on mum's card, but only what little was left from last night. I did get some breakfast and a bottle of vodka mixed with lemonade. Although the vodka was not neat, the bottle was quite generously sized and I was soon wandering around drunk.

I had relapsed and needed a psychiatrist and to get back on my medication but was oblivious to this. I wandered into a park and hid behind a bush. I could see what people were doing but thought they could not see me. I was eventually arrested for exposing myself in public.

I spent some time in a secure unit until I was taken to the psychiatric ward at my local hospital. Medication and therapy soon moved me in a forward direction on my journey to recovery. Although I was well again, I once again had nothing to do with my spare time. My care coordinator suggested I joined a Buddy Scheme, where I would have the opportunity to get paid for telling students my story. Although this was embarrassing, it gave me some pocket money.

I learnt by my mistakes and realized that medication is an important part of recovery and my daily routine. I get on well with my care coordinator and am happy to be well again. I understand that recovery is a journey and although it is uphill, as long as I keep trying, I will eventually go further forwards than I go backwards when I am unwell.

My future looks OK now. I am still involved with the Buddy Scheme and share my narrative and experiences, and lecture on the lived experience at my local university. My future aim is to make the most of the support I have and to eventually use my portfolio to work as a service user consultant.

WORKING IN CREATIVE WAYS WITH SERVICE USERS TOWARDS RECOVERY

WARWICK'S STORY: FAME AND RECOVERY

When we are at school, we all dream of fame. Being a service user doesn't mean I have not achieved this. It means I have a chance to set realistic aims or goals for myself.

1. *Living the dream*. Using mental health services doesn't mean I can't achieve my dream or goal.
2. *Being realistic*. Being a service user gave me the opportunity to be realistic and achieve a goal rather than no goal at all.

3. *Success*. I currently belong to a service user panel at my local university.

Fame is important, but as we get older and know ourselves better, we understand that success, or in the case of mental illness recovery, is more important than fame. (See chapter 35 for more on recovery.)

CREATIVE ARTS THERAPIES

In order to improve the treatment of schizophrenia and psychosis, new and creative interventions are required. NICE 2014 guidelines recommend that creative therapies, including art therapy, dance movement and body psychotherapy, music therapy and drama therapy, should be made available, in particular for the alleviation of negative symptoms. The arts therapies are complex interventions, predominantly emphasizing expression, communication, social connection and self-awareness through supportive interaction. (See chapter 3 for more on therapeutic interaction.) Here we will focus on dance movement psychotherapy and singing for health, as there are interesting developments in the evidence base for these which have implications for mental health practice.

Dance movement psychotherapy

Dance movement psychotherapy has been defined as:

> *an implicit and expressive instrument of communication and expression. Dance Movement Psychotherapy is a relational process in which clients and therapist engage creatively using body movement and dance to assist in the integration process of emotional, physical, social and spiritual aspects of self.*[35]

The approach of dance movement psychotherapy (DMP) and body psychotherapy (BPT) works on the assumption that movement and emotional experiences are biologically and experientially associated.[36] It has long been the case that rhythmic music and dance has been associated with emotional expression and the medium for connectedness with others – from tribal and cultural dance to marching into war. The role of 'mirror neurones' in empathy[37–39] demonstrates that identical sets of neurones can be activated in both parties, as someone witnesses another performing a movement, in terms of expression, emotion or behaviour. This is the basis for understanding the therapeutic processes that occur between a dance movement practitioner and a service user. This empathic reflection or 'mirroring' has been associated with the work of Marion Chase, a dancer and choreographer who used music to stimulate rhythmic synchrony as an outlet for personal expression and re-connection with the world.[40] Chase worked with clients experiencing mental distress in American state psychiatric hospitals in the 1940s, and recognized that tensions and distortions of the body are reflections of traumatic experiences.

There is growing evidence of the efficacy of this therapy for people experiencing emotional withdrawal, blunting of emotions and motor retardation. In one small trial,[36] outpatients with schizophrenia receiving BPT were compared with a matched group receiving a supportive counselling intervention. The service users receiving BPT attended more sessions and had significantly lower negative symptoms than the supportive counselling group. These differences remained at 4-month follow-up. This limited evidence has resulted in a follow-up multi-site trial to test the effectiveness of a manualized BPT intervention group against a control group receiving Pilates.[41] The outcomes of this trial are awaiting publication, but if it shows that BPT and DMP are effective in reducing negative symptoms, it could result in the roll-out of this therapy to service users experiencing psychosis.

Singing for health

The link between music, singing, health and well-being has been explored,[42] and there is a growing evidence base focused on the benefits of choral singing for health and well-being.[43–46] Evidence from a cross-national survey[45] of 1,124 participants from England, Germany and Australia found a 'high degree of consensus' on the positive benefits of choral singing on mood, focused attention promoting relaxation, relief from stress, controlled breathing, social support, cognitive stimulation and motivation. In this study, enduring mental health problems were the most commonly expressed challenge, and singing was described by participants as helpful in the process of recovery.

A follow-up study on the impact of group singing for people with mental health problems was undertaken by Clift and Morrison,[46] using a validated measure of mental distress (CORE-OM Questionnaire) with 42 participants. They found a 'moderate effect' in terms of overall improvement, but significant improvements in dimensions of well-being, problems and functioning. Participants also felt less troubled by negative thoughts and feelings, suggesting that a focus on singing provided distraction from otherwise troubling areas. Interestingly, there was also an improved sense of future orientation. These items are critical in terms of moving forward towards recovery from severe mental health distress. The participants of this research were a community group called the Mustard Seed Singers, who met on a regular basis to sing together, give public performances and be part of a network of seven singing groups. This community innovation is just another example for mental health practitioners of how creative and arts therapies are developing an evidence base showing that these approaches and interventions have significant benefits for mental health service users.

CRISIS RESOURCE MAPPING AND BUILDING SELF-MANAGEMENT

WARWICK'S STORY: RELAPSE

Relapse is a thing that I am aware of. I'll recognize the signs when I begin to stray from my normal routine and when I'm drifting away from the commitments I have to other people. If I have a bad day, I rearrange my activities so that I don't overdo it.

REFLECTION

Think about a crisis or a moment of high stress in your own life.

- Could it have been avoided or minimized if you had discussed a problem with someone beforehand?

- Did you learn something about your own strengths and capabilities?

- Have your thoughts or behaviour changed in some way because of it?

- Did you learn something about the people around you?

This chapter has been aimed at offering the nurse working with a person who is experiencing schizophrenia a conceptual framework, within which a range of resources can be drawn upon to support the person's recovery. The framework needs to be robust for a changing service provision context, and so it was proposed that service users might perceive 'good' nursing as non-judgemental, optimistic and supportive of self-management, regardless of context. The evidence base deployed supports a conceptual framework in which trauma (stress) has interacted with identity to generate an experience of psychosis. All three elements – the trauma, the identity and the illness experience – need to be engaged with, and all three are responsive to creative and psychosocial therapies. The mental health nurse in this model will continue to occupy an ambiguous role – sometimes therapist, sometimes gatekeeper – and requires the skills of reflection to act optimally in both roles. There is a third aspect to the nurse's role which is crucial in the therapeutic alliance: the nurse is one of the key people holding the safety net.

The key question about a safety net might be expressed as: 'Will it break my fall?'

Figures 24.1, 24.2 and 24.3 provide tools for addressing these questions.[47]

Figure 24.1 is a list of 'difficult questions', which nurses can use to reflect on those interactions with a service user in whom a crisis is an overtly or subliminally perceived risk. The list of things is potentially endless, but the reasons for them not being expressed by the service user are most likely to be focused around either a (mis)calculation of the cost of telling versus the cost of not telling, or variations in the service user's awareness of or insight into them.

Figure 24.2, the crisis contract, is similarly a suggestion of how a nurse might approach an issue. Any such contract would need to be approved under local policy.

Figure 24.3, the resource map, is a response to the idea that both the nurse and the person experiencing the crisis can find it difficult to identify the elements of recovery in the crisis.

What am I not being told?	Why am I not being told it?	What can I do to make telling me possible?	What shouldn't I do?
I'm in debt			
I'm back on drugs			
I'm in pain			
My neighbours are harassing me			
Sexual problems			
I'm not taking my medication			
I've broken the law			
Hearing voices			
Abuse perpetrator/victim			
Embarrassing body			
Can't read			

Figure 24.1 Difficult questions.

I am bound by law, policy and professional code to act in your best interest and maintain confidentiality.

You can be dependent on me for some things and also upon others around you.

I will:

- be available
    - at this time ....
    - at this place ....
    - in this way ....
- listen without judgement to what you say
- make an accurate record of events
- act to minimize the number of new people to whom you have to explain everything
- say things that are difficult for me to say and for you to hear
- try your way first
- let you know what the likely outcomes are when making decisions
- advocate the minimum effective use of sedation, deprivation of liberty and loss of dignity
- only involve friends, family, colleagues if you agree
- show you the evidence ...

Signed and dated..

Figure 24.2 Crisis contract.

This is not a crisis rating scale. It is to show what resources there are and how they could be boosted. The higher the score, the greater the depth and range of resources the person has. However, this does not mean the crisis or the risk is any less. Please use approved tools to assess risk.

Date	Rate how much you agree with the following; 1 = Totally disagree 5 = Totally agree	Score 1–5	Comments (what will improve the score)
Personal:	I thrive on adversity		
	I help others when they are in trouble		
	I always bounce back		
	Deep down I'm a strong person		
	I've been here before and recovered		
Social:	I have a lot of good people around me		
	I can identify x number of communities that I belong to		
	I have a clear sense of purpose in my life		
	There are other people in my life who are more important to me than I am		
Cultural:	I have a set of values and I know where they come from		
	There are things I do that make me feel like I belong		
	There are books, music, films that make me feel better (or not alone)		
Professional:	I know who the professionals are who are supporting me, what they do and how to get hold of them (leadership)		
Chemical:	I know what I'm taking, when and why		
	It makes me feel better		
	I can be honest about taking/not taking		

Figure 24.3 Resource map.

CONCLUSION

The tools shown in Figures 24.1, 24.2 and 24.3 address multiple functions – risk management, yes, but also triggers for reflection and means of gathering information – and all have honesty in the therapeutic relationship as a central value. Honesty includes acknowledging the limits of that relationship. A safety net held by just one person is not of great help in any case, and so other, different kinds of relationship will have to be fostered. This potentially is where peer support workers, as suggested in the introduction, are beginning to offer a way forward.

NICE[8] guidelines strongly advocate the inclusion of peer support in service provision that is directed towards service user self-management (while acknowledging the limits of the evidence base at present), and it is certainly consistent with the ethos of this chapter.

Again, the nurse may be a conduit to peer support, although it is increasingly offered within mental health trusts. The types of support offered may include:

- facilitated peer support (where a nurse or others supervise a group which includes the lived experience of others);

- peer-facilitated support (similar to the above, but led by a trained peer support worker);

- buddying/befriending;

- peer mentoring in living skills.

The nurse can enable the peer role by offering supervision to the peer; accessing resources, such as rooms, money or equipment; providing information (with consent) on the service user's situation; safeguarding and lone-working support; identifying an evidence base to support interventions; and helping to open and close the relationship and maintain boundaries within it.

The existence of peer support workers in mental health services is in itself one of the key therapeutic interventions – they are a physical manifestation of the possibility of recovery and self-efficacy. They will walk alongside the first-time traveller, and their very presence proves that the journey can be completed. They are also evidence that some of the values that underpin service provision have been fundamentally changed.

References

1. Barker P. *Psychiatric and mental health nursing: the craft of caring*, 2nd edn. Boca Raton: Arnold, 2009.
2. Britain Thinks. (Ex)aspiration nation. 2013. Available from: http://britainthinks.com/sites/default/files/090713%20Aspiration%20Report%20FINAL%202.pdf [Accessed 30th June 2016].
3. Bee P, Playle J, Lovell K, Barnes P, Gray R, Keeley P. Service user views and expectations of UK-registered mental health nurses: a systematic review of empirical research. *International Journal of Nursing Studies* 2008; **45**: 442–57.
4. Bentall R. Abandoning the concept of schizophrenia. *British Journal of Psychology* 1988; **27**: 303–24.
5. Bentall R. *Madness explained: psychosis and human nature*. London: Penguin, 2003.
6. Rogers A, Pilgrim D. *A sociology of mental health and illness*. Maidenhead: Open University Press, 2010.
7. Romme M, Escher S. *Accepting voices*. London: Mind Publications, 1993.
8. NICE (National Institute for Clinical Excellence). *Psychosis and schizophrenia in adults: treatment and management*. Clinical Guideline 178. London: NICE, 2014.
9. Brimblecombe N, Tingle A, Tunmore R, Murrell T. Implementing holistic practices in mental health nursing: a national consultation. *International Journal of Nursing Studies* 2007; **44**(3): 339–48.
10. Zubin J, Spring B. Vulnerability; a new view of schizophrenia. *Journal of Abnormal Psychology* 1977; **86**: 103–26.
11. Schizophrenia Commission. *The abandoned illness: a report by the Schizophrenia Commission*. London: Re-Think Mental Illness, 2012.
12. DOH. *No health, without mental health: a cross government mental health strategy for people of all ages*. London: HMSO, 2011.
13. Marland R, McNay L, Flemming M, McCraig M. Using timelines in recovery-focused practice in psychosis. *Journal of Psychiatric and Mental Health Nursing* 2011; **18**(10): 869–77.
14. Dudley R, Turkington D. Using normalising in cognitive behavioural therapy for schizophrenia. In: Hagen R, Turkington D, Berge T, Grawe R (eds). *CBT for psychosis: a symptom-based approach*. London: Routledge, 2004: chapter 6.

15. Link B, Phelan J. Stigma and its public health implications. *Lancet* 2006; **367**: 528–9.
16. Angermeyer M, Matschinger H. The stigma of mental illness: effects of labelling on public attitudes towards people with mental disorder. *Acta Psychiatrica Scandinavia* 2003; **108**: 304–9.
17. French P, Hutton P, Barratt S, Parker S, Byrne R. Provision of online normalising information to reduce stigma associated with psychosis: can an audio podcast challenge negative appraisals of psychotic experiences? *Psychosis: Psychological, Social and Integrative Approaches* 2011; **3**(1): 52–62.
18. Meuser KT, Lu W, Rosenberg SD, Wolfe R. The trauma of psychosis: posttraumatic stress disorder and recent onset psychosis. *Schizophrenia Research* 2010; **116**: 217–27.
19. Van Dam DS, Van der Ven E, Velthorst, E, Selten JP, Morgan C, de Haan L. Childhood bullying and the association with psychosis in non-clinical and clinical samples: a review and meta-analysis. *Psychological Medicine* 2012; **42**: 2463–74.
20. Varese F, Smeets F, Drukker M, Lieverse R, Lataster T, Viechtbauer W, Read J, van Os J, Bentall RP. Childhood adversities increase the risk of psychosis: a meta-analysis of prospective and cross sectional cohort studies. *Schizophrenia Bulletin* 2012; **38**: 661–71.
21. Lu W, Mueser KT, Shami A, Siglag M, Petrides G, Schoepp E, Saltz J. Post-traumatic reactions to psychosis in people with multiple psychotic episodes. *Schizophrenia Research* 2011; **127**: 66–75.
22. Cusack KJ, Grubaugh AL, Knapp RG, Frueh BC. Unrecognized trauma and PTSD among public mental health consumers with chronic and severe mental illness. *Community Mental Health Journal* 2006; **42**: 487–500.
23. Read J, van Os J, Morrison AP, Ross CA. Childhood trauma, psychosis and schizophrenia; a literature review with theoretical and clinical implications. *Acta Psychiatrica Scandinavica* 2005; **112**(5): 330–50.
24. Magaud E, Nyman K, Addington J. Cyberbullying in those at clinical high risk for psychosis. *Early Intervention in Psychiatry* 2013; **7**: 427–30.

25. Putts M. Assessment and diagnosis: recognising trauma and posttraumatic stress disorder symptoms in individuals with psychotic disorders. *Journal of Counselling and Development* 2014; **92**: 83–9.

26. Goodman L, Thompson KM, Weinfurt K, Cori S, Acker P, Meuser KT, Rosenberg SD. Reliability of reports of violent victimisation and posttraumatic stress disorder among men and women with serious mental illness. *Journal of Traumatic Stress* 1999; **12**: 587–99.

27. Morrison A, Frame L, Larkin WP. Relationship between trauma and psychosis: a review and integration. *British Journal of Clinical Psychology* 2003; **43**: 331–52.

28. Kilcommons AM, Morrison AP. Relationships between trauma and psychosis: an exploration of cognitive and dissociative factors. *Acta Psychiatrica Scandinavica* 2005; **112**: 351–9.

29. National Centre for PTSD USA. PTSD checklist for DSM-5. Available from: http://www.ptsd.va.gov/professional/assessment/adult-sr/ptsd-checklist.asp [Accessed 2nd August 2016].

30. Grubaugh AL, Zinzow HM, Paul L, Egede LE, Frueh BC. Trauma exposure and posttraumatic stress disorder in adults with severe mental illness: a critical review. *Clinical Psychology Review* 2011; **31**: 883–99.

31. McDonald SD, Calhoun PS. The diagnostic accuracy of the PTSD checklist: a critical review. *Clinical Psychology Review* 2010; **30**: 976–87.

32. Muskett C. Trauma-informed care in inpatient mental health settings: a review of the literature. *International Journal of Mental Health Nursing* 2014; **23**: 51–9.

33. Walsh J, Boyle J. Improving acute psychiatric hospital services according to inpatient experiences; a user-led piece of research as a means to empowerment. *Issues in Mental Health Nursing* 2009; **30**(1): 31–8.

34. APA (American Psychiatric Association). *Diagnostic and statistical manual of mental disorders, 5th edition*. Washington, DC: APA, 2013.

35. ADMP UK (Association of Dance Movement Psychotherapy United Kingdom). Available from: http://www.admt.org.uk/contact-us/ [Accessed 30th June 2016].

36. Röhricht F, Priebe S. Effect of body-oriented psychological therapy on negative symptoms in schizophrenia: a randomized controlled trial. *Psychological Medicine* 2006; **36**: 669–78.

37. Berrol CF. Neuroscience meets dance movement psychotherapy: mirror neurons, the therapeutic process and empathy. *The Arts in Psychotherapy* 2006; **33**(4): 302–15.

38. Winters AF. Emotion, embodiment and mirror-neurons in dance movement psychotherapy: a connection across disciplines. *American Journal of Dance Therapy* 2008; **30**(2): 84–105.

39. McGarry LM, Russo FA. Mirroring in dance movement therapy: potential mechanisms behind empathy enhancement. *The Arts in Psychotherapy* 2011; **38**(3): 178–84.

40. Chalklins S, Schmaus D. The Chace approach to dance movement therapy. In: Lewis P (ed.). *Theoretical approaches to dance movement therapy*, vol. 1. Iowa: Kendall/Hunt, 1986: 17–36.

41. Priebe S, Savill M, Reininghaus U, Wykes T, Bentall R, Lauder C, McCrane P, Rohricht F, Eldridge S. Effectiveness and cost effectiveness of body psychotherapy in the treatment of negative symptoms of schizophrenia – a multi centre randomised controlled trial. *BMC Psychiatry* 2013; **13**(26): 1–8.

42. Stacy R, Britain K, Kerr S. Singing for health: an exploration of the issues. *Health Education* 2002; **102**(4): 156–62.

43. Clift S. Singing for health: a musical remedy. *British Journal of Wellbeing* 2010; **1**(6): 14–16.

44. Clift S, Hancox G, Morrison I, Hess B, Kreutz G, Stewart D. Choral singing and psychological wellbeing: quantitative and qualitative findings from English choirs in a cross-national survey. *Journal of Applied Arts and Health* 2010; **1**(1): 19–34.

45. Clift S, Hancox G. The significance of choral singing for sustaining psychological wellbeing: findings from a survey of choristers in England, Australia and Germany. *Music Performance Research* 2010; **3**(1): 79–96.

46. Clift S, Morrison I. Group singing fosters mental health and wellbeing: findings from the East Kent 'Singing for Health' network project. *Mental Health and Social Inclusion* 2011; **15**(2): 88–97.

47. McLaughlin N. Canterbury Christ Church University, 2012. Developed from Rosen A, Crisis management in the community. *Medical Journal of Australia* 1997; **167**: 633–8.

Further reading

Cabassa L, Nicasio A, Whitley R. Picturing recovery: a photovoice exploration of recovery dimensions among people with serious mental illness. *Psychiatry Online* 2013; **64**(9): 837–42.

Frese F, Knight E, Saks E. Recovery from schizophrenia: with views of psychiatrists, psychologists, and others diagnosed with this disorder. *Schizophrenia Bulletin* 2009; **35**(2): 370–80.

Fukui S, Davidson L, Rapp C. Pathways to recovery, a peer-led group intervention. *Psychiatric Services* 2010; **61**(9): 944.

Maslow A.H. The Maslow Business Reader (ed. D.C. Stephens) John Wiley & Sons, New York, 2000.

Van Gestel-Timmermans H, Brouwers E, van Assen M, van Nieuwenhuizen C. Effects of a peer-run course on recovery from serious mental illness: a randomized controlled trial. *Psychiatry Online* 2012; **63**(1): 54–60.

Relevant web page

www.alpfmedical.info/mental-health/the-thorn-programme
www.behindthelabel.co.uk
Rachel hears voices, sees visions and has other intense experiences.

http://changingminds.org/techniques/questioning/socratic_questions.htm

The person who is extremely distressed and disturbed

JOY A. DUXBURY AND FIONA JONES

LEARNING OUTCOMES

- To be able to define and differentiate between aggression and violence.

- To understand the dynamics of aggression.

- To be able to identify predisposing factors to the development and expression of aggression and violence.

- To be familiar with ways of reducing the potential for aggression and violence in health care settings by promoting caring relationships and environments.

- To understand personal and organizational approaches to working with service users who may and/or do exhibit disturbed behaviour in the form of aggression and/or violence.

- To appreciate the importance of trauma-informed care as a craft within an overall caring milieu.

SUMMARY OF KEY POINTS

- The prevention of distress is a priority for mental health care professionals. For some patients, aggression and/or violence can be one way of communicating unaddressed distress.

- Numerous factors can contribute to the development of aggression and therefore the anticipation of these is essential.

- Therapeutic, caring relationships and environments are hugely important when endeavouring to keep both patients and staff safe.

- To be successful this requires a well-thought-out and proactive multifaceted approach that targets individual and organizational matters and promotes the development of a caring atmosphere.

- Restrictive interventions are rarely seen by patients to be caring and they can often damage the therapeutic relationship. Their use should be minimized as far as possible.

INTRODUCTION

This chapter explores the nature and craft of caring for persons who are extremely disturbed or distressed. The focus in particular is on the prevention and management of aggression and violence using multi-modal indictors and approaches. With a view to adopting a least restrictive approach, personal understandings of the individual who displays distress in this way are explored in the context of the challenges that face both mental health professionals and service users in these settings. Interventions that focus on prevention from an individual and organizational perspective, therapeutic relationships, partnership working and management are identified, using reflection points. The importance of employing strategies that are underpinned by 'trauma-informed care' is highlighted with a view to minimizing the need for reactive and restrictive practices, which can be harmful to both service users and staff alike. Additionally, they can be a significant precursor to the development of distress for individuals in the first place.

Definitions

Aggression: a disposition that may lead to constructive or destructive actions but that usually has long-term negative consequences.

Violence: the harmful use of force or strength. 'Violent person' is generally understood to refer to someone who attacks another.

Trauma-informed care: the development of a culture where staff understand and acknowledge the impact of trauma and their responsibilities in mitigating against retraumatization.

Restrictive interventions: 'deliberate acts on the part of other person(s) that restrict an individual's movement, liberty, and/or freedom to act independently in order to:

- take immediate control of a dangerous situation where there is a real possibility of harm to the person or others if no action is undertaken;
- end or reduce significantly the danger to the person or others;
- contain or limit the person's freedom for no longer than is necessary.'[1] (p.14)

Violence and aggression in health care settings

Violence and aggression are universal phenomena. The frequency of aggression towards professionals in health care settings is a global problem which is well documented in the literature.[2] However, one needs to consider this in the context of broader statistics on societal aggression. It is important that practitioners do not perceive all patients with mental health problems as being or having the potential to be violent, but instead that they recognize the unsettling and unpredictable situation that patients find themselves in when admitted to hospital. Any risk of aggression that does occur, however, can range from verbal abuse through to assault. Historically, aggressive incidents have been under-reported.[3] Although aggression cannot be avoided altogether, its incidence can and should be reduced significantly through the craft of caring that promotes prevention and proactive strategies.

Theories of the causation of violence in health care settings

The reported rise of patient aggression in mental health settings has been of interest to practitioners and researchers for some time,[3] and a number of theories have been developed that endeavour to explain the causes. Research to date demonstrates that some of the characteristics of the socially driven health care environment have a powerful effect in mitigating or precipitating aggression and violence. In particular, aspects of what I refer to as a 'therapeutic triad' of internal, external and contextual factors can be significantly influential and interlinked. The latter includes situational and interpersonal factors that have been drawn from the works of Nijman et al.[4] and Duxbury.[5]

INTERNAL FACTORS

The case for the internal viewpoint has been strong, given the backdrop to mental health. A number of studies, for example, have explored an association between mental illness and violence.[6] This was highlighted in a report from the Royal College of Psychiatrists (RCP), suggesting a number of variables that can be attributed to violence, mental illness being an argued predictor.[7]

EXTERNAL FACTORS

The external stance, in contrast, asserts that it is the environment that leads to aggression and violence. Commonly reported factors include lack of privacy and space, location, treatment regimes, and rules and rituals, including limit setting.[8] The latter points are more about restrictive regimes as opposed to the physical environment. There is significant evidence suggesting that changes to the physical and psychosocial environment can be beneficial, as indicated in the recent Department of Health guidance.[1]

CONTEXTUAL FACTORS

A number of studies have supported the view that non-therapeutic interpersonal styles can affect staff and patient relationships and lead to aggression. Conflict with staff is commonly reported to be contributory.[8] For example,

Kamchuchat et al.[9] suggest that miscommunication is often an underlying cause associated with physical assault.

These multi-modal factors have been identified by a number of authors as contributory both in relation to expressions of frustration and dissatisfaction by service users and in preventing a reliance upon coercive practices.[8,10] While there is some evidence, however, that training and experience in the management of aggression can help reduce negative outcomes, this remains limited, and the more recent focus has shifted somewhat significantly to preventing aggression by improving the therapeutic environment, both personally and organizationally[11] – in other words, through the craft of caring.

> ## REFLECTION
>
> Can you think about things that might contribute to the development of aggression in your workplace? Name four things and decide whether they are internal, external or contextual factors.

Underlying the various theories on the causation of aggression and violence is the need to understand the views of participants, namely patients and health care staff. The experiences and perceptions of both can contribute to the development of aggression, its management and also its consequences.

Staff members' experiences of aggression and violence

Without education, skills training and clinical supervision (see chapter 10), nurses can respond to disturbed or aggressive behaviours as they might outside the work environment. For example, because of the powerful nature of anger as an emotion, people exposed to anger may feel fearful and intimidated. As a result, nurses may avoid patients if they are fearful of them.[12] Conversely, they may 'go in strong' as described by Whittington and Wykes.[13] Clearly, this is neither helpful nor therapeutic for nurse or patient. A number of studies have suggested that staff behaviour can contribute to the development of patient aggression and, indeed, some staff have expressed concerns about the use of restrictive practices. For example, when surveyed, practitioners reported feeling uneasy about the techniques taught in relation to restraint, particularly when trying to balance safety with service users' rights and less invasive procedures.[8] Staff have also raised concerns about injuries resulting in physical and psychological strain, stress, lack of confidence, prolonged sickness and dissonance.[11] The cost to the NHS and allied organizations when staff are injured, under threat or stressed as a result of threatening behaviour is significant and impacts upon staff turnover, burnout and litigation.[14,15]

Patients' experiences of aggression and violence

Similarly, patients may become fearful and/or aggressive in response to their own perceptions of aggressive or controlling behaviours by staff. In a study by Duxbury and Whittington,[8] over 25 per cent of patients surveyed felt that the staff significantly contributed to their aggressive behaviour. Furthermore, certain coercive practices can have negative connotations and outcomes and be perceived to be hostile and non-therapeutic by patients.[16] From a psychosocial perspective, patients can be severely traumatized by the use of some practices and this can affect both their needs and their road to recovery. This will be discussed in more detail later when examining trauma-informed care.

At the extreme, a number of adverse effects have been reported as a result of the use of physical restraint, ranging from service user and staff discomfort to injuries resulting in death. In 2011, in a 'Review of the medical theories and research relating to restraint related deaths in the UK',[17] an analysis was undertaken of what is known about the hazardous nature of the use of restrictive physical interventions, including the use of 'prone restraint'. Duxbury et al.[18] reported a growing evidence base that suggests that there are individuals who may be more at risk of being restrained than others, whether because of bio-physiological, interpersonal, situational or attitudinal factors. These groups are those with serious mental illness or learning disabilities, those from Black and Minority Ethnic communities, those with a high body mass index, men aged 30 to 40 years and young people (under the age of 20).

It is essential that such evidence is used to inform planning around how best to work with people who present behavioural challenges, at both an organizational and an individual service user level.

> ## FIONA'S STORY
>
> During this chapter I am going to try to illustrate various points using the experiences of a colleague of mine who for many years has suffered problems with her own mental health. Her 'journey' through her own illness has been extraordinary, and the subsequent involvement with her local mental health services highlights what can go wrong in services when prevention is not the priority and when restrictive interventions are heavily relied upon. Let me introduce her to you.
>
> Fiona is 40 years old and was first admitted to mental health services when she was 14. She had been living in local authority care in a children's home where she was bullied for being 'odd'. In reality, she had grown up with so much violence in

the home that she was just frightened all the time. Fiona, in desperation, made a very serious attempt on her life and was admitted to an adult acute ward, as there were no other places available. It was a mixed ward and there were dormitories. She was very mixed up and saw this move as further 'proof' that she was indeed 'odd' and didn't fit in anywhere in society except for a psychiatric hospital. Fiona was given medication, mainly to sedate her.

This is what Fiona had to say about her first experience of feeling upset and distressed on a ward and the reasons why she felt this way.

'My first experience of being upset and distressed on the ward was when my parents eventually came to visit. I was allowed out for an hour with them and arrived back at the ward 5 minutes late. The nurse in charge was 'fuming' and told me that all leave was now cancelled. My parents tried to reason with her but they were asked to leave. It had turned into a horrible visit and I became very angry and upset. I was shouting at the nurse, my parents were looking on in horror, all the time trying to reason with her and believing they were to blame. I hadn't seen my parents in 6 months. The staff responded by suddenly, without warning, grabbing me, restraining me and carrying me to the seclusion room. I was crying and screaming but no one came to the door for hours.'

REFLECTION

Ask yourself this question: have you ever been in a situation which gradually spiralled out of your control, and you were on the receiving end of aggressive behaviour from a patient? What led to this situation? Could it have been anticipated? What could have been done differently, particularly with regard to the craft of caring?

FUNDAMENTAL PRINCIPLES IN THE PREVENTION AND MANAGEMENT OF DISTURBED BEHAVIOUR

In the recent Department of Health guidance, *Positive and proactive care*,[1] a number of key principles have been identified as fundamental to fostering a safe and positive caring environment for staff and patients. They include compliance with human rights, understanding people's behaviour and unique needs including their strengths, involvement and participation, the treatment of people with compassion, dignity and kindness, and supporting people to balance safety from harm with freedom of choice.

When endeavouring to prevent the development of aggression and violence in health care settings, each of these principles provides a solid foundation on which to provide care and foster therapeutic environments and relationships. A crucial message here, however, is not to adopt these principles in the face of an aggressive encounter only, although this is clearly advocated, but to interact and communicate with patients and their families in a way that is underpinned by and fosters a therapeutic and caring ethos as a matter of course. Only then can proactivity and prevention be truly possible. Staff should not therefore be focusing their attention on how to manage aggression and violence once it occurs, but how to prevent it in an informed, structured, caring and pragmatic way.

PRIMARY PREVENTION AND PRE-ESCALATION: PROMOTING THE CRAFT OF CARING

In order to promote a culture based on care and prevention as a first-line intervention, staff must be adequately prepared to recognize the symptoms and potential for dysfunctional environments and relationships, and put systems in place to facilitate therapeutic relationships. This I will refer to as pre-escalation. They therefore need to understand the causative factors previously outlined and endeavour to address these before problems arise. This has implications for caring communication styles, understanding the needs of the individual, using good assessment and advance planning tools, and promoting cultures based upon person-centredness, and care as opposed to restriction. (See chapter 3 for more on developing and maintaining therapeutic relationships.) The prevention and management of aggression and violence is an interdisciplinary function, facilitating a multi-faceted approach involving individualized interventions to prevent and then minimize aggressive episodes. Behavioural and environmental strategies are fundamental in maintaining a therapeutic atmosphere.

PREVENTION THROUGH CARE AND PROACTIVITY

It is vital that evidenced-based policies, procedures and training have a high profile in the prevention and management of aggression in all health care organizations. Bowers et al.[19] suggest that a focus on containment, rather than a therapeutic approach, is part of the problem of aggression and violence in clinical settings. Ways of engaging patients proactively to understand their needs and therefore prevent distress are key. Staff training therefore should focus not only upon the use of generic principles of conveying the craft of caring, but also explicitly on philosophies of trauma-informed care, the use of person-centred tools such as advance directives, and the minimization of restrictive practices.

Advance directives

An advance directive is a document used to register advance instructions about future treatment in the event of an incapacitating psychiatric crisis. They are intended to support patients' self-determination at a time when they are vulnerable to loss of autonomy, to help them ensure their preferences are known and to minimize unwanted treatments.[20] The hope is that the very preparation of such documents will promote trust and enhance therapeutic communication and engagement with treatment. However, they are best used as a planning tool for future psychiatric crisis management rather than an intervention to enhance compliance.[21]

Such structured facilitation to complete an advance directive can provide an opportunity for collaboration and exchange and respectful dialogue with a patient about past experiences and preferences for treatment, with a view to making future plans. However, the gap between interest and successful implementation is complex and related to barriers. Some patients find advance directives difficult to understand and the language unfamiliar. For clinicians, service-level barriers are reported, including lack of access to relevant documents, lack of training, lack of communication and lack of time.[20] There is therefore scepticism about their benefit and value. Furthermore, their use has yet to be tested to any great extent in the UK, although they are increasingly advocated.[1]

There is no doubt that strategies for the prevention and management of disturbed behaviour should be discussed with service users on admission to mental health inpatient services, or as soon as possible thereafter, to promote a positive therapeutic alliance and greater communication between staff and patients.[20,22] While research in this area is limited to date, Maitre et al.[23] found in a review of the literature that patients show a strong interest in creating directives of this sort, have a high level of satisfaction when using them, and feel more in control over their mental health care and more respected and valued. Swanson et al.[24] have also reported their value when coupled with dedicated facilitation sessions to help patients complete and use them, with the caveat that system-level policies are required to embed them in practice.

TRAUMA-INFORMED CARE

Trauma-informed care is emerging as an essential value that is seen as fundamental and essential to contemporary, caring mental health practice. It is an integral part of the craft of caring. Jennings[25] argues that effective trauma-informed services are those not just designed to treat symptoms related to abuse; they are services where staff are aware of and sensitive to doing no further harm to survivors. This includes making sure that:

- service users feel connected, valued, informed and hopeful of recovery;
- the connection between trauma and adult psychopathology is known and understood by all staff;
- staff work in mindful and empowering ways with individuals, families and friends and other agencies to promote and protect the autonomy of each individual;
- staff identify and recognize the needs of those who are particularly vulnerable due to personal histories of trauma and past experiences.[25]

The development of a culture and a belief in the value of trauma-informed care, when staff are competent and confident in knowledge of the impact of trauma and the understanding of their responsibilities in mitigating against retraumatization, is key. Hummer et al.[26] found that this awareness needed to start with the orientation of new staff and in staff development with a focus upon therapeutic safety and boundaries; establishing, maintaining and terminating therapeutic relationships; de-escalation; strength-focused care planning; and patient participation and empowerment.[27] The trauma-informed care approach feeds into the 'therapeutic triad', as described earlier, in that a number of simple approaches can be employed to reduce the potential for aggression. For example, a number of studies have demonstrated that simple modifications to the environment can be effective. This can include changes to furnishings to make units more homely, the introduction of colour and olfactory adaptations to promote calm and comfort, and space and 'time out' options to diffuse stress.[28] Features that characterize suboptimal care from a patient perspective include disinterested or disrespectful and non-interactive staff and the use of non-empowering tasks. These are seen to feed previous pervasive patterns of feelings of inferiority and passivity.[29]

Borge and Fagermoen[30] have found that the focus of care in mainstream acute adult inpatient mental health settings is on risk management, illness assessment and medical stabilization – factors clearly aligned with the internal model. Subsequently they state that staff can be preoccupied with medication and coercive practices, a view previously reported by Duxbury.[5,8]

As attention to the impact of trauma has spread, it is increasingly thought that the majority of people accessing mental health services have been exposed to trauma.

To better meet their needs, trauma-informed care has emerged as a key paradigm, particularly in the USA and Australia. Hoda[31] states that trauma-informed care services are those that are cognizant that their services can retraumatize people admitted with trauma histories through the application of coercive practices such as restraint. Admission to inpatient facilities can therefore be equally traumatizing, reintroducing disabling symptoms, loss of autonomy and dislocation from support.

The provision of patient-centred approaches that are based upon sound clinical assessment and judgement is paramount. When planned for and invested in, the time spent can be hugely beneficial. However, circumstances may evolve rapidly in some instances, and deterioration can be speedy. In such circumstances where prevention has either failed as a first resort or been impracticable, de-escalation may be required as a secondary preventative approach.

SECONDARY PREVENTION: DE-ESCALATION

De-escalation can be beneficial when organizational and personal issues have been addressed or planned for but have failed to prevent the escalation of aggression.

De-escalation has been defined as 'the gradual resolution of a potentially violent and/or aggressive situation through the use of verbal and physical expressions of empathy, alliance and non-confrontational limit setting that is based on respect'[32] (p.65).

One could argue that these are also key ingredients for pre-escalation. Nonetheless, de-escalation refers to a range of psychosocial strategies and skills that are employed where a person begins to show signs of agitation and arousal that are believed to be predictive of an impending episode of high-risk behaviours. Most de-escalation strategies are verbal in nature; they are inherently avoidant of confrontation and may on occasions include prompts to service users to move to a low stimulus, private, relaxing area which has been designated for this purpose. When employing the craft of de-escalation, strategies should be individualized and should aim to promote a return to a state of calm. Approaches typically involve establishing rapport and the need for mutual cooperation, demonstrating compassion,

negotiating realistic options, asking open questions, demonstrating concern and attentiveness, using empathic and non-judgemental listening, distraction, redirection to alternate less threatening activities and being sensitive to non-verbal communication.[32,33]

It is important to note that de-escalation is a reactive management strategy. Its sole purpose is to defuse and render the situation safe. It is not appropriate to forensically interrogate or debate the legitimacy of the reasons why a person has become upset or agitated at this point, but instead getting to the root of the concern can be helpful if done in a non-confrontational way. It may be that staff exercise their reflexive muscles and allow co-workers to intervene if it is clear that a one-to-one relationship, for whatever reason, has broken down in some way and/or is noticeably contributing to a level of conflict. Placing demands on people, telling them to stop or telling them that restricted approaches will be used if they do not desist are seldom helpful; verbal exchanges which acknowledge people's state of distress and upset are far more constructive. Prevention is much more valuable than waiting for an incident to occur.

MINIMIZING RESTRICTIVE PRACTICES AS PART OF A TERTIARY PREVENTATIVE STRATEGY

A restrictive practice may be necessary as a proportionate and reasonable response where a person's behaviour places himself or herself or others at imminent risk of significant harm and de-escalation strategies have failed. However, the use of restrictive practices to 'control' aggressive and disturbed behaviour in care settings is an emotive and controversial topic.

Restrictive practices may be employed as a planned intervention, i.e. as part of a pre-arranged strategy informed by risk assessments (chapter 16) and recorded in a care plan (chapter 50). The choice of intervention should be informed by the service user's preference or advance directive (if known), their clinical needs and an appraisal of the immediate environment. Management should begin with those measures that have the least possibility of causing harm. Advance directives (chapter 37) are one way of establishing good foundations to facilitate this. Alternatively, in some

instances they are used in an emergency as a response to a previously unforeseen risk event.

The over-arching term 'restrictive interventions' denotes 'The implementation of a practice or practices that restrict an individual's movement, liberty and/or freedom to act independently without coercion or consequence'[1] (p.14).

Seclusion and restraint are both restrictive approaches sometimes referred to as restrictive physical interventions. They are the practices most commonly referred to in the literature.[1] Combined, they have been described as an integrated intervention directed at managing and controlling a precarious situation.[34–36] They are designed as emergency measures to contain and to deal with situations on a short-term basis.

Restrictive physical interventions should be avoided if at all possible, but where they are used, staff should seek to continue to communicate with service users in order to continually attempt to de-escalate the situation and cease the use of a restrictive physical intervention as soon as possible. Plans and directives should consider which of any prolonged interventions, such as physical or chemical restraint and seclusion, is likely to be least hazardous to the service user.

Individual risk factors, which suggest a service user is more likely to suffer physical and/or emotional trauma, must be recognized and taken into account. This might include, for instance, recognizing that for a female with a history of traumatic sexual abuse, having a male in close proximity may cause added emotional trauma; or for a person who is morbidly obese, being held in a restraint position may cause abdominal pressure to the diaphragm and/or compromise breathing.[17]

Staff undertaking practices such as restraint and seclusion should be mindful of the potential for these interventions to cause significant emotional and physical trauma and, if used as part of a planned intervention, plans should seek to minimize such risks. Effective post-incident debriefing of service users may help, as might supporting service users to record and utilize advance directives about how staff should use restrictive physical interventions if necessary. Knowledge of a patient's background through assessment is crucial. The literature suggests that patients often associate seclusion with punishment, emphasizing the importance of open communication between staff and patients, when someone is secluded, to reduce anxiety and fears associated with confinement.[34,36] This again has implications for trauma-informed care.

REFLECTION

What do you think it would be like to experience a restrictive intervention?

In Fiona's case, a restrictive intervention was used and she felt this could have been avoided.

She felt like violence was the answer to everything. It shaped her future. Fiona became violent from then on and remained in the system until she was 32. She had escaped familial violence, been placed in an unsuitable children's home where she was further bullied and physically attacked, and then, in hospital, dealt with using violence too. Her default setting became 'hit first before they hit you', a stance which has remained with her to a certain extent to this day. When she feels scared, she lashes out. Fiona feels that, without the help of a wonderful care coordinator, who helped her to change her thinking, she would have remained in hospital to this day.

She wishes the staff had just realized that she was frightened, over-medicated, bored and desperate to escape feelings of worthlessness. She says they could have talked to her. They could have gone for a walk with her. She was seriously self-harming and does not understand why nobody took the time to ask why she was so angry and unhappy.

Minimization approaches

Over recent years a number of domestic and international agencies have embraced the use of 'reduction models' in order to reduce reliance on restrictive models of reactive management, and to return to, promote and foster the craft of caring. These effectively focus on well-informed systems of therapeutic relationships and cultures, governance, strong leadership, the use of prevention strategies, a focus on users' rights and ensuring that reflective models support learning from incidents where restrictive interventions are used.

There are some small pockets of evidence of implementation in sectors of the UK, but their use remains far from universal. The strongest evidence base to date is from the international literature. For the purpose of this chapter, I will refer to three specific examples. These are the Six Core Strategies (6CS),[10] Safewards,[37] and, more recently, REsTRAIN YOURSELF (RY).[38]

Multi-component approaches of this sort, which focus on substantial, cultural changes across organizations, seem to be able to demonstrate the most impressive outcomes. For example, studies using a complex intervention approach with a focus on behavioural leadership, service user-centred care and culture shift have reported significantly reduced frequency and duration of restraint and seclusion.[36,39]

A number of recent studies have demonstrated that it is possible to reduce the rate of some restrictive interventions in various settings if an organization is committed to change their approach to aggression/violence management, from reactivity to a more proactive approach.[36,39] All services where staff are trained in the delivery of restrictive practices should have an over-arching strategy to address their minimization.

Some studies have also identified the importance of clear leadership when targeting a reduction in the use of restrictive interventions.[10] Plans should include a mission statement that clearly articulates the organization's philosophy about seclusion and restraint reduction, for example, and describe the roles and responsibilities of all staff in working towards this.

SIX CORE STRATEGIES FOR REDUCING SECLUSION AND RESTRAINT USE

The Six Core Strategies (6CS) were developed in the United States by the National Technical Assistance Center of the National Association of State Mental Health Program Directors just over a decade ago, following extensive evidence reviews and broad consultation with experts in the field.[10] They provide a central multi-element framework for restraint and seclusion reduction through both organizational and practitioner change. The strategies focus on:

- leadership towards organizational change;
- use of data to inform practice;
- workforce development;

- use of restraint and seclusion reduction tools;
- improving service users' role in the inpatient setting;
- vigorous debriefing techniques.

Growing evidence suggests the value and positive impact of this approach in terms of achieving sustained reductions in seclusions and/or restraint episodes, across a range of service types.[35,36,39,40]

SAFEWARDS

More recently Bowers has developed and launched the Safewards Model, derived from his own research and from research conducted by others internationally over many years.[37] Approximately 300 ideas for interventions that could be used to help ward staff reduce levels of conflict and containment were generated. These were then rated by a group of stakeholders, resulting in a list of 16 potential interventions to test in a pilot study on four wards at one hospital. The learning from this resulted in 10 interventions, which were then tested in a single blind cluster randomized controlled trial on 31 wards at 15 different hospitals.[37]

The interventions included using clear mutual expectations, soft words, talk down approaches, positive words, bad news mitigation, ways to know each other, mutual help meetings, calm down methods, reassurance and discharge messages.

A control intervention was introduced on 15 wards, and the 10 experimental interventions on the others. The Safewards interventions produced a 15 per cent decrease in the rate of conflict and a 24 per cent decrease in the rate of containment.

REsTRAIN YOURSELF

A new effort has begun in the north-west of England, called REsTRAIN YOURSELF, which is an adaptation of the 6CS approach. Fourteen acute mental health wards in the north-west region of England are included in the study, with seven wards implementing REsTRAIN YOURSELF and seven comparison wards (control).[38]

The primary aim of the project is to reduce the incidence of harm caused to patients and staff in acute mental health wards as the result of a reduction in physical restraint. The objectives of this effort are to roll out the restraint-related patient safety initiative and to evaluate any changes in patient and staff safety outcomes associated with this implementation.

The immediate process involves implementing the following components:

a. developing leadership for a positive safety culture (leadership-walk arounds);
b. root cause analysis (debriefing);
c. service user-led initiatives (including advance directives);
d. service user and staff experiences;
e. measurements for improvement.

The project implementation plan has four key components:

1. training the trainers;
2. rolling out of training across participating teams;
3. improving collaboration to support learning, sharing and adoption;
4. evaluation.

As part of this project, an over-arching multi-method evaluative design has been adopted.

While this project is ongoing, the principles employed have been tested and positively reported upon in non-UK settings.[11,14,39]

Aligned to the need to explore alternatives to and minimize restrictive practices, a plethora of activity has emerged in the UK over the last 10 years, dating back from a number of high-profile safety incidents in 2003/04 and resulting in the development of guidelines in this area by the National Institute for Health and Care Excellence (NICE).[28] While guidance and strategies were instigated prior to this period, the real impetus began back then. This has continued to increase and the period from 2011 onwards has been a particularly significant time, which has seen a report on restraint-related deaths in the UK,[17,18] the Francis Report on care deficits,[41] Winterbourne,[42] and most recently the 2013 MIND report on crisis in care, which focused on the negative impact of restraint.[43] This latter highlighted the reported use of restraint in a number of trusts across England and has concerned many, resulting in a call for a ban of prone restraint in some circles, however contentious this may be.

Empirical evidence from the UK and North America clearly demonstrates that rate variation in restraint and seclusion is largely influenced by environmental, interpersonal or contextual factors. Unclear policy and guidelines, overcrowding, poor ward design, low or inflexible staff numbers, inexperienced staff, poor staff retention, poor information sharing and service user acuity have all been implicated.[4,28] Unsurprisingly, a number of studies have also shown that various staff characteristics are linked to the development of aggression and violence in mental health service users, including negative interactional styles; provocative, authoritarian behaviour; and poor communication skills,[44–46,8] as highlighted in a previous section. Hence, a substantial body of evidence suggests that many seclusion and restraint episodes may be preventable if these factors are addressed.

Furthermore, variation in the use of restrictive interventions between different areas has been reported, and is likely to be due to a number of factors, including differences in practices; geographical variations in the prevalence and acuity of mental illness; differences in admission policies, with hospitals in some areas treating more acute service users; ward design factors, such as the availability of intensive care and low-stimulus facilities; staff numbers, experience and training; the use of psychotropic medication; the frequent or prolonged seclusion/restraint of service users; and cultural differences among wards and hospitals.[47,48]

CONCLUSION

Patients who express distress/aggression and/or display violence arouse a range of emotions in those who care for them. Staff and patients can experience a sense of powerlessness and frustration. Nurses and their organizations need special personal attributes, skills, education and training to prevent and to intervene when difficult situations arise, safely, therapeutically and in a least restrictive manner. Organizations, however, need to ensure that strategies and clear directives are in place with regard to the craft of caring and the minimization of restrictive practices. Many professionals express unrest with some of the physical intervention techniques taught, particularly when trying to balance safety with service users' rights and less invasive procedures,[8] and with the fundamental act of caring.

In order to care effectively and perfect the craft of caring, open and ongoing communication between all members of the multidisciplinary team is necessary. This is not to say that all violent incidents can be foreseen or even prevented, but that safety concerns for staff and patients can be minimized. Debriefing and post-incident reviews of all incidents of aggression and violence for staff as well as patients is an important component of aggression management. Individuals need opportunities to work through their own feelings and to evaluate the efficacy of nursing interventions, to reduce burnout and to enhance personal and professional growth. Post-incident interviews should be designed to discover exactly what happened and the effects on the participants. They should not be used to apportion blame or to punish those involved.[28]

This chapter has discussed personal, professional and organizational strategies for exploring and addressing patient distress. Ongoing reflection and critique of personal and team practices are significant elements in maintaining therapeutic environments for patients under duress.

Restrictive practices have caused serious trauma, both physical and psychological, and even death in some instances.[27] The use of restrictive practice in its various forms can contradict the intentions behind clinical and educational programmes that are designed to educate and support people. They are viewed as controversial, given their impact and use in 'caring environments'.[49,50]

Restrictive practices should only ever be employed as a last resort. Moves to steer away from reactive crisis management approaches are hugely important and timely in today's climate. In order to achieve this, major environmental, cultural and organizational changes, underpinned by a philosophy of trauma-informed care, are required. Individuals alone cannot prevent or manage aggressive behaviour, and I have outlined current key ideas and approaches to make significant proactive exchanges in order to portray an essence of care and keep both staff and patients safe and to minimize distress. Approaches must be targeted and based upon the perspectives and experiences of those involved. An understanding of factors that can influence the therapeutic triad both positively and negatively is key, and practitioners and their organizations need to work together in order to address the challenges outlined.

Elliot[27] suggests that best practice is to apply universal trauma precautions that nurses routinely use, which are growth-promoting, recovery-focused and less likely to retraumatize those already exposed to interpersonal trauma. Many practices, such as ward rules and restrictions, locked doors, mixed sex facilities and coercive practices such as restraint and seclusion, are experienced by service users as emotionally unsafe and disempowering and therefore traumatizing. Effective trauma-informed care services are those where the staff make it their priority to do no further harm. Trauma-informed care starts with and goes to the heart of the enabling nature of the nurse–patient relationship and the values services place on person-centred care, with a view to reducing conflict and maintaining the 'caring' status quo at all times.

Let Fiona conclude the chapter.

FIONA'S STORY

My life is so much different from what it was before. After that first hospital admission, I went into secure care and, by the time I was 27, I had been in prison and high-secure settings. The turning point for me came when I met a really good nurse who helped me to see the world differently. I am very proud that I have a job and my own house.

I am extremely proud that I now have a role in preventing this type of restraint and seclusion practice and that finally someone is listening to me about why they should not be used. There are many others like me who haven't been able to turn their lives around. Instead, they are still in a perpetual state of feeling scared, misunderstood, in distress and potentially aggressive. Sadly, behaviour of this sort continues to be met with coercion and restriction rather than care and compassion – fundamental skills for the craft of caring.

References

1. Department of Health. *Positive and proactive care: reducing the need for restrictive interventions.* London: DH, 2014.
2. Roche MA, Diers D, Duffield C, Catling-Paull CJ. Violence toward nurses, the work environment, and patient outcomes. *Journal of Nursing Scholarship* 2010; **42**(1), 13–22.
3. Rippon TJ. Aggression and violence in health care professionals. *Journal of Advanced Nursing* 2000; **31**(2): 452–60.
4. Nijman HLI, Muris P, Merckelbach HLGJ, Palmstierna T, Wistedt B, Vos AM, van Rixtel A, Allertz W. The Staff Observation Aggression Scale–Revised (SOAS-R). *Aggressive Behavior* 1999; **25**: 197–209.
5. Duxbury J. An evaluation of staff and patient views of and strategies employed to manage inpatient aggression and violence on one mental health unit: a pluralistic design. *Journal of Psychiatric and Mental Health Nursing* 2002; **9**: 325–37.
6. Steinert T, Wolfe M, Gebhardt RP. Measurement of violence during in-patient treatment and association with psychopathy. *Acta Psychiatrica Scandinavica* 2000; **102**(2): 107–12.
7. RCP (Royal College of Psychiatrists). *Violence in psychiatry.* London: RCP, 1998.
8. Duxbury J, Whittington R. Causes and management of patient aggression and violence: staff and patient perspectives. *Journal of Advanced Nursing* 2005; **50**(5): 469–78.
9. Kamchuchat C, Chongsuvivatwong V, Oncheunjit S, Yip TW, Sangthong R. Workplace violence directed at nursing staff at a general hospital in Southern Thailand. *Journal of Occupational Health* 2008; **50**: 201–7.
10. Huckshorn KA. Reducing the use of seclusion and restraint in mental health systems: a public health prevention approach with interventions. *Journal of Psychosocial Nursing and Mental Health Services* 2004; **42**: 22–33.
11. LeBel J. *The business case for preventing and reducing restraint and seclusion use.* HHS Publication No. (SMA) 11-4632. Rockville, MD: Center for Mental Health Services, Substance Abuse and Mental Health Services Administration, 2011.
12. Smith ME, Hart G. Nurse's responses to patient anger: from disconnecting to connecting. *Journal of Advanced Nursing* 1994; **20**: 634–51.
13. Whittington R, Wykes T. Going in strong: confrontative coping by staff. *Journal of Forensic Psychiatry* 1994; **5**(3): 609–14.
14. LeBel J, Goldstein R. The economic cost of using restraint and the value added by restraint reduction or elimination. *Psychiatric Services* 2005; **56**(9): 1109–14.
15. Sanders K. The effects of an action plan, staff training, management support and monitoring on restraint use and costs of work-related injuries. *Journal of Applied Research in Intellectual Disabilities* 2009; **22**(2): 216–20.
16. Meehan T, McIntosh W, Bergen H. Aggressive behaviour in the high-secure forensic setting: the perceptions of patients. *Journal of Psychiatric and Mental Health Nursing* 2006; **13**: 19–25.
17. Aiken F, Duxbury J, Dale C, Harbison I. *Review of the medical theories and research relating to restraint related deaths.* London: MOJ, 2012.
18. Duxbury J, Aiken F, Dale D. Deaths in custody: the role of restraint. *Journal of Learning Disabilities and Offending Behaviour* 2011; **2**(4): 178–89.
19. Bowers L, Alexander J, Simpson A, Ryan C, Carr-Walker P. Cultures of psychiatry and the professional socialization process: the case of containment methods for disturbed patients. *Nurse Education Today* 2004; **24**(6): 435–42.
20. Papageorgiou A, King M, Janmohamed A, Davidson O, Dawson J. Advance directives for patients compulsorily admitted to hospital with serious mental illness, randomised controlled trial. *British Journal of Psychiatry* 2002; **181**: 513–19.
21. Amering M, Stastny P, Hopper K. Psychiatric advance directives: qualitative study of informed deliberations by mental health service users. *British Journal of Psychiatry* 2005; **186**(3): 247–52.
22. Duxbury J, Wright K. Should nurses restrain violent and aggressive patients? *Nursing Times* 2011; **107**: 9.
23. Maitre E, Debien C, Nicaise P, Wyngaerden F, Le Galudec M, Genest P, Ducrocq F, Delamillieure P, Lavoisy B, Walter M, Dubois V, Vaiva G. Advance directives in psychiatry: a review of the qualitative literature. *Encephale* 2013; **39**(4): 244–51.
24. Swanson JW, Swartz MS, Elbogen EB, Van Dorn RA, Ferron J, Wagner HR, McCauley BJ, Kim M. Facilitated psychiatric advance directives: a randomised control trial of an intervention to foster advance treatment planning among persons with severe mental illness. *American Journal of Psychiatry* 2013; **163**(11): 1943–51.
25. Jennings A. *Models of developing trauma informed behavioural health systems and trauma specific services: a report.* Rockville, MD: Center for Mental Health Services, 2004.
26. Hummer V, Dollard N, Robst J, Armstrong M. Innovations in implementation of trauma-informed care practices in youth residential treatment: a curriculum for organizational change. *Child Welfare* 2010; **89**(2): 79–95.
27. Elliott D, Bjelajac P, Fallot R, Markoff L, Glover Reed B. Trauma-informed or trauma-denied: principles and implementation of trauma-informed services for women. *Journal of Community Psychology* 2007; **33**(4): 461–77.
28. NICE (National Institute for Health and Care Excellence). *Violence and aggression: short-term management in mental health, health and community settings.* London: NICE, 2015.
29. Ashcraft LS, Anthony W. Eliminating seclusion and restraint in recovery orientated crisis services. *Psychiatric Services* 2008; **59**(11): 1198–202.
30. Borge L, Fagermoen M. Patients' own experiences of hospital treatment: wholeness and self worth in time and space. *Journal of Mental Health* 2008; **17**(2): 193–205.

31. Hoda G. *Responding to childhood trauma; the promise and practice of trauma informed care*. Pennsylvania: Pennsylvania Office of Mental Health and Substance Abuse Services, 2006.

32. Cowin LS, Davies R, Estall G, Berlin T, Fitzgerald M, Hoot S. De-escalating aggression and violence in the mental health setting. *International Journal of Mental Health Nursing* 2003; **12**: 64–7.

33. Price O, Baker J. Key components of de-escalation techniques: a thematic synthesis. *International Journal of Mental Health Nursing* 2012; **21**(4): 310–19.

34. Mattson MR, Sachs MH. Seclusion: uses and complications. *American Journal of Psychiatry* 1978; **135**(10): 1210–13.

35. Wale JB, Belkin GS, Moon R. Reducing the use of seclusion and restraint in psychiatric emergency and adult inpatient services: improving patient-centered care. *Permanente Journal* 2011; **15**(2): 57–62.

36. Putkonen A, Kuivalainen S, Louheranta O. Cluster randomized control trial of reducing seclusion and restraint in secured care of men with schizophrenia. *Psychiatric Services in Advance* June 17: pp. 1–6.

37. Bowers L. Safewards: a new model of conflict and containment on psychiatric wards. *Journal of Psychiatric and Mental Health Nursing* 2014; **21**(6): 499–508.

38. LeBel J, Duxbury J, Putkonen A, Sprague T, Rae C, Sharpe J. Multi-national experiences on the use of restraint and seclusion. *Journal of Psychosocial Nursing* 2014; **52**(11): 22–9.

39. McVilly K. *Physical restraint in disability services: current practices; contemporary concerns and future directions*. Victoria, Australia: Department of Human Services, 2008.

40. Azeem MW, Aujla A, Rammerth M, Binsfeld G, Jones RB. Effectiveness of six core strategies based on trauma informed care in reducing seclusion and restraints at a child and adolescent psychiatric hospital. *Journal of Child and Adolescent Nursing* 2011; **24**: 11–15.

41. Francis R. *Report of the Mid Staffordshire NHS Foundation Trust Public Inquiry: executive summary*. London: Stationery Office, 2013.

42. Department of Health. *Transforming care: a national response to Winterbourne View hospital*. London: DH, 2012.

43. Mind. *Mental health crisis care: physical restraint in crisis*. Stratford: Mind, 2012.

44. Bonner G, Lowe T, Rawcliffe D, Wellman N. Trauma for all: a pilot study of the subjective experience of physical restraint for mental health inpatients and staff in the UK. *Journal of Psychiatric and Mental Health Nursing* 2002; **9:** 465–73.

45. Tunde-Ayinmode M, Little J. Use of seclusion in a psychiatric acute inpatient unit. *Australasian Psychiatry* 2004; **12**(4): 347–51.

46. Wynaden D, Chapman R, McGowan S, Holmes C, Ash P, Boschman A. Through the eye of the beholder: to seclude or not to seclude. *International Journal of Mental Health Nursing* 2002; **11**: 260–8.

47. Livingstone A. *Seclusion practice: a literature review*. Victoria, Australia: Victorian Quality Council and Chief Psychiatrist's Quality Assurance Committee, 2007.

48. Stewart D, Bowers L, Simpson A, Ryan C, Tziggili M. Manual restraint of adult psychiatric inpatients: a literature review. *Journal of Psychiatric and Mental Health Nursing* 2009; **16**: 749–57.

49. Paterson B, Bradfley P, Stark C, Saddler D, Leadbetter D, Allen D. Deaths associated with restraint use in health and social care in the UK. The results of a preliminary survey *Journal of Psychiatric and Mental Health Nursing* 2003; **10**: 3–15.

50. Norfolk, Suffolk and Cambridgeshire Strategic Health Authority. *Independent inquiry into the death of David Bennett: an independent inquiry set up under HSG(94)27*. Cambridge: Norfolk, Suffolk and Cambridgeshire Strategic Health Authority, 2003.

Further reading

Bowers L. The Safewards Model. 2014. Available from: http://www.safewards.net/images/pdf/Safewards%20model.pdf [Accessed 23rd May 2016].

Department of Health. *Positive and proactive care: reducing the need for restrictive interventions*. London: DH, 2014. Available from: https://www.gov.uk/government/uploads/system/uploads/attachment_data/file/300293/JRA_DoH_Guidance_on_RP_web_accessible.pdf [Accessed 23rd May 2016].

Huckshorn KA. Reducing the use of seclusion and restraint in mental health systems: a public health prevention approach with interventions. *Journal of Psychosocial Nursing and Mental Health Services* 2004; **42**: 22–33.

NICE (National Institute for Health and Care Excellence). Violence and aggression: short-term management in mental health, health and community settings. London: NICE, 2015. Available from: https://www.nice.org.uk/guidance/ng10 [Accessed 23rd May 2016].

Relevant web pages

http://www.safewards.net/images/pdf/Safewards%20model.pdf [Accessed 8th January 2017]

https://www.gov.uk/government/uploads/system/uploads/attachment_data/file/300293/JRA_DoH_Guidance_on_RP_web_accessible.pdf [Accessed 8th January 2017]

https://www.nice.org.uk/guidance/ng10 [Accessed 8th January 2017]

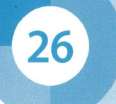

26 The person experiencing bipolar disorder

SALLY HARDY with significant input from an anonymous friend

LEARNING OUTCOMES

- To understand the implications of living and/or working with a diagnosis of bipolar disorder.
- To be aware of the symptoms, characteristics and individual variance associated with a diagnosis of bipolar disorder.
- To be able to identify strategies to help individuals manage mood variations and impulsive behaviours towards minimizing risk and maximizing well-being.

SUMMARY OF KEY POINTS

- The craft of caring for someone with bipolar disorder requires attention being given to individualized experience.
- A range of presenting symptoms, (which may be different at each point of contact), requires understanding a person with a diagnosis of bipolar disorder within the 'here and now'.
- Medication is only one element of treatment options available, with increased evidence revealing that a low–dose approach may be more beneficial and may avoid unwanted, intolerable side effects.
- Maintaining a therapeutic relationship does not equate to being a friend, where boundaries can become compromised and counterintuitive to both persons.
- A mental health promotion approach to managing long-term wellness can be used to sustain and promote recovery.

INTRODUCTION

Men have called me mad; but the question is not settled, whether madness is or is not the loftiest intelligence – whether much that is glorious – whether all that is profound – does not spring from disease of thought – from moods of mind exalted at the expense of general intellect.

Edgar Allan Poe[1]

Through the collaborative writing of this book chapter, we aim to introduce you to a person who is living with and experiencing bipolar affective mood disorder. The experience you have when reading this chapter will be about jumping backwards and forwards between our narrative and material that has been chosen to become part of the book chapter's more formal structure.

As close friends, we feel well placed to share how we have travelled. It felt initially good to share our understanding of the highs and lows of a life experienced through mood changes. It was at an excited point that we agreed to try to capture and explore the consequences of mood changes on our life events, our decisions, our meeting of deadlines and our relationship; all in an attempt to help you, as health care practitioners, understand and therefore interact empathically and therapeutically with others who share this tumultuous experience termed 'bipolar'.

The joint experience of writing this chapter started and halted many times, hit by the excruciating anxiety and concerns of a lengthy low period. We navigated and negotiated during these periods of uncertainty as to how best to include or exclude my friend's significant and very personal contributions. As the various responses to the commitment of a book chapter contribution unfolded, our concerns about this being an invasion of privacy increased. Yet we hope this frustration can in itself be used to help understand what it is like to live and work with bipolar disorder and how this can craft your own approach to caring.

Even the label itself, bipolar disorder, does not capture adequately the extent of highs, middles and lows; the destabilizing process of never quite knowing how to react or respond, never quite knowing with whom you are interacting, or whether your interaction itself can become a further trigger to another change in mood. The anger, frustration, then laughter; intense feelings of love, hatred, fear, loathing; building excitement followed by a crashing of dreams and a shattering of creative ideas. The risks, excitement, adrenaline, then grief, as an inevitability, an acceptance of constant change; not daring to wish for stability in order to achieve our joint task.

Holding on to the pain, anguish, realities of life's disappointments, inevitabilities, situations. Shouldering the blame, hurt and frustrations. Seeking out the person, glimpsing their potential, understanding the delicacy and transparency of human interactions. A living gamble, in that life itself collides and crashes into others along the way.

Living alongside and trying to care for someone with mood changes has replicated the process of trying to write this chapter. The narrative centres on what it is like to live with bipolar disorder through outlining

the relationship we shared. Me, as the friend, the close companion, the academic, the 'stable' one. My friend as the source of the chapter's material, the story yet untold, capturing a lived experience as it continues to unfold. Placing 'you' and your experiences at the centre of the book chapter.

We shared the intention that doing this would help others know more of what it is to live with and exist within (and outside) the system of mental health care – getting the insider viewpoint of a life on the edge, a life lived to the full. A life turned up to high volume, in full Technicolor, three-dimensional, high definition. A life turned upside down, the despair, depression, dread. We also aim to reveal what it is like for the person living within that process of disruption, and to reveal some of the crippling consequences of living within fluctuating mood.

How could we capture all of that in one chapter without patronizing, belittling, othering, stereotyping? Well, this is our attempt to do just that. To take you on the journey of the past 12 months, spanning backwards and pushing forwards, sometimes alone, sometimes in a state of creative harmony.

REFLECTION

Consider for a moment your initial response to what you have read so far about bipolar affective mood disorder. Has the chapter disrupted assumptions of what a book chapter should provide? What do you think might be the deliberate intention behind that disruption, in helping you understand the craft of caring for someone with a diagnosis of bipolar disorder?

Are you confused, reader? That is good. It means we can continue to use the phrase 'disorder' when talking/writing of a destabilizing mental health condition. We were very tempted to shorten the label to just the encapsulating word bi-polar (literally defined as having or relating to two opposite poles or extremities). Hopefully you are now in a place where that sense of 'dis-order' begins to make more sense – not just as a psychiatric label given to a number of characteristics, but more in terms of what it must be like living and experiencing 'bi-polar-dis-order'.

'BI-POLAR DIS-ORDER' (ALSO KNOWN AS MANIC DEPRESSION)

People living with a diagnosis of bipolar affective disorder (estimated as one in 100 people in England), or manic depressive psychosis as it was formerly called – a term first coined by the German psychiatrist Emil Kraepelin (1856–1926) – have to deal with and then pick up the pieces of intense feelings of depression, followed or preceded by extreme feelings of elation, otherwise known as mania.

Living with such mood extremes has consequences. Bipolar disorder impacts on thought patterns, reactions and associated behaviour changes.

During a manic or 'high' episode, thoughts and feelings run to firmly believing there is something special you can do or offer, that other people do not have. Indeed, genius is often associated with the label.[2] Yet in contrast, a depressive or low state can leave a person feeling worthless, meaningless and insignificant. Neither is restricted to a particular time or pattern, although some people are able to recognize what situations may increase the responses that might lead to either a dramatic high or a desperate low.

Many have spoken openly of their personal experience of mania – where the elation, *joie de vivre*, energy and potential are exhilarating, yet despite this 'freedom of enjoyment', mania is often feared. This is due to previous experiences that this period of elation is likely to be followed by intense and prolonged periods of depression; leading often to thoughts of suicide, which in turn are followed by a lengthy period of rebuilding and repairing the damage done, whether financial, relational, criminal or employment-related.

At the lowest point, feelings and thoughts can get to such depths of despair that there are doubts in one's own existence, associated with guilt and self-loathing over either what has or has not happened in their life; fearing for those loved and lost, hurt, let down and even financially and emotionally ruined. These negative thoughts often linger, causing a severe sense of loss, grief and loneliness. These negative thoughts are then exacerbated through social isolation, psychosomatic ailments and physiological side effects that further enhance a sense of self-loathing.

You: I kept having to ask people if I was alive, did I exist in their eyes. It was a scary place to be. Not knowing whether the place I existed was in fact how and where I would end up. A state of nothingness. No sense, no feeling, nothing, look in the mirror, I can see you, therefore you exist. So surreal.

Some people experience what is called a 'mixed state', where both symptoms of depression and mania coexist, within the moment, while others may experience a rapid mood fluctuation. Whatever the individual's experience, such fluctuation causes the person to become unpredictable, volatile, explosive and sometimes violent and aggressive, leading to either hospitalization or criminal convictions, depending on the circumstances.

There are often early warning signs, but it can be difficult to share or even articulate these. Many people speak of not wanting to seek help, particularly as they do not want to hear people's responses to their behaviour, or think about or stop the high, excitable feelings. The opposite of this is dealing with a sense of panic, where feelings cannot and will not go away, leaving the person thinking they simply cannot do anything about anything, particularly when the person is existing in the low depressive state. Thoughts at this time often lead to the conclusion that they just do not deserve to be helped in any way, or just do not need to be alive.

Sleep disturbance can often be the first sign that something is changing. Whether experiencing a high or a low mood state, there are associated sleep pattern changes.

Me: It was the phone calls. I knew if you were high, as I'd get phone calls and texts all times of the night, through into the early morning. This meant you weren't sleeping or able to stop your flow of thoughts. Then I'd get nothing for days on end. I'd send a text and not get a reply. That meant you were struggling and probably literally stuck in your head, stuck in your flat indoors.

You: I could go for days not hearing anything from anyone, then, when someone did ring, I'd be cross at them for not having been in touch when I needed them most. I used to go days on end without leaving the flat, scared to even go into the kitchen. When I did go out, I was overwhelmed with the road signs, car number plates, noise, movements that I could get over-stimulated and start to do crazy things that would then put me back in hospital, so I worked out it was best just to stay inside.

Me: I do remember you ringing me and your sentences would not even make sense, as your mind ran onto the next thing you wanted to tell me. I had to keep my sentences short and to the point. I found myself getting cross. You were still able to laugh but any minute I knew I might say the wrong thing and you'd explode, or sob down the phone. I just had to check you were OK.

You: When the social worker came to section me, with the psychiatrist, I was convinced they were in disguise and it was you. I wasn't going to be fooled.

Me: When I came to see you, the nurse said, 'Oh so Sally does exist!' Then you rang me from hospital that time, and were reading the magazine out to me. I learnt afterwards you'd been sedated because you were being lewd and disinhibited.

You: They gave me an injection in my bum to knock me out. I think it's my brain chemicals. I wish I'd never started on those meds. I got the wrong sort of sleep on those meds. It didn't help. I just wanted to get out.

REFLECTION

- What did you gain from having read chapter 12, 'Classification of mental illness', in terms of understanding the impact of a diagnosis such as bipolar disorder?

- How might chapter 3, 'Developing and maintaining therapeutic relationships', help when considering how you might interact and dialogue with someone who is suspicious of your intention?

SYMPTOMS OF BIPOLAR DISORDER

Many textbooks and articles state that bipolar disorder only occurs in adults. However, it is now estimated that over half of those people who live with bipolar have had their first episode in late teens, or early adulthood. Many leaflets and internet articles state that diagnosing bipolar disorder and getting the right treatment and help are very difficult, largely due to the complicated mix of symptoms. However, these articles often state that, rather like diabetes, bipolar disorder is something that needs to be adapted to and managed in the long term.

Experiencing all or some of the symptoms outlined in Table 26.1 often results in deterioration in a person's ability to function. Children often get into trouble at school, or with their friends and peers. Adults get into difficulty at work, or in their personal and social relationships, and may end up in the judicial system. All of this further

perpetuates a sense of anxiety and depression, as the person fears what and how the symptoms will manifest themselves. (See chapter 19 for further consideration of what it means to have a labelled mental health illness diagnosis.)

However, other people deal with this problem by depersonalizing their situation and end up blaming everyone else for what is happening to them. In turn, this becomes a self-fulfilling prophecy in that they are misunderstood and everyone else just does not understand them and their mental illness properly. This may lead to people with a diagnosis of bipolar disorder ignoring or refusing any offers of help available to them. This may well be because they do not feel anything will be able to help. Perhaps there is no one who can properly understand their particular situation, as it manifests itself and continues to reoccur within them. These thought patterns and resultant behaviours might in turn

Table 26.1 Symptoms of bipolar disorder

Manic/mania	Depressive/melancholia
Mood changes	
Extreme feelings of happiness, energized, on top of the world	Deep sense of sadness, loneliness, emptiness
Extreme irritability – snappy, short-tempered, quick to anger, laughing turns to tears	Extreme sense of hopelessness, suicidal thoughts Feeling guilty, useless, a burden to others, regrets become overwhelming
Cognitive changes	
I can do and achieve anything My life is full of opportunities	I can do nothing well My life is ruined
I have something special to offer	I am not worth anything I might as well be dead
Behaviour changes	
Speaking quickly, rapid thoughts, jumping from one idea to another Being distracted easily Taking on multiple projects at one time, restlessness, lack of concentration for any length of time Unrealistic beliefs in own potential Impulsive buying/spending spree Generosity to a point where others take advantage Not sleeping, or thinking sleep is not needed Repeatedly doing the same thing (unable to switch off) and doing things to excess Engaging in risky behaviours (can be alcohol or drug-related in an attempt to self-medicate) Sexually disinhibited May experience unrealistic thoughts about own skills and abilities, such as having special powers, or being unable to feel pain	Problems concentrating, forgetful Loss of interest in hobbies, friends or going out anywhere Feeling overly tired, slowed down, no energy to do anything Becoming more socially isolated Weight loss or weight gain – through change in eating habits Sleep disturbed, wanting to sleep but not feeling rested Lack or loss of libido Thoughts of death and planning own suicide, attempting suicide May experience paranoia, thinking they have committed a crime or hurt someone May experience obsessive compulsive thoughts and repeated behaviours

lead to a misdiagnosis. Health professionals work with what they observe, often without fully knowing or considering the story behind the immediate situation, or they do not have the chance to make observations over a longer period in order to monitor patterns of thinking and associated behaviours.

Me: What you doing this weekend? Shall I come see you?
You: That would be nice, I miss you.
Me: What time shall I get there?
You: I'm not good in the mornings.
Me: OK, shall I come Sunday afternoon?

You: What will we do?
Me: I don't know, go for a walk, and have some lunch somewhere?
You: I'm getting anxious now.
Me: We can leave it then, if it's going to make you anxious?
You: Don't play games; I've got a mental illness.
Me: I am trying to see what's best for you?
You: It's always what's best for you.
Me: That's not what I said.
You: Good night!

GETTING A DIAGNOSIS

You: It's like looking through a glass darkly.
Me: What is?
You: Psychiatry.

The professional textbooks explain that a doctor or mental health professional should consider ruling out any physical health issues that might be affecting mood or behaviour changes. Think, for example, of the film, *The Madness of King George*. Today, it is recognized that King George III had porphyria, whereas at the time his rapid mood changes, urine discolouration and disinhibited behaviours were considered a 'madness'. Yet analysis of his prolific personal letters has now shown how his sentence construction changed with his mood, revealing that he may indeed have been suffering from 'incessant loquacity' through to severe depression.[3]

Blood tests can help rule out any physical concerns, such as brain bleeds, strokes and tumours pressing on areas of the brain, that might account for severe mood and behaviours changes. A blood test may also help rule out things like thyroid function, or any other metabolic syndromes. As yet, there is no such thing as a blood test that can be used to help determine mental health problems, although science understands more of how the brain functions, and how hormones and enzymes interact with brain cell growth and electrical transmission between synapses.

REFLECTION

- Do you know what the life expectancy is for someone with a severe mental illness diagnosis such as bipolar disorder, compared to the general population?

- What might contribute to a reduced life expectancy for someone with a diagnosed mental illness?

Obtaining a diagnosis of bipolar disorder may only occur after a period of mania, although without careful history taking to reveal depressive states, clinicians may be

left confused, particularly by a presentation of irritability and aggression that can lead to a diagnosis of personality disorder.

There are four frequently used basic types, and then a fifth specific categorization of mood change episodes, that are used to help identify treatment options for the different manifestations of bipolar disorder. These are broadly described as follows:

- *Bipolar I disorder:* This is when a person has experienced a manic, or mixed episode (where feeling low, but also highly energized and excitable), for at least 7 days. Or a first episode of mania that leads to a person needing hospitalization to keep them and/or others safe. This manic episode will often be followed by a 6- to 8-week period of depression, although the length of the mood change experience is not always the same.
- *Bipolar II disorder:* This is more often defined as a pattern of depressive episodes and experience of manic episodes, but not experiencing the extreme mania that requires hospitalization (which differentiates this from type I), or a mixed state.
- *Bipolar disorder (non-specific/not otherwise specified):* This is when there is experience of severe mood changes that do not fall into the specified patterns outlined above, but nevertheless remain outside the person's normal range of behaviours.
- *Cyclothymic disorder, or cyclothymia:* This is described as a milder form of bipolar disorder, where a person experiences cyclical changes in mood over a period of 2 years, but again, not falling into the pattern outlined in the other three categories.
- *Rapid-cycling bipolar disorder:* This is identified when a person has four or more episodes of major mood shifts, or mixed states, within 1 year. Most often, rapid cycling occurs in people who have had their first episode of extreme mood changes as a younger person. Rapid cycling is more frequently seen in women and therefore has been inferred to be linked to hormonal changes associated with menstruation.[4]

RESEARCH INTO BIPOLAR DISORDER

Surprisingly, perhaps, for such a major mental health issue as bipolar disorder, there is limited research in the area. As of April 2015, a search for manic-depressive psychosis in the Cochrane database identified only two studies, and using the search term 'bipolar disorder' brought up 51 reviews, mainly looking at medication efficacy.

With bipolar disorder, genetics are playing a significant part in recognizing how mental illness can be passed down through our family medical history. However, most children with a family history of bipolar disorder will not necessarily develop the illness.[5]

Increasing evidence from neuropsychiatry and neuro-imaging demonstrates that bipolar disorder does show signs of brain function changes that are highly variable and dependent on mood state, but there is no conclusive evidence that any of these brain changes lead to cognitive impairment.[6] Reduced grey matter function has been shown in research on people with schizophrenia, but the evidence is inconsistent in bipolar research. If temporal lobe volume reduction does exist in bipolar disorder, it is highly variable and only found in a small selective group.[7]

In addition to this research, there is a need to consider the role of violence and criminality that occur as a result of mood disorder, and are particularly associated with the mania phase of bipolar disorder. It is crucial to understand the relationship between affective disorders and aggressive behaviour, as violent behaviour is an increased risk for individuals close to the person with bipolar disorder, and there are subsequent increased risks of legal and socioeconomic problems.[8]

It appears that the connection between aggression and mood disorder represents a state of characteristics that sometimes only come to light during a manic phase, and are highly correlated with drug and alcohol consumption (i.e. substance misuse). Depressive states tend to reveal different elements of aggressive behaviour, more frequently irritability, outbursts of anger and hostility.[9]

The risk of impulsive acts in someone with a diagnosis of bipolar disorder has been considered in terms of clarifying whether it is a trait or a state, yet impulsivity is a major component of bipolar disorder,[10] rather than a manifestation of mood state.[11] The notion of impulsivity is well established in bipolar disorder studies, and many have identified this as being the main issue in terms of complications such as substance misuse, violence and suicide.[12] Impulsivity is considered to be a neurophysiologically based inability to conform behaviour and to place behaviours within a social context. As a result, the person does not take into consideration the consequences of impulsivity on situations and/or on others. The associated risks of impulsive acts and behaviours in people with bipolar disorder mean that consideration must be given to whether or not impulsivity can be helped through behavioural, psychological or cognitive strategies to stabilize or limit risk.[10]

People most often seek help for their depressive episodes, rather than for the mania, although, as outlined above, extreme mania can put someone in a position where they can no longer be left alone due to their impulsivity, and are considered at risk of harming themselves, or others.

You: I was really worried that the building had a bomb, so I started guiding the traffic and screaming for people to evacuate. That was when I got picked up by the police and taken to hospital. I've lost my phone, I think I dropped it in the road and it got run over. I lost my belt too, the leather one I like. I think that got lost when they took me to hospital. My clothes were torn too.

Me: Were you scared?

You: I just had this incessant urge that I couldn't let anyone get hurt. At least I know now I wouldn't harm anyone when I'm high.

Me: What about you though, were you harmed?

You: I lose something every time this happens. I've lost so much to this stupid illness. I'm living a life of regrets that is overwhelming sometimes when I look back at what I could have done. You have it so easy in comparison.

Me: It breaks my heart too. I try to offer that arm of friendship, but I know that is nothing really in comparison.

You: Cruel.

Me: What? I am cruel? I don't think that's right.

You: Just imagine what I could have achieved if I'd been in the right place and had your upbringing …

This manic episode had led to a very public spectacle and was recounted as if retelling me about a film they had watched, rather than describing what they were themselves doing. The conversation outlined above came months later, when in a more reflective mode, but getting low – a very lucid and difficult place to be, let alone remain.

Another manic episode followed about 6 months later. Our relationship was strained by now. I was hurting as a result of being called cruel and not knowing quite how to be a friend during this critically reflective mode that merely led to further self-hatred, on both our counts. Yet I could understand the cruelty of being confronted with my 'normality'. This time the mood disturbance (or as the police would call it, public nuisance) arose following several weeks of no sleep, then walking down the high street, and spotting someone they thought they knew in a high-rise window, who looked as though they were going to jump to their death.

This time I noticed even more personal disassociation in the ramblings from the many phone messages being left on my answerphone. The phone calls came at odd times of the day and night when I was not able to respond quickly enough to speak in person. Eventually, we managed to speak. Language was slurred and incomprehensible at first. Eventually I got the flow of what was being said and worked out you were now back in hospital. At one stage, you were just reading to me from a magazine, making comments on the photographs, then reading me more text. The slurred speech I guessed was following some sort of forced injection. I began to get the gist of what had occurred from phrases like; 'they told me I had been disinhibited, sexually lewd'. As if this could not have been possible. Followed by giggles and 'they pricked me in the bum'.

REFLECTION

This chapter explores a friendship and reveals the tensions arising from the impact of changing mood. What are the implications (e.g. ethical and moral) of trying to be a friend to patients when exploring the craft of caring?

TREATMENT OPTIONS FOR BIPOLAR DISORDER

As in the case of diabetes, people living with bipolar disorder are encouraged to consider their illness as a lifelong health condition that requires careful management and includes a personalized self-education programme.

Treatment options need to be used sensitively during the different phases of the bipolar disorder mood state. However, obtaining the right diagnosis can in itself prove elusive, let alone finding the right combination of treatments, as if each manifestation needs to be considered in its own right, with underlying problems being tackled in the longer term.

The most frequently used intervention is medication, although many studies have shown that medication alone is not effective. People often do not remember to take, or sometimes deliberately avoid taking, medications for multiple reasons when in the throes of mood changes.

You: These bloody tablets are making me worse.
Me: You have puffed up like a puffer fish – what are you taking now?
You: They are trying me on lithium sulfate.
Me: You look …
You: I look like Henry the Eighth!
Me: Do you think that's why he needed Hampton Court Palace to live in!
You: Do you think I have his lovely legs?
Me: You know you've got to stick with this for at least 6 months before it levels out?
You: I know.

Mood-stabilizing medication compliance combined with psychosocial and educational interventions have been identified as significant factors to help people with bipolar disorder manage their symptoms, and are often used in order to help decrease the risk of further and repeated hospitalization. As many as one in three people with a diagnosis of bipolar disorder do not take up to 30 per cent of their prescribed medication, which in turn leads to higher risks of substance misuse, rehospitalization and suicide.[13]

It appears, then, that there are few studies that help us understand what and how combination approaches can best be utilized.[14] So what can we do as health care practitioners, keen to enable our patients, friends, family and loved ones to adhere to a treatment pathway that can bring them relief and help them manage their fluctuating health condition?

Optimized personalized treatment options are being explored, with studies showing that low-level lithium, combined with (up to three) other medications to treat psychiatric symptoms (such as depression, psychosis and anxiety, for example) are now more commonly used.[15] See chapters 47 and 48 for further information on psychopharmacology. The study results are inconclusive, except for stating that few of the people involved in the study had managed to maintain low-dose lithium for 6 months at a time. The combination approach showed no statistical differences. They discuss the fact that low-dose lithium led to less need to expose people to additional antipsychotic medications. The average lithium levels in this study were lower than the typical range recommended; however, blood levels remained consistent for those 6 months. They conclude therefore that modest clinical improvement through using low-level lithium highlights 'the persistent and chronic nature of bipolar disorder as well as the magnitude of unmet needs in its treatment' (p.108).

We all move through a continuum of wellness and illness, and react and respond to situations differently, depending on who we are with, how we are feeling, whether we have slept well, eaten properly, exercised, and are generally looking after ourselves to maximize our own mental health and physical fitness. I suggest that each episode and each person needs to be seen within the window of their current state.

IN SUMMARY

I am left feeling inadequate. The research has not revealed an easy answer. My friend has experienced some tragic episodes, and I have mapped and monitored these as if a cold and impassive observer within and outside the writing of this chapter. This is not what I had hoped for. Perhaps we are still considering bipolar disorder as a relatively new term (adopted in the 1980s), yet something we should know more about and understand. We also know the terms mania and melancholia have been in common use for centuries. Therefore, conceptualizing and applying treatment approaches to something that is still not fully fathomed is perhaps just where we are at this point.

How then can I bring this chapter to a close, leaving with a greater understanding, and a sense of hope and optimism for working with and engaging with people with a bipolar dis-ordered life? Well, I think there are several things I have learnt from this experience that I hope will help you too.

1. Engage and explore on a very personal level what the experience (sometimes moment by moment, in their current circumstances), looks and feels like, to help identify steps that can improve and enhance the person where they are. This is called working with the here and now.[16]

2. Discuss with the clinical team what a combined medication and psychological intervention approach would look like for this person, in their current situation. Also look at the longer term, back at their past, and forward to their hopes and aspirations, and consider how treatment options can be used to scaffold and support a more long-term goal-setting approach.

3. Consider the wider context of social support in terms of who the person trusts and speaks honestly with, and who might be willing and able to help with any crisis plans and longer-term goal setting. Chapter 46 considers crisis assessment and resolution and chapter 50 examines collaborative care planning with service users and carers.

4. Plan ahead and know the signs of when changes are occurring. This can be achieved by monitoring patterns of behaviour and mood changes. Work out what triggers any changes, what and where stressful situations occur for the person, and how they react and respond. Sleep pattern changes are often the first sign to watch out for.

5. Discuss and have an agreed crisis plan. It is important for the person to know and understand that help is available and where to seek this out. This can all be identified in a personalized care package, and at case meetings with the full team present, and with those identified as part of the social support (outlined above in element 3). Keep important numbers to hand, and make sure the person who might receive those emergency phone calls at different times of the day and night is able

to respond effectively. Do not be afraid to ask about suicidal thoughts and any plans they have or are making, and continue to assess for suicide risk, whether the person is feeling manic or low, or has changing moods.

6. Begin to know what are the easy-to-eat, healthy options in terms of food and drinks. Eating foods on the go when high, such as an apple with a lump of cheese, or having food that does not require lengthy preparation when feeling low, such as cooked meat and salad items, depending on personal preference, will help to improve nutrition. Monitor exercise, matching food intake as required, and ensure adequate hydration in both high and low states. Refer to chapter 69 for more detail on the importance of physical health care and chapter 70 which looks at health promotion.

7. Good communication is important. Spend time with the person, getting to know their sense of humour, walking together when the person is agitated and full of energy, or being willing to sit (in a peaceful, preferably green space) together when they are lacking energy and enthusiasm. Answer their questions with honesty, and try not to get upset if they say personally hurtful things or get into an argument. Stop trying to make your point over and above theirs. Listen, and be respectful, but also set limits in terms of what language use and turns of phrase you are willing to accept.

8. Be consistent with setting limits to what are acceptable behaviours, and being clear as to the consequences of behaviours that are socially unacceptable. Be realistic with the person in terms of what they can and cannot achieve.

9. Many people react to stress in different ways. Make sure the person with bipolar disorder understands what stress can do to their mind and body, so they can learn to manage their stress response. Undertaking medication, mindfulness (More detail on mindfulness can be found in chapter 44) and dialectical behaviour therapy are all approaches that many people find useful in maintaining a more balanced approach to managing daily hassles and stress.

REFLECTION

How might you use these principles as part of a mental health promotion programme to educate and support others?

CONCLUSION

After the past year's attempt to engage with bipolar, as a personal experience and as a consequence of trying to engage my friend in writing this chapter, I am left feeling that I have not achieved or satisfied the writing of this chapter in close collaboration, as a result of the reality of working alongside someone whose mood and behaviours are in a state of flux. The aim of mutual participation has, I fear, been compromised, yet I am required to deliver on the writing of this chapter as part of my professional role, but also because of a desire to educate and inform others, in their attempts to understand and support people living bipolar dis-ordered lives.

I refer again to the quotation from Edgar Allan Poe at the start of this chapter: my questions are not yet settled.

There is no shame in mental suffering, or in living a life dis-ordered. Despite periods of very public humiliation, a person's life, productivity and intellectual prowess continue unabated. Hope remains for a better future.

References

1. Poe EA. Eleonora. In: *The works of Edgar Allan Poe, the Raven Edition, volume 2*. New York: PF Collier and Son, 1903.
2. Laurance J. You don't have to be bipolar to be a genius – but it helps. *Independent* 3 February 2010.
3. Wolsely L. *Fit to rule*. BBC2, 15 April 2013.
4. Leibenluft E. Issues in the treatment of women with bipolar illness. *Journal of Clinical Psychiatry* 1997; **58**(5): 5–11.
5. Nurnberger JL, Foroud T. Genetics of bipolar affective disorder. *Current Psychiatry Reports* 2000; **2**(2): 147–57.
6. Bearden CE, Hoffman KM, Cannon TD. The neuropsychology and neuroanatomy of bipolar affective disorder: a critical review. *Bipolar Disorder* 2001; **3**: 106–50.
7. Altshuler LL, Bookheimer SY, Townsend J, Proenza MA, Eisenberger N, Sabb F, Mintz J, Cohen MS. Blunted activation in orbitofrontal cortex during mania: a functional magnetic resonance imaging study. *Biological Psychiatry* 2005; **55**(12): 1163–70.
8. Ballester J, Goldstein T, Goldstein B, Obreja M, Axelson D, Monk K, Hickey M, Iyengar S, Farchione T, Kupfer DJ, Brent D, Birmaher B. Is bipolar disorder specifically associated with aggression? *Bipolar Disorders* 2012; **14**(3): 283–90.
9. Dolenc B, Dernovsek MZ, Sprah L, Travcar R, Perugi G, Akiskal H. Relationship between affective temperaments and aggression in euthymic patients with bipolar mood disorder and major depressive disorder. *Journal of Affective Disorders* 2014; **15**(174): 13–18.
10. Peluso M, Hatch J, Glahn D, Monkul E, Sanches M, Najt P, Bowden CL, Barratt ES, Soares JC. Trait impulsivity in patients with mood disorders. *Journal of Affective Disorders* 2007; **100**(1–3): 227–31.
11. Newman AL, Meyer TD. Impulsivity: present during euthymia in bipolar disorder? A systematic review. *International Journal of Bipolar Disorders* 2014; **2**(2).
12. Swann AC, Lijffijt M, Lane SD, Steinberg JL, Moeller FG. Interactions between bipolar disorder and antisocial personality disorder in trait impulsivity and severity of illness. *Acta Psychiatrica Scandinavica* 2010; **121**(6): 453–61.
13. Scott J, Pope M. Self reported adherence to treatment with mood stabilizers, plasma levels and psychiatric hospitalisation. *American Journal of Psychiatry* 2002; **159**: 1927–9.
14. Sajatovic M, Davies M, Hrouda DR. Enhancement of treatment adherence among patients with bipolar disorder. *Psychiatric Services* 2004; **55**(3): 264–9.
15. Neirenberg AA, Friedman ES, Bowden CL, Syvlia LG, Thase ME, Ketter T, Ostacher MJ, Leon AC, Reilly-Harrington D, Iosifescu DV, Pencina M, Severe JB, Calabrese JR. Lithium treatment moderate dose use study (LiTMUS) for bipolar disorder: a randomised comparative effectiveness trial of optimised personalised treatment with and without lithium. *American Journal of Psychiatry* 2013; **170**(1): 102–10.
16. Yalom E. *The theory and practice of group psychotherapy*. New York: Basic Books, 1931.

Further reading

Clarkin JF, Carpenter D, Hull J, Wilner P, Glick I. Effects of psycho-educational intervention for married patients with bipolar disorder and their spouses. *Psychiatric Services* 1998; **49**(4): 531–3.

Kraepelin E. *Manic depressive insanity and paranoia*. Edinburgh: E & S Livingstone, 1921.

Leader D. Bipolar memoirs: what have I done? *Guardian*, 26 April 2013. Available from: https://www.theguardian.com/books/2013/apr/26/human-touch-in-bipolar-times [Accessed 25th July 2016].

Poe EA. *The complete stories and poems*. New York: Doubleday and Company Inc., 1984.

Rea MM, Thompson MC, Miklowitz DJ, Goldstein MJ, Hwang S, Mintz J. Family focused treatment versus individual treatment for bipolar disorder: results of a randomised controlled trial. *Journal of Consulting and Clinical Psychology* 2003; **71**(3): 482–92.

Relevant web pages

MIND. Bipolar disorder. http://www.mind.org.uk/information-support/types-of-mental-health-problems/bipolar-disorder/

NHS Choices. Bipolar disorder. www.nhs.uk/conditions/bipolar-disorder/Pages/Introduction.aspx

Rethink Mental Illness. Bipolar disorder. www.rethink.org/diagnosis-treatment/conditions/bipolar-disorder

Royal College of Psychiatrists. Bipolar disorder. www.rcpsych.ac.uk/healthadvice/problemsdisorders/bipolardisorder.aspx

Stephen Fry: the secret life of the manic depressive. 2006. www.imdb.com/title/tt0808482/

Time to Change. Bipolar disorder: blogs and personal stories. www.time-to-change.org.uk/category/blog/bipolar

The person with a personality disorder

CHRISTOPHER ALEC GORDON

LEARNING OUTCOMES

- To have a broad understanding of what personality disorders are.

- To begin to understand the impact of personality disorders on the individual, the nurse, health services and society.

- To be aware of the aetiology or causes of personality disorder.

- To understand the development and context of the diagnoses.

- To have an awareness of policy guidance.

- To understand the relevance of attachment difficulties and trauma.

- To know the general principles of nursing people with personality disorder.

- To know the general principles of nursing people with personality disorder in specific settings including community mental health and inpatient mental health settings.

- To understand why clinical supervision is so important.

SUMMARY OF KEY POINTS

- Personality disorders are common and complicated conditions; they influence the way people feel and think about themselves and how they interact with others. Adverse experience and genetic and neurobiological factors are all considered to play a part in causing personality disorder.

- They pose considerable treatment and management challenges to health care professionals; equally service users and carers experience challenges in accessing effective services.

- Borderline personality disorder is the type most likely to be encountered in a health care setting, as there is

- a relatively high prevalence and these individuals are more likely to seek help.
- A relatively long period of assessment is recommended with several meetings over a period of weeks. It is important to identify and treat any comorbid conditions in the first instance.
- Risk needs to be addressed and managed from the onset of involvement with mental health services; along with crisis planning, this forms a central part of treatment.

- General mental health treatment can be as beneficial as specialist psychosocial treatments, provided guiding principles are adhered to.
- Clinical supervision is important in helping to reflect objectively and make use of any strong emotional reactions evoked by service users; this ensures good, safe clinical practice, better clinical outcomes and reduced staff burnout.

INTRODUCTION

This chapter is concerned with the treatment and management of personality disorders and is written in a style that makes it accessible to a general audience with a wide range of knowledge and skills. It aims to provide accurate information and practical guidance and support. It is not an academic paper but will provide key references to support evidence-based care and for further reading.

The chapter is contextualized throughout with contributions from an expert by experience. The term 'expert by experience' refers to those who have experienced personality disorder and who also have experience of accessing and using mental health care services. Amongst others, the term includes patients, clients and service users and, for the purposes of this chapter, the term 'service user' will be used throughout.

Nursing has been broadly defined as 'the therapeutic use of self',[1,2] and in this context nursing people diagnosed with personality disorder presents unique challenges and rewards. The 'craft of caring'[3] for people with personality disorder is more concerned with 'being with' than 'doing to', and the relationship is key to the success of any form of treatment or management. The challenges and rewards therefore lie in that relationship for both parties.

This places the emphasis on the 'therapeutic relationship' and developing collaborative partnerships with service users, working alongside them on their needs.[4] This process is dependent on trust, which as we will see is a difficult issue for most people diagnosed with personality disorder (see chapter 3).

In essence, personality disorders are relational conditions which affect an individual's experience and perception of others, themselves and the world around them. They are considered dimensional or on a continuum, in that we all have personalities and, as part of this, personality disorder traits to some degree or another. The actual diagnoses lie at the severe end of the spectrum and are persistent, pervasive and problematic.

This chapter will explore the diagnostic criteria and living experience of personality disorder, the prevalence and impact of personality disorder, the development and causes or aetiology, assessment and diagnosis, and treatment and supervision.

Simple reference to psychological models and concepts will be used throughout, particularly attachment theory, in order to provide a structure to explore understanding and reflection and as a model to assist in treatment and management.

WHAT ARE PERSONALITY DISORDERS?

SERVICE USER'S PERSPECTIVE

Having a personality disorder [PD] is very difficult for everyone involved. At my worst I behaved like a petulant 6 year old with no boundaries and no understanding of the word 'NO'. All normal reasoning goes out of the window and you live for the moment with no regard for the consequences. My family never understood my PD. They had lived with it for so long that they thought it was just that I was a badly behaved person, with no care for anyone. Friends were oblivious to the majority of my illness, as they just assumed that that was who I was. The strain of my PD has lost me many relationships and I was powerless to prevent this, but trying to make amends was futile as generally people do not understand it, and how can you justify your actions when you don't truly understand them yourself?

Personality disorders are now generally perceived to be relatively common and complicated conditions with a heterogeneous mixture of symptoms which pervasively influence the way people think and feel about themselves and the way in which they interact with others. They may behave in ways that challenge the accepted norms of society. Individuals frequently experience high levels of distress, which often impacts on their families, friends and the general community. It is suggested that people who attract the diagnosis of personality disorder operate predominantly within a world of feeling which is usually unpleasant and distressing. There is a wide spectrum of diversity, severity and disability which is coupled with high rates of comorbidity, including depression, psychosis, self-harm and substance misuse. The onset of the disorder is generally within early adulthood. However, it can be apparent in childhood and adolescence, or emerge later in life. Personality disorders pose considerable treatment and management challenges to health care professionals, and accessing effective services presents equal challenges to service users and carers.

Personality disorders are broadly defined as:

> *An enduring pattern of inner experience and behaviour that deviates markedly from the expectations of the individual's culture, is pervasive and inflexible, has an onset in adolescence or early adulthood, is stable over time, and leads to distress or impairment.[5] (p.685)*

There are currently 10 types of personality disorder, each with its own specific set of diagnostic criteria, shown in Table 27.1. These criteria are set out within two main diagnostic manuals: the recently revised *Diagnostic and statistical manual* (DSM-5)[6] and the *International classification of disorders* (ICD-10)[7] which is in the process of revision (see chapter 12). Although there are parallels between the manuals, there are differences in what the types of personality disorder are called and how they are classified and described. Due to the cross-over of some of the personality disorders, the DSM-5 uses a clustering system.

Each of the individual types has distinctive patterns of relating, which are broadly described in Table 27.2.

The type of personality disorder most likely to be encountered within health care settings is borderline personality disorder (BPD), as there is a relatively high prevalence in comparison to the other types, and because service users with BPD are more likely to seek help than those with other types. When health care staff refer generally to personality disorder, it is most likely that they are referring to BPD.

It is referred to as 'borderline' not because it is nearly or not quite something, as commonly misperceived, but because it includes psychotic symptoms (problems associated with a loss of reality, such as dissociation or paranoia) and neurotic symptoms (affecting mood, such as anxiety or depression). The symptoms of BPD are summarized in Box 27.1.

Table 27.1 Personality disorder diagnoses

Classification system	DSM-5 *The diagnostic and statistical manual of mental disorders* (American Psychiatric Association, 2013)		ICD-10 *The international classification of mental and behavioural disorders* (World Health Organization, 1992)
Classification of personality disorder	*Cluster A* Odd, bizarre, eccentric	• Paranoid • Schizoid • Schizotypal	• Paranoid • Schizoid • Histrionic

	Cluster B Dramatic, erratic	• Histrionic
		• Antisocial
		• Narcissistic
		• Borderline
			• Dissocial
			• Emotionally unstable
			  – Impulsive type
			  – Borderline type

	Cluster C Anxious, fearful	• Obsessive–compulsive • Dependent • Avoidant	• Anankastic • Dependent • Anxious (avoidant)

Table 27.2 Personality disorder patterns of relating

Personality disorder	Pattern of relating
Paranoid	Tend to distrust others and are suspicious that others' motives will cause them harm.
Schizoid	Are detached from social relationships and tend to have a very restricted range of emotional expression.
Schizotypal	Are acutely uncomfortable in close relationships, have odd perceptual distortions, and eccentric behaviour.
Antisocial	Tend to disregard and violate the rights of others.
Borderline	Are unstable in interpersonal relationships, have poor self-image, rapidly changing moods, and are highly impulsive.
Histrionic	Tend to be superficial with excessive emotionality and need for attention.
Narcissistic	Are grandiose, need admiration and respect, and lack empathy towards others.
Avoidant	Are socially inhibited, feel inadequate, and are hypersensitive to criticism.
Dependent	Tend to be submissive with clingy behaviour, and need to be taken care of.
Obsessive–compulsive	Are preoccupied with order and control, and are perfectionists.

BOX 27.1: THE SYMPTOMS OF BORDERLINE PERSONALITY DISORDER (BPD)

- Fear of rejection and abandonment
- Deliberate self-harm and suicidality
- Unstable interpersonal relationships
- Impulsive and self-defeating acts
- Feelings of emptiness and numbness
- Identity problems
- Intense anger
- Paranoia
- Dissociated or 'cut-off'

Source: American Psychiatric Association, *Diagnostic and statistical manual of mental disorder: fifth edition (DSM-5)* (2013).[5]

THE IMPACT OF PERSONALITY DISORDERS

Estimates of prevalence suggest that 5.8 per cent of the general population have a diagnosable personality disorder.[8] In terms of the prevalence of the individual types, this is difficult to tell due to the variance in findings. Obsessive–compulsive appears high while dependent and schizotypal are relatively low.[9] Prevalence is considered particularly high within health care settings, including 50 per cent of mental health inpatients, 40 per cent of psychiatric outpatients and 25 per cent of GP attendees. Borderline represents a high proportion of these figures as service users with BPD tend to seek help more than those with other types.[10] The lifetime prevalence of BPD is considered to be 1 per cent.[11] The prevalence of personality disorder is highest in prison populations, with estimates of up to 80 per cent, including high levels of antisocial personality disorder.[12]

Personality disorder is associated with increased mortality (Standard Mortality Rate [SMR] = 4.2) with a reduced life expectancy of 18.7 years for women and 17.7 years for men. The highest rates of mortality (SMR 10.0) are in the younger age groups.[13]

Rates of self-harm are high and suicide rates are significant and comparable to that of depression.[14]

In 2007, the economic impact of people with personality disorder in contact with primary care in England was estimated to be £704 million, and, if lost employment costs are included, £7.9 billion, set to increase to £12.3 billion by 2026.[7]

REFLECTION

How many patients within your nursing environment might be experiencing the symptoms of personality disorder?

WHAT CAUSES PERSONALITY DISORDERS?

SERVICE USER'S PERSPECTIVE

My family were also unable to accept that my PD may have been born from something from my childhood, which they would have had to address or acknowledge.

The aetiology or causes of personality disorder continue to be a source of debate. They are considered to be influenced by a number of factors, including genetic factors, neurobiological factors and adverse experience. The general consensus is that they are a combination of either a genetic predisposition or biological vulnerability together with some form of childhood trauma or emotional, mental or social development difficulty.[15] Most people with a diagnosis of personality disorder report significant childhood traumas such as neglect, abandonment, loss and abuse.[16] A high proportion of people with BPD report childhood sexual abuse. However, not everyone who experiences abuse as a child develops personality disorder; it is considered to be the poor response to the abuse which makes people vulnerable.

In combination with this, personality disorders are strongly associated with attachment difficulties and most people with personality disorder are considered to have a childhood history of insecure attachment with their main carers. Approximately 95 per cent of people with BPD are coded as insecure.[17]

Early relationships with their main carers play a vital part in the development of how people learn to recognize and manage their emotions (or not), particularly difficult emotions, and how they see themselves and perceive and interact with others.

Prolonged exposure to negative interactions and relationships and poor and abusive experiences as children with those whom they are dependent upon or those who are in positions of power or authority are likely to result in psychological difficulties and unhealthy or unproductive patterns of relating to themselves, others and their culture and environment, which persist into adult life.

A typical pattern seen in people with a diagnosis of BPD is 'attach and attack'. This is often seen in mental health care settings, where the service user will have a strong need for a service but once this is secured will reject or denigrate it. The pattern in this instance is the need for another person to help manage difficult emotions, but not trusting that individual with this vulnerability, which in turn arouses further difficult feelings and the need for attachment. This 'push and pull' dynamic is equally frustrating for help-seeker and help-provider, and a lack of understanding of this can lead to extremes of exclusion and rejection, or a provision of idealized care that is prescriptive and fosters dependence.

REFLECTION

With a colleague, consider how the attach/attack dynamic might be happening with someone you are nursing with BPD.

HOW HAS THE DIAGNOSIS OF PERSONALITY DISORDER COME ABOUT?

SERVICE USER'S PERSPECTIVE

Unless you go into psychosis, then PD really does just present to those who know no better as a person with little respect for rules and reckless behaviour.

Compared to other mental health diagnoses such as schizophrenia or depression, the diagnosis of personality disorder is relatively new and first entered the diagnostic classification systems in the 1980s. This was largely as a result of increased clinical interest and an awareness of service users presenting with common psychiatric problems who appeared more resistant to treatment if they had certain types of personalities: co-existing (or comorbid) personality disorders. However, personality disorder is not a new concept; it has been apparent since the early stages of psychiatry, and has been described in various forms throughout the ages.

When the diagnosis was first introduced, many mental health professionals either refused or were very reluctant to work with people with personality disorders, because they believed that they were untreatable and their services had nothing to offer, they had no resources, or they lacked the skills and training required.

Staff in generic psychiatric services often reported feeling overwhelmed and confused by the complex and demanding nature of the difficulties presented by people with a diagnosis of personality disorder, leading to negative judgements and exclusionary practices and high sickness rates and absence.

Service users with a diagnosis of personality disorder who experienced secondary mental health care services commonly reported sub-standard care, discrimination and rejection. The use of derogatory labels by psychiatric staff such as 'difficult', 'bad', 'manipulative', 'time-wasters' and 'attention seekers' was said to be common.

Markham and Trower[18] found that service users with a label of BPD attracted more negative responses from nursing staff than those with a label of schizophrenia or depression. Staff reported less sympathy and optimism towards these service users and rated their experiences of working with them as more negative. These results confirm earlier findings[19] that nurses decreased their positive interactions with personality disordered service users and replaced them with disparaging comments and disconfirming responses/comments compared to service users with other diagnoses.

Many people working in mental health services, and service users, say that personality disorder became a diagnosis that effectively excluded people from mainstream mental health services.[20]

REFLECTION

Do you or your colleagues respond to challenging behaviour differently depending upon diagnosis? If so, why?

POLICY GUIDANCE FOR PERSONALITY DISORDER

SERVICE USER'S PERSPECTIVE

Mental health services are only relatively recently becoming aware of PD and learning to cope with them. They are not given the respect other more prominent illnesses are, as mostly they are just seen as bad or attention-seeking behaviour.

In 2003, the Department of Health and National Institute of Mental Health England (NIMHE) set out to address exclusionary practice and discrimination by issuing Policy Implementation Guidance on personality disorder, called *Personality disorder: no longer a diagnosis of exclusion*.[21] This guidance set out a vision both for the development of new services for people with personality disorders and for supporting existing local services in their work through education, training, consultation and support. A Capabilities Framework for staff called *Breaking the cycle of rejection* was produced to support this work.[22]

The key purpose of the guidance was to provide accessible and appropriate management and care for people with personality disorder who experience significant distress or difficulty, and placed a requirement upon all general mental health trusts to establish either specialist multidisciplinary community teams or specialist day services.

The guidance in itself challenged commonly held beliefs that personality disorders are not treatable by providing evidence that certain psychosocial approaches are effective.

The guidance did not specify the use of any particular approach, but advocated the guiding principles common to these treatments, including:

- being well-structured;
- devoting effort to achieving adherence;
- having a clear focus;
- being theoretically coherent to both mental health care worker and service user;
- being relatively long-term;

- being well integrated with other services;
- having a clear treatment alliance between mental health care worker and service user.[21]

These proposed implementations were set to be introduced into a culture in which many mental health professionals are sceptical about the effectiveness of treatment and hence inclusion of people with personality disorder in mainstream mental health services. It was suggested at the time that general adult mental health services 'are not yet organized to allow patients with personality disorders easy access, and practitioners lack the necessary skills to implement effective treatment'[23] (p.425).

This was particularly true for mental health nurses, and still remains so for some. Faced with attempting the therapeutic use of self with inadequate and inappropriate service structures and no psychological model or training to know how, when, how much and what part of self to use, treatment attempts were doomed to fail, with service user and staff casualties alike.

The principles outlined in the policy guidance were reinforced in 2009 by National Institute for Health and Care Excellence (NICE) guidelines for borderline and antisocial personality disorder, which included further guidelines and evidence to support treatment and management, which will be referred to in the remainder of the chapter.[24,25]

A competencies framework[26] has been developed which addresses the workforce issues and requirements for effective treatment and management, and it is recommended that the reader reviews this document.

REFLECTION

In consideration of the increased awareness and prevalence of personality disorders, to what extent have your training needs been met? Discuss any unmet need with a senior nursing colleague.

THE RELEVANCE OF ATTACHMENT THEORY

SERVICE USER'S PERSPECTIVE

I found trusting staff in mental health to be very difficult and was always very wary. However, once I had spent significant time with the same person and confided in them or leant on them, then I did become attached, although didn't realise it at the time. When I lost my CPN [Community Psychiatric Nurse] after many years, I went through a bereft mourning period. In hindsight, having a PD meant that I saw a relationship that wasn't there but held an unhealthy attachment to it. This can be very damaging and very hard to break. The feeling of imagined rejection, when the staff member moved on, did, at times, trigger a relapse in my mental health.

Although attachment theory in itself is too simplistic to explain the complexity of the nature and causes of personality disorders, it does offer a relatively simple model to begin to understand personality disorders and provide a framework for considering treatment. As a universal theory, it is relatively easy to reflect upon and apply to others empathically.

It can be argued that attachment theory should be a key consideration of any nurse in any health care setting, yet it is barely touched upon in nursing training, if at all. Attachment is considered particularly important in mental health care, and nowhere more so than in the understanding, treatment and management of personality disorders.[27]

Attachment theory was developed by John Bowlby[28-30] and postulates a universal human need to form close affectional bonds. At its core is the reciprocity of early relationships, which is a precondition of normal development in all mammals, including humans. Bowlby suggested that we are not born with the capacity to regulate our own emotions and we learn to manage this through attachment to our main caregivers. The attachment behaviours of the human infant (proximity seeking, smiling, clinging, crying) are reciprocated by adult attachment behaviours (touching, holding, soothing, cooing) and these responses strengthen the attachment behaviour of the infant towards that particular adult. The overall goal of the attachment system is the experience of security; a regulator of emotional experience or 'secure base'. The infant's experience of this secure base is then internalized into a working model for managing emotions in later life (thought to happen between 1 and 2 years of age). Attachment or proximity–seeking behaviour is often triggered in adults by 'threat, illness or fatigue' and this is when attachment becomes highly relevant to all nursing disciplines. Failed or pathological attachment in early childhood gives rise to the repetition of maladaptive attachment patterns in adulthood. Approximately 40 per cent of the general population are classified as insecurely attached. Attachment and relational difficulties are frequently seen in and reported by those who experience adult mental health problems, particularly disorders of the personality. Health care professionals can be seen in terms of attachment figures, which raises the question of whether people with personality disorder are attachment seeking rather than attention seeking.

REFLECTION

Consider the development of 'therapeutic relationships' in the context of attachment theory.

HOW PERSONALITY DISORDERS ARE ASSESSED AND DIAGNOSED

NICE guidelines state that personality disorders should be formally assessed by secondary care community mental health teams.[23]

Assessing personality disorder can be a complex process and a relatively long period of assessment is recommended, with several meetings over a period of weeks. Personality disorder has historically been considered as a secondary diagnosis, i.e. other mental illnesses are considered first. Personality disorder often sits alongside comorbidity, so it is important to identify and treat comorbid conditions in the first instance. However, one of the pitfalls for this approach is that treatments prescribed for other mental health problems might be contraindicated for personality disorder. For instance, there are no recommended drugs to treat personality disorder; therefore a review of medication is an important part of the assessment process.

An extended assessment is a process of assessment over 4 weeks and provides a collaborative means of capturing the service user's history with them (and carers where appropriate) to begin to recognize and formulate difficulties, identify strengths and coping mechanisms, and identify needs and treatment options. The process complements the Integrated Care Programme Approach (ICPA) (see chapter 37), and, with permission, the assessment is shared with the service user's clinical and service network, and family and carers. The extended assessment can also include a formal assessment of personality disorder such as Structured Clinical Interview for DSM-IV Personality Disorders II,[31] the International Personality Disorder Examination[32] or the Standardised Assessment of Personality.[33] The extended assessment process requires relatively little training. However, although the process of capturing and recalling someone's history can be a validating experience, it can also be a painful one if it includes trauma. Therefore, it is recommended that the process is clinically supervised by an expert.

Where there is a history with mental health services, a review of the clinical records can be a helpful part of the assessment process. It is particularly helpful when a service user with a complex presentation has become 'stuck' or is in a 'revolving door' situation with services. It is also appropriate where service users are unable or unwilling to work collaboratively. A complex case note review involves a member of the team reviewing all clinical records to assist services to learn from past interventions, to review the efficacy of treatment to date and to help plan future interventions and ways forward.

The diagnosis is concerned with meeting specific criteria which are *persistent* (at least a year), *pervasive* (affecting all aspects of a person's life) and *problematic* (causing significant distress). Considering the spectrum of diversity and severity, diagnosis should always be considered within the context of these 'three Ps'.

Any mental health professional can diagnose personality disorder if they are trained and competent to do so. Even without specific training, the nurse has a valuable role in helping service users to understand the diagnosis.

The differences in the diagnostic criteria between DSM-5 and ICD-10[5,6] can cause confusion to nurses and other health professionals and service users and carers alike. It is therefore important to be clear about terms and specific criteria when exploring the diagnosis, and to break down the descriptions into lay terms, exploring each of the criteria in the context of the service user's own life, experiences, culture and understandings. It is recommended that both diagnostic manuals are reviewed in detail and that information is provided to service users and their families and carers as appropriate.

Educational and awareness workshops are also effective ways of exploring the diagnosis for service users and their families, friends and carers.[34]

Caution is advised in applying the diagnosis to young people, whose personality is still considered to be forming. Adolescence is also a transitional period in life and can appear similar to some of the diagnostic criteria, particularly for BPD. There is a tendency to use the term 'emerging personality disorder' (EPD) where there is some diagnostic certainty. The benefit of early recognition and diagnosis is early treatment and prevention.

It is recognized that the term 'personality disorder' is contentious and causes offence to some service users. The views of service users who do not wish to be labelled should be respected. All diagnoses need to be recorded clearly in the clinical notes with a comment about the service user's view.

> ## REFLECTION
>
> Is there someone you are currently nursing with a diagnosis of personality disorder? If so, what does it mean to them?

RISK ASSESSMENT AND MANAGEMENT

> ## SERVICE USER'S PERSPECTIVE
>
> Self harm [SH], for me, was about pain. I burned myself severely. I had to find a way to stop my emotions and immense pain achieved that for me. I also used it as a punishment to myself if I felt I had failed. Honestly, at times I also used SH (when I was an inpatient) as a means of manipulation. I could control certain areas of my care and staff by self-harming.

Issues of risk need to be addressed and managed from the onset of involvement with mental health services. Risk assessment and management and crisis planning are a central part of treatment. As part of this process, a risk matrix is created; this is a collaborative tool that helps service users and staff to identify protective as well as risk factors.[35]

The role of medication PDs

> ## SERVICE USER'S PERSPECTIVE
>
> Medication was not helpful to me; while it dealt with some of the anxiety behaviours, it was not productive and more of a managing tool, for me and those trying to deal with me.

NICE guidelines[23] state that there are no effective medications for BPD or for the individual symptoms, and that specific medication should only be used in the short term to manage crises. However, a recent audit in England[36] found widespread and combined use of antipsychotics, antidepressants, benzodiazepines and mood stabilizers. This can partly be explained by the treatment of comorbid conditions; however, inappropriate polypharmacy may be a causal factor in reduced life expectancy.

RECOMMENDED TREATMENTS FOR PERSONALITY DISORDER

SERVICE USER'S PERSPECTIVE

Psychological therapies I have found to be impossible. The core nature of my illness means that I do not trust or wish to comply. At the first signs of difficulty in opening up and the subsequent emotions that brings, my PD fights any productive resolution.

There is a growing body of evidence to show that personality disorders can be effectively treated and managed. However, there remains some uncertainty about what works for what type of personality disorder.

Considerable advances have been made in the last two decades in developing specialist psychosocial treatments for personality disorders and developments have been particularly apparent for Borderline Personality Disorder. NICE-recommended specialist treatments[23] include mentalization-based therapy (MBT), dialectical behaviour therapy (DBT), cognitive analytic therapy (CAT), cognitive behavioural therapy (CBT), inter-personal therapy (IPT) and transference-focused psychotherapy (TFP).

However, the majority of people who seek treatment will receive this from general mental health services rather than specialist centres or teams. Research examining specialist treatment versus certain general mental health treatment provides good evidence that general mental health services which use certain principles can provide effective treatment for some personality disorders; and in some cases, such as BPD, are as beneficial as specialist treatments.[37]

The reasons for this are unclear, but it is a reasonable hypothesis that the benefits may be more concerned with the attachment to the clinician(s) rather than the type of treatment employed.

The benefits of these generalist treatments are that they draw upon the existing skills of practitioners, such as mental health nurses, and only modest training and supervision are required in order to be effective, as opposed to learning new and specific skills required for specialist interventions which can be lengthy and expensive. Generalist treatment approaches are therefore the most pertinent and appropriate treatment approach for mental health nurses to consider and adopt.

The four main types of evidence-based general treatments are: structured clinical management (SCM), which produced good results when compared to MBT;[38] general psychiatric management (GPM), which was compared to DBT and found to be equally effective;[39] good clinical care (GCC), which was found to be equally effective as CAT;[40] and supportive psychotherapy (SP), for which a general equivalence was found with TFP and DBT with adolescents with borderline features.[41]

Each of these approaches shares very similar guiding principles, including: staff who are willing, hopeful and optimistic about working with people with personality disorder; staff who are empathic and validating with a shared consensus and collaborative agreement about treatment goals; clinicians who actively engage the service user; well-structured and consistent treatment that is relatively long-term; a treatment model that has a clear and theoretically underpinned focus which is coherent to staff and service users; and a clinical team that is well trained and supervised. The organization of treatment needs to be well structured, coordinated, integrated with other services and, most importantly, understood by service users and carers.

SCM summarizes the processes of treatment in the following way:

- careful assessment;
- giving the diagnosis;
- information about diagnosis;
- crisis planning;
- risk assessment and management;
- development of a hierarchy of therapeutic areas;
- agreement of clinician and service user responsibilities;
- development of motivation and establishment of therapeutic alliance;
- stabilization of drug misuse and alcohol abuse;
- development and agreement of comprehensive formulation;
- involvement of families, relatives, partners and others.[37]

In addition to these approaches, there is a new whole systems approach called relational recovery,[42] which shares the principles and treatment approaches of generalist models such as SCM but is guided throughout by a collaborative formulation framework known as guided formulation (GF). Relational recovery is currently being evaluated in the context of the whole system including in comparison to evidenced-based psychological therapies in primary and secondary mental health care.

The role of the relational recovery team is to provide specialist training, consultation, support and supervision to the frontline workforce in inpatient and community settings, as well as providing clinical care.

Relational recovery combines a structured and psychologically informed approach. The emphasis is on collaboration and it recognizes the importance of relationships and people's unique strengths in recovering from serious mental health problems. Chapter 3 has information on developing and maintaining therapeutic relationships.

Guided formulation is central to the relational recovery care pathway. It is a collaborative process, which helps service users, carers and staff make sense of difficulties by pulling together past and present difficulties, identifying relational patterns, reflecting upon feelings and behaviour and identifying recovery goals. See chapters 35 and 36 for more detailed information on recovery. The guided formulation informs treatment choices, risk management and crisis plans (see chapter 46), and the care plan in general (see chapters 8 and 50). The guided formulation is owned by the service user and shared with families and carers and the wider clinical network as appropriate. The process can take up to 12 weeks and should only be undertaken by staff who have been specifically trained in this approach and who are specifically supervised (the guide; that is, the member of staff supervising the person carrying out the guided formulation).

One of the many benefits of guided formulation is that it helps the service user to begin to think and reflect about themselves in a psychological way, and can be an important prelude to specialist therapies. Alternatively, it can inform a decision not to pursue or to delay further in-depth treatment.

Guided formulation is primarily a collaborative process. However, by its very nature, it can be challenging for some, and there may be occasions when the service user is unable or unwilling to engage, when the team might undertake a guided formulation to assist in planning care and managing risks without the service user's involvement.

SERVICE USER'S PERSPECTIVE

Guided formulation has not been beneficial to me due to the structure and timeframe for completion. I found with my PD, I needed to have a trusting relationship to be able to work with someone and the timeframe was not conducive to that. When you are in the throes of PD, then you do not want help ... equally when you are on the better side of your PD, you do not think you need help.

The evidence for effective treatments of personality disorder is generally best for borderline types; the other types are considered to benefit, but the evidence base is not as strong. Antisocial personality disorder tends to respond better to less emotive approaches such as CBT (see chapter 40), while avoidant types do not respond well to the generalist approach.

As part of a generalist approach, other helpful interventions can include:

- *practical and social care interventions:* housing, finances, employment, education, occupation, etc.;
- *making and maintaining links:* support networks and other services;
- *guided self-help:* assistance with self-help books and courses, websites, etc.;
- *service user and carer workshops:* educational workshops on the diagnosis, NICE guidelines, etc.;
- *psycho-educational groups:* identifying, understanding and managing diagnoses;
- *skills-based groups:* anxiety management, emotional regulation.

Nidotherapy is a relatively new concept in the treatment of personality disorder and other persistent mental health problems[43] and is particularly relevant to nurses. It involves a collaborative assessment and a change of the environment. The term derives from the word *nidus*, which is Latin for 'nest'. Therapy is concerned with making change in the external environment, as opposed to other treatments for personality disorder, such as psychotherapy (see chapters 42 and 43 for more information on psychodynamic approaches), which aim for internal change. This therapy is often employed for treatment-resistant personality disorders, and is suitable for most types, but particularly paranoid, schizoid, schizotypal, avoidant and dependent types. The therapy targets relevant family and friends, neighbours, health and social services, housing, police and others to promote understanding and tolerance of the service user's eccentricities and a lifestyle to fit their needs. Problem solving and goals can often be more the concern of the therapist or team than the service user. Formulation is a useful tool for identifying problem areas in the environment and providing an understanding of these. This approach is growing in popularity and provides an effective treatment choice for people who are unable to, or choose not to, access psychological interventions. The approach can also be used in parallel with other treatments and can be particularly helpful as part of generalist approaches. The approach is relevant to all areas of nursing, and the model works particularly well in assertive outreach teams.

REFLECTION

Consider your team's approach to personality disorder and how this might fit with the principles of a generalist approach such as SCM.

THE ROLE OF INPATIENT MENTAL HEALTH CARE

SERVICE USER'S PERSPECTIVE

Inpatient mental health care should never be a place for someone with PD unless they are a danger to themselves. The behaviour I displayed was very difficult to manage on an inpatient ward and disruptive to all those around me. Being an inpatient, against my will, made my PD far more prominent. The PD is like having the mindset of a very naughty child. When you are told that you cannot do something and have to abide by structure and rules, then the bad behaviour linked to the PD will take control and prove far more dangerous than being left in the community with support. Being an inpatient with PD should ever only be a safeguard and temporary measure.

The role of inpatient treatment in the care of people with personality disorder is tenuous and is considered unbeneficial, if not harmful. This appears true for most types of personality disorder, although there is some evidence that obsessive–compulsive, avoidant and dependent types may gain some benefits.[44] In spite of providing little to no clinical benefits, admission can be a life-saver. The most frequent reason for admission to mental health units for people with personality disorder is a high risk of suicide and self-harm. Short admissions to manage crisis can be helpful in managing such risks. Ideally, these should be considered and agreed on beforehand in the form of a crisis plan. NICE guidelines for borderline personality disorder[23] suggest a period of no more than 3 days. Short-term admission can also be helpful for reviewing medication, for treating comorbidity such as depression and dual diagnosis, and for managing ruptures in community treatment. Various reasons have been explored to explain why people with personality disorder respond poorly to inpatient treatment. One of the main difficulties is managing consistencies in approach by a large number of caregivers. The service user is faced with multiple attachment figures who have different attachment and caregiving styles. The role of the key worker is essential in providing a key attachment figure. The development of nursing key workers in the 1950s was a direct result of attachment research. However, this is challenging in a system that provides 24-hour care in shifts. Clearly agreed goals need to be specified in the care plan, as this is often the one remaining constant.

ENDINGS AND TRANSITIONS

Due to the attachment difficulties associated with personality disorder, particularly the strong fears of abandonment in BPD, all predictable endings or transitions with or between staff or services should be discussed and planned for. It is also important to manage staff absence by giving notice of staff unavailability, including leave, and having a back-up plan for staff sickness.

THE IMPORTANCE OF CLINICAL SUPERVISION

Clinical supervision is an essential aspect of the treatment and management of personality disorders because they tend to cause strong emotional reactions in carers. The supervisor can provide a buffer to such reactions and objectively help to reflect on and make use of emotional reactions. Chapter 10 explores clinical supervision in some detail.

As care providers, our internal experience (thoughts and feelings) of and reactions (behaviours) to people with personality disorder are often very telling, and may provide a clue to or a reflection of their early relational patterns. There may be a strong feeling of wishing to rescue the service user by striving to provide ideal care, or an equally strong feeling of anger and rejection, and a tendency to overlook or neglect. This may represent the service user's early experiences of neglect, loss or abuse, or be an unconscious invitation to staff to replicate this abusive pattern of relating, or it might be an attempt to fill the void of childhood unmet need. Different members of the nursing team may have opposing views, which may lead to conflict and inconsistencies of care. It is commonly said that service users with personality disorder split or divide the team; this is probably less a result of any conscious attempt on behalf of the service user and more likely to be a result of the service user finding an existing difference within the team. This may reflect the inner conflict (needing an attachment but not trusting one) of the service user or may say something about a conflict in their early experiences (inconsistencies in parental care).

Nursing people with personality disorder calls upon the carer to consider their own style of attachment and caregiving. It may touch upon their own early experiences, some of which might painfully reflect those of service users. There is no other area where clinical supervision is so essential.

The payoff of regular clinical supervision is good, safe clinical practice and better clinical outcomes, as well as reduced staff burnout, sickness and absence.

CONCLUSION

Considerable advances have been made in the field of personality disorder in the last two decades, and there is a growing body of evidence to support a number of effective treatments and approaches. However, it is still unclear exactly what works for whom. The debate about the causes of personality disorder continues. Traditional medical approaches appear to offer little. Access to specialist services and teams is growing, and the need to support health care professionals in the therapeutic use of self with good training and supervision is becoming better understood.

ACKNOWLEDGEMENT

The author would like to thank Jo Gibson, Service Evaluation Assistant, for her help with this chapter.

References

1. Peplau H. *Interpersonal relation in nursing*. New York: Putnam, 1952.
2. Uys LR. Towards the development of an operational definition of the concept 'therapeutic use of self'. *International Journal of Nursing Studies* 1980; **17**: 175–80.
3. Barker P. *Psychiatric and mental health nursing: the craft of caring*, 2nd edn. London: Hodder Arnold, 2009.
4. Barker P, Whitehill I. The craft of care: towards collaborative caring in psychiatric nursing. In: Tilley S (ed.). *The mental health nurse: views of practice and education*. Blackwell Science: Oxford, 1997.
5. American Psychiatric Association. *Diagnostic and statistical manual of mental disorders (DSM-IV-TR)*. Washington DC: American Psychiatric Association, 2000.
6. American Psychiatric Association, *Diagnostic and statistical manual of mental disorders: fifth edition (DSM-5)*. Washington DC: American Psychiatric Association, 2013.
7. WHO (World Health Organization). *International classification of diseases*. Geneva: WHO, 1992.
8. McCrone P, Dhanasiri S, Patel A, Knapp M, Lawton-Smith S. *Paying the price: the cost of mental health care in England in 2026*. London: Kings Fund, 2008.
9. Singleton N, Bumpstead R, O'Brien M, Lee A, Meltzer H. *Psychiatric morbidity among adults living in private households, 2000*. London: Stationery Office, 2001.
10. Moran P, Mann A. The prevalence and 1-year outcome of cluster B personality disorders in primary care. *Journal of Forensic Psychiatry* 2002; **13**(3): 527–37.
11. Grant BF, Chou SP, Goldstein RB, Huang B, Stinson FS, Saha TD, Smith SM, Dawson DA, Pulay AJ, Pickering RP, Ruan WJ. Prevalence, correlates, disability and comorbidity of DSM-IV borderline personality disorder: results from the wave 2 National Epidemiologic Survey on Alcohol and Related Conditions. *Journal of Clinical Psychiatry* 2008; **69**: 533–45.
12. Singleton N, et al. *Psychiatric morbidity among prisoners in England and Wales*. London: Stationery Office, 1998.
13. Fok MLH, Hayes RD, Chang CK, Stewart R, Callard FJ, Moran P. Life expectancy at birth and all-cause mortality among people with personality disorder. *Journal of Psychosomatic Research* 2012; **73**: 104–7.
14. Gerson J, Stanley B. Suicidal and self-injurious behaviour in personality disorder: controversies and treatment directions. *Current Psychiatry Reports* 2002; **4**(1): 30–8.
15. Coid J. Aetiological risk factors for personality disorders. *British Journal of Psychiatry* 1999; **174**: 530–8.
16. Bierer LM. Abuse and neglect in childhood: relationship to personality disorder diagnoses. *CNS Spectrums* 2003; **8**(10): 737–54.
17. Levy KN. The implications of attachment theory and research for understanding borderline personality disorder. *Development and Psychopathology* 2005; **17**: 959–86.
18. Markham D, Trower P. The effects of the psychiatric label 'borderline personality disorder' on nursing staff's perceptions and causal attributions for challenging behaviour. *British Journal of Clinical Psychology* 2003; **42**: 243–56.
19. Fraser K, Gallop R. Nurses' confirming/disconfirming responses to patients with borderline personality disorder. *Archives of Psychiatric Nursing* 1993; **7**(6): 336–41.
20. Dinos S, Stevens S, Serfaty M, Weich S, King M. Stigma: the feelings and experiences of 46 people with mental illness. *Journal of Psychiatry* 2004; **184**: 176–81.
21. NIMHE (National Institute for Mental Health England). *Personality disorder: no longer a diagnosis of exclusion*. Leeds: Department of Health, 2003.
22. NIMHE (National Institute for Mental Health England). *Breaking the cycle of rejection: the personality disorder capabilities framework*. Leeds: Department of Health, 2003.
23. Bateman A, Tyrer P. Services for personality disorder: organisation for inclusion. *Advances in Psychiatric Treatment* 2004; **10**: 425–34.
24. NICE (National Institute for Health and Care Excellence). *Borderline personality disorder: treatment and management. Clinical Guideline 78*. London: NICE, 2009.
25. NICE (National Institute for Health and Care Excellence). *Antisocial personality disorder: treatment, management & prevention. Clinical Guideline 77*. London: NICE, 2009.
26. Roth AD, Pilling S. Using an evidence-based methodology to identify the competences required to deliver effective cognitive and behavioural therapy for depression and anxiety disorders. *Behavioural and Cognitive Psychotherapy* 2008; **36**(2):129–47.

27. Fonagy P, Target M, Gergely G. Attachment theory and borderline personality disorder: a theory and some evidence. *Psychiatric Clinics of North America* 2000; **23**(1): 103–22.

28. Bowlby J. *Anxiety*. New York: Basic, 1969.

29. Bowlby J. *Separation*. New York: Basic, 1973.

30. Bowlby J. *Loss*. New York: Basic, 1980.

31. First MB, Gibbon M, Spitzer RL, Williams JBW, Benjamin LS. *User's guide for the structured clinical interview for DSM-IV Axis II Personality Disorders*. Washington DC: American Psychiatric Press, 1997.

32. Loranger AW, Janka A, Sartorius N (eds). *Assessment and diagnosis of personality disorders: the International Personality Disorder Examination (IPDE)*. Cambridge: Cambridge University Press, 1996.

33. Mann AH, Raven P, Pilgrim J, Khanna S, Velayudham A, Suresh KP, Channabasavanna SM, Janca A, Sartorius N. An assessment of the Standardized Assessment of Personality as a screening instrument for the International Personality Disorder Examination: a comparison of informant and patient assessment for personality disorder. *Psychological Medicine* 1999; **29**(4): 985–9.

34. Carter C, Sired S, Gordon C. Evaluation of borderline personality disorder awareness workshops for service users and carers. *Mental Health Practice* 2015; **19**(2): 26–31.

35. Yeandle J, Gordon C, Challis E, Fawkes L. Risk assessment and management of people with personality disorders. *Mental Health Practice* 2013; **17**(2): 21–3.

36. Royal College of Psychiatrists. *Prescribing observatory for mental health audit*. London: Royal College of Psychiatrists, 2012.

37. Bateman AW, Krawitz R. *Borderline personality disorder: an evidence-based guide for mental health professionals*. Oxford: Oxford University Press, 2013.

38. Bateman A, Fonagy P. Randomized control trial of outpatient mentalization-based treatment versus structured clinical management for borderline personality disorder. *American Journal of Psychiatry* 2009; **166**: 1355–64.

39. McMain S, Links PS, Gnam WH, Guimond T, Cardish RJ, Korman L, Streiner DL. A randomised control trial of dialectical behavioural therapy versus general psychiatric management for borderline personality disorder. *American Journal of Psychiatry* 2009; **166**: 1365–74.

40. Chanen AM, Jackson HJ, McCutcheon LK, Jovev M, Dudgeon P, Yuen HP, Germano D, Nistico H, McDougall E, Weinstein C, Clarkson V, McGorry PD. Early intervention for adolescents with borderline personality disorder: quasi-experimental comparison with treatment as usual. *Australian and New Zealand Journal of Psychiatry* 2009; **43**: 397–408.

41. Clarkin JF, Levy KN, Lenzenweger MF, Kernberg OF. Evaluating three treatments for borderline personality disorder. *American Journal of Psychiatry* 2007; **164**: 922–8.

42. Pack S, Wakeham S, Beeby R, Fawkes L, Yeandle J, Gordon C. Management of borderline personality disorder. *Nursing Times* 2013; **109**(15): 21–3.

43. Tyrer P. Nidotherapy: a new approach to the treatment of personality disorder. *Acta Psychiatrica Scandinavica* 2002; **105**: 469–71.

44. Bartak A, Spreeuwenberg MD, Andrea H, Holleman L, Rijnierse P, Rossum BV, Hamers EF, Meerman AM, Aerts J, Busschbach JJ, Verheul R, Stijnen T, Emmelkamp PM. Effectiveness of different modalities of psychotherapeutic treatment for patients with cluster C personality disorders: results of a large prospective multicentre study. *Psychotherapy and Psychosomatics* 2009; **79**(1): 20–30.

Further reading

Department of Health. *Meeting the challenge – making the difference: a new practitioner's guide*. London: DH, 2014. Available from: http://www.emergenceplus.org.uk/news-from-emergence/507-meeting-the-challenge-making-a-difference-a-new-personality-disorder-practitioner-guide.html [Accessed 8th September 2016].

Relevant web pages

American National Association for Personality Disorder – Treatment and Research Advancements (TARA). http://www.tara4bpd.org/dyn/index.php

BPD World. http://www.bpdworld.org/
   This charitable organization works to reduce the stigma of Borderline Personality Disorder (BPD).

Emergence. http://www.emergenceplus.org.uk/
   This national user-led organization provides information about all aspects of personality disorder.

Mental Help. Personality disorders. http://www.mentalhelp.net/poc/center_index.php?id=8
   This charity provides a wealth of information about personality disorder.

MIND. Personality disorders. http://www.mind.org.uk/information-support/types-of-mental-health-problems/personality-disorders

National Education Alliance for Borderline Personality Disorder. http://www.borderlinepersonalitydisorder.com/
   This American site provides lots of information, including video and audio links.

NHS evidence search on self-harm with links to NICE guidelines. http://www.evidence.nhs.uk/search?q=self-harm

NICE (National Institute for Health and Care Excellence). Antisocial personality disorder: prevention and management. http://www.nice.org.uk/guidance/CG77

NICE (National Institute for Health and Care Excellence). Borderline personality disorder: recognition and management. http://www.nice.org.uk/guidance/cg78

Personality disorder. http://personalitydisorder.org.uk/
   This is a comprehensive site managed by a national personality disorder development team.

Royal College of Psychiatrists. Personality disorder. http://www.rcpsych.ac.uk/healthadvice/problemsdisorders/personality-disorder.aspx

Samaritans. http://www.samaritans.org/

28 The person experiencing disturbing voices, ideas and beliefs

CHERYL FORCHUK, ELSABETH JENSEN AND NATALIE FARQUHAR

LEARNING OUTCOMES

- To understand psychosis.
- To be able to define delusions and hallucinations.
- To know how to distinguish disturbing from non-disturbing instances of psychosis.
- To understand how interpersonal relationships may aid the nurse in caring for clients.
- To have a working knowledge of common forms of treatment for psychotic symptoms.

SUMMARY OF KEY POINTS

- Delusions and hallucinations are the most common symptoms of psychosis.
- When these or other symptoms of psychosis are experienced, they may be disturbing to the client or their friends and family.
- In these cases, the client is brought into contact with the mental health care system.

- Nurses should care for clients in the context of therapeutic relationships.
- Once the therapeutic relationship is established, there are a variety of treatments that may be used to address the underlying condition.

INTRODUCTION

This chapter is written from the perspectives of two nurse academics with decades of clinical experience, as well as a student nurse who has personally experienced psychosis. The personal illustrations and content of this chapter reflect these points of view. Many of the experiences discussed in this chapter fall under the broad category of psychosis. Psychosis is a break with reality, and may indicate the existence of an underlying psychiatric disorder, though not always. Nurses must always carefully assess clients experiencing a psychotic episode, particularly if it is the client's first episode. Both the client and their family may find the experience of psychosis to be difficult, as they would find many health challenges. Because of this the nurse should cultivate a well-developed sense of self-awareness regarding his or her potential reactions to psychotic symptoms, and should be equally prepared to address any issues of stigmatization. There are two primary features of psychosis: disturbing beliefs and perceptions.

BOX 28.1: DSM-5 DEFINITION OF DELUSIONS

Delusions are fixed beliefs that are not amenable to change in light of conflicting evidence. Their content may include a variety of themes (e.g., persecutory, referential, somatic, religious, grandiose)… The distinction between a delusion and a strongly held idea is sometimes difficult to make and depends in part on the degree of conviction with which the belief is held despite clear or reasonable contradictory evidence regarding its veracity[23] (p. 87).

BOX 28.2: DSM-5 DEFINITION OF HALLUCINATIONS

Hallucinations are perception like experiences that occur without an external stimulus. They are vivid and clear, with the full force and impact of normal perceptions, and not under voluntary control. They may occur in any sensory modality, but auditory hallucinations are the most common in schizophrenia and related disorders … The hallucinations must occur in the context of a clear sensorium; those that occur while falling asleep (*hypnagogic*) or waking up (*hypnopompic*) are considered to be within the range of normal experiences. Hallucinations may be part of religious experience in certain cultural contexts[23] (pp. 87–8).

Common symptoms of psychosis include delusions (a belief not held by others, with evidence suggesting that the belief is false) and hallucinations (a perception not observed by others, where evidence suggests that the perception is without stimulus) (see Box 28.1). Delusions and hallucinations can occur alone or in combination with other signs and symptoms of mental illness. They are features of several psychiatric diagnostic categories, including, but not limited to, schizophrenia, depression, psychotic depression, mania, schizo-affective disorder, anorexia nervosa, bulimia, delusional disorder, psychosomatic disorder, paranoid personality disorder, schizotypal personality disorder, and a variety of substance abuse disorders.[1] For more information on the classification of mental illnesses, see chapter 12. The experience of childhood abuse is also a factor in the development of delusions in adults with mental illness. In studying people with delusions, Read and Argyle[2] found that 50 per cent had a history of childhood sexual abuse or a history of childhood physical abuse, and an additional 29 per cent had experienced both forms of abuse. So, in one form or another, 79 per cent of individuals experiencing delusions were abused as children. Chapter 29 has information on the experience of sexual abuse.

Many people hold false beliefs about themselves, their health, and the world. There are times when false, or groundless, beliefs can interfere with health and functioning. When a person's beliefs have the potential to cause them to harm themselves or another person, by commission or by omission, the beliefs are defined as disturbing. These beliefs may not disturb the person holding them, but they often disturb other people. The term 'delusion' is used to describe these cases. A delusion is a rigidly held, irrational belief that persists in spite of evidence that it is not true. Usually people will have a cluster of beliefs that are groundless and extreme. This is referred to as a 'delusional system'.

Hallucinations, like delusions, may or may not be considered disturbing. When hallucinations are understood as culturally appropriate, they may not result in distress for the individual who experiences them or for others. In some cases, a hallucination may also comfort the person by functioning as their only friend and confidante. Hallucinations may be disturbing when they are unwanted and are not culturally appropriate (see Box 28.2).

An important part of the craft of caring requires understanding that everyone experiences false beliefs from time to time. Consider the following example. Alcock[3] contracted a sore throat while travelling in Asia. He was offered an antibiotic and a Chinese herbal remedy based on snake bile. He accepted the antibiotic but declined the snake bile. Within a few days he was better, concluding that the antibiotic had worked. Later he learned his infection was viral, and that it had simply run its course. Had he chosen the snake bile, he could just as easily have believed in its effectiveness, as the infection would have cleared in the same number of days.

Beliefs, simply defined, are convictions or opinions held as truths in the mind of the believer.[4] Many beliefs are supported by facts, while others are held on faith. The common feature is that the believer holds their beliefs to be true. Spiritual beliefs are based on faith and may be quite contrary to facts and evidence based on science. However, they are known to contribute to good health. Even healthy people hold beliefs that contradict facts and scientific evidence. And strong beliefs may not be given up easily. How often have you heard someone say, 'I have no friends', or 'I am so overweight', when the evidence is quite contrary? Or have you ever avoided walking under a ladder? Even educated people behave superstitiously at times.

REFLECTION

Have you ever experienced a belief or perception that those around you would not agree with or support? Using the definitions above, would these be considered 'false'?

DISTURBING BELIEFS AND HALLUCINATIONS

How do beliefs develop? Alcock[3] describes beliefs as our 'expectations about our world' (p.48). Beliefs derive from four sources: direct experience, observation, logical thought and authority. They are developed out of direct experience and are based on observed patterns in the world. When two events occur together, they become associated. The feeling of hunger is associated with unpleasantness, while being fed leads to feelings of satisfaction. When parents tell their children that they are either bright or stupid, beliefs about the self form: 'I have the ability, I can do this', or 'I'm stupid, I'll never be any good.' Authority figures may also teach us about the world: 'Don't trust strangers', 'This is how we do (or don't do) it in our family' (see case study 2 later in this chapter).

Hallucinations are perceptual experiences, and are distinct from beliefs. Frequently nurses encounter people who are hearing disturbing voices. 'Hearing voices' usually describes an auditory hallucination; however, hallucinations can involve any sense. For example, in addition to auditory hallucinations, there are visual hallucinations, olfactory hallucinations, taste hallucinations and tactile hallucinations.

Another distinction is sometimes made between a hallucination and an illusion. Both phenomena involve perceiving something that is not perceived by others. However, an illusion is based on the apparent misperception of something that can be seen by others. For example, a person may see something more sinister in a shadow – but others can see the shadow.

Disturbing beliefs

Muse[4] observed that, 'The same type of delusion has caused certain persons to be canonized as saints in the early Christian period, persecuted as witches in the middle ages, and confined in an institution in the 20th century' (p.320). This observation alerts us to the social context of beliefs. Cultural ignorance in health care providers can result in misunderstandings and incorrect assessments. (See Box 28.1 for the DSM-5 definition.) Disturbing delusions are so extreme they defy credibility. The nurse may infer the existence of such delusions via direct communication with the client, or may infer it from their behaviour; for example, eyeing other people with suspicion and mistrust. Delusions can interfere with relationships, work and self-care. They are of particular concern when they jeopardize the person's safety, or the safety of others.

Beliefs may function to reduce anxiety, and increase structure and consistency in the person's day-to-day dealings with the world. They result from processing information in both hemispheres of the brain. There is some evidence that delusions can result when the left hemisphere receives incomplete information from the right, or if the interpreter function of the left hemisphere is malfunctioning. Neuroscience provides some evidence that disturbing beliefs, or delusions, are at least modestly associated with impairment of the central nervous system.[5]

Delusions have also been reported as a feature of disorders of the central nervous system. Examples of this include Capgras syndrome and dementias resulting from substance abuse. Capgras syndrome causes the person to believe that identical doubles or robots have replaced people close to them. This condition has been linked to diffuse or localized lesions, especially of the right hemisphere.[6]

> ## REFLECTION
>
> What do you think about when you hear the term 'delusion'?

Experiences with hallucinations

Not all auditory hallucinations are disturbing. An early study[7] found that the relationship one had with an auditory hallucination, or the 'voice', affected the course of the illness. People who live with their voices for a long time sometimes develop a positive relationship with them. Miller, O'Connor and DiPasquale[8] found that the majority of clients reported some positive effects of their hallucinations. These attitudes did not change after treatment, but those who reported positive experiences were more likely to continue hallucinating after treatment. Romme[9] compared clients who heard voices to non-clients, and found that non-clients were more likely to report a positive experience with the voices. They concluded that hearing voices lies on a continuum with normal functioning.

In another study Forchuk[10] asked individuals with chronic mental illnesses about their social support. Almost all of the 124 clients in the study reported very small social networks (friends to whom they could turn for help). In some situations, the clients' only supports were the nurse and their 'voices'. Others reported that their only supports were the nurse and a pet. So, although the nurse or others may perceive the auditory hallucination as a *symptom*, the client may perceive it as a close friend. (See Box 28.2 for the DSM-5 definition of hallucinations, and case study 1.)

Not all auditory hallucinations are disturbing – but does that mean they are not problems? The nurse must ask: who are the 'voices' a problem for? Consider the following personal illustration.

CASE STUDY 1

Dr Fairchild is a 59-year-old physicist, admitted after his wife had taken him to the family doctor for an evaluation of strange behaviour. She discovered he had spent a large amount of money on laboratory equipment for the basement. When she asked him about this, he had told her that he had discovered time travel. She was told not to worry, as he had access to unlimited wealth through his discovery. On checking with his Dean, she confirmed that her husband had suffered a number of grant rejections, had been reported by a number of his students for bizarre grading of exam papers, and as a result, the university was considering suggesting early retirement.

Dr Fairchild's beliefs are not disturbing to him. They are disturbing to his wife, who sees the family resources dwindling. The beliefs are also disturbing to his Dean, who is concerned about productivity and performance. Dr Fairchild is at risk of squandering his resources and of damaging the relationships he has with his wife and his employer.

PERSONAL ILLUSTRATION (PROVIDER)

A client I worked with spent all day in her room. It was difficult to encourage her to get off her bed for meals or to go to the washroom. Eventually, when discussing the issue, she described why she spent so much time in bed; she was listening to a centuries-old conversation among several angels, and sometimes, if she was lucky, she would hear God as well. They were discussing plans for the great flood. Details about the animals and the geography kept her fascinated for hours on end. How could she leave for lunch and miss the possibility of hearing God's input to the conversation? Were these voices a problem? On one hand, she had lost contact with almost all her family and her level of functioning on a day-to-day basis was dramatically reduced by her constant focus on the voices. On the other hand, she saw herself as an important person, and involved in an important process. She felt that without her voices she would be 'nothing'. Not all auditory hallucinations interfere with functioning or with the person's activities of daily living. These things need careful evaluation together with the client.

Some hallucinations are horrifically disturbing. Clients have described hearing screaming, tortured voices pleading with them for relief. Others have described taunting, insulting voices that can issue commands (called command hallucinations) such as to jump off a bridge or strangle a friend. Frequently, disturbing voices list every fault of the client and tell them that they are worthless or evil. Experiencing multiple disturbing voices makes contact with others very difficult. Sometimes, in these situations, there are insulting voices and friendly voices all speaking at once. The nurse trying to speak is simply one more voice competing for attention.

Understanding delusions and hallucinations can be difficult for a beginning practitioner. While delusions and/or hallucinations are a feature of many conditions, not every person with that diagnosis will suffer from them. It is important to assess the person, and to identify the presence or absence of these experiences. If they are present, they are not all the same. Depending on their characteristics, they may require different interventions.

REFLECTION

What do you think about when you hear the term 'hallucination'? Have you ever had an experience where you thought you 'heard' or 'saw' something that no one else heard or saw?

INTERPERSONAL APPROACHES

Interpersonal approaches emphasize the importance of therapeutic, trusting relationships in the primary intervention. Developing interpersonal relationships is an important aspect of the craft of caring, because it is within these relationships that therapeutic progress can be made. Hildegard Peplau[11,12] suggests that nursing interventions reverse the process that occurred when the hallucinations developed. To do this, it is first important to identify the phase of hallucination development. The nurse then helps the individual identify and name the anxiety. In order to mitigate the loneliness the client may be experiencing, the nurse provides regular opportunities to interact with people.

At this time, the nurse also needs to consider her or his comfort and confidence in working with people with delusions and/or hallucinations. Depending on the nature of the delusions, nurses have found that extended contact can lead to impatience and anger.[13] In nursing people who experience hallucinations, the nurse must cultivate self-awareness regarding any potential sources of discomfort that might prevent appropriate care. Peer consultation, or consultation with the multidisciplinary team, can be an important source of support for the nurse.

While Peplau originally proposed four phases in the therapeutic relationship, she later described three phases – orientation, working (with two sub-phases) and resolution. Each phase is an important part of the craft of caring.

The *orientation phase* is the first phase, where the nurse and the client get to know each other, develop understanding, work through each other's preconceptions, set parameters, and agree on the focus of the therapeutic relationship. This phase can take up to a year or longer to work through, when the problems have been present for a long time and the client finds it hard to trust others. At this time the nurse will begin the assessment of the person and their experiences. If trust is not established, it is best for another nurse to take the client on.[14]

It is critical to carry out assessment throughout the therapeutic process. Assessment may be conducted using a validated tool.[15,14] In assessing, the nurse works from the perspective of a participant-observer and makes inferences through identifying themes and forming hypotheses. Finally, the nurse collaborates with interventions in the nurse–client relationship that will effect changes favourable to the client.[16]

Problems can only be identified and explored in the *working phase*, the phase in which therapeutic work is done. Whether the client is believed to be suffering from delusions or hallucinations, it is important to find out as much as possible from the client, family, friends, associates, the interdisciplinary team, spiritual advisors and any other sources of information. For more information on developing and maintaining therapeutic relationships, see chapters 13, 14 and 15 for information on assessments.

Interpersonal approaches to nursing the person with delusions

Peplau[17] defined delusions as one of several possible responses to repeated frustration. Fixed responses, such as delusions, occur after repeated frustrations that produce anxiety. The beliefs cannot be given up, as this would cause overwhelming insecurity in the person.[5] It is important to know that there is often a thread of truth at the core of most delusions, and that these often serve as a way of dealing with underlying anxiety;[18,13] hence it is important to understand the delusion(s).

The underlying core of the delusion must be decoded before the underlying need can be understood.[18] Only when the underlying need is met in a healthier way can the delusion be given up. This can only happen in the context of a safe and trusting relationship. Donner[18] cautions that the delusion should never be interpreted directly to the client – neither should it be confronted, as this will only escalate the client's anxiety. The same points can be made for hallucinations.

Safety is always a concern. To ensure everyone's safety, the clients may be on close or intensive observation. Whenever safety precautions are taken, the content of the delusion should be considered. For a person such as Mikel (case study 2), who fears people in uniforms, it would be unwise to have a uniformed person provide close observation. In Willow's case (case study 3), her 'monster' is a 'he'. She will experience less anxiety if observed by a woman. These suggestions may seem so obvious that the reader wonders why they are made explicit, yet there are many examples in the real world of problems arising from failure to consider the obvious.

Rosenthal and McGuinness[13] caution against agreeing with delusions. Agreement is as unhelpful as disagreement. Logic and debate are inappropriate, as this frustrates the client and escalates his or her anxiety. Instead, the nurse should focus on the client's feelings, as this validates the client's reality. To avoid either agreeing *or* disagreeing with the delusional content, the nurse may look for what is *true to the listener*, and then support or agree with that. For example, when Willow says she is frightened of the snake, the nurse can agree with Willow's fear: 'It sounds like you are feeling very afraid of what is happening.' The nurse should not say, 'It sounds like that snake in you is really frightening', since that would reinforce the delusion. Similarly, a statement like, 'Don't you realize a snake would be killed by the acid in your stomach?' would be seen as argumentative and risks failure to establish trust in the nurse. At times, a client will directly ask whether or not the nurse believes what the client is describing. In order to agree with the truth and avoid reinforcing or confronting the delusion, the nurse could say, 'I don't feel or see the snake, but I believe it is real to you' (see case study 3).

PERSONAL ILLUSTRATION (CLIENT)

The therapeutic relationships formed with staff were key to my recovery. I was so scared when I entered the hospital. There was one nurse who really alleviated my fear and anxiety, making me feel safe. He did just what I needed; with patience he listened to me. He did not deny or confirm my hallucinations, just comforted me and empathized with my emotions. At this point I still wanted to hide my disturbing thoughts and beliefs from the world as much as I could. I would cry and not explain the reasons for my sadness because part of me knew my thoughts were not rational. Once the staff were no longer strangers to me and trust was formed, I began to feel more comfortable opening up about the details of my distorted beliefs, thoughts and hallucinations. This made it easier for the staff to provide me with the help I needed because now we were working collaboratively. It was at that point that I began to decipher reality more purposefully with the medical support team.

CASE STUDY 2

Mikel is a 25-year-old man admitted for assaulting the postman. He is under close observation as he is still potentially violent. As he speaks, his eyes move about, scanning his environment constantly. He sits forward on a chair in the dayroom, talking in a low voice.

Mikel: 'I don't know why I am here. I am not crazy. I don't like to be locked up'.

Nurse: 'Can you tell me what happened just before you came here?'

Mikel: 'A policeman came. He said he wasn't, but he had the uniform on. I know them. I tried to protect myself, then others came. They took me here. What will happen to me?'

Nurse: 'You say you "know them"; have you had other experiences with the police?'

Mikel: 'They came after me. The police, I don't trust them. They take people, and you never see them again. They beat me, left me for dead. I came to this country. I thought I would be safe here, but they are everywhere. Now they found me, and brought me here.'

He continues to look anxiously about the room as they talk.

In Mikel's delusion, people wearing any kind of uniform are police and are the enemy. He sees his efforts to protect himself as legitimate, because he is a victim of the horrors of war. The beliefs about danger were formed in the past, and are out of place in the present. His belief that he needs to protect himself from the non-existent threat makes him dangerous to others, especially those wearing a uniform.

CASE STUDY 3

Willow is a 15-year-old student, admitted for depression and delusions involving snakes. Her schoolwork has deteriorated over the past 6 months and she has gained weight. She looks downward, avoiding eye contact and her clothes are plain and very baggy. Willow is depressed and believes she is dying. Obviously, no snake could survive inside the human body, yet this is her belief. She is clearly troubled. By stating she wishes she could get the snake out, Willow alerts the nurse to the possibility that she might do something that would result in self-harm. The content of the delusion should also alert the nurse to the possibility of sexual abuse. Should the issue of sexual abuse arise, it will be important for the nurse to be empathic and non-judgemental. However, the nurse should not introduce the topic.

Willow: 'The snake is eating me. I am going to die.'

Nurse: 'Tell me more about the snake.'

Willow: 'It's inside me. It's eating everything.' Tears flow. 'The monster put a snake in me because I was bad. He said it was my fault. He said the snake would eat me and I would die because I was bad. I'm not supposed to tell. But I'm scared, I don't want to die, but I'm bad. I have to die. The snake will kill me by eating me from the inside.'

Nurse: 'You sound afraid.'

Willow: 'I'm scared. I don't want to die. I wish I could get it out.'

Her head is low. Her voice is barely audible.

It can be tempting at times to try to talk someone out of a delusion. This tends to result in the client either not trusting the nurse's motivation or coming up with a more elaborate explanation to account for the reasons presented by the nurse. When working with a client over a long period of time, the nurse will observe periods of both wellness and difficulty. If the delusion is not experienced, then it may be possible to discuss the delusional content. It is often helpful for clients to learn to recognize early signs of difficulty, to prevent relapse.

PERSONAL ILLUSTRATION (PROVIDER)

A nurse case manager worked with a particular client for 3 years during which the client had several relapses. When this client was psychotic, he always had a delusion that his food was poisoned. He would eventually refuse all food and drink and be hospitalized for 4 to 6 weeks in order to recover both physically and mentally. The nurse case manager and client were able to establish that the early signs of trouble were finding that his food seemed to have a metallic taste. This client learned to alert the case manager when this occurred, so he could have an early assessment and readjustment of medication. This strategy was successful in breaking the pattern of regular re-hospitalizations.

Three major types of delusions are encountered.[4,13] These are *delusions of persecution*, *delusions of grandeur*, and *negative delusions* (see Box 28.3). Other categories may be encountered, including referential (the belief that comments and other environmental cues are directed at the experiencer), somatic (preoccupation regarding bodily health or organ functioning), erotomanic (a false belief that someone is in love with the believer) and nihilistic (a belief, without good evidence, that a major catastrophe will occur) (see Box 28.3).

BOX 28.3: THREE MAJOR TYPES OF DELUSION

Delusions of persecution
Delusions of persecution involve the belief that others are out to get the person, and that he or she is at risk of being harmed by these persecutors. These delusions can be dangerous. People may try to defend themselves from the danger that they believe is present. In the process, they can harm or even kill others. These occur more commonly in people who may have experienced danger from others at some point in their life, and in abusers of some drugs, such as amphetamines. See case study 2.

Delusions of grandeur
The person with delusions of grandeur holds exaggerated beliefs about their abilities, status, worth or accomplishments. These delusions are likely to be boastful or egotistical. Others who know the individual do not substantiate the contents of the belief system. The behaviour resulting from the delusions is disturbing to others around the individual. See case study 1.

Negative delusions
Negative delusions usually occur in people who are depressed. They are mood congruent and involve themes of despair, inadequacy and hopelessness. These beliefs are disturbing as they can result in self-harm or suicide. The delusions also interfere with the person's ability to get on with his/her life tasks.

As with other delusions, it will take time for the individual to feel safe enough to begin to share the issues that are at the core of their beliefs. Although it may be tempting simply to point out the seemingly obvious, this action will only aggravate the individual and raise their anxiety even more. The two main approaches to helping people with disturbing beliefs are the interpersonal nurse–client relationship, and appropriate medical evaluation and treatment. See case study 1 for an example from practice.

PERSONAL ILLUSTRATION (CLIENT)

Although some of my delusions persisted, in the hospital it seemed as though I would have a new disturbing delusion each morning that would go away by lunch, only to wake up the next day to a new distorted belief. Although many people's delusions of grandeur are disturbing to others and not to the client, I perceived mine as deeply negative. My uncle, who suffered from depression, took his life when I was four. I believed that before he died he saw into the future and knew that one day I would want to commit suicide. So, to protect me from my demise he cut his life short. Having the delusion that his death was for me, and therefore my fault, was very disturbing. As much as the thoughts of suicide were racing through my head, I did not attempt to hurt myself because of the belief that I was physically incapable of successful completion of suicide due to him saving me.

Interpersonal approaches to nursing the person with auditory hallucinations

Peplau also described the potential interpersonal development of auditory hallucinations. She believed that hallucinations could develop to avoid anxiety and to mitigate loneliness. In order to treat hallucinations interpersonally, Peplau suggests that nursing interventions reverse the process that occurred when the hallucinations developed.[11,12] Her approach develops in four stages,[1,12] which are further elaborated by Clack.[19] The nurse can only begin to address issues presented by disturbing hallucinations in the working phase of the therapeutic relationship.

Peplau's stages of hallucinations are:

1. *Comforting.* The individual feels lonely and/or anxious and finds that focusing on comforting thoughts relieves the discomfort. At this stage the thoughts are clearly understood to be one's own.
2. *Condemning.* The person continues to court similar relief and increasing reliance on illusory figures to meet their needs. The individual gradually puts themselves into a 'listening' mode and becomes unable to control their own awareness.
3. *Controlling.* There is a marked loss of ability to focus awareness, indicated by withdrawal from others in order to interact with the hallucination. The person gives up trying to combat the hallucination and may feel lonely when the voices leave.
4. *Conquering.* The voices become increasingly threatening, particularly when commands are not followed.

There is a failure of strategies to conceal ongoing inter-actions with hallucinations. There is a continued loss of control over concentration and awareness.

Clack[19] suggests several strategies to assist people with hallucinations:

1. The first step is always to establish a therapeutic rela-tionship, show acceptance and listen.
2. Next, the nurse should look and listen for cues or symptoms of the hallucination, focusing on the cue and eliciting the individual's observation and description.
3. Then, the nurse should identify if the hallucination is emotionally or toxically based (e.g. street drugs). Clack suggests that, if asked, the nurse should acknowledge that he or she is not experiencing the hallucination.
4. Next the nurse should follow the direction of the client and help them observe and describe the hallucination. Eliciting observations of current and past hallucina-tions is part of the process of establishing trust, as well as assisting in understanding what the person is expe-riencing. This helps the person in determining why the hallucinations are occurring. The individual is to be encouraged to observe and describe thoughts, feelings and actions. According to Clack's theory, the person should observe or describe needs that may be underly-ing the hallucinations in order to see what needs it may be serving.
5. The nurse then suggests and reinforces meeting needs through interpersonal relationships and explores other behaviour concerns.

We now have many more medications to assist the indi-vidual than when Clack's paper was written. This means a person may recover from the symptoms much more quickly, even though recovery involves more than managing symp-toms. Clack's interventions, which include listening, accept-ing and being patient, also support recovery. If the individual is obtaining secondary gains from the hallucinations, they may be unwilling to continue the medication. Therefore, understanding whether additional needs are being met by the hallucination is as important today as it was 1962.

PERSONAL ILLUSTRATION (PROVIDER)

A colleague recently discovered, to her amaze-ment, that the young man she had admitted *was* indeed a successful rock star, with a Porsche, a mansion and a large bank account, even though he was poorly dressed, penniless and dishevelled on admission. In this case, family members were available to validate his story. Had they not been available, he might easily have found himself under treatment for delusions!

REFLECTION

What do you think it would be like to experience the symptoms of psychosis?

UNDERSTANDING PSYCHOSIS THROUGH OTHER APPROACHES TO CARING

Voices as a symptom of psychosis

Understanding psychosis is an essential part of car-ing for clients who experience it, and there are many reasons why people experience psychosis. For exam-ple, Beyerstein[20] stated that: 'Anything that prompts a move from word based thinking to imagistic or pic-torial thinking predisposes a person to hallucinating.' He further states that things which bias 'the brain's representational system towards memory images at the expense of sensory information can also predispose to hallucinating' (p.1).

When assessing a client, the nurse may simply ask the individual if they are hearing any unusual voices or see-ing any unusual phenomena. If they are, the nurse may ask if the client perceives the experiences as a problem. Occasionally, a person experiencing psychosis will deny this, or be unable to confirm this due to language or cogni-tive difficulties (case study 4).

Although there are many causes of psychosis, mental health nurses will encounter this symptom most commonly among people who have been diagnosed with schizophrenia.

CASE STUDY 4

Michael sat alone in the TV room on the inpatient psychiatric ward. 'No, no, no! I will not do that! Now you leave me alone! Shut up! Get out of here!'

A student nurse, Donovan, stood in the door-way. Michael was his assigned client for the day. How should he approach him?

Donovan needs to remember that the first steps are always to listen and to work on establishing a therapeutic relationship. Since this is a new cli-ent assignment, it would be unlikely that Michael would trust Donovan immediately. So patience is required. Donovan would need to introduce him-self and let Michael know he is available.

'Michael, my name is Donovan. I am a student nurse and will be with you today … I heard you talking a moment ago and you sounded pretty upset. Perhaps you could tell me about that …'

Someone with schizophrenia is generally not psychotic all the time. They typically have periods of wellness between acute psychotic episodes. The pattern of psychosis and wellness varies considerably among individuals. For a few people, the symptoms of psychosis are chronic in nature and do not fluctuate with acute periods followed by periods of wellness. (See chapter 24 for a more in-depth discussion of schizophrenia.)

Disturbing voices are commonly experienced by people diagnosed with dissociative identity disorder (previously known as multiple personality disorder).[21,22] This condition is usually a consequence of serious, life-threatening sexual abuse early in life. During periods when one personality is in charge, the voices of one or more other personalities can still talk, sometimes to each other. Some voices can be frightening and the voice(s) may suggest self-harm or suicide (see chapter 27).

Spiritual and cultural approaches

Cultural and spiritual approaches begin with the recognition that a cultural or spiritual issue may be present. Within many traditions, it is considered normal to be able to communicate with the dead. The DSM-5[23] distinguishes between bizarre and non-bizarre delusions: 'Delusions are deemed *bizarre* if they are clearly implausible and not understandable to same-culture peers and do not derive from ordinary life experiences' (p. 87). Similarly, many cultures would value communication with a spiritual power, spiritual guide, angel or higher being. It is extremely important in these situations to be aware of cultural and family norms and not to pathologize a spiritual situation. For a detailed discussion of cultural issues that may arise in the assessment of clients, and for access to the Cultural Formulation Interview (CFI), see the DSM-5.[23]

Pharmacological approaches to caring

Following admission into a hospital, health professionals will evaluate the client, test which medication will be of best benefit, and titrate the dosage. These medications

PERSONAL ILLUSTRATION (CLIENT)

My definition of recovery is that it does not have a finish line, and is a never-ending journey to be higher on the spectrum of mental health. I believe myself to be completely symptom-free. However, what one interprets as a symptom can vary. One 'hallucination' that still is present in my life is one based on faith and is the ability to hear God's voice. My perceived 'voice of God' does not control or interfere with my life, and most importantly does not negatively affect my health or functioning. This belief that I can hear God when I need Him is a positive aspect of my life, bringing me comfort in difficult times. My nurse and physician agree that this is not a symptom. Thankfully I have spiritually and culturally sensitive practitioners who are understanding and don't pathologize my spirituality.

are not curative and thus do not eliminate the underlying thought disorder. Rather they may allow the client to function in a supportive environment.[24] The nurse's responsibilities include monitoring and documenting side effects and therapeutic effects, educating the client and family about the medication to promote compliance, minimizing the impact of side effects, and providing support for clients experiencing adverse side effects. Nurses are also responsible for communicating their observations to the other members of the team, administering prescribed medications, and reporting the person's responses. It is necessary for the nurse to have a good knowledge of the classes of medications usually prescribed for persons with disturbing beliefs (see chapters 47 and 48 for more information). Benefits and side effects can only be identified through careful observation. Some side effects are minor, while others may be transient. Knowledge of strategies for dealing with side effects such as dry mouth and blurred vision can be very reassuring to the client.

STRATEGIES TO ASSIST WITH COPING

People who continue to experience hearing problematic voices often develop specific coping strategies to deal with the problem. Understanding when the voices occur may help in identifying appropriate coping strategies. For example, many people report that the voices are worse when they are alone. They may need to structure their time carefully to include ample opportunity for interacting with others. Some people have found that listening to something else helps to block out the voices, and will use headphones and a portable audio player such as a smartphone. It is useful to explore with each individual the pattern of when the voices are most problematic and when they seem to fade away.

The craft of caring can be supported by a variety of approaches to coping. Buccheri et al.[25] summarized several strategies: self-monitoring of the hallucinations; reading aloud and summarizing; talking with someone; watching and listening to television; saying 'stop' and naming objects; listening to music with headphones; listening to relaxation tapes with headphones; wearing a unilateral ear plug; and humming a single note. They found that, among all participants, at least one strategy relieved the distress associated with auditory hallucinations. In a later study, Buccheri et al.[26] found that 82 per cent of participants continued to use at least one strategy.

Frederick and Cotanch[27] asked research participants to report self-help techniques they had found useful for coping with auditory hallucinations. The responses were grouped into physiological approaches to reduce arousal (relaxing, lying down, sleeping, calm music, alcohol, extra medication); physiological approaches to increase arousal (loud music, walking, pacing, jogging); cognitive approaches (acceptance of voices, reduced attention to voices); and behavioural changes (leisure or work activity, seeking interaction, isolating oneself).

New technologies may also assist people in coping with delusions and hallucinations by identifying them early on. Forchuk et al.[28] showed that smartphones with specific apps for self-monitoring are a promising resource for clients with psychotic or mood disorders. Clients reported that the use of a smart health record enhanced their sense of control by monitoring moods and early personal signs of psychosis. A small exploratory study on the use of smart technology to support independent living for people experiencing schizophrenia and related disorders has also shown promising results.[29] Chapter 72 explores in more detail the use of health care technology and mental health nursing.

> ## REFLECTION
>
> How do you cope with challenging situations?

CONCLUSION

We all hold some beliefs that others would disagree with and have had experiences that disturbed us. Experiences with delusions and hallucinations are extreme examples of this. While some delusions and/or perceptions may be innocuous, others may be very disturbing and can place the individual at risk. The nurse needs to help the person feel as comfortable as possible, to be honest about concerns, to listen carefully to what is being said, to assess the severity of problems, to monitor the client's response to treatment, and to work with the client on mutually agreed goals. To communicate best with the person experiencing disturbing beliefs and/or perceptions, the nurse should support and listen to the client without reinforcing or directly confronting the content of the client's disturbing experiences.

References

1. APA (American Psychiatric Association). *Diagnostic and statistical manual of mental disorders*, 4th edn. Washington, DC: APA, 1994.
2. Read J, Argyle N. Hallucinations, delusions, and thought disorder among adult psychiatric inpatients with a history of child abuse. *Psychiatric Services* 1999; **50**(11): 1467–72.
3. Alcock JE. Alternative medicine and the psychology of belief. *Scientific Review of Alternative Medicine* 1999; **3**(2): 45–52.
4. Muse MB. *Psychology for nurses*. Philadelphia: WB Saunders, 1926.
5. Butler RW, Braft DL. Delusions: a review and integration. *Schizophrenia Bulletin* 1991; **17**(4): 633–47.
6. Buckwalter KC. Are you really my nurse, or are you a snake sheriff? *Journal of Psychosocial and Nursing Mental Health Services* 1993; **31**: 33–4.
7. Benjamin L. Is chronicity a function of the relationship between the person and the auditory hallucination? *Schizophrenia Bulletin* 1989; **15**: 291–310.
8. Miller L, O'Connor E, DiPasquale T. Patients' attitudes towards hallucinations. *American Journal of Psychiatry* 1993; **150**: 584–8.
9. Romme M. Listening to the voice hearers. *Journal of Psychosocial Nursing and Mental Health Services* 1998; **36**: 40–4.
10. Forchuk C. The orientation phase of the nurse–client relationship: Testing Peplau's theory. *Journal of Advanced Nursing Practice* 1994; **20**: 532–7.
11. Peplau HE. Anxiety, self and hallucinations. In: O'Toole AW, Welt SR (eds). *Interpersonal theory in nursing practice: selected works of Hildegard E. Peplau*. New York: Springer, 1989: 270–326.
12. Peplau HE. Interpersonal relations and the process of adaptation. *Nursing Science* 1963; **1**(4): 272–9.
13. Rosenthal TT, McGuinness TM. Dealing with delusional patients: discovering the distorted truth. *Journal of Mental Health Nursing* 1986; **8**: 143–54.
14. Forchuk C, Westwell J, Martin ML, Bamber-Azzapardi W, Kosterewa-Tolman D, Hux M. The developing nurse–client relationship: nurses' perspectives. *Journal of the American Psychiatric Nurses Association* 2000; **6**(1): 3–10.
15. Forchuk C, Brown B. Establishing a nurse–client relationship. *Journal of Psychosocial Nursing* 1989; **27**(2): 30–4.
16. Peplau HE. Themes in nursing-safety. In: Mereness D (ed.) *Psychiatric nursing: developing psychiatric nursing skills*, 2nd edn. Dubuque, IW: WC Brown, 1971: 142–7.
17. Peplau HE. *Interpersonal relations in nursing*. New York: GP Putnam, 1952.
18. Donner G. Treatment of a delusional patient. *American Journal of Nursing* 1969; **69**: 2642–4.
19. Clack J. An interpersonal technique for handling hallucinations, in nursing care of the disoriented patient [Monograph 13]. *American Nurses Association Publication* 1962; 16–29.
20. Beyerstein B. Believing is seeing: organic and psychological reasons for hallucinations and other anomalous psychiatric symptoms. *Medscape Mental Health* 1996; **1**(11): 1–10.
21. Putnam FW. *Diagnosis and treatment of multiple personality disorder*. New York: Guilford Press, 1989.
22. Stafford LL. Dissociation and multiple personality disorder: a challenge for psycho-social nurses. *Journal of Psychosocial Nursing and Mental Health Services* 1993; **31**: 15–20.
23. APA (American Psychological Association). *Diagnostic and statistical manual of mental disorders, 5th edition*. Washington, DC: APA, 2013.
24. Mycek M, Harvey RA, Champe PC, Fisher B, Cooper C. *Pharmacology*. Philadelphia: Lippincott-Raven, 1997.
25. Buccheri R, Trystad L, Kanas N, Waldron B, Dowling G. Auditory hallucinations in schizophrenia: group experience in examining symptom management and behavioural strategies. *Journal of Psychosocial Nursing and Mental Health Services* 1996; **34**: 12–25.

26. Buccheri R, Trystad L, Kanas N, Dowling G. Symptom management of auditory hallucinations in schizophrenia: results of 1-year follow-up. *Journal of Psychosocial Nursing and Mental Health Services* 1997; **35**: 20–8.

27. Frederick JA, Cotanch P. Self-help techniques for auditory hallucinations in schizophrenia. *Issues in Mental Health Nursing* 1994; **16**: 213–24.

28. Forchuk C, Rudnick A, Reiss J, Hoch J, Donelle L, Corring D, Godin M, Osaka W, Campbell R, Capretz M, Reed J, McKillop M. Mental health engagement network: an analysis of outcomes following a mobile and web-based intervention. *Journal of Technologies in Society* 2015; **11**(2): 1–10.

29. Corring D, Campbell R, Rudnick A. Cognitive remediation for inpatients with schizophrenia or schizoaffective disorder using 'smart' technology in a simulated apartment: a feasibility and exploratory study. In: Abdulrazak B, Giroux S, Bouchard G, Mokhtari M, Pigot M (eds). *Toward useful services for elderly and people with disabilities*. Berlin and Heidelberg: Springer, 2011: 286–9.

Further reading

Davidson L, Johnson A. Providing safety in the midst of psychosis: an interpersonal dimension of recovery. *Psychosis* 2012; **6**(1): 77–9.

This is a first-person account of psychosis in the form of a dialogue between a client with psychosis and a person who is trying to understand their experience. The topic is how a positive interpersonal dynamic was established from the perspective of a client.

Forchuk C, Jewell J, Tweedell D, Steinnagel L. Reconnecting: the client experience of recovery from psychosis." *Perspectives in Psychiatric Care* 2003; **39**(4), 141–50.

This article addresses the client experience of psychosis and recovery.

Forchuk C, Jewell J, Tweedell D, Steinnagel L. Role changes experienced by clinical staff in relation to clients' recovery from psychosis. *Journal of Psychiatric & Mental Health Nursing* 2003; **10**: 269–76.

This article discusses the experience of psychosis and recovery from the perspective of clinical staff.

Garety P, Hemsley D. Characteristics of delusional experience. *European Archives of Psychiatry and Neurological Sciences* 1987; **236**(5): 294–8.

This quantitative study attempts to characterize the dimensions of delusions (including such dimensions as dismissability and absurdity) and concludes that delusions are extremely variable. In general, the only dimension all delusions have in common is conviction.

Hayward M. *Overcoming distressing voices*. London: Robinson, 2012.

This book discusses auditory hallucinations and how they may be distressing or not distressing. It has five components: understanding, changing response to voices, changing beliefs and relationships, looking to the future and carers. It approaches these topics using a CBT model. It is useful for voice-hearers, and includes many case studies of personal experiences of hearing voices.

Larsen J. Finding meaning in first episode psychosis: experience, agency, and the cultural repertoire. *Medical Anthropology Quarterly* 2004; **18**(4): 447–71.

This article explores how patients respond to their first episode of psychosis by creating a framework of meaning or a narrative explanation for it. It suggests that cultural context plays a major role in how patients explains their psychosis to themselves.

Lobban F, Barrowclough C. *A casebook of family interventions for psychosis*. Chichester: Wiley-Blackwell, 2009.

This is a practical guide for clinicians assisting families with loved ones who are experiencing psychosis. It contains information on how to stage a successful intervention.

Maher B. The relationship between delusions and hallucinations. *Current Psychiatry Reports* 2006; **8**(3): 179–83.

This article defines delusions and hallucinations. It examines co-occurrence of delusions and hallucinations and suggeststhat hallucinations may cause delusions. It is useful for clinicians.

Rhodes J, Jakes S. Perspectives on the onset of delusions. *Clinical Psychology & Psychotherapy* 2010; **17**(2): 136–46.

The authors discuss various factors that influence the onset of delusions and suggest that it may be useful for clinicians to determine a narrative describing the social and emotional context of the client when they experienced the onset.

Royal B. An emergency plan for schizophrenia relapse. *Psychosis* 2014; **7**(1): 92–5.

One woman writes about her experience living with schizophrenia and her personal emergency response plan that she developed to better cope with relapses.

Thomas NS, Rossell S, Farhall J, Shawyer F, Castle D. Cognitive behavioural therapy for auditory hallucinations: effectiveness and predictors of outcome in a specialist clinic. *Behavioural and Cognitive Psychotherapy* 2010; **39**(2): 129–38.

This study suggests that cognitive behavioural therapy is effective for the treatment of positive symptoms of psychosis, although it is much less effective for negative symptoms of psychosis. It also suggests that CBT can be effective for auditory hallucinations, even when the client has a lack of insight into their condition.

Tweedell D, Forchuk C, Jewell J, Steinnegal L. Families' experience during recovery or nonrecovery from psychosis. *Archives of Psychiatric Nursing* 2004; **18**(1): 17–25.

This article discusses families' experiences of psychosis, recovery and non-recovery.

Relevant web pages

Alzheimer Society of Canada. Delusions and hallucinations. http://www.alzheimer.ca/en/Living-with-dementia/Understanding-behaviour/Delusions-and-hallucinations

Canadian Mental Health Association. Get informed: psychosis. https://www.cmha.bc.ca/get-informed/mental-health-information/psychosis

Canadian Mental Health Association. Hallucinations and delusions: how to respond. http://www.cmha.bc.ca/files/6-hallucinations_delusions.pdf

Children's Hospital of Eastern Ontario. Helping children and youth with psychosis: information for parents and caregivers. http://www.cheo.on.ca/uploads/psychosis/psychosis%20eng.pdf

Government of Canada. About mental health. http://healthycanadians.gc.ca/healthy-living-vie-saine/mental-health-sante-mentale/improving-mental-health-ameliorer-sante-mentale/what-quoi-eng.php

NHS Choices. Psychosis. http://www.nhs.uk/conditions/Psychosis/Pages/Introduction.aspx

The person with experience of sexual abuse

ROXANE AGNEW-DAVIES AND PHOEBE

LEARNING OUTCOMES

- To be aware of different categories and types of abuse.
- To be able to reflect on your attitudes and practice.
- To know how to recognize and help overcome barriers to disclosure.
- To be able to promote safe conversations about violence.
- To know how to ask questions about past and current abuse.
- To understand how to respond positively to disclosures of abuse.
- To be able to offer support to people experiencing the effects of abuse.
- To be able to signpost to agencies that can help.

SUMMARY OF KEY POINTS

- The craft of caring rests on good self-care. If you need support in relation to your own childhood (or later) experiences of sexual abuse, or to support other people, further reading or website links at the end of this chapter might help.
- Expectations about who will be harmed and who will harm them will influence nurses' capacity to identify and support people at risk.
- It is not enough to ask questions. Your response and action after a disclosure can make a big difference for years to come. Admission can afford a safe respite. Discharging a victim of abuse has implications for safeguarding.

- Separate the person from what has been done to them.
- Practising asking questions about abuse builds confidence.
- Responding positively when someone discloses is really important to the craft of caring.
- Safety is a top priority. Victims may be abused by more than one person. Before information is shared, proper risk assessment is needed to safeguard a person from further harm.
- You will talk to experts by experience. Never assume you know better than they do about what is best for them. Be careful about what you say and do because it can be understood differently to what

you intend. Offering a tissue can be taken to mean 'Stop making a fuss.'

- There are stages in the process of healing that people need help to work through, including acknowledging what happened, believing that it was not their fault, working through feelings or reactions, building trusting, healthy relationships and making sense of it

all, before they might feel free to concentrate on the present and to move on.

- Signposting to local services is part of the craft of caring.
- Victims want help to talk about abuse safely and to be treated with respect.

INTRODUCTION

Roxane

I worked as a clinical psychologist for 15 years in various settings: psychology departments, an inpatient psychiatric unit, a community mental health team and primary care. In 2000, I began to manage six refuges and the national helpline for Refuge, a national charity for women and children escaping domestic violence. During the next 4 years, more than 500 women talked to my staff and me about their experiences of physical, sexual and psychological abuse. As this hidden world unfolded, I struggled emotionally, mentally and socially to understand what I heard, to find ways to support people to heal from their trauma, and to look after myself and my staff in the process. I rewrote basic psychological materials as I became aware of the danger of medicalizing and pathologizing an individual for a global social problem and as I realized the dangers of victim blaming when the real problem was the abuse, not the survivor.

About a quarter of the women who experienced domestic violence as adults had suffered sexual and/or physical abuse from childhood. When they needed loving supportive partners to help them outgrow the pain, they got the opposite – further abuse, betrayal and blame by someone they had trusted. They asked unanswerable questions such as 'Why me?' or 'What have I done wrong?' I learned that even when I felt sad and helpless to undo the past, women appreciated the chance to talk and our willingness to hear and believe them rather than deny their experience.

What is one of the worst punishments for a human being? Solitary confinement: being imprisoned alone. I began to equate the experiences of victims of domestic violence with those of hostages; after all, many victims of domestic violence describe experiencing what Amnesty International terms the defining features of torture. I discovered that one in seven wives were raped by their husbands and 90 per cent told no one at the time. I believe that, if health professionals do nothing else, at least we can break the isolation if someone is assaulted in the most intimate way possible, and that is important in itself. To illustrate, Brian Keenan and John McCarthy were held hostage in Lebanon for over 4 years. Having spent long years alone, both have described the importance of the months they were held together –neither could escape, but

it helped tremendously that another shared and understood their experience. I realized that, although I couldn't change the past, I could enter the room and bear witness as a victim of sexual abuse described their experiences. As I encouraged people to share their thoughts and feelings, and listened to what happened, we discovered a way to break the abuser's power – the victim was no longer alone, no longer controlled and no longer silenced. This underpins my work as an expert witness in immigration tribunals, trying to give a voice to victims trafficked for sexual exploitation. This chapter reflects some of what these women taught me.

Phoebe

I am a survivor of long-term physical and sexual abuse which began when I was a child and continued through adulthood. I was abused by a neighbour and his 'friends', most of whom held positions of authority within society. From the onset of the abuse, it was as though I lived two separate lives as I chose to hide what was being done to me. There was no single reason for this, but more a culmination of factors which made it feel impossible to reach out to anyone. The longer the abuse carried on, the more I blamed myself for having been stupid enough to trap myself in the situation. On top of all this, I had also gone through completely separate incidences of sexual abuse which left me feeling like 'Rape me' was permanently etched across my forehead.

As a young adult, unsuccessful suicide attempts and complete self-loathing resulted in repeated psychiatric admissions for depression. I was faced with disbelief, judgement, anger and accusations when I tried to tell what I was going through. When it was discovered that my abuser was in a position of power, I was accused of having a crush on him and luring him into my bed. I never disclosed the full extent of the abuse because I couldn't face more disbelief or judgement. My abusers were threatening me and had carried out some of their threats to show me that things could get a lot worse if I didn't shut up.

By my early twenties, I chose to live my life as though the abuse wasn't occurring. After each assault, I would just carry on as if nothing had happened. I cut off emotionally and most of the time was quite numb. I would sometimes try to ring helplines to try to release some of the pain anonymously, if it started to push through, but I found it too difficult to speak. By my mid-twenties, the abuse had escalated to the degree that I had to have several hospital admissions for physical and sexual injuries they'd inflicted on me. I made several attempts to escape but they continually tracked me down. I walked away from everything I owned and lived on the streets in an attempt to escape them. Though I had a brief period of about 6 months when I managed to elude them, they inevitably caught up with me. I was gang-raped, beaten and left haemorrhaging and close

to death. After hospital treatment, I spoke to the police but later withdrew my statement as I was accosted and threatened the same day I spoke to them and I had no faith in a successful police investigation.

I moved to London, seeking out anonymity in its vast population. I was accepted into a refuge for women suffering domestic violence. Though it wasn't the first time that I had been treated with respect, belief and support by professionals, it was the first time that it was consistent, and the acts of the majority of staff were offered in a manner that I found myself able to accept.

WHAT IS SEXUAL ABUSE?

How we think about sexual abuse will influence what we look for and how we ask questions. For example, if our understanding of sexual abuse is limited to vaginal penetration, how will we help victims of female genital mutilation or a gay man talk about their experiences? Sexual abuse is not confined to service users, but happens to our colleagues, family and friends. Many people do not associate their experiences with sexual abuse and yet will readily agree that they went along with sex, to keep the peace, even when they did not want to. A nurse who is gentle and patient, and takes time to explain what sexual abuse means and to ask questions about various types of sexual abuse, can help people define their experiences and validate their reactions, which is a therapeutic process in its own right. We might even help people to recognize a pattern of behaviours when they have not yet identified it as abusive.

Childhood sexual abuse means pressuring, forcing, coercing or tricking a child (under 16) into participating in any kind of sexual activity. It can include showing children pornography, telling them explicit sexual stories, touching them sexually or asking them to make sexual touches. In the UK, about 5 per cent of children have experienced contact sexual abuse and 5 per cent of children on the child protection register had experienced sexual abuse.[1] About a third of all rapes and a third of all sexual crimes in the UK are committed against children under 16.

Sexual abuse of children (and adults) can be associated with harmful traditional practices in some cultures, such as *female genital mutilation (FGM)*, which is defined by the World Health Organization as:

all procedures involving partial or total removal of the external female genitalia or other injury to the female genital organs for non-medical reasons. It has no health benefits and harms girls and women in many ways. It involves removing and damaging healthy and normal female genital tissue, and hence interferes with the natural function of girls' and women's bodies. The practice causes severe pain and has several immediate and long-term health consequences, including difficulties in childbirth also causing dangers to the child.[2]

Over 20,000 girls in the UK could be at risk of FGM.[3]

In a *forced marriage*, one or both spouses are forced to marry under duress (physical and/or emotional abuse).[4] This is very different from arranged marriages where the couple have choices about accepting the arrangement. Forced marriage can be driven by family efforts to control unwanted behaviour and sexuality, including perceived promiscuity or coming out as LGBT. Forced marriage often results in repeated sexual abuse of the person who did not want to marry, or vulnerable people, such as those with disability.

Sexual assault of an adult is any kind of intentional sexual touching of somebody else without their consent, including any part of their body, clothed or unclothed, either with the body or an object. Rape is specifically defined under the Sex Offences Act[5] as penile penetration of the mouth, anus or vagina. Causing a person to engage in any sexual activity without consent, or administering a substance with that intent, is also sexual abuse. Non-penetrative sexual abuse includes sexual harassment, inappropriate touching, indecent exposure, and being photographed or forced to watch or enact sexual acts without consent. Consent is not reluctant agreement or silence; a person only consents if he or she agrees by choice and has the freedom and capacity to make that choice.[6]

Trafficking for sexual exploitation means the recruitment, transportation, transfer, harbouring or receipt of persons by threat, force, coercion or deception. It involves the abuse of power over a person in a position of vulnerability or payments for the purpose of exploiting that person. Exploitation includes forced prostitution or other forms of sexual exploitation, forced labour or services, or practices similar to slavery.

Often these different types of abuse overlap. For instance, a victim of childhood abuse may become sexually abused as a teenager, or a victim of trafficking (VoT) may be recruited through her family or a 'partner' who promises a new life and opportunities. Sixty per cent of women trafficked for sex report being physically and/or sexually abused before they were trafficked, and 95 per cent of women report physical and/or sexual violence while in the trafficking situation.[6]

Double or multiple victimization can entrap victims and make it more difficult to escape. For example, a woman brought to the UK under a spousal visa who discloses sexual and physical abuse by her husband and in-laws may be told by her parents that she must stay for the so-called 'honour' of the family. I try to explain that it is the abuse, or the people who collude with it, not the victim, that is the problem. I remember that when I work with a victim of abuse, I am not alone in the room; the shadow of the abuser(s), along with others, hangs over us and I work hard to hold them, not the victim, accountable.

> ## REFLECTION
>
> If you had not heard of one of the listed types of sexual abuse, read one of the relevant references or explore a website listed at the end of this chapter.

WHICH PEOPLE SUFFER FROM SEXUAL ABUSE AND HOW COMMON IS IT?

On average, Rape Crisis reports that 85,000 women are raped every year across England and Wales and over 400,000 women are sexually assaulted. Among the general public, most people think that rapists are strangers who attack women in public places or break into their homes. In fact, most victims are attacked in private by someone they know. A British Crime Survey[7] found that 45 per cent of rapists were a husband or partner, 9 per cent were an ex-husband or ex-partner and another 29 per cent were known to the victim. Only 17 per cent were strangers. We need to understand that sexual assaults most commonly happen at home, by people whom victims trust.

Sarah Payne,[8] who consulted many victims of rape, reported: 'Everyone I spoke to felt strongly that these attitudes need to be challenged as they affect the whole process the victim goes through' (p.10).

Here is what one woman said: 'You often see screaming tabloids about attacks on men, women and children from a stranger but you very rarely see a headline about violence from a family member or someone in the home' (Focus Group i)[8] (p.10).

As the statistics above indicate, adults vulnerable to sexual abuse may be victims of domestic violence. The Home Office[9] has defined domestic violence as:

> *any incident or pattern of incidents of controlling, coercive, threatening behaviour, violence or abuse between those aged 16 or over who are, or have been, intimate partners or family members regardless of gender or sexuality. The abuse can encompass, but is not limited to:*
>
> * *psychological*
> * *physical*
> * *sexual*
> * *financial*
> * *emotional*

Although 14 per cent of men are victims of domestic violence over their lifetime, women are more likely to be injured, need medical attention, be afraid and be raped.[10] Victims of domestic violence in safe houses run by Refuge UK reported many types of sexual abuse during research funded by the Department of Health:

* Oral rape
* Vaginal rape
* Forced prostitution
* Disfiguring of breasts
* Refusal to practise safe sex
* Forced into pornography
* Forced sex after childbirth/operations
* Threats to get compliance
* Religious prohibitions ignored
* Anal rape
* Penetration with objects
* Forced sexual acts with others
* Chemicals poured into labia
* Refusal or forcing contraception
* Filming without consent
* Infection with STI/HIV
* Female genital mutilation (FGM)
* Sexual insults

Each year, 600,000 to 800,000 men, women and children are trafficked across international borders. Approximately 80 per cent are women and girls. Up to 50 per cent are minors.[11] Within the UK, 2,255 people were identified as potential VoTs in 2012, of which 35 per cent of the adults and 28 per cent of the children reported sexual abuse.[12] In 3 months during 2013, 394 people from 59 countries including Albania and Nigeria were referred to the NRM (National Referral Mechanism), which is a process that aims to identify VoTs. Two men and 138 women were identified as VoTs for sexual exploitation, with many other cases still being investigated.

SEXUAL ABUSE IS HARD TO TALK ABOUT

It takes two to speak the truth – one to speak and another to hear.

Henry David Thoreau, 1849[13] (p.283)

Who has the responsibility to ask or to tell: the worker or the person? Phoebe said that she 'chose to hide it'. Should it be the responsibility of a child to speak out, even if they are abused by an adult they trust? What should they do, for example, if they are disbelieved by their parents? Many victims believe that if the professionals wanted to know, they would have asked. After all, when we assess people at intake, we ask hundreds of other questions, often personal. However, only 10 to 30 per cent of recent violence is asked about and identified in clinical practice.[14] Barriers reported by professionals include lack of confidence, knowledge and competence, along with anxieties about the consequences of asking (see Figure 29.1).[15]

However, if the discussion does not happen, people cannot access help to recover from abuse. NSPCC research[1] has shown that many children do not get support to help them come to terms with their experiences. More than one in three children (34 per cent) who experienced contact sexual abuse by an adult and four out of five children (82.7 per cent) who experienced contact sexual abuse from a peer did not tell anyone else about it at the time.

The disclosure might only be made when the person feels unable to cope any longer, or when they complete

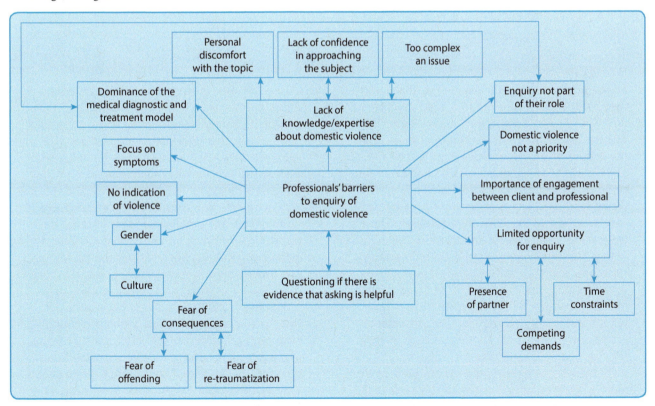

Figure 29.1 Professionals' barriers to enquiry about domestic violence. Reproduced from Howard *et al.*, Barriers and facilitators of disclosures of domestic violence by mental health service users: qualitative study. *Brit J Psychiat* 2011; **198**(3): 189–194 with permission.

questionnaires that ask direct questions about abuse. The following extract is from a conversation with a woman in the UK, aged 35 years, who experienced 10 years in an abusive relationship that included sexual assault, and who was living in a safe house at the time of interview.[16]

Woman: Yeah, yeah, the sexual abuse came out when I basically called the police for harassment because he was phoning me at like 2 or 3 o'clock in the morning every night, you know basically threatening suicide and so I phoned up the police to basically go for harassment to stop it and I had to fill in a questionnaire at the end for domestic violence, and erm, one of the questions were has he ever forced himself upon you for sex and I just burst into tears. So it came out that way rather than …

Interviewer: Right, so something you'd endured at the time but didn't …

Woman: No, I never really spoke to them.

Interviewer: … didn't want to talk about.

Woman: No.

Interviewer: So the questionnaire sort of really triggered that for you?

Woman: Yeah yeah, like I say I didn't think about it until they asked that question and it all came flooding back.

Interviewer: So they were able to put you in contact with the [sexual abuse counselling centre] were they?

Woman: Yeah yeah, they put me in contact with them, like I say I got counselling and they also put up, because obviously once it had come out I was fearful so they put a bobby van, the scheme, which is all the alarms on the windows and doors and stuff and the [service] also helped me with dealing with my housing association to get new lights put up, security lights and stuff. But they were very good. [16]

When this woman disclosed, she valued the practical support that she was offered to promote her safety as well as the therapeutic support to recover her well-being. See chapter 3 on developing and maintaining relationships. I often think of this process as two stages, akin to a house on fire. We cannot start rebuilding the house until the fire is put out. In other words, the first stage of the craft of caring for someone is to promote their safety from further harm. This might include legal action, changes in accommodation, improved security or practical support that depends on referrals to other agencies and/or good multidisciplinary team work. In contrast, bad practice would be to refuse to work with a victim at current risk until the situation changes, or to put the victim at increased risk. Phoebe describes mixed responses of staff below.

PHOEBE'S STORY

At the age of 15, my GP recognized that I was depressed and referred me to a child psychiatry unit where I was admitted as an inpatient. This was the first point in my life where I believe that the actions of professionals, alongside their reactions to what I said or did, played a significant role in both my present and future well-being. The varied work ethics of nurses within the unit was very apparent to me even as a teenager. There were some nurses who came to me a half hour before the end of their shift to question me about my mood and then write up their report. Others would perhaps ask me a couple of times during the day, though still asking quite clinical questions about mood and appetite. The conversation would usually end quite abruptly as soon as they felt they had the information they required.

Of course, there were other nurses who cared more than what they needed to write up their report at the end of the day. They would take time to talk and try to get to know me. Some kept very distant, never speaking of themselves. It would

always be very much a one-sided conversation. Although they were trying to be caring and compassionate, I found myself neither able nor wanting to open up to them. The nurses that I did open up to were the ones who showed a more human side to themselves. They would talk to me about day to day things in a friendly manner. They might ask me what I had for lunch, saying that they'd had sandwiches. We might talk about a television show that had been on the night before or something that was going on in the town. They showed their human side, without ever having to disclose any of their personal history, so I found myself able to open up to them.

However, I didn't immediately disclose the abuse I was going through. I guess without realizing it, I was testing the water. I told them of other things that were going on in my life. Perhaps due to realizing that the problems I was talking to them about were not the main cause of my depression, they brushed them aside as if they were inconsequential. For instance, I spoke about being bullied in school and was told not to worry as in a few years I'd be at university and all those problems would be behind me. Their reactions to what were very real problems to me left me feeling more isolated and terrified than before as I realized that if they weren't even able to help me come up with solutions to these smaller issues, then how could they ever help me escape the men who were abusing me, who were threatening to kill me and hurt the people I loved, if I ever spoke up?

There was one nurse that took the time to get to know me and, in the space of just one or two conversations, she had gained my trust. She didn't demean my problems or what I had to say. For the first time since the abuse began, I felt it might be safe enough to reach out for help and I started

to cry. I cried for 3 or 4 hours, fighting an internal battle; wanting to speak up so the abuse would stop but also terrified of the threats and riddled with shame about what I'd allowed to be done to me. The bits that I told came out fragmented. I felt dirty and ashamed for trying to put the abuse into words. I didn't have the vocabulary or the knowledge to explain easily my experiences. And my fear kept stopping me mid-sentence and I would clam up again. I didn't admit being abused by more than one person and I refused to give up a name as I was too scared. The nurse was patient and kind. She repeatedly told me that it wasn't my fault and that trying to tell someone about it didn't make me a bad person.

REFLECTION

Many factors make it difficult for people to disclose, e.g. being afraid of the abuser's threats, because it is hard to put into words, or because of shame. Is it safe to tell you about sexual abuse? What will you do with that information? The craft of caring requires us to be aware that our attitudes and beliefs will be conveyed to victims, even if that is not our conscious intention. What are your attitudes and beliefs around sexual abuse and what emotions does it bring up for you?

THE EFFECTS OF SEXUAL ABUSE

Physical consequences of sexual abuse can be clustered under acute injuries, chronic infections and psychological distress. Phoebe was diagnosed with depression by her GP. I explore the relationship between sexual violence and depression through a number of aspects:

- chronic psychological abuse or grooming so that over time the victim comes to believe what the abuser tells them;
- sadness consequent on the experiences of abuse;
- disruption to normal daily function at home, school/ work, and socially, which damages mood and self-esteem;
- the impact of violence and abuse on guilt, shame or self-blame.

I think that depression is a natural reaction to what victims of sexual violence have endured. Victims of sexual abuse mostly present with moderate or severe symptoms of depression and post-traumatic stress. Phoebe referred to fear, numbing and low mood, all of which are symptom clusters in post-traumatic stress. Some are afraid that they 'are going mad', that there is something wrong with them and that poor mental health is a character flaw.

Suicidal ideation is a common means by which victims think of escaping from the abuse. I have learned to explain the difference between wanting to kill yourself

and wanting the abuse to stop, and to say, 'I believe you have the right to live safely without fear or abuse.' Victims have told me that nursing staff have often been unsympathetic to self-harm, suicide attempts or problematic substance use. I think that, as part of the craft of caring, it is important to see these behaviours as indicators of abuse, and to understand that, unless the abuse is recognized and the safety of the person improves, they are forced into maladaptive coping mechanisms to numb the pain or to escape. Chapters 22 and 23 have further detail on self-harm and suicide respectively.

REFLECTION

'Why don't they leave?'

Imagine an aircraft carrying passengers held hostage by terrorists with guns. Why do the hostages not get off the plane? Why do they not stand up to the terrorists? Why did they choose to fly in that plane with terrorists?

Your answers will parallel some of the reasons for the behaviours of people who experience sexual abuse.

LEARNING ABOUT EXPERIENCES OF SEXUAL ABUSE

The first step is to increase your awareness, through reading this chapter, by going to training on abuse, by completing an e-learning module (e.g. the Social Care Institute for Excellence (SCIE) e-learning package – see 'Relevant web pages') or by reading a consultation with survivors.[8,17,18] If you broaden your understanding of people's experiences of sexual abuse, you will be much better equipped to ask relevant questions, to support people to disclose details and to act as a safe listener. For more general information on assessment refer to chapters 13 and 14.

Focusing on the aetiology of symptoms and showing concern about the real, external danger, rather than just treating the symptoms, is central to the craft of caring. By asking about violence, you are giving important messages: you care about their safety; the problem is not too shameful to discuss; their distress is understandable; you hope the situation can change; abuse is wrong and not the responsibility of the victim; they are not alone.

It can help to have an introductory sentence to explain why you are asking questions, such as 'Many people have experienced abuse, which affects not only their physical health but also their psychological well-being.' Then specific questions about sexual abuse could include:

- Did anyone hurt you sexually as a child?
- Did anyone cut or stitch you down below?

- Has anyone called you sexual names, like 'whore' or 'fag'?
- Do you have to go along with sex to keep the peace?
- Has anyone made you have sex when you were sick, or when it was painful?
- Has your partner made you have oral or anal sex when you didn't want to?
- Has s/he used an object in a sexual way that you didn't like?
- Has s/he made you perform sexual acts when you didn't want to?
- Did they make you watch porn or copy porn in a way you didn't like?
- Has s/he refused to practise safe sex or use birth control?
- Has s/he had affairs or talked about other partners to make you feel bad?
- Many victims of abuse have gynaecological or health problems. Has anyone infected you with HIV or STIs?

REFLECTION

If you ask someone with a black eye, 'How did you get that?', who are you holding responsible? Would a victim feel less blamed or ashamed if you asked, 'Who hurt you?'

THINKING ABOUT HOW YOU RESPOND TO A DISCLOSURE

What you say in response to a disclosure can have a profound impact on the person who has experienced sexual abuse. They may not have told anyone else. They may not only remember and think about what you say, but it can influence whether they will take the risk to trust anyone else again. Here is one person commenting on attitudes that imply 'contributory negligence':[8] 'The advertising we've had so far puts all the onus on the victim, it's "don't go out and get drunk, you might get raped". The onus needs to be on the man, to stop women feeling shameful' (Focus Group iii)[8] (pp.10–11).

In general, people who have experienced sexual abuse want:

- to be believed;
- to be treated with dignity;

- to be reassured that it was not their fault;
- to feel safe and comforted;
- not to feel like a 'victim';
- services that support them and their family;
- to feel in control;
- to be able to make informed choices.[8]

The person is the expert on what they need and what should happen next. They are the only person with all the information about their situation. As such and as part of the craft of caring, you need to be guided by them. Asking 'What do you need right now?' is a means to empower them and find out about their priorities and concerns.

WHAT CAN BE OFFERED TO HELP?

What services can help? In the craft of caring, it is important that you find out about local services that support victims of sexual abuse or domestic abuse, and be ready to offer to refer people on different occasions, depending on their safety and journey of healing. A sexual assault referral centre (SARC) may be most appropriate immediately after an assault, while a referral to Rape Crisis or a specialist traumatic stress service may be most appropriate further down the line. In general, you can empower people by ensuring that they are aware that help is available and that they do not have to cope alone.

Your response can help the person to recognize their experience as abusive and lift the self-blame many victims feel (not least because the abuser tells them they are responsible). In the craft of caring, it is important to let them know that no one deserves to be treated that way. You could also reassure the person about confidentiality and that it is safe to talk to you (within the confines of your policies on safeguarding). You might say, for instance:

- I'm sorry to hear that has happened to you.
- Thank you for trusting me and having the courage to tell me. What do you need?
- Many people tell me they feel embarrassed or ashamed. I think that the shame lies with the people who hurt you. The problem is the abuse, not you.

- You did not deserve to be treated that way. It's not your fault.
- Their behaviour towards you is wrong and against the law.
- Nothing you say or do can give a person the right to violate you/your personal space in the way that has been done to you.
- You did what you needed to do to survive and now you can begin to heal.
- It takes a lot of courage to speak about what has happened to you the way that you have. Courage is not being fearless; it's doing something despite being afraid.

PHOEBE'S STORY

The morning after I first disclosed to the nurse that I had been sexually abused, the psychiatrist came and told me, rather officiously, that an appointment had been arranged for my mother to come to be told what I had revealed to them the night before. I couldn't believe it. I broke down pleading with her not to; I pointed out that they had promised not to repeat to my parents anything that I told them unless I said it was OK. She dismissed this by saying that they had legal obligations. When they were trying to gain my trust and made those promises, they meant that 'as much as possible' things would be kept between them and me. But this was the first that I heard of it. I had fully believed I was talking to them in confidence. She wouldn't discuss it. She immediately left my room, saying my mother was coming an hour later. All I could do was keep begging as she walked away. I became completely enveloped in shame and terror.

In the following days, the doctors would claim that the way they had dealt with things had been 'for the best'. 'It's like ripping off a plaster,' they said. 'Your parents had to be told and it's best to get it over and done with straight away without discussion or debate.' Ripping off a plaster is a short sharp

pain that can't be avoided and that causes no lasting damage. They hadn't ripped off a plaster. They had taken a sledgehammer to my trust in them, which was akin to a sheet of fragile thin glass, and smashed it into a million pieces, irreparably. I felt stupid for thinking that anyone would listen to me or take my concerns seriously. I felt naïve for believing their promises and opening up to them, and violated by the way they had stripped me of all control over what happened next.

Looking back, I can see that they had to inform my parents that I had been sexually abused. I think, even at the time, I realized that to a certain degree. But the way they chose to strip me of any say in the matter, disregarding promises they made to me on my admittance to the unit and their refusal to discuss it at all with me did insurmountable damage to my ability to trust anyone in authority or, for that matter, any other human beings at all. That day, I decided that confidentiality is meaningless, trusting is foolish, and speaking up puts you in danger and leaves you feeling more violated and vulnerable than the abuse itself. Over a decade passed before I came even close to trusting in a professional again.

'Treat me like a human being'

When asked what advice they would give professionals about how to respond to people with experiences of sexual or domestic violence, problematic substance use and/or mental ill-health, most people said the most important need was to be valued as a human being.[19] For example:

Asking for help is the most difficult thing you can ever do. And when you do that, you just want someone to say 'Look, it's not your fault, and we're going to get you some help, and you are

not this worthless human being...' That's the first thing you need, then practical help. But what you really need is for someone to treat you like you're worth something, you're not just something out of the gutter.

Nottingham, interviewee[19] (p.5)

Some survivors also highlighted the importance of small acts of respect and kindness – for example, workers calling if they are late for an appointment, being offered a cup of tea, and for one survivor, simply 'a friendly face and a hug can mean a lot' (Nottingham, survey respondent)[19] (p.5). A significant number of women described workers as good because they were patient, listened, were not judgemental and did not force survivors to take steps for which they were not ready. These are all necessary attributes in the craft of caring.

In contrast, survivors of sexual violence affected by problematic substance use tended to experience stigma and negative responses, such as being told by a drugs worker 'if you are able to stand on a street corner, you can collect your [methadone] script'[19] (p.5).

Another woman commented:

> *I find people can be a bit judgmental. It might be my perception, but … it's like in the hospital, you choose it, you chose to take an overdose … but I was feeling crap. The nurse got a bit moody like she didn't want to be with me.*
>
> **Nottingham interviewee[19] (p.9)**

PHOEBE'S STORY

When someone speaks to you about abuse they went through, it can be difficult to know how to show support without interrupting what they are saying and, I find, people often resort to physical contact. It is as though we have a need to reach out to support others when we can see they are in pain but it isn't always helpful. Often, when I speak about my past, the person I'm speaking to will rub my arm. I know that it is done as a gesture of support, solidarity and compassion but, in my head, I'm just thinking, 'I'm not a cat who is comforted by being stroked.' It feels patronizing, invasive and uncomfortable. And then I feel ungrateful for feeling that way when I know that they are trying to be supportive.

One day, when speaking to Roxane about some of what I was escaping, she gently reached out her hand. She didn't quite touch mine; she left the decision to make contact up to me. It was empowering to be given the choice whether or not to reach out to accept that support. I felt no pressure to and wasn't worried that I'd feel guilty if I didn't. I took it as a sign that she was telling me that although she wasn't there when I was going through what I was speaking to her about, she was there to support me through the horror of the memory of it. What may seem like such a small, insignificant gesture can, in fact, mean a great deal. As I took hold of her outreached hand, it broke down a barrier within me that I hadn't realized existed because it was the first time in many years that I didn't feel completely alone in my pain.

Don't disappear

Offering another appointment contributes to the craft of caring, as it shows your understanding that sexual or physical abuse causes trauma, and that you are willing to talk about it and committed to supporting the person. A clear message that 'You can talk to me again' or questions about progress in follow-up meetings helps convey the message that you know it takes a while to recover from abuse and that neither you nor the person can overcome the trauma in one session.

Help with childcare

To safeguard children and help parents recover from experiences of abuse, they need help to talk freely. One interviewee remarked: '[Gaps in services are] advice for mothers, things they can take their children to… even with the crisis team it was hard to talk about how I was feeling in front of my daughter'[19] (p.13).

CONCLUSION

People with experiences of sexual abuse have increased contact with health care services, but the abuse may not always be identified as a causal factor in their physical and mental health problems. To improve your practice and craft of caring, here are some key things to try:

- Build into your daily working life your understanding that people you see may have experienced some form of sexual abuse.
- Ask people specific questions about sexual abuse in private, when they cannot be overheard.

- Be positive and supportive in your response to disclosures of abuse.
- Give information or refer to agencies or services that can help (know what services are available within your area for survivors of sexual abuse).
- Keep an accurate record that may help the person in the future, e.g. with housing or legal rights.
- Take care of confidentiality and information sharing to safeguard the person.
- Follow up the conversation and talk about it with the person again.

References

1. Radford L, Corral S, Bradley C, Fisher H, Bassett C, Howat N, Collishaw S. *Child abuse and neglect in the UK today*. London: NSPCC, 2011.
2. WHO (World Health Organization). Female genital mutilation. Available from: http://www.who.int/topics/female_genital_mutilation/en/ [Accessed 25th July 2016].
3. GOV.UK. Improving the lives of girls and women in the world's poorest countries. 2013. Available from: https://www.gov.uk/government/policies/improving-the-lives-of-girls-and-women-in-the-worlds-poorest-countries/supporting-pages/helping-to-end-female-genital-mutilation-for-girls-and-women-in-africa [Accessed 24th May 2016].
4. Foreign & Commonwealth Office. *Dealing with cases of forced marriage: practice guidance for health professionals*, 1st edn. London: FCO Services Publishing, 2007.
5. Sexual Offences Act (2003). Available from: http://www.legislation.gov.uk/ukpga/2003/42/contents [Accessed 24th May 2016].
6. Zimmerman C, Hossain M, Yun K, Roche B, Morison L, Watts C. *Stolen smiles. The physical and psychological health consequences of women and adolescents trafficked in Europe*. London: London School of Hygiene & Tropical Medicine, 2006.
7. Walby S, Allen J. *Domestic violence, sexual assault & stalking: findings from the British Crime Survey*. Home Office Research Study 276. London: Home Office, 2004.
8. Payne S. *Rape: the victim experience review*. London: Home Office, 2009.
9. Home Office. Domestic violence and abuse. Available from: https://www.gov.uk/guidance/domestic-violence-and-abuse [Accessed 25th July 2016].
10. Howarth E, Feder G. Prevalence and physical impact of domestic violence. In: Howard LM, Feder G, Agnew-Davies R (eds). *Domestic violence & mental health*. London: Royal College of Psychiatry, 2013, ch. 1.
11. US Department of State. Trafficking in persons report. 2014. Available from: http://www.state.gov/j/tip/rls/tiprpt/2014/ [Accessed 25th July 2016].
12. UKHTC (United Kingdom Human Trafficking Centre). A strategic assessment on the nature and scale of human trafficking in 2012. Serious Organised Crime Agency (SOCA) Intelligence Assessment, 2013.
13. Thoreau HD. *The writings of Henry David Thoreau, vol. 1: A week on the Concord and Merrimack Rivers*. Boston: Houghton & Mifflin, 1906.
14. Howard LM, Trevillion K, Khalifeh H, Woodall A, Agnew-Davies R, Feder G. Domestic violence and severe psychiatric disorders: prevalence and interventions. *Psychological Medicine* 2010; **40**: 881–93.
15. Rose D, Trevillion K, Woodall A, Morgan C, Feder G, Howard L. Barriers and facilitators of disclosures of domestic violence by mental health service users: qualitative study. *British Journal of Psychiatry* 2011; **198**(3): 189–94.
16. Evans M, Agnew-Davies R, Sardinha LM, Feder G. Women's experiences of meaningful change following domestic abuse. Unpublished raw data, 2014.
17. Women's National Commission. Still we rise. 2009. Available from: http://wnc.equalities.gov.uk/work-of-the-wnc/violence-against-women/news-and-updates/276-launch-of-together-we-can-end-violence-against-women-and-girls-a-strategy.html [Accessed 25th July 2016].
18. Women's National Commission. A bitter pill to swallow. 2010. Available from: http://wnc.equalities.gov.uk/work-of-the-wnc/violence-against-women/news-and-updates/309-a-bitter-pill-to-swallow-report-from-the-wnc-focus-groups.html [Accessed 25th July 2016].
19. Stella Project. *'Treat me like a human being, like someone who matters': findings of the Stella Project Mental Health Initiative Survivor Consultation*. London: AVA, 2012. Available from: http://avaproject.org.uk/wp-content/uploads/2016/03/Treat-me-like-a-human-being-SPMHI-survivor-consultation-report-June-2012.pdf [Accessed 25th July 2016].

Further reading

Bass E, Davis L. *The courage to heal: a guide for woman survivors of child sexual abuse*. New York: Collins Living, 2008.
Davis L. *The courage to heal workbook: for adult survivors of child sexual abuse*. New York: Collins Living, 1990.
Foa EB, Rothbaum BO. *Treating the trauma of rape*. New York: Guilford Press, 1998.
Howard LM, Feder G, Agnew-Davies R (eds). *Domestic violence & mental health*. London: Royal College of Psychiatry, 2013.
NICE (National Institute for Health and Care Excellence). *Domestic violence and abuse: how health services, social care and the organisations they work with can respond effectively*. NICE public health guideline 50, 2014.
Trevillion K, Agnew-Davies R, Howard LM. Healthcare professionals' response to domestic violence. *Primary Health Care* 2013; **23**(9): 34–42.
WHO (World Health Organization). *Responding to intimate partner violence and sexual violence against women: WHO clinical and policy guidelines*. Geneva: WHO, 2013.

Relevant web pages

Foreign and Commonwealth Office. www.fco.gov.uk
Forward. www.forwarduk.org.uk
Men's Advice Line (for male victims of abuse). www.mensadviceline.org.uk
NICE (National Institute for Health and Care Excellence). Domestic violence guidelines. www.nice.org.uk/guidance/PH50
Rape Crisis (free helpline (lunch, eves.) 0808802 9999). www.rapecrisis.org.uk
Refuge. www.refuge.org.uk
Respect. http://respect.uk.net/
Social Care Institute for Excellence (SCIE). Sexual health and abuse e-learning package. http://www.scie.org.uk/publications/elearning/sexualhealth/index.asp
Stop the Traffik. http://www.stopthetraffik.org/real-life-stories
Womens Aid Federation of England. https//www.womensaid.org.uk/

30 The person with an eating disorder

GILLIAN TODD AND ROSEMARY MARSTON

LEARNING OUTCOMES

- To understand how to develop and maintain a therapeutic alliance using motivational interviewing skills.

- To understand what enables and maintains an eating disorder.

- To be able to integrate the concepts of the recovery model as part of the 'craft of caring'.

- To understand and be able to reflect on the development and consequence of high expressed emotion in the multidisciplinary team when treating these patients.

- To have a template to develop a skills-based training approach for all carers, family carers and professional carers.

- To develop a motivational clinical supervision model which is informed by research and compassion.

- To know the diagnostic criteria for eating disorders (see chapter 12 for information on classification).

SUMMARY OF KEY POINTS

- Understanding eating disorders requires the clinician to understand the complex interactions between physical, psychological and social factors with which the service user struggles.

- Treating an eating disorder is not only about food, weight and shape and refeeding practices. It is about seeing the 'whole person' and understanding their challenges and their strengths, particularly in terms of helping them make and sustain relationships in a self-compassionate manner.

- Supporting the social network of service users of all ages through emotional intelligence teaching is vital for assisting the transition from clinical care to independent living.

- Time for motivational supervision and a space for self-reflection for staff are prerequisites for coping with the tense emotional climate generated by a disorder which challenges normal survival instincts and philosophical and spiritual beliefs.

- The lack of early detection, the absence of a swift treatment response and flexible treatment options by services which are difficult to access, and treatment delivery which can be coercive and has seemingly arbitrary rules can produce the iatrogenic effect of unwittingly maintaining an eating disorder.

- Families and staff who are not educated or supported to understand the complex nature of the disorders also contribute to maintaining the disorders.

INTRODUCTION

This chapter proposes a new way of developing the nursing and multidisciplinary therapeutic relationship with the service user who has an eating disorder, in order to establish a working alliance in all treatment settings.

We propose the integration of family carers at all levels of treatment. We recommend that all carers, including all clinicians in the multidisciplinary team (MDT), develop their interpersonal skills and knowledge base by understanding the service user's perspective, and applying health behaviour change theories to their relationships with the service user and each other. Treatment and care should provide an ongoing shared learning environment for service users, carers and clinicians.

We will try to illustrate how to reframe the power imbalance between service users, nurses and all clinicians, in line with the Tidal Model, the recovery model, self-determination theory, motivational interviewing and motivational enhancement theory.

Not eating poses major ethical, conceptual and existential problems for the whole MDT in delivering treatment. Service users believe that having to eat regularly in a controlled fashion deprives them of their liberty, identity and autonomy, and they see their relationship with food as vital for helping them to manage their emotions and their lives. Food for them is 'the enemy'.

The first steps in treatment are to assess the physical and psychological risks generated by the eating disorder and then to focus on ordered eating. Many inpatient and day-patient programmes leave the management of feeding to the nursing staff. Sometimes these service users are held under the Mental Health Act, but the majority are not.

REFLECTION

Developing a therapeutic alliance with and providing psychological support to the service user, while also persuading and sometimes forcing them to eat, be weighed, and have their liberty curtailed due to the process of feeding, is a challenge not currently supported by ongoing specialist training. In your eating disorder work, how do you help reluctant service users to accept treatment?

CURRENT TYPES OF TREATMENT AND PROGNOSIS

In the UK eating disorders are treated mainly in psychiatric services: in specialist psychiatric eating disorder (ED) services, or generic psychiatric services for people of all ages. There is a shift in treatment focus at the age of 18, when people move from child and adolescent mental health services (CAMHS) to adult psychiatric services. In CAMHS, the evidence for family engagement is clear and families are routinely involved in both therapy and management meetings. In adult settings the evidence is less clear, and confidentiality is cited as a reason not to include families, who would have been an integral part of the care team in CAMHS, and who will continue to provide care. This exclusion results in a lack of information for the treatment team and a sense of abandonment and sometimes anger felt by carers. Recently, psychological services attached to general practitioner (GP) settings have begun to provide some outpatient care.

The National Institute for Health and Care Excellence (NICE)[1] guidelines recommend that most people with an eating disorder be managed on an outpatient basis initially, as most of them are aged 15 to 24 and live at home, and this causes the least disruption to their lives. Outpatient treatment is often 1 hour per week, with the family providing the main care.

The overall prognosis for anorexia, as reported in the 2004 NICE guidance, is that '43% of people recover completely, 36% improve, and 20% develop a chronic disorder'[2] (p.16). Sufferers are mainly female. The mortality rate for anorexia is the highest of all psychiatric illnesses, at 10 to 20 per cent.[2]

In the case of bulimia the average age of onset, at 18 to 19 years, is slightly higher than that for anorexia, which is 16 to 17 years. Bulimia sufferers, 60 per cent of whom are female, are mostly successfully treated in an outpatient setting with cognitive behaviour therapy–enhanced (CBT-E). Other psychosocial interventions include dialectical behaviour therapy (DBT) for impulsive, self-harming behaviour. About 50 per cent of people will recover, 30 per cent will have relapses and remissions and 20 per cent will remain fully symptomatic.[1]

Binge eating disorder (BED) is more common in adults (in their 30s and 40s) and there are equal numbers of male and female sufferers. The physical risk is mainly due to becoming obese, and the psychological risk is associated with clinically significant depression (chapter 21) and anxiety (chapter 20). Treatment is similar to that for bulimia, that is, CBT-BED, or interpersonal therapy (IPT) for BED[3] (p.155). Sufferers with BED may eat large amounts of food in secret, and may have long periods of starving, which makes the likelihood of a binge much greater. Treatment should cover self-esteem issues, anxiety and depression, and should link feelings of a lack of control to the drive to eat as though ravenous.

Treasure et al.[4] suggest that on average an eating disorder will last 5 to 6 years, often spanning adolescence to adulthood. These authors summarize prognosis as: 'Effective treatment early in the ... illness, which (has lasted) less than 3 years, leads to a good outcome in 90% of cases' (p.21); the caveat to this is that successful treatment is most often seen in those aged 18 years and under. They also state that 'Restoring weight to a normal level in hospital, by itself, does not ensure ... that the outcome is good' (p.22). They suggest that treatment, along with aiming to establish weight restoration and/or less disorganized eating, should also address 'understanding and unpicking the association of food and weight issues with emotions, styles of thinking and relationships'[4] (p.23).

Current studies of eating disorders span environmental factors, genetic factors, maturational development factors and cognitive constructions which may occur because of starvation or due to the intermittent delivery of nutrition caused by the disorders and which may also be part of an epigenetic profile, a bio-psychosocial matrix.

THE RECOVERY MODEL ETHOS AND THE TIDAL MODEL

The Mental Health Foundation website[5] explains the recovery model as promoting several relational factors (see also chapters 35 and 36). The one which most often defeats service users, in our experience, is being able to develop 'resilience to possible adversity or stress in the future'.

Other factors highlighted by people as supporting them on their recovery journey include:

- being believed in;
- being listened to and understood;
- getting explanations for problems or experiences;
- having the opportunity to temporarily resign responsibility during periods of crisis.[5]

Treasure[6] states that for the purposes of treatment it may not be helpful to focus on a specific cause of the eating disorder. She describes the view of the sufferer as 'a vulnerable individual, in the wrong place at the wrong time' as a more helpful construction for care.

A nurse-generated model of care which promotes and outlines the idea of nursing care as a 'craft' is the Tidal Model.[7] The authors mention six key philosophical assumptions: 'the virtue of curiosity', 'the power of resourcefulness', 'the person's wishes', 'the paradox of crisis', the fact that 'goals must belong to the person', and lastly, 'pursuing elegance', by which they suggest keeping things (for example, language) simple.

> ### REFLECTION
>
> Every interaction with a service user should honour these six key philosophical assumptions of the Tidal Model as a mark of respect to them. In your practice, how can you integrate these principles?

MOTIVATIONAL INTERVIEWING (MI) AND SELF-DETERMINATION THEORY (SDT)[8]

Motivation interviewing (MI) can be used in order to focus on developing a respectful, listening relationship which clearly overlaps with the Tidal Model, and promotes the development of a sense of personal curiosity, encouraging the service user to ask: 'How did I get here?'[6] Chapter 39 contains more information on MI.

These theories make an assumption 'that humans have an innate tendency for personal growth towards psychological integration'. People are far less likely to change if the pressure to do so comes from an external source. They may do so for pragmatic reasons – for example, to keep a job, or to get out of hospital – but they will not continue to maintain the change of their own volition.[8]

Self-determination theory (SDT) explains why people change (or not),[8] and MI explains how to establish the therapeutic conditions needed to elicit and direct changes in health behaviour. The Tidal Model[7] outlines a philosophical stance of respectful caring that underlines the necessary qualities of the nursing therapeutic alliance.

The MI model also focuses attention on the 'spirit' and quality of empathy in the therapeutic relationship (see chapter 3). Miller and Rollnick's *Motivational interviewing: helping people change* (3rd edn) proposes that if there is negative tension in the relationship it should be called 'discord', rather than 'resistance', suggesting that both parties have contributed to the development and possible maintenance of this 'discord'.[9]

> ### REFLECTION
>
> Discord in the relationship between the nurse and the service user can require positive reframing, away from criticism and blame of the service user. Consider how you handle this discord, and reflect on where you believe the responsibility for the quality of the relationship lies.

MI emphasizes the fundamental importance of specific communication skills, 'listening' to the service user and helping them to move in the direction of change experiments. MI is a 'conversation style' rather than a therapy. It directs responses to enhance self-esteem and self-confidence to try to improve resilience to experiment with change strategies.

A useful acronym for listening skills is 'OARS':

- *Open* questions are questions which provide practice for 'bigger picture' thinking, a move away from too much detail. However, a battery of questions will stop people from engaging.
- *Affirmations* are an acknowledgement of the efforts, intentions and strengths of the person. Ideally, with practice, the service user will learn to give themselves praise, thus raising their self-esteem.
- *Reflections* are speech patterns which focus on the words used by the patient, by repeating them or paraphrasing them, or include speculation regarding the patient's unspoken emotions. A complex reflection might also involve the use of paradox by emphasizing the negative or playing down the negative, using a stronger or quieter tone of voice, for example, 'You feel making new friends is never going to happen', or 'You feel that it will take a little longer than you hoped to make new friends.'
- *Summaries* are a gathering of ideas/points every few minutes to check out with the service user what was heard.

Put together, the process of engagement should look like this: *Listen*, *Offer* seeds to plant (either through asking permission to give advice or through strategically reflecting on the service user's strengths and intentions (using OARS)), and then *Listen* to the reply (LOL); this pattern should be repeated. The service user should talk more than the nurse (or other clinician). Questions of any sort must be kept to a minimum, as repeated questioning can be experienced as an attack.

Attention should be paid to language, being positive and not critical. Turning negatives into positives becomes an intervention skill; for example, 'You need to learn some boundaries' could become 'You are very clear about which rules and direction you will follow, in the face of great pressure to do otherwise.' The service user's skills of determination and seeking an identity are seen as a positive, as it is these skills and this energy which will support change.

The service user is directed to a position where they are willing and able to attempt 'actions', 'goals' or 'experiments' towards change, thus strengthening their sense of self-efficacy and promoting a sense of personal agency.

Using ambivalence

The 'mixed message', or ambivalence, from the disorder requires exploration: 'on the one hand you want to look after yourself and manage your relationships and on the other hand you find the eating disorder does a good job of caring for you as long as you remain isolated'. A thoughtful

process of working through this ambivalence helps people to move in the direction of expanding their repertoire of coping behaviours. We work on 'planting seeds' with discussion and information about how change happens more generally for anyone.

The MI intervention positions the expert role with the service user. This stance is based on regarding service users' reactions to change as 'normal'; that is, applying health psychology concepts which suggest that all people maintain behaviours because they gain benefit from these behaviours, even though significant others disagree, and recognizing that people move through stages of change in relation to their preparedness to act.[10]

Service users' attachment to the eating disorder is strong, as the disorder has many positive functions.[11] Among other things, it can be relied upon, it gives an identity, it gains attention, it halts sexual development, it prevents the pain of strong emotions[12] and it helps manage boredom.[13]

REFLECTION

- People with an eating disorder have a very limited repertoire of achieving human desires and establishing a sense of control; they only have the eating disorder. Through developing self-reflection skills and emotional intelligence about relationships, they can learn to tolerate change.

- How can you integrate as a treatment target supporting the natural human desires to control areas of our lives, have an identity, manage our sexual status, dampen strong emotions, find reliable relationships, and so on? How can you help the service user to develop a variety of ways to facilitate this sense of control?

Timing is crucial; when we are pushed too quickly to change, we cling to what we know best – in other words, the status quo – regardless of any negative effects.[14]

REFLECTION

- It is a fundamental principle of engagement to believe that service users can learn and tolerate change. Trust and sometimes blind faith are also components in equal relationships.

- We hold the 'hope' for our service users. How do you demonstrate this in your practice?

MOTIVATIONAL ENHANCEMENT THERAPY (MET)

During the last 20 years a model for working with all carers, which can also be applied to MDTs, has been developed by Treasure et al.[4] This is a motivational skills model for

all carers, for service users of all ages and for all eating disorder conditions, called the motivational enhancement therapy model (MET).

MET requires the nurse to understand the bio-psycho-social causation mix, while also delivering a care package that is rooted in the recovery model (see chapters 35 and 36 for more detail on the recovery model). MET is an amalgam of the maintenance and cognitive models of eating disorders and MI. There are natural overlaps with SDT, the recovery model and the Tidal Model.

THE MAINTENANCE MODEL

A cognitive-interpersonal maintenance model, initially discussed in 2006 by Treasure and Schmidt[15] and revisited in 2013[16] by the same authors, proposes four areas which contribute to maintaining an eating disorder. These include genetic factors, which 'account for over 50% of the risk in eating disorders'[17] (p.15); emotional dispositions (service users 'tend to be more sensitive than others to perceived threat')[17] (p.16); thinking styles which are related to a detail-focused rigidity when processing information; and interpersonal factors. 'Social avoidance can be a core feature'[16] (p.4), ranging from being unable to detect emotions in others to being super-sensitive to emotions in others. Both stances leave the service user alone and unconnected, thus lowering their self-esteem. Learning to cope with emotions can be made more difficult by intense emotional responses from close others.

The behaviour that needs to be targeted to help ameliorate the effects of weight restriction, purging, bingeing, vomiting, and so on, is the interpersonal style of the service user, i.e. the forming, building and maintaining of relationships (see chapter 3).

THE COGNITIVE WORLD OF PEOPLE WITH EATING DISORDERS

Studies evaluating the cognitive world of people with eating disorders inform the nurse of the attentional bias differences in these service users. This information is helpful in explaining how and why service users seem to choose to remain anxious, fearful, angry and critical of all attempts to make them see the logic of changing.

In a study exploring social reward and rejection sensitivity, Cardi et al.[18] found 'an attentional bias to rejecting faces and a difficulty disengaging their attention from these stimuli' among service users with eating disorders, and they also had a 'sustained attentional avoidance of accepting faces' (p.1). Service users acknowledge that they are more sensitive than other people and believe that they are unlikeable. Often they believe that they are being manipulated and lied to because this is what they deserve.

Service users do not notice attempts at looking friendly or accepting, and miss out on the soothing rewards of positive relationships. Consequently, they behave as though they do not trust and cannot self-soothe, and their self-esteem becomes further diminished.

Service users can be taught to understand and manage their 'attention to the negative' thinking style, in different ways. One method of doing this is by using cognitive remediation therapy developed for eating disorders by Tchanturia and discussed in her 2014 paper.[19] Simply put, this is training the brain to be flexible and to move from a detailed focus to 'bigger picture' thinking.

Cardi et al.[20] also studied rank perception and self-evaluation, showing clearly that people with eating disorders 'had higher levels of unfavourable social comparison, submissive behaviours, and external and internal shame than healthy controls' and 'Heightened sensitivity to social rank related cues, [and] impaired self-evaluation at an automatic level of processing' (p.1).

Examples of maintenance of eating disorders

The relationships role modelled by the MDT, when they are based on historical ways of delivering care and are not grounded in respect for the service user, contain the damaging maintaining effects of high expressed emotion. This directs criticism, blame and scapegoating towards the service user and team members. However, it is possible for high expressed emotion to be reframed in a way that is positive for the service user (see Table 30.1).

REFLECTION

In social interactions the 'attentional bias' refers to the fact that service users learn to focus on negative responses from others, and consequently may behave in ways that elicit these predictable and easily identifiable negative responses, thus strengthening their low self-esteem. Notice when MDT clinical interactions are negative and critical of each other – these are the role models service users will learn from, thus promoting the eating disorder as a way to manage negative emotions.

Clinical hierarchies often promote rank as value, with health care assistants, nurses and service users frequently positioned at the lower end of the scale of the 'power to make decisions'. Nurses are chided by other team members for not managing to 'feed patients', or 'having no boundaries' particularly when they attempt to see the service user's perspective and work collaboratively. These types of personal, negative, responses can be construed as

Table 30.1 Reframing high expressed emotion

High expressed emotion	The reframe
Paranoia	Learning to trust is difficult.
Criticism	No one is perfect.
Grandiose self-belief	I have confidence in myself and need to learn to have confidence in others.
Smothering and intrusiveness	I believe that others can and will learn to care for themselves.

a consequence of the absence of self-reflection and compassion, both for the criticizer and for others in the wider caring team. This power play is experienced by service users as demonstrating how unimportant they are, and that their views and values do not matter.

REFLECTION

In this critical atmosphere, all parties become negative, frustrated, hopeless and submissive, and they sabotage any attempt to change, preferring the predictability of the status quo. This lowers self-esteem and diminishes the motivation of everyone involved. When you feel under emotional pressure, how do you resolve it and maintain your positivity and hopefulness?

CASE STUDY 1: IN THE DINING ROOM

A service user asks for pepper. The staff member asks if there are rules about using pepper. The service user looks around at others, raises her eyebrows and sighs. The service user next to her says quietly, 'Staff should know what they are doing.' There are sighs all round and rolling of eyes. The staff member responds: 'I don't appreciate everyone belittling my question and suggesting nurses should know better.'

The service users immediately respond by retreating into the eating disorder. One says: 'It is inappropriate to talk to us like that.' Another says: 'Why are you picking on X? That is not fair.' X, near to tears, says: 'You shouldn't be talking to me like that. It's not fair and it's unprofessional.' The staff member says: 'I was not picking on you' (X was not either the patient who spoke under her breath

or the patient who asked for pepper), and then becomes upset and irritable.

This results in hurt feelings and anger all round. The meal is much harder to finish, although there is a sense of martyrdom and heightened critical excitement in the patient group. The staff member is then left with a sense of dread that anything they do or say could result in disciplinary action. The ward sister removes the staff member from the patient support group.

A motivational response to the situation outlined in case study 1 would need to be measured and neutral in tone, and is not a natural way of speaking.

CASE STUDY 1 (CONTINUED): A MOTIVATIONAL RESPONSE

Staff member: 'I need to check about handing out the pepper as I guess there are rules about using it.'

Patients roll their eyes.

Staff member: 'I detect some unhappiness about my question. I need some help to know how to check out what the guidance is here. I guess it would be very unsettling for everyone to realize that not everyone knows what to do for the best. I feel upset that asking for the information causes some of you to think the nursing staff are useless.'

The ward sister publicly organizes a post-meal discussion. This might open a dialogue later in a group setting about how asking for information, especially around food, can develop into an argument, with everyone feeling irritated for different reasons.

A MODEL FOR SELF-REFLECTION

Treasure et al.[4] (pp.93–112) use animal metaphors to provide simple non-threatening examples of unwitting accommodating and enabling behaviours from all carers, to explain how caring responses can perpetuate rigid, inflexible thinking in service users.

The animal models are intended to help self-reflection in all carers in a non-threatening manner.

- Jellyfish – having heightened emotional responses and can indulge in blaming others; also appears critical and unpredictable. They find it difficult to separate the person from the illness. This can lead to the service user feeling fearful, angry and/or let down.

- Kangaroo – over-protective and enmeshed, appears to want to control and 'fix'. This can lead to feelings of helplessness and fear in the recipient and get the confirming message that they are not able to grow up.
- Ostrich – lacking self-belief, does not value their own input, appears self-effacing and weak. This can lead to a feeling that no one cares, they are 'too much' to cope with and not worth the effort.
- Rhinoceros – wanting to compete and defeat the illness with logic and control, appearing arrogant and self-absorbed. This can lead the service user to feel angry, aggressive, submissive and hopeless.
- Terrier – constantly nagging and trying to head off problems. Appears thoughtless and controlling. This can lead to the service user wanting to 'trick' and dissemble to ward off this constant criticism.
- St Bernard – calm, caring, reliable. This can lead to the service user feeling trusted and quietly develop confidence. When the service user feels valued, compromise becomes acceptable.
- Dolphin – watchful, caring, thoughtful. This can lead to the service user considering taking risks and discussing their own opinions and tolerating compromise.

NURSING AND RELATED TREATMENT ISSUES

Nursing staff report feeling uncomfortable especially in the dining room, as though their task is akin to being a gaoler. Long et al.[21] asked service users with anorexia nervosa their perspectives of inpatient mealtimes. The resulting qualitative analysis had three emerging themes: first, 'Mealtime delivery (logistical factors influencing meals)'; second, 'Individual outcomes (cognitions, emotions, behaviours and physical sensations during meals)'; and third, 'Mealtime characteristics (including disengagement, perceived battlegrounds, and a desire for involvement in mealtimes)' (p.419). The study team asked for ideas from these service users relating to what may improve the process and atmosphere at mealtimes. The service users said 'they would like to take a more active role in the decision making and implementation of meals'. They wanted 'goals set within safe, supportive environments so that meals would be challenging and new skills relating to eating could be learned'. They also said that 'they were given insufficient autonomy and that this left them unprepared for continuing their improved eating away from the ward' (p.424). This paper provides an insight into the conflicts experienced by service users and staff in a dining room situation, as well as making suggestions for improvements for individual service users.

Service users should be involved in the organization of the delivery of their care, alongside learning how to cope with their fears and anxieties when that delivery is not perfect or does not suit everyone. Chapter 50 has more information on collaborative care planning. Tolerating compromise promotes resilience. Staff planning before and evaluation after meals is essential, and it is recommended that specific feeding teams are developed to include all members of the MDT. Mindfulness practice for all before and after meals is essential for service users and staff (chapter 44).

A RECOVERED SERVICE USER'S PERSPECTIVE

It is vital to understand the service user's insight into their illness and the background of its development.

In the dining room staff carry the weight of a lot of expectations from service users. They have the responsibility to create as safe an environment as possible in supporting people to do that which they have avoided for large parts of their lives. Emotions always run high and mealtimes can seem like a war zone. Service users are conflicted when confronted with food. They know that this is an unavoidable part of treatment and are ambivalent in their acceptance of it. This inner ambivalence can sometimes be mirrored unwittingly by the treating team.

Feeding generates memories of being forced or cajoled to eat at home, which is meant to be good for you but which we really hate! Saying that you should eat it because they tell you so is not going to work. Staff will experience the turmoil that parents face at family mealtimes, multiplied by the number of service users eating together.

Service users are often high achievers who live by hard and fast rules. When a service user comes from a background of having high expectations placed upon them, the tendency to think that whatever they do will never be good enough leads them to believe they are unworthy of compassion. If this is the case at home, how can they trust a virtual stranger to guide them safely through the conflict created by eating? Sometimes it can seem that the staff are ruining a good therapeutic relationship by insisting that they eat. It is never helpful for staff to compare either the amount or type of food from one patient to another and/or to compare food size and type from one meal to another for the individual patient, and trading with service users over the quantity of food on their plates rarely works.

Service users can make progress in terms of their eating and weight gain, and then when physical changes start taking place the anxiety becomes too much to contend with mentally, and progress slows down or even goes backwards. It is always two steps forward, one step back when things are going well.

Staff in the dining room can help by diverting attention from the food itself. A focus on personal needs and goals, bigger picture thinking, and removing the emphasis from making arbitrary comparisons with others can give the encouragement needed to fight the internal and negative influence of the anorexic voice.

Here are two examples of the nursing influence in my own treatment, one of which was good and the other which felt damaging. I also provide an example of the domino effect which can be created in the dining room when one service user feels aggrieved and others become drawn into the situation.

My symptoms were restriction and over-exercise. I never suffered binge/purge symptoms. On arriving for inpatient treatment, part of me felt some sense of relief that I would be taken care of, but another part would question whether I deserved any help at all. I felt guilty at all the damage I had caused to others and found the compassion of the nurses difficult to accept, especially in the dining room. My sense of needing to be punished was pervasive.

Scenario 1
This guilty feeling was overwhelming and I just looked at my food and bolted from the dining room. I couldn't cope with the thought of eating and felt I didn't deserve it. One of the nurses left the dining room and came to find me. I was crying uncontrollably and I felt that all the bad things I had done could never be forgiven and I was better off dead. I said this aloud, and the response from the nurse was that she had no idea what it was I had done to make me think so badly of myself but that, whatever it was, she couldn't watch me punishing myself. She said that whatever had happened in my past must have been devastating if my answer to dealing with it was to starve myself. She told me that nobody deserved this sort of life and that she felt I deserved to be treated better than I was treating myself. With that, I went back to the dining room and I felt that I might have a better chance

of making an informed choice about whether my life was worth living at some point in my future. I had no idea what she saw in me that seemed so deserving but I felt I wanted to find out for myself.

Scenario 2
I had graduated from the supervised table to the unsupervised table. A staff member was there, which was unusual because we were considered to be more advanced in treatment and not in need of supervision, but perhaps this was an exception to that rule. She asked me why I didn't have the things which a person of my age normally would expect to have. She listed some of those things – a home of my own, a husband, a good job – and she did this in earshot of everyone at the table. At that point in time, I found it impossible to continue to eat and I was fighting back my tears. The other service users tried to support me but the damage had been done. Instead of reminding me of my progress in treatment, she managed to humiliate me and remind me of all the deficits in my life. This had a devastating effect on me and was something that I replayed over and over in my mind for the remainder of that admission and beyond.

Scenario 3
This example illustrates the domino effect that can be created when conflict arises in the dining room. The setting was the serving of a morning snack in the dining room, which included a milky drink. I was sitting next to a girl who was bulimic and she always drank her mug of coffee very quickly and in one gulp. This fascinated me because not only was the drink made with full fat milk but it was boiling hot, and it took me about 10 minutes to start sipping it. The nurse supervising snacks asked her whether she would keep her drink down or would she vomit when we left the dining room. She was stunned at being asked this question. I was infuriated that she had been singled out and humiliated in this way and instantly leapt to her defence. She became very tearful and upset and the other service users reacted furiously. Some saw this as an opportunity to retaliate and make accusations against staff about similar experiences, while others saw this as an opportunity to challenge other service users whom they felt would also be likely to use compensatory behaviours.

The outcome was chaotic and was not confined to the dining room. There was a polarization in the service user group and created a 'them versus us' stand-off. This type of altercation left many of us questioning just how much staff as a whole understood what it was like to have an eating disorder, and there was a real breach of trust. That a member of the nursing team could be so judgemental, in such a public way, raised a number of issues which threatened the notion of the team being compassionate and non-judgemental for quite some time. Did the staff really care about the difficulties we faced in the dining room or were they just bullies?

Integrating food into living

Hospital can lead to institutionalization and life upon discharge can feel very threatening. Safety around food and how to maintain weight restoration is an important issue, and finding ways to spend unstructured time feels very challenging.

In my role I accompany people out for snacks or meals. There is a lot of anxiety for service users in doing this. When a staged approach is used, service users begin to feel more confident in making a public appearance with food in cafes and restaurants. Being prepared to make the effort to integrate with the wider population takes significant courage, and the rehearsal gives a sense that practice eating can be worthwhile.

The danger of returning to restricting food intake is ever-present, particularly in the early stages of recovery, and developing new interests and skills is vital prior to discharge. Exploring voluntary work options, joining social clubs or looking at education and study options are all things to consider before discharge from any treatment.

Rosemary Marston

CONCLUSION

This chapter has aimed to provide a framework that supports the service user with an eating disorder in becoming resilient to the demands of life. Resilience is about learning to tolerate not being perfect; construing failure as a necessary, valuable process; and learning when to trust and when to take calculated risks. Collaboratively caring for someone requires all parties to tolerate compromise.

The ability to self-reflect and develop emotional intelligence about ourselves as clinicians is the precise skill we want the services users to learn. We want them to 'put themselves in others' shoes', to experiment with tolerating flexible decisions when not everyone is happy with the outcome, and for all to move away from a 'one size fits all' therapy culture.

Maintaining a therapeutic stance which honours the service user's rights and freedoms not to change may paradoxically give the space to plant the seed that change is possible. When a service user says, 'I can't do this', a good response would be, 'I know you can't do this, at the moment.' Feeling heard and believed is a crucial building block in a therapeutic relationship. Pushing too hard in one direction forces the person to push in the other direction.

Attending to any behaviours we do not like makes those negative behaviours stronger and more embedded.

REFLECTION

Can you practise giving attention to behaviours you want to see more of and reducing your attention and subsequent negativity to behaviours you do not like? What message does this send to the service user?

Structured educational timetables throughout the day, providing information about current research and skills practice on social communication skills and emotional intelligence, is essential. Calmness, a neutral tone of voice and a total lack of criticism embody the 'spirit' of care that is required. Seeing the service user as we see any individual – as someone with hopes, dreams, aspirations and challenges – will help them to tolerate change. Nurses are curious, resourceful, creative and in a pivotal position to model and embed this philosophy in all treatment settings.

References

1. NICE (National Institute for Health and Care Excellence). *Eating disorders, core interventions in the treatment and management of anorexia nervosa, bulimia nervosa and related eating disorders. Clinical Guideline 9.* London: NICE, 2004.
2. Arcelus J, Mitchell AJ, Wales J, Nielsen S. Mortality rates in patients with anorexia nervosa and other eating disorders: a meta-analysis of 36 studies. *Archives of General Psychiatry* 2011; **68**(7): 724–31.
3. NICE (National Institute for Health and Care Excellence). Eating disorders, core interventions in the treatment and management of anorexia nervosa, bulimia nervosa and related eating disorders: summary of identification and management. 2004. Available from: https://www.nice.org.uk/guidance/cg9/resources/algorithms-547648093 [Accessed 31st October 2016].
4. Treasure J, Smith G, Crane A. *Skills-based learning for caring for a loved one with an eating disorder: the new Maudsley method.* London: Routledge, 2007.
5. Mental Health Foundation. What supports recovery? Available from: http://www.mentalhealth.org.uk/a-to-z/r/recovery [Accessed 28th October 2016].
6. Treasure J, personal communication, 2005.

7. Buchanan-Barker P, Barker PJ. The Tidal Commitments: extending the value base of mental health recovery. *Journal of Psychiatric Mental Health Nursing* 2008; **15**: 93–100.

8. Markland D, Ryan RM, Tobin VJ, Rollnick S. Motivational interviewing and self-determination theory. *Journal of Social and Clinical Psychology* 2005; **24**(6): 811–31.

9. Miller WR, Rollnick S. *Motivational interviewing: helping people change*, 3rd edn. New York: Guilford Press, 2013.

10. Prochaska JO, Di Clemente CC. Transtheoretical therapy: toward a more integrative model of change. *Psychotherapy: Theory, Research and Practice* 1982; **19**(3): 276–88.

11. Serpell L, Treasure J, Teasdale J, Sullivan V. Anorexia nervosa: friend or foe? *International Journal of Eating Disorders* 1999; **25**: 177–86.

12. Serpell L, Teasdale JD, Troop NA, Treasure J. The development of the P-CAN, a measure to operationalize the pros and cons of anorexia nervosa. *International Journal of Eating Disorders* 2004; **36**(4): 416–31.

13. Gale C, Holliday J, Troop NA, Serpell L, Treasure J. The pros and cons of change in individuals with eating disorders: a broader perspective. *International Journal of Eating Disorders* 2006; **39**(5): 394–403.

14. Prochaska JO, Di Clemente CC. Stages and processes of self-change of smoking: toward an integrative model of change. *Journal of Consulting and Clinical Psychology* 1983; **51**(3): 390–5.

15. Schmidt U, Treasure J. Anorexia nervosa: valued and visible. A cognitive-interpersonal maintenance model and its implications for research and practice. *British Journal of Clinical Psychology* 2006; **45**: 343–66.

16. Treasure J, Schmidt U. The cognitive-interpersonal maintenance model of anorexia nervosa revisited: a summary of the evidence for cognitive, socio-emotional and interpersonal predisposing and perpetuating factors. *Journal of Eating Disorders* 2013; **1**: 13.

17. Treasure J, Smith G, Crane A. *Skills-based caring for a loved one with an eating disorder: the New Maudsley Method*, 2nd edition. Abingdon: Routledge, 2016.

18. Cardi V, De Matteo R, Corfield F, Treasure J. Social reward and rejection sensitivity in eating disorders: an investigation of attentional bias and early experiences. *World Journal of Biological Psychiatry* 2012; Early Online, 1–12.

19. Tchanturia K, Eli D, Fleming C. Effectiveness of Cognitive Remediation and Emotion Skills Training (CREST) for anorexia nervosa in group format: a naturalistic pilot study. *European Eating Disorders Review* 2014; **22**: 200–5.

20. Cardi V, De Matteo R, Gilbert P, Treasure J. Rank perception and self-evaluation in eating disorders. *International Journal of Eating Disorders* 2014; **47**(5):543–52.

21. Long S, Wallis D, Leung N, Meyer C. 'All eyes are on you': anorexia nervosa patient perspectives of in-patient mealtimes. *Journal of Health Psychology* 2012; **17**: 419–28.

Further reading

Care Services Improvement Partnership and National Institute of Mental Health. *New ways of working for everyone in mental health*. London: Department of Health, 2007.

Department of Health. *The National Service Framework (NSF) for adults with mental health problems*. London: Department of Health, 1999.

Department of Health. *Mainstreaming gender and women's mental health – implementation guidance*. London: DH, 2003.

Department of Health. *Refocusing the Care Programme Approach: policy and positive practice guidance*. London: DH, 2008.

Deprivation of Liberty Safeguards 2009. Available from: http://webarchive.nationalarchives.gov.uk/+/www.dh.gov.uk/en/socialcare/deliveringadultsocialcare/mentalcapacity/mentalcapacityactdeprivationoflibertysafeguards/index.htm [Accessed 28th October 2016].

Mental Capacity Act 2005. Available from: http://www.legislation.gov.uk/ukpga/2005/9/contents [Accessed 28th October 2016].

Mental Health Act 2007. Available from: http://www.legislation.gov.uk/ukpga/2007/12/introduction [Accessed 28th October 2016].

RCP (Royal College of Psychiatrists). *MARSIPAN: Management of Really Sick Patients with Anorexia Nervosa. College Report CR162*. London: RCP, 2010.

Royal College of Psychiatrists. *Guidelines for the nutritional management of anorexia nervosa*. 2005. Available from: http://www.rcpsych.ac.uk/files/pdfversion/cr130.pdf [Accessed 7th October 2016].

Schmidt U, Wade TD, Treasure J. The Maudsley Model of Anorexia Nervosa Treatment for Adults (MANTRA): development, key features and preliminary evidence. *Journal of Cognitive Psychotherapy: An International Quarterly* 2014; 28(1): 1–25.

Social Exclusion Unit. *Mental health and social exclusion report*. London: Social Exclusion Unit, 2004.

Relevant web pages

B-EAT (Beating Eating Disorders). http://www.b-eat.co.uk
Formerly the Eating Disorder Association (EDA). This is the UK's largest national eating disorder charity.

CARED (Caring About Recovery from Eating Disorders). http://www.caredni.org
This is a newly formed charity in Belfast, N. Ireland.

King's College London. Eating disorder research pages. http://www.kcl.ac.uk/ioppn/depts/pm/research/eatingdisorders/resources/index.aspx

FEAST (Families Empowered and Supporting Treatment of Eating Disorders). http://www.feast-ed.org

New Maudsley Approach. http://www.thenewmaudsleyapproach.co.uk

Royal College of General Practitioners. Eating disorders. http://www.rcgp.org.uk/clinical-and-research/clinical-resources/nutrition/eating-disorders.aspx

Succeed Foundation. http://www.succeedfoundation.org
This is a UK-based charity, set up in 2010.

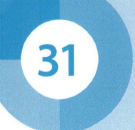

31 The person experiencing mental health and substance misuse problems

PHILIP A. COOPER AND GRAHAM NAUGHTON

LEARNING OUTCOMES

- To understand the key issues for people with mental health and substance misuse concerns.
- To be familiar with the latest evidence regarding engagement, persuasion, treatment and interventions.
- To be aware of service user perspectives and be able to reflect on your own practice.
- To be aware of screening and assessment tools to aid the engagement and treatment process.

SUMMARY OF KEY POINTS

- Mental health and substance misuse issues are complex, and understanding the relationship between mental health and substance misuse can help to build trusting relationships.
- Assisting with practical problems, including accommodation, welfare benefits and social activity, can be more important in the early phases of engaging a person to persuade them to access treatment than directly addressing mental health and substance misuse.
- Effective assessment and engagement are essential if subsequent interventions are to be successful by seeking out the views of the expert by experience (the person you are seeing).
- If a person is unable to achieve a change in their behaviour on the first occasion, this does not mean that future interventions will be unsuccessful; it means lessons can be learned that will help in the next attempt to change.
- Take time to engage the person from the start, and build a respectful, trusting, non-judgemental relationship in an atmosphere of hope and optimism. Be direct in your communications and use a flexible and motivational approach.

INTRODUCTION

The chapter will highlight key issues for the person experiencing co-existing mental health and substance misuse issues. It will build on the evidence base about this subject, alongside the views of a service user who has experienced co-existing mental health and substance misuse issues. In addition, it will explore some of the main approaches and processes involved in facilitating natural change behaviour in mental health nursing practice for people with mental health issues who misuse substances, including practical examples of screening and assessment tools. To do this, an understanding of the nature of change and working with people in realistic timescales over the long-term is required.

Unrealistic expectations of change can prove frustrating for professionals and service users. The nature of the therapeutic relationship is crucial in engaging with people and beginning the processes of change behaviour.

THE IMPORTANCE OF CO-EXISTING MENTAL HEALTH AND SUBSTANCE MISUSE ISSUES

The diagnosis, care and treatment of people who have severe mental health issues and who misuse substances is a challenge to health and social care services because people in this group:

- are at a higher risk of relapse (in terms of both substance misuse and mental health problems), including readmission to hospital, risk of serious self-harm and suicide, depression, demoralization and poor physical health;[1]
- often have a delayed diagnosis of severe mental illness combined with misuse of substances, or their condition

worsens due to an interaction between the misused drugs and prescribed medications;[2]
- often have wider health and social needs due to the condition itself or high-risk behaviours such as sharing syringes, and may be at an increased risk of cardiac or respiratory diseases and blood-borne diseases;[2]
- may have an increased likelihood of social isolation, unstable housing or unemployment.[2]

WHAT'S IN A NAME?

SERVICE USER'S PERSPECTIVE

I am not a diagnosis, I am Graham (see chapter 19). Dual diagnosis workers helped me get the right intervention for the first time. I should be easy to access help for both mental health and substance misuse but it isn't.

Numerous terms have been used to describe the co-existence of severe mental health and substance misuse issues. The term 'dual diagnosis' began to emerge in the US literature in the mid-1980s.[3] There is a wide diversity of the people who broadly have any mental health problem and misuse a variety of substances. This diversity can hinder the process of research, as studies incorporate very different research cohorts in varying study settings, and may limit studies to areas of mental health or substance misuse separately. There is the potential difficulty where 'dual diagnosis' describes people who may have two or more conditions that may be present at the same time, constituting a multiple diagnosis.[4] The term 'dual diagnosis' suffers from a lack of conceptual clarity and is prone to conceptual blurring, because 'dual diagnosis' is a relatively new term, although it has drawn attention to co-existing mental health and substance misuse issues.[5]

Mental health services in the UK have been mandated to follow a categorization system (see chapter 12) which places people in clusters of mental health distress, including specific clusters for 'psychosis and affective disorder (high substance misuse and engagement)' and 'psychosis and affective disorder – difficult to engage' (see Box 31.1). A cluster is a global description of a group of people with similar characteristics, as identified from a holistic assessment and rated using the Mental Health Clustering Tool.[6]

BOX 31.1: UK MENTAL HEALTH AND SUBSTANCE MISUSE CLUSTERS

Care Cluster 16. Psychosis and Affective Disorder (High Substance Misuse and Engagement). Includes people with enduring, moderate to severe psychotic or bipolar affective symptoms with unstable, chaotic lifestyles and co-existing problem drinking or drug taking. They may present a risk to self and others and engage poorly with services.

Care Cluster 17. Psychosis and Affective Disorder – Difficult to Engage. Includes people with moderate to severe psychotic symptoms with unstable, chaotic lifestyles. There may be some problems with drugs or alcohol not severe enough to warrant care associated with cluster 16. This group have a history of non-concordance, are vulnerable and engage poorly with services.

REFLECTION

Addressing both mental health and substance misuse at the same time has many benefits. Adults and young people who have a mental health issue and misuse substances are among the most vulnerable in society. They experience some of the worst health, well-being and social outcomes, and treating issues at the same time seems entirely logical. How would you recognize substance misuse in people who experience psychosis?

PREVALENCE OF CO-EXISTING PROBLEMS

An explanatory model has been proposed that suggests people with mental health issues are more likely than the general population to use substances.[7] There appears to be some evidence in the USA to support this view, although it does not apply to all substances and has not been clearly demonstrated outside the USA.[8] It is not clear how many people in the UK have a mental illness and misuse substances (dual diagnosis), due to several factors:

- differences in how 'dual diagnosis' is defined;
- difficulties with diagnosis; for example, substance misuse may 'mask' an underlying mental illness or vice versa, or people may come to acute services with unrelated health problems and any 'dual diagnosis' may be missed;
- the fact that people in this group may not be using services or receiving relevant care;
- a lack of national data.[2]

Research has indicated that between 22 and 44 per cent of adult psychiatric service users in hospitals in England also have substance misuse problems. Urban populations have higher rates of dual diagnosis than rural areas, and despite over 60 per cent of service users in high secure facilities having a history of substance misuse, only 20 per cent are receiving treatment specifically for their substance misuse.[9] The prevalence of co-existing mental health and substance misuse problems may affect between 30 and 70 per cent of those presenting to health and social care settings.[10] Improving screening and assessment of substance misuse among those with mental health issues will continue to be crucial in addressing the complex needs that present to practitioners. The emergence of new psychoactive substances (NPSs) that appear to mimic more established substances has been a concern. In 2014, 101 new psychoactive substances (previously called 'legal highs' in the UK prior to the Psychoactive Substances Act 2016 where the production and supply of psychoactive substances, which are often referred to as legal highs, is now against the law) were detected for the first time, and it is interesting to note that the new drugs coming on to the market are mainly synthetic cannabinoids, stimulants, hallucinogens and opioids that mirror the established substances.[11]

REFLECTION

In the UK, NPSs are becoming increasingly prevalent in assessments. How can you stay up to date with NPSs that are being developed? What do you think are the problems for practitioners in assessment for those using NPSs?

APPROACHES TO TREATMENT

In the UK, there has been a focus on integrating care in one place, yet this does not seem to have been implemented in many areas of practice. There is a mix of people being treated for one issue and then accessing treatment for the other problem (serial models), and people being treated for both issues at the same time but by different services (parallel models).[12] A variety of services in the UK have lead workers or champions with an interest in mental health and substance misuse;[13] or there are identified practitioners in substance misuse or mental health services who provide care to deal with both issues at the same time in community mental health settings[14] or in specialist dual diagnosis clinics.[15] There appears to be a movement towards using the expertise from both services to bring about high quality interventions.[16]

THE FOUR-STAGE MODEL

A four-stage treatment model for people with mental health and substance misuse issues has been developed to allow practitioners working with people over the long term to offer timely and appropriate treatment interventions.[17] The stages are:

- *Engagement* – developing and maintaining a therapeutic relationship between the person and the practitioner using warmth, genuineness and accurate empathy to provide the optimum environment for change to take place using a non-judgemental and non-confrontational approach.[18] Graham expressed the view that 'building a positive relationship with workers helped me have a lot of trust'.
- *Persuasion* – using the principles of motivational interviewing by examining any ambivalence and motivation to change.[19] Graham expressed the view that 'being given lots of options about what was possible gave me hope'.
- *Active treatment* – realistic goal setting by the person and not the practitioner will facilitate natural change behaviour, whereas unrealistic goals will produce failure and reduce self-belief in the person trying to address substance misuse issues.[19] Graham expressed the view that being asked to take part in 'teaching workers helped me understand about setting goals that I could achieve and not keep failing, it was a way for me to learn and helped me change'.
- *Relapse prevention* – identifying high-risk situations for relapse and rehearsing alternative coping strategies to cope in anxiety-provoking situations.[20] Graham expressed the view that 'learning different ways to cope really helped and we had a laugh doing it; keep your interactions humorous at every opportunity'.

When working with adults and young people with known or suspected psychosis and co-existing substance misuse, take time to engage the person from the start, and build a respectful, trusting, non-judgemental relationship in an atmosphere of hope and optimism. Be direct in your communications, use a flexible and motivational approach, and take into account the following:

1. Stigma and discrimination are associated with both psychosis and substance misuse.[21]
2. Some people will try to conceal either one or both of their conditions.[21]
3. Many people with psychosis and co-existing substance misuse fear being detained or imprisoned, being given psychiatric medication forcibly or having their children taken into care, and some fear that they may be 'mad'.[21]

SCREENING AND ASSESSMENT

SERVICE USER'S PERSPECTIVE

Look past the substance and see the person. Asking about the link between mental health and substance misuse was useful, not being told off or criticized.

Identifying and assessing both areas of mental health and substance misuse is the first goal of any service in either field and can be used to establish the engagement process (see chapter 13). Assessing both areas requires drawing together areas of mental health (see chapter 13) and substance misuse over a period of time, including four core areas that are relevant to both:

• measurement of the nature, duration and frequency of issues;
• clarification of how, when and where the issues occur;
• explanation of the impact of the issues for the person;
• variation of possible changes in the pattern of the issues that occur.[22]

Essential substance misuse information needed for assessment includes: what substances are being used, how much and how often the person is using, the route of ingestion of each substance, the length of time substances have been used and the places where substances were used, who they use substances with and times substances are used, patterns of substance misuse over time (stable or unstable), any withdrawal symptoms and any accidental or deliberate overdoses when using substances.[23] Every question should

be phrased in a way that is aimed at engaging the person. The health care professional should be interested and seek out knowledge; do not be frightened of not knowing about substances or mental health issues, as the expert in front of you will tell you about it.

Health care professionals in all settings should routinely ask adults and young people with known or suspected psychosis about their use of alcohol and/or prescribed and non-prescribed (including illicit) drugs.[21] In addition, they should conduct an assessment of dependency[24,25] and seek corroborative evidence from families, carers or significant others, where possible, if permission is given.

In the UK, a number of assessments are recommended to assess substance misuse, including the Alcohol Use Disorders Identification Test (AUDIT),[26] the Severity of Alcohol Dependence Questionnaire (SADQ),[27] the Clinical Institute Withdrawal Assessment (CIWA-AD),[28] and the Leeds Dependency Questionnaire.[29] A self-assessment of a person's readiness to change their use of substances can be really useful to prioritize the substance to be worked on and in which order (see Box 31.2).[30]

REFLECTION

The emphasis should be on engaging and using the assessment as a means to get a second opportunity to go through the information being gathered. Why do you think that going through any assessment report with the servicer user may be useful?

BOX 31.2: READINESS TO CHANGE MEASURE (ADAPTED FROM: CENTER ON ALCOHOLISM, SUBSTANCE ABUSE, AND ADDICTIONS RESEARCH DIVISION)

Using the scale below, indicate how ready you are to change (cut down or stop) your use of any of the substances listed.

Substance used	Not ready to change	Unsure	Ready to change	Trying to change
	1 2 3	4 5	6 7 8	9 10

ENGAGEMENT

SERVICE USER'S PERSPECTIVE

I only started telling you [mental health services] the truth after a few years as I told you what I thought you wanted to hear; not addressing both issues meant that I thought you could not help.

Health care professionals' values, attitudes and beliefs can affect the quality of care provided, and the process of engagement will be adversely influenced by negative attitudes.[22] There are a number of necessary personal attributes for any health care professional who is working to engage with people who have mental health and substance misuse issues. These include being committed, having a good knowledge base and skills in motivational approaches to facilitate natural change behaviour, an ability to build trusting relationships, effective communication skills and acceptance, which is crucial to remaining non-judgemental and positive about change taking place and for treating each individual with respect.[18] Encouraging service users to take part in delivering education sessions is a great way to equalize the power difference between worker and service user. It can serve another purpose: to deliver education to the service user who is attending part of the course. Service users attending dual diagnosis courses as students has enabled them to help themselves and others in peer support situations.

REFLECTION

Engagement is concerned with understanding the perspectives of those you are working alongside and exploring options to respond to identified needs; for example, finding somewhere to live (instead of a house) or dealing with finances may be more important than addressing substance misuse or mental health issues initially. Why do you think this is the case? Would you always offer a drink to or accept one from a service user at a first assessment to enhance engagement?

BEHAVIOUR CHANGE AND THE CYCLE OF CHANGE

Change occurs naturally, and practitioners can be the catalyst to facilitate the process of change behaviour. Change is strongly influenced by interpersonal interaction; the relationship between the practitioner and service user is crucial, as most examples of change behaviour occur in the first few sessions.[19] The practitioner has an effect on treatment dropout, retention, adherence and outcome. An empathic counselling style seems to facilitate change (its absence may deter change), and people who believe they are more likely to change do so.[19] Service users whose health care professionals believe they are likely to change do so, and those who are told they are not likely to improve do not, so health care professionals' comments about change are important. Motivation for and commitment to change predicts subsequent behaviour, and people who argue against change (resistance) produce less change.[19]

REFLECTION

People who use substances change their behaviour all the time; for example, someone who does not have enough money for vodka will drink a cheaper alternative, and the same applies to all other substances. The ability to change is not in doubt. The timescale is the element that is not known, so consider the factors that have influenced change in your own life.

BOX 31.3: STAGES OF CHANGE

This model introduces the idea of clinical interventions as procedures involving a distinct sequence of changes over time.

Pre-contemplation (not thinking about change). A person does not have a problem and does not think they want to change.
Contemplation (thinking about change). A person is beginning to become aware that a problem exists.
Decision making (planning change). A person has decided that they are ready for change and has committed themselves to this process.
Action (making changes). A person has actively started to change their behaviour or their environment.
Maintenance (keeping it going). A person has changed and made significant gains but is either slipping or help is needed to prevent a relapse or maintain the gains.
Lapse or relapse. A person has slipped back into a brief bout of substance use or has begun to use the substance again after previous achievements in maintaining changes.[31]

INTERVENTIONS AND TREATMENT

SERVICE USER'S PERSPECTIVE

Your job is to get me to explore the solutions that I have within myself. There were a number of times when I did not want to be involved with mental health services. Positive and optimistic contacts with a dual diagnosis practitioner helped me to get to a position where I considered changing what I did; using my views of using substances and not the worker's was much more useful. I had been told loads of times to stop and how bad substance misuse was, but that had not stopped me before.

BOX 31.4: PROS AND CONS OF USING SUBSTANCES[19]

What's good about using substances?
Any concerns about using substances?

BOX 31.5: EXAMPLES OF BRIEF INTERVENTIONS

- Provide advice and information tailored to meet the needs of the individual.
- Ask the person to consider the positive and negative consequences of substance misuse in relation to physical, social and psychological and spiritual needs.
- Consider discussion of consequences of intoxication, binge drinking and/or excessive substance misuse.
- Give practical advice on how to reduce substance misuse.
- Provide written or electronic information during interventions to complement the one-to-one session, including details of local substance misuse service support.

Source: Adapted from Cooper.[22]

A useful tool to begin the engagement process is to ask about the good elements about using any substance and then asking if there were any concerns about the substances being used (see Box 31.4).

Brief interventions

Using brief interventions is a less time-intensive approach (5–10 minutes) which may be crucial when building a trusting relationship with people experiencing a range of complex issues in their lives[22] (see Box 31.5). Using an assessment report to check the accuracy of information gathered and as a brief intervention can be a useful means to build trust. Opportunistic contacts with people who are not seeking treatment can be particularly appropriate occasions to use brief interventions when working with people with complex needs (see chapter 41). The clinical activities listed in Box 31.5 use talk-based interventions targeting change behaviour for substance misuse and associated health issues. The components of brief interventions entail easy-to-understand, structured advice, using written or electronic information where appropriate, and using a flexible motivational approach. Brief interventions are often based on a series of ingredients using the acronym FRAMES:[32]

- **Feedback** – provides feedback on the individual's assessments;
- **Responsibility** – the individual is responsible for change;
- **Advice** – provides advice on changing behaviour;
- **Menu** – provides a variety of options for change;
- **Empathy** – warm, genuine, empathic and understanding approach;
- **Self-efficacy or self-belief** – encourages optimism about changing behaviour.

Persuasion

SERVICE USER'S PERSPECTIVE

Working with a dual diagnosis practitioner who was consistent in their attempts to get me to think about what I was doing from my perspective made me realize that I needed to do something about my own situation.

Motivational interviewing (MI; see chapter 39) has a growing evidence base to support treatment interventions for people with mental health and substance misuse issues.[21,33] MI is a therapeutic intervention which uses specific skills and an interpersonal style when working alongside people with mental health and substance misuse issues.[19] The skills used include reflective listening to understand the person's perspective, and using this elicited information to increase a person's motivation for positive change. The approach is person-centred but identifies areas to work on, including providing information and encouraging the person to put forward their own reasons for making a change. The motivational interviewer should at the same time avoid direct persuasion or giving advice that is not requested, and avoid labelling behaviours as problematic and confrontation.[19] There are four main principles involved in MI:

- expressing empathy – being interested in and wanting an understanding of the person's perspective using reflective listening;
- supporting self-efficacy/belief – focusing on the person's strengths and efforts with a view to helping them to talk about past successes;
- rolling with resistance – viewing resistance as a sign to change tactics and make attempts to reflect and empathize with resistant statements;
- developing discrepancy – helping the person to identify contradictions between current behaviour and what they want to achieve in the future.

The best ways of implementing motivational approaches incorporate open-ended questions to avoid yes or no answers. Using positive statements to encourage and support the person can be used and practitioners can then reflect and summarize their interpretation and check the interpretation is correct with the service user. MI is a useful approach to engage people in treatment interventions, exploring resistance to change and facilitating natural change behaviour.[33] To better help dually diagnosed service users sustain treatment involvement, MI practitioners should pay special attention to recovery accomplishments, values, abilities and self-esteem, while linking these attributes to service participation where appropriate, and creating a safe, valuing atmosphere that is conducive to self-disclosure.[34]

Active treatment

SERVICE USER'S PERSPECTIVE

I used to set myself unrealistic goals and did not achieve them. Realistic goal setting for me was vital so I did not feel like a failure.

Cognitive behaviour therapy integrated treatment (C-BIT) is a manualized treatment approach designed to enhance health care professionals' skills and confidence in working alongside people collaboratively to prompt and maintain behaviour change[35] (see chapter 40). The rationale is to encourage people with mental health and substance misuse issues to self-manage the issues that present at any point in time and work on different phases of treatment.[17]

Harm minimization or reduction are approaches used in substance misuse services, and it has been identified that such approaches focus on reducing drug-related harms rather than drug use for those still using substances.[36] The use of such approaches for people with mental health and substance misuse issues appears logical, as realistic long-term goals can be framed around such approaches to improve engagement phases of treatment, retaining people in service contact while using individual approaches that accept the possibility that people may perceive a benefit from using substances when they experience mental health issues.

Peer support or mutual aid group dual-focused interventions for people with mental health and substance misuse issues have been associated with reductions in substance misuse and increased adherence to medication and attendance at 12-step groups. Self-help groups may have a particular advantage for those attending, because they can provide a safe and comfortable environment to discuss issues that may attract stigma elsewhere.[37]

REFLECTION

How do you think you could encourage peer support networks with the people you know?

Relapse prevention

SERVICE USER'S PERSPECTIVE

I have learned that whenever a slip-up takes place I can never be back to 'square one', as I will have learned things along the journey to maintaining abstinence.

There are a number of potential factors that can contribute to a relapse in substance use, including an increase in mental health distress, peer pressure from others to use substances, living in areas where there is easy access to substances and having little support in community settings, not having meaningful activities, and having arguments with significant people.[38] If these factors are not considered during treatment, then one of the most likely outcomes is relapse. Substance misuse and mental illness rarely affect only one individual, and a person's social network, including their partner, children and other significant individuals in their life, should play an active part in recovery by accessing support to help facilitate and maintain change behaviour where possible. Support and education for families and carers about substance misuse and mental health can be matched to their relative's stage of change and can help to avoid confrontation, allowing more positive results.

CONCLUSION

People with mental health issues using substances continue to constitute a complex area of practice. The craft of caring includes a major focus on engaging a trusting, therapeutic relationship rather than focusing on substance misuse change. Assessing both mental health and substance misuse effectively can aid engagement and potential treatment options. Optimism about the possibility of change is crucial, because change is always happening, and the role of the practitioner is to facilitate the natural change process. Every meeting is an opportunity, and a long-term, realistic perspective must always be maintained.

References

1. Mueser KT. Working with people with mental health-substance use. In: Cooper DB (ed.). *Mental health-substance use: introduction to mental health-substance use.* London: Radcliffe, 2010: 107–19.
2. NICE (National Institute for Health and Care Excellence). *Dual diagnosis: community-based services to meet people's wider health and social care needs when they have a severe mental illness and misuse substances.* London: NICE, 2014.
3. Bachrach LL. Young adult chronic patients: an analytical review of the literature. *Hospital and Community Psychiatry* 1982; **33**: 189–97.
4. Crome IB. An exploration of research into substance misuse and psychiatric disorder in the UK: what can we learn from history? *Criminal Behaviour and Mental Health* 2007; **17**: 204–14.
5. Smith GL, Morris P. Dual diagnosis: what does it mean? *Mental Health and Substance Use: Dual Diagnosis* 2010; **3**(2): 162–5.
6. Department of Health. *Mental Health Clustering Booklet (V3.0) 2013–2014.* London: Department of Health, 2013.
7. Mueser KT, Noordsy DL, Drake RE, Fox L. *Integrated treatment for dual disorders: a guide to effective practice.* New York: Guilford Press, 2003.
8. Phillips P, Johnson S. Explanatory models for dual diagnosis. In Phillips P, McKeown O, Sandford T (eds). *Dual diagnosis: practice in context.* Chichester: Wiley-Blackwell, 2010; 13–26.
9. Mental Health Network NHS Confederation. *Factsheet September 2011. Updated figures and statistics: key facts and trends in mental health.* London: NHS Confederation, 2011.
10. Crome L, Chambers P, Frisher M, Bloor R, Roberts D. *The relationship between dual diagnosis: substance misuse and dealing with mental health issues.* London: Social Care Institute for Excellence, 2009.
11. EMCDDA (European Monitoring Centre for Drugs and Drug Addiction). *European drug report 2015: trends and developments.* Lisbon: EMCDDA, 2015.
12. Department of Health. *Mental health policy implementation guide: dual diagnosis good practice guide.* London: Department of Health, 2002.
13. Edwards R. The development of dual diagnosis link workers in a mental health trust: reflections from clinical practice. *Advances in Dual Diagnosis* 2011; **4**(2): 75–83.
14. Progress – National Consortium of Consultant Nurses in Dual Diagnosis and Substance Use. *5 Boroughs Partnership NHS Dual Diagnosis (03/08/15; 28/09/15).* Available from: http://www.dualdiagnosis.co.uk/news/Progress100601.ink [Accessed 24th May 2016].
15. Progress – National Consortium of Consultant Nurses in Dual Diagnosis and Substance Use. *Manchester Dual Diagnosis Service (05/08/15; 28/09/15).* Available from: http://www.dualdiagnosis.co.uk/news/Progress100602.ink [Accessed 24th May 2016].
16. Cooper DB. Setting the scene. In: Cooper DB (ed.). *Mental health-substance use: intervention in mental health substance use.* London: Radcliffe, 2011: 1–7.
17. Osher FC, Kofoed LL. Treatment of patients with psychiatric and psychoactive substance abuse. *Hospital and Community Psychiatry* 1989; **4**(10): 1025–30.
18. Watkins D, McCormick F, Cuff R. Engaging the individual and family. In: Cooper DB (ed.). *Mental health-substance use: care in mental health substance use.* London: Radcliffe, 2011: 74–88.
19. Miller W, Rollnick S. *Motivational interviewing helping people change*, 3rd edn. New York: Guilford Press, 2013.
20. Hsu SH, Marlatt GA. Relapse prevention in substance use. In: Cooper DB (ed.). *Mental health-substance use: practice in mental health substance use.* London: Radcliffe, 2011: 203–17.
21. NICE (National Institute for Health and Care Excellence). *Psychosis with coexisting substance misuse: assessment and management in adults and young people.* London: NICE, 2011.
22. Cooper PD. The person who experiences mental health and substance use problems. In: Barker P (ed.). *Psychiatric and mental health nursing: the craft of caring*, 2nd edn. London: CRC Press, 2009: 252–61.
23. Kipping C. Communicating harm reduction. In: Cooper DB (ed.). *Mental health-substance use: responding in mental health substance use.* London: Radcliffe, 2011: 203–17.
24. NICE (National Institute for Health and Care Excellence). *Drug misuse – opioid detoxification. NICE guidelines [CG52].* London: NICE, 2007.
25. NICE (National Institute for Health and Care Excellence). *Alcohol-use disorders: diagnosis, assessment and management of harmful drinking and alcohol dependence. NICE guidelines [CG115].* London: NICE, 2011.
26. Saunders JB, Aasland OG, Babor TF, de la Fuente JR, Grant M. Development of the Alcohol Use Disorders Identification Test (AUDIT): WHO collaborative project on early detection of persons with harmful alcohol consumption. *Addiction* 1993; **88**: 791–804.
27. Stockwell T, Murphy D, Hodgson R. The severity of alcohol dependence questionnaire: its use, reliability and validity. *British Journal of Addiction* 1983; **78**(2): 145–55.
28. Sullivan JT, Sykora K, Schneiderman J, Naranjo CA, Sellers EM. Assessment of alcohol withdrawal: the revised Clinical Institute Withdrawal Assessment for Alcohol scale (CIWA-AR). *British Journal of Addiction* 1989; **84**: 1353–7.
29. Raistrick D, Bradshaw J, Tober G, Weiner J, Allison J, Healey C. Development of the Leeds Dependence Questionnaire (LDQ): a questionnaire to measure alcohol and opiate dependence in the context of a treatment evaluation package. *Addiction* 2006; **89**(5): 563–72.

30. Hesse M. The Readiness Ruler as a measure of readiness to change poly-drug use in drug abusers. *Harm Reduction Journal* 2006: 3.

31. Di Clemente CC, Schumann K, Greene PA, Earley DA. Transtheoretical Model perspective on change process-focussed intervention. In: Cooper DB (ed.). *Mental health-substance use: intervention in mental health substance use.* London: Radcliffe, 2011: 69–87.

32. Lock C, Kaner E, Heather N. Brief interventions: mental health-substance use. In: Cooper DB (ed.). *Mental health-substance use: intervention in mental health substance use.* London: Radcliffe, 2011: 102–13.

33. Hettena JE, Kirsch J. Motivational interviewing: mental health substance use. In: Cooper DB (ed.). *Mental health-substance use: intervention in mental health substance use.* London: Radcliffe, 2011: 88–101.

34. Glassman S, Kottsieper P, Zuckoff A, Gosch EA. Motivational interviewing and recovery: experiences of hope, meaning, and empowerment. *Advances in Dual Diagnosis* 2013; **6**(3): 106–20.

35. Tobin D. Cognitive Behavioural Integrated Treatment (C-BIT). In: Cooper DB (ed.). *Mental health-substance use: care in mental health substance use.* London: Radcliffe, 2011: 175–87.

36. Phillips P. Reducing drug related harm among mentally ill people. In: Phillips P, McKeown O, Sandford T (eds). *Dual diagnosis: practice in context.* Chichester: Wiley-Blackwell, 2010: 51–7.

37. Rosenblum A, Magura S, Laudet AB, Vogel H. *Mutual aid groups.* In: Cooper DB (ed.). *Mental health-substance use: intervention in mental health substance use.* London: Radcliffe, 2011: 207–24.

38. Drake RE, Wallach MA, McGovern MP. Future directions in preventing relapse to substance abuse among clients with severe mental illnesses. *Psychiatric Services* 2005; **56**(10): 1297–302.

Further reading

Barrowclough C, Haddock G, Wykes T, Beardmore R, Conrod P, Craig T, Davies L, Dunn G, Eisner E, Lewis S, Moring J, Steel C, Tarrier N. Integrated motivational interviewing and cognitive behavioural therapy for people with psychosis and comorbid substance misuse. *British Medical Journal* 2010; **341**: c6325.

Cooper DB. *Mental health-substance use: care in mental health-substance use.* London: Radcliffe Publishing, 2011.

Cooper DB. *Mental health-substance use: developing services in mental health-substance use.* London: Radcliffe Publishing, 2011.

Cooper DB. *Mental health-substance use: intervention in mental health-substance use.* London: Radcliffe Publishing, 2011.

Cooper DB. *Mental health-substance use: introduction to mental health-substance use.* London: Radcliffe Publishing, 2010.

Cooper DB. *Mental health-substance use: practice in mental health-substance use.* London: Radcliffe Publishing, 2011.

Cooper DB. *Mental health-substance use: responding in mental health-substance use.* London: Radcliffe Publishing, 2011.

Montanari L, Pasinetti M, Thanki D, Vicente J. Co-morbid substance use and mental disorders in Europe: a review of the data. European Monitoring Centre for Drugs and Drug Addiction, 2015. Available from: http://www.emcdda.europa.eu/attachements.cfm/att_220660_EN_TDAU13002ENN.pdf [Accessed 24th May 2016].

Phillips P, McKeown O, Sandford T (eds). *Dual diagnosis: practice in context.* Chichester: Wiley-Blackwell, 2010.

Relevant web pages

Dual Diagnosis. www.dualdiagnosis.org [Accessed 9th January 2017]

Dual Diagnosis Website. http://users.erols.com/ksciacca/

Home Office (2016) Psychoactive Substance Act (UK). Home Office London. https://www.gov.uk/government/collections/psychoactive-substances-bill-2015 [Accessed 9th January 2017]

MIND (UK) www.mind.org.uk

National Consortium of Consultant Nurses in Dual Diagnosis and Substance Abuse. www.dualdiagnosis.co.uk [Accessed 9th January 2017]

32 Sexuality and gender

AGNES HIGGINS AND LIZ BROSNAN

LEARNING OUTCOMES

- To be aware of the complexities that surround the language used to describe people's gender identity and sexual orientation.

- To understand how gender impacts on people's expression of mental distress and on the care they receive within mental health services.

- To be aware of the impact of lesbian, gay, bisexual, transgender and intersex (LGBTI) identities on mental health.

- To be able to respond to people's sexuality and gender in an informed and sensitive manner.

KEY POINTS

- Sexuality is a core dimension of humanness and encompasses gender identity and sexual orientation, among other elements.

- The history of sexuality and people's experience of mental health problems has largely been a history of misunderstanding, misconception, stigma and myth.

- Gender has a significant impact on the way mental distress is experienced and understood by the person.

- Mental health policies and services are gender-blind, perpetuating gender stereotypes and health disparities between men and women.

- Mental health practitioners' professional thinking continues to be influenced by gender biases and stereotypes which impact negatively on health outcomes and slow people's journey toward recovery.

- Exploring people's concerns around sexuality, identifying specific problems and meeting information and support needs form a core dimension of high quality recovery-oriented service, and are central to the craft of caring.

- Mental health practitioners need to develop gender-sensitive and LGBT-affirmative approaches to care that take the unique needs of each individual into consideration.

INTRODUCTION

Mental health practitioners working within a recovery ethos will recognize the importance of creating a space that acknowledges the centrality of the person's life story and their identity in any healing relationship. Central to the craft of caring is a recognition of the importance of the person's story.[1] An integral part of that story is the person's experiences and expression of sexuality, gender identity and sexual orientation. Indeed, gender is a critical determinant of mental health, as it impacts on women and men's socio-economic positions, roles and status, as well as their ability and willingness to access resources and supports. When men and women enter the mental health system, gender also impacts on the way practitioners interpret and respond to their mental distress. Similarly, sexual orientation and the expression of one's sexual orientation is a core aspect of sexuality, and a part of one's existence that can be life-affirming by promoting intimacy, pleasure, self-esteem and human connection. Paradoxically, it can also be a source of personal pain and distress.

This chapter explores some of the issues that surround sexuality, gender and sexual orientation, with a view to enabling mental health nurses to respond to people's expressions of sexuality in a more informed and sensitive manner. Before we discuss some of our thoughts around sexuality, gender and mental health, we would like to position ourselves, the authors, in the context of the topic under discussion. Firstly, we are both women who have been shaped in very different ways by a heteronormative society that privileges heterosexual relationships and views same-sex relationships as less valid; consequently, our experiences of living and expressing our sexuality are remarkably different. One of us gives expression to their sexuality through a long-standing heterosexual relationship that is empowering, nurturing and loving. The other author expresses fluid sexuality and gender in a rejecting or exploitative heteronormative society which has resulted in silencing, rejection, abuse and pain. This had mental health consequences, resulting in 13 years of service use. Throughout that period no attempt was ever made by mental health professionals to discuss or address significant childhood abuse or sexual orientation. The healing and resolution only occurred once a break with mental health services was achieved. Secondly, as we are both women, we cannot speak of men's sexualities except as 'outsiders' of their experiences or as 'insiders' from the perspective of women who have been in relationship with men. It is the combination of these two lives that form the backdrop to some of the issues discussed in this chapter. It is beyond the scope of this chapter to discuss every issue; therefore, emphasis is placed on gender and sexual orientation. In writing this we were also conscious of the need to avoid reinforcing the very real disparities of power and expectations around disclosure that collaboration between 'service-user and professional' frequently entails. In particular we were mindful of the identity management work required of user-practitioners/academics, rarely demanded of other professionals who conceal their own vulnerabilities. In addition, control over one's own story and how it can be appropriated by others is an area of growing debate, albeit beyond the remit of this chapter.[2,3]

AN EXPLORATION OF CONCEPTS AND LANGUAGE: SHIFTING LANDSCAPES

> ### REFLECTION
>
> - What do you understand by the following terms: sex, gender, sexual orientation and sexuality?
> - What are your beliefs about male and female gender roles?
> - How did you come to acquire those beliefs?

Before we consider the complex interface between sexuality, gender, sexual orientation and mental health, there is a need to examine some key concepts and binary categories that are frequently taken for granted. The term 'sex' has two general meanings. Firstly, it is used to describe the physical 'sexual act'. Secondly, it is used to identify a person's designation at birth as male or female based on their anatomy (genitalia/reproductive organs) or biology (sex chromosomes and/or hormones).[4] The short biblical statement 'Male and Female, He created them' (Genesis 5:2) exemplifies the normative binary division that is reinforced by traditional biological science wherein XX chromosomes denotes 'female' and XY chromosome pairing 'male'. When XX and XY chromosome pairings come together, the resulting offspring is most likely XX or XY, a baby with visible 'male' or 'female' genital features. However, a review of the literature challenges the simplicity of the biologically determined male and female binary, as we now know that at least 2 per cent of the population are intersex. Intersex means the person is born with a reproductive or sexual anatomy that falls outside the accepted norms of male or female.[5] An intersex person may be born with ambiguous genitalia, or have elements of both male and female anatomy, or have anatomical features and/or different hormonal levels that are inconsistent with chromosomal sex. These conditions may be identified at birth (in cases where genitalia are obviously ambiguous), at puberty (when a person fails to develop secondary sex characteristics or develops characteristics that are not expected), in adulthood (when fertility difficulties present) or upon autopsy. Using the examples of intersex conditions and the ability to surgically change one's sex, Hird[6] (p.137) challenges the essentialist interpretation of the term 'sex', arguing that 'if it is possible to become a "sex", then surely there can be no such thing as a natural "sex"' – thus concluding that the term 'sex' is a social construction.

Based on the assumption of the existence of only two mutually exclusive sex typologies (male and female), the presence (or absence) of sexual organs also provides a convenient means of classification for assigning one to a certain gender (masculine, feminine). The term 'gender' refers to the socially constructed roles, behaviours, activities and attributes that a given society considers appropriate for men and women and, as an extension, denotes the social ordering of relations between men and women.[7] While masculine and feminine ideologies can vary and change over time, normative masculinity positions men as self-reliant, tough, competitive, emotionally in control if not emotionally inexpressive, and dominant. By contrast, western feminine ideologies view women as emotional, caring, compassionate, and more passive and maternal than men.[8] Today, writers also challenge essentialist interpretations of gender and some argue for the decoupling of gender from biological sex (male, female). For example, Butler[9] argues that it is repetitive norms and practices that produce and stabilize sex and gender, and, as such, gender is not a fixed attribute of a person. She states that 'when the constructed status of gender is theorized as radically independent of sex, gender itself becomes a free-floating artifice, with the consequence that man and masculine might just as easily signify a female body as a male one, and woman and feminine a male body as easily as a female one'[9] (p.137). Today, the alignment of gender exclusively to the physical body and the person's genitals is also challenged by people whose gender identity and/or gender expression differs from the sex assigned to them at birth. Transgenderism is an inclusive term for many gender identities that crosses socially constructed gender norms, and is inclusive of transsexualism (people whose gender identity is opposite to the sex assigned to them at birth); cross-dressers or transvestites (people who wear clothing, accessories or make-up not stereotypically associated with their assigned gender); and androgynous (people whose gender identity is both female and male, or neither female or male) or other differently gendered people.[10]

The term 'sexual orientation' refers to a person's physical, emotional or romantic attraction to another person. Sexual orientation should be viewed on a spectrum or continuum rather than as a dichotomy, as people can be attracted to the opposite sex (heterosexual), the same sex (lesbian or gay), both sexes (bisexual) or neither. However, working from the premise that there are just two sexes and that sexual attraction to the opposite sex (heterosexual) is the norm and an indisputable fact of nature, a heteronormative world view dominates.[11] Heteronormativity holds that people fall into distinct and complementary genders (men and women), with a natural alignment between biological sex, gender identity and gender roles in life. Thus a heteronormative view organizes all patterns of thought, all relations, and all social institutions around a heterosexual model of male/female social relations and through a lens of heterosexuality.[12] A heteronormative social climate is damaging and alienating for those who do not conform, as it marginalizes, silences and denies different experiences. It can also leave people, especially vulnerable children and young people, exposed to homophobic and transphobic bullying and violence.

The term 'sexuality', although sometimes used to refer to sexual activity, is a much more encompassing term, and refers to a set of ideas, meanings and social practices which surround sexual activity.[4,13] Sexuality is a highly individualized and personal concept that is unique to each person; consequently, it cannot be easily defined or categorized. The most frequently used definition of sexuality within the health care literature is the World Health Organization (WHO)[14] definition, which suggests that sexuality is:

> *a central aspect of being human throughout life and encompasses sex, gender identities and roles, sexual orientation, eroticism, pleasure, intimacy and reproduction. Sexuality is experienced and expressed in thoughts, fantasies, desires, beliefs, attitudes, values, behaviours, practices, roles and relationships. While sexuality can include all of these dimensions, not all of them are always experienced or expressed. Sexuality is influenced by the interaction of biological, psychological, social, economic, political, cultural, legal, historical, religious and spiritual factors.*[14] *(p.5)*

This definition not only highlights the all-encompassing and dynamic nature of sexuality, but emphasizes the social, cultural, political, legal, moral, spiritual and psychological issues and variations that influence our understanding of sexuality. Indeed, the study of sexuality (and gender) is a meeting point (and veritable battleground of ideas) for many different disciplines and approaches. While they debate the extent to which biology and biological determinism shade social construction, they all share a consensus 'that desire and sexual practice are the variable products of culture; that sexual identity is unstable and surprising … and that gender inequality remains a challenge'[13] (p.vii).

GENDER AND MENTAL HEALTH

REFLECTION

- How does the differing position and status of men and women impact on their mental health?

- How does gender (both your own and the other person's) impact on how you interpret and respond to people's distress?

This section considers the complex issues of gender and mental health. According to the WHO report on mental health at the international level: 'Gender runs like a fault line, interconnecting with and deepening the disparities associated with other important socio-economic determinants such as income, employment and social position'[15] (p.2). In other words, gender difference has significant explanatory power for why men and women experience different mental health issues and how they are treated differently both within and outside mental health services.

Gender and gender role enforcement

Throughout history, women's mental health has been subjected to a more pathologizing discourse than men's, perpetuated by a belief that women are irrational, mentally weak and the more vulnerable sex.[8,16,17] Over the years, a number of feminists have critiqued psychiatric care in relation to the care and treatment of women and have shone a light on the link between mental health services and gender role enforcement (See chapter 65 for more information on services for women).[8,18,19] These writers argue that, within a patriarchal society, women who rejected socially constructed gender norms and revolted against the traditional modernist view of femininity were at greater risk of being labelled as mentally ill. Indeed, the classic 1970 study by Broverman et al.[20] illustrated how dominant notions of masculinity and femininity were internalized by mental health professionals and formed part of their diagnostic framework. Other more recent researchers have highlighted how women who demonstrated behaviours that were inconsistent with feminine sex-role stereotype[21] or demonstrated behaviours that was considered to have 'left-leaning tendencies'[22] (p.214) were also deemed pathological. Crabtree's[23] ethnographic study in Malaysia also found that suspicion of sexual promiscuity in women commonly led to forced admission to psychiatric hospital, as sexual promiscuity in women was seen as a revealing sign of mental illness. Issues of gender are also reflected in international debates on the need to develop both health policy and services that are gender-sensitive and responsive to the specific needs of men and women.[24–27] Cutting's[28] argument that 'women's expression of distress is very different from men's', and as a consequence 'their presentation, patterns of onset, causal reasons … outcome/prognosis, responses to treatment, and the consequences of their distress are all specific to them' (p.11) can just as easily be reversed and applied to men's experiences of distress.

Gender, causation and mental distress

Evidence indicates that the impact of gender is compounded by its interrelationship with social, structural and economic determinants of health, such as income, education, housing and employment. Many of the negative experiences that expose women to mental health issues arise from their unequal position and status within society, which has led to subjugation, discrimination and violations of their rights, including sexual and reproductive rights.[29,30] In addition, socially determined roles and responsibilities place women, far more frequently than men, in situations where they have very little control over important decisions concerning their lives. Women in paid work receive significantly lower wages than their male counterparts and are more likely to occupy lower-status jobs, work part-time or work in poorly regulated sectors, such as the service industry. In addition, women tend to be more involved in caring roles (for children and ageing parents), as well as carrying the burden of housework, which limits their employment and educational opportunities, with consequent risk of poverty. Indeed, women constitute 70 per cent of the world's poor, and lone mothers with children are the largest group of people living in poverty.[15,29] Poverty is also a contributing factor to homelessness, leading women to become financially dependent and more likely to remain in abusive or violent relationships. The severity and duration of exposure to violence is also highly predictive of mental health problems.[31] Men report other forms of adverse events, such as workplace violence and serious financial issues, with the loss of paid work due to unemployment having particular negative effects on men's masculinity and mental health.[32]

Gender and diagnosis

Today, men and women are understood to be affected by mental health problems in equal proportion, but their experiences of problems (and, as a consequence, the types of diagnoses they receive) are different. Women are more likely to be diagnosed with panic disorder, generalized anxiety disorder, obsessive–compulsive disorder and post-traumatic stress disorder. They are also more likely to engage in self-harm behaviours. In addition, women receive a diagnosis of depression at twice the rate of men, with anorexia, bulimia and personality disorder being overwhelmingly diagnosed in young women.[32,33] Other diagnoses are specific to women – for example, post-partum psychosis and post-natal depression; the linking of mental health problems to the emotional elements of menstruation and menopause are, however, highly contentious.[8] Because women tend to live longer than men, prevalence rates for dementia and depression are also higher among older women. On the other hand, men are twice as likely to be affected by substance misuse (alcohol and drugs), with a lifetime prevalence rate of 20 per cent compared to 8 per cent for women.[33] Men are more likely to be diagnosed with antisocial personality disorder, to receive a diagnosis of sexual addiction and to die by suicide.[32] Although some diagnoses (schizophrenia and bipolar disorder) are not gendered, schizophrenia is diagnosed 5 years earlier in young men than women, with some studies reporting that women experience a higher frequency of hallucinations than men.[29] Similarly, while there is no difference in the rates of diagnosis between men and women for bipolar disorder, women are reported to develop more rapid cycling forms of the 'illness' and are more likely to be hospitalized during the manic phase.[30]

While the above research suggests a gender difference in some diagnoses, the current gender diversification of mental illnesses is not static and changes in social dynamics could see different gendered expressions as time moves on. For example, Busfield[8] suggests that, given moves towards greater equality for women within the workplace and the family setting, gender role confusion might increase among men, with a resultant susceptibility towards depression. Rates of eating disorders are also increasing among young men, with an increase in prevalence reported among gay and bisexual men in comparison to heterosexual men.[34] Likewise, increasing alcohol and drug use by women (relative to past norms) may also result in higher rates of female dependency in the future.[32]

Gendered nature of emotional expression and help-seeking

Gender differences are not only present in the determinants of mental distress and type of diagnosis men and women receive, but are also evident in emotional expression and patterns of help-seeking. Busfield[8] points out that it is generally considered acceptable for women to talk about their feelings, and as a consequence it is not surprising that women are more likely to seek help from their primary care physician. On the other hand, social norms of traditional masculinity, which discourage men from displaying or discussing emotions, make help-seeking more difficult; consequently, they are often seriously distressed before they access professional services.[35,36] Having said this, it is important not to stereotype either gender, as all help-seeking behaviour involves an ongoing dialogue between the person's individual circumstances and the benefits and risks of seeking help. While a number of barriers to help-seeking are common to both men and women, such as fear of stigma, being labelled and being prescribed medication, others are unique to context. For example, women who are mothers report fear of losing custody of their children as a barrier to help-seeking,[37,38] and gay men report a reluctance to seek help for fear of their sexual orientation being pathologized.[39,40]

Gendered nature of treatment

Studies also reveal gender difference in the type of treatment and care offered to men and women. Busfield[8] argues that because gender biases and stereotyping permeate professional thinking, it is not surprising to see gender difference in the type of treatment offered. Once women seek help from their primary physician, in comparison to their male counterparts, they are more likely to leave the practitioner with a prescription for medication and are less likely to be referred to a speciality mental health service. Thus, it is estimated that women throughout Europe and North America are prescribed twice as many psychotropic drugs as men.[33] This statistic suggests that the focus is on treating women's symptoms, as opposed to the root cause of the problem.

There is a risk that our emphasis on women and mental health may gloss over the circumstances that make some men particularly vulnerable to coercive psychiatric treatment. Men are more likely to be admitted to a mental hospital, detained in high security units and detained 'involuntarily' under the Mental Health Act. Race is another factor which interacts with gender positions to make some men – for example, black men – more likely to be diagnosed and treated coercively by mental health services. These rates of admissions might be related to society's gendered perceptions of men, and particularly black men, as being more dangerous and in need of control.[17]

SEXUAL DIVERSITY: LESBIAN, GAY, BISEXUAL AND TRANSGENDER ISSUES

For the vast majority of people, their sexuality, sexual identity and sexual orientation are an integral part of their identity that can be celebrated, demonstrated and spoken about in an open manner. However, in a world where heteronormativity prevails, the sexual identity of people with an LGBT (lesbian, gay, bisexual and transgender) identity continues to be constructed as 'other'.[11] While many LGBT people develop positive coping strategies to deal with the many forms of prejudice and discrimination rooted within the heterosexist structures of society, others are not so fortunate and experience significant mental health issues compared to their heterosexual counterparts. This is not to suggest that LGBT people are in any way more prone to mental distress, but it recognizes that the stress of living as a member of an oppressed minority group can result in what is commonly referred to as 'minority stress'.[41] The minority stress model suggests that psychological distress is an outcome of both enacted and felt stigma. In other words,

REFLECTION

John is 54 years of age, married since he was 24 years of age, with three grown-up children. He says his wife is a wonderful woman and mother, and he loves her deeply but he is not sexually attracted to her. He is questioning his sexual orientation and thinks he may be gay, saying that women never really excited him. He has tried to put the thought out of his mind for years, but as he gets older it is getting increasingly difficult to ignore these thoughts. On a few occasions, he has visited a gay club when he was travelling with work, but has never had a sexual encounter with another man. In the past 3 years, he has tried to take his own life on two occasions, and he says "life is such a mess and full of turmoil he cannot go on". How might you respond to his distress and concerns? How might the multidisciplinary team assist you in responding to his distress and concerns?

the stigmatization, prejudice, harassment and discrimination associated with being from a minority group creates a hostile and stressful social environment. This environment, compounded by the internalization of society's negative attitudes and sexual identity concealment (or 'staying in the closet'), increases the rates of psychological distress.

There is now a large, international, empirical body of evidence indicating higher rates of depression, anxiety, self-harm and overall psychological distress among the LGBT population, with high rates of suicide attempts among GB men and transgender men and women.[42–46] In addition, research on health-related behaviours has shown elevated levels of smoking, alcohol consumption and recreational drug use, with some suggestions that the use of alcohol and drugs is a means of coping with the stigma and prejudice.[47,48] Many international studies also report on the hate crimes and violence perpetrated against the community, with research highlighting the more intense reactions towards transgendered men and women due to transphobia.[49,50] Although many LGBT people will present to mental health services with distress that is peripheral or unrelated to their sexual orientation or gender identity, there are a range of LGBT-specific stressors that can impact on mental health, and practitioners should be aware of these. Box 32.1 provides examples of LGBT-specific stressors.

LGBT people are diverse and varied and experience similar fears to the heterosexual population around accessing and utilizing mental health services, including the stigma that surrounds mental 'illness'; the fear of being labelled, medicated or having a mental health problem entered into their medical records; not liking to talk about personal life; hearing about bad experiences from others; and the cost of therapy. In addition, LGBT people report a deep

distrust of the mental health service and identify a number of barriers to receiving LGBT-affirmative care (Box 32.2). LGBT people's fears and anxieties are not surprising, as psychiatry has a long history of pathologizing people whose sexual behaviours or identities do not conform to

BOX 32.1: LGBT-SPECIFIC STRESSORS THAT CAN AND DO IMPACT ON MENTAL HEALTH

- Difficulty accepting LGBT identity.
- Fear of 'coming out' or telling others they are LGBT or being unable/not wanting to come out for fear of rejection from family, friends and other loved ones.
- Experience of rejection by family and friends when LGBT identity is revealed.
- Homophobic bullying, harassment or violence in school, work or other environments.
- Exposure to negative messages about being LGBT, including stigmatization, prejudice and stereotyping.
- Disenfranchised or unacknowledged grief following death or relationship break-up of partner.
- Hiding and concealment of sexual orientation; for example, an LGB person who is in a heterosexual marriage/relationship or a transgender person who hides their preferred gender.

BOX 32.2: BARRIERS TO ACCESSING MENTAL HEALTH SERVICES

- Practitioners' assumption that all people using services are heterosexual.
- Practitioners' use of heterosexist language that adds to people's feeling of isolation.
- Practitioners using inappropriate language when discussing a transgender client's gender.
- Practitioners' hesitancy to enquire about sexuality and sexual orientation.
- Practitioners' lack of understanding of LGBT health issues.
- Practitioners pathologizing people's LGBT identities or assuming all mental health problems relate to the person's LGBT identity.
- Insensitivity, prejudice and discrimination from other people who use services, in the form of homophobia, biphobia, transphobia and heterosexism.[39,40,51]

traditional heterosexual norms or identities. Indeed, these sexual identity groups have been (and remain) subjected to numerous harmful treatments in the guise of 'cures' and have been the recipients of official and unofficial eugenic policies because their experiences and identities lie outside mainstream norms.[11]

RESPONDING TO PEOPLE'S SEXUALITY AND GENDER IN AN INFORMED AND SENSITIVE MANNER

Developing a gender-sensitive mental health service

> **REFLECTION**
>
> - What causes men and women to have different experiences of mental health services?
> - To what extent do you consider the service you work in to be gender-sensitive?

Mental health practice can perpetuate, exacerbate or challenge inequalities between men and women. However, internationally, the vast majority of mental health policies and services are still very much gender-blind, thus perpetuating gender stereotypes and health disparities between men and women, impacting negatively on health outcomes and slowing people's journey towards recovery. Internationally, there is a call for all mental health services to adopt a gender-sensitive approach to service planning and delivery.[24,25] A gender-sensitive approach takes the unique needs of both men and women into consideration in the care planning process, and is consistent with the values and practices underpinning the craft of caring.[1] Central to the craft of caring is the development of a collaborative relationship (see chapter 3 on developing and maintaining therapeutic relationships and chapter 50 on collaborative care planning with service users and carers). Box 32.3 provides some examples of gender-sensitive practices that you may wish to consider.

Creating a safe context for disclosure and discussion

> **REFLECTION**
>
> - What it is about your practice, the team or the environment you work in that may communicate to service users that it is safe to disclose their sexuality and past traumas?
> - What it is about your practice, the team or the environment you work in that may communicate to service users that it is unsafe to disclose their sexuality and past traumas?

The development of a safe and supportive environment is core to mental health nursing and the craft of caring,[1] and central to any discussion on sexuality. Research on

> **BOX 32.3: GENDER-SENSITIVE PRACTICES**
>
> - Services have policies that acknowledge the different needs of men and women in the cause and experience of mental distress.
> - Services provide education to staff on gender issues and gender-sensitive care.
> - Practitioners interrogate their own gender stereotypes and have confidence to challenge gender stereotyping within the team that is exploitative or harmful.
> - Practitioners consider how gender roles may impact on the person's mental health and their understanding of their distress.
> - Care and treatment models address the realities of the differences between women and men and use gender-disaggregated data (data showing difference between men and women) in planning services.
> - Practitioners review research evidence when planning care and treatment approaches to consider if findings are equally applicable to men and women. For example, does the evidence consider how gender impacts on metabolism of prescribed medication or does evidence support gender-specific group programmes for people who have experienced sexual trauma?
> - Practitioners create a therapeutic context that promotes shared power, control and decision making between men and women.
> - Practitioners respect people's requests to have a person of the same gender looking after them or not to stay within mixed-sex accommodation.[52,53]

sexuality within the mental health context is sparse, highlighting a distinct lack of knowledge and provision of care in this area. What research is available clearly indicates that, for people who experience mental distress, the expression of sexuality continues to be an important part of their lives.[54–57] However, researchers continually highlight how infrequently mental health professionals offer people an opportunity to discuss the sexual and relationship aspect of their lives[58,59] or enquire about past sexual history, including history of sexual violence.[60] Yet this is what service users consistently report they want from their health care practitioners.[61,62]

A second hallmark of professional caring is the establishment of a close, confiding relationship[l] and, as mental health nurses, it is important to create safe spaces for people to discuss issues of sexuality, including both positive and negative sexual experiences. People who use the mental health service may fear disclosing their mental health issue to new partners for fear of rejection, or have anxiety around initiating intimate relationships or negotiating safe sexual boundaries or practices. Service users may also have concerns about sexual side effects of psychotropic medication or the safety of taking medication during pregnancy or the postnatal period.[57,63,64] Further information on psychopharmacology can be found in chapters 47 and 48. In addition, research suggests that both women and men with a diagnosis of mental health problems report higher rates of sexual coercion, sexual exploitation and sexual abuse compared to those without a diagnosis, and require sensitive support if healing is to commence.[65,66]

Exploring people's concerns around sexuality, identifying specific problems and meeting information and support needs is not the prerogative of any one discipline, but an important dimension of holistic care provided by the multidisciplinary team. While there are a number of frameworks provided within the literature for assessment and intervention,[67] there is no easy formula (see chapters 13, 14 and 15 for more general information on assessment). Engaging in a conversation on issues of love, intimacy, desire, sexual needs, sexual orientation and sexual trauma requires practitioners to have skills in listening, empathy, presence and emotional connection. However, central to listening and bearing witness is the ability to create a safe space for the person's story to emerge; the therapeutic and emancipating value of talking frankly about feelings and experiences

should not be underestimated. While including issues of sexuality within the horizons of practice requires a proactive approach, it must be remembered that people choose whether they are comfortable with discussing and disclosing sexuality issues. If people do not wish to talk, not only is that their choice, which must be respected and honoured, but there is a need to reflect on the possibility that there may be something within the situation/environment that makes the person feel unsafe or vulnerable. Practitioners need to be consciously alert to the inherent power differential within relationships and fine-tune their self-reflective practice so that they are consciously aware of how gender roles and heteronormativity may influence interactions and interpretations.[68] Chapter 11 addresses issues of critical reflection.

Developing LGBT-affirmative practices

REFLECTION

Before reading the next section, take a few minutes to reflect on the following scenarios.

- Susan, a female service user, comes to complain that another service user (Kate), who is a lesbian female, is using the female bathroom. She states she is uncomfortable having to share the bathroom with a lesbian. How would you deal with this conflict?

- Joshua, a transgender man, tells you that one of your colleagues continues to call him by his female name and refers to him as 'her', even though he has requested that he be called by his correct name and gender. How would you respond?

BOX 32.4: LGBT-AFFIRMATIVE PRACTICES

- Service policies make a clear statement of inclusiveness of LGBT people and services display signs highlighting a policy of inclusive practice.
- Documentation and assessment forms use language which is inclusive of LGBT people and their families.
- Mental health information includes reference to LGBT people, for example, reference to questioning sexual orientation, fear of coming out and homophobic bullying, disenfranchised grief and gender transitioning.
- Information leaflets include information on local LGBT services, LGBT helpline numbers or other specific LGBT supports.
- Practitioners are informed and educated on LGBT issues, including gender and sexual identity

development, 'coming out' issues and gender transition.
- Practitioners ask inclusive questions when talking to a person and do not assume people are heterosexual (for example, 'Do you have a partner?' rather than 'Are you married?').
- Practitioners are aware of the debates around language and ask the person which term they prefer to use.
- Practitioners reassure people that all personal information disclosed is confidential.
- Practitioners respond sensitively and supportively when people disclose their LGBT identity.
- Practitioners do not assume that young people are only going through a phase or are too young to be aware of or declare a sexual orientation or gender identity.[69,70]

Professional anti-gay bias and the invisibility of LGBT identities within health care frequently result in LGBT people receiving sub-optimal care and experiencing direct or indirect discrimination when they use health services. Within the context of developing LGBT-affirmative nursing practice, nurses need to take an LGBT-affirmative approach and challenge anti-LGBT bias, both within themselves and within their service. They also need to be mindful that any person who comes to the service may identify as an LGBT person. Box 32.4 provides some examples of LGBT-affirmative practices that help to indicate to LGBT people that they are welcome within the service, that they are not at risk of discrimination should they disclose their sexual orientation or gender identity, and that they are welcome to discuss issues related to being an LGBT person.

CONCLUSION

The history of sexuality and people with mental health problems has largely been a history of misunderstanding, misconception, stigma and myth, with mental health services incorporating traditional gender stereotypes into their diagnostic frameworks and practices, and taking on a control and regulator function in relation to sexual behaviour.[11] At a time when people's rights are increasingly being emphasized, evidence suggests that within today's services the gender and sexual dimension of people's lives are being ignored or minimized. Holistic, recovery-oriented care, which is the core of mental health nursing and the craft of caring,[1] is predicated on the value of personhood and the uniqueness of each individual. Central to this is the need to develop gender transformative policies and practices that challenge existing inequalities between men and women; recognize the different experiences and needs of men and women; address issues of sexual orientation, gender preference and sexual trauma in a sensitive and evidence-based manner; and develop strategies to support the rights of each man or woman as a sexual citizen.

References

1. Barker P. *Psychiatric and mental health nursing: the craft of caring*, 2nd edn. London: Hodder Arnold, 2009.
2. Costa L, Voronka J, Landry D, Reid J, Mcfarlane B, Reville D, et al. "Recovering our stories": a small act of resistance. *Studies in Social Justice*. 2012; **6**(1): 85–101.
3. Russo J, Beresford P. Between exclusion and colonisation: seeking a place for mad people's knowledge in academia. *Disability & Society* 2015; **30**(1): 153–7.
4. Mauthner M. Understanding sexuality. In: Madoc-Jones B, Coates, J (eds). *An introduction to women's studies*. Oxford: Blackwell Publishers, 1996: 132–55.
5. Blackless M, Charuvastra A, Derryck A, Fausto-Sterling A, Lauzanne K, Lee E. How sexually dimorphic are we? Review and synthesis. *American Journal of Human Biology* 2000; **12**(2): 151–66.
6. Hird MJ. *Sex, gender, and science*. New York: Palgrave Macmillan, 2004.
7. Jackson S, Scott S. *Gender: a sociological reader*. London and New York: Routledge, 2002.
8. Busfield J. *Men, women and madness: understanding gender and mental disorder*. London: Macmillan, 1996.
9. Butler J. Feminism and the subversion of identity. In: Butler J. *Gender trouble*. London and New York: Routledge, 1990: 1–25.
10. APA (American Psychological Association). *Report of the APA Task Force on Gender Identity and Gender Variance*. Washington, DC: APA, 2009.
11. Higgins A. Sexuality and gender. In: Barker P (ed.). *Psychiatric and mental health nursing: the craft of caring*. London: Hodder Arnold, 2009: 618–25.
12. Bloodsworth-Lugo M. Heteronormativity. In Eadie J (ed.). *Sexuality: the essential glossary*. London: Arnold, 2004: 84–95.
13. Eadie J. *Sexuality: the essential glossary*. London: Arnold, 2004.
14. WHO (World Health Organization). *Defining sexual health: report of a technical consultation on sexual health, 28–31 January 2002*. Geneva: WHO, 2006. Available from: http://www.who.int/reproductivehealth/topics/gender_rights/defining_sexual_health.pdf [Accessed 5th September 2016].
15. WHO (World Health Organization). *Gender disparities in mental health*. Geneva: WHO, Dependence DoMHaS, 2001. Available from: http://www.who.int/mental_health/media/en/242.pdf [Accessed 5th September 2016].
16. Appignanesi L. *Mad, bad and sad: a history of women and the mind doctors from 1800*. London: Hachette, 2011.
17. Prior PM. *Gender and mental health*. Basingstoke and London: Macmillan Press, 1999.
18. Showalter E. *The female malady: women, madness and English culture 1830–1980*. London: Virago, 1985.
19. Chesler P. *Women and madness: revised and updated for the first time in thirty years*, 2nd edn. New York: Palgrave Macmillan, 2005.
20. Broverman IK, Broverman DM, Clarkson FE, Rosenkrantz PS, Vogel SR. Sex-role stereotypes and clinical judgments of mental health. *Journal of Consulting and Clinical Psychology* 1970; **34**(1): 1–7.
21. Crosby J, Sprock J. Effects of patient sex, clinician sex, and sex role on the diagnosis of antisocial personality disorder: models of unpathologizing and overpathologizing biases. *Journal of Clinical Psychology* 2004; **60**(6): 583–604.
22. Read J, Beavan V. Gender and psychosis. In: Read J, Dillon J (eds). *Models of madness: psychological social and biological approaches to psychosis*, 2nd edn. London and New York: Routledge, 2013: 210–19.
23. Crabtree SA. Strategies of social and sexual control of Malaysian women in psychiatric institutional care. *Health Care for Women International* 2004; **25**(6): 581–95.
24. Payne S. How can gender equity be addressed through health systems? Joint Policy Brief 12. Copenhagen: WHO Regional Office for Europe, 2009. Available from: http://www.euro.who.int/__data/assets/pdf_file/0006/64941/E92846.pdf [Accessed 8th September 2016].
25. Bergin M, Wells JS, Owen S. Towards a gendered perspective for Irish mental health policy and service provision. *Journal of Mental Health* 2013; **22**(4): 350–60.
26. Women's Health Council. A guide to creating gender-sensitive health service. Ireland: Women's Health Council Ireland, 2007. Available from: http://health.gov.ie/wp-content/uploads/2014/03/gender_manual.pdf [Accessed 8th September 2016].

27. Australian Women's Health Network. Women and mental health. 2012. Available http://awhn.org.au/wp-content/uploads/2015/03/100_AWHNWomenMentalHealthPositionPaper2012.pdf [Accessed 8th September 2016].

28. Cutting P. The problem with psychiatry – a woman's perspective. In: Henderson C, Smith C, Smith S, Stevens A (eds). *Women and psychiatric treatment: a comprehensive text and practical guide.* London: Routledge, 2013: 9–21.

29. WHO (World Health Organization). Women's mental health: an evidence based review. 2000. Available from: http://whqlibdoc.who.int/hq/2000/WHO_MSD_MDP_00.1.pdf?ua=1 [Accessed 5th September 2016].

30. WHO (World Health Organization). *Gender and mental health.* Geneva: WHO, Health DoGaWs, 2002. Available from: http://www.who.int/gender/documents/mental_health/a85573/en/ [Accessed 5th September 2016].

31. Afifi M. Gender differences in mental health. *Singapore Medical Journal* 2007; **48**(5): 385–91.

32. Wilkins D, Payne S, Granville G, Branney P. *The gender and access to health services study: final report.* Department of Health (UK), Men's Health Forum and Univeristy of Bristol: 2008.

33. Rogers A, Pilgrim D. A sociological view of mental health and illness. In: Gask L, Lester H, Kendrick T, Peveler R (eds). *Primary care mental health.* London: Royal College of Psychiatrists, 2009: 40–56.

34. Feldman MB, Meyer IH. Eating disorders in diverse lesbian, gay, and bisexual populations. *International Journal of Eating Disorders* 2007; **40**(3): 218–26.

35. Addis ME, Mahalik JR. Men, masculinity, and the contexts of help seeking. *American Psychologist* 2003; **58**(1): 5 –15.

36. Möller-Leimkühler AM. Barriers to help-seeking by men: a review of sociocultural and clinical literature with particular reference to depression. *Journal of Affective Disorders* 2002; **71**(1): 1–9.

37. Begley C, Higgins A, Lalor J, Sheerin F, Alexander J, Nicholl H, Lawler D, Keenan P, Tuohy T, Kavanagh R. *Women with disabilities: barriers and facilitators to accessing services during pregnancy, childbirth and early motherhood.* Dublin: National Disability Authority, 2009.

38. Diaz-Caneja A, Johnson S. The views and experiences of severely mentally ill mothers. *Social Psychiatry and Psychiatric Epidemiology* 2004; **39**(6): 472–82.

39. King M, McKeown E. *Mental health and social wellbeing of gay men, lesbians and bisexuals in England and Wales. A summary of findings.* London: MIND, 2003.

40. McFarlane L. *Diagnosis homophobic: the experience of lesbians, gay men and bisexuals in mental health services.* London: PACE, 1998.

41. Meyer IH. Prejudice, social stress, and mental health in lesbian, gay, and bisexual populations: conceptual issues and research evidence. *Psychological Bulletin* 2003; **129**(5): 674–97.

42. King M, Semlyen J, Tai SS, Killaspy H, Osborn D, Popelyuk D, Nazareth I. A systematic review of mental disorder, suicide, and deliberate self harm in lesbian, gay and bisexual people. *BMC Psychiatry* 2008; **8**: 70.

43. Maguen S, Shipherd JC. Suicide risk among transgender individuals. *Psychology & Sexuality* 2010; **1**(1): 34–43.

44. Chakraborty A, McManus S, Brugha TS, Bebbington P, King M. Mental health of the non-heterosexual population of England. *British Journal of Psychiatry* 2011; **198**(2): 143–8.

45. Bockting WO, Miner MH, Swinburne Romine RE, Hamilton A, Coleman E. Stigma, mental health, and resilience in an online sample of the US transgender population. *American Journal of Public Health* 2013; **103**(5): 943–51.

46. Pompili M, Lester D, Forte A, Seretti ME, Erbuto D, Lamis DA, Amore M, Girardi P. Bisexuality and suicide: a systematic review of the current literature. *Journal of Sexual Medicine* 2014; **11**(8): 1903–13.

47. Marshal MP, Friedman MS, Stall R, King KM, Miles J, Gold MA, Bukstein OG, Morse JQ. Sexual orientation and adolescent substance use: a meta-analysis and methodological review. *Addiction* 2008; **103**(4): 546–56.

48. McCabe SE, Bostwick WB, Hughes TL, West BT, Boyd CJ. The relationship between discrimination and substance use disorders among lesbian, gay, and bisexual adults in the United States. *American Journal of Public Health* 2010; **100**(10): 1946–52.

49. Lombardi EL, Wilchins RA, Priesing D, Malouf D. Gender violence: transgender experiences with violence and discrimination. *Journal of Homosexuality* 2002; **42**(1): 89–101.

50. Stotzer RL. Violence against transgender people: a review of United States data. *Aggression and Violent Behavior* 2009; **14**(3): 170–9.

51. Shipherd JC, Green KE, Abramovitz S. Transgender clients: identifying and minimizing barriers to mental health treatment. *Journal of Gay & Lesbian Mental Health* 2010; **14**(2): 94–108.

52. Women's Health Council. *Women's mental health: promoting a gendered approach to policy and service provision.* Dublin: Women's Health Council, 2005.

53. Victorian Women and Mental Health Network. *Increasing safety and gender sensitivity in mixed sex psychiatric units.* 2009. Available from: http://www.wwda.org.au/wp-content/uploads/2013/12//vwmhn1.pdf [Accessed 5th September 2016].

54. McCann E. The expression of sexuality in people with psychosis: breaking the taboos. *Journal of Advanced Nursing* 2000; **32**(1): 132–8.

55. McCann E. Exploring sexual and relationship possibilities for people with psychosis – a review of the literature. *Journal of Psychiatric and Mental Health Nursing* 2003; **10**(6): 640–9.

56. McCandless F, Sladen C. Sexual health and women with bipolar disorder. *Journal of Advanced Nursing* 2003; **44**(1): 42–8.

57. Davison J, Huntington A. 'Out of sight': sexuality and women with enduring mental illness. *International Journal of Mental Health Nursing* 2010; **19**(4): 240–9.

58. Higgins A, Barker P, Begley CM. 'Veiling sexualities': a grounded theory of mental health nurses responses to issues of sexuality. *Journal of Advanced Nursing* 2008; **62**(3): 307–17.

59. Quinn C, Happell B, Browne G. Talking or avoiding? Mental health nurses' views about discussing sexual health with consumers. *International Journal of Mental Health Nursing* 2011; **20**(1): 21–8.

60. Read J. Childhood adversity and psychosis: from heresy to certainty. In: Read J, Dillon J (eds). *Models of madness: psychological social and biological approaches to psychosis,* 2nd edn. London and New York: Routledge, 2013: 249–75.

61. Crawford MJ, Shaw T. Psychiatric out-patients' views on talking about sex. *Psychiatric Bulletin* 1998; **22**: 365–7.

62. Dillon J, Bullimore P, Lampshire D, Chamberlain J. The work of experience-based experts. In: Read J, Dillon J (eds). *Models of madness: psychological social and biological approaches to psychosis,* 2nd edn. London and New York: Routledge, 2013: 305–18.

63. Higgins A, Nash M, Lynch AM. Antidepressant-associated sexual dysfunction: impact, effects, and treatment. *Drug, Healthcare and Patient Safety* 2010; **2**: 141–52.

64. Quinn C, Happell B, Browne G. Sexuality and consumers of mental health services: the impact of gender and boundary issues. *Issues in Mental Health Nursing* 2011; **32**(3): 170–6.

65. Chen LP, Murad MH, Paras ML, Colbenson KM, Sattler AL, Goranson EN, Elamin MB, Seime RJ, Shinozaki G, Prokop LJ, Zirakzadeh A. Sexual abuse and lifetime diagnosis of psychiatric disorders: systematic review and meta-analysis. *Mayo Clinic Proceedings* 2010; **85**(7): 618–29.

66. Spataro J, Mullen PE, Burgess PM, Wells DL, Moss SA. Impact of child sexual abuse on mental health. Prospective study in males and females. *British Journal of Psychiatry* 2004; **184**: 416–21.

67. Higgins A. All of me: embracing sexuality as a dimension of care. In: Cooper J, Cooper D (eds). *Palliative care – mental health*. London: Radcliffe Publishing, 2012: 126–46.

68. Hammersley P, Reads J, Bullimore P. *Asking the question: starting the journey: childhood sexual abuse and trauma – enquiry and response. A workbook for mental health care workers*. Auckland: Auckland Rape Crisis and the Department of Psychology, Auckland University, New Zealand, 2013.

69. Higgins A, Allen O. *Gay, lesbian and bisexual people: a good practice guide for mental health nurses*. Dublin: Irish Institute of Mental Health Nursing and GLEN, 2010.

70. American Psychological Association. *Practice guidelines for LGB clients: guidelines for psychological practice with lesbian, gay, and bisexual clients*. Washington DC: American Psychological Association, 2012.

Further reading

Apfel RJ, Handel MH. *Madness and loss of motherhood: sexuality, reproduction and long-term mental illness*. Washington DC: American Psychiatric Press, 1993.

Department of Health (Victoria Australia). *Promoting sexual safety, responding to sexual activity, and managing allegations of sexual assault in adult acute inpatient units: Chief Psychiatrist's guideline*. Melbourne: Victorian Government, 2012. Available from: https://www2.health.vic.gov.au/mental-health/practice-and-service-quality/safety/promoting-sexual-safety-in-inpatient-settings/sexual-safety-in-inpatient-settings-service-response [Accessed 8th September 2016].

Department of Health (Western Australia). *Responding to an allegation of sexual assault disclosed within a public mental health service*. Western Australia: WA Health, 2012. Available from: http://www.mentalhealth.wa.gov.au/Libraries/pdf_docs/Sexual_Assault_Guidelines_Final_Completion_22022012__2__2.sflb.ashx [Accessed 5th September 2016].

Hellman R, Drescher J. *Handbook of LGBT issues in community mental health*. New York: Haworth Medical Press, 2004.

Higgins A, Sharek D, McCann E, Sheeran F, Glacken M, Breen M, McCarron M. *Visible lives: identifying the experiences and needs of older lesbian, gay bisexual and transgender people in Ireland*. Dublin: GLEN, 2011. Available from: http://www.glen.ie/attachments/Visible_Lives_Main_Report_Final.pdf [Accessed 5th September 2016].

Levine SB, Risen CB, Althof SE. *Handbook of clinical sexuality for mental health professionals*. London: Routledge, 2011.

LGBT Youth Scotland. *Life in Scotland for LGBT young people: health report*. LGBT Youth Scotland, 2013. Available from: https://www.lgbtyouth.org.uk/files/documents/Life_in_Scotland_for_LGBT_Young_People_Health_Report.pdf [Accessed 5th September 2016].

Lucksted A. Raising issues: lesbian, gay, bisexual, & transgender people receiving services in the public mental health system. Unpublished report, available from the author or at http://www.rainbowheights.org/downloads/FINAL_VERSIONAlicia%20Lucksted.pdf [Accessed 8th September 2016]. A summary of this report was also published in the *Journal of Gay and Lesbian Psychotherapy* 2004; **8**(3/4).

Maycock P, Bryan A, Carr N, Kitching K. *Supporting LGBT lives: a study of the mental health and well-being of lesbian, gay, bisexual and transgender people*. Dublin: Gay and Lesbian Equality Network/ BeLonG to Youth Service, 2009. Available from: http://www.glen.ie/attachments/SUPPORTING_LGBT_LIVES_-_Main_Report.pdf [Accessed 5th September 2016].

Mental Health Commission. Lesbian, gay, bisexual and transgender service users: guidance for staff working in mental health services. 2013. Available from: http://www.mhcirl.ie/File/LGBT_SU_Guide_for_staff.pdf [Accessed 5th September 2016].

Ministry of Health (New South Wales) *Sexual safety of mental health consumers guidelines*. Sydney: NSW Government, 2013. Available from: http://www0.health.nsw.gov.au/policies/gl/2013/pdf/GL2013_012.pdf [Accessed 5th September 2016].

National Centre on Domestic Violence, Trauma & Mental Health. *Responding to domestic violence: tools for mental health providers. Chicago: Domestic Violence & Mental Health Policy Initiative*. Austin TX: National Centre on Domestic Violence, Trauma & Mental Health, 2004. Available from: http://www.nationalcenterdvtraumamh.org/wp-content/uploads/2012/01/Responding-to-DV-Tools-for-MH-Providers.pdf [Accessed 5th September 2016].

NCICP (National Center for Injury Prevention and Control). *Sexual violence: facts at a glance*. Atlanta, GA: NCICP, 2012. Available from: http://www.cdc.gov/violenceprevention/pdf/sv-data-sheet-a.pdf [Accessed 5th September 2016].

Preves SE. *Intersex and identity: the contested self*. New Brunswick: Rutgers University Press, 2003.

Rosenstreich G. *LGBTI people: mental health and suicide*. Sydney: National LGBTI Health Alliance, 2011. Available from: http://lgbtihealth.org.au/sites/default/files/Biefing_Paper_FINAL_19_Aug_2-11.pdf [Accessed 5th September 2016].

Transgender Equality Network Ireland. *A coming out guide for trans young people*. Glasgow: LGBT Youth Scotland, n.d. Available from: http://www.teni.ie/attachments/664c0589-3011-46a5-a6a3-28269015b71b.PDF [Accessed 5th September 2016].

Victorian Mental Illness Awareness Council Australia. *Zero tolerance for sexual assault: a safe admission for women*. Brunswick East: Victorian Mental Illness Awareness Council Australia, n.d. Available from: http://www.abc.net.au/reslib/201305/r1115028_13591277.pdf [Accessed 5th September 2016].

Relevant web pages

Look aftter Yourself - Mental health Info for LGBT People: http://www.lgbtmentalhealth.ie [Accessed 9th January 2017]

Mental Health Foundation: http://lgbt.foundation/information-advice/mental-health/

The History of psychiatry and homosexuality: http://wwwaglp.org/gap/ [Accessed 9th January 2017]

WHO (World Health Organization). Defining sexual health. http://www.who.int/reproductivehealth/topics/sexual_health/sh_definitions/en [Accessed 9th January 2017]

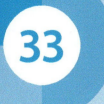

33 The person with dementia

JULIA WOOD AND JACQUIE NUNN

LEARNING OUTCOMES

- To be able to define dementia and describe its prevalence and the process of diagnosis.

- To have an overview of the specific ethical issues relating to the care of people with dementia.

- To understand the challenges in communication and be able to develop appropriate approaches.

- To recognize behavioural and psychological symptoms as an attempt to communicate.

- To acknowledge the role of family members and carers as part of the team.

- To accept that with the right support it is possible to live a good life with dementia.

SUMMARY OF KEY POINTS

- Dementia is an umbrella term for a number of progressive diseases or conditions of the brain with similar symptoms. It is characterized by problems with cognitive function which can present as behavioural and psychological symptoms.

- People with dementia often lack mental capacity to make some decisions, but by concentrating on residual strengths rather than defects a person's autonomy and independence can be maximized.

- Informal carers are our partners in the care of people with dementia and we have responsibilities to consider their well-being.

- There are some useful strategies that can be used to support communication with a person with dementia.

- With the right support people can live well with dementia.

INTRODUCTION

Most dementias are progressive and are currently incurable,[1] and therefore the nurse must provide care which will support the person living with dementia and those close to them to live the best lives they can. Dementia is increasing worldwide as the population ages, with estimates suggesting that 35.6 million people live with dementia, and this is set to double by 2030.[2] The World Health Organization (WHO)[2] considers it a public health priority. Dementia is a psychiatric disorder appearing in ICD-10 while in DSM-5 the term 'dementia' has been replaced by 'major and mild neurocognitive disorder'.

Only since the 1990s has the discourse on dementia changed from a medical model where people were sufferers of their psychiatric disorders to a more person-centred approach.[3] The voices of the person with dementia and those close to them are now being listened to and actively sought.[4] Although this demonstrates a marked improvement, care of people with dementia remains, too frequently, suboptimal.[5]

DEMENTIA AND ITS DIAGNOSIS

Dementia is a syndrome due to disease of the brain, usually of a chronic or progressive nature, in which there is disturbance of multiple higher cortical functions, including memory, thinking, orientation, comprehension, calculation, learning capacity, language, and judgement. Consciousness is not clouded. Impairments of cognitive function are commonly accompanied, and occasionally preceded, by deterioration in emotional control, social behaviour, or motivation. This syndrome occurs in Alzheimer's disease, in cerebrovascular disease, and in other conditions primarily or secondarily affecting the brain.[6] *(p.46)*

Dementia is not a normal part of ageing;[7] most people will never develop dementia even if they live into very old age (see Table 33.1).

Table 33.1 Prevalence of dementia (%)

Age (years)	Male	Female
60–4	0.4	0.4
65–9	1.6	1
70–4	2.9	3.1
75–9	5.6	6.0
80–4	11.0	12.6
85–9	12.8	20.2
90+	22.1	30.8

Source: Revised from Aktar et al.[8] (p.78).

Before dementia can be diagnosed, people experiencing symptoms need screening for reversible causes. Tests should include routine haematology; biochemistry, including

This chapter aims to offer some information, refers to some necessary skills and reports on some personal experiences which together can help you to care for a person with dementia.

electrolytes, calcium, glucose, renal and thyroid function; serum B12 and folate levels; and a midstream urine test if delirium is suspected. Depending on clinical presentation and the person's history, tests for HIV, syphilis, chest X-ray and electrocardiography may be appropriate. Further considerations are: other psychiatric disorders, specifically depression and psychosis; brain tumour; medication or side effects; and pain management.[9]

The most common type of dementia is Alzheimer's disease, accounting for approximately 62 per cent of people with dementia.[10] The brain of a person with Alzheimer's contains multiple amyloid plaques and neurofibrillary tangles caused by abnormal processing of proteins in the brain; these lead to the death of neurones and the atrophy of the cerebral cortex.[11] Although not routine investigations, MRI scans can show brain atrophy and PET scans amyloid plaques,[12] while the FDG-PET when showing a decrease in glucose metabolism is a strong indicator of early stage Alzheimer's.[13]

Vascular dementia accounts for about a further 17 per cent of people with dementia.[10] It results from strokes that affect parts of the brain responsible for memory and intelligence and normally follows a step-wise progression, often demonstrating major deficits in some areas of cognition while sparing others.[14]

Other common types of dementia include mixed Alzheimer's and vascular, dementia with Lewy bodies, and frontotemporal lobe dementia, which is the most common dementia in people under 65.[7]

There is no cure for common types of dementia. Drug treatments are available for Alzheimer's disease which have shown some improvements, but these improvements are limited.[15] At present, concentration needs to be on non-pharmaceutical interventions and care and support for people living with dementia and those caring for them.

FAMILY CARER'S PERSPECTIVE: DIAGNOSIS

My husband is one of the 0.4 per cent to be diagnosed with dementia at the age of 60. The diagnosis came after a period of increasingly worrying symptoms for my husband and even inappropriate treatment following misdiagnosis. Because the early signs of dementia can be confused with other physical illnesses, or with depression, it took 4 years to eliminate other possibilities. While Alzheimer's disease is commonly associated with memory loss, the most noticeable early symptoms are frequently marked changes in behaviour as the individual loses their capacity to make sound judgements. That was our experience and, as in many families, the period pre-diagnosis were dark days, with family tensions and distress that were the consequence of coping with new personality traits and surprising and unfamiliar patterns of behaviour. Although there is no cure for dementia there are treatments and it is essential to understand the options and to make early interventions when possible. For that reason to hear the consultant's devastating words 'In my opinion you have Alzheimer's disease' came almost as a relief.

It was only once we had the diagnosis that we could begin to understand the present reality and to plan for the future. Our experience is typical of people with early-onset dementias, who may be struggling to cope in the work environment and where the diagnosis may lead to major life-style changes. And when I say 'we' that is deliberate. Learning to live with dementia has had profound consequences, not just for Tony but for me and our two sons.

REFLECTION

Why is it important for someone with dementia to receive a diagnosis?

ETHICAL ISSUES IN DEMENTIA

Many of the ethical issues in dementia are similar to those in the care of others with mental health difficulties. Mental capacity is important, as those in a caring role aim to keep a person safe and well cared for, while allowing them to have as much independence and self-determination as they desire. This difficult balancing act is common in the care of people who have fluctuating mental capacity, regardless of symptoms and diagnosis. Historically it was believed that serious mental illness would automatically mean that the person lacked capacity, at least for major decisions such as consenting to medical treatment.[16] This view has been reconsidered, with autonomy becoming an important principle in medical ethics.[17–19] See chapter 2 for a consideration of ethics and mental health nursing, and chapter 67 looks at mental health, the law and human rights. Social exclusion is widely considered a problem experienced by people with mental health problems,[20] and supporting people to be socially included is an important role for health care professionals.[21]

Other mental health issues can be temporary, sometimes with long periods free from symptoms. However, dementia is a progressive condition, so it is unlikely that there will be any marked improvement but it will become worse. It is also a condition that largely (although not exclusively) affects older people. Ageism is a reality in many

societies and, as Nelson[22] reports, in the United States older people become marginalized and stripped of power and responsibility. People with dementia suffer the dual prejudice against their age and their condition.

The carer of the person with dementia can improve their quality of life and sometimes functional capacity through focusing on their strengths.[23] Residual abilities and talents can be tapped and interests from the past reinstated. It can be valuable for people diagnosed with dementia to make advance decisions about their life and care after they lose capacity.[24] People can make decisions about how, where and by whom they would like to be cared for and by whom decisions should be made on their behalf as their symptoms progress.[25] Plans can be made about the types of treatment they would or would not want, but there are also issues about finance and property to consider. Depending on the jurisdiction in which the person lives, some of these decisions may be legally binding, while others can help guide those who must decide. In England and Wales the Mental Capacity Act 2005 governs decision making, with best interests being the guiding principle for a person who lacks capacity. Similar principles apply in other jurisdictions, some governed by statute, others by accepted ethical principles.[26,27]

FAMILY CARER'S PERSPECTIVE: ETHICAL ISSUES

Here again, diagnosis was crucial because it meant that we could draw up Lasting Powers of Attorney both for Health and Welfare and for Financial Affairs. In the former case it meant that we could talk together about some very difficult choices

about clinical interventions and end-of-life care and that my husband could set down his wishes at a time when he was still capable of expressing them. Whenever possible it is of course crucial to ensure that the person feels they are understood and their preferences taken seriously, however progressive brain failure inevitably compromises autonomy. In our own experience and that of new-found friends in our dementia support group it has become evident that people with dementia are often poor witnesses for their ability to care for themselves or to report reliably on pain or discomfort. Ethical issues are a minefield for family carers in day-to-day living. Innocuous items of mail can, for example, cause a catastrophic reaction, such as the time when an estate agent's circular led Tony to believe I had put our house up for sale. For his peace of mind we now screen all of our post. The yardstick for the family in relation to ethical issues is to ask ourselves in every instance, 'What is in Tony's best interests?'

CARERS

Unpaid carers play an important part in supporting people with dementia. They may be a partner, a relative or a friend providing practical physical and/or emotional support, helping a person to retain independence and advocating on their behalf. Caring often has a negative impact on their own physical and mental health and well-being. This can lead to unnecessary hospitalization and residential care for the person with dementia.[28] NHS England[29] has made a commitment to carers, aiming to ensure carers are listened to and provided with the support they need to enable them to continue caring while having their own needs met. Working with people with dementia comes with the additional responsibility of caring for their carers.

Best practice should include the people close to those in our care. Although it is important to listen to a person with dementia, often they may not be able to give an accurate report of their abilities and needs. They may feel unsafe or insecure in the unfamiliar environment where care is delivered, and a familiar person may be able to help with these feelings. Carers often know the person well and are skilled and experienced in delivering care and able to share their knowledge and help us to give the best personalized care.

Carers in England have legal rights.[30] Among others, they have the right to receive an assessment of their own needs by the social services department of the local authority. This assesses the help and services the carer needs, which may include respite care. The family doctor should book appointments at appropriate times or provide home visits to people with caring responsibilities. Whatever the law dictates in a given jurisdiction, caring for the carer is part of holistic care, and helping them to access appropriate services and resources is an important part of the health and social care professionals' role. The carers' role can also be supported if the community is 'dementia friendly', enhancing inclusion and quality of life for the person with dementia.[31]

FAMILY CARER'S PERSPECTIVE: THE ROLE OF FAMILY CARERS AND DEMENTIA-FRIENDLY COMMUNITIES

The move to make communities 'dementia friendly'[31] is admirable, but in our experience probably a long way from being achieved. We have learned rapidly that society is much better adapted to the needs of individuals with physical disability than to those of people with a major cognitive disability. This is a particular issue for my husband as he has early-onset dementia and appears fit and well. Simple things like easy access to disabled toilets (we have braved disapproving glares) and shared changing rooms would make life very much easier. Travelling brings its own difficulties – in order to be eligible for the special assistance service at airports Tony has to agree to be pushed in a wheelchair that he does not need. I have learned over time that it pays to be open about the problem, once a waiter understands that my husband cannot read the menu, or a shopkeeper realizes that he can no longer manage money, then people have been kind and encouraging.

Being there in a support role that is as unobtrusive as possible is a key to being a family carer and it is thrown sharply into focus in health care settings. Whether we are at the GP or in a hospital my hope as carer is that I am seen as being in a sense 'part of the team'. On the one hand I can be an advocate for my husband and help the professionals understand his condition and needs. Equally I can ensure that once we get home I can support the professionals by checking that he takes medication, monitoring his progress or ensuring that he does not injure himself because he has not understood the instructions of a physiotherapist.

COMMUNICATION

Communication is key in the care of people with dementia, but there are significant challenges. Verbal skills are affected by dementia, as is understanding of spoken and written language. People with dementia can often be living in a different reality as more recent memories fade. Communication is about an interaction with an individual, and the importance of putting the person first was recognized by the influential work of Tom Kitwood.[32] He describes the psychological tasks in dementia care as the generation and continuation of positive interactions. He recognizes the high level of skill needed to facilitate positive communication.

Many people describe people with dementia as being like children. This shows disrespect for the person, their history and experience. Research has shown that infantilizing communication leads to resistance to care,[33] which is often considered 'challenging behaviour', which can be easily explained by a person feeling they are being spoken to disrespectfully and their dignity is being undermined. Kitwood[32] suggests that many people underestimate the ability of people with dementia to communicate and understand. However, communication does need to be amended, and Stokes[34] offers some guidance on how this can be appropriately achieved (see Table 33.2). Chapter 3 has information on developing and maintaining therapeutic relationships.

Communication with people with dementia requires flexibility and adaptation. There are no right and wrong ways, as each person is unique. However, this general advice is a starting point, and, through learning about the person and their reactions, meaningful communication can be achieved.

Language matters; it affects the person with dementia and how others perceive them (see Table 33.3).

Behavioural and psychological symptoms in dementia

All behaviour can be considered a form of communication. However, many behavioural and psychological symptoms are described as 'challenging behaviour' and some behaviours can be very challenging to carers and professionals. These symptoms often occur due to unmet needs, when the person lacks the ability to communicate more conventionally.[35] Stress also leads to agitation and even aggression. As short-term memory fails but older memories can remain intact, people with dementia may find themselves surrounded by 'strangers' in an unfamiliar place.[36] A bio-psychosocial approach[37] helps understanding of the person and their needs. Considering these needs can develop care that reduces behaviour that distresses the person and those caring for them. Good empathic communication and looking at non-verbal cues and behaviour to understand the person's needs is a valuable technique to reduce behavioural and psychological symptoms.

Table 33.2 Communication

Keep it simple.	Go slowly, and use short, simple sentences. Use proper names for people and objects rather than 'it' or 'she'.
Do not contradict.	Use of validation is more useful than constantly trying to bring the person in to the present.
Be patient.	Give them time to respond; try not to finish their sentences or show frustration.
Look for meaning behind behaviours.	All behaviours can be considered attempts at communication, particularly when verbal ability is lost.
Make a meaningful connection.	Behaviour may be associated with past life and experience; understanding this can help meaningful engagement. Talk about things that interest them, explore happy memories, know and value the individual.

Source: Revised from Stokes.[34]

Table 33.3 Use of language

Commonly used terms	What can be perceived	Better terms
Challenging behaviour	The person is intentionally behaving in a way that will challenge other people.	Psychological and behavioural symptoms
Cot sides	The person is like a baby.	Bed rails
Feeding	The person is helpless like a baby or an animal which needs to be fed.	Helping a person to eat
Wandering	The walking is aimless.	Frequent/constant walking
Pushing fluids	The power and responsibility is with the carer rather than partnership.	Offering drinks
Good boy/girl/man/woman	Affirmation of a desired behaviour as is done to improve a child's behaviour.	Thank you for ...

FAMILY CARER'S PERSPECTIVE: COMMUNICATION, BEHAVIOUR AND PSYCHOLOGICAL SYMPTOMS

Difficulties in communication are the hardest and most painful part of caring for a partner with dementia. In the early stages it was often possible to work out what my husband was trying to say but soon much of his communication became reduced to strings of words that made less and less sense. To all intents and purposes the person he was has gone, and in his case the memories of the past are just as muddled as those of more recent events. At this stage the only way to cope is to hold on to what remains. Though the words may have gone, he is still able to appreciate music, to watch a sunset or to laugh at an episode of *Fawlty Towers*. In the context of health care, increasingly it becomes important to be acutely aware of non-verbal communication – facial expression, being distracted, and 'switching off'. At these times we have been helped by health care professionals who are sensitive to the signals and adapt their practice, for example, by allowing me as his carer to supply the details for form filling. Being unable to recall your address or your full name and date of birth is humiliating and makes Tony feel vulnerable and threatened.

The vulnerability of living with Alzheimer's also contributes to unusual behaviour patterns. My husband compensates for his sense of 'losing it' by hiding precious things: tea towels, socks, keys, garden tools and random food supplies all get stashed in some very unusual places. He gets up at 5am to get ready for work in the job he had to give up several years ago. He constantly worries that he has not heard recently from his parents who are both long dead. Each day reveals new and strange manifestations of the ravages of dementia and Tony is dependent for all routine aspects of day-to-day living. The only way to cope is to follow the rule of 'one day at a time' and as far as possible to give him the reassurance that his problems are small and that he is making perfect sense.

REFLECTION

Why is communication so important in the care of people with dementia?

Reminiscence

Reminiscence can be valuable for people with dementia. It is a psychosocial intervention using the assumption that older memories remain until the later stages of dementia and reminiscence is used as a form of communication.[38] Reminiscence involves discussion about past experiences, events and activities with another person or group, often prompted by photographs, familiar objects, music, sounds or smells from the past.[39] Reminiscence is popular in dementia care, with participants and staff rating it highly.[39] The aims can be merely to provide an enjoyable activity in the company of others or to improve mood and well-being, promote positive communication, enhance personal identity and further individualized care and/or stimulate memories.

Reminiscence may be used in any number of ways. Dempsey et al.[40] suggest that, if used appropriately, it can lead to more positive mental health, enhanced self-esteem and improved communication skills. However, staff require support, training and supervision to use the techniques for best results. The Cochrane review[39] and a more recent review[41] suggest that reminiscence has positive effects, but evidence is limited. Different ways of using reminiscence require full definition and randomized controlled trials to assess the efficacy of various approaches.

Validation

Reality orientation (RO) was a commonly used approach in the 1960s and 1970s, but many people with dementia were uncomfortable with reminders that they were so out of touch with the world around them.[42] It is particularly hard if people are reminded that loved ones have died, as they relive a bereavement which may be far into their past. This led to validation, which involves acceptance of the different reality and truth of a person with dementia.[43]

Developed by Naomi Feil, validation is a therapy using behavioural and psychotherapeutic approaches for communicating with older people diagnosed with dementia.[44] Validation incorporates values that include treating everyone as an individual, recognizing their value and exploring the reasons behind behaviour without judgement. It recognizes the importance of empathic engagement to build trust, restoring dignity and reducing anxiety. The techniques map with generally accepted good communication with people with dementia.[34] The techniques must be tailored to the person's stage of dementia.

As a therapy, the Cochrane review[43] found insufficient evidence to draw conclusions about efficacy due to the lack of large, good quality randomized controlled trials. They suggest that the positive effects of studies may not be specifically due to validation but the result of structured intervention or increasing the attention given to individuals. However, even if the therapy may be of dubious efficacy, the principles of person-centred care and empathizing with the person's own reality is an approach that can facilitate good communication and trusting relationships.

Moving from reality orientation to cognitive stimulation therapy

RO has often been applied mechanistically with insensitivity to individual needs.[45] The intention is to present information relating to time, place and person by either continuously reminding people of reality throughout the day, or classroom type RO where groups meet regularly and take part in structured reality based activities. A Cochrane review of classroom type RO[45] found evidence for some positive effects on behaviour and cognition, but it was unclear which features of RO are effective and whether positive effects remain after the programme ends.

Cognitive stimulation therapy (CST) was developed in response to the apparent advantages of RO. Spector et al.[46] describe an evidence-based structured programme consisting of 14 twice-weekly 45-minute group sessions:

> *The programme included a 'reality orientation board', displaying both personal and orientation information, including the group name (chosen by participants). The board was to provide a focus, reminding people of the name and nature of the group, and creating continuity. Each session began with a warm-up activity, typically a softball game. This was a gentle, non-cognitive exercise, aiming to provide continuity and orientation by beginning all sessions in the same way. Sessions focusing on themes (such as childhood and food) allowed the natural process of reminiscence but had an additional focus on the current day. Multisensory stimulation was introduced when possible. Sessions encouraged the use of information processing rather than factual knowledge. For example, in the 'faces' activity, people were asked, 'Who looks the youngest?' 'What do these people have in common?', with factual information as an optional extra. A range of activities for each session enabled the facilitator to adapt the level of difficulty of the activities to take into account the group's cognitive capabilities, interests and gender mix.[46] (p.249)*

In this randomized controlled trial, significant improvements were found in cognition, quality of life and communication in the intervention versus the control group. The Cochrane review[47] found consistent improvement in cognition in people participating in CST programmes, also finding promising improvements in self-reported quality of life and well-being. The encouraging results concluded that CST may be more cost-effective than treatment as usual.[48] As a relatively new psychological treatment for people with dementia, it requires more investigation, but will probably prove useful under the wider umbrella of person-centred care and communication.

FAMILY CARER'S PERSPECTIVE: REMINISCENCE, VALIDATION AND CST

While reminiscence is currently at the forefront of therapeutic approach to dementia, perhaps it should be used cautiously and with an awareness of the risk of stereotyping. In our case talking about his own past is certainly helpful in establishing Tony's sense of identity and his garbled memories of childhood and early adulthood are grounded by talking about photographs and handling objects such as the 'custard jug' that came out every Christmas when he was a small child. However, as a person with early-onset dementia born in 1950 he is outraged by the idea that he wants no more than to sit and listen to Vera Lynn. As family carers we rapidly developed our own version of 'validation therapy' which entailed focusing strongly on reassurance and encouraging Tony's sense of confidence by ignoring mistakes and allowing as much freedom as possible. If he empties the dishwasher and puts all the dirty plates into the cupboard then it's a case of 'Oh, thanks for the help!' and clearing up the mess later. Constantly to note the bizarre aspects of some of his behaviour and to reinforce his awareness of the extent of the damage to his mind would be pointless and cruel. The limitation to the approach has to come in matters of health and safety – insisting that he was still fit to drive and refusing to take his prescribed Donepezil being two instances when it has been in his best interests to over-ride his impaired judgement.

Forms of CST and gentle 'reality orientation' are also helpful approaches and ones which we have perhaps adopted instinctively. It would be cruel to remind Tony constantly that his parents are dead, as each time he hears it the news brings fresh grief. However, helping him to keep track of the day, the month, what is in the news, and giving him the opportunity to be involved in activities such as those offered by organizations such as Dementia Adventure or the Royal Academy's In Mind programme have made an immense difference to his sense of self and shown that he has a continuing capacity to learn and engage with others.

LIVING WELL WITH DEMENTIA

As a progressive syndrome, without cure, inevitably dementia is viewed negatively, and feared by many. However, people can still live well with the right support and understanding. Research with people living with dementia and those close to them[49] has identified six themes as key to living a good life, relating to identity, happiness and fulfilment, which have long been linked to human well-being.[50] People with dementia have the same needs and are as different from each other as everyone else. What is different in dementia is the support needed to fulfil these needs. The six themes are discussed below.

1. Respecting identity

Dementia diagnosis does not mean a person loses their individuality. Labels can be unhelpful, as people with dementia are not a homogeneous group, and it must be the person who is cared for, not their dementia. They have a history, relationships, preferences and aspirations. Waiting for dementia to take over can stop the person living a full life. Support is needed to enable them to find happiness through maintaining their strengths and to continue to grow as a person, remembering and celebrating their history and individuality. Tom Kitwood[51] recognized that, with the right support and care, personal growth in people with dementia was possible. Far from being the end, a diagnosis of dementia can be the beginning of a new phase in a person's life.

2. Embracing now

Reminiscence is much used as a way of engaging with people with dementia. It can bring pleasure, as everyone enjoys remembering the best parts of their life, and it is important in maintaining identity. However, we also enjoy experiences in the here and now, and this should not be forgotten because a person has dementia. Facilitating people to continue having experiences, allowing people to live in the moment can be fulfilling and may become even more important as coherent memory diminishes. Memory-based activity needs to be balanced with enjoying the moment.

3. Sustaining relationships

A link has been identified between social relationships and social activities and the self-rated quality of life in older people.[52] Meaningful relationships are no less important after the onset of dementia. There is a danger that dementia can lead to social isolation as a person loses some of their abilities to interact in the social world as they did before. Relationships are best maintained when dementia is recognized as one of many human imperfections, while recognizing potential benefit from meaningful adult social interactions. Embracing change enables positive relationships to continue.[49] Communication goes beyond words, and emotions can be expressed and recognized by people with dementia beyond the loss of verbal communication. Recognition that people with dementia need not only social contact but also to participate and give pleasure to others can help sustain relationships.

4. Valuing contrast

One of the things that makes one appreciate the good things in life is that there is a balance between happiness and sadness, exciting and mundane, good and bad. This is normal life, and the idea that we can protect a person with dementia from negativity is not only unrealistic but unhelpful. Everyone is entitled to experience a full range of emotions to maximize their experience of life. If a person is sad at times, this is not a failure of care; it is normal, and facilitating all types of experience can lead to a more fulfilled life.

5. Supporting agency

Autonomy is a term much used in medical ethics.[e.g.17] Under many definitions of autonomy, older people in need of care, especially those with dementia who may lack capacity to make certain decisions, are unlikely to be considered autonomous.[53] However, this does not mean that the person should not be making decisions where they can and taking risks. Risk is a part of everyday life and can also be a need.[54] Deprivation of the opportunity to take risks can significantly detract from a person's well-being. There is an understandable desire to keep a person safe, but too much control detracts from maximal independence and basic rights may be affected. Facilitating people to take some risks can enable the individual to live as they choose in the time remaining to them.

6. Maintaining health

Maximization of health (physical, social, emotional, psychological and spiritual) is an important part of anyone's well-being. As the majority of people with dementia are older, comorbidity is common. There is often a view among people with dementia, those who care from them, and even health care professionals that problems are due to their dementia and treatment would be futile. A diagnosis should not stop investigation of problems that anyone else would receive; for example, depression frequently coexists with dementia but is often overlooked.[55] Ensuring that appropriate care and treatment are offered for physical or psychological conditions will enable the person to live a more complete and fulfilling life. Chapter 69 considers physical health care and chapter 70 on health promotion.

The ESRO[49] report highlights three key strategies to overcome the barriers preventing people living a good life with dementia. The first is timely *diagnosis without fear*, enabling receipt of the right support to live well with dementia. Next is *increasing public awareness of dementia*. With better understanding, fear can be reduced and people with dementia can retain their place in their community and reduce isolation. Finally, living a good life can be facilitated by improving the *flexibility of care*. Person-centred care is a common mantra but needs to become a reality for everyone and every time. People with dementia and those caring for them need to receive the support that is right for them to maximize quality of life.

These ideas are not new, but they highlight what is needed to ensure that all people with dementia live the best life they can. Dementia has many negative aspects, but that does not mean that people with dementia and those close to them cannot enjoy many good things in their lives.

FAMILY CARER'S PERSPECTIVE: LIVING WELL WITH DEMENTIA

When Tony was diagnosed with Alzheimer's it was like hitting a wall. We felt as though we had lost our future and every day was filled with the grief of bereavement. The idea of 'living well with dementia' seemed far-fetched and was a challenge for the whole family. However, things have changed. There have certainly been losses for Tony: his professional identity, his love of reading and the theatre and his freedom to choose how to spend his time. However, through a concerted effort by us all he has been able to retain a sense of self and in fact to establish a new identity through 'embracing the now'. He has begun to paint and his art work shows a remarkable sense of pattern and colour. Without a doubt he has developed new skills, in spite of his disability. We have been supported by a small group of family and friends, although there are some who find communicating with Tony in his state of dementia too difficult. We have a new friendship group of people similarly affected by early-onset Alzheimer's and who have shared information and encouragement. As a family we have learnt too that in spite of our best efforts Tony is sometimes lost in the distress and fear of 'losing his mind'. We try to respect those times and to allow him to grieve and at the same time protect him from our own frustrations and misery. Acknowledging his emotions is an important aspect of supporting his sense of agency, as well as putting in place the arrangements to make it possible for him to enjoy cycling, swimming and supported travel and visits. There is much to look forward to and with proper support it is definitely possible to have a good quality of life while living with dementia, at least in the early and middle stages of the disease.

All health care professionals should be under no illusions about the huge impact, not just on the patient, but on the whole family of a diagnosis of dementia, and without direct experience it is hard to understand the day-to-day realities of living with Alzheimer's. However, they should never underestimate the extent to which they can make a difference through responding sensitively to the needs of the patient and showing an understanding of the role of family members as partners in care.

REFLECTION

What strategies will you adopt to help a person live well with dementia?

CONCLUSION

In this chapter we have given an overview of dementia and its impact on people who live with the condition. While facts and tips on working with people with dementia are important, understanding the person and those close to them is crucial. Jacquie's perspective helps to illustrate what life is like for her and her family living with Tony's dementia. The experience cannot be generalized, as every individual and their family will encounter 'their' dementia in a unique way. What I hope it can do is to identify the person rather than a condition or a role, helping the reader to interpret facts and guidelines in the lived experience of people with dementia.

References

1. Alzheimer's Association. What is dementia? 2014. Available from: http://www.alz.org/what-is-dementia.asp [Accessed 25th May 2016].
2. WHO (World Health Organization). Dementia: a public health priority. 2012. Available from: http://apps.who.int/iris/bitstream/10665/75263/1/9789241564458_eng.pdf?ua=1 [Accessed 25th July 2016].
3. Gilmour JA, Brannally T. Representations of people with dementia – subaltern, person, citizen. *Nursing Inquiry* 2009; **17**(3): 240–7.
4. Brooker D. *Person-centred dementia care: making services better.* London: Jessica Kingsley, 2006.
5. England E. Improving the management of dementia. *British Medical Journal* 2006; **332**(7543): 681–2.
6. WHO (World Health Organization). *ICD 10.* 2007. Available from: http://apps.who.int/classifications/apps/icd/icd10online2007/index.htm?gf00.htm+ [Accessed 25th May 2016].
7. Draper B. *Understanding Alzheimer's disease and other dementias.* London: Jessica Kingsley, 2011.
8. Aktar S, Rani M, Nordin M, Rahman J, Aris M, Rathor M. Dementia prevalence and risk factors. *International Review of Social Sciences and Humanities* 2012; **2**(2): 176–84.
9. NICE (National Institute for Health and Care Excellence). Dementia: supporting people with dementia and their carers in health and social care. 2006. Available from: https://www.nice.org.uk/guidance/cg42?unlid=9429054072016126125418 [Accessed 25th July 2016].
10. Alzheimer's Society. Demography. 2013. Available from: http://www.alzheimers.org.uk/site/scripts/documents_info.php?documentID=412 [Accessed 25th May 2016].
11. Dash P, Villamarrete-Pittman N. *Alzheimer's disease.* New York: Demos Medical Publishing Inc, 2005.
12. Drzezga A. Amyloid-plaque imaging in early and differential diagnosis of dementia. *Annals of Nuclear Medicine* 2010; **24**: 55–66.
13. Cason E, Treglia G, Fagioli G. Leading role of ¹⁸F-FDG-PET imaging in early diagnosis of Alzheimer's disease: an overview. *Research and Reports in Nuclear Medicine* 2011; **1**: 11–19.
14. Maj M, Sartorius N. *Dementia*, 2nd edn. Chichester: Wiley, 2002.
15. NICE (National Institute for Health and Care Excellence). Donepezil, Galantamine, Rivastigmine and Memantine for the treatment of Alzheimer's disease: review of NICE technology appraisal. 2011. Available from: https://www.nice.org.uk/Guidance/ta217K12 [Accessed 25th July 2016].
16. Cairns R, Maddock C, Buchanan A, David A, Hayward P, Richardson G, et al. Reliability of mental capacity assessments in psychiatric in-patients. *British Journal of Psychiatry* 2005; **187**: 382–7.
17. Beauchamp T, Childress J. *Principles of biomedical ethics*, 6th edn. Oxford: Oxford University Press, 2009.
18. Edwards SD. *Nursing ethics: a principle-based approach*, 2nd edn. Basingstoke: Palgrave Macmillan, 2009.
19. Gillon R. Ethics needs principles – four can encompass the rest – and respect for autonomy should be 'first among equals'. *Journal of Medical Ethics* 2003; **29**: 307–12.
20. Morgan C, Burns T, Fitzpatrick R, Pinfold V, Priebe S. Social exclusion and mental health. *British Journal of Psychiatry* 2007; **191**: 473–83.
21. Lloyd C, Tse S, Deane F. Community participation and social inclusion: how practitioners can make a difference. *Australian e-Journal for the Advancement of Mental Health* 2006; **5**(3): 1–10.

22. Nelson TD. Ageism: prejudice against our feared future self. *Journal of Social Issues* 2005; **61**(2): 207–21.

23. Gottleib LN. *Strengths-based nursing care*. New York: Springer, 2012.

24. Nuffield Council on Bioethics. Dementia ethical issues. 2009. Available from: http://nuffieldbioethics.org/project/dementia/ [Accessed 25th May 2016].

25. Wood J. Perspectives of decision making in a UK care home: a grounded theory study [PhD Thesis], Kingston University, London, 2012.

26. Lautrette A, Peigne V, Watts J, Souweine B, Azoulay E. Surrogate decision makers for incompetent ICU patients: a European perspective. *Current Opinion in Critical Care* 2008; **14**(6): 714–19.

27. Buchanan A. Mental capacity, legal competence and consent to treatment. *Journal of the Royal Society of Medicine* 2004; **97**(9): 415–20.

28. Department of Health. Assessment, eligibility and portability for care users and carers. 2012. Available from: https://www.gov.uk/government/uploads/system/uploads/attachment_data/file/136450/IA-Annex-C-assessment-and-eligibility.pdf [Accessed 25th May 2016].

29. NHS England. NHS England's commitment to carers. 2014. Available from: http://www.england.nhs.uk/wp-content/uploads/2014/05/commitment-to-carers-may14.pdf [Accessed 25th May 2016].

30. NHS Choices. A guide to carers' rights. Available from: http://www.nhs.uk/CarersDirect/guide/rights/Pages/carers-rights.aspx [Accessed 25th May 2016].

31. Alzheimer's Society. Dementia-friendly communities. 2014. Available from: https://www.alzheimers.org.uk/dementiafriendlycommunities# [Accessed 25th July 2016].

32. Kitwood T. *Dementia reconsidered: the person comes first*. Buckingham: Open University Press, 1997.

33. Williams KN, Herman R, Wilson K. Elderspeak communication: impact on dementia care. *American Journal of Alzheimer's Disease and Other Dementias* 2009; **24**(1): 11–20.

34. Stokes G. Tackling communication challenges in dementia. *Nursing Times* 2013; **109**(8): 14–15.

35. Hotchhalter AK, Stevens AB, Burgio L. Rates of resident needs-driven behavior and nursing assistant skill use in nursing homes. *Long Term Care Interface* 2007; **8**(2): 36–40.

36. Bonner C. *Reducing stress-related behaviours in people with dementia*. London: Jessica Kingsley, 2005.

37. Sabat SR. A bio-psycho-social approach to dementia. In: Downs M, Bowers B (eds). *Excellence in dementia care: research into practice*. Maidenhead: Open University Press, 2008: 70–84.

38. Norris A. *Reminiscence with elderly people*. London: Winslow, 1986.

39. Woods B, Spector AE, Jones CA, Orrell M, Davies SP. Reminiscence therapy for dementia: review. *Cochrane Database*. Wiley Online Library, 2009.

40. Dempsey L, Murphy K, Cooney A, Casey D, O'Shea E, Devene D, et al. Reminiscences in dementia: a concept analysis. *Dementia* 2014; **13**(2): 176–92.

41. Cotelli M, Manenti R, Zanetti O. Reminiscence therapy in dementia: a review. *Maturitas* 2012; **72**(3): 203–5.

42. Waite J, Harwood RH, Morton IR, Connelly DJ. *Dementia care: a practical manual*. Oxford: Oxford University Press, 2009.

43. Neal M, Barton Wright P. Validation therapy for dementia. *Cochrane Database*. Wiley Online Library, 2009.

44. Feil N. *The validation breakthrough: simple techniques for communication with people with 'Alzheimer's type dementia'*. Baltimore, MD: Health Promotion Press, 1993.

45. Spector A, Orrell M, Davies S, Woods B. Reality orientation for dementia: review. *Cochrane Database*. Wiley Online Library, 2000.

46. Spector A, Thorgrimsen L, Woods B, Royan L, Davies S, Butterworth M, et al. Efficacy of an evidence-based cognitive stimulation therapy programme for people with dementia: randomised controlled trial. *British Journal of Psychiatry* 2003; **183**: 248–54.

47. Woods B, Aguirre E, Spector AE, Orrell M. Cognitive stimulation to improve cognitive functioning in people with dementia: review. *Cochrane Database*. Wiley Online Library, 2012.

48. Knapp M, Thorgrimsen L, Patel A, Spector A, Hallam A, Woods B, et al. Cognitive stimulation therapy for people with dementia: cost-effectiveness analysis. *British Journal of Psychiatry* 2006; **188**: 574–80.

49. ESRO. A good life with dementia. 2014. Available from: http://fabrica.org.uk/wp-content/uploads/2015/08/A_Good_Life_with_Dementia.pdf [Accessed 25th July 2016].

50. Wang S. *Aquinas and Satre: on freedom, personal identity, and the possibility of happiness*. Washington DC: Catholic University America Press, 2009.

51. Kitwood T. Positive long-term changes in dementia: some preliminary observations. *Journal of Dementia Care* 1995; **4**(2): 133–44.

52. Bowling A. *Ageing well: quality of life in old age*. Maidenhead: Open University Press, 2005.

53. Agich G. *Dependence and autonomy in old age*. Cambridge: Cambridge University Press, 2003.

54. Zinn JO. *Social theories of risk and uncertainty*. Blackwell: Oxford, 2008.

55. Theison AK, Geisthoff UW, Förstlf H, Schröder SG. Agitation in the morning: symptom of depression in dementia? *International Journal of Geriatric Psychiatry*. Wiley Online, 2008. Available from: http://www.gnmhealthcare.com/pdf/09-2008/09/1638914_Agitationinthemorningsymp.pdf [Accessed 25th May 2016].

Further reading

Brooker D. *Dementia care*. Abingdon: Routledge, 2013.

Healey E. *Elizabeth is missing*. London: Penguin, 2014.

Hughes JC. *How we think about dementia*. London: Jessica Kingsley, 2013.

Relevant web pages

Alzheimer's Society. http://www.alzheimers.org.uk/

SCIE (Social Care Institute for Excellence). Dementia. http://www.scie.org.uk/publications/dementia/index.asp [Accessed 9th January 2017]

Section 4

Care planning and approaches to therapeutic practice

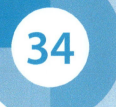

34 Admission of a person in acute distress

ANGUS FORSYTH AND MARION JANNER

LEARNING OUTCOMES

- To understand the context of the acute care pathway and the role of the acute inpatient unit in providing recovery-focused interventions.

- To appreciate the experiences of people who present to acute services in acute distress.

- To be able to evaluate the culture of the acute inpatient ward's therapeutic milieu in providing recovery-focused interventions.

- To apply the principles of positive risk taking and building resilience to individual risk formulation and risk mitigation strategies.

- To explore the challenges to client collaboration in the acute setting and how to overcome these barriers.

SUMMARY OF KEY POINTS

- Service users access acute care in times of acute crisis at a vulnerable time in their lives.
- Assessment of service user need should involve a holistic assessment and focus upon the service user's strengths.
- The therapeutic environment of adult acute wards needs to focus upon building resilience and facilitating recovery with service users.

- Utilizing the framework of trauma-focused care can facilitate mental health nurses to reflect on the effects of restrictive interventions on service users.
- Clinical supervision and person-centred formulations of care can lead to positive engagement strategies with service users.

INTRODUCTION

The provision of adult acute inpatient care needs to be considered with respect to the overall acute care pathway where individuals present in crisis and the severity of presentation and the risk to the individual or others is too great to be safely managed within a community setting. Modern models of acute care have demonstrated that recovery is more effective when it occurs in the community setting and utilizes the community resources that are available to

Table 34.1 Tensions in providing care in acute mental health settings

	Recovery-centred approaches	Coercive approaches
Decision making	Service user involvement	Prescribed by team
Expectations/rules	Mutually derived	Organizationally driven
Interventions	Focus on self-management and advance directives for care; strengths-based	Focus on observation, medication and restraint; symptom-based
Power	Shared	With team
Restrictive practices	Individually care planned	Blanket restrictions; ward driven
Language/discourse	Empowerment, collaboration, involvement; service user centred	Emphasis on compliance and control, symptom management

maintain the individual's contact with their local community and reduce the likelihood of stigma from developing. This means that the provision of adult acute inpatient care requires the stabilization of acute distress and support for the safe discharge of individuals, with support of community services, in a timely way. The goal of acute inpatient care is to provide safe and effective care[1] that is characterized by a comprehensive assessment of mental, social and physical health care needs. Acute inpatient mental health care is also characterized by a range of competing tensions. For example, individuals who present in acute distress are more likely to be detained under a section of the Mental Health Act, have increased risks to self or others[2] and can present challenges to the role of the mental health nurse in providing either an engagement[3] or observational approach[4] for individuals in acute distress. Table 34.1 highlights the tensions in providing recovery-focused care in comparison to coercive approaches in acute mental health care.

This can present challenges to the mental health nurse in working collaboratively to empower clients or to implement containment strategies to manage acute distress. Such approaches underpin a need to control and contain individual distress and can result in the disempowering of individuals in acute distress.[5] Service user views of acute inpatient care also highlight the challenges in providing person-centred care in clinical environments that are characterized by a reliance on increasing observation levels; chaotic

ward environments; and overuse of restraint, resulting in the service users describing their experience of acute care as inhumane, traumatizing and coercive.[6] These interventions can be the antithesis of a recovery-based approach,[7] which is characterized by the development of a collaborative relationship that is hope-inspiring and empowering, together with optimism for recovery from the current episode of distress, and which utilizes individual goals, strengths and resources. Additional reading with regard to developing a recovery-focused approach can be found in chapter 35, and information on incorporating this within a risk management approach can be found in chapter 36. The craft of caring is enhanced when the mental health nurse is able to maintain (and at times repair possible ruptures in) the therapeutic relationship at times when the service user is unable to self-manage and presents risks to either themselves or others.

REFLECTION

Using Table 34.1, explore the ways in which care is provided within your team and whether there are dominant trends. For example, how are service users involved in treatment decisions? What is the dominant language used in care meetings with regard to recovery or symptom management? Can you identify areas where practice needs to change?

THE EXPERIENCE OF ACUTE DISTRESS

The nature of acute distress is a unique and idiosyncratic experience and the threshold for admission to the acute inpatient unit varies across care settings. Acute distress can manifest itself in many ways. It may involve an individual with low mood who lacks motivation to get out of bed, with considerable weight loss, is no longer eating or drinking and is developing pressure sores due to lack of movement and personal care. They are acutely suicidal, feel that life is not worth living and may well have formulated a plan to end their life. It may also involve the expression of self-harm, the inability to

cope with further urges to self-harm and feeling out of control. More on self-harm can be found in chapter 22. The person who is suicidal is discussed in chapter 23. Acute distress may also manifest itself within the individual who is unable to cope with the intensity of relationships and can feel abandoned by others, resulting in impulsivity and anger directed towards themselves and characterized by the experience of intense emotions, feelings of worthlessness, profound self-harm and thoughts of wanting to die. The individual who experiences excessive anxiety constantly seeks reassurance from family members, regularly checks and monitors their health, feels out of control and may develop rituals to reduce their anxiety, but this only prolongs their anxiety and makes it worse. There are also individuals who are guarded and mistrustful of others, and who may also hear voices and hold strong beliefs that others are going to cause them some harm and this may result in both avoidance and hypervigilant behaviours to 'expose' the perpetrators. Extremes of mood may also be present in acute distress where the individual, who is elated in mood, is unable to take rest, is overactive, overtalkative to the extent that they are unable to express their words or that they experience accelerated thought processes that result in poor concentration and their attention switching from one topic to another. Due to the grandiose nature of their beliefs, they may also make elaborate plans,

and believe that they are extremely wealthy, resulting in lavish spending sprees that can leave them financially destitute.

Despite the individual nuances in the presentation of acute distress, the therapeutic relationship is the mainstay of the therapeutic arsenal at the disposal of the mental health nurse. The development of a sound therapeutic alliance provides the mental health nurse with a solid foundation to build the delivery of interventions such as administering medications, providing psychological interventions, and providing health and well-being advice and specific interventions for relapse prevention. A sound therapeutic alliance epitomizes the craft of caring by the mental health nurse, and is also essential in working collaboratively to identify the needs of the individual and the goals of the admission. These subjects will now be explored.

ASSESSMENT OF NEED

The important role of assessment in the craft of caring is underlined and further explored in chapter 13. However, within the inpatient setting, the holistic assessment of the individual by the mental health nurse will incorporate the following elements.

- *Mental state presentation.* That is, key risks from the mental state examination together with strategies to treat, improve and monitor symptomatology. This may include specific symptom rating scales for depression, anxiety, psychosis and mania.
- *Physical health and well-being.* Issues related to comorbidity, such as obesity, diabetes, coronary heart disease and respiratory disorders and their management; together with preventative strategies to optimize health, such as dietary advice, lifestyle factors and exercise and smoking advice. Issues of physical health care and health promotion are considered in chapters 69 and 70.
- *Risk assessment and risk mitigation.* A risk formulation should be developed for each risk factor to show the degree of risk and the precipitating and predisposing factors, as well as the prolonging and protective factors. This should also contain a summary of how the presenting risks will be managed and mitigated.
- *Service user strengths.* A strengths-based assessment is service user centred and is facilitated in a therapeutic conversation with the mental health nurse. It focuses upon their current life situation and their connectedness to others, the roles that they perform and the strengths that help them to keep going when things get tough, and this may include support from others and personal values and beliefs. There is also a focus upon their personal goals and individual hopes and dreams for the future. Past coping history to adverse events is also explored, and reflection on or learning from past events can lead the service user to new evaluations of self. This is also facilitated by exploring valued social roles and how others view the service user

and a review of personal gifts or unique aspects of the individual, which all contribute toward enabling the development of a personal narrative that is not limited and bound by professional diagnostic codes and labels but provides a story which is about the future and is hope-inspiring.

- *Medication concordance.* An assessment of concordance should be undertaken to ascertain whether the individual understands the medications that are prescribed and whether they are being taken correctly. Reasons for non-concordance may relate to the complexity of prescribed medications, side effect tolerance, product choice, individual involvement in decision making, personal beliefs about medication, incorrect knowledge about the effects of medication, lack of insight into the need for medication, previous experience of medication and identification with the diagnosis and the limitation that this may have on the individual's lifestyle, due to stigma and the side effects of medication. Chapters 47 and 48 discuss psychopharmacology.
- *Social inclusion.* Usual social routines should be identified, as well as any barriers to social inclusion which may involve housing issues, debts, financial issues, occupational factors, relationships and connectedness to others, hobbies and interests. Identifying interventions to overcome barriers will promote recovery and facilitate discharge from hospital.
- *Therapeutic activities.* Boredom and lack of structure are two of the main triggers for the expression of aggression and self-harm within an acute inpatient ward. An activity checklist can be used to assess the service user's strengths and interests to enable the development of a personalized activity plan for the individual to utilize during their inpatient stay.
- *Psychological interventions.* These should be based upon a formulation of service user need and used to improve coping and control over identified problem areas and reduce distress. This may involve coping strategy enhancement approaches for people who experience

voices; behavioural activation for people with low mood; mindfulness-based meditation for those with difficulty in coping with emotional distress (see chapter 44).

- *Carer/nearest relative involvement.* Assessment should identify the principal carer, together with any relevant issues which may contribute to carer distress. Some of the issues that may need to be addressed with carers, subject to service user consent, are leave and discharge arrangements, medication issues, early signs monitoring and carer support meetings.
- *Barriers to discharge.* At the earliest opportunity any potential barriers to discharge – such as housing, lack of family support, other agency involvement or safeguarding issues – should be clearly identified and incorporated

into the multidisciplinary team planning process to facilitate safe and timely discharge from the unit. See chapter 37 on the care programme approach and chapter 50 on collaborative care planning with service users and carers.

> ### REFLECTION
>
> Review the assessment documentation used within your team/department and identify the main focus of intervention. What are the areas that are given priority? How are the service user and carer involved in this prioritization? Are there any gaps in the process?

THE ACUTE INPATIENT WARD'S THERAPEUTIC MILIEU

In recent times several sources of discourse have influenced the development of the therapeutic culture and milieu of the adult acute inpatient ward. The aforementioned acute policy implementation guide, which identified the key standards of care within acute mental health wards, became the health care regulator's currency for evaluation of the quality of services provided within these environments.[8] Building upon this, an innovative service-user-led initiative known as Star Wards[9] developed a framework for improving the therapeutic culture of inpatient wards, and this involved 75 standards. Wards were able to opt into the programme and work towards implementing these standards.

Building further upon these definitions of standards for adult acute inpatient care, the Royal College of Psychiatrists developed the Accreditation for Inpatient Mental Health Services (AIMS)[10] which consists of three standard levels, with the core standard of safety being a prerequisite for accreditation, while the remaining two standard levels highlight excellence in acute care. This includes the physical and psychological environment, the care pathway, and the provision of therapeutic activities and interventions. Accreditation is achieved through the triangulation of a series of data, including self-review by the unit, service user and carer feedback, staff feedback and independent peer review.

Despite the positive effects of these approaches, concerns about the safety of service users on acute mental health wards emerged following the death of a service user from a BME background after the use of prone restraint,[11] and the findings of the Winterbourne View Inquiry,[12] on a case involving widespread abuse of residents with a learning disability, being cared for in an independent hospital, found that staff used physical restraint on a frequent basis and that it was used as a first rather than a last resort. Additional findings from service users found that the use of restraint varied across acute inpatient wards in England, and that restraint was not always used as a last resort.[13] These high-profile cases have called into question the use of restraint and its role as an effective intervention in acute and residential settings, and led to the publication

of Department of Health guidance[14] on the use of restrictive practices, which effectively prohibited the use of prone restraint. In addition, the Department of Health guidance recommended that a method of restraint should be the least restrictive possible, and only used as a last resort, and only in the care and management of service users detained under the Mental Health Act. The continued use of restrictive practices can present a significant challenge to the craft of caring from the mental health nurse, leading to a reduction of trust from the service user, and can also contribute to the erosion of personhood and alienation of the service user.

Seclusion, restraint, observation levels and as required medications are examples of containment strategies utilized by mental health staff to manage conflict within acute mental health wards. See chapter 25 for further information on caring for the extremely distressed and disturbed person. These have been studied extensively to produce the *Safewards* model,[15] to help understand why conflict and flashpoints occur. This has resulted in the development of 10 key interventions, which have been rigorously evaluated, to reduce conflict in the acute ward. These include mutual expectations, talk down tips, bad news mitigation, positive discharge messages and other interventions to reduce the potential for aggression within the ward setting.

Sensory integration approaches have been used extensively in the USA as an alternative to restraint and seclusion in psychiatric inpatient settings.[16] Sensory modulation has been defined as a clinical intervention that focuses on the use of environments, equipment and activities to regulate individuals' sensory experience and optimize physiological and emotional well-being.[17] The use of sensory modulation approaches has seen the use of sensory rooms in acute wards which provide individuals in acute distress with the opportunity to reduce their arousal with the use of alternative sensory inputs, such as weighted blankets, rocking chairs, meditation, aromatherapy, light projections, comforting music, different textured materials and brushing techniques, to name but a few.

TRAUMA-INFORMED CARE

There is evidence to support the linkage between early childhood trauma and later adverse mental health outcomes. The concept of trauma-informed care was developed to acknowledge that the majority of people who use mental health services had been previously exposed to a traumatic event at some time in their lives. Furthermore, the controlling and coercive nature of adult mental health care that relied upon restrictive interventions such as restraint and seclusion, as well as authoritarian approaches which centred upon enforcing ward rules and routines, meant that these individuals then experienced further trauma.[18–20] There have also been examples where the use of restraint has resulted in the development of post-traumatic stress disorder in service users with no previous experience of trauma.[21]

Interventions utilized to inform the implementation of trauma-informed care have initially focused upon the eradication of restraint and seclusion, but research from the USA has identified six key interventions to support a trauma-informed culture of care.[22] These include clear clinical leadership support about the key principles and modelling these approaches with staff; collection of data on restraint incidents; debriefing and problem analysis of restraint events and selection of alternative strategies; trauma-informed education and skills development for staff; trauma assessment scales and self-management skills; and lastly, but most importantly, the inclusion of service users at all levels of care. The use of coproduction methods and in particular the inclusion of service users' stories of their experience of restraint or seclusion are powerful means of facilitating attitude change among professional staff, and enable critical reflection on their previous assumptions about the use

of those specific care approaches. See chapter 11 for further information on critical reflection.

REFLECTION

Think about the rules and routines currently in place in the ward where you work, and identify which aspects are related to a controlling or trauma-informed culture of care. What would it be like to experience those aspects of care? What would you change?

Inherent within the trauma-informed model of care is the use of the safety plan, which is a tool that is collaboratively constructed with the service user and provides a shared understanding of the situations or trigger events that could result in the experience of intense emotion or acute distress to the individual. This is also accompanied by a behavioural description of how the service user would appear to others, as (for example, due to dissociative reactions) the service user may not be able to articulate their feelings or needs and may appear unresponsive and withdrawn. It is therefore essential that a concrete description of the experience is captured, along with a range of coping strategies that have been previously formulated with the service user and have been found effective in coping with the distress. The safety plan also enables the exploration of previous experience and any previous exposure to restraint and the reasons for this. This helps to prevent potential risk situations from occurring but also provides a clear plan of intervention should distress escalate for the service user.

DEVELOPING RESILIENCE IN ACUTE MENTAL HEALTH CARE SETTINGS

Most of the discussion in this chapter thus far has focused on developing interventions to improve the culture of care on acute wards to ensure that service users experience a personalized and person-centred approach to their presenting acute distress. I will now focus upon individualized approaches to accentuate the craft of caring for people with acute distress using a strengths-based resilience-enhancing approach.

REFLECTION

Before reading further, please review the assessment documentation in use on your ward, and reflect upon the language used. Is it problem-focused or strengths-based? How is this information shared with the service user? How are they involved in the care planning process? Are interventions 'done to' the service user, or do service users have an active role in self-management?

The service user who presents with acute distress has usually experienced a personal crisis in their lives which has brought them into contact with mental health services and they may well feel bewildered about navigating their way through the acute care pathway. While admission to hospital can sometimes be a frightening experience, it also provides an opportunity for the service user to reflect on the key issues that contributed to the current crisis, and can often be viewed as an opportunity to further determine their future goals. According to the Department of Health's guidance *Best practice in managing risk*,[23] risk occurs when client risk factors outweigh the protective factors presented by the client. Dynamic risk factors are amenable to change – for example, stress, low mood, alcohol use, low self-esteem, conflict in relationships, etc. – and help to guide interventions. In addition, the role of protective factors is also important when attempting to modify risks presented by individuals. Figure 34.1 provides an overview of protective factors and is adapted from

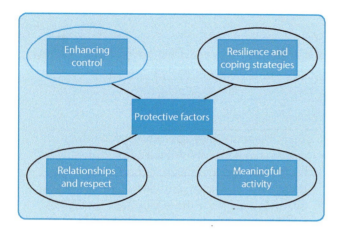

Figure 34.1 Protective factors.

health and well-being initiatives,[24] but it is relevant to the development of resilience to mental health vulnerabilities.

Enhancing control

This dimension is concerned with promoting individual autonomy over one's mental health and well-being. The more engaged an individual is with taking personal control over their care and strategies to reduce risk factors, the greater their likelihood of improving coping and recovery from current problems or challenges that they experience. This dimension helps clients to identify those things they can influence and their degree of belief that they can implement strategies to enhance their recovery.

Relationships and respect

An empathic supportive relationship is a prerequisite for building an effective therapeutic alliance,* which provides a platform for building effective therapeutic interventions. Supportive relationships can enhance recovery, while expressed emotion in relationships can result in additional stress and deterioration in mental health. The building of effective and supportive relationships may involve:

- maintaining contact with family and friends;
- one-to-one sessions with the mental health nurse;
- overcoming personal barriers to engaging with others, e.g. because of stigma;
- promoting hope and optimism;
- empathic understanding;
- building on personal strengths;
- genuineness and warmth;
- promoting unconditional positive regard.

The therapeutic alliance is characterized by three key components: a sound therapeutic relationship, goals set by the service user, and interventions or strategies designed to achieve those targets.

Resilience and coping strategies

Helping individuals to develop a range of coping strategies in response to the stressors that they experience will help to reduce stress and improve resilience and control over these stressors. These relate to addressing dynamic factors which may arise out of the assessment of needs. Examples include self-esteem, negative thoughts, emotional reactions or the use of alcohol or drugs. In essence, dynamic factors relate to those factors that are amenable to change. Coping strategies may include but are not limited to the following:

- CBT interventions;
- solution-focused approaches;
- problem-solving techniques;
- self-monitoring with diaries;
- psycho-education;
- regulating feelings;
- relaxation;
- anxiety management approaches;
- mindfulness;
- motivational interviewing;
- behavioural experiments;
- graded exposure techniques;
- group work;
- assertiveness;
- overcoming low self-esteem;
- coping strategy enhancement;
- distraction;
- skills rehearsal.

Meaningful activity

Meaningful activity provides a clear structure and purpose to a person's life. Activity helps to contain difficult feelings and can also be a meaningful intervention to activate mood and reduce negative symptoms. Meaningful activity centred on social participation also helps to reduce stigma and alienation, and can contribute towards building positive self-esteem and further influence resilience and coping strategies. This may include the following approaches:

- scheduling pleasant activities;
- ward diversional activities;
- behavioural activation approaches;
- group work;
- community meetings;
- leisure clubs;
- gardening;
- occupational therapy groups;
- community groups;
- vocational experiences;
- walking groups;
- creative writing;
- music;
- art;
- Star Wards activities;
- hobbies;
- computer games;
- interactive video games;
- discussion groups;
- exercise.

CASE STUDY 1

Gillian is a 34-year-old woman who was admitted to the inpatient unit following an overdose of 30 paracetamol tablets after drinking a bottle of vodka. Gillian has a small but close circle of friends. She is an only child and lives with her parents, who are very concerned about her. She works in a local factory as a production assistant, she has no current relationship and prior to her admission her social life mainly consisted of going out with her friends to local pubs and nightclubs. The main trigger for her overdose was being asked by a friend to make a false statement about a work colleague's behaviour, which Gillian refused to do, and this resulted in her friend taking an overdose, for which Gillian felt responsible. Since admission to the ward, progress has been slow and Gillian has found it difficult to engage with her care plan, stating that if she leaves the ward she will kill herself, resulting in anxiety among the multidisciplinary team and also a therapeutic impasse for Gillian. A risk formulation is provided in Table 34.2.

Formulation

With regard to the maintaining factors, Gillian currently finds it difficult to move forward, and this is linked to being blamed for not complying with her friend's request to make a false statement, and the fact that she was made to feel responsible for her friend taking an overdose. This may have compounded her low self-esteem associated with her being overweight and being bullied at school for this. Gillian's self-worth appears to depend upon what others think of her, and she uses alcohol whilst at home to manage her emotional arousal, but this also puts her in vulnerable situations. According to Gillian, she was sexually assaulted while drunk on two occasions, and she states that she does not wish to be alive. Gillian is currently not able to fully engage with her care plan. Due to these factors she is currently avoiding leaving the ward and re-engaging with her life, as she perceives that she is unable to cope with her feelings. Gillian's

Table 34.2 Summary of risk and protective factors

Triggers	Predisposing factors
• Concerns about being asked by a friend to make a false statement • Feeling responsible for a friend's suicide attempt • Recurrent negative thoughts about being blamed for the above • Not being trusted by family members to keep herself safe at home, which led to her admission to the ward • Alcohol abuse (56 to 90 units per week as evidenced by the Psychiatric Liaison nurse report; this increased to 100 units in 2012, according to Gillian) • Suicide attempts have occurred at night time, around 10pm	• Being bullied at school when overweight ('massive', in Gillian's words) • Previous self-harm in the form of cutting herself with a razor to help her feel her emotions • Alcohol abuse and putting herself in vulnerable situations • Rupture in her relationships with friends • Feelings of low self-worth, where worth depends upon what people think of Gillian • Core beliefs involve evaluating herself as a 'fat, disgusting, waste of space', which can affect her mood and result in her feeling angry, sad and frustrated, and increase her drinking and isolation from others • Gillian reports being sexually assaulted on two occasions in the past 3 years
Protective factors	**Maintaining factors**
• Being in hospital • Support of family • Support of friends who visit the ward	• Alcohol abuse/misuse • Being on close observations • Remaining in hospital • Fear of meeting friends when out of the ward and avoidance of going home • Emotional avoidance and seeking help from others • Avoidance of leaving the ward • Limited collaboration and engagement in treatment plans

CASE STUDY 1 (continued)

behaviour is one of attachment to the ward and an avoidance of acknowledging and working on her problems by maintaining her dependence by being an inpatient. During the past 2 months she has made one attempt to kill herself by placing a ligature around her neck.

Model of protective factors

Enhancing control. It is useful for Gillian to identify the areas that she is able to control and let go of the areas she is unable to control. For example, she is unable to control how others think about her, but able to exert control over her own behaviours (such as testifying in court). Therefore letting go of past evaluations of others and concentrating on her own strengths would be useful. Use of a responsibility pie chart is helpful to facilitate this process.

Relationships and respect. Developing a wider range of supportive social relationships will increase recovery and reduce suicidal thinking, but this is difficult to achieve due to her being in hospital. Action: work with her parents to gradually increase time out of the ward and refer her to an occupational therapist and independent sector agency to increase social activity. Liaise with her employers about support for going back to work.

Resilience and coping strategies. Skills and strategies to develop resilience should be developed by enabling Gillian to regulate her feelings and tolerate discomfort. Mindfulness meditation is helpful in this area, as is use of the sensory room equipment. Use of behavioural experiments could help Gillian re-evaluate her feelings about leaving the ward and allay concerns that others will always criticize her. Also discussed with Gillian was the possibility of working with a psychotherapist as a long-term strategy to facilitate her ongoing recovery.

Meaningful activity. Opportunities to undertake regular activity which provides achievement and pleasure, and acts as a container for emotional reactions, are currently limited for Gillian due to her being in hospital. Action: work with an activity coordinator to engage in an individual activity plan to help activate her mood and also look at activities out of hospital, for example, attending the gym of which Gillian is a member.

Commentary

In developing the above case formulation, it was important to involve Gillian within the process. As mentioned, Gillian was initially reluctant to participate in the planning process, due to her fear and anxiety associated with leaving hospital, with the prospect of meeting her former colleagues and friends who made her feel scared, vulnerable and sad. Following a collaborative and structured model initially focusing on facts – for example triggers, type of overdose, consequences of overdose – Gillian was able to participate and elaborate her feelings associated with the events which led to her admission to the ward. Through a psycho-educational approach using cognitive behaviour therapy, Gillian was able to identify and acknowledge the links between her physiological arousal patterns, thoughts and behaviours, and understand the safety behaviours associated with the ongoing inpatient stay. This was like a vicious circle – the longer she stayed in hospital, the more anxious she became about leaving the ward, and the more her suicidal thoughts would increase. Gillian began to understand that the function of her suicidal thoughts was to protect her from feeling anxious. This was gradually substituted for graded leave periods from the ward with staff and family members, which enabled Gillian to reconceptualize the possible consequences of discomfort rather than the inevitability that she would meet her friends, or that they would criticize and reject her. With increased practice, Gillian's confidence and resilience improved to the extent that she was able to go on overnight leave and then weekend leave; eventually she was discharged. This was achieved through the development of a therapeutic relationship built upon mutual trust, the participation and involvement of Gillian, acknowledgement of the emotional context of Gillian's difficulties, the setting of clearly constructed collaborative goals and a joint reconceptualization of the graded leave periods, together with practical skills in emotional regulation through cognitive restructuring and graded exposure and problem solving associated with practical issues. A more in-depth analysis of the craft of caring for an individual who self-harms can be found in chapter 22, and for an individual who is suicidal in chapter 23.

BARRIERS TO SERVICE USER COLLABORATION IN THE ACUTE SETTING

Acute inpatient wards, by their very nature, can seem busy and focused more on task completion than on providing person-centred care. This can pose significant challenges to the craft of caring. The development of a sound therapeutic relationship in an acute inpatient setting can be negatively influenced by a range of factors, for example the sudden and unpredictable increased acuity of service users on the ward, which can result in staff interventions being directed to providing containment strategies, such as observation and restraint. Other factors which can interrupt therapeutic relationships can include staff availability, reliance on the use of agency and bank staff, and the burden of paperwork, which can hinder therapeutic engagement with service users.

Despite these external influences on the mental health nurse's attempts to develop therapeutic relationships, it is also important to acknowledge the internal cognitive factors of the mental health nurse which may also influence these attempts. While I was observing practice in the acute inpatient ward, I was struck by the ways in which mental health nursing staff explained service user behaviours. For example, when a service user had engaged in self-harm, or another had returned from ward leave with signs of alcohol intoxication, this was usually explained in terms of whether the service user was in control of their behaviour and this in turn influenced the degree of empathy and warmth displayed by the nurses when discussing nursing interventions. Service users who were thought to be in control of their actions received more routine and less empathic responses from staff who subsequently attended them. Further observation and refection revealed that this was also more likely to occur in the case of those service users who were well known to services and were frequent users of the service. Nurses were also observed to express more frustration in nursing handovers when discussing the care of these service users. It was clear from these accounts that staff were categorizing service users and that these categories further influenced the therapeutic relationship.[25] These reactions of nursing staff could be explained with reference to Weiner's attributional model of helping,[26] which states that helping is dependent upon the attributional framework of the helper. In this case, the attributional framework consisted of the dimensions of controllability and stability to the individual presentation. When beliefs are embedded in a ward's culture, they become taken-for-granted assumptions and unwritten rules on how to intervene with service users. Additional commentary exploring the craft of caring in developing and maintaining therapeutic relationships can be found in chapter 3.

The craft of caring is enhanced when interventions enable staff to become more aware of these assumptions and rules, which can be uncovered through the process of reflection. Reflective capacity is a necessary precursor for effective clinical supervision. Use of a structured reflective model enables practitioners to become aware of their feelings associated with the experience of the service user who, for example, repeatedly engages in self-harm, highlighting practitioners' feelings of frustration and anxiety about how to offer helpful interventions. Further guided exploration aimed at understanding the service user's experiences may identify that they have had a series of traumatic early experiences, characterized by intense feelings of hopelessness and abandonment by others, and that self-harm is a way of communicating their distress to others and also a way of connecting to others. The nurse can use this information to plan new interventions of showing concern and warmth when assisting the service user with her wounds. Such unconditional and non-judgemental positions are important for building trust and open up new possibilities to relate with the service user.

The use of a structured clinical supervision model enables the team to develop a formulation of the service user's needs,[27] and this will usually identify the presenting issues – for example, self-harming behaviours, thoughts and beliefs, emotional reaction of the service users, relationships with others, and high-risk behaviours such as suicide attempts. This will also help to identify the frequency, intensity and duration of the thoughts, feelings and behaviours, and the circumstances in which they occur. Reflection and clinical supervision are therefore important tools to enable the mental health nurse to become more self-aware, to obtain feedback from others and to critically examine taken-for-granted assumptions to enhance their craft of caring for service users.

The case formulation should also explore the relationship between the individual's thoughts, feelings and behaviours, obtained from the assessment. For example, the triggers for self-harm may include occasions when the individual has been out with friends and compares self to others, after conflict with others, when alone, or after having seen an account of abuse on TV. This may result in thoughts of inadequacy, of not being good enough or a failure. These beliefs may give rise to feelings of overwhelming anxiety and frustration, in the form of an increased heart rate, palpitations, rapid breathing, chest pain, light-headedness and headache. The service user may further interpret this as evidence of impending loss of control, resulting in self-harming behaviour in the form of lacerations of the arms and legs, which can ensure a feeling of calm and serve to shift attention away from the distressing thoughts, images and feelings that were previously present. A useful model to use here is the cognitive model of Padesky and Mooney,[28] which explains the relationship between environmental factors and resulting cognitions, physical sensations and emotional and behavioural reactions.

An effective case formulation should also identify the links between past experiences and the here-and-now presentation. While much attention has been given to early traumatic experiences, it is important to remember that such experiences are painful for the service user to disclose and may not therefore be forthcoming. However, as part of a trauma-informed culture of care, it is important to 'ask the question', as it imparts to the service user that the team understands the relationship between previous trauma and current experience, and allows permission for the service user to approach nursing staff later and disclose any aspect of their previous experience(s). The role of nursing staff during any disclosure is to utilize their therapeutic skills of active listening, empathizing and providing non-judging support during the process, with signposting to other services, such as psychotherapy.

An effective case formulation will also help to explain to the team the factors which predispose the individual service user's vulnerability to their mental health crisis, as well as the precipitating factors in the here and now. The formulation will show the prolonging factors and, taken as a whole, will provide opportunities to intervene with the service user. The interventions may be given in terms of a therapeutic modality, for example from cognitive behavioural (chapter 40), psychodynamic (chapter 42) or systemic perspectives, but need to support service user recovery. The case formulation should be developed and shared with the service user and carers (subject to consent), and can be an effective platform for moving care forward, particularly when service users, carers and staff feel that the current care plan has reached an impasse.

> ## REFLECTION
>
> How are case formulations utilized in your practice with complex presentations? What is the mental health nurse's role in the case formulation process? What additional resources does the team need to enhance this area of care? How is the case formulation recorded in the care programme approach?

CONCLUSION

The service user who presents in acute distress will use acute inpatient mental health services at times of crisis to stabilize their distress, and to further promote their recovery in a community setting when it is safe to do so and at the earliest opportunity. This is important to maintain links within their local community and also to reduce the likelihood of stigmatizing beliefs from others. While the therapeutic milieu of adult acute inpatient wards has seen much transformation by way of service-user-focused and academic practice development initiatives, there remain concerns about the use of restrictive practices such as observation, restraint and as required medication. Utilizing strengths-based and trauma-informed care frameworks can facilitate the mental health nurse and colleagues to reflect on and question the impact of such interventions on the pathway to recovery for service users in acute distress. Such approaches will also optimize the craft of caring within adult acute inpatient wards and enhance the service user experience.

SERVICE USER COMMENTARY

Angus describes so accurately the issues and dynamics most clearly at play on mental health wards. After 12 years of a punishing mental illness (the dreaded borderline personality disorder), quite a few admissions (mainly voluntary!) and 10 years of running Star Wards, I've concluded that there is one over-arching factor that should be uppermost in people's minds – self-esteem: how good, or otherwise, people feel about themselves.

For service users, being on a ward is of course a time of great darkness, and most of us are feeling seriously crap about ourselves, our lives, and probably about being in hospital, especially if we've been sectioned. Making substantial, sustainable changes while in hospital is highly ambitious but small things can really help, brighten the moment and perhaps set things on a better trajectory. Arguably everything that happens (activities, conversations, care planning, therapy) should be in the context of what is most likely to have a positive effect on people's sense of self-worth. Wards are super-creative about this, whether it's generous, hand-created Welcome Bags[29] or recognizing how hard it is for us to be separated from family and pets and making thoughtful arrangements to keep us connected.

One of the most memorable experiences for me was a quiet, gentle, highly empathetic nurse who promised to come and say goodbye before the end of her shift as I was leaving the next day. When 10pm came and she didn't, I recognized that the ward was so busy and she'd got so much on her mind that it just wasn't possible. But at 10.15 – there she was! This made a disproportionate difference to me and to how I felt she valued our relationship, my recovery and indeed me.

There aren't many jobs tougher than working on a mental health ward. Staff are heroic – selfless, stoic, skilled. Saintly, frankly. But it's inescapable that many are inadequately supported, especially health care assistants (HCAs). A recent *Guardian* blog[30] expressed this perfectly: 'It's a cruel paradox that HCAs spend the most time out of all health professionals with patients, but have the least amount of training and supervision. We must, and can, do much more

to value HCAs and to invest in them.' We developed Ward Stars[31] as a professional development and validation scheme for HCAs, but the single most important thing is for managers (and colleagues and when possible service users and visitors) to notice and express appreciation. Thinking: 'Wow. That was very thoughtful of Ania' is a good start, but it needs to be conveyed to Ania. A simple 'thank you!' makes a big difference.[32]

When service users feel better about ourselves, we are more open to doing other stuff that will help our recovery. As leadership guru and enthusiastic Star Wards supporter Henry Stewart says: 'People work best when they feel good about themselves.'[33] Simple acts of appreciation by others are the ultimate gift – and sustainable even in times of financial crisis!

REFLECTION

Coproduction involves service users in the delivery of training and education programmes. How are service user experiences and stories utilized in the training and education of inpatient staff? What areas of training would benefit from this approach? How would coproduction influence the value base for interventions and the craft of caring for mental health nurses?

References

1. Department of Health. *Mental health policy implementation guide: adult acute inpatient care provision*. London: Department of Health, 2005.

2. Rethink Mental Illness. *Behind closed doors: acute mental health care in the UK: the current state and future vision of acute mental health care in the UK*. London: Rethink Mental Illness, 2004.

3. Cutcliffe JR, Barker P. Considering the care of the suicidal client and the case for 'engagement and inspiring hope' or 'observations'. In: Cutliffe J, Ward M (eds). *Key debates in psychiatric/mental health nursing*. Edinburgh: Elsevier, 2006: 142–256.

4. Ward M, Jones J. Close observations: the scapegoat of mental health care? In: Cutliffe J, Ward M (eds). *Key debates in psychiatric/mental health nursing*. Edinburgh: Elsevier, 2006: 257–71.

5. Pilgrim D. *Key concepts in mental health*, 3rd edn. London: Sage; 2014.

6. MIND. *Listening to experience: an independent inquiry into acute and crisis mental healthcare*. London: MIND, 2011.

7. Bonney S, Stickley T. Recovery and mental health: a review of the British literature. *Journal of Psychiatric and Mental Health Nursing* 2008; **15**: 140–53.

8. Commission for Healthcare Audit and Inspection. *The pathway to recovery: a review of NHS acute inpatient mental health services*. London: Commission for Healthcare Audit and Inspection, 2008.

9. Star Wards. Available from: www.starwards.org.uk [Accessed 5th August 2016].

10. Royal College of Psychiatrists. *Standards for acute inpatient services for working-age adults – 5th edition*. London: Royal College of Psychiatrists, 2014.

11. Blofeld J. *Independent inquiry into the death of David Bennett*. Cambridge: Norfolk, Suffolk and Cambridgeshire Strategic Health Authority, 2003.

12. Pope-Smith A. Winterbourne View – a compendium of key findings, recommendations and actions. Dudley Metropolitan Council, 2012. Available from: http://www.2gether.nhs.uk/files/Winterbourne_View[1].pdf [Accessed 5th August 2016].

13. MIND. *Mental health crisis care: physical restraint in crisis*. London: MIND, 2012.

14. Department of Health. *Positive and proactive care: reducing the need for restrictive interventions*. London: Department of Health, 2014.

15. Bowers L. Safewards: a new model of conflict and containment on psychiatric wards. *Journal of Psychiatric and Mental Health Nursing* 2014; **21**(6): 499–508.

16. Champagne T, Stromberg N. Sensory approaches in inpatient psychiatric settings: innovative alternatives to seclusion and restraint. *Journal of Psychosocial Nursing and Mental Health Services* 2004; **42**(9): 34–44.

17. Sutton D, Nicholson E. *Sensory modulation in acute mental health wards: a qualitative study of staff and service user perspectives*. Auckland, New Zealand: Te Pou o Te Whakaaro Nui, 2011.

18. Regan K. Trauma informed care on an inpatient pediatric psychiatric unit and the emergence of ethical dilemmas as nurses evolved their practice. *Issues in Mental Health Nursing* 2010; **31**(3): 216–22.

19. Harner H, Burgess AW. Using a trauma-informed framework to care for incarcerated women. *Journal of Obstetric, Gynecologic and Neonatal Nursing* 2011; **40**(4): 469–76.

20. Muskett C. Trauma-informed care in inpatient mental health settings: a review of the literature. *International Journal of Mental Health Nursing* 2014; **23**(1): 51–9.

21. Frueh BC, Knapp RG, Cusack KJ, Grubaugh AL, Sauvageot JA, Cousins VC, Yim E, Robins CS, Monnier J, Hiers TG. Special

section on seclusion and restraint: patients' reports of traumatic or harmful experiences within the psychiatric setting. *Psychiatric Services* 2005; **56**(9): 1123–33.

22. Azeem MW, Aujla A, Rammerth M, Binsfeld G, Jones RB. Effectiveness of six core strategies based on trauma informed care in reducing seclusions and restraints at a child and adolescent psychiatric hospital. *Journal of Child and Adolescent Psychiatric Nursing* 2011; **24**(1): 11–15.
23. Department of Health. *Best practice in managing risk*. London: DH, 2007.
24. National Mental Health Development Unit. *The mental wellbeing impact assessment toolkit*. London: NMHDU, 2010.
25. Forsyth A. The effects of diagnosis and non-compliance attributions on therapeutic alliance processes in adult acute psychiatric settings. *Journal of Psychiatric and Mental Health Nursing* 2007; **14**(1): 33–40.
26. Weiner B. *Judgments of responsibility: a foundation for a theory of social conduct*. New York: Guilford Press, 1995.
27. Persons JB. *The case formulation approach to cognitive-behavior therapy*. London: Guildford Press, 2012.

28. Padesky CA, Mooney KA. Clinical tip: presenting the cognitive model to clients. *International Cognitive Therapy Newsletter* 1990; **6**: 13–14.
29. Arriving and leaving. *Wardipedia*. Available from: http://www.wardipedia.org/37-arriving-and-leaving/ [Accessed 4th June 2016].
30. Anonymous. We healthcare assistants are the least trained but most hands-on NHS staff. *Guardian* Healthcare Network blog. 2015. http://www.theguardian.com/healthcare-network/2015/mar/12/healthcare-assistant-nhs-mental-health-patients [Accessed 29th November 2016].
31. Ward Stars. Available from: www.wardstars.org [Accessed 4th June 2016].
32. Appreciative culture. *Wardipedia*. Available from: http://www.wardipedia.org/34-appreciative-culture/ [Accessed 4th June 2016].
33. Stewart H. People work best when they feel good about themselves. Available from: http://happymanifesto.com/resources/henry-stewart-people-work-best-when-they-feel-good-about-themselves/ [Accessed 4th June 2016].

Further reading

Allen JG. *Traumatic relationships and serious mental disorders*. Chichester: Wiley, 2001.
Callaghan P, Playle J (eds). *Mental health nursing skills*. Oxford: Oxford University Press, 2009.
Gross JJ. *Handbook of emotional regulation*, 2nd edn. New York: Guilford Press, 2015.

Pilgrim D, McCranie A. *Recovery and mental health: a critical sociological account*. Basingstoke: Palgrave McMillan, 2013.
Weinstein J. *Mental health, service user involvement and recovery*. London: Jessica Kingsley, 2010.

Relevant web pages

Happy Manifesto. http://www.happy.co.uk/the-happy-manifesto-10-steps-to-a-great-workplace/
This website provides key strategies to enhance the workplace to increase staff well-being.
Safewards. http://www.safewards.net/
This website provides further information and resources on the conflict and containment model.

Sensory modulation. http://www.ot-innovations.com/content/view/29/58/
This website provides a comprehensive literature review and resources for developing sensory approaches in mental health settings.

35 What does the recovery approach really mean?

JULIE REPPER AND RACHEL PERKINS

LEARNING OUTCOMES

- To be able to define recovery from the perspective of people using services.
- To understand the ways in which personal recovery differs from clinical recovery.
- To be aware of ways in which services can support the recovery of the people they support.
- To be able to consider changes you can make to your own role to improve the recovery focus of your own practice.
- To appreciate the various approaches and interventions that help to inspire hope, enable people to take back control of their lives, and facilitate access to opportunities.
- To be able to explore the ways in which you can implement a rights-based approach in your own practice.

SUMMARY OF KEY POINTS

- Recovery is user-defined, and it is difficult to arrive at a universal definition of a process that is individually determined.
- The experience of recovery results in changing expectations of services and of self.
- Mental health workers can support people in their recovery by:
  - using their own lived and life experience in their practice;
  - changing the balance of power in their relationships with people facing mental health challenges;
  - inspiring hope in the people they support and a belief in their own potential;
  - facilitating control over life, mental health challenges and in keeping themselves well through personal recovery planning, recovery education, joint crisis planning, collaborative care planning and negotiated safety planning;
  - enabling people to access opportunities to do the things they want to do in life; taking a social disability and rights approach;
  - identifying barriers to these opportunities and focusing on providing the adjustments and supports that will enable people to overcome these barriers and do what they want to do, rather than focusing on what they can do without support.

INTRODUCTION

The term 'recovery' has been used in health services for many years. It has traditionally referred to the restoration of functioning, an eradication of symptoms and a return to a former state of health. However, towards the end of the last century, people diagnosed with psychiatric conditions reclaimed the term and redefined it to refer to their own circumstances and experiences. Hence they objected to professionals' negative prognoses and pessimism about their chances of recovery. They claimed that recovery was an alien concept in mental health services, and a term rarely used by professionals in relation to people who have serious mental health problems.[1] Instead they proclaimed their right to recovery of a meaningful life even in the continued presence of symptoms; they demonstrated that they can achieve control over their own lives and destinies[2] by both minimizing the deleterious effects of the condition on their own lives *and* campaigning against the social and political barriers (prejudice, discrimination and marginalization) that have even more disabling effects upon their life chances.[3]

It is not surprising that the redefinition of a familiar term has led to some confusion about the meaning of recovery. Nor is it surprising that recovery has come to mean all things to all people, as new treatments and approaches are claimed to effect 'recovery' by reducing symptoms,[4] while empowering approaches are equally heralded as recovery-focused by virtue of their impact on people's confidence and social relationships.[5] Professionals, seeking to respond to the wishes and preferences of those using services, have renamed their services as recovery teams; professional training courses now profess to teach recovery; pharmaceutical companies report on their success in achieving recovery … and people who themselves are striving towards their own recovery are once again finding that professionals are defining recovery for them and many are understandably protesting against this.[6] Pilgrim and McCranie[7] have written a comprehensive sociological critique of recovery and mental health, drawing attention to the various definitions of recovery, the different meanings attached to it, the potential for it to appear unrealistically optimistic and the problems associated with its individualized and subjective nature. Deegan[8] offers a response to such an appraisal:

Perhaps the phenomenon is elusive precisely because it is so fundamental. Perhaps it is because the recovery process cannot be described with traditional scientific, psychiatric, or psychological language. Although the phenomenon will not fit neatly into natural scientific paradigms, those of us who have been disabled know that recovery is real because we have experienced it. (p.12)

This chapter will explore what recovery means to those diagnosed with a psychiatric condition and consider the ways in which people working in mental health services can support their journeys of recovery by inspiring hope, enabling them to take back control, and facilitating access to opportunities to achieve their life goals.

WHAT DO PEOPLE WITH MENTAL HEALTH CONDITIONS MEAN BY RECOVERY?

The concept of Recovery refers primarily to a person … reclaiming his or her right to a safe, dignified and personally meaningful and gratifying life in the community … It emphasises self-determination and such normal life pursuits as education, employment, sexuality, friendship, spirituality and voluntary membership in faith and other kinds of communities beyond the limits of both disorder and the mental health system and consistent with the person's own values, preferences and goals.[9] (p.464)

This is a useful description of what recovery means that does not fall into the trap of offering a universal definition. The meaning of recovery differs from person to person and changes over time, because those things that are valuable or meaningful differ both across individuals and across time. When a number of people on an acute ward where we work were asked what recovery meant to them, they replied with a range of answers, including:

- 'When life doesn't hurt any more'
- 'When I think I might be happy one day'
- 'When I can go out on my own'
- 'When I can sleep at night'
- 'When I feel able to see my friends again'.

People further along in their recovery journey, employed as peer support workers in the same service as those above, were asked the same question and replied in different ways:

- 'Being in work and feeling that I am contributing something.'
- 'Being able to manage my own condition and knowing when to ask for help.'
- 'Living with my partner with a child was always my dream of recovery. Now I have got there but I realise that I find life a lot harder than many other people.'
- 'Just when I think I am truly recovered and can manage all of my symptoms well enough, another sort of experience knocks me off my feet and I realise this journey will go on for ever.'

What do people with mental health conditions mean by recovery?

35

Perhaps the most commonly quoted definition of recovery was written by Bill Anthony[10] in a paper that synthesized the core elements of survivor narratives of recovery:

> *Recovery is a deeply personal, unique process of changing one's attitudes, values, feelings, goals, skills and/or roles. It is a way of living a satisfying, hopeful, and contributing life even with limitations caused by the illness. Recovery involves the development of new meaning and purpose in one's life as one grows beyond the catastrophic effects of mental illness. (p.15)*

Anthony[10] captures the personal nature of recovery reflected in the quotations from individuals listed above. However, this personal journey is not one travelled alone: it occurs within a social and political context. Anthony's definition lacks the reference to rights that is present in Davidson's[9] description, and ignores the reality of the prejudice, discrimination and exclusion that can have such a significant impact on our journeys. However, Anthony does refer to a change of attitude, values and feelings. This shift is part of the process of moving towards recovery.

REFLECTION

Think back to an event in your own life that was distressing, shocking or saddening.

- How did you feel at that time?
- How did your feelings change over time?
- What helped you to understand what had happened?
- What helped you to rebuild your confidence?
- How did this affect your own self-belief, your ambitions and your relationships?

You have just reflected on your own experience of recovery. You will find that some of your own experiences will concur with those of the people you support. This should not be surprising. We are all human beings, and we share needs, emotions, responses and ambitions. Recovery is a shared experience and drawing on our own experiences will help us to work in a more empathic, humanistic, reflective manner.

Our own experiences of what has been diagnosed as mental illness are reflected in the accounts of many others. When these disturbances first begin, they are often frightening, shocking and isolating. It is hard to believe that anyone else could have felt the same way, and it is impossible to articulate what is happening to you and how it makes you feel. On the one hand you are afraid that others will instantly know that you are 'mad' and judge you as such; on the other hand, they may just normalize your experiences, minimizing feelings that are terrifying and very different from anything you have felt before. There is a period of time when you question how others who have experienced similar feelings have managed to cope with them or even survive them. You try to deny them, find ways of coping, pretend that you are all right, or avoid contact with others. If things become utterly unbearable, either you or people close to you are likely to seek help from 'expert professionals' – people whom you believe (or hope) will be able to make things better. Having sought solutions in clinical treatment, you then wait for these to 'work'. The shift that Anthony refers to (above) comes when you realize that all of the treatments and interventions offered by others come at a cost and none provides all of the answers. First, you give up, to others, the right to define your own reality. Your experience is reduced to diagnostic and symptomatic labels that fail to reflect the full complexity of your experience. Second, while we may wish treatments and interventions to 'turn the clock back' – to restore us and our lives to how they used to be – this is not possible. We are changed by our experiences. While there is a way forward, there is no way back and, as most mental health conditions fluctuate, or leave us with continuing challenges, we have to, for better or worse, accept them as part of who we are. Many, if not most, of our mental health challenges fluctuate, or are, to a greater or lesser extent, ever present. We grow as much from the bad things that happen to us as from the good things. Third, there may well be unwanted and distressing side effects from some treatments. Fourth, the situation that triggered the problem in the first place is still there (for example, difficult relationships, unresolved trauma, grief or stress), and additional challenges may be added as a consequence of becoming a 'mental patient'.

Recovery involves a change of mind-set in which you begin to make sense for yourself of what is happening, start to take responsibility for your own recovery and recognize that you have a large part to play in keeping yourself well and asserting your rights. As one woman we worked with explained:

> *It took 36 years for me to realise. I have been using mental health services since I was 6 years old and I have screamed for someone to do something. I even set fire to myself in the 136 suite because I so desperately wanted someone to help. Now I realise. I wept when the penny dropped. You can't make me better, it is only me who can do that. I have to work it out for myself.*

This sounds harsh, but ultimately it is empowering and strengthening to recognize that you can do something for yourself, that you are not entirely dependent on others' expertise, that you can work out what helps you and what makes things worse, that only you know what sort of treatment, support and experiences make you feel better. This is the beginning of recovery. As another woman we know said: 'My recovery started when I realized that the professionals did not have all the answers.'

REFLECTION

- It can be difficult to conceive of a professional role when we do not need to provide answers and solutions – yet that is what we need to do if we are to support recovery.

- How do you feel about encouraging people to make their own decisions and supporting them to implement their own decisions even if you do not agree with them?

- If you were finding your own way back into life following a crisis, would you want someone else to try to fix you (with tablets or therapy), or would you want to find out how you can manage your condition (including treatment) so that you can play a larger part in keeping yourself well?

Too often the negative images that are present in wider society are reinforced within mental health services where the dominant narratives are of deficit and dysfunction, risk, fading life chances and rigid boundaries between 'them' and 'us', the 'staff' and 'patients', the 'mad' and the 'sane'.

[E]ven the briefest perusal of the current literature on schizophrenia [shows] … that this collection of problems is viewed by practitioners almost exclusively in terms of dysfunction and disorder. A positive or charitable phrase or sentence rarely meets the eye … Deficit-obsessed research can only produce theories and attitudes which are disrespectful of clients and are also likely to induce behaviour in clinicians such that service users are not properly listened to, not believed, not fairly assessed, are likely treated as inadequate and are also not expected to be able to become independent and competent individuals in managing life's tasks.[11] (pp.xii–xiii)

It is clear from the life of Peter Chadwick (an academic psychologist with a diagnosis of schizophrenia), and many, many other personal narratives of recovery,[12–17] that despite such stereotypes, recovery of a life that is personally valued, meaningful, contributing and satisfying is possible, even for those who continue to experience disabling cognitive and emotional problems. Such personal stories not only provide evidence of the possibility of recovery; they also provide an invaluable guide for mental health workers and mental health services seeking to support people in their recovery journey.

HOW CAN MENTAL HEALTH WORKERS SUPPORT PEOPLE IN THEIR RECOVERY?

The first principal of a recovery-focused approach is the recognition that we, as mental health workers, cannot 'do' recovery; we can only support people in their journey. This means that, just as people experiencing mental health problems have to recognize that they can take more responsibility for their own well-being, mental health workers have to shift their position from 'fixer' or 'expert' to supporter or resource. That is not to say that mental health workers are redundant. We may have many different tools and strategies that could be helpful, but rather than using these as we see fit to achieve our goals, we need to make these available for the person we are supporting to use as they wish, to achieve their own goals. Thus, a recovery-focused approach is not about a professional expert and a passive recipient, but about a relationship between two experts. One is an expert through professional training and experience, and the other is an expert through personal experience.

This egalitarian relationship begs questions about our role in caring for people. We contend that promoting recovery is about mental health professionals respecting, empowering, supporting and ultimately enabling people rather than caring for them. As professionals, we should aim to care about them as fellow human beings, as people with whom we share emotional experiences, and so have empathy; we may have ideas and expertise in approaches and strategies which could help them; we may have understanding of their vulnerability, distress and disability. However, what we do with this is less about a craft of caring than about demonstrating compassion (defined as 'shared suffering' rather than 'pity for the misfortunes of others') and inspiring them to believe in their own possibilities.

Very often, professionals have their own experience of recovery – from trauma, bereavement, physical or mental illness – and need to consider how these life experiences can be used safely and effectively in their practice. Increasingly, services are employing people who have used mental health services as peer workers who are trained to use their own experiences explicitly to support others facing similar challenges. Evidence suggests that this brings significant benefits to the peer workers themselves, to the people whom they support, and to the culture of the services in which they work.[18,19] It appears that the most important characteristics of the peer-to-peer relationship are reciprocity, mutuality and hope – a recognition that recovery is possible ('if they can do it then it must at least be possible for me'). This begs questions about the role of professionals and the nature of their relationships with

How can mental health workers support people in their recovery?

35

those whom they support. Hierarchies of power and divisions between 'us' and 'them' need to be broken down if people are to be enabled to take back control and responsibility.

Personal recovery narratives describe the skills, qualities and characteristics of mental health workers and approaches that people find useful, and thus they offer the key to providing effective recovery-focused support. Leamy et al.[20] systematically reviewed 97 papers to identify five processes that are fundamental in recovery:

1. *Connectedness* – the importance of relationships and social support (including support from others who have similar experiences), and being part of the community;
2. *Hope and optimism about the future* – believing in the possibility of recovery and having the motivation to take on the challenge; having dreams and aspirations and valuing personal achievements;
3. *Identity* – overcoming stigma and discrimination, rebuilding and/or redefining a positive sense of identity;
4. *Meaning in life* – rebuilding a meaningful and valued life with social goals and roles, understanding and finding meaning in what has happened – often with reference to spirituality;
5. *Empowerment* – taking personal responsibility and control over life, focusing on strengths and assets.

REFLECTION

Think about these five characteristics of recovery and consider their importance in your own life:

- *Connectedness.* How important is it for you to have friends who have similar views to your own?

- *Hope.* Do you generally believe that your life brings possibilities and opportunities?

- *Identity.* Who are you? What do you do? What do you believe in? Are you satisfied with the answers to these questions? Do you feel your identity is important to you?

- *Meaning.* Do you feel there is a point to your life? Do you make a difference? Do you have ambition?

- *Empowerment.* Can you make changes in your own life? Can you make your views heard?

Once again, reflection on these points draws attention to the similarities between those of us who have experience of mental distress and those who do not. At the core of our relationships with people we support is our shared humanity.

Repper and Perkins[3] drew on personal experiences and accounts of recovery to identify three inter-related components that are critical: hope, control and opportunity/participation. These constructs are now widely used in recovery documentation and policy in various countries around the world, and they explicitly embrace the processes identified by Leamy et al.[20]

First, *hope* – the belief that things will get better, that a meaningful life is possible, lays the foundation for recovery.

> *The turning point in my life was ... where I started to get hope. Dr. Charles believed that I could. And Rev Goodwin believed that I could. Certain people believed that I could ... and held that belief even when I didn't believe in myself.[21] (p.75)*

It is hard to believe in yourself when you are finding everyday activities so difficult; it is hard to believe in a future when feelings of distress are overwhelming; it is incredibly difficult to take on the challenge of recovery if you cannot see a possibility of improvement and all the messages you receive from others are of doom and gloom. The challenge for mental health workers, while recognizing the enormity of the challenges facing the person, is both to hold on to the belief that recovery is possible for everyone, and to inspire that same belief in the person themselves.

> *Hope is at the heart of recovery. Just as the person must hold on to hope in the journey of recovery, the practitioner must hold onto hope that recovery-orientated system change is possible and powerful.[22] (p.10)*

Second, taking back *control* is essential for the person to have an active role in their recovery. This involves them recognizing their own skills and resources, sources of meaning and value, and using these to manage their condition and building on them in order to achieve their ambitions and dreams.

> *To me, recovery means I try to stay in the driver's seat of my life. I don't let my illness run me. Over the years I have worked hard to become an expert in my own self-care.[23] (p.10)*

The role of the mental health worker lies in helping a person to make sense of what has happened, grieve for what they have lost and begin to move forward with their life; inspiring confidence by pointing out their abilities, skills, experience and resources; helping them to develop ways of coping so that they are ready to take back control.

Taking back control is not confined to managing symptoms. Recovery is about rebuilding a meaningful life, so the person also needs to be supported to identify their own ambitions, to think about the steps needed to achieve these and the sort of help they would like, to ensure they have the best chance of succeeding.

Third, having access to *opportunities* to do the things you want to do in life is essential for recovery. Citizenship – access to those opportunities that all citizens have a right to expect – is central to everyone's identity. This includes being a valued member of their communities, having access to the opportunities that exist in those communities and having the opportunity to contribute to those communities. Being able to give – to do things for others – is critical in fostering self-worth and well-being and connecting people to their communities. If mental health workers are to facilitate access to opportunities, they need to see their role extending beyond services and into the world of the people whom they support; helping them to access roles, relationships, activities and resources that exist in their neighbourhood so that they can achieve their own goals; facilitating access to material resources including benefits, wages, housing and reasonable living facilities; and helping them to maintain the roles and relationships that they value as well as developing new ones.

WHAT DOES ALL THIS MEAN FOR PRACTITIONERS?

How can mental health workers inspire hope?

It is perhaps easier to think of all the things that we might do to diminish hope, such as focusing on the person's problems and deficits, telling them what they should not do, that this will be a long process, or that they are very ill, or expecting them to fit into existing routines and block rules on an inpatient ward (for example, no phones or personal radios being allowed for 3 days after admission, all bedrooms being locked between 9am and 5pm, only being allowed outside when a member of staff is available, no hot drinks being allowed after midnight). If we are to inspire them to believe in their own possibilities, we need to value them for who they are, the challenges they face and what they have to offer.

We need to see and have confidence in their skills, abilities and potential. We need to ask them how we can help them, what we can do so that they feel safe. We need to listen carefully to their experiences and demonstrate that we have heard them; we need to believe what they say they are feeling. We have the challenge of demonstrating that we appreciate how bad they feel now and at the same time show them that we believe that things will get better. We need to accept and appreciate that their ideas, goals and feelings might change, and that they may have setbacks but these can serve to help them work out what they are ready to take on and what might be a step too far at the moment.

The importance of focusing on the person's strengths, interests and potential rather than their problems is illustrated by a mother speaking of her son's progress:

In the old days, David's life consisted of sitting and staring into space, chain smoking, walking a lot, listening to his beloved folk music and coming home for dinner once a week. Today he still smokes and walks a lot, but he also works at a restaurant for an hour a day, gets himself to a clubhouse for lunch every day, and has learned to ride buses so that he can get to his music and pottery lessons each week … I do not believe these changes came about because of the possibility for schizophrenia to improve over the years. Nor do I believe that the newer medications played a role, since he had been taking them for many years before these positive changes occurred. David's changes came about rather quickly when professionals and family members began to focus on his considerable strengths instead of his illness … In the old days the emphasis was on his treatment, aside from medication, this was helping with his abysmal 'daily living skills' – helping him to learn to ride the buses, take a shower, make eye contact and so on. But where should he go on the bus? For whom should he have a shower? With whom should he make eye contact? … this approach got nowhere. A few years ago … the psychiatrist said 'I don't want to hear all that again. That's his illness and we have not been able to change that for years. Tell me about his strengths; we would do better to work on those.'[24] (p.24)

However, inspiring hope is not just about building on strengths in order to survive; it is about growth and flourishing, and working towards the achievement of goals, aspirations and dreams. This will only be successful if the person is working towards goals that are in line with their own aspirations – not the priorities or goals of the mental health worker. Traditionally, it was believed that people must be encouraged to 'be realistic' and work towards 'achievable' goals so that they do not have to suffer the consequences of failure. One mother expressed her frustrations about this: 'Our experience of the mental health world is that expectation falls quickly into the hole of "we mustn't set him up to fail". This, like so much else, is a blanket, one size fits all, attitude which has the potential to keep everyone safely in a world of lowest common denominator'[25] (p.4).

If we are to work in genuinely respectful and collaborative relationships, then we need to support people to pursue their own goals, however ambitious they may appear. We should recognize that we are all motivated by our 'big dreams' but achieve these in 'small steps': even if the final goal is not achieved, much can be gained and learnt along the way. For example, a person who aims to go to university will first need to look into the courses available, research what qualifications are necessary and consider undertaking an access course, fill in application forms, prepare for an interview and so on. All of these activities will be valuable and may lead onto a successful university place, but if not, the person may decide to go into further education for a different type of qualification. By comparison, advising a person that they are unlikely to succeed in their ambition risks reducing their enthusiasm, motivation, confidence – and hope.

How can we enable a person to take back control?

Once again, it is not difficult to see how traditional modes of supporting people with mental health problems have sapped their confidence and reduced their sense of control over their own condition. Professionals are trained to give answers, solve problems, prescribe treatment and provide a cure. Patients are socialized into believing that when they are feeling bad they should turn to an expert for advice, help and treatment. The problem is that this erodes their belief in the possibility of their management of their own condition or their own life. If they do not understand what is happening or why it might be happening, then they may well start to avoid taking any risks in life in the fear that symptoms may re-occur or worsen. If they have no idea how their own behaviour and decisions impact on their well-being, then they can neither reduce the likelihood of setbacks, nor change behaviours quickly when early signs are occurring. It can all feel very frightening and out of control.

At the heart of recovery-focused relationships is genuine 'shared decision making'. This is a process in which the person receiving support and the practitioner work collaboratively, bringing together the expertise and experience of both of them, accessing further evidence if they wish, to come to a decision that meets the person's preferences. In this way people are given the information and support that they need to take control (see chapter 50 for more on collaborative care planning). Shared decision making is formally defined by the King's Fund Foundation for Informed Medical Decision Making as:

> *a process in which clinicians and patients work together to select tests, treatments, management or support packages, based on clinical evidence and the patient's informed preferences. It involves the provision of evidence-based information about options, outcomes and uncertainties, together with decision support counselling and a system for recording and implementing patients' informed preferences.*[26] *(p.vii)*

Most research into shared decision making has focused on treatment decisions in relation to medication, where it is reported to result in greater treatment engagement, higher satisfaction with services and better quality decision making.[27] However, the same collaborative, negotiated process is applicable to all decisions that are made with regard to a person using services. For example, it has been used in the development of joint crisis plans where the patient, their care coordinator, a psychiatrist and an intermediary carefully negotiate a plan expressing the person's wishes and preferences in case of a crisis. This process has been shown to lead to a reduction in inpatient days and significantly less likelihood of compulsory admission.[28]

Similarly, a collaborative approach can be used to develop a negotiated safety plan rather than a professionally-led risk assessment (see chapter 36 for more on risk and recovery). Traditional approaches to risk focus on professionals' views of previous negative events and current potential for harm, and expect the professional to 'manage' these risks. Person-centred safety planning starts with an evaluation of risks from the perspective of the individual and those close to them, as well as professionals. It emphasizes the strengths, resources and preferences of people with mental distress and works to enhance their capacity to develop self-directed plans to manage risk in the pursuit of valued life goals. Responsibility for promoting safety is shared between the person and the professionals: what the person can do to keep him-/herself safe and what staff can do to help. It has been shown that shared documentation and 'transparency' is possible in forensic services[29] and that a more recovery-oriented approach to risk assessment and management through negotiated safety planning can reduce the use of seclusion and restraint in crisis services.[30] Chapter 46 has more information on crisis assessment and resolution.

The Health Foundation funded a shared decision-making project in four child and adolescent mental health services, which resulted in a new approach to the conduct of all conversations from the point of first contact onwards.[31] The project reported benefits for the young people using the services as well as for staff. Young people felt a greater sense of engagement and empowerment that enriched their experience of care and allowed them to take ownership of their treatment and begin to understand the reasons behind the clinical work being done with them. Clinicians felt that the shared decision-making approach helped to make sure their interventions were meeting the needs of young people and their families. They also said that getting rapid feedback from service users became a valuable part of decision making and treatment planning. At the inpatient unit, anecdotal evidence from nurses suggested that shared decision making led to fewer incidences of aggressive behaviour.[32] The less hierarchical collaborative relationship at the heart of shared decision-making is central in recovery-focused practice. Whether developing a person-centred care plan, asking what a person wants to wear or eat, or deciding what treatment is most acceptable and effective for them and how, when and how much is preferred, everything needs to be done in such a way that the person themselves is the final arbiter in decision making whenever possible.

It is easy to accede to a person's wishes if their judgement concurs with ours; however, sometimes there are formal rules governing what we can and cannot allow the person to do (as, for example, when they are compulsorily detained or when they have been formally assessed as lacking capacity). However, even where these rules exist, we can offer maximum choice within the boundaries imposed by the rules – for example, choice about timing of leave, what time someone wants to get up in the morning, route of medication and so on.

Care plans and safety plans, developed via a process of shared decision making, should explicitly support the person to take back control over their problems and their life. One very personal tool that can be useful in enabling a person to take back control of their problems is the personal recovery plan. The personal recovery plan belongs to the individual: it can be developed without help from, or reference to, others; it is a learning plan to assist people to become experts in looking after themselves and rebuilding their lives. Mary Ellen Copeland devised the first Wellness and Recovery Action Plan (WRAP)[33] and many others have adapted it. WRAP is a format that includes:

- A list of things that the person can do to stay well and help themselves feel better: things that they enjoy doing and make them feel good, like eating well, sleeping well, exercise, seeing friends, walking, praying or being in nature.
- A daily maintenance plan which includes a description of how they are when they feel well, and a list of things they need and like to do every day to stay well.
- A list of the things that upset them or make them feel bad (triggers), such as overwork, seeing people whom they find difficult, anniversaries of sad events, getting over-tired, drinking too much alcohol, spending too much time alone, family friction or financial difficulties.
- A list of the way they feel when things are not right (early warning signs), such as feeling anxious or nervous, feeling slower or faster than usual, avoiding people, increased irritability or tearfulness. This is followed by a list of things they could do to cope with these feelings or reduce them, such as doing things that they enjoy, speaking to a close friend, making a point of reducing activity and getting to sleep early.
- A description of how they know when things are breaking down; the signs that show them that they need to take action, ask for help or change their plans, and adopt behaviours to stop things getting worse. These signs might include not sleeping for a (specified) period of time, being obsessed with negative thoughts, avoiding eating, avoiding seeing people, seeing or hearing things that are not there or suicidal thoughts. This is followed by a plan of what they can do to help themselves when things are breaking down, such as calling their care coordinator, arranging for someone to come and stay with them for a while, spending time doing relaxation or exercising each day, or taking time off work.

Copeland, who devised WRAP, describes the process whereby she took control of her own experiences by using a personal recovery plan.[34] However, while it is possible for people to develop their own recovery plan, they may well find it helpful to discuss it with others, maybe a family member or friends, or someone who has developed their own recovery plan – a peer worker, or with a mental health worker who has ideas that they might not have thought of. However, it belongs to them and they can use it, change it and develop it in the ways they find most helpful.

It should be emphasized that recovery is not just about managing your problems – it is about rebuilding your life. This has been recognized in some personal recovery plans which also include a plan for identifying and pursuing aspirations.[35]

Further approaches to enable people to take back control include self-management education or attending recovery courses at a Recovery College.[36] The goal of these educational approaches is to give the person an understanding of their condition that enables them to manage it better for themselves. Essentially, they raise confidence and competence in living with a mental health condition. Recent research into Recovery Colleges (of which 32 now exist in England alone) suggests that people attending courses benefit in other ways as well.[37] All courses bring together the expertise of professional and lived experience: they are co-produced and co-facilitated by a mental health worker and a peer trainer. Students learn from others who have been through similar struggles, and they learn alongside others who continue to face similar challenges. It is this mutual support that gives them the greatest sense of possibility. In addition, their social networks increase and they gain friends with whom they can progress to mainstream opportunities.

How can mental health workers enable people to access opportunities and participate in their communities?

A central part of supporting someone in their journey of recovery is actively helping them to explore what they want to do, access opportunities they value within their communities (such as education, employment, social or spiritual activities) and participate as valued citizens. For most of us, it is much harder to establish new roles, relationships and activities than to hold on to what we already have. This means that, from first contact with a person, the mental health worker can help by finding out what the person already does; with whom, when and where; and which of these responsibilities, activities and relationships they value. Together they can then work out how to keep these going through a crisis. This might involve thinking about who can take care of their day-to-day responsibilities; letting friends and families know what has happened – a letter, a phone call, an email, a text message (they do not need to make decisions about how much to disclose at this stage; they can just send a note to say they are unwell, until they feel able to consider what and whether to tell people about their mental health problems); cancelling appointments and engagements; sending a sick note to an employer or college; supporting people who are important to the person to understand what has happened.

Although it can be helpful to have a respite from activities and relationships during a crisis, it is important to resume roles, relationships and responsibilities as the crisis abates. Too often it is assumed that a person has to be 'fully better' to return to work, college, clubs and hobbies. The result is that all confidence is lost, the routine loses its meaning, friends drift away, jobs are lost, college courses move on and there is too much catching up to do. The reality is that the longer someone is away from something, the more difficult it is to go back. It can be helpful to start as soon as possible, perhaps by sorting out any problems caused by the crisis, saying thank you to those who helped and apologizing to those who might have borne the brunt of the person's irritability. Then it is possible to start making a plan to resume relationships and activities gradually, and think about the sort of support that might be helpful to ensure this is successful. If the person has been admitted, this process can, and should, start while they are still an inpatient.

One of the biggest challenges for mental health workers lies in encouraging, supporting and inspiring people to believe in their own possibilities and identify life goals for themselves. Various approaches can help in this (see chapter 3 for more on therapeutic relationships). Life coaching courses at the local Recovery College may be a useful way to work alongside peers over several weeks to share misgivings and generate ideas and ambitions together. Alternatively, it can be helpful to remove boundaries and encourage them to dream: what would they do if they won the lottery? What were their teenage dreams? If they were someone else, what would their ambition be? This sort of exercise can free them up from their perceptions of their own limitations and begin to make planning more fun.

There are two ways of thinking about enabling a person to access the opportunities they value and be equal citizens in their communities. Traditionally, within mental health services we have adopted what might be described as a 'clinical' approach. This focuses on promoting inclusion by changing the person so they 'fit in' via treatment, therapy, confidence building, skills training and so on. However, in the broader disability world, a 'social' approach has been adopted, combined with a rights perspective.[38–42] This focuses on changing the world so that it can accommodate the person. For example, if you have a broken spine, while clinical treatment may be important, the primary focus is not on making you able to walk again but on support and adjustments you need to be able to live a full and contributing life (a wheelchair, ramps, lower work surfaces and so on). Back in 1992, Patricia Deegan[43] argued that a similar approach might be more fruitful in the mental health arena:

> if we think about it, having a psychiatric disability is, for many of us, simply a given. The real problems exist in the form of barriers in the environment that prevent us from living, working and learning in environments of our choice … [the task is] to confront, challenge and change those barriers and to make environments accessible. If we remember that environments are not just physical places but also social and interpersonal environments, then it is clear that those of us with psychiatric disabilities face many environmental barriers that impede and thwart our efforts to live independently and gain control over our lives and the resources that affect our lives. (p.11)

Adopting a social and rights-based approach means we need to think beyond 'service land', recognizing the resources available within communities and using our skills to support both individuals and organizations in the community. In this regard, we need to ask different questions. Instead of focusing on 'what is wrong with the person', we should ask:

- What does the person value/want to do with their life?
- What are the barriers that prevent participation (social, cultural, physical; assumptions, attitudes)?
- How can we get around these barriers (providing support, making adjustments, changing expectations, breaking down prejudice, changing attitudes)?
- How can we help people to assert their rights to participation and freedom from discrimination?

INCLUSION, RIGHTS AND CITIZENSHIP

It is a social model that underpins the United Nations Convention on the Rights of Persons with Disabilities (UNCRPD) (ratified by the UK and 227 other countries) and the UK Equality Act. The UNCRPD demands a move from:

> viewing persons with disabilities as 'objects' of charity, medical treatment and social protection towards viewing persons with disabilities as 'subjects' with rights, who are capable of claiming those rights and making decisions for their lives based on their free and informed consent as well as being active members of society.[43] (p.1)

It requires that disabled people, including those facing mental health challenges, have the right to the same opportunities as other citizens (at home, at work and as members of the community) and the right to the support and adjustments (based on their own preferences and choices) that they need to participate as equal citizens. The UK Equality Act (again including people with mental health conditions) outlaws discrimination and requires the providers of goods or services (including education and employment) to make 'reasonable adjustments' to enable participation. (See chapter 67 on mental health, the law and human rights.) Reasonable adjustments in the arena of mobility and sensory impairments are widely understood: wheelchairs, ramps, hearing loops, personal assistants and so on. The question that all mental health workers and those who face mental health challenges need to explore is: what are the equivalent adjustments and supports required by people with mental health challenges? Examples might include flexible working hours, a buddy to provide support during unstructured times such as breaks and meal times, extra time or feedback, or a mentor.

Just as recovery is not about the absence of symptoms but about living well, achieving goals is not necessarily about doing things unaided but about having the support you need to do the things you want to do; success is not whether a person can manage without support but what they can manage with support.

> *Inclusion and citizenship are not about 'becoming normal' but creating inclusive communities that can accommodate all of us. Not about 'becoming independent' but having the right to support and adjustments (in line with our choices and aspirations) to ensure full and equal participation and citizenship.*[44] *(p.14)*

CONCLUSION

If we are to facilitate the recovery of people whom we support, we first have to value them as fellow human beings, as people who have the ability and the right to live meaningful, valued lives in which they receive the support that they need to do the things they want to do. At the centre of our work are the relationships that we build with people: trusting conversations in which they are given time and acceptance to work out ways of understanding what has happened

to them, explore ways in which they can begin to manage their own well-being and take back control of their lives, build up the belief that they have the potential to move forwards in the faith that someone will be there to encourage them, and help them to pick up the pieces if things do not go to plan. Essentially, we have to be prepared to work with them in ways in which we would want to be supported if we were in their position.

References

1. Coleman R. *Recovery, an alien concept.* Port of Ness: Working to Recovery, 2011.
2. Chamberlin J. *On our own.* London: Mind Publications, 1988.
3. Repper J, Perkins R. *Social inclusion and recovery: a model for mental health practice.* Edinburgh: Baillière Tindall, 2003.
4. Whitaker R. *Anatomy of an epidemic: magic bullets, psychiatric drugs, and the astonishing rise of mental illness in America.* New York: Crown Publishing Group, 2011.
5. Ryan P, Ramon S, Greacon T (eds). *Empowerment, lifelong learning and recovery in mental health towards a new paradigm.* Basingstoke: Palgrave Macmillan, 2012.
6. Rismiller DJ, Rismiller JH. Evolution of the antipsychiatry movement into mental health consumerism. *Psychiatric Services* 2006; **57**(6): 863–6.
7. Pilgrim D, McCranie A. *Recovery and mental health. A critical sociological account.* Basingstoke: Palgrave Macmillan, 2013.
8. Deegan PE. Recovery: the lived experience of rehabilitation. *Psychosocial Rehabilitation Journal* 1988; **9**(4): 11–19.
9. Davidson L, Roe D. Recovery from versus recovery in serious mental illness: one strategy for lessening confusion plaguing recovery. *Journal of Mental Health* 2007; **16**(4): 459–70.
10. Anthony WA. Recovery from mental illness: the guiding vision of the mental health service system in the 1990's. *Psychosocial Rehabilitation Journal* 1993; **16**(4): 11–23.
11. Chadwick P. *Schizophrenia: the positive perspective.* London: Routledge, 1997.
12. Lapsley H, Nikora LW, Black R. *'Kia Mauri Tau!' Narratives of recovery from disabling mental health problems.* Report of the University of Waikato Mental Health Narratives Project. Wellington, New Zealand: Mental Health Commission, 2002.
13. Brown W, Kandirikirira N. *Recovering mental health in Scotland.* Edinburgh: Scottish Recovery Network, 2007.
14. Davidson L, Lynn L. *Beyond the storms, reflections on recovery in Devon.* Exeter: Recovery Devon, 2009.
15. LeCroy CW, Holschuh J. *First person accounts of mental illness and recovery.* Oxford: John Wiley & Sons, 2012.
16. Romme M, Escher S, Dillon J, Corstens D. *Living with voices, 50 stories of recovery.* Ross-on-Wye: PCCS Books in association with Birmingham City University, 2009.
17. Adshead G. *Their dark materials: narratives and recovery in forensic practice.* London: Royal College of Psychiatrists, 2012.
18. Repper J. *Peer support workers: theory and practice.* Implementing Recovery for Organisational Change (ImROC) briefing paper 5. London: Centre for Mental Health, 2013.
19. Trachtenberg M, Parsonage M, Shepherd G, Boardman J. *Peer support in mental health care. Is it good value for money?* London: Centre for Mental Health, 2013.
20. Leamy M, Bird V, Le Boutillier CL, Williams J, Slade M. Conceptual framework for personal recovery in mental health: systematic review and narrative synthesis. *British Journal of Psychiatry* 2011; **199**: 445–52.
21. Vincent SS. Using findings from qualitative research to teach mental health professionals about the experience of recovery from psychiatric disability. In: *Proceedings of the Harvard University Graduate School of Education, 4th Annual Student research conference.* Cambridge, MA: Harvard University Press, 1999: 72–81.
22. Tondora J, Miller R, Slade M, Davidson L. *Partnering for recovery in mental health. A practical guide to person-centred planning,* Chichester: Wiley, 2014.
23. Deegan P. Recovering our sense of value after being labeled. *Journal of Psychosocial Nursing* 1993; **31**(4): 7–11.
24. Wasow M. *Coping with schizophrenia: a survival manual for parents, relatives, and friends.* Palo Alto, CA: Science & Behavior Books, 1982.

25. Scottish Recovery Network. Stories and experiences. Available from: http://www.scottishrecovery.net/stories-experiences/ [Accessed 23rd August 2016].

26. Wasow M. Strengths versus deficits or musician versus schizophrenic. *Psychiatric Services* 2001; **52**(10): 1306–7.

27. Kreyenbuhl J, Nossel IR, Dixon LB. Disengagement from mental health treatment among individuals with schizophrenia and strategies for facilitating connections to care: a review of the literature. *Schizophrenia Bulletin* 2009; **35**(4): 696–703.

28. Henderson C, Flood C, Leese M, Thornicroft G, Sutherby K, Szmuckler G. Effect of joint crisis plans on use of compulsory treatment in psychiatry: single blind randomised controlled trial. *British Medical Journal* 2004; **329**: 136.

29. Horstead A, Cree A. Achieving transparency in forensic risk assessment: a multimodal approach. *Advances in Psychiatric Treatment* 2013; **19**: 351–7.

30. Ashcraft L, Anthony W. Eliminating seclusion and restraint in recovery-oriented crisis services. *Psychiatric Services* 2008; doi:10.1176/appi.ps.59.10.1198.

31. Law D. Shared decision making in child and adolescent healthcare. 2011. Available from: http://www.health.org.uk/areas-of-work/programmes/closing-the-gap-through-changing-relationships/related-projects/promoting-choice-and-collaboration-in-child-and-adolescent-mental-healthcare/ [Accessed 26th August 2016].

32. Health Foundation. Closing the gap. 2012. Available from: www.youngminds.org.uk/assets/0000/3753/Closing_the_Gap_Report.pdf [Accessed 26th August 2016].

33. Copeland M-E. *Wellness recovery action plan*. Brattleboro, VT: Peach Press, [1997] 2001.

34. Copeland M-E, Mead S. *Wellness recovery action plan and peer support. Personal, group and program development*. Brattleboro, VT: Peach Press, 2004.

35. Perkins R, Rinaldi M. *Taking back control. A guide to planning your own recovery*, London: South West London and St George's Mental Health NHS Trust, 2007.

36. Perkins R, Repper J, Rinaldi M, Brown H. *Recovery colleges*. Implementing Recovery through Organisational Change (ImROC) briefing paper. London: Centre for Mental Health, 2012.

37. McGregor J, Repper J, Brown H. 'The College is so different from anything I have done'. A study of the characteristics of Nottingham Recovery College. *Journal of Mental Health Education, Training and Practice* 2014; **9**(1): 3–15.

38. Chamberlin J. Psychiatric survivors: are we part of the disability movement? *Disability Rag and ReSource* 1995; March/April: 4–7.

39. Chamberlin J. Psychiatric disabilities and the ADA. An advocate's perspective. In: Gostin LO, Beyer HA (eds). *Implementing the Americans with Disabilities Act*. Baltimore: Brooks, 1993.

40. Beresford P, Nettles M, Perring R. *Towards a social model of madness and distress? Exploring what service users say*. York: Joseph Rowntree Foundation, 2010.

41. Perkins R. UK mental health policy development: a counter-argument deriving from users' experiences. In: Phillips P, Sandford T, Johnston C (eds). *Working in mental health: practice and policy in a changing environment*. Oxford: Routledge, 2012: chapter 2.

42. Repper J, Perkins R. Recovery: a journey of discovery for individuals and services. In: Phillips P, Sandford T, Johnston C (eds). *Working in mental health: practice and policy in a changing environment*. Oxford: Routledge, 2012: chapter 7.

43. United Nations. Convention on the Rights of Persons with Disabilities. 2006. Available from: www.un.org/disabilities/convention/conventionfull.shtml [Accessed 26th August 2016].

44. Slade M, Amering M, Farkas M, Hamilton B, O'Hagan M, Panther G, Perkins R, Shepherd G, Tse S, Whitley R. Uses and abuses of recovery: implementing recovery-oriented practices in mental health systems. *World Psychiatry* 2014; **13**(1): 12–20.

45. Deegan P. The Independent Living Movement and people with psychiatric disabilities: taking back control over our own lives. *Psychosocial Rehabilitation Journal* 1992; **15**: 3–19.

Further reading

Chamberlin J. *On our own*. London: Mind Publications, 1988.

Davidson L, Tondora J, Lawlwaa MS, O'Connell M, Rowe M. *A practical guide to recovery-orientated practice*. Oxford: Oxford University Press, 2009.

Leamy M, Bird V, Le Boutillier CL, Williams J, Slade M. Conceptual framework for personal recovery in mental health: systematic review and narrative synthesis. *British Journal of Psychiatry* 2011; **199**: 445–52.

LeCroy CW, Holschuh J. *First person accounts of mental illness and recovery*. Oxford: John Wiley & Sons, 2012.

Repper J, Perkins R. *Social inclusion and recovery: a model for mental health practice*. Edinburgh: Baillière Tindall, 2003.

Romme M, Secher S, Dillon J, Corstens D. *Living with voices, 50 stories of recovery*. Ross-on-Wye: PCCS Books in association with Birmingham City University, 2009.

Sayce L. *From psychiatric patient to citizen: overcoming discrimination and exclusion*. London: Macmillan, 2000.

Relevant web pages

Implementing Recovery through Organisational Change (ImROC). www.imroc.org
ImROC provides resources, papers, presentations and access to training, conferences and workshops about recovery.

Scottish Recovery Network. www.scottishrecovery.net
This website provides all kinds of papers, narratives, training materials, films and details of events relating to recovery.

36 The recovery approach and risk management

JESS HOLLEY AND DEAN PEARSEY

LEARNING OUTCOMES

- To understand what is meant by a recovery-oriented care approach and how it can be adopted in practice in order to support individual recovery.

- To recognize the progression of routine risk management, from a preoccupation with public safety through to a more collaborative approach that runs parallel to recovery-oriented care.

- To understand how a positive risk taking approach can be a key mediator in helping people to move forward in their recovery.

- To be critically aware of the impact risk adversity and professional accountability can have upon the implementation of recovery-oriented care.

SUMMARY OF KEY POINTS

- The concept of individual recovery has become an important principle to help service users maximize their potential despite mental illness. As such, recovery-oriented care is a guiding principle in the delivery of mental health services.

- There is, however, a pre-existing culture of risk management practice which may impact upon the provision of mental health services supporting recovery-oriented care.

- In more recent modifications to risk management practice – where there are attempts to move away from the more traditional conceptualization of risk to a more collaborative, positive approach – service users are encouraged to identify risks which are salient to them whilst building upon their strengths in order to move forward in recovery.

- Mental health professionals may experience role-conflict when service users' right to live independently needs to be weighed carefully against the likelihood of harm arising.

> *If recovery is the person's responsibility, then how come I get the blame when things go wrong?*
>
> **Larry Davidson[1] (p.642)**

INTRODUCTION

Recovery has developed a specific meaning in mental health and is defined as: 'A deeply personal, unique process of changing one's attitudes, values, feelings, goals, skills and/ or roles. It is a way of living a satisfying, hopeful and contributing life, even with limitations caused by the illness'[2] (p.527). Recovery-oriented care (ROC) is an approach that has been introduced into mental health services in order to explicitly support individual recovery. There have, however, been concerns about the implementation of recovery-oriented approaches, alongside mental health professionals' responsibility to reduce and manage service users' exposure to risk. This chapter will provide a critical overview of literature exploring how understandings of ROC and risk management practice (RMP) are represented in mental health policy and research and how they are enacted in day-to-day practice.

A RECOVERY APPROACH IN MENTAL HEALTH SERVICES

The concept of individual recovery first emerged in the National Service Framework for Mental Health[3] through its emphasis on information, empowerment, partnership, community-based care, family support and health promotion.

Mental health policies advocating a recovery-oriented approach in mental health care provision focus on a perceived need to create a more optimistic and positive approach to care for those who use mental health services.[4] This was an attempt to move away from previously held assumptions that the long-term nature of symptoms inhibited service users in taking control of their lives and recovering. Policies that advocate ROC state that 'people who use mental health services will be involved, as equal partners and at every level, to ensure the new services make sense'[4] (p.5). This links with wider health and social care initiatives for chronic disease management and the promotion of 'the expert patient' in other chronic illnesses such as arthritis, multiple sclerosis and diabetes.[5]

ROC policies do not only focus on self-management and choice of treatment and care. In 2007, the Department of Health published a 'commissioning framework for health and well-being' which stressed the importance of mental health services to provide direct support to people to function as full citizens in their communities.[6] Furthermore, the Department of Health's most recent strategic paper, *No health without mental health*,[7] builds on previous evidence which has identified many factors that help people recover and lead the lives they want to lead, stating:

> *More people who develop mental health problems will have a good quality of life – greater ability to manage their own lives, stronger social relationships, a greater sense of purpose, the skills they need for living, working, improved chances in education, better employment rates and a suitable and stable place to live. (p.21)*

ROC policies are therefore used as a vehicle for nurses to implement the craft of caring in two forms, both the problem-focused/situation-specific, and the more holistic, which concerns the person's life and how it is lived.[8]

What does the recovery approach look like in practice?

It has been suggested that adopting a recovery-oriented approach has profound implications for mental health services, in which the goals of mental healthcare are re-shaped around the individual's life goals and that service users' rights are respected when making decisions about all aspects of their recovery.[9] Claire Boutillier and colleagues[10] carried out a qualitative analysis of 30 international documents on recovery-oriented practice policy guidelines. The four main practice domains were:

1. *Promoting citizenship.* Guidance provided in New Zealand[11] indicated that, in order to promote citizenship, mental health professionals should adhere to human rights principles by respecting the rights of individual service users and their families. Additionally, a practice guidance document from Devon, UK,[12] suggested that mental health professionals need to work closely with mainstream organizations in order to promote service users' social integration into the community. This will help to accommodate people's needs for community supports by helping them access housing, education, financial independence and participation in community life.[13]

2. *Organizational commitment.* A number of documents outlined mental health professionals' role in encouraging service users' and their families' involvement in service development and evaluation in order to improve the quality of service provision.[13,14] One practice-based document reported by the National Institute of Mental Health in England[15] states that it is an essential requirement for mental health professionals to be committed to work outside their usual working hours in order to ensure service users are able to move in and out of the system as required and therefore enable them to direct their own recovery process.

3. *Supporting personally defined recovery.* Traditional mental health services primarily focused upon the mental health worker making decisions with regard to identifying realistic goals and treatment choices for the service user – also known as a detached relationship.[14] Mental health professionals can support personally defined recovery by providing service users with timely and accurate information in order for service users to have personal preference, choice and involvement in decision-making processes about their care.[16] This is also known as a shared decision-making approach.[14]

4. *Working relationship.* Mental health professionals are encouraged to formulate partnerships with service

users by providing coaching to them in order to facilitate their involvement in all aspects of their care. One way this can be achieved has been outlined in a number of practice documents,[17,18] which describe how mental health professionals can foster hope and optimism in their daily practice by valuing service users' own abilities to move forward in recovery.

For further detail on the recovery approach, please see chapter 35.

RISK IN MENTAL HEALTH SERVICES

The concept of risk is most commonly interpreted in mental health care culture as the likelihood of an event happening with potential harmful outcomes for oneself and others.[19] In 1994 the Department of Health brought out guidance on the discharge of people with mental health disorders and their continuing care within the community.[20] The main aims of these guidelines were to provide advice for mental health professionals working within the community on assessing and managing risks which service users may present to themselves or others, stating that: 'Risk is a prime consideration in discharge decisions'[20] (p.3). The focus of reducing risk for newly discharged service users was a response to adverse events and failures in community mental health care; the concept of risk was highlighted through high-profile cases of murder, suicide and self-harm involving people with severe mental health problem.[21] The official inquiries into these incidents emphasized the importance of risk assessment as a mechanism that identifies and controls individuals who are at risk to themselves and others.[22] These adverse incidents also brought about a preoccupation with 'public safety' and resulted in mental health services seeking means to exert control over patients, especially ensuring their compliance with treatment.[23]

Care planning and routine risk management

Prior to 1994, risk assessment was based on a non-structured clinical approach whereby information was gathered non-systematically through service users' ongoing clinical assessment. This approach was seen as vulnerable to mental health professionals' subjectivity, bias and theoretical interests, while possibly ignoring relevant information that may have contributed to the occurrence of untoward incidents.[24] More consistent approaches to assessment and management of risk were introduced into the Care Programme Approach (CPA) in the mid-1990s.[23]

The CPA was first introduced in 1990 as a framework to plan personalized care for mental health service users.[25] The CPA's four basic elements were:

1. to systematically assess service users' health and social care needs;
2. to agree a recorded written care plan between mental health professionals, service users and carers;
3. to allocate a key worker whose role is to remain in close contact with service users while continuously monitoring the care programme;

4. to be regularly reviewed alongside service users' progress in relation to their health and social care needs.[26]

When the CPA was initially introduced in England, there was no mention of risk.[25] The CPA was extended in the early 1990s to incorporate a more structured approach to risk work, following on from issues raised by public, policy and professional agendas.[20] In this structured approach, professionals are required to conduct risk assessments and develop a risk management plan for people discharged from hospital.[20]

Since formal RMP procedures were introduced into the CPA in the early 1990s, service users became increasingly defined in terms of the risk they were seen as presenting, 'rather than in terms of their needs and rights'[26] (p.2). Changes were made to the CPA by the government in 1999 in order to make it a more effective and efficient system of care coordination.[27] One of these changes meant that risk should not simply be considered an assessment of danger that an individual poses to themselves and others. As such, mental health professionals need to take into account the user's social, family and welfare circumstances, as well as the need for positive risk taking.[27] For further detail on the CPA, please see chapter 37 and for collaborative care planning with service users and carers see chapter 50.

> ## REFLECTION
>
> When developing a care plan with a service user, in what way do you allow the service user to take the lead?

A collaborative approach to risk

In 2007 the Department of Health published a framework of principles underpinning best practice of RMP in all mental health settings.[28] In this policy document, risk management was defined as 'developing flexible strategies aimed at preventing any negative event from occurring or, if this is not possible, minimising the harm caused'[28] (p.13). In risk management, the assessment of risk factors – personal characteristics or circumstances that are linked to a negative event and that cause or facilitate an event occurring – need to be carried out in order to identify ways of reducing the likelihood of their occurrence.[28]

The philosophy underpinning this framework was one that 'balanced care needs against risk needs'[28] (p.4) by emphasizing: positive risk management; collaboration with service users and others involved in service users' care; the importance of building service users' strengths in order to move forward in recovery; the organization's role in risk management alongside individual mental health professionals' role. Promoting openness and transparency through effective decision making and communication between service users and mental health professionals were essential, as 'the risk management plan has no purpose if it is not shared between the relevant parties and used as a basis for joint action'[28] (pp.28–9). Please see chapter 50 for further information on collaborative care planning.

Mental health professionals' role in communicating risk to service users can be a complex matter, giving rise to a number of practical and attitudinal problems. In one study, interviews were conducted with mental health professionals working on inpatient wards to explore their attitudes towards discussing risk with service users.[29] Mental health professionals expressed concerns about the impact which informing service users of risks could have on service users' identities, which could cause them to assign stigmatizing labels to themselves and develop lower self-esteem.[29] It has been suggested that this may cause difficulties for mental health professionals in adopting a collaborative approach to risk management. In turn, the problems that arise when communicating risk may also be disempowering for service users by decreasing their perceived competence towards an involvement in risk decisions.[30]

Positive risk taking

The current guidance on best practice in managing risk[28] also emphasizes positive risk taking (also known as positive risk management). Positive risk taking is described as an important component of ROC whereby service users are encouraged to take risks which enable them to move forward in recovery.[19] It has been suggested that this approach may be a key mediator in how people move forward in recovery, while enabling them to discover new meaning in their lives by learning by experience what works best for them.[31] The approach involves mental health professionals:

> *weighing up the potential benefits and harms of exercising one choice of action over another. Identifying the potential risks involved (i.e. good risk assessment), and developing plans and actions (i.e. support for safety) that reflect the positive potentials and stated priorities of the service user (i.e. a strengths approach).[32] (p.6)*

These broader understandings of risk and risk management suggest that mental health workers should not be solely concerned with the need to reduce service users' direct risk of harm to self and others, but should also consider those wider 'chronic' risks that impact negatively on individual recovery. As such, a positive risk taking approach could be considered an important factor in the craft of caring, as it incorporates recovery into risk management not only by remedying or ameliorating distress, but by also exploring ways to help the person develop and grow in day-to-day life.[8]

One study conducted qualitative interviews with mental health professionals in order to evaluate the effectiveness of adopting a positive risk management approach with mental health service users who present high risks to themselves or others.[33] Findings indicated that service users were more likely to be a risk to themselves than to others, particularly with regard to risks such as self-harm and social isolation. These findings indicated that, when formulating a risk management plan, the focus should be widened from high-risk concerns to low-risk concerns which are salient to service users.[33] This was further supported by Sarah Birch and colleagues,[34] who explored the implementation of a positive risk taking approach through an audit of self-harm across three women's mental health units over a period of 3 years. The mental health professionals provided a suitable environment for service users to self-harm in order to reduce actual harm. Service users were offered support, reassurance, acceptance and a sense of communalism in the hope of diminishing their need to self-harm. Results showed that adopting a positive risk taking approach significantly reduced incidences of self-harm over 6 months.[34]

Although there are obvious benefits to positive risk taking in supporting a ROC approach, there are also concerns that the 'term is easily misunderstood and often confused with casual, permissive or reckless attitudes'[31] (p.8). It has also been suggested that there is a lack of differentiation between positive risk taking, which service users might be encouraged to experience, and risks which need to be minimized.[35]

REFLECTION

Think about a time when you implemented a positive risk taking approach. In what ways did the potential beneficial outcomes outweigh the potential negative outcomes?

RISK ADVERSITY AND PROFESSIONAL ACCOUNTABILITY

Mental health professionals' responsibility to manage risk has been associated with their being accountable if anything should go wrong in situations involving service users'

care. Some health care professionals have referred to this as a culture of blame.[36] This, as described previously in this chapter, arose in response to a number of adverse incidences in community mental health care in the early 1990s which resulted in a preoccupation with public safety, whereby mental health services wanted to exert control over service users in order to reduce harm to themselves and others.[23] It is argued that service users' right to live independently needs to be weighed carefully against the likelihood of harm arising.[37] A risk-averse culture in mental health services has resulted in mental health professionals becoming excessively focused upon documentation and defensive practice, which can undermine service users' needs.[38] There is therefore a fine balance between mental health professionals' responsibility to empower service users on the one hand, and their duty to protect service users on the other.

It has been suggested that the notion of professional autonomy is shaped by the idea of specialist knowledge that is central to the professional role.[39] For example, mental health professionals' knowledge and expertise in managing risk restricts their professional jurisdiction.[38] Literature surrounding patients' choice in psychiatry has indicated that issues of professional jurisdiction can often restrict the amount of involvement that service users have in their own care.[40,41] In particular, with regard to mental health professionals' role in managing and reducing risk, Glenn Roberts and colleagues[41] have argued that the parameters of service users' choice and responsibility are set by mental health professionals' judgement on service users' exposure to risk and levels of mental capacity. In situations where the service user is at high risk of harming themselves or others, personal preferences for their care can often be displaced by considerations of risk.[40]

Beate Schrank and Mike Slade[9] have argued that the values and attitudes of staff may have to shift, so that instead of defining their roles as 'outside experts' for people with mental illness, they define their roles as helpers on people's paths of life, accepting an equal partnership with the service users regarding their care. This shift in the balance of power may, however, be challenging for professionals. For example, adopting a positive risk taking approach in mental health services is not always straightforward. A recent study explored mental health professionals' experiences of supporting positive risk taking in mental health and learning disability outreach settings.[42] Mental health professionals described how risk management influenced their approaches to risk taking. A common theme was that 'Staff negotiate a balance of control over risk-taking with the service user, mindful that misjudging this balance could ultimately result in service responses shaped by rare, adverse incidents rather than by the everyday risks faced by most service users'[42] (p.147).

The findings of the study concluded that some mental health professionals felt a lack of support and reassurance from other mental health professionals in their team who resorted to more conservative practices of risk management. These more conservative approaches to risk management encouraged coercion between mental health professionals and service users and therefore undermined the therapeutic relationship when undertaking positive risk taking.[43,42]

> ## REFLECTION
>
> Think about how you and the rest of your team discuss situations regarding service users' care that may result in adverse outcomes. In what way do you come to a decision?

CONCLUSION

In summary, more recent modifications to RMP – which involve attempts to move away from the more traditional conceptualization of risk to a more collaborative, positive approach – may be central to developing ROC.[44] There are, however, long-standing concerns over risk-adversity in mental health services which may undermine meaningful clinical decision making, while making engagement with service users more difficult.[45] It has been suggested that it is important to learn how people with mental health problems view and cope with risk; this may help mental health workers to address not only their own concerns about risk but also those of service users.[46] As such, this chapter will end with a personal reflection from someone who has lived experience, particularly illustrating what individual recovery means to them and how issues of risk have impacted upon their recovery journey.

> ## SERVICE USER'S PERSPECTIVE: RECOVERY, RISK AND REFLECTION
>
> To me, recovery means leading a life you want to lead. Being comfortable within yourself. Being able to be with your family and those close to you again without a degree of separation. It means the rampaging elephant in the room has been poached for ivory, is no longer a threat, and is now adorning your wall as a reminder of what makes you stronger.
>
> I in no way endorse hunting.
>
> But I digress.
>
> Recovery is an individual thing. It is not an enviable task, traversing this line between risk

management and running the risk of wrongly categorizing someone who has simply gone off track as a potential threat to society.

I remember, shortly after my illness became so pronounced I could scarce leave the house, my father took me to the hospital. There I was, an ostensibly grown man, wailing like a newborn, because the world around me terrified me. I did not know what was going on. I was in immense pain, but a threat to no one. Eventually, a care team was sent to my home, and they tried to assess the situation. The thing I remember most clearly was being asked if I had any weapons or any intentions to harm anyone. This jolted me, sent me deeper down. Was I one of *them*?

Now, I understand, this may well have been a formality, but it was clumsy, at best; inappropriate, more accurately; and downright offensive, if you want to get a little carried away.

Assessing and managing risk may well be necessary, but a focus from the industry on prevention of something that is thankfully rare, rather than cure of something that is sadly all too common, is, to my mind, almost something from the realm of science fiction. The stigmas that exist, like stereotypes, may well exist for a reason, but just as I would not accept a politician actively employing racial stereotyping in their industry, I don't think these stigmas should be encouraged and employed as part of a carer's trade.

A more optimistic and positive approach to risk can in no way be a bad thing, but is this just an idea? The key, of course, is the people working within the services. They need to be nothing short of extraordinary, with regard to patience, sensitivity and *humanness*. They need to be able to approach every service user as what they are: an individual. For me, I am blessed with a strong family unit, and so this was one of the reasons I never felt completely lost. To be candid, I remember

telling myself, *if I can't get through this, then no one can*. It is already implied that I know this family unit I speak of is a rarity in today's society. So, the care worker needs to be able to assess the situation based upon *who the service user is*.

If the service user does not harm themselves or another, they should be able to live whatever life they would like to lead. The care worker should, in my opinion, work with the service user in order to identify achievable goals and implement a structure which will allow the service user to attain these goals.

I am pleased to say that my experience with the services has, on the whole, been very positive. Many of the things I have spoken of, we did; we discussed my goals and identified what I needed to change in my life, and I have, on the whole, faced nothing but patience, sensitivity and humanness from the professionals who have aided my recovery.

A pivotal moment was a risk which I took against all advice. When my illness became awful, I had just finished my first year of university. In my mind, it was crucial for me to return and complete my studies, yet, understandably, my care worker strongly advised me not to. I chose not to take this advice. I returned to university, and endured the hardest 6 months of my life.

But then it got better.

Had I not taken this step, I am not sure who I would be today.

The wellness of the service user should always supersede this notion of risk prevention. I have known a fair few 'mentally ill' people in my time, and they have posed less of a threat to society than some of the supposedly 'mentally well' people I have encountered.

If I had been stopped from returning to university, because an individual made the judgement that I was a threat, then I think it is very unlikely I would have been in a position to be asked to write these words. It is strange how our world works.

References

1. Davidson L, O'Connell M, Tondora J, Styron T, Kangas K. The top ten concerns about recovery encountered in mental health system transformation. *Psychiatric Services (Washington, D.C.)* 2006; **57**(5): 640–5.

2. Anthony WA. Recovery from mental illness: the guiding vision of the mental health system in the 1990s. *Psychosocial Rehabilitation Journal* 1993; **16**(4): 11–23.

3. Department of Health. *Report of the Expert Committee: Review of the Mental Health Act 1983.* London: Stationery Office, 1999a.

4. Department of Health. *The journey to recovery – the government's vision for mental health care.* London: HMSO, 2001a.

5. Department of Health. *The expert patient: a new approach to chronic disease management for the 21st century.* London: Department of Health, 2001b.

6. Department of Health. *Commissioning framework for health and well-being.* London: Department of Health, 2007a.

7. Department of Health. *No health without mental health: a cross-government mental health outcomes strategy for people of all ages.* London: Department of Health, 2011.

8. Barker P, Whitehill I. The craft of care: towards collaborative caring in psychiatric nursing. In: Tilley S (ed). *The mental health nurse: views of practice and education.* Oxford: Blackwell Science, 1997: 15–27.

9. Schrank B, Slade M. Recovery in psychiatry. *Psychiatric Bulletin* 2007; **31**(9): 321–5.

10. Boutillier C, Leamy M, Bird V, Davidson L, Williams J, Slade M. What does recovery mean in practice? A qualitative analysis of international recovery-oriented practice guidance. *Psychiatric Services* 2011; **62**(12): 1470–6.

11. O'Hagan M. *Recovery competencies for New Zealand mental health workers*. Wellington: New Zealand Health Commission, 2001.

12. Devon Partnership NHS Trust. *Putting recovery at the heart of all we do: what does this mean in practice?* Exeter: Devon Partnership National Health Service Trust, 2008.

13. Lloyd C, Waghorn G, Williams P. Conceptualising recovery in mental health rehabilitation. *British Journal of Occupational Therapy* 2008; **71**: 321–8.

14. Slade M. *Personal recovery and mental illness: a guide for mental health practitioners*. Cambridge: Cambridge University Press, 2009.

15. NIMHE (National Institute of Mental Health in England). *Emerging best practices in mental health recovery: guiding principles*. London: NIMHE, 2004.

16. Farkas M. The vision of recovery today: what it is and what it means for services. *World Psychiatry* 2007; **6**: 68–74.

17. Shepherd G, Boardman J, Rinaldi M, Roberts G. *Supporting recovery in mental health services: quality and outcomes: briefing paper*. London: ImROC, 2014.

18. Boardman J, Craig T, Goddard C, Henderson C, McCarthy J, McInerny T. *Recovery is for all: hope, agency and opportunity in psychiatry*. London: South London and Maudsley NHS Foundation Trust and South West London and St George's Mental Health NHS Trust, 2010.

19. Morgan S. Risk-making or risk-taking? *Openmind* 2000; **101**: 16–17.

20. Department of Health. *Guidance on discharge of mentally disordered people and their continuing care in the community*. London: HMSO, 1994.

21. Moon G. Risk and protection: the discourse of confinement in contemporary mental health policy. *Health & Place* 2000; **6**(3): 23–50.

22. Alaszewski A, Alaszewski H, Ayer S, Manthorpe J (eds). *Managing risk in community practice*. London: Baillière Tindall, 2000.

23. Department of Health. *Modernising mental health services: safe, sound and supportive*. London: TSO, 1998.

24. Ryan T. Perceived risks associated with mental illness: beyond homicide and suicide. *Social Science & Medicine* 1998; **46**(2): 287–97.

25. Department of Health. Caring for People. *The Care Programme Approach for people with a mental illness referred to specialist mental health services*. Joint Health/Social Services Circular. C(90)23/LASSL(90)11, 1990.

26. Langan J, Lindow V. *Mental health service user involvement in risk assessment and management*. Bristol: Policy Press, 2004.

27. Department of Health. *Effective care co-ordination in mental health services: modernising the care programme approach – policy booklet*. London: Crown Copyright, 1999b.

28. Department of Health. *Best practice in managing risk: principles and guidance for best practice in the assessment and management of risk to self and others in mental health services*. London: Department of Health, 2007b.

29. Langan J. Involving mental health service users considered to pose a risk to other people in risk assessment. *Journal of Mental Health* 2008; **17**(5): 471–81.

30. Mitchell W, Glendenning C. *A review of the research evidence surrounding risk perceptions, risk management strategies and their consequences in adult social care for different groups of service users*. York: SPRU, 2007.

31. Boardman J, Roberts G. *Recovery, risk and safety: implementing recovery through organisational change, briefing paper 9*. London: ImROC, 2014.

32. Morgan S. *Positive risk-taking. Practical ways of working with risk*. A Practice Based Evidence production for Hampshire Partnership NHS Foundation Trust, 2011.

33. Kaliniecka H, Shawe-Taylor M. Promoting positive risk management: evaluation of a risk management panel. *Journal of Psychiatric and Mental Health Nursing* 2008; **15**(8): 654–61.

34. Birch S, Cole S, Hunt K, Edwards B, Reaney E. Self-harm and the positive risk taking approach. Can being able to think about the possibility of harm reduce the frequency of actual harm? *Journal of Mental Health* 2011; **20**(3): 293–303.

35. Boardman J, Craig T, Goddard C, Henderson C, McCarthy J, McInerny T. *Recovery is for all: hope, agency and opportunity in psychiatry*. London: HMSO, 2010.

36. Sawyer A. Risk and new exclusions in community mental health practice. *Australian Social Work* 2008; **61**(4): 327–41.

37. SCIE (Social Care of Excellence Institute). *Enabling risk, ensuring safety: self directed support and personal budgets*. London: SCIE, 2010.

38. Clifford P. Evidence and principles for positive risk management. In: Whittington R, Logan C (eds). *Self-harm and violence: towards best practice in managing risk in mental health services*. Chichester: John Wiley & Sons, 2011: ch. 11.

39. Waring J, Currie G. Managing expert knowledge: organizational challenges and managerial futures for the UK medical profession. *Organization Studies* 2009; **30**(7): 755–78.

40. Samele C, Lawton-Smith S, Warner L, Mariathasan J. Patient choice in psychiatry. *British Journal of Psychiatry* 2007; **191**(1): 1–2.

41. Roberts G, Dorkins E, Wooldridge J, Hewis E. Detained – what's my choice? Part 1: discussion. *Advances in Psychiatric Treatment* 2008; **14**(3): 172–80.

42. Robertson JP, Collinson C. Positive risk taking: whose risk is it? An exploration in community outreach teams in adult mental health and learning disability services. *Health, Risk and Society* 2011; **13**(2): 147–64.

43. Brown S, Calana M, Scrivener A, Szmukler G. Trust in mental health services: a neglected concept. *Journal of Mental Health* 2009; **18**(5): 449–58.

44. Roberts G, Boardman, J. Becoming a recovery-oriented practitioner. *Advances in Psychiatric Treatment* 2014; **20**(1): 37–47.

45. Morgan JF. *Giving up the culture of blame: risk assessment and risk management in psychiatric practice*. London: Royal College of Psychiatrists, 2007.

46. Eriksson BG, Hummelvoll JK. People with mental disabilities negotiating life in the risk society: a theoretical approach. *Journal of Psychiatric and Mental Health Nursing* 2008; **15**(8): 615–21.

Further reading

Boardman J, Roberts G. *Recovery, risk and safety: implementing recovery through organisational change, briefing paper 9*. London: ImROC, 2014.

Davidson L, O'Connell M, Tondora J, Styron T, Kangas K. The top ten concerns about recovery encountered in mental health system transformation. *Psychiatric Services (Washington, D.C.)* 2006; **57**(5): 640–5.

Department of Health. *Best practice in managing risk: principles and guidance for best practice in the assessment and management of risk to self and others in mental health services*. London: Department of Health, 2007.

Holley J, Chambers M, Gillard, S. The impact of risk management practice upon the implementation of recovery-oriented care in community mental health services: a qualitative investigation. *Journal of Mental Health*, in press.

Morgan S. Risk-making or risk-taking? *Openmind* 2000; **101**: 16–17.

Roberts G, Boardman J. Becoming a recovery-oriented practitioner. *Advances in Psychiatric Treatment* 2014; **20**(1): 37–47.

Relevant web pages

ImROC (Implementing Recovery through Organisational Change). http://www.imroc.org/latest-news/publications/imroc/

Scottish Recovery Network. http://www.scottishrecovery.net/

Tidal Model. http://www.tidal-model.com/

37 Using the care programme approach

MARTIN WARD

LEARNING OUTCOMES

- To understand the nature of the Care Programme Approach (CPA) and how it fits with whole systems care.
- To appreciate the problems faced by service users who are in recovery.
- To be able to apply the CPA to individualized service user care.
- To be able to evaluate the effectiveness of good discharge planning and inter- and multidisciplinary collaboration.
- To understand the necessity for service user involvement in every stage of the care process.

SUMMARY OF KEY POINTS

- The CPA is a modified version of case management that is designed to support service users with mental health problems receiving care from secondary services.
- It is designed for the most vulnerable and at-risk individuals.
- It requires a multidisciplinary/agency approach.
- Patients receive CPA if they require complex support from more than one agency or professional group.
- Service users are assessed for risk, health and social care needs.
- Each service users has a multidisciplinary care plan which they help develop.
- A care coordinator is appointed to facilitate the delivery of the care plan.
- The care plan must be reviewed at regular intervals.

INTRODUCTION

Imagine that you find a plot of land, with wonderful views and the potential for a great home. You make your plans and build your dream house, move your furniture in and sit back to enjoy your good fortune. Then, it rains, and you realize the builder did not install a roof. Everything gets ruined and in a short time you are left with a shattered dream, no money, just rubble. You are worse off than before you started because you have seen what the future could have held. Although this scenario is not real, the sad fact is that, all too often, through bad planning or lack of knowledge, we spoil things that may have improved our lives in some way.

To a certain degree health care follows a similar pattern to this scenario. Investment is made in new technologies, infrastructure and staff education. From admission to discharge, the service user's journey is organized, logical and effective. Yet it only takes one piece of the jigsaw to be missing and all this effort is wasted, with service users left feeling cheated by the eventual failure of a system that was intended to change their lives for the better. Perhaps significantly, this only becomes apparent once the service user has been discharged from inpatient care back into a community setting where they are expected to resume a successful and rewarding lifestyle or at least to exercise a degree of independence and autonomy. Historically, the link between inpatient and community care has been that missing component, meaning that skills and recovery processes learnt while under supervision were not practised once service users returned home. The result was often the absence of a 'roof' and a complete waste of resources for services, and a disheartening, sometimes damaging, conclusion for the service user. Further information on recovery can be found in chapters 35 and 36.

During this chapter I am going to try to illustrate various points using the experiences of Tony, an old friend of mine who for many years suffered problems with his own mental health. His 'journey' through his own illness, and the subsequent involvement with his local mental health services, provide a not uncommon commentary on many people's perception of 'being cared for', eventually highlighting the application of the craft of caring at its best. The illustrations come from discussions between him and me while writing this chapter.

Tony's story is similar to that of many people around that time. They felt very much that being discharged home was simply the start of another cycle of illness and readmission – a merry-go-round, as Tony puts it. Nothing seemed to fill the in-between times when they felt reasonably well. Worse still, there was always the promise of help, both

SERVICE USER'S PERSPECTIVE

Tony is 55 years old and has suffered long-term mental health problems for about 25 of those years. In the early 1990s he was admitted to and discharged from his local psychiatric hospital at least a dozen times. He is married with two grown-up boys. He was unemployed for nearly 10 years but has been in full-time employment since 2003.

When I used to be admitted to hospital, it was because the world became too confusing for me. I could not concentrate and the voices in my head made it impossible to make any sense of things. I would get a week or two of help and then usually just be told I was being discharged on the Friday or whatever. They always said that someone would contact me to come and visit me at home. Well, it was usually the same chap, a young community psychiatric nurse. Nice bloke. We would have a cup of tea and he would give me a number to ring if I needed anything from him. I never did ring. Trouble was, when I should have called him, I didn't because I was not well enough to think about it. So, I usually went back into hospital. It was like a merry-go-round.

before they left hospital and once discharged, but inevitably it never materialized. In effect, the 'roof' was promised but never built.

BACKGROUND TO THE CPA

It was to address the perceived failure of the support mechanisms for people with long-term and enduring mental health problems that in 1991 the Care Programme Approach (CPA) was launched.[1] It came about as a result of the Spokes enquiry, where none of the professional disciplines could agree on the right course of action in the care and after-care of a mental health service user, Sharon Campbell.[2] To a degree, it was based on the US system of Case Management introduced in the 1970s. The CPA's main aims were to introduce a framework to generate continuity of care in secondary mental health services, to promote multi- and interdisciplinary team working, to involve service users in all aspects of their care process and to utilize effective assessment, treatment and evaluative processes to ensure the appropriateness of the care offered. It was originally divided into two levels:

1. standard CPA, for individuals who were supported by only one agency, were able to manage their own mental health problems effectively and who could, if necessary, maintain the link between themselves and the care agency;

2. enhanced (often referred to as complex) CPA, designed for people utilizing more than one care agency, with complex needs, and who were assessed as being at risk of relapse.

It was operationalized at a time when radical changes were taking place in UK community mental health services. A massive hospital closure programme, with significantly reduced inpatient beds, was driving the agenda for service users to be discharged and supported more in the community. However, it was apparent that in many instances hospitals were closed before the corresponding community infrastructure was put in place, leaving discharged service users with limited or no support and without the possibility of being re-admitted. Discharge planning was still in its infancy, with few scales being used to assess levels of ability, competency or mental health status. It would be several years before the Health of the Nation Outcome Scales[3,4] and a plethora of risk assessment tools began to bridge the gaps and make inpatient discharge a controlled and more robust activity, and several more years before the CPA itself was fully implemented across all services linking health and social care.

At the heart of the CPA was the introduction of a 'key worker', an individual whose job it was to monitor a caseload of service users and ensure they coordinated care to meet their needs across disciplines, agencies and services. Guidance was put in place to establish a care plan for each service user, with set review times, to ensure that they did not fall between the gaps in service provision, and the roles and responsibilities of care coordination for the key worker. In 1999 further refinements were introduced to increase the range and scope of the assessment schedules, to include risk assessment and management, employment, leisure and accommodation requirements and the necessity to devise plans that actually met service user needs.[5] Later, provisions were set which altered the way community mental health care was configured,[6] with specialist teams working with service users with specific needs. In 2008 the CPA was overhauled completely, providing more transparent working processes, including key workers being renamed as case managers, then as care coordinators, and reducing both the

administrative bureaucracy and the number of people who would need to receive 'complex' CPA.[7]

Inevitably, with scarce resources and limited budgets, health services had to find ways to prioritize who should, and should not, receive long-term care. This has led to some critics perceiving the CPA as a failed initiative.[8-10] Simpson[11] went as far as to suggest that the introduction of the CPA had reduced the capability of community psychiatric nurses to deliver effective psychosocial interventions because they had to spend additional time in administrative duties. However, the reality is that, as legislation and policy developments have linked themselves to the CPA, and depended upon it to be able to function – for example, the National Service Framework for Mental Health,[12] the NHS Plan,[13] Good Psychiatric Practice[14] and the Mental Health Act 2007[15] – it has become pivotal to the provision of targeted care for people most at risk within secondary care services. (One of the most comprehensive reviews of CPA and its development and implementation is *Refocusing the Care Programme Approach: policy and positive practice guidance*.[7])

HOW DOES THE CPA WORK?

Quite simply, the CPA is a system to enable health and social care staff to provide care to people with mental health illness, living in the community, according to their individual needs. Fine words, but the devil is in the detail. It is one thing to say that the right people will be targeted, will work with the care coordinator to devise their own support system and then be evaluated on a regular basis to ensure that everything possible is being done to meet their specific needs, but it is another to operationalize that process for every member of the secondary care mental health population. The best way to understand how the CPA works is to break it down into its component parts, which will be discussed in turn in the rest of this section.

An assessment meeting is convened for all health care disciplines potentially involved in the care of the individual

In the case of a service user who is currently an inpatient, this is the starting point for the CPA. It should be undertaken during the individual's stay in care, and in plenty of time to plan for his/her discharge properly. In the case of someone who is living within the community, either a person who has previously been in contact with mental health services or someone who is new to them, this should be part of their assessment process to determine if they are suitable for CPA. The service user can bring with them to the meeting an advocate, such as a member of their family, a primary carer or a close friend, to give them support.

Those professionals attending the meeting would act as representatives of their respective disciplines/agencies. If the decision is ultimately made to offer CPA to the service user, they might then act as one of the care providers, depending upon the needs of the patient.

Decisions are made concerning information gathered about the service user, or directly from him or her

These include physical, mental and social needs; social, gender, spirituality, educational and leisure issues; and will also consider risk and risk management factors. Additional information concerning housing, accommodation, employment and cultural needs should also be collected.

The decision as to whether or not the service user is suitable for the CPA, or warrants it at the enhanced level, is made by the team

Not all service users need the intensity associated with the CPA. Lower levels of care may be offered, but these will be delivered either by representatives of single disciplines/agencies members or others co-opted specifically to meet the needs of the patient; that is, the service user's primary health care physician (GP) may be asked to review the patient's medication and general mental health status on a regular basis.

A care coordinator is appointed from within the team

The care coordinator may be from any discipline and their appointment will be based on several factors – their availability, their relationship with the service user (see chapter 3 for details on developing and maintaining therapeutic relationships), their ability to be able to coordinate others involved in the care process and their specific skills in relation to the service user's needs. They have several roles. The most important of these is acting as the link between the service user and the care team. They will monitor the impact of the CPA against care targets set out within a care plan and facilitate the involvement of all other members of the team. It is vital that the coordinator has regular contact with the service user so that they can establish the effects of the care being offered, re-assess care needs and try to ensure collaboration and treatment adherence with the individual. The coordinator can be any member of the care team, but in most cases the individuals who best suit this role are either psychiatric/mental health nurses[1] or social workers.[2]

A written multidisciplinary care plan is constructed

The coordinator is responsible for taking the lead on this. Based on the needs identified by the assessments, there may be any number of other personnel involved in delivering care, so it is necessary for the coordinator to ensure that they know who is doing what, and when (see chapter 50 for more detail on collaborative care planning). The plan must reflect other health and social requirements to ensure that it is not biased towards one or the other, in effect creating a deficit that may exacerbate the service user's condition. The plan must be agreed by all those responsible for care delivery to ensure it is carried out properly, including the service user, and must list every aspect of the care to be provided, including medications, talking therapies, indicators to help the patient know when he is becoming unwell again, arrangements for physical health and the contact details of all concerned. Targets are set for each of the identified needs (on a priority basis), and the personnel or discipline responsible for them measure their input based upon these. However, wherever possible, the service user must be involved in this activity as something of a priority – the issue of service user collaboration is discussed in further detail later in the chapter. Others who could be involved include representatives of the person's religious faith, primary carers, teachers and, in the case of someone who will be discharged from inpatient care, the patient's GP. This is particularly important, as physical health needs must be monitored and dealt with as and when they arise, to optimize the patient's general health status and ability to recover.

Care is delivered based on the care plan requirements

This may sound like a strange thing to say, given that the care plan is in place, the service user is in a position to receive the care or work with individual care providers and the system is designed to meet identified needs. Nonetheless, it must be remembered that the CPA came about as a result of a lack of coordination among care providers, with individuals slipping through the net of care provision, sometimes with serious consequences. It is the major task of the care coordinator to ensure that everything agreed in the care plan is delivered as requested, and at the time and place designated.

The care plan is reviewed regularly

The plan is compared against the service user's health and social need status. The care coordinator is responsible for monitoring not just the service user's health care status but also the designated care evaluation meeting times. Each of the care providers will provide feedback concerning their own input. There are two types of review. The first is undertaken by the coordinator (or in most cases a single care provider, such as a community psychiatric nurse (CPN)) on a regular basis to ensure that things are going according to plan.

This review may result in the team being called for a full meeting if something needs to be changed or modified. The second relates more to those receiving long-term support and will bring together every involved member of the team at approximately 6-monthly intervals. As in the case of the initial assessment and review meeting, the service user and any other key stakeholders, specifically primary and secondary carers, should also be present at this review (see chapter 13). However, it is important to remember that exposing service users to large groups of professionals and being questioned on their care and health needs can be a daunting proposition. In such a threatening environment many may not be able to express themselves fully, thus creating the wrong impression, with subsequent care running the risk of being inappropriate or unnecessary. It is essential that service users' involvement is handled sensitively and within their ability.

For many service users their first impressions of being involved in the CPA in those early developmental days came as both a shock and a pleasant surprise – shock, because previously they had never been followed up properly once they left hospital, and surprise because no one actually explained to them what the CPA was. Service users who were being seen solely by a CPN, or the representative of only one agency, were at first also considered for the CPA. This also caused some confusion, because many of these individuals felt that their community support was adequate. It was when things went wrong and they found themselves without the help of their CPN that they felt stranded. In effect this was the problem. Services could cope with the complexity of community care as long as everything went along smoothly. Of course, life is not like that, for anyone, and particularly for people with complex mental health issues. If staff were not in a position to recognize need, the craft of caring itself became impossible to apply. The expression 'slipping through the net' was used to describe those individuals who had either avoided contact with health and social care services, for whatever reason, or were simply unknown to them. Those who had regular contact with their CPN or social worker could be more

carefully monitored but, when things became complicated for them, they could easily miss meetings or sessions, and the care worker would not necessarily know there was anything wrong until a cry for help materialized.

WHO SHOULD RECEIVE THE CPA?

So far we have established that individuals who have a complex set of needs, which require that two or more care professionals work with them, are suitable to be selected for CPA provision. However, there are guidelines for the team making this assessment that provide a template to help selection (see chapters 13, 14 and 15 for more information on assessment). The most up-to-date checklist can be found on the NHS Choices website[16] which provides information for both care professionals and patients alike as to the selection criteria. The following are those items that would, potentially, place an individual within the CPA parameters. They may be:

- being diagnosed as having a severe mental disorder;
- being at risk of suicide, self-harm or harm to others;
- a history of violence or self-harm;
- being neglectful of themselves and not taking treatment regularly;
- being vulnerable;
- misusing, or having misused, drugs or alcohol;
- relying significantly on the support of a carer, or have their own caring responsibilities;
- having recently been detained under the Mental Health Act;
- having parenting responsibilities.

However, this is just a checklist and some of these items need further development in order to make sense. For example, on the face of it, having a severe mental disorder might sound straightforward enough. But it is the measure of the ongoing debilitation suffered by the individual as a result of the condition that is important here, not the diagnosis itself. Someone who, because of their mental health problems, loses independence and self-determination, becomes reliant upon others for basic needs or simply is too unwell to lead an independent lifestyle, is more likely to be considered. A service user diagnosed with a long-term psychotic illness might seem like an obvious choice, but if they are leading a stable life, adhere to their medication or treatment programme, manage their symptoms (especially hearing voices) effectively and have good informal carer support, it is unlikely that they would need the CPA. This would be even more the case if they did not fit any of the other criteria on the list. Conversely, someone with a long-term anxiety disorder that gives them panic attacks and related phobias, or someone whose symptoms of post-traumatic stress disorder create intolerable and sometimes volatile behavioural problems, might be more suitable. In fact, irrespective of their diagnosis, an individual who met two or more of the criteria on the list would almost certainly be selected.

Self-neglect may not initially seem like a suitable criterion for CPA. However, the negative symptoms associated with many mental health challenges, psychosis in particular, often mean that, left untreated, individuals may be at risk of serious physical health complications on top of ever-increasing psychiatric ones (see chapter 69 for more on physical health care). They become at risk simply because of their non-adherence to treatment, leading to social withdrawal and a steady decline in general health status. Similarly, vulnerability may seem like a strange criterion, but that is because it needs to be unpicked a little for it to make sense. Vulnerability could mean anything from being at risk or unsafe because of their own behaviour, to being helpless or defenceless with an inability to make decisions about their own personal security. It is their susceptibility to danger and their general failure to address its consequences that places them on the CPA list. Their vulnerability may take different forms, such as physical or emotional abuse, or financial difficulties.

Vulnerability comes in many forms, and for the purposes of CPA selection each one needs to be considered on its own merit. Factors that may be significant include those who are isolated from family, friends or neighbours and thus cannot be monitored in terms of their health status. Some people have a mental health condition that creates memory problems (other than those experienced as the effects of dementia) and therefore inhibits their potential for treatment adherence. Some people cannot communicate well, either because of social withdrawal or because their symptoms interfere with normal thought processes. Some people have problems with their informal, primary carers – for example, if the carer is dependent upon them for providing financial support, a home or emotional verification, the individual's

stability in maintaining these is paramount. Likewise, if the individual has a poor relationship with their carer or simply does not get on with them, this can diminish his or her life to the point where he or she becomes not only vulnerable but possibly even suicidal. This can be exacerbated in the case of carers who have problems of their own to deal with, such as drug and alcohol difficulties. Ultimately, individuals who become highly dependent upon someone else for the running of their own lives and cease to be able to take care of themselves or protect themselves against significant harm or exploitation would be regarded as being vulnerable from a mental health standpoint.

Detention under the UK Mental Health Act, either for assessment or treatment purposes, suggests that the individual is going through a period of volatility health-wise and may be particularly at risk, either to themselves or to others. Having parenting responsibilities, in and of itself, is not necessarily a problem unless it is combined with other factors on the list, especially vulnerability and neglect. The remaining points on the list are relatively self-explanatory. However, it is important to remember that it is more likely to be combinations of these that will suggest suitability for CPA, particularly as many of them overlap in some way.

REFLECTION

Mental health problems, no matter how small they appear to outsiders, always present huge challenges to the individuals who suffer from them. They are far more complex than simply evaluating a set of pre-ordained criteria. Ask yourself these questions.

1. How often have I faced a difficult situation and not been able to resolve it, at least not straight away? What did this do to my own mental health status, and how did it affect other aspects of my life?

2. Did other people really understand what was going on inside my head, and the emotional turmoil that I experienced?

The CPA may not, in itself, be a panacea for intervention activities for people with severe mental health problems, but at least it provides a mechanism that requires constant evaluation and demands that action be taken whenever circumstances require it. As such it means that care staff tasked with providing care are better positioned to understand the nature of the problems being experienced, thus potentially enhancing their own craft of caring because it becomes more focused on the individual.

SERVICE USER'S PERSPECTIVE: WHY I WAS ACCEPTED FOR THE CPA

The trouble with me was that I had so many problems! I was in a mess. I was doing practically nothing for myself, was dependent on my wife for pretty much everything, both around the house and out of it. I didn't go out, didn't meet with anyone else, hardly spoke to the kids, except to shout at them, and spent most of my days either in bed or watching awful daytime TV. Worst of all, I was hearing voices all the time, no stopping them. I knew they weren't for real, but they interfered with my ability to think straight. Sometimes I would just shout out loud to tell them to stop. They didn't. I had no job, no money coming in except for benefits and my wife was threatening to leave. We argued a lot, or at least she did. I would just go and hide when she got angry. That last time, I had to go into hospital. I had not been taking my meds for as long as I can remember. It was terrifying.

REFLECTION

It is perhaps amazing that some people are able to tolerate a large number of problems and still somehow manage to lead a form of independent life. Tony was lucky in the sense that his wife stayed with him and supported him as best she could. His hospitalization periods were almost a respite for her when she could regain her strength and take some time out to look after herself. But the quality of Tony's life generally was extremely poor.

Ask yourself this question.

- Have you ever been in a situation which gradually spiralled out of your control, to the point where the quality of your life deteriorated and you found yourself locked into negative feeling and an absence of any ideas of how to resolve your situation successfully? If the answer is 'no', you are lucky, because at times most of us have problems which drag us down in some way and affect our ability to solve them. If you did not experience this yourself, what about a friend or close relative?

- If the answer is 'yes', how did you manage to turn things around?

The big question is:

- Did you, or your friend or relative, manage to do this for yourself, or was there help from a third party?

We can see from Tony's personal account that he met several of the criteria for acceptance onto the CPA. These included:

- a worsening serious mental health condition;
- vulnerability;
- social withdrawal;
- personal neglect;
- non-adherence to medication;
- having parenting responsibilities;
- financial difficulties;
- poor communication;
- deterioration of his relationship with his primary carer (his wife).

Tony was eventually placed on the CPA, though at first he did not realize it. It was the late 1990s and, as we will see in the next section, not all health and social care staff

knew how to use the framework properly. He was admitted to his local psychiatric hospital. As he explained earlier, a young staff nurse kept asking him questions he had never had to answer before and he gradually began to think that maybe there was something different about this admission. However, in those early days there was something missing from much of the process of assessment and it led to confusion on the part of the service user and disjointed care on the part of the care professionals. This was service user involvement.

SERVICE USER INVOLVEMENT

One of the key considerations of the CPA is the service user's role. As mental health care has become more enlightened over the years, it has been recognized that simply telling a person to do as they are told in terms of their treatment, medication or even lifestyle only produces minimal success. Indeed, it is quite demeaning to be told what to do by someone else without ever being able to say what you think yourself. This approach, known

universally as 'compliance', usually only works when the person telling the individual what to do is present. In their absence the person tends to do their own thing – just as most of us do in our everyday lives. It is human nature to have self-determination concerning what we do and how we lead our lives. It gives us dignity and self-respect. We tend to share responsibility for our daily lives with others, but having the final say on decisions about what we will do is our prerogative. We collaborate with others on a regular basis, and more recently health care has adopted a similar approach using this collaborative approach. In certain instances this has been extended even further, to the point where service users have almost total control over their own care process, an approach known as concordance – where two or more people work together on a chosen care activity but only one, the service user, makes the final decisions.

To be able to appreciate what sort of a difference this makes to service users' lives, it is useful to look at the research. In the early years of the CPA, there were several significant studies that presented a variety of outcomes. Both McDermott[17] and Phillips[18] found that service users felt excluded from the care process, even though the system was designed to involve them, with Allen[19] reporting that carers also felt the same way. They also felt intimidated by the professional meetings that were held to evaluate care, and were generally dissatisfied with the outcomes of these events. On the other hand, Alexander and Brady[20] stated that the service users in their sample felt that the CPA had made a positive difference to their lives. In particular they highlighted their involvement in care decision-making activities, and the ability to foresee problems before they occurred, as being useful. Conversely, a study undertaken by Anthony and Crawford[21] showed that some mental health nurses were uncomfortable with allowing service users more involvement in their own care. Even quite recently service users have complained that they are misunderstood and excluded from the CPA.[22]

In Tony's case, on the admission described above he stayed slightly longer than usual – 5 weeks in fact. But before he left he was asked to attend a meeting where he met people he did not know, along with the psychiatrist and care staff, including the young staff nurse. He says he felt intimidated by this, but because everyone was 'nice' to him he answered their questions as best he could and tried to focus on what they were telling him.

> ### SERVICE USER'S PERSPECTIVE
>
> They were all watching me, like I was in a zoo or something. I sat in the middle of this big circle of people, half of whom I had never met before. I don't think I did well answering their questions but I tried to. They nodded their heads and smiled a lot. When I came out, I was not really sure what had happened. No one came out to tell me so I guessed they would do so later. No one did. About a week later Raymond, the young nurse, came to speak to me and said everything was set for my discharge and he had been asked to be my key worker, or something like that. He said he would come and visit me at home the day I left and we would discuss what was going to happen. Guess what, he did too!

It was not until several years later that Tony realized what the CPA was all about. By that time he had changed his care coordinator for a new one, who explained everything to him in detail. He also became active in his own care process and, although he had two more admissions, his care coordinator eventually started to brief him about what was to happen and in the team meetings he was asked what it was he wanted to happen, and even for his advice on the best way to achieve it. In 2010 he was taken out of the CPA because he had resumed a meaningful and stable life with his wife, a job and one married son. Most of the items in his original acceptance criteria were no longer issues for him. He still hears voices, but he has learnt to control this with the help of a specialist psychologist. His CPN (also his care coordinator) visits him still, but mostly just for that cup of coffee and a chat. His road to recovery was hard. More information on recovery can be found in chapters 35 and 36.

CONCLUSION

The CPA is not a panacea for all mental health problems, especially those in secondary care. But as with the case of Tony it can provide a framework that, if coordinated effectively, is able to martial resources in support of service users' needs and ensure that they have the opportunity to take part in their own recovery, or at the very least maintain themselves in the community with some degree of independence. Having their health status monitored regularly, changing care plans to reflect their actual requirements and access to specialist individuals who are able to meet their needs appropriately are things that characterize an approach that is a long way away from the early days of community mental health care. For psychiatric and mental health nurses, the craft of caring needs mechanisms in place that offer the potential for individual creativity. It is not people themselves who have changed over the years, but the methods of organizing them. Let Tony conclude the chapter.

SERVICE USER'S PERSPECTIVE

It was not really till a couple of years ago that I realized just how bad my life had been in those early days of my illness. Since they started me on the CPA, and when I really knew what it was about, I began to turn things around with the social worker who got me additional benefits and help for Christine [my wife] with child care; the psychologist who put me in touch with the hearing voices network, my GP who sorted out a lot of my chest and muscle pains, but most of all Kevin [my second care coordinator] who has stuck by me these past 12 years. Christine even attended a couple of the review meetings with me. Without them, and especially Kevin, I think there is a possibility Christine would have left me, and I would probably have ended my own life. I owe them so much. I feel in control these days and have started helping others who are in the same situation as me at a special club in the health centre. I even enjoy my job. How many people can say that, I wonder?

References

1. Department of Health Caring for People. *The Care Programme Approach for people with a mental illness referred to specialist mental health services.* Joint Health/Social Services Circular. C(90)23/LASSL(90)11. London: Department of Health, 1990.
2. Department of Health and Social Security. *Report of the Committee of Inquiry into the Care and After Care of Sharon Campbell (Chairman: J. Spokes).* London: HMSO, 1988.
3. Wing JK, Curtis RH, Beevor AS. *HoNOS: Health of the Nation Outcome Scales: report on research and development July 1993–December 1995.* London: Royal College of Psychiatrists, 1996.
4. Ganeshalingam Y, Chang D, Dunn, N. The evidence for effective psychiatric admissions as measured by an audit of Health of the Nation Outcome Scales recording. *Journal of the Evaluation of Clinical Practice* 2010; **16**(1): 196–8.
5. Department of Health. *Effective care co-ordination in mental health services: modernizing the Care Programme Approach – a policy booklet.* London: Department of Health, 1999.
6. Department of Health. *Community mental health teams. Mental health policy implementation guide.* London: Department of Health, 2002.
7. Department of Health. *Refocusing the Care Programme Approach: policy and positive practice guidance.* London: Department of Health, 2008.
8. Audit Commission. *Finding a place: a review of mental health services for adults.* London: HMSO, 1994.
9. Bindman J, Beck A, Glover G, Thornicroft G, Knapp M, Leese M, Szmulker G. Evaluating mental health policy in England. Care Programme Approach and Supervision Registers. *British Journal of Psychiatry* 1999; **175**: 327–30.
10. Simpson A, Miller C, Bowers L. The history of the Care Programme Approach in England: where did it go wrong? *Journal of Mental Health* 2003; **12**: 489–504.
11. Simpson A. Community psychiatric nurses and the care co-ordinator role: squeezed to provide 'limited nursing'. *Journal of Advanced Nursing* 2005; **52**(6): 689–99.
12. Department of Health. *National Service Framework for Mental Health: modern standards and service models.* London: Department of Health, 1999.
13. Department of Health. *The NHS Plan* (Cmnd 4818–I). London: Department of Health, 2000.
14. Royal College of Psychiatrists. *Good psychiatric practice*, 2nd edn. Council Report CR125. London: Royal College of Psychiatrists, 2004.
15. HMSO. *The Mental Health Act 2007.* London: HMSO, 2007.
16. NHS Choices. *Care Programme Approach.* Available from http://www.nhs.uk/CarersDirect/guide/mental-health/Pages/care-programme-approach.aspx [Accessed 1st August 2016].
17. McDermott G. The Care Programme Approach: a patient perspective. *Nursing Times* 1998; **94**(8): 57–9.
18. Phillips P. The Care Programme Approach: the views and experiences of service users. *Mental Health Care* 1998; **1**(5): 166–8.
19. Allen C. The Care Programme Approach: the experiences and views of carers. *Mental Health Care* 1998; **1**(5): 160–2.
20. Alexander H, Brady L. What does receiving the Care Programme Approach mean for service users? *Health Bulletin* 2001; **59**(6): 412–16.
21. Anthony P, Crawford P. Service user involvement in care planning: the mental health nurses' perspective. *Journal of Psychiatric and Mental Health Nursing* 2000; **7**: 425–34.
22. Rogers B, Dunne E. A qualitative study on the use of the Care Programme Approach with individuals with borderline personality disorder: a service user perspective. *Journal of Psychosocial Nursing and Mental Health Services.* 2013; **51**(10): 38–45.

Further reading

NHS Choices. Care Programme Approach. Available from: http://www.nhs.uk/CarersDirect/guide/mental-health/Pages/care-programme-approach.aspx [Accessed 16th September 2016].

Relevant web pages

Rethink Mental Illness. CPA. https://www.rethink.org/search?s=CPA

38 Providing culturally safe care

ANTHONY J. O'BRIEN, RUTH DeSOUZA AND MARIA BAKER

LEARNING OUTCOMES

- To understand the various meanings given to the term 'culture'.

- To be aware of the range of cultural identities of individuals.

- To be able to identify the possible impacts of cultural issues on mental health and mental health care.

- To understand the need to reflect on one's own cultural identity as the basis for culturally safe care.

- To be aware of the concept of cultural safety.

- To be able to identify strategies for providing culturally safe mental health services.

SUMMARY OF KEY POINTS

- To provide therapeutic care nurses need to understand the cultural needs of service users.

- Culture can include many aspects of identity, such as ethnicity, religion, spiritual practices and gender, among others.

- Ethnicity can influence the pathway to care, the responses of nurses and mental health services, and the outcomes of care.

- Cultural safety is a framework for providing care that recognizes both the nurse's and the service user's cultural identities.

- Cultural safety supports the philosophy of recovery in mental health care.

- Culturally specific services aim to provide safe services that address the problem of cultural domination in mainstream services.

- Global population movements contribute to the need for nurses to be responsive to the needs of service users from a wide range of cultural backgrounds.

INTRODUCTION

The encounter between a nurse and a service user and their family and community may involve an interaction between two or more people with multiple and very different identities. For the nurse, the service user, their family and community, a wide range of beliefs, experiences, norms and values will influence perceptions of mental health and mental health care. The therapeutic relationship (see also chapter 3) is influenced by a multiplicity of cultural beliefs and values – those of the nurse and those of the service user. The role of the nurse is to develop a relationship which recognizes and respects the service user's cultural and spiritual identity, and the influence of cultural identity on the therapeutic encounter. We wish to affirm the shifting and multiple nature of cultural identity, rather than to propose a model of identity as fixed and unchanging.

Here, we shall discuss the issue of *culture* as it relates to mental health nursing. Our definition of culture includes spiritual identity, given the increasing spiritual diversity of many Western countries, and the recognition of the need for psychiatry to develop partnerships with faith-based organizations.[1] Global population movements challenge our traditional views of culture[2] and require culturally informed responses from mental health nurses. We aim to provide a basis for mental health nurses to reflect on their own cultural identities and those of the people they care for. We shall not provide prescribed responses for engaging with people whose cultural and spiritual identities are different from one's own. Rather, we shall suggest a process of reflection on cultural and spiritual identity, and on the impact of cultural difference on interactions between nurse and service user. Although the term 'culture' is most frequently used to refer to ethnic culture, it can usefully be applied to a range of differences, including those of gender, sexuality, physical ability, age and religion. Here, 'culture' refers only to ethnic culture, or ethnicity, another term that is not always used consistently.[3] We recognize that the discussion may also have relevance to various forms of group *belonging,* such as social class, religion and gender. The terms 'religion' and 'spirituality' require some clarification.

> ### REFLECTION
>
> How would you define yourself culturally? Would you give priority to ethnicity, religious beliefs, gender, sexuality, or some other aspect of culture?

Religion and spirituality

Before psychiatry emerged as a discipline, 'mental illness' was viewed as a consequence of religious or moral breaches. More recently, the religious and spiritual dimensions of life have been ignored by mental health professionals and services which are largely 'white' institutions and adhere to secular scientism.[4] In line with the less technocratic notion of cultural safety which requires that a safe space is provided for cultural issues and identities, religious safety would mean providing a safe space for religious issues and identities which can be integrated into a plan of care.[5] We include religion and spirituality in considerations of cultural safety, although we note that these are aspects of human experience that carry their own requirements for safe practice (for more on spirituality and mental health nursing, see chapter 9). Increasingly spiritual assessments are being incorporated into care, as part of routine assessments and integrated into care plans[6] (see chapter 50 for more on collaborative care planning). The idea of religious competence as an aspect of cultural safety acknowledges that people hold values and beliefs that impact on mental health – such as those related to alcohol consumption, sleep and diet (for example, fasting). Mental health nurses need to be aware of both interiorized practices (that is, private beliefs and practices such as prayer) and institutionalized practices conducted in the community, and support these needs to be met in a respectful and safe manner.

> ### REFLECTION
>
> - Consider faith and belief. Do you have spiritual beliefs that help you cope with stress?
>
> - *Importance:* What role do your beliefs have in regaining health?
>
> - *Community:* Are you part of a religious or spiritual community? If so, does this provide support to you and how?
>
> - *Address in care:* As a health care provider, how could you address these issues when providing care for service users?

Research and theory on the 'need for nursing'[7] provide a theme which integrates this chapter with other sections of this book. Among the needs identified by this body of work is the need for cultural respect and affirmation. As with other human needs, cultural needs do not immediately show themselves to the nurse, and should not be identified independently by the nurse. Instead, service users should be engaged in identifying those needs. The need for engagement as a basis for providing culturally safe care recognizes the relationship between nurse and service user as central to the process of providing appropriate care. Without a relationship of empathy and trust, service users are not likely to identify cultural needs, and so will not be able to avail themselves of opportunities for support in meeting those needs.

We draw on New Zealand experiences in the development of the concept of cultural safety, a concept that has been given wide international recognition.[8-10] Consistent with the view that reflection on cultural identity is the basis for providing culturally safe care to others, the chapter should be seen in light of the authors' cultural identities and context.

- Anthony O'Brien is a Pakeha* male academic and clinical practitioner.
- Ruth DeSouza is an East African Goan New Zealander resident in the lands of the Kulin Nations in Victoria, Australia.
- Maria Baker is a Māori† mental health nurse, of Ngapuhi, Te Rarawa tribal descent.

We work in postcolonial New Zealand and Australia, societies that are meeting the challenges of restoration and redress for past events, and of the neocolonization process of globalization.[11] In this chapter, the authors locate their scholarship in the context of Aotearoa and Australia as colonized white settler nations, where indigenous people were removed from their lands and resources to facilitate colonial settlement. The mental health of communities cannot be considered without addressing the social determinants of health,[12] including the consequences of colonialism for the health of indigenous communities. The authors propose a view of mental health within a systems (rather than individualistic) perspective, whereby the lens of care is widened beyond the individual to consider service users in the context of their families and communities and in the context of social and structural inequities in order to provide care that is safe, innovative and holistic. Using an approach that focuses on social determinants of health allows consideration of 'the circumstances in which people are born, grow up, live, work and age, and the systems put in place to deal with illness. These circumstances are in turn shaped by a wider set of forces: economics, social policies, and politics'.[13]

A range of research and literature provides an international perspective. While the model of cultural safety we outline is considered to be applicable in the New Zealand context, like models of nursing and mental health care, it needs adaptation to local contexts if it is to fully acknowledge the realities of individual nurses and service users.

RACE, ETHNICITY AND CULTURAL IDENTITY

The concept of race has its origins in anthropologists' attempts to classify human beings on the basis of observable differences in physical attributes. Many early writings on race, including those of prominent theorists of psychiatry, reflect views of the innate superiority of white people over other races.[14] Because of these associations, the term 'race' is used less often currently.[3] The term refers to human groupings based on biologically determined racial characteristics, and a set of associated social and political processes sometimes termed 'racialization'.[15] Recent genetic evidence questions previous assumptions of biologically distinct races, lending further support to the idea of race as a social construction.[16] In the health sciences it is now more common to speak of 'ethnicity', a term that implies a sense of group belonging, which is self-claimed and not imposed on the basis of observable physical attributes. However, the concept of ethnicity recognizes the biological basis of physical characteristics of ethnic groups. The terms 'race' and 'ethnicity' are sometimes used interchangeably.

Culture can be defined as a set of traditions, beliefs, values and practices shared by members of a social group.[14] While it is commonly thought that culture and ethnicity are synonymous, the concepts are not identical. A person is born with particular characteristics, some of which are attributable to ethnicity, in the biological sense discussed above. Frequently, individuals are influenced by characteristics of more than one ethnic group. For instance, a person's physical characteristics may reflect Asian and Caucasian ancestry. Indeed, individuals may not be aware of all the influences on their ancestry. Physical attributes are subject to interpretation, and so do not have fixed or stable meanings. If we wish to understand a person's beliefs, values and behaviour, we need to know about the group affiliations of that person, or their culture.

Members of a single ethnic group will have different experiences of what it means to be a member of that group. However, the language used to describe ethnicity reflects the tendency to make generalizations, which have the potential to become stereotypes. The term 'Asian' has been criticized for its tendency to obscure differences between specific ethnic groups in the USA, Canada, the UK, and Australia and New Zealand. Differing uses of 'Asian' within the UK include or exclude ethnic Indians or Chinese in different surveys and do not always reflect individuals' self-perceived ethnic identities. A similar issue is found in New Zealand where differing constructions of 'Asian' are employed. Popular discourse and the media employ a racially based construction that includes only East and Southeast Asian peoples, while another construction, increasingly used in health research, includes people from East, South and Southeast Asia, but excludes people from the Middle East and Central Asia. In health, such broad categories can mask high health needs of groups within the category, resulting in services being targeted inappropriately. In clinical practice, service users may not identify with broad categories such as 'Asian', creating the

---

* The term 'Pakeha' is used in New Zealand to refer to people of Anglo, Celtic or Caucasian ancestry.
† Māori are the indigenous people of Aotearoa/New Zealand.

potential for miscommunication. To make sound clinical decisions about the mental health needs of members of this group, it is necessary to recognize its diversity. Within ethnic groups other forms of group belonging will influence individuals' perceptions of health. As Shattell and Hogan[17] note, within different cultures there are differences in the way health encounters are experienced. Furthermore, for some people religion represents a world view that is a more defining marker of identity than ethnicity. Nurses need to recognize that 'culture' can be a form of imposition, in which a nurse classifies a service user based on the nurse's belief or expectations of that person's cultural identity. This is especially so if the nurse's classification is based solely on characteristics such as name, skin colour or facial features rather than the person's expressed cultural identity. Box 38.1 summarizes the results of New Zealand research documenting clinical nursing practice in the area of identification of cultural needs.

BOX 38.1: SUMMARY OF RESEARCH FINDINGS

In an audit of case notes in 11 out of 22 mental health services in New Zealand,[18] it was found that, in 65 per cent of cases, service users were not given the opportunity to identify their cultural needs. In addition, 28 per cent of service users were not offered support for those cultural issues they did identify. Encouragingly, in 65 per cent of cases Māori cultural advisors were consulted regarding the care of Māori service users. However, only 23 per cent of Māori service users were offered cultural assessment in accordance with the requirement of the New Zealand Mental Health Standard.[18] For the purposes of this study, identification of ethnicity by the nurse was not considered to represent an opportunity to identify cultural needs. Assessment is a key aspect of nursing care and is crucial to planning appropriate care. Without an opportunity to identify cultural needs, service users are not able to access cultural support, and this is likely to have an adverse effect on their engagement with and response to care. (Chapter 13 provides more information on assessment.) Providing an opportunity to identify cultural needs is dependent on the establishment of rapport, and it should be negotiated with the service user.

CULTURAL DIFFERENCES IN CLINICAL PRACTICE

Psychiatry is a system of practices firmly set within a Western scientific tradition. Consideration of the impact of culture on clinical practice therefore begins with a review of the culturally determined nature of Western psychiatry. The individualistic illness model of mental distress is a construct developed by Western psychiatry, but one which contrasts sharply with collectivist ways of thinking, such as those of Indian, African, Asian and Polynesian cultures.[19] Also, Western models of mental health care are based on the ideal of disengagement of the self, so that the search for mental health becomes a search for an ideal individual self. This is reflected in models of psychotherapy and treatment, which assume a universal self, free of the influences of culture.[20] This approach does not recognize paradigms of collectivist cultures. For example, Māori cultural beliefs see good mental health as an outcome of harmony with oneself, one's family, community, ancestors, creator and the environment.[21] Within Western models of mental health, culture and religion are considered to provide the content (thoughts, perceptions, feelings) associated with mental illness, while the form (depressed mood, psychosis) is considered to be culture-free. Leff[22] presents evidence from studies in a wide range of countries which suggests that functional psychosis is a universal human experience.

However, he cautions that this conclusion should be interpreted carefully, as the instruments used in the studies 'were constructed in the West and may have imposed a cultural stereotype on the patient populations examined' (p.42).

Whatever the influence of culture on the content or form of mental illness, when people come into contact with mental health services, culture plays a significant role. Evidence suggests that ethnicity influences presentation to services, assessment, and decisions about care and treatment.[23] Ethnicity has also been found to influence pathways to care, diagnosis, prescribing patterns, and use of electroconvulsive therapy.[24] In New Zealand, Māori people are 2.9 times more likely than non-Māori to be placed on community treatment orders.[25] While there are many factors that may mediate the influence of ethnicity (such as age, social isolation, gender, socio-economic status or severity of illness), it seems that ethnicity is a significant factor in service users' involvement in mental health care. It is also possible that aspects of a person's presentation that are ascribed to culture are actually related to other aspects of their identity, such as religion. While ethnicity may be evident to an observer, religious beliefs are not usually obvious. Both cultural and religious identity will influence the acceptability and appropriateness of mental health services.

Working at the 'care face'[7] of mental health brings nurses into close contact with service users, in situations where ethnic difference may play a crucial role in shaping relationships. One area of nursing practice that has been influenced by ethnicity is nurses' perceptions of dangerousness. When behaviour is perceived to be dangerous, there are a number of responses available to nurses. These range from 'one to one' intervention and supported time out, to coercive measures such as seclusion and restraint. Nurses' responses to perceived dangerousness may be influenced by the ethnicity of the service user. In a study of violence in inpatient units, there was no difference, based on ethnicity, in rates of compulsory detention.[26] However, the same study reported that non-violent black patients were four times more likely than non-violent whites to be admitted to a locked unit. Another study found that restraint was almost four times more likely to be used following violence by black than white service users,[27] suggesting that nurses may have a lower tolerance of violence by blacks than by whites.

While there is clear evidence that rates of diagnosis and decisions about treatment and care are influenced by clinicians' perceptions of ethnicity, there is also concern that insufficient attention may be given to the influence of biological differences between different ethnic groups. Metabolism of psychoactive medications, development of side effects and adverse effects, and thresholds of effectiveness have all been shown to have some variability related to ethnicity.[28] The incidence of metabolic syndrome, a disorder associated with use of second generation antipsychotic agents, is also more prevalent in some ethnic groups.[29] The effects of these differences may be further compounded by cultural differences in help-seeking, expression of symptoms and patterns of communication.[30] Nurses need to be familiar with the specific effects of psychoactive medications on different ethnic groups, and of cultural differences in patterns of response. (Chapters 47 and 48 provide more information on psychopharmacology and medicines management.)

DEVELOPING EFFECTIVE RESPONSES TO CULTURAL DIFFERENCE

Nurses learn, through therapeutic relationships, to respond effectively to the emotional distress of service users. Part of this process involves reflection on the experiences, assumptions and skills the nurse brings to the therapeutic relationship. The increasing ethnic diversity of countries in which mental health nursing is practised suggests a need for reflection on cultural identity as part of the process of development of nursing skills. Reflection should include consideration of power differences in the nurse–patient relationship, placing the onus for recognizing and responding to cultural difference with the nurse, rather than the service user. Clinical supervision can provide opportunities to reflect on the influence of cultural identity on clinical practice.[31]

REFLECTION

Consider a clinical situation you have observed where there was a difference in the cultures of a nurse and a service user. This could be an initial assessment, a home visit, administration of medication or any common clinical situation. How did cultural differences impact on that situation? How did cultural identities of the nurse and the service user influence the power differences between them? Can you suggest how the nurse could address these differences to provide culturally safe care?

The diverse cultural needs of users of health services require that nurses develop approaches to care that recognize and respect the culture of service users. Box 38.2 summarizes terms used in the nursing literature to describe models of cultural awareness as they relate to clinical practice.

BOX 38.2: MODELS OF CULTURAL AWARENESS

Cultural sensitivity is 'an ongoing awareness of cultural differences and similarities among populations'[32] (p.162). It involves awareness of cultural difference and knowledge of some of the culturally specific beliefs and practices that may influence service users' engagement with care.

Cultural competence is defined as 'respect for, and understanding of, diverse ethnic and cultural groups, their histories, traditions, beliefs and value systems'[33] (p.177). This recognizes the need for nurses to be sensitive to the culture of service users, and to respond to cultural diversity within the service user group. Wells[34] has identified the need for cultural competence to extend beyond the individual, and embrace institutional change.

Cultural proficiency begins with examination of cultural biases, those 'cultural values and beliefs that are internalized through the socialisation process'[34] (p.193), and includes organizational change within educational institutions and health services. The concept of cultural safety meets Wells's[34] criteria for cultural proficiency, but also requires reflection on the particular history of the society in which health care is provided.

CULTURALLY SAFE CARE

Cultural safety differs from cultural sensitivity, cultural competence and cultural proficiency by envisaging a process of change from sensitivity, through awareness, to safety. Although it originated in New Zealand, cultural safety has been applied to a range of social contexts.[8,9]

Cultural safety has been defined as:

> *The effective nursing practice of a person or family from another culture, and is determined by that person or family. Culture includes, but is not restricted to, age or generation; gender; sexual orientation; occupation and socioeconomic status; ethnic origin or migrant experience; religious or spiritual belief; and disability.*
>
> *The nurse delivering the nursing service will have undertaken a process of reflection on his or her own cultural identity and will recognise the impact that his or her personal culture has on his or her professional practice. Unsafe cultural practice comprises any action which diminishes, demeans or disempowers the cultural identity and well-being of an individual.*[35] *(p.7)*

Although cultural safety was originally developed as a response to the disproportionate health problems of Māori, the concept is applicable to all cultures. Within a dominant culture, indigenous peoples and those seen as different by the dominant culture are potentially at risk and require culturally safe care. This is also important for immigrant groups, such as Pacific Island people in New Zealand, Vietnamese in Australia, West Indians in the UK, and North African immigrants to European countries.

Cultural safety begins with analysis of the historical relationships between the different groups that make up a society. The focus of cultural safety is on the social positions of these groups, rather than solely on their distinctive cultural beliefs or practices, as a basis for developing culturally safe relationships with service users. On this basis, health is placed in a political and historical context. Cultural safety focuses on the social, economic, political and historical influences on health. Because the political and historical context of each society is unique, cultural safety needs to be given specific meaning within local contexts. The principle of recognition of the histories of different cultures within different societies, the historical relationships between different cultures and, in particular, issues of power differences between cultures is a significant extension of concepts such as cultural sensitivity and cultural competence.

Nurses learning to be culturally safe practitioners begin with reflection on their own cultural identity and history, and move, through guided education, to commitment to personal and political change. Wood and Schwass[36] depict this process of change as occurring in three stages: *dualism, relativism* and *evolving commitment.* The model of change is outlined in Box 38.3, followed by an example of development of cultural safety in the process of assessment.

BOX 38.3: DEVELOPING CULTURAL SAFETY IN THE PROCESS OF ASSESSMENT

Stage one: dualism

At this stage of development nurses rely on authority to provide answers to questions of cultural difference. They typically look to literature and the opinions of experts to guide their thinking, although their own beliefs are strongly held. A statement characteristic of this stage is 'Culture doesn't matter to me. I treat everyone the same regardless of their culture.' The nurse at this stage is not aware that she cannot step outside her own culture, and that her interactions are, in part, culturally determined.

Stage two: relativism

This stage involves awareness of the diversity of cultural perspectives, but the nurse may feel that all views have equal validity. Authorities, including cultural authorities, are simply one more opinion. There appears to be no basis for action that is better than another. A nurse might say: 'We all have our own views, but none of us can claim to be right. Even members of the same culture might have different views. We should try to respect them all.' This statement recognizes diversity both between and within cultures, but that diversity is seen as invalidating actions that are committed to a particular cultural perspective.

Stage three: evolving commitment

The nurse at this stage is able to both recognize diversity of cultural perspectives, and commit to a course of action. The action is informed by the realities of the nurse's culture, his or her place in the power relationships of health care, and the realities of the culture of the service user. Commitment is demonstrated in the statement: 'People don't always feel safe to identify their cultural needs. We need to create a safe environment in which needs can be expressed, and provide the right supports so that those needs can be met.' The nurse making this statement is aware that factors outside the individual nurse–patient relationship influence the health care encounter, and consciously uses the power of his or her position to benefit the patient.

Source: Adapted from Wood and Schwass.[36]

Stage one: clinical example

The nurse conducts an assessment interview and records the service user's ethnicity after asking the patient to select ethnicity from a list provided on the assessment form. There is no discussion of whether the categories available reflect the person's cultural identity. The nurse believes that while it is important to acknowledge cultural identity, this can be achieved on the basis of ethnicity. There may be an assumption that the person will make any special needs known, and so no inquiry about special cultural needs is undertaken. Any requests regarding cultural needs are responded to on the basis of the same treatment to all patients regardless of particular cultural needs.

Stage two: clinical example

As part of the assessment interview the service user is asked to identify their ethnicity, but is also asked if the available categories accurately reflect their cultural identity. Additional comments or issues are recorded after discussion with the service user. The nurse is aware that ethnicity does not determine cultural beliefs, and asks if there are any particular cultural needs. Specific needs will be addressed if the resources for doing this are immediately available. If there are no resources immediately available, this is simply recognized as a limitation of the system.

Stage three: clinical example

The nurse creates a safe environment for the assessment interview, perhaps by involving members of the service user's family, with consent of the service user. The service user self-identifies his ethnicity, and is given an opportunity to identify any specific needs or concerns. When specific needs are identified by the service user, the nurse talks to colleagues and members of the service user's cultural group to establish ways of providing appropriate cultural support. Support is provided only in consultation with the service user. The nurse reflects on the impact of social processes on the health care encounter and uses the experience to further his or her own knowledge of resources and supports available, and to make that knowledge available to other nurses in the service.

CULTURAL SAFETY AND COLLABORATIVE CARE

The process of psychiatric and mental health nursing involves establishing collaborative therapeutic relationships with service users on the basis of their need for nursing care. (Therapeutic relationships are also discussed in chapter 3). Barker's[37] Tidal Model of mental health nursing stresses the need for the person's experience of mental distress or illness to be understood by the nurse. It also emphasizes provision of 'support and services a person might need to live an ordinary life' (p.234). However, development of understanding between nurses and service users is influenced by differences that must be negotiated by the nurse.[38] In cross-cultural encounters, the paradoxical nature of nursing is apparent. After researching nurses' experiences of cross-cultural caring, Spence[39] concluded that 'Trying to be oneself in a way that enables others to be themselves, under circumstances that are intrinsically never fully knowable, is unlikely to be free of tension' (p.629). For indigenous or ethnic minority nurses the issues may be even more complex. A study of Māori mental health nurses found that these nurses needed to call upon their indigenous cultural knowledge as well as knowledge of the professional culture of nursing, resulting in the experience of 'bridging two worlds'.[40]

Nurses who are focused on establishing a therapeutic relationship will consider both their own cultural identity and those of service users. Making sense of the experience of mental distress or illness requires understanding of the influence of culture on that experience. Because of the diversity of service users' cultural identities in relation to that of the nurse, it will not be possible for nurses to understand all the possible cultural influences the nurse and the service user bring to the therapeutic relationship. Such an approach, while demonstrating cultural sensitivity, assumes that racism is the product of ignorance and that, by learning about other cultures, people will be educated out of their prejudice.

Nurses also need to provide an opportunity for service users to make their cultural needs known. Additional strategies include developing partnerships with cultural intermediaries, or developing roles for cultural support workers. Collaborative care relies on therapeutic communication, which reflects the cultural backgrounds of nurses and service users. Communication patterns are influenced by culture, with many communication patterns being culturebound.

In a study of Chinese service users' communications patterns with nurses, unique cultural influences were identified.[41] While the nurses were aware that Chinese culture had a significant effect on therapeutic communication, their communication strategies tended to reflect the Western models of their nursing education. The authors concluded that 'to be therapeutic with clients from diverse backgrounds, nurses need to understand the intricacies of different cultures' (p.34). The researchers recommended that Chinese service users would benefit from nurses' improved understanding of culturally bound communication strategies. We would add that understanding the culture of others does not involve becoming an expert or authority on those cultures.

The dominant interpersonal model of mental health nursing is a Western construct, having been developed within a North American cultural context and then adopted in other Western and non-Western countries. However, the practice of mental health nursing needs to be responsive to the realities of the diverse cultures in which it takes place, in order to provide care that service users experience as culturally safe.

RECOVERY AND SERVICE USER INVOLVEMENT

Recovery recognizes the fact that an individual cannot fully heal in an environment that supports racism, homophobia, sexism, and colonization. Developing a healthy society can be seen as recovery on a collective scale.[42]

Recovery is a central tenet of mental health nursing practice, its emancipatory focus placing the service user at the centre of care and in doing so returning the possibility of dignity, self-determination, connection and healing to those whose lives have been changed by mental distress and illness (additional information on recovery can be found in chapters 35 and 36). Originating in the antipsychiatry movement which was also shaped by feminism and other liberation movements, recovery provides an alternative framework to the professionalization and pathologization of mental illness.[43] A recovery framework for psychiatric nursing must explicitly take into account social and structural inequities such as colonization and racism, in addition to individual factors such as empowerment, hope and autonomy (keeping in mind that these notions are also problematic). Bringing cultural and religious identities to the centre of mental health nursing practice can assist practitioners in achieving broader emancipatory aims wrought by feminism, postcolonialism and other social justice movements. Contact with the mental health care system is a result of diverse experiences and therefore mental health nurses must consider what people might be 'recovering from' and consider the need for the expansion of support services beyond the health system to include other social supports and structural changes as well.

It can be useful to consider issues of culture in the context of involvement of service users in the planning, provision and evaluation of mental health services. Mental health services have traditionally been organized around the needs of service providers, rather than service users,[44] and have reflected the cultural values of the provider group. However, users of services are disproportionately members of minority cultures, whose values are not always recognized in the services provided. Involvement of service users means that nurses have to consider how their practice can best meet the needs of the people they care for. One way of meeting the needs of culturally diverse groups is to involve those groups in the provision of services. Service users can be involved in direct care roles or in advisory roles aimed at promoting the cultural safety of the service. Nurses can expect to work alongside service users and can learn from both the service experience and the cultural experience this group has to offer.

Involvement in services can extend to managing service provision. Pierre[45] describes the role of a company formed by service users to provide services to ethnic minority service users in Liverpool. In providing services, the company seeks to create a nonracist environment which challenges institutional processes encountered by ethnic minorities in mainstream services. Pierre concludes that 'user involvement is not an impossible dream, but a necessary possibility and a desirable antidote to the uncaring, unhelpful and unwanted image of psychiatry currently portrayed among black users'[45] (p.256).

The cultural safety model calls for changes at an institutional level in order that mental health services are safe for members of all cultures. It also draws attention to issues of power in the provision of mental health services. Service users from overrepresented ethnic groups can be involved in the provision of mainstream services (those which are available to all members of the community), or in the development of culturally specific services to members of their own communities.

> ### REFLECTION
>
> - How do staff working in the services in which you are employed reflect the cultural backgrounds of those who use the services?
>
> - Do service users have the option of seeking care from clinicians of their own culture?

CULTURALLY SPECIFIC SERVICES

Another response to the overrepresentation of service users from minority cultures is the development of services provided by members of those cultures for service users of their own culture.[46] Culturally specific services aim to overcome the problem of cultural domination often experienced in mainstream services, and to meet the needs of service users in ways that are consistent with their cultural beliefs. New Zealand has developed a model of *kaupapa* Māori ('using a Māori approach') services for Māori service users.[47] While the same range of treatment options available in mainstream services is available in Māori services, the staff are all Māori, and are committed to observing Māori protocol in providing services.

Staff of culturally specific services may be nurses or other health professionals, or they may be employed especially for their cultural knowledge and skills. This includes traditional and contemporary cultural knowledge. Culturally skilled staff work alongside clinical staff, providing treatment programmes that are likely to include cultural activities and incorporate cultural protocols within standard forms of treatment.

While culturally specific services may be useful for members of overrepresented minorities, caution needs to be exercised in offering service users choice in participating in culturally specific services. We have already discussed the important issues of choice in cultural identity, and the same caution needs to be exercised in offering culturally specific care. If clinicians ascribe culture on the basis of ethnicity, then there may be misunderstandings in offering culturally specific care.

Culturally specific services have the potential to offer a real alternative to service users, which challenges the dominant Western values of mental health services. Nurses from marginalized ethnicities need educational opportunities aimed at developing the unique combination of cultural and clinical skills necessary to provide culturally specific care. They need to recognize that culturally safe care requires structural change supported by allocation of resources in order to address the effects of historical processes.

Huarahi Whakatu – Dual Competency Programme

In New Zealand, a Nursing Council accredited programme called Huarahi Whakatu is available to Māori registered nurses. It offers a dual competency-based professional development programme which recognizes Māori cultural knowledge and skills possessed alongside nursing competencies.[48,49] The programme assists Māori nurses to identify and enhance the distinct elements they bring to their practice. The notion that underlies this pedagogy is that Māori nurses affirm that nursing care aligns well with Māori cultural values and the principles of caring for others.[50] Located within a Māori developmental ethos, the programme is informed by the principles of adding value to an indigenous workforce, by asserting the importance of being Māori, with the validation of contemporary Māori cultural worldviews.[51,52]

This example of indigenous health workforce development is one of a number of cultural competency-based programmes in New Zealand established by Māori.[53] The concept of cultural safety and that of cultural competency has been advanced by Māori in New Zealand as a strategy to address the inequities experienced by Māori. By doing so, such programmes integrate the paradigms of Māori cultural identity while addressing the barriers in the health and education system to proactively build the capacity of the Māori health workforce.

> **REFLECTION**
>
> What cultural skills and knowledge do you bring to your role as a mental health nurse? How can you draw on the cultural skills and knowledge of your colleagues?

FUTURE DEVELOPMENTS

Ethnic diversity in Western countries continues to increase at an unprecedented rate. In addition, minority ethnic groups have become more vocal about maintaining their cultural identity and practices. Global political events have led to religious diversity becoming more visible in Western countries. Combined with increased immigration from non-traditional source countries, this has led to increased societal anxiety and the desire to address issues of cohesion and national identity. Increasing diversity is likely to continue through continuing population movements throughout the twenty-first century. This will place demands on individual nurses to reflect on the nature of their own cultural identity and the implications of cultural differences for their encounters with service users.

Nurses will also need to develop a broad range of cultural skills and knowledge, although they cannot be expected to become experts in the cultures of service users. Services will need to consider how to recruit and retain nurses from marginalized ethnic groups, and may need to provide culturally specific services for some populations. The value of mental health services working with faith-based organizations has been signalled as something with great potential in mental health care. Individual, institutional and social change is necessary to meet the challenges of cultural diversity.

While much of the responsibility for addressing issues of providing culturally safe care rests with service managers and funders, individual nurses can also take action to improve their responsiveness to service users from cultures different to their own. *Clinical supervision* offers an opportunity for reflection on cultural issues, including cultural identity, power and the nurse's ability to respond to cultural needs (see chapter 10 for more on clinical supervision).

Supervision with nurses from different cultures is one way of facilitating this, either as supervisors or as participants in group supervision.[28]

Opportunities to develop cultural knowledge and skills may also present themselves in the form of service development and education, liaison with cultural services and discussion with colleagues and service users. Nurses need to focus on development of cultural awareness and skills as part of their professional development, and as part of their commitment to meeting the full range of needs of service users.

CONCLUSION

Cultural safety in mental health nursing is not merely a polite recognition of one aspect of a service user's identity. By recognizing and responding to the multiple identities of service users, we seek to engage more deeply in interpersonal relationships, with the aim of providing therapeutic care. To achieve a deeply interpersonal level of engagement, mental health nurses need first to reflect on their own cultural identities, on the social and historical contexts of mental health care, and on the implications of cultural difference for power in the therapeutic relationship.

The continued relevance of interpersonal models of mental health nursing depends on their capacity to respond to the demands of increasing cultural diversity. Without

awareness of cultural identity, therapeutic relationships in mental health nursing are simply one more form of professional relationship in which care, treatment and services are provided to service users without recognition of their full identities.

The nursing relationship has been described as frequently 'one-way traffic'. Concepts such as collaborative care mark nursing's commitment to know and respond to the other, recognizing that the capacity to know another person is limited by the nurse's perceptions of 'otherness'. For nurses to offer themselves more fully to service users, the cultural dimension of the nursing relationship needs to be acknowledged and explored.

References

1. Leavey G, Dura-Vila G, King M. Finding common ground: the boundaries and interconnections between faith-based organisations and mental health services. *Mental Health, Religion and Culture* 2012; **15**(4): 349–62.
2. Bhugra D, Gupta S (eds). *Migration and mental health*. Cambridge: Cambridge University Press, 2010.
3. Drevdahl DJ, Philips DA, Taylor JY. Uncontested categories: the use of race and ethnicity variables in nursing research. *Nursing Inquiry* 2006; **13**(1): 52–63.
4. Crossley D. Secular psychiatry and the self. *Mental Health, Religion and Culture* 2011; **14**(1): 31–4.
5. Whitley R. Religious competence as cultural competence. *Transcultural Psychiatry* 2012; **49**(2): 245–60.
6. Gomi S, Starnino VR, Canda ER. Spiritual assessment in mental health recovery. *Community Mental Health Journal* 2014; **50**(4): 447–53.
7. Barker P, Jackson S, Stevenson C. The need for psychiatric nursing: towards a multidimensional theory of caring. *Nursing Inquiry* 1999; **6**: 103–11.
8. Brascoupé S, Waters C. Cultural safety exploring the applicability of the concept of cultural safety to Aboriginal health and community wellness. *International Journal of Indigenous Health* 2009; **5**(2): 6–41.
9. Doutrich D, Arcus K, Dekker L, Spuck J, Pollock-Robinson C. Cultural safety in New Zealand and the United States looking at a way forward together. *Journal of Transcultural Nursing* 2012; **23**(2): 143–50.
10. Racine L. The enduring challenge of cultural safety in nursing. *CJNR (Canadian Journal of Nursing Research)* 2014; **46**(2): 6–9.
11. Mohammed SA. Moving beyond the 'exotic': applying postcolonial theory in health research. *Advances in Nursing Science* 2006; **29**(2): 98–109.
12. Lauder W, Kroll T, Jones M. Social determinants of mental health: the missing dimensions of mental health nursing? *Journal of Psychiatric and Mental Health Nursing* 2007; **14**(7): 661–9.
13. WHO (World Health Organization). What are social determinants of health? Available from: http://www.who.int/social_determinants/sdh_definition/en/ [Accessed 7th October 2016].
14. Fernando S. *Mental health, race and culture*, 3rd edn. Basingstoke: Palgrave Macmillan, 2010.
15. Anderson JM. Reflections on the social determinants of women's health exploring intersections: does racialization matter? *CJNR (Canadian Journal of Nursing Research)* 2006; **38**(1): 7–14.
16. Culley L. Transcending transculturalism? Race, ethnicity and health-care. *Nursing Inquiry* 2006; **13**(2): 144–53.
17. Shattell M, Hogan B. The problem of miscommunication. *Journal of Psychosocial Nursing and Mental Health Services* 2005; **43**(10): 29–32.
18. O'Brien TP, O'Brien AJ, Morrison-Ngatai L, McNulty N, Skews G, Ryan T. *Clinical indicators for mental health nursing standards of practice. Report to Health Research Council of New Zealand.* Wellington: Health Research Council of New Zealand, 2002.
19. Wendt DC, Gone JP. Rethinking cultural competence: insights from indigenous community treatment settings. *Transcultural Psychiatry* 2012; **49**(2): 206–22.
20. Carnevale FA. Toward a cultural conception of the self. *Journal of Psychosocial Nursing and Mental Health Services* 1999; **37**(8): 26–31.
21. Durie M. Indigenizing mental health services: New Zealand experience. *Transcultural Psychiatry* 2011; **48**(1–2): 24–36.
22. Leff J. *Psychiatry around the globe. A transcultural view.* London: Gaskell, 1988.
23. Alarcón RD. Culture, cultural factors and psychiatric diagnosis: review and projections. *World Psychiatry* 2009; **8**(3): 131–9.

24. Pi EH, Simpson GM. Psychopharmacology: cross-cultural psychopharmacology: a current clinical perspective. *Psychiatric Services* 2005; **56**(1): 31–3.
25. Ministry of Health. *Office of the Director of Mental Health. Annual report 2013*. Wellington: Ministry of Health, 2014.
26. Noble P, Rogers S. Violence by psychiatric inpatients. *British Journal of Psychiatry* 1989; **155**: 384–90.
27. Bond CF, DiCandia CG, McKinnon JR. Responses to violence in a psychiatric setting: the role of patients' race. *Personality and Social Psychology Bulletin* 1988; **14**: 448–58.
28. Campinha-Bacote J. Becoming culturally competent in ethnic psychopharmacology. *Journal of Psychosocial Nursing and Mental Health Services* 2007; **45**(9): 27–33.
29. Salsberry PJ, Corwin E, Reagan PB. A complex web of risks for metabolic syndrome: race/ethnicity, economics, and gender. *American Journal of Preventive Medicine* 2007; **33**(2): 114–20.
30. Ghali S, Fisher HL, Joyce J, Major B, Hobbs L, Soni S, Chisholm B, Rahaman N, Papada P, Lawrence J, Bloy S, Marlowe K, Aitchison KJ, Power P, Johnson S. Ethnic variations in pathways into early intervention services for psychosis. *British Journal of Psychiatry* 2013; **202**(4): 277–83.
31. DeSouza R. Multicultural relationships in supervision. In: Wepa D (ed.). *Clinical supervision in the health professions: the New Zealand experience*. Auckland: Pearson Education, 2007: 96–109.
32. Majumdar B, Browne G, Roberts J, Carpio B. Effects of cultural sensitivity training on health care provider attitudes and patient outcomes. *Journal of Nursing Scholarship* 2004; **36**(2): 161–6.
33. Bush CT. Cultural competence: implications of the Surgeon General's report on mental health. *Journal of Child and Adolescent Psychiatric Nursing* 2000; **13**(4): 177–8.
34. Wells MI. Beyond cultural competence: a model for individual and institutional cultural development. *Journal of Community Health Nursing* 2000; **17**: 189–99.
35. Nursing Council of New Zealand. *Guidelines for cultural safety, the Treaty of Waitangi and Maori health in nursing education and practice*. Wellington: Nursing Council of New Zealand, 2011.
36. Wood PJ, Schwass M. Cultural safety: a framework for changing attitudes. *Nursing Praxis in New Zealand* 1993; **8**(1): 4–15.
37. Barker P, Buchanan-Barker P. *The Tidal Model: a guide for mental health professionals*. London: Brunner-Routledge, 2005.
38. Walsh C. Negotiating difference in mental health nursing in New Zealand. In: Tilley S (ed.). *The mental health nurse. Views of education and practice*. Oxford: Blackwell, 1997: 172–85.

39. Spence DG. Hermeneutic notions illuminate cross-cultural nursing experiences. *Journal of Advanced Nursing* 2001; **35**: 624–30.
40. Wilson D, Baker M. Bridging two worlds: Māori mental health nursing. *Qualitative Health Research* 2012; **22**(8): 1073–82.
41. Arthur D, Chan HK, Fung WY, Wong KY, Yeung KW. Therapeutic communication strategies used by Hong Kong clients with their Chinese clients. *Journal of Psychiatric and Mental Health Nursing* 1999; **6**: 29–36.
42. Ida DJ. Cultural competency and recovery within diverse populations. *Psychiatric Rehabilitation Journal* 2007; **31**(1): 49.
43. Slade M. Mental illness and well-being: the central importance of positive psychology and recovery approaches. *BMC Health Services Research* 2010; **10**(1): 26.
44. Repper J. Adjusting the focus of mental health nursing: incorporating service users' perspective of recovery. *Journal of Mental Health* 2000; **9**: 575–87.
45. Pierre SA. Psychiatry and citizenship: the Liverpool black mental health users' perspective. *Journal of Psychiatric and Mental Health Nursing* 2000; **7**: 249–57.
46. Bhui K, Sashidharan SP. Should there be separate psychiatric services for ethnic minority groups? *British Journal of Psychiatry* 2003; **182**: 10–12.
47. Clements J, Blissett W. Culture and mental health in Aotearoa, New Zealand. In: Moodley R, Ocampo M (eds). *Critical psychiatry and mental health: exploring the work of Suman Fernando in clinical practice*. East Sussex: Routledge, 2014: 227–36.
48. Te Rau Matatini. Huarahi Whakatū Professional Development and Recognition Programme. 2014. Available from: http://teraumatatini.com/sites/default/files/Huarahi%20Whakatu%20Pamphlet%20_.pdf [Accessed 3rd November 2016].
49. Baker M, Levy M. E Toru Ngā Mea. *Pimatisiwin* 2013; **11**(3): 471.
50. Simon V. Characterising Māori nursing practice. *Contemporary Nurse* 2006; **22**(2): 203–13.
51. Smith LT. *Decolonizing methodologies: research and indigenous peoples*, 2nd edn. New York: Zed Books, 2010.
52. Pihama LE. *Tīhei mauri ora: honouring our voices: mana wahine as a kaupapa Māori: theoretical framework* (Unpublished doctoral thesis). University of Auckland, 2001.
53. Ratima MM, Brown RM, Garrett NK, Wikaire EI, Ngawati RM, Aspin CS, Potaka UK. Strengthening Māori participation in the New Zealand health and disability workforce. *Medical Journal of Australia* 2007; **186**(10): 541.

Further reading

Bhui K. *Racism and mental health: prejudice and suffering*. London: Jessica Kingsley, 2002.

Burnard P, Gill P. *Culture, communication and nursing*. Abingdon: Routledge, 2015.

Centre for Social Justice. *Mental health: poverty, ethnicity and family breakdown*. London: Centre for Social Justice, 2011.

Fernando S. *Mental health, race and culture*. Basingstoke: Palgrave Macmillan, 2010.

Fernando S, Keating F (eds). *Mental health in a multi-ethnic society: a multidisciplinary handbook*. London and New York: Routledge, 2008.

McCarthy A, Coleborne C (eds). *Migration, ethnicity, and mental health: international perspectives, 1840–2010*. Abingdon: Routledge, 2012.

Rogers A, Pilgrim D. *A sociology of mental health and illness*. Maidenhead: McGraw-Hill Education (UK), 2014.

Sewell H. *Working with ethnicity, race and culture in mental health: a handbook for practitioners*. London: Jessica Kingsley, 2009.

Wepa D (ed.). *Cultural safety in Aotearoa New Zealand*. Cambridge: Cambridge University Press, 2015.

Relevant web pages

Black Mental Health UK (England). http://www.blackmentalhealth.org.uk/
This website was developed to raise awareness and address the stigma associated with mental illness.

Flinders University. Shannon's journey. http://www.flinders.edu.au/nursing/mental-health-and-culture/shannons-journey/
Shannon is an Australian aboriginal woman experiencing postpartum psychosis.

Flinders University. Sui's journey. http://www.flinders.edu.au/nursing/mental-health-and-culture/sui/home.cfm
Sui is an Asian Australian woman with cognitive decline.

He Kokonga Ngakau – Mo wai Te Matauranga (Roots of resilience) (New Zealand). https://www.mcgill.ca/resilience/
Dr Pam Bennett's research confirms that for Māori, Māori methods of treating mental health are preferable to Western models.

Healthtalk. http://www.mentalhealth.org.uk/help-information/mental-health-a-z/b/bme-communities/
This website, hosted by the University of Oxford (UK), is devoted to providing free reliable information about health issues. This page provides information about mental health issues experienced by the black and ethnic minority (BME) community.

Māori digital stories about whanau (family) caregiving. https://www.youtube.com/watch?v=G9zXJOnRuEl&feature=youtu.be

Māori mental health nursing oral history project. http://www.maorinursinghistory.com/

Mental Health Commission of Canada. http://www.mentalhealth-commission.ca/English/focus-areas/diversity
This page covers issues of cultural diversity in mental health services.

Mental Health Foundation (England). Black and ethnic minorities. http://www.mentalhealth.org.uk/help-information/mental-health-a-z/b/bme-communities/

Multicultural Mental Health Resource Centre (Canada). http://www.multiculturalmentalhealth.ca/
This website provides access to resources to support culturally safe and competent mental health care.

39 Motivational interviewing

ELIZABETH HUGHES

LEARNING OUTCOMES

- To understand the fundamental philosophy, principles and skills of motivational interviewing (MI).

- To explore therapeutic interactions where MI can be usefully applied.

- To understand how MI can fit in with other therapeutic approaches, such as cognitive behavioural therapy (CBT).

- To be aware of the evidence base for MI across a range of health conditions.

- To be able to apply MI to specific examples of therapeutic interactions and reflect on your own skills and limitations in being able to make MI a tool in the craft of caring.

SUMMARY OF KEY POINTS

- People are best persuaded by their own reasons for change (not ours).
- The best conditions for change occur when the practitioner listens, reflects and does not judge people's choices.
- Most people are ambivalent about whether to change or not (rather than in denial).
- MI has been used successfully in mental health settings to promote healthy lifestyle choices (e.g. smoking, substance use, medication adherence).

INTRODUCTION

When we take people merely as they are, we make them worse; when we treat them as if they were what they should be, we improve them as far as they can be improved.

Goethe, 1749–1832[1]

Motivational interviewing (MI) is a therapeutic interaction that helps people think about change. According to Miller and Rollnick,[2] 'it is a collaborative conversation style for strengthening a person's own motivation and commitment to change' (p.12). As practitioners, it is important to bear in mind that we are not equipped with special powers to *make* people change. All we can do is ensure that we have created the optimum environment in which people feel safe to explore their options and choices without feeling judged or 'nagged'. MI focuses on the exploration and resolution of ambivalence about change. It aims to find out a person's unique reasons for wanting to change, their readiness and ability to change, and their perceived or actual barriers that prevent this change from happening. MI has taken various forms and names, including motivational enhancement therapy,[3] compliance therapy[4] and treatment adherence therapy.[5]

Miller and Rollnick[2,6] originally developed MI in the context of working with people with alcohol and drug services. The therapeutic approach is person-centred at its heart (heavily influenced by Carl Rogers'[7] person-centred therapy) and was developed as a response to the confrontational and challenging approach to addiction treatment that existed in the 1980s and 1990s. The prevailing model at the time was the 'Minnesota Model' that had been developed in the 1950s; it was based on the principle of Alcoholics Anonymous (AA) that addiction was a chronic and relapsing illness. While the philosophy of the Minnesota Model and the AA was based on compassion, the development of a confrontational style in the treatment of addictions became the norm. Practitioners used to consider people with addictions as being 'in denial' and therefore saw their role as

shattering this denial and helping people to recognize that they had a problem. Bill Miller found that a confrontational approach led to poor outcomes, and he developed MI with Steven Rollnick as an alternative approach, which quickly became established in Europe and Australia.

Over the years, MI has been adapted and applied beyond the treatment of addictions because of its utility in helping people consider healthy choices and changes to their lifestyle. MI has been used in the wider field of health care for both mental health and physical problems, including alcohol misuse, cannabis and other drug use, smoking, sexual health, bulimia, diet and exercise, treatment compliance, gambling, emotional well-being and parenting practices.[8] The aim of this chapter is to describe the key principles, processes and skills of MI, and to illustrate its application in mental health with some examples and reflection points. Although the examples in this chapter draw on real people's experiences and therapeutic interactions, they do not describe one actual person.

FUNDAMENTAL CONCEPTS IN MI

How do people change?

Before we begin to discuss MI, it is important to consider the process that people go through when changing behaviour. We all know that changing is *hard* and we can all think of something we have attempted to change but struggled to put our intentions into action, or something that we managed to change but it was not long before we went back to our old ways. This is part of the normal process of change. Most people typically lapse several times before finally cementing the changes. For others, the hurdles to change can sometimes be insurmountable.

> ### REFLECTION
>
> Consider a behaviour that you successfully managed to change for some time. This behaviour could be health-related, e.g. overeating, or could be related to work, e.g. procrastinating. Ask yourself:
>
> * What circumstances led you to make the change?
> * How did you do it?
> * What difficulties did you come across in trying to make the change?
> * What helped you make the change?
> * What helped you sustain the change?

There are four key ingredients required for change: Desire, Ability, Reason and Need (DARN).[9]

* *Desire:* People are motivated by a dream or a wish they have for things to change for the better. To put it simply: change has got to be 'worth it'. It is important for people

to make their dreams and wishes explicit, and to understand how a change, such as adopting a healthy habit or dropping an unhelpful or destructive behaviour, can get them closer to their dream or wish. Desire focuses on the feelings that the thoughts of change create: these thoughts should be exciting (and maybe a bit scary!).
* *Ability:* People need to have the means and behavioural skills to support their desire for change. Willpower alone is not sufficient. If people perceive that change is beyond their capabilities, they may not even try. Self-efficacy is a concept introduced by Bandura,[10] referring to the belief or confidence in one's own ability to achieve change.
* *Reason:* This is the rationale that people give for making a change, based on weighing the benefits of change against staying the same.
* *Need:* This reflects the idea that change is necessary and urgent in order to avoid the negative consequences that may ensue if the person stays the same.

Sustain talk vs. change talk

The DARN ingredients for change are often revealed when people are allowed the time and space to talk about it. This is known as 'change talk'. Here is an example of change talk from someone who wants to give up smoking:

* Desire: 'I would like to breathe more easily.'
* Ability: 'I know I can do it because I managed to quit in the past.'
* Reasons: 'I want to be healthier and save money.'
* Needs: 'With my asthma, I can't continue smoking or I will not be able to breathe.'

When people are feeling uncertain about change, we will hear 'sustain talk', which is the opposite of change talk.

Sustain talk is characterized by content related to desire, ability, reason and need to stay the same (maintain the status quo). Here is an example of sustain talk for the same person as above:

- Desire: 'I really love to smoke, it's my one naughty pleasure.'
- Ability: 'I've tried quitting so many times and always relapse.'
- Reason: 'I like smoking as it gives me something to do when I am bored.'
- Need: 'If I didn't smoke, I don't know how I would manage my anxiety.'

REFLECTION

Consider something that you would like to change in your everyday life and think through the DARN ingredients that could motivate you:

- You have a real *desire* for things to be different, i.e. you could see a new way of doing things, and you could see the benefits and outcomes of that change.

- You recognize that you have the *ability* to change, i.e. you have the skills, resources and support to be able to change.

- You have good *reasons* to change, i.e. you can justify making the change because of the advantages of it against the advantages of staying the same.

- You recognize your *need* to change, i.e. you have a sense of urgency about change to avoid the consequences that may happen if you stay the same.

Now write down some change talk statements under the acronym DARN:

- *Desire:* If I change, then I will …

- *Ability:* I know I am able to change because … / I can help myself change by … / I can get help and support to change by … / I am already doing … to help myself change.

- *Reason:* I am ready to change because … / I want to change because …

- *Need:* If I didn't change then … / I have to change now because …

Motivation in a state of constant motion

Motivation is a constantly shifting state rather than a dichotomous concept (motivated versus not motivated). People can leave a consultation session with a practitioner feeling very motivated, but their motivation can quickly change in an instant in the face of temptation. People are often 'ambivalent' about change, rather than being completely against any change. Our task as practitioners is to explore the nature of this ambivalence and help the person identify their own reasons for change and the strategies that may help them. People are more likely to be driven to change by their own motives, and not the ones imposed externally. People will vary in how willing and able they are in terms of adopting new behaviours. Some have very clear *desire*, *reason* and *need* to change, but lack the confidence in their *ability* to implement and maintain this change. Others are confident, but lack the urgency of needing to change at the current time, because they have other priorities and/or do not see that change is that important or relevant to them.

A common challenge that is often identified by practitioners is what to do about the 'unmotivated service user'. The first step is to challenge this label: no one is actually 'unmotivated' but they are rather not willing to adopt the viewpoint and goals suggested by the practitioner. This is known as discord. As part of MI, practitioners seek to develop a shared agreement with the service user around the problem and strategies for change. Discord is usually highest at the start of a therapeutic relationship (when the service user is likely to be more defensive and less interested in change talk) and should decrease over time if the practitioner uses strategies appropriate to the service user's stage of change. Minimizing discord between the practitioner and the service user is crucial as it is associated with high treatment dropout rates, and reduces the likelihood of productive change talk.

PRINCIPLES AND PROCESSES OF MI

MI is based on *compassion* and *acceptance*, which are fundamental principles underpinning any therapeutic interaction in the craft of caring for people who are vulnerable and in need. Compassion is the deliberate commitment to pursue the welfare and best interests of others, and it is not about suffering or identifying with others, or feeling sorry about them. Also see chapter 3 on developing and maintaining therapeutic relationship, as these principles are very important for creating an atmosphere conducive to the consideration of change. Acceptance refers to what the service user brings or holds as important, and it is not necessarily the practitioner's acceptance of the service user's behaviour. In the context of MI, the practitioner's personal approval (or disapproval) of the service user's behaviour is irrelevant and unhelpful.

The following approaches would not be considered MI-compliant. Try to avoid using the following strategies to help convince people change by:

- inciting fear, e.g. emphasizing what would happen if they did not change: 'If you don't give up alcohol, you will die …'
- preaching, e.g. repeatedly telling them what they have to do: 'You have to take your medication at the same time every day, we have been through this several times'
- blaming, e.g. telling them it is their fault: 'I am not surprised that you keep getting respiratory infections because you continue to smoke'

However, information and advice still have an important place in helping people to consider change. It is the process through which the information is offered or invited that is a subtle difference.

Here are the same scenarios addressed in a more MI-compliant way:

- 'I wonder if you would be interested in hearing more about alcohol and its impact on health?'
- 'You have recognized there is an issue with taking your medication every day; I can offer some time to talk about how medicines work and what that means for your routine – would this be of interest?'
- 'You've noticed that you have had a lot of respiratory infections recently, and you are feeling really poorly. I wonder if it would be useful to have a chat about this and consider how to help reduce this happening?'

Note that the difference here is that rather than narrowly focusing on the target behaviour, the options for discussion are opened up. Once a conversation is flowing, then information can be offered in a simple and non-judgemental way.

Over the years, there has been an increasing focus in MI research and practice on developing specific skills, perhaps at the expense of maintaining the underlying philosophy,

or 'spirit', of MI; therefore, it is as important to consider MI as a therapeutic stance as much as a set of skills. In other words, in MI, it is not only *what* you do, but also *how* you do it. The 'spirit of MI'[9] comprises three concepts: *collaboration*, *evocation* and *autonomy*.

Collaboration: One of the key aspects of the spirit of MI is that an intervention is not *done to* the service user but is rather *done with* them. MI holds that each party brings their own expertise; the service user is an expert on their own life, motives and difficulties, whereas the practitioner brings their knowledge and insights from having worked with people who experienced similar difficulties. This requires that the practitioner is self-aware and self-monitors their aims, preconceptions and motives, because these may lead to a one-way conversation or to questions with value-added judgements.

Evocation: This is the process of finding out what goals, values, dreams, strengths and skills service users have and trying to use these as a stepping-stone for a potential behaviour change. It is the opposite of a deficit-focused process, in which we are trying to give service users what they lack, whether it is knowledge, skills or chemicals, in order to help them overcome their problems.

Autonomy: This aspect of MI is about respecting the right of the person to decide their own direction, choices and lifestyle, even when we think that these are not in their best interests. Valuing the service user's autonomy over and above a 'positive' change may appear counterintuitive for a conscientious practitioner, especially in the current outcome-driven health care system. Still, telling someone what to do, or what they cannot do, usually provokes a reaction in the opposite direction and can be counterproductive for engagement and collaboration. Paradoxically, respecting a service user's autonomy not to change is likely to make them think about change.

SKILLS IN MI

There are four important skills which underpin the practitioner–service user interaction in motivational interviewing; these make up the acronym OARS:[9] Open-ended questioning, *Affirmation*, *Reflection* and *Summarizing*.

Open-ended questioning

By asking open-ended questions, we allow people to tell their story; for example: 'Can you tell me about a typical day when you …', or 'Can you start by telling me about the time when you started using alcohol as a way of coping?' Closed questions are often answered with a 'yes/no' or a single-word response; e.g. 'Do you drink alcohol as a way of coping?' or 'You were very young when you started using

drugs, weren't you?' It is important to allow time for people to answer the question before moving on to another, and we can encourage people to talk by following up their answer with prompts such as 'Can you elaborate on this so that I understand where you are coming from?' or 'I'd be interested in hearing more about this.'

Affirmation

Affirmation is recognizing people's strengths, and acknowledging what they are able to achieve, often under difficult circumstances. Affirmation requires genuineness and not just giving compliments for the sake of it. It is also about being supportive of a person's decisions and life choices without being patronizing or falsely positive. Here is an example of using affirmation:

Service user: 'Waking up in hospital after getting drunk and taking those pills freaked me out … It was an eye-opener and I want to change, for myself and my family …'
Practitioner: 'I respect and support your idea that this last alcohol binge and overdose is an opportunity for you to make some changes and consider what is really important. What sorts of things are important in your life that are worth giving up drinking for?'

Reflection

It is essential to be able to listen effectively so that we can understand the meaning of what the service user tells us and accurately paraphrase and repeat this back to them. Reflection of content is essential to allow the service user to hear their own story, gain some insights, and make sense of what has happened. Reflection is not just repeating information parrot-fashion; it requires that we 'read through the lines' and are able to verbalize the service user's feelings or thoughts, which can sometimes be implicit in what they are telling us. In MI, we listen carefully for both change talk and sustain talk and we reflect this back to the person. For example:

Service user: 'I want to give up smoking but I cannot do it at the moment. I am very stressed at work now and my partner also smokes at home … I am fed up with trying.'
Practitioner: 'OK, you feel frustrated because you have a battle going on between wanting to give up smoking but finding it almost impossible at the moment because of the situation at work. You are also battling alone because your partner smokes, is this right?'

Summarizing

We use reflection throughout an MI conversation to highlight important messages and verbalize hidden issues and unspoken emotions as they are happening at a given moment. We use a summary at the end of an MI conversation by collecting the main messages to a cohesive narrative with the view to deciding what to do next. Summarizing is a good way of bringing a subject to a close and helping the conversation move on. Rollnick, Miller and Butler[9] describe summarizing as the process of collecting flowers and making a bouquet to offer to service users: the flowers are the person's own change talk statements and the bouquet is made up of these statements. In the end, the person can hear an accumulation of their own desires, abilities, reasons and needs as motives for change. A summary should conclude with asking the service user what the next step might be. Here is an example of a practitioner giving a summary of the service user's change talk statements:

'Let me see if I understood everything right. You have many reasons to want to stop drinking. You mentioned being able to enjoy life, to save money and to stop arguing with your partner. You worry that if you don't stop drinking you will end up very ill and lose your partner. You have tried in the past and stayed sober for a while, but it was difficult to keep going without a drink. Did I miss anything important? So, we know where we want to get to: to stop drinking and be able to carry on with your life without falling back into the drink. Now let's decide together how we can achieve this and what the next step should be.'

MI AS A TOOL IN THE CRAFT OF CARING

Like in all therapeutic approaches, to become a competent practitioner in MI requires training and ongoing supervision. The Motivational Interviewing Network of Trainers (MINT) is an international group of MI-trained therapists who are committed to the dissemination of the MI evidence base and good practice. The MINT website is a useful resource for practitioners, service users and the public, as it includes rich information, links, videos, training resources and updated research.

Practitioners who do not have specific training in MI can still use it as a tool in the craft of caring by incorporating some of its principles and skills within a framework that addresses three important elements of change: (a) motives and readiness; (b) ambivalence and barriers; (c) self-efficacy and capacity (see Figure 39.1). These elements are

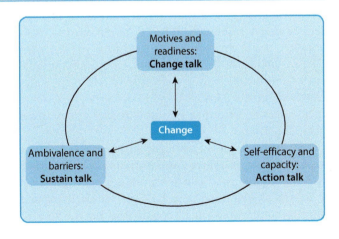

Figure 39.1 A framework for using MI in the craft of caring.

interlinked and the conversation between a practitioner and a service user may shift from one element to another. For example, after assessing the service user's motives and readiness for change, the practitioner may stumble upon barriers and ambivalence, which the service user may be willing to address if their belief in their ability to change increases (self-efficacy).

Motives and readiness: 'change talk'

The objective here is to generate and promote change talk by identifying the service user's reasons and readiness for change and the importance they attach to change. It is also useful to explore people's value-base, as this is often very powerful in stimulating change. For instance, if someone attaches importance to spending time with their grandchildren, then their desire to stay healthy and fit to be able to look after their grandchildren will be a powerful motivator but not immediately recognized as such. Change talk can help us arrive at goals that are congruent with the person's own motives, values and stage of readiness.

We can start change talk with open-ended questions:

- 'So what makes you feel that it might be time for a change?'
- 'If you had a magic wand and you could stop drinking overnight, how will your life change for the better?'
- 'If you could change, what difference will this make to your family/those close to you?'
- 'Is there anything that you worry may happen if you did not change/if you carried on in the same way? What are your thoughts about what could happen if you didn't change?'

Following on from this, we can use reflection and affirmation to acknowledge people's motives for changing and the fact that have thought about what may happen if they did not change, in terms of looking after themselves, and especially if change is motivated by concern for others.

The next step is to explore the importance that the service user attaches to change. A useful exercise is to consider 'importance of change' (reason, need) and 'confidence' (ability, skills, support, etc.). Using a sliding scale is a useful way of eliciting really helpful information and clarifying in the person's mind where they are at, what they want, and what they may need to do to achieve their goals and desires.

We would first start with 'importance' and ask: 'On a scale from 1 to 10, where 1 is not at all important and 10 is extremely important, how important would you say it is for you to stop using cannabis?' Further clarifying and eliciting questions should be used to draw out the detailed information, such as, 'Why that score?', 'What made you give that score?', 'Why not lower?' and 'What would have

to be different for you to move up two points?' Once this has been exhausted, we move on to 'confidence', and we consider the person's own idea of their ability to make the change successfully (if they so wish). The aim is to elicit a view of self-efficacy.

In a similar format, we would then ask: 'On a scale of 1 to 10, where 1 is not at all confident to 10 where you feel confident that you could easily make the change immediately, where would you place yourself now?' We can then follow up on the service user's answer by asking them to explain their score: 'Can you tell me why you placed yourself there?' We can also use further prompts to draw out more detail such as: 'What else makes you think that you are a "7" in terms of confidence?' and 'What would help you move from a 7 to a 9 in terms of confidence?'

This exercise can generate a lot of useful information, including DARN, as well as some practical barriers and issues that might need to be tackled before the target behaviour itself can be approached. You will find that some people have placed a lot of importance on the change, but lack the confidence (typically if the change is a new one, or if they have a lot of experience of previous failure): 'I would love to stop drinking, I know it's ruined my life, but what's the point? I always end up going back to it.' Conversely, some people have plenty of confidence but no change talk: 'Yeah, I can easily give smoking up any time I want, I just don't need to do this right now.'

Enhancing self-efficacy is important not only at the outset but also throughout people's journey towards change. Affirmation is a form of reflection where we focus on people's strengths and successes. It can be used to continuously enhance someone's sense of self-efficacy by focusing on their achievements but also their efforts. Even when people do not manage the change or they relapse, MI practitioners need to maintain therapeutic optimism and a sense of hope and try to instil this in the service user, their carers and other professionals. For example: 'I am amazed at how you have found the strength to keep going with the detox, even though it's been really tough for you recently with your relationship breaking down. Under the circumstances, having a set-back tells us that we need to change our strategy and not give up altogether.' If someone has a history of failed attempts to change, goals should be small, realistic and achievable in order to increase a person's sense of mastery and personal control.

Ambivalence and barriers: 'sustain talk'

The objective here is to recognize and understand sustain talk by validating and exploring the person's ambivalence and perceived barriers to change. When working with people with multiple needs and mental health problems, it is important to acknowledge that change may be more challenging (although it is also important to retain hope and optimism). For instance, feeling hopeless about the future because of depression, or smoking cannabis as a way of managing symptoms of mental illness, will be significant barriers to considering making a lifestyle change. It is helpful to acknowledge the challenges and be optimistic and hopeful, as well as using affirming strategies to reflect back successes and strengths (no matter how small they seem). We also have to be careful that while we are trying to understand and validate the service user's ambivalence, we are not inadvertently being drawn into the service user's sustain talk and getting trapped in therapeutic nihilism.

Discord between practitioner and service user

Discord is a mismatch between goals and objectives around care or treatment plan. In order to work with a truly person-centred approach, we need to be mindful of how our personal hopes, wishes and agenda can affect how we work with someone in the process of health behaviour change. We should recognize our own frustrations around direction of travel and 'progress'. If we notice that discord is escalating, then it is time to stop and think about how our approach is fuelling this discord. For example, are we pushing a specific agenda, are we preaching, judging, being confrontational, making all the suggestions and not listening? If this is happening, it is time to 'back off and come alongside'. We need to work with people where *they* are (not where we expect them to be). Reflecting back what is happening during the conversation can stimulate a more useful discussion.

Practitioner: 'You seem to be getting quite angry when we talk about alcohol.'
Service user: 'Well, you just seem to bang on about it all the time and I'm sick of it.'
Practitioner: 'OK, that's fair enough; it sounds as though you don't want to talk about alcohol at all, and we can avoid the subject altogether.'
Service user: 'Well I wouldn't go as far as that, I know I have problems, just don't want to be reminded of them every time we talk.'

Here are some traps that practitioners can fall into which may lead to discord:

- being the 'expert' ('In my professional opinion, you should use nicotine gum to stop smoking');
- taking control away ('Well, actually, I am sorry to say that you don't have any choice, you really have to …');
- misjudging the service user's level confidence or readiness for change (premature focus) ('I think you should go in for a detox now that you have admitted that you have been drinking heavily …');
- meeting force with force (argument, challenge, confrontation) ('Cannabis makes your illness worse, and I know you are still using it, even though you deny it').

To get back on track after being trapped in discord, we can use the following strategies:

- Convey to the service user that they have choice and control ('At the end of the day ultimately the choice to use drugs is yours'). This is a really powerful and empowering strategy.
- Reassess the service user's readiness and confidence ('Maybe we need to revisit how ready you feel, rather than continue talking about this plan').
- Try to shift the focus of the conversation to an area that the service user is more likely to engage with ('Perhaps we should use today's session to discuss all the things you enjoyed doing when you felt well in yourself').
- Reframe your statements into something neutral without using loaded words to talk about the problem ('Perhaps I could have put that better; what I meant to say is that I want to understand what makes your illness worse, whether this is cannabis, stress or other things').

REFLECTION

As health professionals, we all share a desire to be helpful and solve people's problems. This is a perfectly reasonable intention, but it may sometimes lead us to impose our own ideas about what is best for a person and what changes that person should make; this is known as the 'righting reflex'. If you feel like you are doing all the problem solving or you are generating reasons and solutions, then you are probably in 'righting reflex' mode. To be effective in MI, we should be aware of our 'righting reflex' and try to curb it.

Think about the tone of the conversations you usually have with service users:

- Are you giving advice without the person asking for it?

- Are you making suggestions about why the person should change, rather than eliciting from them their own reasons for change?

- Are you blaming them for not changing (either directly or subtly)?

- Are you feeling like a 'stuck record' giving the same health advice over and over again?

- Are your 'helpful' suggestions being met with 'yes, but …' statements?

If this happens, then it is time to *stop*, start listening to what the person is actually saying and come alongside them rather than trying to push or pull them in a certain direction.

EVIDENCE BASE FOR MI

Good quality evidence as to whether MI works, and for whom, come from four seminal MI-specific meta-analyses,[11–14] which have been helpfully summarized in a practice-friendly review.[8] These meta-analyses drew on randomized controlled trials (RCTs) comparing MI with either 'passive' alternatives, such as no treatment, waiting lists, and treatment as usual and information giving, or with 'active' interventions, such as cognitive behavioural therapy (CBT), person-centred therapy or a 12-step programme. See chapter 6 for further information on evidence-based practice in mental health care.

Based on the above sources, the strongest evidence in support of MI is for the problem for which it was originally designed: alcohol misuse. The general message, across all the different areas to which MI has been applied, is that MI is more effective than passive alternatives in bringing about change in symptoms, well-being, behaviours or functioning, but it is as good as other active interventions. The advantage of MI over equally effective active interventions is that it is on average briefer, and therefore more efficient. MI's effects are stronger at immediate rather than distant follow-ups, and tend to fade away over time; however, its effects have been shown to be durable for up to 3 years (Project MATCH).[15]

In support of combining MI with other interventions, in particular CBT, a recent meta-analysis[16] found small but significant effects on reducing depressive symptoms and alcohol consumption in people with depression and alcohol misuse when they used MI plus CBT compared to treatment as usual or other interventions (such as 12-step or person-centred therapy). This conclusion partially applies to people with psychosis and substance misuse; a large and seminal RCT[17] found a reduction in alcohol consumption following CBT plus MI, (compared to usual care alone) but no difference in psychotic symptoms, hospital admissions or functioning.

MI has been delivered in various ways, for example, in one-to-one sessions or in a group setting, and by a therapist, who may or may not use a manual, or by a computerized programme. One meta-analysis[13] found group MI to be less effective compared to individual MI, or to combined group and individual MI. The use of a manual for therapists to deliver MI could weaken its effects,[12] at least in comparison to other active treatments.[8] This may be because the standardization of MI in a manual may inadvertently lead therapists to push service users towards a certain direction or goal, which goes against the spirit of MI. On the contrary, standardization works in favour of MI when it is combined with CBT and is delivered via a computer, with larger effects noted on depressive symptoms[16] and drug use[18] for MI plus CBT by a computer against the same by a therapist. More information on CBT is available in chapter 40.

CONCLUSION

With the rise in mortality and morbidity related to preventable 'lifestyle'-related disease, health behaviour change is everyone's business. Every health care interaction is an opportunity for change interventions to take place. Using MI skills, especially open-ended questions, affirmation, reflection and summarizing (OARS), we can help service users change by: (a) identifying and using their own motives and readiness for change ('change talk'); (b) exploring and managing their ambivalence and barriers for change ('sustain talk'); and (c) identifying and enhancing their self-efficacy and capacity to change ('action talk'). With MI we 'go alongside' the service users rather than 'pushing or pulling' towards a certain direction. Nurses and other practitioners within multidisciplinary teams often feel under pressure to persuade someone to change for the better, but paradoxically, the determined pursuit of this can be counterproductive. The *real craft of caring* comes with the realization that no practitioner, no matter how skilled and experienced they are, can persuade someone to change *unless* the person is willing, ready and able to do it for themselves.

SERVICE USER COMMENTARY

Bobby Swift

In the process of helping people change and move forward in their personal journey, I have found MI an effective technique. Good, sustainable, long-term outcomes often start with an MI process. Working with people who suffer from mental illness or who lack confidence or have poor self-esteem that find it difficult to make positive changes can be frustrating for the person who tries to help them, whether a professional, a family member or a friend. There is a real temptation to want to solve quickly and fix immediately the person's problems. Many years of experience have taught me that this approach only provides short-term fixes that do not effect any long-term change and benefit to people. I have found that, by offering a process that has acceptance and compassion at its core, it is easier to build trust and rapport. A caring profession can work effectively by providing people with a safe space in which they can explore their problems, rather than trying to incite fear as motivation for change. Evoking a clear image of what people want to be, how they want to progress, and making sure this is done using personal, unique ideas, features, colours and emotions, is very powerful. Respecting people's autonomy and ability to create this changed image of their life is an important aspect of MI and is central to the acceptance and tolerance offered by this technique. I would also agree that reflecting back the service user's comments and ideas is vital to creating a viable action plan. It is important to draw a light to the positive motivations that will propel people forward, and to acknowledge that people themselves will *always* create a better blueprint for change than a professional ever could.

Bobby Swift is a patient, carer and public involvement representative for Northumbria University at Newcastle, UK.

References

1. Goethe, JW von (1749–1832). *Wilhelm Meister's apprenticeship. Book VIII*, Chapter IV, paragraph 8. New York: P.F. Collier & Son, 1917; New York: Bartleby.com, 2000. Available from: www.bartleby.com/314/ [Accessed 25th May 2016].
2. Miller WR, Rollnick S. *Motivational interviewing: preparing to change addictive behavior*, 2nd edn. New York: Guilford Press, 2002.
3. Miller WR, Zwebden, A, DiClemente CC, Rychtarik RG. *Motivational enhancement therapy manual: a clinical tool for therapists treating individuals with alcohol abuse and dependence. Project MATCH*. Monograph series, vol. 2. Rockville, MD: US Department of Health and Human Services Institute on Alcohol Abuse and Alcoholism, 1992.
4. McIntosh A, Conlon L, Lawrie S, Stanfield AC. Compliance therapy for schizophrenia. *Cochrane Database of Systematic Reviews* 2006; 3.
5. Staring AB, Van der Gaag M, Koopmans GT, Selten JP, Van Beveren JM, Hengeveld MW, Loonen AJ, Mulder CL. Treatment adherence therapy in people with psychotic disorders: randomised controlled trial. *British Journal of Psychiatry* 2010; **197**(6): 448–55.
6. Miller WR, Rollnick S. *Motivational interviewing: preparing people people for change*. New York: Guilford Press, 1991.
7. Rogers CR. A theory of therapy, personality, and interpersonal relationships as developed in the client-centered framework. In: Koch S (ed.). *Psychology: a study of a science. Study 1, volume 3: formulations of the person and the social context*. New York: McGraw-Hill, 1959: 184–256.
8. Lundahl BW, Burke B. The effectiveness and applicability of motivational interviewing: a practice-friendly review of four meta-analyses. *Journal of Clinical Psychology: In Session* 2009; **65**: 1232–45.
9. Rollnick S, Miller WR, Butler CC. *Motivational interviewing in health care: helping service users change behaviour*. London: Guildford Press, 2008.
10. Bandura A. *Self-efficacy: the exercise of control*. New York: Freeman, 1997.
11. Burke BL, Arkowitz H, Menchola M. The efficacy of motivational interviewing: a meta-analysis of controlled clinical trials. *Journal of Consulting and Clinical Psychology* 2003; **71**(5): 843–61.
12. Hettema J, Steele J, Miller WR. Motivational interviewing. *Annual Review of Clinical Psychology* 2005; **1**: 91–111.
13. Lundahl BW, Tollefson D, Kunz C, Brownell C, Burke B. Meta-analysis of motivational interviewing: twenty five years of research. *Research on Social Work Practice* 2010; **20**(2): 137–60.
14. Vasilaki EI, Hosier SG, Cox WM. The efficacy of motivational interviewing as a brief intervention for excessive drinking: a meta-analytic review. *Alcohol and Alcoholism* 2006; **41**(3): 328–35.
15. Project MATCH Research Group. Matching alcoholism treatments to client heterogeneity: Project MATCH three-year drinking outcomes. *Alcoholism: Clinical and Experimental Research* 1998; **23**: 1300–11.
16. Riper H, Andersson G, Hunter SB, de Wit J, Berking M, Cuijpers P. Treatment of comorbid alcohol use disorders and depression with cognitive-behavioural therapy and motivational interviewing: a meta-analysis. *Addiction* 2014; **109**: 394–406.
17. Barrowclough C, Haddock G, Wykes T, Beardmore R, Conrod P, Craig T, Davies L, Dunn G, Eisner E, Lewis S, Moring J, Steel C, Tarrier N. Integrated motivational interviewing and cognitive behavioural therapy for people with psychosis and comorbid substance misuse: randomised controlled trial. *British Medical Journal* 2010; **24**: 341, c6325. doi: 10.1136/bmj.c6325.
18. Kay-Lambkin FJ, Baker AL, Lewin TJ, Carr VJ. Computer-based psychological treatment for comorbid depression and problematic alcohol and/or cannabis use: a randomized controlled trial of clinical efficacy. *Addiction* 2009; **104**(3): 378–88.

Further reading

Miller WR, Rollnick S. *Motivational interviewing: helping people change*, 3rd edn. New York: Guilford Publications, 2013.
This is a seminal textbook by the developers of MI, Miller and Rollnick, which demonstrates how the four-process MI model – engaging, focusing, evoking, and planning – can be put into practice via case vignettes and examples of structured dialogues.
Schumacher JA, Madson MB. *Fundamentals of motivational interviewing: tips and strategies for addressing common clinical challenges*. New York: Oxford University Press, 2014.
A useful textbook for professionals across disciplines which provides a clear overview of the principles and methods of MI. The different chapters apply MI to a series of clinical challenges, including service user non-adherence, disengagement, high expectations, slow progress or relapse, and practitioner over-identification or frustration with a service user.

Relevant web pages

Cardiff Motivational Interviewing Workshops. http://www.micardiff.co.uk
This is a useful website for those seeking training opportunities in MI. It offers information on ongoing workshops, seminars and summer courses, which are supported by Miller and Rollnick.
MINT (Motivational Interviewing Network of Trainers). http://www.motivationalinterviewing.org
This website has been developed and is run by an international organization of trainers in MI. It has a wealth of open access information and resources for practitioners to use in their day-to-day work, including assessment and intervention manuals, literature and video demonstrations.

MITRIP (*Motivational Interviewing: Training, Research Implementation, Practice*). http://www.mitrip.org/ojs/index.php/mitrip
This journal's articles are open access and can be downloaded as PDF files. There is a search function for the journal's content to retrieve articles on MI with a specific focus (e.g. addiction, training).

40 Cognitive behaviour therapy (CBT)

LINA GEGA

LEARNING OUTCOMES

- To become familiar with the historical milestones that led to the development and evolution of cognitive behaviour therapy (CBT) as an umbrella term for different approaches and interventions.

- To be able to list the types of problems and populations for which CBT has an evidence base and the different modalities by which CBT can be delivered.

- To understand the key concepts underpinning CBT theory and practice, with an emphasis on the role of cognition.

- To recognize important therapeutic processes and techniques used in CBT, with a focus on cognitive restructuring techniques.

- To be able to reflect on one's skills and limitations in making CBT a tool in the craft of caring.

SUMMARY OF KEY POINTS

- Cognitive behaviour therapy (CBT) is an umbrella term that encompasses many different therapeutic approaches and techniques, whose common aim is to help people change the way they feel by changing the way they think or behave.

- CBT has historically evolved in three waves, starting from behaviour therapy followed by cognitive therapy and concluding with third wave therapies.

- Beck's cognitive therapy model assumes three levels of thinking: negative automatic thoughts, rules for living and core beliefs (schemas). Each level manifests in a 'cognitive triad', i.e. what people think about themselves, others and the future.

- Cognitive restructuring is the key method in cognitive therapy; it takes the form of strategic questions (guided discovery) that aim to identify and understand unhelpful and destructive thoughts and then generate and reinforce more helpful alternatives.

- Key techniques in cognitive restructuring include: capturing and recording negative thoughts, examining the evidence for and against a negative thought, challenging unhelpful rules for living, and reconstructing distressing images.

INTRODUCTION

An individual's affect and behaviour are largely determined by the way in which he structures the world.

Beck et al.[1] (p.3)

Cognitive behaviour therapy, or CBT, aims to reduce the symptoms and distress manifesting as part of a problem by helping people change how they think and behave in response to certain situations and experiences that can maintain the problem. The term 'cognitive' relates to 'thoughts'; these can take the form of words or images and have to do with processes by which we understand and interpret the world, such as perception, attention and memory. The term 'behaviour' refers to people's mental and physical 'actions', such as habits, rituals, avoidance and reassurance seeking. Therapists affiliated to either the cognitive or the behavioural schools of CBT often use similar techniques but a different rationale to explain how interventions work: behaviour therapy by helping people unlearn unhelpful behaviours and re-learn helpful ones, and cognitive therapy by helping people recognize and change their misinterpretations and unhelpful beliefs.

CBT has an extensive evidence base for a broad range of emotional, behavioural and mental health problems,[2,3] such as anxiety problems,[4] depression,[5] severe mental illness,[6]

eating disorders[7] and physical symptoms.[8,9] Beyond clinically defined populations, CBT has been adapted to suit people with specific needs or social and demographic characteristics, such as carers[10] and people from culturally diverse backgrounds[11] and those with intellectual disabilities.[12] CBT can be delivered in a variety of formats: individually or in a group,[13] therapist- or self-guided,[14,15] via a computer,[16] or by telephone[17] or using virtual reality.[18] More on evidence-based practice in mental health care can be found in chapter 6.

This chapter opens with a brief history of how CBT has evolved through the years, starting with behaviour therapy, followed by cognitive therapies, and more recently third wave therapies. Nowadays, CBT is not simply 'one' intervention but rather it is an umbrella term that includes many different approaches, all of which share the same premise: that the way we feel is shaped by the way we think about, and respond to, certain situations and experiences. CBT interventions work by breaking the vicious cycle of negative thoughts, unhelpful behaviours and troubling emotions. This chapter will focus on the traditional cognitive therapy as developed by Beck and colleagues,[1] whose main therapeutic method – called cognitive restructuring – aims to change unhelpful ways of thinking and reinforce more helpful alternatives. This chapter will demonstrate how cognitive restructuring can be used in the craft of caring for people who feel anxious, distressed, sad or hopeless.

HISTORICAL CORNERSTONES OF CBT

First wave: 'Changing the way we feel by changing the way we act'

Behaviour therapy, the earliest form of CBT, is based on the clinical application of learning theories, which state that people's behaviour is determined by the rewards or the relief they experience or expect as a consequence of this behaviour. The main contributors to the development of behaviour therapy in the 1950 and 1960s were Joseph Wolpe[19] in South Africa, Hans Eysenck[20] in the UK and B. F. Skinner in the USA.[21] The cornerstone method of behaviour therapy was first described as 'systematic desensitisation'[19] but has evolved into what is today known as 'exposure therapy', an evidence-based intervention used for a wide range of anxiety disorders.[22] Exposure therapy is the gradual confrontation of a feared object or situation until anxiety and fear subside over time, while refraining from any physical and mental actions that may artificially decrease anxiety – what is known as safety behaviours (e.g. medication, relaxation or reassurance).[23] Other established evidence-based methods of behaviour therapy include behavioural activation,[24,25] progressive or applied muscle relaxation[26,27] and habit reversal.[28,29]

Second wave: 'Changing the way we feel by changing the way we think'

Aaron Beck and Albert Ellis in the USA, originally psychoanalytical psychotherapists, identified limitations in behaviour therapy and suggested that emotional problems stem largely from the way people think about themselves, others, the world around them, their life and their future. This set the foundations for an approach that focused on helping people change how they think as a way of overcoming their emotional problems. Ellis first developed rational psychotherapy,[30] later to become rational emotive behaviour therapy (REBT),[31] while Beck later developed cognitive therapy.[1] Both REBT and cognitive therapy emphasize cognitive change as the key process underpinning emotional change, but they also incorporate behavioural techniques as a way of testing and reinforcing cognitive change. By the early 1980s, behaviour and cognitive therapies were brought together under the umbrella term 'CBT', which is now used to describe the collective evidence base[2] and professional capabilities[32] underpinning all the different interventions included within this type of psychological therapy.

Third wave CBT: 'Accepting and letting go of the way we feel, think and act'

Several variants and extensions of CBT have been developed over the last 20 years – the so-called 'third wave' therapies.[33] While traditional CBT focuses on changing unhelpful patterns of thinking and behaviours that maintain a problem, third wave CBT assumes a more flexible stance in redefining what a 'problem' is and sometimes accepting rather than changing certain ways of thinking and acting within the context of the person's life, relationships and values. Third wave therapies feature in the specialist interest groups of the UK's leading organization for CBT, the British Association for Behavioural and Cognitive Psychotherapies (BABCP),[34] and are included in the clinical guidelines by the National Institute for Health and Care Excellence.[35,36] Examples of evidence-informed third wave therapies include acceptance and commitment therapy (ACT),[37,38] dialectical behaviour therapy (DBT),[39,40] mindfulness-based cognitive therapy[41,42] and compassion-focused therapy.[43,44]

Nurse training in CBT: from nurse behaviour therapists (NBTs) to Improving Access to Psychological Therapies (IAPT)

The first training programme in the UK for nurses to practise behaviour therapy was founded 40 years ago by Professor Isaac Marks at the Maudsley Hospital,[45] and was continued by Professor Kevin Gournay at the Institute of Psychiatry[46] in London. This was an innovative and even controversial programme at the time, given that psychiatrists and psychologists had the monopoly in delivering therapies, which were furthermore dominated by psychoanalytical and psychodynamic approaches. Isaac Marks demonstrated that nurse behaviour therapists were as effective as,[47,48] and more cost-effective than,[49,50] psychiatrists and psychologists in treating people with anxiety problems. More recent seminal studies supported that nurses can be more effective than psychologists in delivering CBT for health anxiety in medical settings[51] and can produce significant therapeutic gains for people with severe mental illness following minimal CBT training.[52]

In 2008, the English government announced the Improving Access to Psychological Therapies (IAPT) Programme, whose aim was to train thousands of CBT practitioners and establish first-point-of-contact therapy services in primary care.[53] Nurses form a large part of this IAPT workforce. Integral to the IAPT Programme is monitoring symptom improvement and return to work for all the people who access IAPT services, with national outcomes being reported regularly.[54] Both the ethos of IAPT, in terms of being a well-evaluated training programme with clear objectives embedded within health services, and the national IAPT curriculum[55,56] have drawn on the original nurse behaviour therapy training; so the long tradition of nurses disseminating evidence-based CBT continues 40 years after it was first pioneered by Isaac Marks.

KEY CBT CONCEPTS

Consider the following scenario: a mother, a father and their daughter sit at the table talking. Their daughter makes an announcement: the mother feels sad and bursts into tears, and the father feels angry and storms out of the room. They have both heard the same announcement, yet reacted in different ways; how could this be? The cognitive model explains how someone's physiological and behavioural responses to an event are determined by how the individual feels at the time and how they perceive and interpret the event.

The cognitive triad

The view that we hold about (a) ourselves, (b) the world/others and (c) our future/life has been described as a 'cognitive triad'.[1] Figure 40.1 gives an example of a cognitive triad for a person who is depressed and their views are negative and hopeless. This is expressed by statements such as 'I'm useless', 'others are better than me' and 'the future is bleak'. For another person who is anxious, the cognitive triad may include statements such as 'I am weak and can't cope', 'others are ready to judge me' and 'my life is a disaster'.

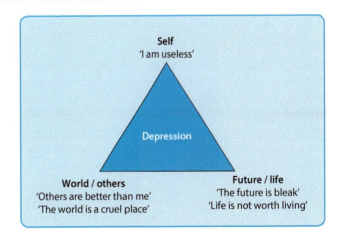

Figure 40.1 The cognitive triad.

The three levels of cognition

The cognitive model describes three levels of cognition: negative automatic thoughts (NATs), rules for living and core beliefs (Figure 40.2).

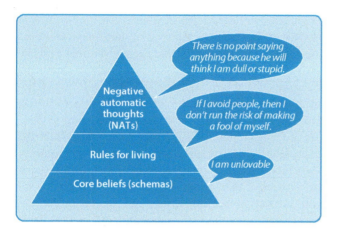

Figure 40.2 Levels of thinking.

CORE BELIEFS

Adverse early childhood experiences are thought to influence the development of negative core beliefs, or schemas, about the self, others and the world. Core beliefs are absolute statements that underpin the way we view and interpret what happens in the world around us (e.g. situations, relationships) and within us (e.g. physical sensations and emotional states). For example, someone can have the following core beliefs: 'I am unlovable', 'other people are better than me' and 'the world is a dangerous place'. These core beliefs may make the person interpret a criticism from a partner as confirmation that they are indeed unlovable, a missed deadline at work as a sign that others are better, and an accident as proof of a threatening and dangerous world.

RULES FOR LIVING

Rules for living are self-statements that follow this format: 'If … then' or 'Unless … then'. Common themes for rules for living include achievement, acceptance and control. Here are some examples:

- Achievement: '*If someone is better than me at something, then I am a failure*'; '*Unless I do something perfectly, it's not worth doing at all*'
- Acceptance: '*If someone does not like me, then there is something wrong with me*'; '*Unless people always approve of me and praise me, I am worthless at my job*'
- Control: '*If I ask for help or admit that I cannot do something, then it means I am useless or weak*'; '*Unless I control what I say all the time, I will make a fool of myself*'

What is the relationship between core beliefs and rules for living? Core beliefs shape rules for living and, in turn, rules for living reinforce the veracity of core beliefs. For example, if someone's core belief is that they are worthless or unlovable, a subsequent rule for living would be: '*If people disapprove of me or are critical of me, then I am worthless and unlovable.*' This traps the individual in an unhelpful pattern of behaviour trying to please everyone, but as it is impossible to please everyone all the time, any hint of displeasure or criticism from others only serves to reinforce the person's core belief that they are worthless and unlovable.

NEGATIVE AUTOMATIC THOUGHTS (NATs)

NATs are experienced as a constant stream of words or images in our minds that reflect the meaning of the things around us. The characteristics of NATs are that they are automatic and pop into our mind every time we are making a judgement about a situation or trying to interpret what people say or do. For example: '*There is no point in doing this*' or '*I am worried that people think I am stupid.*' NATs are fleeting in nature and tend to come and go if they are not important or meaningful to us; however, if we pay attention and attach meaning to NATs, they become powerful and persistent. In the moment, NATs feel plausible and rarely do we stop and question their accuracy or meaning. The adage '*It's the thought that counts*' is important when it comes to NATs: it is not a situation or an experience that makes us feel upset, sad, angry or anxious, but it is the way we think about it and what this situation or experience tells us about ourselves that determines our emotional state in response to it.

REFLECTION

A friend passes you by on the street without saying hello.

- How would that make you feel?
- What would run through your mind?
- What would you do?

Consider the same scenario for someone who is depressed or socially anxious. In this case, they may take this situation to heart and assume that their friend does not like them and that no one would want to give them the time of day because they see themselves as boring and uninspiring. They may feel sad, rejected, worried or angry, and then avoid contacting other friends in fear of further rejection or negative evaluation.

The take-home message is that when we are feeling depressed, anxious or distressed, our perception of an event is often distorted, irrational and unhelpful for our emotional state.

Table 40.1 Typical thinking errors: definitions and examples

Type of thinking error	Definition	Example
Catastrophizing	Expecting that the worst will happen and overestimating the probability of it happening	'I'll be out on the street and destitute if I make a mistake at work, get fired and cannot keep up with mortgage payments.'
Emotional reasoning	Using feelings to guide our judgement; confusing how things feel with how things really are	'I feel bad so I must have done something wrong.'
All-or-nothing/black-or-white thinking	Thinking in absolute terms, not considering the 'grey areas' or middle ground	'It is wrong to lie and, if someone lies to you, you can never trust them again.'
Arbitrary inference	Jumping to conclusions, making judgements without evidence, believing that we know what others are thinking	'I know my boss is thinking that I'm not up to the job and it's just a matter of time before I'm fired.'
Generalizing	Making sweeping statements based on single incidents, overestimating the importance of isolated events	'I will never be able to teach again because I froze last time I had to give a lecture.'
Personalizing	Assuming that one has responsibility for everything, blaming ourselves over things that we have little control or influence on	'My daughter did not do well at her exams and it's all my fault because I should have helped her more to revise.'
Selective attention/filtering	Focusing on the negative and discounting the positive; looking for evidence to back up our ideas and disregarding evidence which challenges them	'I passed my exams this time, but it was just luck'; 'I must be stupid and ignorant because I had nothing interesting to say when my colleagues were talking in the canteen the other day.'
Fixed rules	Using commands rather than wishes and options as the driving force for our behaviours, such as 'I should' and 'I must', rather than 'I would like to' or 'I would prefer it'	'I should always meet deadlines, otherwise I am incompetent.'

Thinking errors

Having stated above that 'It's the thought that counts' in the context of CBT, an important CBT strategy is to move away from *what* we think (content) to *how* we think (process). Unhelpful, self-defeating and destructive cognitive processes are known as 'thinking errors'; these shape the content of our thoughts, be they NATs, rules for living or core beliefs. In CBT, before we explore the content of our thoughts, we need to understand what thinking errors lie behind these thoughts. Definitions and examples of typical thinking errors are displayed in Table 40.1.

KEY THERAPEUTIC PROCESSES IN CBT

Therapeutic relationship and collaboration in CBT

The role of the therapeutic relationship in the craft of caring for nurses is discussed in detail in chapter 3. In reference to psychological therapies, practitioners are expected to possess effective interpersonal skills, as described by Carl Rogers:[57] expressing empathy, warmth, genuineness and unconditional positive regard towards the person receiving therapy. These skills have a consistent and significant, albeit moderate, impact on outcomes with CBT,[58] but also regardless of therapy type.[59] Unique to the therapeutic relationship in CBT is the concept of collaborative empiricism.[60] This considers that the therapist and the service user are experts in their own right and are working together on equal footing to develop a shared understanding of the problems (case formulation), make joint decisions about the agenda of each therapy session, and utilize strategies that encourage autonomy for the service user to eventually become their own therapist.

Case formulation

A CBT formulation is a shared understanding between the therapist and the service user of what maintains a problem. Several condition-specific models can be used as templates for the formulation of individual problems. All these models provide a diagrammatic illustration of how thoughts, feelings and behaviours interact to maintain a problem. For example, Clark's[61] model of panic disorder suggests that people attend to specific bodily sensations (e.g. feeling dizzy, out of breath or having palpitations) that they misinterpret as 'dangerous' (e.g. they fear that they will have a heart attack or pass out). These misinterpretations cause more anxiety, which feeds into people's bodily sensations (e.g. making their heart beat faster), subsequently making them run away from the situation or engage in safety behaviours (e.g. sitting down, holding on to a friend). These safety behaviours prevent people from discovering that they will not pass out or not have a heart attack even if the frightening bodily sensations are there, thereby trapping people into a vicious circle of misinterpretation, anxiety/fear and safety behaviours. Similar condition-specific CBT models have been developed for social phobia,[62] post-traumatic stress disorder,[63] obsessive-compulsive disorder,[64] psychosis[65] and eating disorders.[66]

Setting goals in CBT

A goal in CBT is a statement about what a person would like to be able to do – and under what circumstances – so that they are convinced that their problem has improved. Goals need to be SMART – Specific, Measureable, Achievable, Realistic and Time-limited (which is similar to goals in motivational interviewing, as discussed in chapter 39).

Let us take, for example, a student who seeks CBT because they are depressed, they lack motivation and energy, they do not manage to do any work and their grades are dropping. The student may set out to achieve the following SMART goal by the end of therapy: '*To be able to spend 1 hour, without interruption, doing homework every day for 2 weeks*'. Some questions to help us elicit a SMART goal in the context of CBT are:

- '*What would you like to be able to do in the near future that you cannot do now because of the problem?*'
- '*If you woke up tomorrow and the problem was gone, how would you know?*'
- '*How could your family and friends tell if your problem improved?*'
- '*If you were to feel better, what would you do differently on a day-to-day basis?*'

It is helpful to include potential or actual obstacles and difficulties in achieving our goals, and to identify what support or resources could assist or smooth our progress towards achieving our goal. For example, a person's family may be a source of support, but it can also be an obstacle if family members collude with a person's thoughts and behaviours that maintain the problem. For example, if someone is depressed, their family may provide them with emotional and practical support by doing everything for them, but they may also prevent the person from taking opportunities to be active and achieve things for themselves.

Homework in CBT

CBT places emphasis on activities completed outside therapy sessions; this is commonly referred to as 'homework'.[67] Examples of such activities include completing a thought diary or a sleep diary, doing physical exercise for a certain amount of time, or confronting feared situations such as looking at a picture of a spider or going up an escalator. Homework tasks serve various purposes: they test out the formulation in the light of events that occur between sessions and they help gather information or rehearse skills.[68]

Structure of CBT sessions

Cognitive behavioural therapy is time-limited and usually brief, typically six to 20 therapy sessions;[36] however, up to 40 sessions over an extended period are recommended for more complex problems such as anorexia nervosa or borderline personality disorder.[35] Therapy sessions follow a specific structure. First, a collaborative agenda is set to make best use of time during the therapy session. The therapist encourages the service user to contribute items to this agenda by asking them: '*What would you like us to focus on today?*' or '*Is there anything that happened since we last spoke that you would like us to include in our discussion today?*' Part of the agenda for each session is to review the service user's mental state and any escalation of risk, which should take precedence over other issues. Homework assignments are reviewed at the beginning of the session and new homework is agreed towards the end of the session.

REFLECTION

Think of a few things that you would like to change because they make you unhappy, frustrated or anxious. This could be related to health (e.g. eating too much, not exercising enough), or work (e.g. avoiding or delaying doing things that you consider difficult or boring), or home (e.g. shouting at your children or arguing with your parents or your partner).

1. Compose appropriate SMART goals for each of the things that you would like to change.

2. Set homework tasks to do every day to be able to achieve your goals.

3. Every day, monitor the completion of your homework tasks (not completed, partially completed, fully completed).

4. At the end of the week, rate how close you are to achieving your goal (0 = not at all, 10 = completely).

This exercise can help you understand the CBT process and how it may work in practice. Think about the following questions:

- What resources and support does someone need to be able to complete their CBT homework and achieve their goals?

- What type of difficulties may someone face when trying to complete their homework?

- How may someone feel if they achieve their goal?

- How may someone feel if they do not manage to complete their homework?

CBT TECHNIQUES

Cognitive restructuring is the key method of cognitive therapy. It is not as much about challenging how people think as it is about identifying and understanding unhelpful and destructive thinking, and then generating and reinforcing more realistic and helpful alternatives. This is achieved through a process called 'Socratic questioning' or 'guided discovery': a series of strategic questions – rather than giving advice or instructions – that the therapist uses to allow the service user to discover by themselves new insights and alternative perspectives. This section describes a small selection of techniques commonly used in cognitive restructuring, focusing on 'verbal reattribution' techniques, i.e. structured and purposeful conversations during a therapy session. Apart from discussion-based techniques, cognitive restructuring also incorporates behavioural experiments,[69] i.e. exercises and tasks that the person carries out to test and reinforce their new way of thinking in specific situations.

Monitoring NATs

Cognitive restructuring begins with identifying salient NATs that are central to the maintenance of a problem. Learning to identify NATs is the first step towards being able to see and experience more realistic perspectives. NATs are captured by tuning into sudden changes in emotion and asking questions to help bring tacit thoughts to the forefront of one's mind. A helpful way of capturing NATs is to go through a recent incident when the person experienced strong emotions or severe symptoms associated with their problem. Here are some examples of questions that could help elicit NATs about an incident:

- *'When was the last time that you felt miserable/angry/anxious/scared?'*
- *'Looking back over the past week, which was the worst day for you? What was happening at the time that made it so bad?'*
- *'What was going through your mind at the time? What were you saying to yourself?'*
- *'Before you felt this way, what was running through your mind, what thoughts or images did you notice?'*

It is important to capture NATs as they happen. To this end, service users are encouraged to write down their thoughts, the situation and emotional reaction, as they happen, using a thought record or diary. If not recorded, NATs can be quickly forgotten and all is left is distress, anxiety or sadness. Not only do the thought records increase awareness of NATs, but they also help identify a pattern of occurrence, demonstrate the link between thoughts, feelings and behaviours, and finally highlight the importance and meaning that the person attaches to them. Thought records help the service user make sense of their distress, so that they can look back at an incident, question their NATs that caused distress, and develop new perspectives that could help alleviate their distress.

It is interesting to mention here that, in the third wave therapies, there is a strong move away from traditional Beckian cognitive restructuring. NATs and intrusive images are treated as passing cognitive events which the service user is not a 'participant in' but an 'observer of'. This is achieved by encouraging the service user to notice and acknowledge the thoughts, but then let the thoughts drift in and out of their mind without trying to control, analyse, justify or change them. A metaphor often used is standing on the railway platform, watching the trains (thoughts, images, sensations) arrive, stop for a while and then pull away from the station, without boarding any of them.

Examining the evidence for and against a thought/belief

The first step to challenging NATs is to examine the evidence for and against them. It is not possible to challenge every single NAT that arises from various incidents in our everyday lives, so how do we know which NATs to target? While keeping a thought record, we can help the service user identify which thoughts are the most potent and salient ones by asking this question: *'If we could make one or two thoughts go away, which ones would you choose in order to make a real difference in the way you feel?'* The evidence that supports the thought is discussed first: *'What makes you think that this thought is true?'* or *'What evidence do you have that supports this thought?'* In this way, the therapist seeks to understand the service user's existing beliefs before examining the counter-evidence and generating new perspectives.

It is difficult for service users to readily see the evidence against a NAT because naturally one of the processes maintaining an NAT is selectively attending to the evidence that supports it. The therapist needs to guide the service user through a thinking process that allows new evidence to be discovered and new perspectives to be generated, so that NATs are eventually replaced by more helpful alternatives. This process is known as 'Socratic questioning' or 'guided discovery'. Examples of questions to use within guided discovery to produce evidence against NATs and generate alternatives are:

- *'You said that you believe this NAT to be 50/80/99 per cent true; what is the other 50/20/1 per cent?'*
- *'If you didn't feel depressed/stressed/angry/scared/insecure at the time, what would you think about the situation?'*
- *'If you felt happier/relaxed/calm/reassured/confident at the time, how would you respond to the situation?'*
- *'When this happened, you thought that it meant that you/others/your life would … What else could it be? What alternative explanations/interpretations would someone else suggest?'*

Point, counter-point or role reversal is another technique to generate evidence for and against a thought, in which the therapist argues in favour of a thought and the service user assumes the role of the therapist and argues against the thought. The service user and therapist physically swap chairs and the service user takes notes or uses a flipchart as the therapist usually does. In the end, patient and therapist assume their original positions and discuss the learning outcome of the exercise. In this way, the therapist demonstrates an understanding of the service user's point of view and the service user steps into a different role and gains some distance from their emotional state to be able to generate new perspectives.

Questioning rules for living

Let us consider the following example. John, a 28-year-old accountant, has the following key rules for living: 'If I don't do things perfectly, I will have failed' and 'If I fail, it means I'm useless'; 'Therefore I must do everything perfectly'. Because John is scared of making a mistake, he procrastinates and goes over and over his work multiple times before he submits it to his employer. The unintended consequence of this is that John misses deadlines and receives negative feedback from his employer, which inadvertently brings on the very thing that he is afraid of and is trying to prevent: a sense of failing and of being useless.

How do we identify and question those unhelpful rules for living? In John's case above, one strategy is to ask a series of questions whose answers have the format 'If … then' or 'Unless … then'. For example:

- *'If you made a mistake, what would be so bad about it? What would that say about you?'*
- *'Unless you do things perfectly, what do you fear may happen?'*

Once we identify the rule for living, we take an inquisitive stance towards it:

- *'What's your idea about how this rule for living developed?'*
- *'In what way is this rule of living understandable or helpful?'*
- *'In what way is this rule of living unhelpful, counterproductive or distressing?'*
- *'What are the advantages and disadvantages of living by this rule?'*
- *'If you no longer believed and acted as if this rule for living was true, what would be an alternative rule to hold?'*

Considering the advantages and disadvantages of holding a certain belief could elicit useful information not about its factual accuracy but about how helpful or unhelpful it is in light of the person's difficulties and needs. This could be very important for engaging a service user to consider alternatives when their beliefs are associated with cultural or religious norms. In this case, considering alternatives is not because the beliefs are 'flawed' but because they are unhelpful for the specific problem we are addressing. Alternative ideas, which could be more helpful in overcoming the problem or meeting people's needs, are then considered within the same cultural and religious framework.

Reconstructing images

Thoughts and beliefs for many of us do not take the form of words, but occur in a pictorial form, as images. Unpacking the meaning of an image is as important as exploring verbal expressions of our beliefs. Service users may acknowledge their beliefs as irrational in their minds, but they may say that these beliefs feel true in their hearts. Imagery reconstruction specifically taps into this 'felt sense' of a belief being true. To retrieve an important image associated with a core belief, we can ask the service user to recall when they first remembered feeling this way and to form an image of the situation, e.g. it could be as a child being chastised by their parent. Using guided discovery, the memory and meaning of the image is explored, e.g. by bringing the adult-self into the picture to talk to the child-self. This enables the service user to make links between the described experience and the formation of the core belief. The content of the image is discussed and then re-scripted and replayed in the imagination, so that a new, helpful and constructive image is put in place.

REFLECTION

- Cognitive restructuring of negative beliefs can be challenging because the therapist can readily see the alternatives; however, they cannot advise or tell the service user how to think and what to do, but they need to help the service user arrive at alternatives by themselves.

- Imagine a friend whose relationship has just broken down coming to you in tears; they blame themselves, saying that they are unattractive and unlovable, that everyone else is in a happy relationship except them, and that they will never find anyone else to be happy with. Instinctively, you would want to reassure them, remind them of all their qualities that make them lovable, point out how many people are not in relationships and have gone through the same thing your friend

is going through, and of course tell them that sooner or later they will meet someone else. This is the sort of conversation we would naturally have with a friend, giving them advice, telling them what is obvious to us and trying to convince them they should not feel sad or blame themselves.

- If the same conversation had to take place in the context of cognitive restructuring using guided discovery, what questions would you ask your friend to help them arrive at the same conclusions?

CONCLUSION

In this chapter we have discussed different therapeutic techniques under the CBT umbrella, whose common aim is to help people change the way they feel by changing the way they think or behave. In CBT practice, it is usually difficult to know whether someone's symptoms and distress improve because they have changed the way they think or because they have changed the way they behave; often, any changes in behaviour influence one's thinking and any changes in thinking are reflected in one's behaviour. The benefits and drawbacks of taking medication alongside

CBT is also an important issue: some literature suggests that combining therapy and medication can be better than each of those alone, but our service user's perspective suggests that medication could interfere with one's ability to access emotions and engage in therapy. CBT should always be considered within the wider framework of patient care, which may need to include a risk assessment and management. CBT interventions can be a useful tool in the craft of caring, but must be applied with supervision and within the limitations of one's professional competence.

SERVICE USER COMMENTARY

Carolyn Asher

As a service user I have not had much CBT, given that medication is often seen as the only solution to my issues by the team. Because I am usually symptomless when on medication, I have not been able to work on the issues that surface when I fully believe in my unhelpful thoughts. However, as I do have plenty of NATs, rules for living, thinking errors and core beliefs, I can work on these. Being asked 'how I feel about something' is a stumbling block as the medication dampens my emotions so that it is difficult to get in touch with one's feelings. Remembering how I felt when

something happened or indeed remembering what happened clearly is also a challenge. I liked the idea of writing down NATs as they happen, as memory is often poor after the event. This and the other techniques highlighted in the text make for a positive way to deal with the issues that many service users face. The chapter is a useful source as a brief overview of CBT.

Carolyn Asher is a patient, carer and Public Involvement and Engagement Coordinator and Service User Research Assistant for Southern Health NHS Foundation Trust at the Research and Development Department, Southampton, UK.

References

1. Beck AT, Rush JA, Shaw BF, Emery G. *Cognitive therapy for depression.* New York: Guilford Press, 1979.
2. Roth A, Fonagy P. *What works for whom? A critical review of psychotherapy research,* 2nd edn. New York: Guilford Press, 2005.
3. Hofmann SG, Asnaani A, Vonk IJJ, Sawyer AT, Fang A. The efficacy of cognitive behavioral therapy: a review of meta-analyses. *Cognitive Therapy and Research* 2012; **36**(5): 427–40.
4. Olatunji BO, Cisler JM, Deacon BJ. Efficacy of cognitive behavioral therapy for anxiety disorders: a review of meta-analytic findings. *Psychiatric Clinics of North America* 2010; **33**(3): 557–77.
5. Cuijpers P, Berking M, Andersson G, Quigley L, Kleiboer A, Dobson KS. A meta-analysis of cognitive-behavioural therapy for adult depression, alone and in comparison with other treatments. *Canadian Journal of Psychiatry* 2013; **58**(7): 376–85.
6. Jauhar S, McKenna PJ, Radua J et al. Cognitive-behavioural therapy for the symptoms of schizophrenia: systematic review and meta-analysis with examination of potential bias. *British Journal of Psychiatry* 2014; **204**: 20–9.
7. Murphy R, Straebler S, Cooper Z, Fairburn CG. Cognitive behavioral therapy for eating disorders. *Psychiatric Clinics of North America* 2010; **33**(3): 611–27.
8. Williams AC, Eccleston C, Morley S. Psychological therapies for the management of chronic pain (excluding headache) in adults. *Cochrane Database of Systematic Reviews* 2012; **11**: CD007407.
9. Price JR, Mitchell E, Tidy E, Hunot V. Cognitive behaviour therapy for chronic fatigue syndrome in adults. *Cochrane Database of Systematic Reviews* 2008; **3**: CD001027.

10. Turner W, Macdonald GM, Dennis JA. Cognitive-behavioural training interventions for assisting foster carers in the management of difficult behaviour. *Cochrane Database of Systematic Reviews* 2005; **2**: CD003760.

11. Pan D, Huey SJ, Hernandez D. Culturally-adapted versus standard exposure treatment for phobic Asian Americans: treatment efficacy, moderators, and predictors. *Cultural Diversity and Ethnic Minority Psychology* 2011; **17**(1): 11–22.

12. Vereenooghe L, Langdon PE. Psychological therapies for people with intellectual disabilities: a systematic review and meta-analysis. *Research in Developmental Disabilities* 2013; **34**(11): 4085–102.

13. Jónsson H, Hougaard E. Group cognitive behavioural therapy for obsessive-compulsive disorder: a systematic review and meta-analysis. *Acta Psychiatrica Scandinavica* 2009; **119**(2): 98–106.

14. Coull G, Morris PG. The clinical effectiveness of CBT-based guided self-help interventions for anxiety and depressive disorders: a systematic review. *Psychological Medicine* 2011; **41**(11): 2239–52.

15. Cuijpers P, Donker T, van Straten A, Li J, Andersson G. Is guided self-help as effective as face-to-face psychotherapy for depression and anxiety disorders? A systematic review and meta-analysis of comparative outcome studies. *Psychological Medicine* 2010; **40**: 1943–57.

16. Hedman E, Ljótsson B, Lindefors N. Cognitive behavior therapy via the Internet: a systematic review of applications, clinical efficacy and cost-effectiveness. *Expert Review of Pharmacoeconomics and Outcomes Research* 2012; **12**: 745–64.

17. Turner CM, Mataix-Cols D, Lovell K, Krebs G, Lang K, Byford S, Heyman I. Telephone cognitive-behavioral therapy for adolescents with obsessive-compulsive disorder: a randomized controlled non-inferiority trial. *Journal of the American Academy of Child and Adolescent Psychiatry* 2014; **53**(12): 1298–307.

18. Opriş D, Pintea S, García-Palacios A, Botella C, Szamosközi Ş, David D. Virtual reality exposure therapy in anxiety disorders: a quantitative meta-analysis. *Depression and Anxiety* 2012; **29**(2): 85–93.

19. Wolpe J. The systematic desensitization treatment of neuroses. *Journal of Nervous and Mental Disease* 1961; **132**: 189–203.

20. Eysenck H. The effects of psychotherapy. *Journal of Consulting Psychology* 1952; **16**: 319–24.

21. Skinner BF. *Science and human behavior.* New York: Macmillan, 1953.

22. Ougrin D. Efficacy of exposure versus cognitive therapy in anxiety disorders: systematic review and meta-analysis. *BMC Psychiatry* 2011; **11**(1): 200.

23. Marks IM. *Fears, phobias & rituals.* Oxford: Oxford University Press, 1987.

24. Lewinsohn PM, BiglanT, Zeiss A. Behavioral treatment of depression. In: Davidson P (ed.). *Behavioral management of anxiety, depression, and pain.* New York: Brunner/Mazel, 1976: 91–146.

25. Ekers D, Webster L, Straten A. Van, Cuijpers P, Richards D, Gilbody S. Behavioural activation for depression, an update of meta-analysis of effectiveness and sub group analysis. *PloS One* 2014; **9**(6); e100100.

26. Jacobson E. *Progressive relaxation,* 2nd edn. Chicago: University of Chicago Press, 1938.

27. Ost L-G. Applied relaxation: description of a coping technique and review of controlled studies. *Behaviour Research and Therapy* 1987; **25**(5): 397–409.

28. Azrin NH, Nunn RG. Habit-reversal: a method of eliminating nervous habits and tics. *Behaviour Research and Therapy* 1973; **11**(4): 619–28.

29. Woods DW, Miltenberger RG. Habit reversal: a review of applications and variations. *Journal of Behavior Therapy and Experimental Psychiatry* 1995; **26**(2): 123–31.

30. Ellis A. Rational psychotherapy. *Journal of General Psychology* 1958, **59**: 35–49.

31. Dryden W, Branch R. *The fundamentals of rational emotive behaviour therapy: a training handbook,* 2nd edn. Chichester: Wiley, 2008.

32. Hool N. *BABCP Core Curriculum Reference Document.* BABCP, 2010. Available from: http://www.babcp.com/files/About/BABCP-Core-Curriculum-V2–190913.pdf [Accessed 11th January 2016].

33. Ost L-G. Efficacy of the third wave of behavioral therapies: a systematic review and meta-analysis. *Behaviour Research and Therapy* 2008; **46**(3): 296–321.

34. BABCP. *Special Interest Groups within BABCP.* Available from: http://www.babcp.com/Membership/SIG/SIG.aspx [Accessed 11th January 2016].

35. NICE (National Institute for Health and Care Excellence). *Borderline personality disorder: recognition and management: NICE guidelines [CG78].* London: NICE, 2009.

36. NICE (National Institute for Health and Care Excellence). *Common mental health problems: identification and pathways to care. [CG123].* London: NICE, 2011.

37. Hayes SC, Strosahl KD, Wilson KG. *Acceptance and commitment therapy: an experiential approach to behavior change.* New York: Guilford Press, 1999.

38. Ost LG. The efficacy of Acceptance and Commitment Therapy: an updated systematic review and meta-analysis. *Behaviour Research and Therapy* 2014; **61**: 105–21.

39. Linehan MM. *Cognitive–behavioral treatment of borderline personality disorder.* New York: Guilford Press, 1993.

40. Panos PT, Jackson JW, Hasan O, Panos A. Meta-analysis and systematic review assessing the efficacy of dialectical behavior therapy (DBT). *Research on Social Work Practice* 2014; **24**(2): 213–23.

41. Segal ZV, Williams JMG, Teasdale JD. *Mindfulness-based cognitive therapy for depression: a new approach to preventing relapse.* New York: Guilford, 2001.

42. Gotink RA, Paula Chu, Busschbach JJV, et al. Standardised mindfulness-based interventions in healthcare: an overview of systematic reviews and meta-analyses of RCTs. *PLoS One* 2015; **10**(4): e0124344.

43. Gilbert P. Introducing compassion-focused therapy. *Advances in Psychological Treatment* 2009; **15**: 199–208.

44. Leaviss J, Uttley L. Psychotherapeutic benefits of compassion-focused therapy: an early systematic review. *Psychological Medicine* 2015; **45**: 927–45.

45. Marks IM, Connolly J, Hallam RS. Psychiatric nurse as therapist. *British Medical Journal* 1973; **3**(5872): 156–60.

46. Gournay K, Denford L, Parr A-M, Newell R. British nurses in behavioural psychotherapy: a 25-year follow-up. *Journal of Advanced Nursing* 2000; **32**: 343–51.

47. Marks IM, Hallam RS, Philpott R, Connolly JC. Nurse therapists in behavioural psychotherapy. *British Medical Journal* 1975; **3**(5976): 144–8.

48. Marks I. Controlled trial of psychiatric nurse therapists in primary care. *British Medical Journal (Clinical Research Edition)* 1985; **290**(6476): 1181–4.

49. Ginsberg G, Marks I. Costs and benefits of behavioural psychotherapy: a pilot study of neurotics treated by nurse-therapists. *Psychological Medicine* 1977; **7**(4): 685–700.

50. Ginsberg G, Marks I, Waters H. Cost-benefit analysis of a controlled trial of nurse therapy for neuroses in primary care. *Psychological Medicine* 1984; **14**(3): 683–90.

51. Tyrer H, Tyrer P, Lisseman-Stones Y, McAllister S, Cooper S, Salkovskis P, et al. Therapist differences in a randomised trial of the outcome of cognitive behaviour therapy for health anxiety in medical patients. *International Journal of Nursing Studies* 2015; **52**(3): 686–94.

52. Turkington D, Kingdon D, Turner T, Insight into Schizophrenia Research Group. Effectiveness of a brief cognitive-behavioural

therapy intervention in the treatment of schizophrenia. *British Journal of Psychiatry* 2002; **180**: 523–7.

53. Clark DM. Implementing NICE guidelines for the psychological treatment of depression and anxiety disorders: the IAPT experience. *International Review of Psychiatry* 2011; **23**(4): 318–27.

54. DH (Department of Health). *IAPT three-year report. The first million patients.* London: DH, 2012. Available from: http://www.iapt.nhs.uk/silo/files/iapt–3-year-report.pdf. [Accessed 11th January 2016].

55. DH (Department of Health). *Improving access to psychological therapies implementation plan: curriculum for low-intensity therapies workers.* London: DH, 2008. Available from: http://www.iapt.nhs.uk/silo/files/implementation-plan-curriculum-for-low8208intensity-therapies-workers.pdf [Accessed 24th January 2016].

56. DH (Department of Health). Improving access to psychological therapies implementation plan: curriculum for high-intensity therapies workers. London: DH, 2008. Available from: http://www.iapt.nhs.uk/silo/files/implementation-plan-curriculum-for-high8208intensity-therapies-workers.pdf [Accessed 24th January 2016].

57. Prochaska JO, Norcross JC. *Systems of psychotherapy: a transtheoretical analysis.* New York: Thompson Books/Cole, 2007.

58. Keijsers GP1, Schaap CP, Hoogduin CA. The impact of interpersonal patient and therapist behavior on outcome in cognitive-behavior therapy. A review of empirical studies. *Behavior Modification* 2000; **24**(2): 264–97.

59. Martin DJ, Garske JP, Davis MK. Relation of the therapeutic alliance with outcome and other variables: a meta-analytic review. *Journal of Consulting Clinical Psychology* 2000; **68**(3): 438–50.

60. Dattilio FM, Hanna MA. Collaboration in cognitive-behavioral therapy. *Journal of Clinical Psychology* 2012; **68**(2): 146–58.

61. Clark DM. A cognitive approach to panic. *Behaviour Research and Therapy* 1986; **24**(4): 461–70.

62. Clark DM, Wells A. A cognitive model of social phobia. In: Heimberg RG, Liebowitz MR, Hope DA, Schneier FR (eds). *Social phobia: diagnosis, assessment, and treatment* New York: Guilford, 1995; 69–93.

63. Ehlers A, Clark DM. A cognitive model of posttraumatic stress disorder. *Behaviour Research and Therapy* 2000; **38**: 319–45.

64. Salkovskis RM. Obsessive-compulsive problems: a cognitive behavioural analysis. *Behaviour Research and Therapy* 1985; **23**: 571–83.

65. Garety PA, Kuipers E, Fowler D, Freeman D, Bebbington PA. Cognitive model of the positive symptoms of psychosis. *Psychological Medicine* 2001; **31**: 189–95.

66. Fairburn CG, Cooper Z, Shafran R. Cognitive behaviour therapy for eating disorders: a 'transdiagnostic' theory and treatment. *Behaviour Research and Therapy* 2003; **41**: 509–28.

67. Kazantzis N, Abate L (eds). *Handbook of homework assignments in psychotherapy: research, practice, and prevention.* New York: Springer, 2007.

68. Kazantzis N, Deane FP, Ronan KR. Homework assignments in cognitive and behavioral therapy: a meta-analysis. *Clinical Psychology: Science and Practice* 2000; **7**(2): 189–202.

69. Bennett-Levy J, Butler G, Fennell M, Hackmann A, Mueller M, Westbrook D (eds). *Oxford guide to behavioural experiments in cognitive therapy.* Oxford: Oxford University Press, 2004.

Further reading

Grant A (ed.). *Cognitive behavioural interventions for mental health practitioners.* Exeter: Learning Matters, 2010.

This is a clear, concise and nurse-focused book that addresses CBT within contemporary contexts, explains the fundamentals of CBT and describes CBT applications for different populations and clinical problems, including anxiety, depression, schizophrenia and personality disorders.

Hawton K, Salkovskis PM, Kirk J, Clark DM. *Cognitive behaviour therapy for psychiatric problems.* Oxford: Oxford University Press, 1989.

An 'old' but classic textbook and a comprehensive practical guide for students and practitioners who want a more substantial understanding of CBT models and methods across a wide range of mental health problems. The book covers a historical overview of behavioural and cognitive treatments, and provides detailed guidelines and case examples on CBT assessment strategies, formulation and treatment techniques.

Wright JH, Turkington D, Sudak DM, Thase ME. *High-yield cognitive-behavior therapy for brief sessions: an illustrated guide.* Arlington, VA: American Psychiatric Publishing, 2010.

A substantial but user-friendly book that will appeal to professionals who have limited time with service users and wish to offer structured but powerful CBT interventions. The guide includes video illustrations with role plays of how to implement brief CBT in practice. It covers depression, anxiety, psychotic symptoms, suicidal ideas, sleep problems, substance misuse and physical problems.

Relevant web pages

BABCP (British Association for Behavioural & Cognitive Psychotherapies). www.babcp.com

This is the leading body for CBT in the UK. Its aims include maintaining professional standards and disseminating information. The public can access CBT resources and find an accredited therapist through an online register.

Get Self Help. www.getselfhelp.co.uk

This website offers free downloads of CBT self-help information, resources, diaries, worksheets and handouts to use as part of self-guided therapy, with the use of a CBT book (see www.overcoming.co.uk) and support from a therapist.

IAPT (Improving Access to Psychological Therapies). http://www.iapt.nhs.uk

This website includes guidance documents, learning resources and examples of materials used for CBT training and service delivery in the context of the IAPT Programme. It includes some example videos of therapist–client interactions in a typical CBT session (http://www.iapt.nhs.uk/workforce/iapt-older-peoples-training).

MindEd. www.minded.org.uk

This website is funded by the Department of Health and is an educational resource for adults who look after or work with children and young people with mental health problems. It gives authoritative and comprehensive information and training packages for a range of symptoms and risk factors associated with mental health and behavioural and emotional problems experienced by children and young people.

Overcoming. www.overcoming.co.uk

This website complements www.getself.co.uk because it provides a list of authoritative self-guided therapy books which could be used by individuals to follow a structured CBT programme by themselves, with or without support from a therapist.

41 Using solution-focused approaches

SIMON PROUDLOCK AND SONIA SANGHVI

LEARNING OUTCOMES

- To have a basic understanding of what solution-focused therapy (SFT) is.

- To understand that there needs to be a shift in your thinking in order to become more solution-focused.

- To know how to move from working with problems to working with solutions.

- To know how to build solutions with service users by utilizing non-problem talk, reframing, compliments, goal setting, the miracle question, exceptions and scaling.

- To understand how versatile SFT is in a variety of different settings.

- To be able to see how SFT has impacted on care for one service user.

SUMMARY OF KEY POINTS

- SFT is a versatile therapeutic intervention that can be easily incorporated into everyday nursing, enhancing the craft of caring.

- SFT is a strengths-based approach to working with service users, and as such is highly regarded by service users.

- One barrier most professionals need to overcome is how to work in a solution-focused way rather than focusing on problems.

- SFT helps professionals connect with service users by discovering what it is they need to see differently in order to better manage their mental health.

- SFT helps service users discover their preferred future, and the miracle question is a great tool to facilitate this.

- SFT has proved to be useful in working with service users in a variety of settings, including mental health (both inpatient and outpatient), schools, drug and alcohol services, crisis resolution and home treatment teams, employee assistance programmes and social work settings.

INTRODUCTION

As an introduction to solution-focused therapy, let me see if I can get you thinking about solutions rather than problems with an exercise adapted from Steve Freeman[1]:

- Take a blank piece of A4 paper and divide it into two halves.
- On the left-hand side, write down a problem that is real and current or something you would like to change.
- On the right-hand side, write down your resources, skills, expertise, your own and others' experience in solving problems, anyone that could help, etc.
- Before you finish off, what would the person who knows you best add to the list?
- Tear down the centre, so you have two pieces of paper – one with the problem, and one with the solutions.
- Now, throw away the part you don't want.

If you have thrown away the problem, you have just taken your first step to becoming solution-focused. Focusing on the strengths and resources of the service user instead of the problem is in essence what SFT is all about. In this chapter I hope to show you how versatile SFT can be and how easily you can incorporate it into the craft of caring.

WHAT IS SFT?

SFT simply shifts the focus from talking about the problem to talking about solutions, focusing on the present and the future rather than the past. Service users focus on recovering and creating solutions rather than talking about their problems. SFT has little or no interest in gaining an understanding of the problem, believing that the majority of service users know a considerable amount about their problem and have already been mulling over ways around the problem for a long time before they contemplated seeking help.

Steve de Shazer and Insoo Kim Berg are credited with developing solution-focused brief therapy together with their colleagues at the Brief Family Therapy Centre in Milwaukee, Wisconsin, USA, in the 1980s. Developed inductively rather than deductively, de Shazer and colleagues spent many hours observing a variety of therapy sessions to see what therapist activities were most useful. As a result, SFT is not theory-based but developed pragmatically, grounded on the optimistic assumption that people are healthy and competent and have the ability to construct solutions.

The philosophy of SFT emphasizes the need for practitioners to adopt a stance of not knowing, leaving their assumptions at the door. The majority of professionals have been trained to focus on problems and then to work with service users to alleviate those problems. Within the medical model, we are trained to move from assessment to diagnosis to treatment. Professionals in this context are seen as the experts – we are the ones who will fix your problem.

As we will discover, building solutions with service users is a fascinating experience, utilizing non-problem talk, reframing, compliments, goal setting, the miracle question, exceptions and scaling – all simple but highly effective tools to help service users identify and achieve a preferred future.

CENTRAL PHILOSOPHY OF SFT

REFLECTION

How useful would the central philosophy of SFT be to you and your friends?

Simple but pivotal to the workings of SFT, and integral to the craft of caring, is its central philosophy (taken from Berg and Miller[2]):

1. If it ain't broke don't fix it.
   SFT's philosophy is to not go looking for problems. By following the key elements and basic assumptions, SFT sees the service user as the expert, allowing them to tell us what they need help with. They are the ones who know what is broken and needs fixing. Only when the service user realizes that there is a problem does it become a problem.
2. Once you know what works, do more of it.
   It may seem like simple common sense, but similar to the previous point, once the service user has identified what does work, SFT encourages them to do more of it. The practitioner works with them to identify their role in making something work. We help them see what part of the solution they are responsible for; what part they are in control of – but more importantly, how they can make that solution, or part of it, happen again.
3. If it doesn't work, then don't do it again; do something different.
   The final part of the philosophy suffers from a case of 'Easier said than done'. To start with we don't usually realize that our strategies of old for solving problems aren't working.

At one stage they did work, and giving up on that involves the risks associated with doing something different. Not only does the thought of abandoning old coping strategies cause stress, but the majority of times we don't know what the 'something different' consists of.

Take, for example, an individual who has always had a couple of drinks to cope with stress. Initially this was highly effective – the alcohol would relax the individual and the stress would subside. But over time, as the individual drinks more and more, the original solution becomes part of the problem. But the individual still clings to the hope that his strategy for drinking will work again and relieve stress. As they are so invested in their 'solution', there is a natural reluctance to stop using it.

The job of SFT practitioners is to help service users realize that their tried and tested methods of solving problems may no longer be working. Once this has been achieved, you move on to the harder task of searching for something different that may work. Although there is no guarantee that the 'something different' will work, what we do know is that what they are currently doing is not working. Helping service users to realize that they will be no worse off by doing something different can facilitate an individual to experiment with alternative ways of solving their problems. As Steve de Shazer[3] put it, 'All that is necessary is that the person involved in a troublesome situation does something different' (p.7).

WHAT ABOUT THE PROBLEM?

A common misperception about SFT is that it ignores the problem. We would struggle to form any type of therapeutic relationship with the service user if we ignored the very essence of what brings them to seek help. Being solution-focused doesn't mean we have to ignore the problem; it just means we focus our attention and energies on discovering how the service user would like to see their life if the problem disappeared. By taking this strengths-based, positive approach, we strengthen our relationship with the service user and empower them to tackle not only their current problem but problems that occur in the future (see chapter 3 for more detail on developing and maintaining therapeutic relationships). This difference between a problem-focused approach and a solution-focused approach is innovatively described by Bannink:[4]

Suppose you are hungry and decide to eat in a restaurant. After having waited for some time, you are invited to take a seat and the manager introduces himself. He asks you questions regarding your hunger: 'How hungry are you? For how long have you been preoccupied with this feeling? Were you hungry in the past? What role did hunger play at home with your family or with other relatives? What disadvantages and possible advantages does hunger have for you?' After this, having become even hungrier, you ask if you can now eat. But in addition the manager wants you to complete some *questionnaires about hunger (and perhaps about other issues that the manager finds important). Once everything is finished, a meal is served to you that you did not order, but that the manager claims is good for you and has helped other hungry people. What are the chances of you leaving the restaurant feeling satisfied? (p.87)*

Allowing service users the opportunity to simply offload their problems can be invaluable. Unfortunately, I feel professionals sometimes don't get given enough credit for actively listening to a service user's concerns – many of the outcome measures we are required to do don't seem to recognize active listening as an intervention. But sometimes, due to the magnitude of what we are being told, any other intervention except listening simply wouldn't be appropriate. In these circumstances, building solutions may not be advisable.

However, in my experience, after approximately 30 minutes of offloading, services users start to repeat themselves, telling you the same problems but in slightly different language. When this happens, and as long as you have acknowledged the situation and the distress it may be causing, there may be an opportunity to refocus and reframe to solution talk. Initially, the service user may be resistant and persist in talking about the problem, but if done respectfully, most service users will welcome the opportunity to start building solutions.

FROM PROBLEMS TO SOLUTIONS

Changing from being problem-focused to being solution-focused is not an easy process. Practitioners seem to struggle to throw caution to the wind, take that leap of faith, and stop paying so much attention to the problem. I suppose it feels wrong not to ask problem-solving questions. It feels like we are short-changing our service users. Here they are, coming to us for help with their problems, and all we want to do is talk about solutions. How can this be right?

Table 41.1 highlights some of the differences between being solution-focused and being problem-focused. This is

Table 41.1 Differences between being problem-focused and being solution-focused

Problem-focused	Solution-focused
Interest in the past	Interest in the present and future
Goals of the service	Service user's goals
The professional is the expert	The service user is the expert
Deficits	Resources and strengths
Disability	Ability
Pathology	Competence
Resistance	Cooperation

intended to show how different ways of working may affect the conversations you have with service users.

LINES OF ENQUIRY

Think for a moment about the last time you met a service user for an initial assessment. How many of these questions focused on the strengths of the service user? Did you ask how they were coping already? About what they wanted? Or the service user's best hopes in seeking help?

Many of our questions are designed to gather as much information as possible about the person and their situation, and, as a result, are mainly problem-focused. As well as trying to obtain a full history, we are trying to assess any risk factors or issues that may warrant safeguarding concerns. Also, by obtaining as much information about the

Table 41.2 The language of problems and the language of solutions

Language of problems	Language of solutions
What I *don't* want	What I *do* want
When things *go wrong*	When things *go right*
Forces *beyond* my control	Forces *within* my control
I'm *stuck*	I am *progressing*
I expect *more troubles* to come	I see some positive *possibilities*

SFT emphasizes the language we use when we talk to service users. Once we start in a problem-focused way, it can be difficult to move the conversation to one where we want to talk about strengths, resources and solutions. Simply changing how we talk to service users can influence how quickly we can help them find solutions (see Table 41.2).

service user as possible, we feel more empowered and confident to help them.

For me, a good initial assessment uses a combination of problem-focused questions and solution-focused questions. SFT questions can be used to assess clinical risk, and the use of non-problem talk (see below) allows us to connect better with the service user while discovering possible solutions for follow-on meetings. Starting with 'What are your best hopes for coming here today?' or 'What would you like to see different if this meeting was successful?' opens the conversation to solution talk.

CHANGING THE FOCUS OF THE PRACTITIONER

REFLECTION

- To what extent do you feel you utilize a solution-focused approach in your own life?

- What may get in the way of using a solution-focused approach in your own practice, or within your team or environment?

The switch to being solution-focused starts with ourselves. On the whole we can be very negative and critical of ourselves, but by starting to the see the strengths, achievements and positives in our own lives, we can open our minds to searching for and recognizing similar solutions in the lives of service users.

Start by discovering your best self, by noting down what your greatest achievements are, what your best friend would

say about you, what skills, talents and abilities shine out in you, what you are passionate about and what you like best about yourself. Then move to focusing on your strengths at work and what you do differently to your colleagues; think about what the service users you support say about you; and what you would need to do to do your job that little bit better.

The next stage of changing your focus is to leave your assumptions at the door. It can be hard to embark on any interaction with a service user without having a whole host of preconceived ideas about them and their problems. We can probably all describe the general characteristics of someone who is depressed. But by doing so we miss the person behind the diagnosis. Instead of listening and observing and finding out about the client in front of us, we sometimes use our own perceptions, baggage, experiences and training to cloud what the service user may be telling us. As a result, we won't be finding out about *their* solution.

SFT encourages you to embrace this stance of not knowing by searching for the *person* behind the problem to help them find *their* solutions. Use what the service user tells you to build solutions and behavioural experiments, and never assume your experience and understanding of what they are saying is the same as that of the client. In summary, become a toddler again, learning about the service user's world with gentle probing: 'Why?' or 'How come?'

BUILDING SOLUTIONS

REFLECTION

- What might get in the way of someone fully engaging in building solutions?

- If you were to ask yourself the miracle question, what would you answer?

Solutions can come from many different directions. In this section I hope to show you how you can assimilate some of the SFT tools and techniques into your practice as a nurse, adding to the craft of caring. By doing so you can help service users find their own solutions, highlighting what will be discussed in chapter 50 on collaborative care planning. It is important to remain solution-focused and not solution-forced, guiding service users to achieve their preferred future.

Although we generally need to steer away from advice giving, SFT stays true to the premise that the client is the expert by simply offering insights into possible solutions as suggestions. The whole issue of advice giving in SFT is adequately discussed by de Shazer and Dolan,[5] where Insoo Kim Berg simply asks: if, as a solution-focused practitioner, you knew something that would help a service user, why would you not share that with them?

1. Non-problem talk

Many service users seek help because they feel that they are drowning in their problems. Unable to see anything else about themselves but their problem, the conversation quickly becomes saturated with problems. As long as the conversation stays stuck with problem talk, service users will be unable to see solutions.

Sometimes referred to as 'problem-free talk', non-problem talk can be the first step in identifying solutions. Although to the untrained eye these conversations can resemble simple small talk, the correct use of non-problem talk can do more than just put the person at ease and help build rapport. The simple chit-chat that occurs allows the practitioner to catch a glimpse at possible future solutions.

Some examples of non-problem talk are shown in Box 41.1. I have always been pleasantly surprised by how a session can change just by focusing on the person and not their problem – a heavily depressed and suicidal man who

BOX 41.1: NON-PROBLEM TALK: EXAMPLE QUESTIONS

- I know very little about you apart from what brings you here today. What would you feel happy to tell me about yourself?
- What are you interested in?
- What do you enjoy doing? How about before the problem started?
- What are you good at?
- Tell me a little more about your family?
- How would your best friend describe you?

starts to look up and smile as I connect with him on his passion for fine rum and cigars; and the excessively anxious and traumatized lady who, when asked what her family thought about her cooking, dryly replied, 'Well, I haven't killed them yet.'

2. Reframing

Reframing simply encourages the service user to think differently about their problems. By helping them generate new descriptions about their problems, potential solutions can be revealed. This new description reduces the hold of a problem, and when things are seen differently, they can become resources in creating solutions, sometimes stopping the service user seeing from everything in negative, absolute ways.

Some examples may help to clarify:

Service user: 'I've been so depressed I can't seem to do anything.'

Practitioner: *'But you made it here today – how did you manage that?'*

Service user: 'It feels like we've done nothing but argue for the last few months.'

Practitioner: *'But last time we met you told me about what a good time you both had had for your birthday? What was different then?'*

Service user: 'There's no point in even trying – you can't help me!'

Practitioner: *'Yet you still made it to our appointment – I'm wondering if part of you does feel there is a point in trying?'*

Service user: 'I feel depressed all the time.'

Practitioner: *'I know it sometimes feels that way. But I'm wondering if there was any time in the last few days when things seemed a little better?'*

3. Compliments

Compliments play a big part in SFT. They are used to genuinely express admiration to the service user and as a way to reinforce their strengths, resources and solutions. Used consistently and genuinely, compliments are a fundamental way in which we collaborate with the service user to build solutions.

As practitioners, we are not going out of our way to look for something to compliment our service users on. All we are doing is simply bringing to the forefront of our service users' experience the personal qualities and strengths that may have been hidden beneath the problem. In the course of our conversations, when they start to identify or show us resilience, a sense of humour, evidence of hard work, compassion or any other quality that may enhance the solution we are working towards, we bring this to their attention.

4. Goal setting

A large part of SFT uses goal setting as a way of maintaining solutions. Goals can come in many different formats – some goals direct us towards something we want, others evolve from being driven away from something we don't want. SFT uses a mix of both – we pick an end point, a preferred future, and work towards that.

It is important to help our service users realize that goals are adjustable. As we experience life, what is important to us can change. Our vision of our preferred future changes as we move along our journey. The actual goal is far less important than how important it is to you and how you can go about achieving it. Without goals, individuals lack direction in their lives, struggling to make any long-lasting changes, lacking an incentive to change.

SFT identifies the following principles when using goal setting:

- *The goal must be important to the client.*
- *Keep goals small, achievable and realistic.*
- *Make goals concrete, specific and behavioural.* Service users will often tell us very generic goals such as 'to be normal, to just live a normal life' or 'to no longer be depressed'. Although there is nothing wrong with these goals, it can be hard to work towards a solution. Follow-up questions encourage them to express these goals in more behavioural terms. As SF practitioners we want to know what they will be doing when they are living this normal life and are no longer depressed.

- *Goals express the presence of something or a behaviour, rather than an absence.* SFT encourages us to look at goals as doing something different, and hence the presence of 'something else' rather than stopping something. For example, for those who want to lose weight, rather than expressing the goal as 'stopping eating all the junk food', a solution-focused practitioner would gently enquire as to what they would be eating instead. To make the goal even more concrete, we would ask them what they would be doing once they had lost their desired weight.
- *Goals are expressed as beginnings rather than endings.* When we ask service users to tell us how they will know when their problems are solved, they usually describe the finish line – how their life will look when everything is better. Effective goal setting encourages them to look at what the first step might look like. This helps to break what can seem like an inordinate task into a more achievable set of tasks.
- *Goals are realistic and achievable within the context of the service user's life.*
- *The client sees the goal as involving hard work.*

5. The miracle question

The miracle question is a pivotal part of SFT, and it has almost become its trademark. It is one of the most useful and creative starts to the process of eliciting a description of a *preferred future*.

The standard formulation of the miracle question looks something like this:

Suppose that tonight, while you are asleep, a miracle happens, and all the problems that brought you here today disappeared. As this miracle occurs while you are sleeping, you do not immediately know that it has happened. When you wake up, what will be the first small signs that you will notice that will tell you that the miracle has happened?

By asking the miracle question, the practitioner can gain valuable insight into how the service user would like to see themselves if they were free of their problems. The miracle question gives the client the *permission* to start to fantasize about an ideal future – a life without their problems. Rarely do we allow ourselves the opportunity to think how good our lives could be if we could just get over our current difficulties. The miracle question opens up that opportunity.

Service users tend to experience pleasant emotions during replies, enhancing their experience of seeking help, leading to another exception to their current state. Creative thinking is stimulated, allowing them to come up with new goals or ambitions. Each response is as individual as the service user, reminding me that they really are the expert on themselves.

I have had many miracles involving winning the lottery. And why not? – a great thing to wish for. This type of answer allows the practitioner to work with the service user to formulate a more realistic preferred future. One way of responding to this type of answer could be to emphasize what a great miracle it would be to win the lottery, and then to ask *how* winning the lottery would make a difference. By gently exploring this difference, a bigger picture of the preferred future is generated.

Another common response from service users who have lost someone significant is that their miracle would involve them returning. Responses such as 'My wife would be lying next to me' or 'He wouldn't have had the affair that ended our marriage' are just two examples. Like the response about winning the lottery, they are great responses to what a miracle might look like.

Similarly, though, service users are very realistic and know that the loss cannot be undone. The majority of people whom I see trying to cope with a loss have already exhausted all means possible to reverse the loss. As in the case of the dream of winning the lottery, the practitioner carries on in much the same way, exploring with the service user what would be different for the client if their loved one was back.

Finding solutions out of grief and loss is a hard process for both service user and practitioner. The miracle question helps us to gauge how far they have got with their grief. Some will be so full of grief that the miracle question has allowed them to share a little more of what their loved one meant to them.

As a practitioner, allow them to expand on what that loss means. Encourage them to tell you more about what their loved one meant to them, and what this person would want for the service user today. Eventually, explore how ready they may be for solution talk by asking, 'How will you know when it is time to stop grieving and start to do something, even the smallest thing, differently?'

NOW THAT I'VE GOT YOU BELIEVING IN MIRACLES …

Once you have explored their miracle in as much depth as possible, and discovered who in their life would notice the most if this miracle had happened, ask them to identify which parts of the miracle are happening already. Typically, a significant part of the miracle is already happening. Then, referring back to the central philosophy of SFT, ask what they can do to keep this happening, and what the first step is to make more of this miracle happen, focusing the conversation on what they would *do* differently, rather than simply describing how they would *feel* differently.

6. Exceptions

Another major component of SFT is the use of exceptions. Exceptions are not remarkable or unique; they are happening all the time. They are occasions when their problems could have occurred but did not – or at least were less severe. For example, an exception can be seen as an occasion when a socially anxious service user is able to attend a social event and their anxiety is not as problematic as it usually is. Some examples are given in Box 41.2.

When working with exceptions, the focus is usually placed on the Who? What? When? and Where? of exception times. We want to elicit the intimate details of what was going on when the exceptions were happening. Our goal is to help the service user identify what was different when the exception was happening, in order for them to replicate all or part of that exception. As exceptions are identified, strengths are uncovered, leading to a sense of achievement.

> ## BOX 41.2: IDENTIFYING EXCEPTIONS: USEFUL QUESTIONS
>
> - Tell me about times when the problem is not happening, or when it is less severe.
> - You mentioned earlier that some times are better than others. What is it like during these times?
> - Over the last couple of weeks, when would your partner say you might have been feeling a little bit better?
> - Are there times when you are able to resist the urge to drink? How come you managed not to drink this time compared to others?
> - Are there times when you could have lost your temper but didn't? How did you manage to do that?
> - Since we met last, have there been times when you and your partner didn't argue? What was different about these times?

7. Scaling

The use of scaling is an invaluable tool for practitioners to use in SFT. In its simplest form, scales encourage clients to put a numerical figure on where they are when describing a particular problem. As De Jong and Berg[6] state, 'Scaling is a useful technique for making complex aspects of a client's life more concrete and accessible to both practitioner and client' (p.108).

Many service users find increased clarity when they are able to allocate a number to their problem. It allows them to channel their thoughts into defining the problem as it is now to how much worse it could be and how good things could be. I am genuinely surprised at the rating service users give themselves. They will express in great detail their problem situation and how they are not able to handle the level of distress the problem has caused them. Then when

I ask a scaling question to try to determine how well they are coping, I am expecting to hear a 0 or a 1 and they come back with a 3 or a 4. Expressing this surprise opens up the opportunity for a compliment.

Some examples of scaling questions are given in Box 41.3.

Once the service user has taught us about their scale and how they see themselves now, we continue by asking them to tell us what needs to happen to move them one place up the scale. In doing so, we are on the right path to helping our services users do something different that will enable them to find their solutions.

BOX 41.3: EXAMPLES OF SCALING QUESTIONS

- On a scale of 0–10, where 0 is the worst you've been feeling, and 10 is the best, where would you put yourself today?
- What could be the first thing you could do to move one point higher up the scale?
- What is it that you are doing that keeps it at a 4?
- On a scale of 0–10, how committed are you to reaching your goals and making these changes we have been talking about? What do you think might get in the way? What would need to be different for you to be more committed?

- What are you doing that stops it getting any lower?
- How will you know you've moved as far up the scale as you need to go?
- How long do you think it might take you to move one point up your scale?
- Where do you need to be on your scale in order to not have to come back and see me again?

ADAPTABILITY AND AREAS OF USE

REFLECTION

- Are there any areas that you can think of where a solution-focused approach may not be appropriate?

- What do you think prevents SFT from being used more widely?

SFT is a very versatile way of working. I have used it with the most complex of services users to those experiencing less severe symptomology. Within the crisis resolution and home treatment team (CRHTT), I have gradually been training the whole multidisciplinary team in how to incorporate the ethos of SFT into their practice. Even in the face of a mental health crisis, SFT has proved invaluable in helping service users see that there could be a preferred future other than taking their own life. More

general information on crisis assessment and resolution can be found in chapter 46.

One area where it has proved invaluable is in group work. Within the CRHTT we facilitated a 6-week SFT group (see Proudlock and Wellman[7]). Despite each service user coming into crisis for a very individual reason, the feedback at the end of the group was that everyone felt connected with each other as they could all relate to each other. Instead of the group being problem-focused, the goal was to achieve a preferred future; some sort of miracle.

Within the field of rehabilitation, SFT works well for those struggling with alcohol and drug addictions. Instead of striving for abstinence, it has faith in the service user, searching for a preferred future which may include using substances in a more controlled way. When working with children and young people, turning into a solution detective can be more engaging than focusing on the problem. Regardless of the age, culture or diagnosis of the service user, SFT can be incorporated into your work.

FINAL TIPS

Try to incorporate SFT into your work rather than seeing it as an alternative. Ask the service user what type of support they need at this time. You are a witness to their change, not part of it. Let them be the expert.

Try asking 'What's been better?' rather than 'How are you?' Lead by being one step behind – the service user is

the navigator, you are the driver. If what you are doing as a practitioner isn't working, stop doing it and do something different.

Smile. Relax. Have some fun with SFT. Create the most wonderful of solutions with service users.

CONCLUSION

SFT can be easily incorporated into more traditional ways of working and is a useful way of working to enhance any nurse's craft of caring with a wide variety of service users. It has many similarities to motivational interviewing (discussed in chapter 39) and can complement cognitive behavioural therapy (discussed in chapter 40), especially with those service users who may be initially slightly harder to engage. As my co-author's contribution below suggests, the service user's response is generally very positive towards SFT, if not at times challenging. I would strongly encourage all nurses, once qualified, to take further training in SFT to learn just how versatile and powerful solution-focused therapy can be.

SERVICE USER COMMENTARY

Sonia Sanghvi

To have a professional start with the view that you as a service user have insight and understanding into the problem is refreshing and exciting (as well as terrifying), as it almost puts you in the driving seat and makes you an active participant in recovery/therapy. More often than not, it is so much more beneficial to look at ways of dealing with and resolving the issues that lead to the behaviour that has led you to ask for help, rather than focusing on the problematic behaviour itself.

It is incredibly helpful to get someone thinking about the skills/knowledge/resources they already have to solve a problem (especially someone who doesn't believe they have any of these resources) rather than continuing to focus on the behaviour they want to change. As a service user, it is hard to accept that someone believes that you are capable of finding a solution, and it can be a very uncomfortable situation to find yourself in, but knowing that even just one person believes in you is incredibly powerful.

Having seen different professionals, it makes a refreshing change for me to see someone with a background in SFT who takes the *stance of not knowing*. It is obvious when a professional believes that they are the expert and this makes the therapeutic relationship difficult from the start. When this happens, it can at times lead to the service user depending on the practitioner to solve the issue rather than working through it together.

The *central philosophy of SFT* for a service user is scary and uncomfortable. 'If it doesn't work, then don't do it again, do something different.' To be told this, and then to come to this conclusion yourself, is very powerful. You can see that your tried and tested coping mechanisms aren't working, but because they are the only thing that ever has, you are reluctant to make a change. This is incredibly hard to hear and accept but it is also a very enlightening realization.

Giving the service user time to *offload the problem* is important but cannot be the only focus of the session. It's no wonder that service users choose to do this, especially when we may not have anyone else who can or does listen to us or when we feel that we are unable to talk to anyone we know about things. As a service user it is easy to get into the habit of offloading without realizing that there is a point at which it stops being helpful/positive. In my experience, having the discussion move from problem-focused to solution-focused once any distress has been acknowledged can very quickly change the way I have been looking at a problem.

Reframing really does make you look at the situation differently. At times I have felt as if I have stopped caring about anything but questions like those shown above have shown me that there are actually things that I do still care about. And *compliments* are sometimes tough for service users to hear – I find it easy to shrug compliments off, but when they have been 'teased' out of me through chit-chat/small-talk, they become much harder to dismiss and ignore.

Exceptions are hard to recognize, as they are often small things you find yourself doing on a daily basis. It is just as hard to admit to them, as it proves that you do have skills and resources to deal with situations you may have thought impossible. Once you find an exception, it is difficult to recognize what made that situation different, which is why using this approach is so helpful.

A solution-focused approach allows you as a service user not only to utilize your own resources but to acknowledge that you do have these in the first place. It can be incredibly easy to find yourself in a situation where you become dependent on the care being provided and expect a professional to solve the problem.

In my experience, SFT is uncomfortable because you start to own the problem and realize that the solution is in your control; that you may be the one standing in the way of your own recovery. This is difficult to accept; it is so much easier to believe that external factors are to blame (and they may indeed be part of the problem).

References

1. Freeman S (2006) Solutions Focused Approaches – PowerPoint presentation downloaded from www.ukasfp.org.uk July 2008.

2. Berg IK, Miller SD. *Working with the problem drinker: a solution focused approach.* New York: Norton, 1992.

3. de Shazer S. *Keys to solutions in brief therapy*. New York: W.W. Norton, 1985.
4. Bannink FP. Solution focused brief therapy. *Journal of Contemporary Psychotherapy*. 2007; **37**: 87–94.
5. de Shazer S, Dolan Y. *More than miracles*. Philadelphia: Haworth Press, 2007.
6. De Jong P, Berg IK. *Interviewing for solutions*. California: Brooks/Cole Thomson Learning, 2002.
7. Proudlock S, Wellman N. Solution focused groups: the results look promising. *Counselling Psychology Review* 2011; **26**(3): 45–54.

Further reading

Berg IK, Miller SD. *Working with the problem drinker: a solution focused approach*. New York and London: W.W. Norton, 1992.
Berg IK, Reuss NH. *Solutions step by step: a substance abuse treatment manual*. New York and London: W.W. Norton, 1997.
Fiske H. *Hope in action: solution focused conversations about suicide*. New York: Routledge, 2008.
Henden J. *Preventing suicide: the solution focused approach*. Chichester: Wiley, 2008.
Macdonald A. *Solutions-focused therapy, theory, research and practice*. London: Sage, 2007.
Nelson T. *Doing something different: practices in solution focused brief therapy*. London: Routledge, 2010.
O'Hanlon B, Bertolino B. *Even from a broken web: brief, respectful solution-orientated therapy for sexual abuse and trauma*. New York and London: W.W. Norton, 2002.
Proudlock SM. *The solution focused way: incorporating solution focused therapy tools and techniques into your everyday work*. London: Speechmark, 2011.
Sharry J. *Solution focused group work*. London: Sage, 2007.

Relevant web pages

Institute for Solution Focused Therapy. http://www.solutionfocused.net/
MacDonald A. Solution-focused brief therapy evaluation list. http://www.solutionsdoc.co.uk/sft.html
UK Association of Solution Focused Practice. http://www.ukasfp.co.uk/
Solution-focused practice toolkit: helping professionals use the approach when working with children and young people. http://www.nspcc.org.uk/services-and-resources/research-and-resources/solution-focused-practice-toolkit/
US Solution Focused Brief Therapy Association. http://www.sfbta.org/

42 Psychodynamic approaches with individuals

ANGELA COTTON AND DINA POURSANIDOU

LEARNING OUTCOMES

- To understand key psychodynamic developments and concepts.
- To appreciate the considerable influence of psychoanalytic and psychodynamic approaches upon contemporary mental health care with individuals.
- To realize the importance and value of some of these concepts to mental health nursing practice.
- To understand some of the theoretical background and interventions used in post-Freudian (relational) psychodynamic counselling and psychotherapy.
- To be able to think critically about some of the possibilities and limitations of psychodynamic approaches.

SUMMARY OF KEY POINTS

- Psychodynamic approaches appreciate the need to understand past experiences to enable the resolving of present distress.
- It is important to acknowledge the role of the unconscious and its influence upon behaviours and relationships.
- There is increasing recognition of the usefulness of psychodynamic concepts within diverse psychotherapeutic approaches.

INTRODUCTION

It has been suggested that psychodynamic psychotherapy, with its roots in psychoanalysis, 'is the most ambitious of all therapies in terms of its scope and aims'[1](p.6). Since the original ideas and practices proposed and developed by Dr Sigmund Freud and his close colleagues more than 100 years ago, psychoanalysis has undergone considerable changes to its methods and interventions, and it continues to have significant influences upon most of the 'talking therapies'. The ideas have been taken up, interrogated and critiqued within disciplines as diverse as psychology, sociology, cultural studies, education and literary criticism. The focus of this chapter is an exploration of the psychodynamic approach to working with individuals. Consideration will be given to key concepts associated with this approach, along with an appreciation of their contemporary significance within mental health care. The chapter will present discussion of some psychodynamic interventions, illustrated with examples from contemporary mental health care practice. Acknowledgement is also made of and appreciation expressed for the particular historical and cultural milieu within which early psychoanalysis developed. There is an associated recognition of the period towards the end of the nineteenth and beginning of the twentieth century as being one of considerable transformations. Such issues constitute, for psychodynamic approaches, a particular location, where Cartesian philosophies of science and the Enlightenment were juxtaposed with considerable moral and religious constraint in the West. Psychoanalysis thus emerged amid the boom of the human sciences and, likewise, it also strove to differentiate itself clearly from the other disciplines, having as its unique object of knowledge, psychic reality.

THE DEVELOPMENT OF THEORIES AND INTERVENTIONS

The psychodynamic approach has its beginnings in the study of human experience, motivations and development at the beginning of the twentieth century. Freud, a medical doctor in Vienna, began to develop his ideas while working with the psychiatrist Josef Breuer in the 1880s and 1890s. Freud studied for 3 years in Paris prior to this, under Jean-Martin Charcot, Professor of Neuropathology, who was exploring the use of hypnosis in treating what was termed 'hysteria' (paralysis of some part of the body or loss of one of the senses for which no physiological cause was apparent). These experiences influenced Freud's thinking in three ways:

- the significance of hypnosis for appreciating the power of the unconscious (a 'hidden' part of the personality where repressed memories are located);
- the observation of attachment developed as a consequence of hypnosis, 'magnetic passion', sometimes filial, sometimes maternal or sometimes erotic (the beginnings of ideas on transference);
- some connections between sexuality and 'neurosis' ('libido' as psychic energy compelling behaviour).

Freud's thinking advanced and evolved over some 40 years and his work came to dominate psychotherapy in the twentieth century. His ideas have become interwoven, albeit not without tensions, with cultural beliefs in the West. For example, concepts such as ego, libido, fixation, catharsis and repression have become part of everyday discourse, integrated within the popular imaginary as well as being well established within discourses of psychodynamic psychotherapies. Psychodynamic theories propose that dynamic inner forces control and regulate human behaviour: 'the assumption that there are unconscious mental processes, the recognition of the theory of resistance and repression, the appreciation of the importance of sexuality and of the Oedipus complex – these constitute the principal subject-matter of psychoanalysis and the foundations of its theory'[2] (p.145).

Freud came to believe, in contrast to the thinking of the time, that behaviour is often irrational and that much of our behaviour has reasons which are not in our conscious awareness. The struggles in the mind, a consequence of battles of instinct, reason and conscience, he named 'psychodynamic'. The premise of all such approaches to therapy is that the client is not aware of the motivations for their behaviour, which are rooted in the unconscious; a further element is the importance of infantile experience. Instinctual drives and their associated 'psychic energy', which may be difficult to express, become evident in symptoms of distress, with the original emotion becoming embedded in the unconscious. In view of this, childhood experiences, repressed erotic feelings and unconscious conflicts can become manifest in adult behaviour.[3] 'Psychoanalytic theory is built up on the perception of the resistance exerted by the patient when we try to make him [sic] conscious of his unconscious'[4] (p.161).

Nowadays the term 'psychodynamic' is used to refer to a broad approach to explaining psychological phenomena with reference to unconscious mental processes, including intrapersonal and interpersonal.

THE STRUCTURAL MODEL OF THE MIND

Freud's structural model proposed that the human mind could be thought of as being organized around three psychic agencies, or themes: the id, the ego and the superego.[2] The id represents instinctual drives concerned with meeting sexual, aggressive and bodily needs. Irrational and impulsive, (subject to the *pleasure principle*), the id's processes (the libido) are largely unconscious and not amenable to social restrictions, but create tensions which require release through real solutions or fantasy. The earliest mental processes of infants are those of the id:

> *the dark, inaccessible part of our personality ... we call it a chaos, a cauldron full of seething excitations ... It is filled with energy reaching it from the instincts, but it has not organisation, produces no collective will, but only a striving*

to bring about the satisfaction of the instinctual needs subject to the observance of the pleasure principle.[5] (pp.105–6)

Freud proposed that the ego emerges as the baby develops and begins to adapt to the *reality principle* where satisfaction of needs have to wait. The ego is the conscious, rational aspect of the personality which responds to the outside world. The superego represents what is 'right' and 'wrong' according to the cultural environment, and has both conscious and unconscious elements. There are two aspects of the superego, the *ego ideal* (which relates to what is 'proper' virtuous behaviour) and the *conscience* (concerned with censoring immoral impulses from the id). Conflicts between the id and the ego give rise to the experience of anxiety; the person tries to resolve this anxiety by using defence mechanisms, these include the following:

- repression ('pushing' back unacceptable or unwanted feelings, thoughts and/or memories into the unconscious mind; 'motivated forgetting');
- regression (returning to/using coping strategies from an earlier stage in one's life where no conflict was present);
- projection (inadmissible feelings are attributed, 'projected' onto others);
- denial (distancing or disavowal of an idea, refusing to accept reality);
- reaction formation (the replacement of anxiety-provoking feelings with their opposite);
- displacement (redirecting feelings/behaviour onto a substitute object because it is not possible to face the real target);
- splitting (demonstrating an inability to reconcile negative and positive attributes of self or others);
- sublimation (unacceptable impulses are channelled into socially appropriate activity, e.g. sexual desire channelled into artistic/creative endeavours – perceived as a positive defence mechanism);
- rationalization (constructing an acceptable reason for behaviour that is really about another, less acceptable reason);
- conversion (development of physical symptoms as an outlet for intra-psychic conflict, e.g. paralysis, blindness).

Defence mechanisms are reversible and can be adaptive, as well as problematic. Adaptive use of defence mechanisms helps people to achieve their goals in acceptable ways. Defence mechanisms become problematic when they interfere with functioning, relationships and orientation to reality.

Examples of defence mechanisms

- *Sublimation*: A nurse who has feelings of anger and hostility toward his line manager sublimates those feelings by working out vigorously at the gym.
- *Projection:* A young adult blames his substance abuse on his parents' refusal to buy him a new car.
- *Splitting:* A client tells a nurse that she is the only one who cares about her, yet the following day, the same client refuses to talk to the nurse.

REFLECTION

- Can you identify times when you might find yourself using any of the defence mechanisms listed above?
- What unconscious conflict might you be protecting yourself from?
- Could you see how using defence mechanisms could be useful?
- How could such use become problematic?

UNCONSCIOUS, PRECONSCIOUS, CONSCIOUS

The topographical metaphor of an iceberg has been employed to understand the relationship between the conscious, the preconscious and the unconscious. The largest aspect is the 'underwater ice': the 'unconscious is a particular realm of the mind with its own wishful impulses, its own mode of expression and its particular mental mechanisms which are not in force elsewhere'[6] (p.249). The preconscious, which contains thoughts and memories which are accessible to us, and the conscious, all of the thoughts and feelings we are aware of at a given time, are both thought to interact with, and be influenced by, the deeper inaccessible unconscious.

The psychodynamic approach works on assumptions that feelings and ideas arising from actual events become repressed into the unconscious and manifest themselves as 'symptoms', dreams, slips of the tongue (parapraxis) and jokes.[7] The related uses of defence mechanisms as a protection against anxiety or guilt require considerable psychic energy: 'repression demands a persistent expenditure of force, and if this were to cease, the success of the repression would be jeopardised, so that a fresh act of repression would be necessary'[8] (p.151).

It is important to acknowledge that short-term use of defence mechanisms is believed to be an adaptive strategy for coping with pressures; it is when they become more habituated and are perhaps interfering with relational processes that they may be deemed problematic. Exploring such defences is an aspect of the psychodynamic approach; the intention is that the client becomes aware of their limitations, with a view to developing more useful, adaptive strategies.

REFLECTION

- The defence mechanism of denial involves keeping external events from awareness; the situation that is too much to handle is 'refused' – not experienced.

- Can you think of situations within your nursing practice where denial may be a protective defence?

- Can you think of examples where denial may be less useful, or actually contribute to a person's distress?

- Reaction formation can take a person beyond denial; conscious (ego) feelings are expressions of their opposite unconscious (id) ones. An example might include deliberate generosity and kindness where anger and fear might be present. From your experiences in mental health nursing, identify further possible illustrations of this defence mechanism.

Dreams

'The interpretation of dreams is the royal road to a knowledge of the unconscious activities of the mind'[9] (p.769). Freud believed that dreams were motivated by repressed wishes and urges, and contained unconscious 'hidden messages' as expressions of intra-psychic conflict. Analysis of the content and symbolism of dreams was thought to rediscover and resolve such conflict.

Introspection/free association

This psychoanalytic technique is foundational; the patient is encouraged to talk about whatever comes to mind, no matter how inappropriate it may seem. 'In the therapeutic session itself we might choose the use of free association … in the encouragement to the client to be more spontaneous, and to the therapist to listen with that free-floating attention which Freud saw as the counterpart to free association'[7] (p.150). Introspection and the putting into words of all thoughts, images, perceptions and feelings are viewed as central to such 'free association'. Particular patterns may then be discerned by the analyst who then offers suggestions about hidden desires, the identification of which would promote recognition and relief.

Transference

Transference refers to feelings towards the therapist/clinician which have their origin in an earlier relationship, usually with an early caregiver. One of the objects of psychoanalysis is to interpret these feelings and to deal with the resistances which may be associated with such symbolisms. Greenson has defined transference as:

the experiencing of feelings, drives, attitudes, fantasies and defences toward a person in the present, which do not befit that person but are a repetition of reactions originating in regard to significant persons of early childhood, unconsciously displaced onto figures in the present. The two outstanding characteristics of a transference reaction are: it is a repetition and it is inappropriate.[10] (p.155)

Countertransference

Countertransference is concerned with the responses of the therapist within the psychodynamic encounter. Aiyegbusi speaks of 'feelings that are stirred up in the clinician which may be best understood as a response to the patient's transference feelings in combination with the clinician's internal world'[11] (p.25). This phenomenon has been characterized as 'the identifications and tendencies belonging to an analyst's personal experiences and personal development which provide the positive setting for his analytic work and make his work different in quality from that of any other analyst'.[12]

The compulsion to repeat

The psychodynamic approach has as a starting point the assumption that how we relate to others is influenced by

REFLECTION

- Transference and countertransference are now well-established concepts within the therapeutic (nurse–patient) relationship.

- A transference example within mental health nursing: within the working phase of the relationship (see chapter 3) the person in care sees you (in your role as primary nurse) as a nurturing parental figure and responds to you as overly responsible for their recovery, excessively deferring decisions to you.

- Countertransference has implications for mental health nursing. Particular individuals may remind you of someone for whom you have or had strong feelings (positive or negative). Patient care may be influenced by an over-identification with them; there may be similarities with our own characteristics or issues that we have resolved in the past. There may be feelings of over-protection or sexual attraction, with the need to carefully identify within supervision just where these emotions 'belong'.

our earliest childhood experiences. These early relationships become internalized and become patterns for relating to others throughout our lives. This 'compulsion to repeat' has the effect that behaviours in relationships may be less effective because the patterns established may be less than helpful.

POST-FREUDIAN (RELATIONAL) PSYCHODYNAMIC APPROACHES: OBJECT RELATIONS

Post-Freudian psychoanalysts have continued to develop and extend understandings of human psychic experiences. These practitioners, including Melanie Klein and some of those she educated – Wilfred Bion, Betty Joseph, Herbert Rosenfeld and Hanna Segal – have made creative and original psychoanalytic contributions. Object relations theory extends and develops Freud's notions of the unconscious and proposes a model that views humans as relationship-seeking from birth. In particular, the mother, or key parental figure, and infant relationship plays a critical role in the baby's development of self and identity, distinct and separate from the mother/key caregiver. 'The rise of object relations theories in psychoanalysis was associated with a shift of interest towards developmental issues … the individual's experience of himself or herself, and …increasingly concerned with relationships'[13] (p.81). Klein, through her approach to analysis of babies and children, came to view mental structures as arising out of a variety of internal objects leading to unconscious 'phantasy' and culminating in an integrated self.[14]

The ideas of Donald Winnicott, one of the early proponents of object relations theory, have continued influence within psychodynamic approaches. He developed language which was arguably more simple and homely: 'Winnicott repeatedly uses a handful of idiosyncratic terms to communicate his ideas: holding, using, playing, feeling real, illusion and disillusion, true and false self, going on being' and foreground the baby's relationship with an actual mother 'holding and handling' and 'being a good-enough mother'[15] (p.111). Winnicott proposed the notion of maternal ambivalence in relation to her new baby (the coexistence of hate alongside love) and how such ambivalence exists in all human relationships, not least the psychoanalytical therapeutic relationship. In view of this, working with the transference (the therapist coming to symbolize a significant person in the individual's life) and the countertransference (the patient invoking feelings in the therapist that may symbolically represent another) becomes a central aspect of the therapeutic work. Thus the analytic setting for Winnicott is the opportunity for growth that may have been absent for the patient earlier in life; the restoration of an environment to resume and facilitate necessary development.[10] Such notions of psychological containment and boundaries are themes which continue to have centrality within contemporary psychodynamic approaches. Psychic change is thought to occur when past and current knowledge are allowed to be part of the ego and is possible when the ego is less restrictive, when it is open to new experience. Therefore, the ego must tolerate conflicted feelings and thoughts about the self and others for knowledge to be allowable and accessible. 'Knowledge gained in the psychoanalytic situation is the cornerstone of the working through process. Working through consists of the conscious aspect of insight combined with the more unconscious aspects of … be(ing) able to endure, accept, and eventually integrate new knowledge about the self and its internalized objects'[16] (p.xvi). As Britton observes: 'we want to love, to hate and to know our objects, and we also need to be loved, fear being hated and want to be understood', illustrating something of the psychological conflict regarding these wishes and desires.[17] Psychological containment and the need for therapeutic boundaries are both central to notions of the therapeutic relationship and may be read as integral to the nurse–patient relationship (see chapter 3).

PSYCHODYNAMIC CONCEPTS IN MENTAL HEALTH NURSING PRACTICE

Psychodynamic approaches have had considerable influence within contemporary mental health care, and there is a diversity of allegiances among the fields of therapeutic endeavour. Some practitioners align themselves with the psychoanalytic tradition while others 'prefer to use the psychoanalytic as a base from which to move critically towards an integrative position … [making] their own use, some extensively and some minimally, of Freud's principles and concepts, in some cases without recognising their source'[7] (p.149).

Terms which originated in psychoanalysis have now come to be embedded within therapeutic discourses in contemporary mental health care: projection, repression, displacement, denial, transference and countertransference are present in conversations between therapists, in clinical supervision, and in everyday discourse.

There have been endeavours to explore how unconscious influences make an impact within mental health care. The seminal work of Isabel Menzies Lyth continues to have relevance in understanding how defences against anxiety underpin nursing work. She applied Klein's theories and Bion's work on organizations, and illustrated (controversially at the time) how the stresses of nursing, and the intimate relationship it demanded with patients, impacted on the organization of care. She observed that nurses, who were close to people who were ill and caring for those who were dying, were experiencing emotional pressures which they struggled to defend against. She identified how nurses' and health care managers' use of defence mechanisms against anxiety within care settings enabled them to 'survive' extreme emotional circumstances.[18]

The influences of the psychodynamic approach to working with individuals is evidenced within an array of mental health care settings. An example of such work is within forensic mental care. Within forensic mental health care there is recognition that nurses 'must manage highly complex, intensive relationships day in, day out'[11] (p.36). Here, the psychodynamic approach has been perceived as 'a useful way of capturing the richness of clinical nursing experience in forensic services', and has been utilized as a framework to provide a way to work effectively within forensic mental health care 'by offering a language for the complex emotional and behavioural phenomena that can often feel puzzling or indeed overwhelming'[19] (p.11).

Mental health practitioners have found that such a framework can inform therapeutic activity, and can be a way for mental health nurses to work effectively with complex interpersonal phenomena. Having knowledge of and being informed by an awareness of unconscious processes is perceived as crucial. A psychodynamic appreciation of the emotional impact of forensic nursing, along with integration of other theoretical frameworks, can strengthen clinical nursing practice.[11] An appreciation of the defences stirred up by interpersonal work, the requirement that nurses have to process intense projections from a complex client group, and the concomitant sensitive acknowledgement and addressing of countertransference within psychodynamically oriented supervision and reflective practice are central.[11]

Kay speaks of how 'in the current climate, unconscious counter-transference reactions are more likely to be seen as "mistakes" made by the nurse rather than clues to understanding more about the patient'[20] (p.34). His psychodynamic approach situated within forensic mental health care advocates: 'The nurse who can adopt an attitude of free-floating attention, who can observe from a distance or listen with a "third ear" to discover what may be behind a surface communication can tune in to the patient and begin to understand what may seem incomprehensible'[20] (p.34). Themes from psychodynamic approaches which have significance for all mental health practitioners include attention to unconscious process, an appreciation of and relevance of the past, and issues concerning the mental health practitioner's involvement in the process of care.[21] The usefulness of psychodynamic insights more broadly within nursing practice has been the focus of the work of Tew, Rafferty and Paget.[22] Their view is that psychosocial events in nursing can be understood through a psychodynamic perspective, which echoes Aiyegbusi in that it can 'offer nurses a significant way of explaining why they feel the way they do. Such understanding can lead to insights, which inform responses, thereby enhancing the capacity to practice with integrity'[22] (p.2).

COGNITIVE ANALYTICAL THERAPY

Psychodynamic approaches are becoming increasingly influential and integrated with cognitive models. Cognitive analytic therapy (CAT) is a collaborative and relational approach to therapeutic change.[23,24] CAT draws on object relations theory[25,26] and personal construct theory[27] and proposes that representations of self, others and the world are socially formed by early reciprocal interactions with significant others.[24] The influence of the theorists Vygotsky and Bakhtin (notions of putting experiences into words through dialogue and 'voice') is apparent, along with the recognition of the interplay of biological and social influences on psychological distress.[28,29] Thus a dialogical perspective on the self is central for CAT. The dialogical-self has implications for therapy in that learning takes place through the development, use and internalization of language, cultural signs and tools.[30]

A further development within contemporary mental health practice has been the growing significance of psychodynamic phenomena within broader psychotherapeutic endeavours; for example, there is increasing acknowledgement and exploration of transference and countertransference within both therapeutic and supervision processes for cognitive behaviour therapy.[31,32] The feelings and reactions within therapy are thus seen as a valuable source of information about a patient's (and therapist's) inner world.

CONCLUSION

We are all tangled within contradictory and over determined psychodynamic forces.[33] *(p.528)*

As this chapter has shown, there has been a proliferation of theories of the self within the field of psychotherapy. Such theories endeavour to address, or in some way bear on, traditional philosophic questions about the self from as far back as Aristotle. In view of such theories, psychodynamic psychotherapy may be positioned as an exploration or treatment of the self, or, following Michel Foucault, psychotherapies may be said to be 'technologies of the self'. The implications here are that such 'regimes of truth' within the culturally shared discourses[34] of psychoanalysis enable particular practices for care of the self: 'Whether the ultimate therapeutic goal is autonomy, symptom relief, character change, or something else, the means of getting there is thought to be discovery of the "real" or "true" self or, as some would say, the integration of the self'.[35] From such thinking it is evident that Sigmund Freud laid the groundwork for much of contemporary thinking about care of the self. While there are acknowledged differences within the field – even conflicts between those psychoanalysts who give importance to internally generated experiences and those who place a greater emphasis on the interpersonal environment, such ideas continue to have resonance. For mental health nursing, it may be useful to think of such resonance within the context of the 'craft of caring': the embracing and blending of art and science in the integration of psychodynamic skills and concepts within meaningful, values-based nursing.[36] Understanding and giving human responses to distress may certainly be enhanced by acknowledging the significance of the unconscious to our psychic realities, and its potential impact upon nurse–patient encounters in everyday practice and promoting recovery. Within such a perspective, making a space for and valuing psychodynamic approaches would be part of what Barker has suggested as lifelong practice: 'Genuine caring

needs the same intimacy, quiet, care, attention and sensitivity to create the conditions … for healing and recovery'.[36]

Within this chapter, then, we have presented an overview of some of the observations, theories and psychodynamic interventions which began with Freud, and can still be seen as making a significant contribution to contemporary mental health practice, counselling and psychotherapy. The influence of psychoanalysis continues:

> *it is that quest for understanding – even though his understanding has in some respects been shown to be time-bound – which still appeals to many therapists and clients, who likewise may puzzle about what makes them the persons they are. It is that aspect of puzzling over mysteries that remains his [Freud's] lasting legacy in the field of therapy.[7] (p.3)*

In psychodynamic approaches to working with individuals, we must recognize that we are all subject to the unconscious, and there is the expectation and acceptance that 'there is no definitive answer, more a moving towards something, as yet unknown'[37] (p.65).

References

1. British Psychoanalytic Council. Making sense of psychotherapy and psychoanalysis 2014. Available from: https://www.bpc.org.uk/sites/psychoanalytic-council.org/files/Mind-opt.pdf [Accessed 10th September 2016].
2. Freud S. *The ego and the id*. London: Penguin Freud Library vol. 11, 1923.
3. Friedman HS, Schustack MW. *Personality: classic theories and modern research*. Boston: Allyn and Bacon, 1999.
4. Fodor N, Gaynor F. *Freud: dictionary of psychoanalysis*. New York: Philosophical Library, Inc., 1950.
5. Freud S. *New introductory lectures on psychoanalysis*. London: Penguin Freud Library vol. 2, 1933.
6. Freud S. *Introductory lectures on psychoanalysis*. London: Penguin Freud Library vol. 1, 1916–17.
7. Jacobs M. *Sigmund Freud*, 2nd edn. London: Sage, 2003.
8. Freud S. *Repression*. London: Penguin Freud Library vol. 11, 1915.
9. Freud S. *The interpretation of dreams*. London: Penguin Freud Library vol. 4, 1900.
10. Greenson RR. *The technique and practice of psychoanalysis*. London: Hogarth Press, 1967.
11. Aiyegbusi A. Clarke-Moore J. The nurse–patient relationship with offenders: containing the unthinkable to promote recovery. In: Aiyegbusi A, Clarke-Moore J (eds). *Therapeutic relationships with offenders: an introduction to the psychodynamics of forensic mental health nursing*. London: Jessica Kingsley, 2009: 15–32.
12. Winnicott DW. Hate in the counter-transference. *International Journal of Psychoanalysis* 1949; **30**(2): 69–74.
13. Fonagy P. *Attachment theory and psychoanalysis*. London: Karnac, 2004.
14. Klein M. A contribution to the psychogenesis of manic-depressive states (1935). In: *The writings of Melanie Klein*. London: Hogarth, 1975, 23–89.
15. Minsky R. *Psychoanalysis and gender. An introductory reader*. London: Routledge, 1996.
16. Waska R. *Love, hate, and knowledge: the Kleinian method and the future of psychoanalysis*. London: Karnac, 2010.
17. Britton R. *Belief and imagination: explorations in psychoanalysis*. London: Routledge, 1998.
18. Menzies Lyth I. Social systems as a defense against anxiety. An empirical study of the nursing service of a general hospital. *Human Relations* 1960; **13**: 95–121.
19. Aiyegbusi A. Introduction. In: Aiyegbusi A, Clarke-Moore J (eds). *Therapeutic relationships with offenders: an introduction to the psychodynamics of forensic mental health nursing*. London: Jessica Kingsley, 2009: 9–14.
20. Kay M. Managing hate: the nurse's counter-transference. In: Aiyegbusi A, Clarke-Moore J (eds). *Therapeutic relationships with offenders: an introduction to the psychodynamics of forensic mental health nursing*. London: Jessica Kingsley, 2009: 33–42.
21. Higdon J. *Psychodynamic theory for therapeutic practice*, 2nd edn. Basingstoke: Palgrave MacMillan, 2012.
22. Tew L, Rafferty M, Paget M. *Nurses and their patients: informing practice through psychodynamic insights*. Keswick: M&K Update, 2009.
23. Kerr IB. Cognitive analytic therapy. *Psychiatry* 2005; **4**(5): 28–33.
24. Ryle A, Kerr IB. *Introducing cognitive analytic therapy: principles and practice*. Chichester: Wiley, 2002.
25. Ogden TH. The concept of internal object relations. *International Journal of Psychoanalysis* 1983; **64**(2): 227–41.
26. Ryle A. The value of written communication in dynamic psychotherapy. *British Journal of Medical Psychology* 1983; **56**: 361–6.
27. Kelly GA. Personal construct theory and the psychotherapeutic interview. *Cognitive Therapy and Research* 1977; **1**(4): 355–62.
28. Vygotsky LS. *The collected works of LS Vygotsky: problems of the theory and history of psychology*, 3rd edn, ed. Rieber RW, Wollock J. New York: Plenum Press, 1997.
29. Bakhtin MM. *The dialogic imagination: four essays*. Austin: University of Texas Press, 2010.
30. Leinman M. The concept of sign in the work of Vygotsky, Winnicott and Bakhtin: further integration of object relations theory and activity theory. *British Journal of Medical Psychology* 1992; **65**(3): 209–21.

31. Prasko J, Diveky T, Grambal A, Kamaradova D, Mozny P, Sigmundova Z, et al. Transference and counter-transference in cognitive behavioral therapy. *Biomedical Papers* 2010; **154**(3): 189–98.

32. Prasko J, Vyskocilova J. Countertransference during supervision in cognitive behavioral therapy. *Activitas Nervosa Superior Rediviva* 2010; **52**(4).

33. Parker I. Reflexive social psychology: discourse analysis and psychoanalysis. *Free Associations* 1994; **4**(4): 527–48.

34. Foucault M. *Discipline and punish*. New York: Vintage/Random House, 1979.

35. Erwin E. *Philosophy and psychotherapy*. London: Sage, 1997.

36. Barker P. The nature of nursing. In: Barker P (ed.). *Psychiatric and mental health nursing. The craft of caring*, 2nd edn. London: Edward Arnold, 2009: 3–11.

37. Taylor M, Loewenthal D . Researching a client's experience of preconceptions of therapy. A discourse analysis. *Psychodynamic Counselling* 2001; **7**(1): 63–82.

Further reading

Bion W. *Elements of psycho-analysis*. London: Heinemann, 1963.

Casement P. *On learning from the patient*. London: Tavistock, 1991.

Casement P. *Further learning from the patient: the analytic space and process*. London: Routledge, 2002.

Jacobs M. *Psychodynamic counselling in action*, 4th edn. London: Sage, 2010.

Klein M. *The psychoanalysis of children*. London: Hogarth, 1932.

Lacan J. *The four fundamentals of psycho-analysis*. London: Penguin, 1979.

Leiper R, Maltby, M. *The psychodynamic approach to therapeutic change*. London: Sage, 2004.

Segal H. *The work of Hanna Segal: a Kleinian approach to clinical practice*. London: Jason Aronson, 1981.

Spillius E. *Encounters with Melanie Klein: selected papers of Elizabeth Spillius*, ed. Roth P, Rusbridger R. New Library of Psychoanalysis. London: Routledge, 2007.

Symington N. *The analytic experience: lectures from the Tavistock*. London: Free Association Books, 1986.

Waska R. *Real people, real problems, real solutions: the Kleinian psychoanalytic approach with difficult patients*. New York: Brunner-Routledge, 2005.

Wittgenstein L. *Philosophical investigations*. Oxford: Blackwell, 1958.

Relevant web pages

British Psychoanalytic Association. http://www.psychoanalysis-bpa.org

British Psychoanalytic Council. http://www.bpc.org.uk

British Psychotherapy Foundation. http://www.britishpsychotherapyfoundation.org.uk

Institute of Psychoanalysis. http://www.psychoanalysis.org.uk

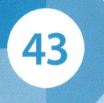

43 Psychodynamic approaches to working in groups

ANTONY FROGGETT AND STEVE DELANEY

LEARNING OUTCOMES

- To understand the psychodynamic approach to groups.
- To be aware of the importance of 'dynamic administration' issues when setting up a group.
- To understand the role of the 'conductor' in the group.
- To be aware of some of the challenges that can arise when conducting a group.
- To know how to find out more about groups and to get further training.
- To be stimulated to explore the possibility of running a group.

SUMMARY OF KEY POINTS

- The psychodynamic approach to groups offers a different way of understanding psychological difficulties – one that emphasizes the importance of communication and relationships.
- There are many different types of groups (for example, structured/unstructured; open/closed) that work in different ways.
- Planning and dealing with practicalities (i.e. *dynamic administration*) are an important part of creating a therapeutic environment.
- Groups are often effective when they combine a high degree of support with a high degree of challenge.

- The therapist's role is to create a *culture of enquiry* rather than to provide solutions to problems.
- Difficulties are inevitable in groups. Sometimes these can be opportunities for group members to try new ways of dealing with problems.
- A group approach can be used to support staff teams and to understand the problems that occur in organizations.
- Supervision, training and being part of a network are essential for developing one's skill in running groups.

INTRODUCTION

The widespread use of therapeutic groups emerged during the Second World War as a practical response to the needs of soldiers with psychiatric conditions. The Northfield experiments in the 1940s were led by senior medical officers who were to become key figures in psychoanalysis, group analysis and the development of therapeutic communities in the UK.[1] The group approach was a radical departure from what had preceded it, and today it retains both its element of pragmatism and its sense of adventure.

Practitioners have taken a psychodynamic approach to groups and applied it to a wide range of patients – such as people with eating disorders, people who self-harm, people with depression, and people with a diagnosis of a personality disorder. Groups are appealing to mental health practitioners because they offer the possibility of being able to treat a larger number of people than with one-to-one therapies. Groups are also able to help patients who are difficult to engage in individual therapies, such as those with addictions or those in forensic settings. Groups are often appealing to service users because they offer a sense of togetherness and support, which can increase motivation for change and reduce feelings of isolation. However, the idea of a therapy group can also be unsettling for both patients and staff. There can be anxieties about it not being 'real' therapy, about the lack of confidentiality or about the difficult dynamics that can arise in groups.

The purpose of this chapter is to help you think about the craft of conducting a group and to encourage you to find out more about whether this is a useful approach that could help patients.

PSYCHODYNAMIC APPROACH TO WORKING WITH GROUPS

People are group animals. We only survive – individually and as a species – by being part of a group. Human beings are social to the very core. We depend upon others from the moment of birth, for both our physical and our emotional needs.

Most psychological approaches start with the notion of the individual. However, each person is emotionally and psychologically entwined with others – our families, our communities, and the rest of humanity. We are only 'individual' because we have language, meanings and values that we share with others. Our identity is defined by our relationship to groups. We can say, for example, that we are a parent, a nurse or British, and it is by showing that we share something with others that we express what is unique about ourselves. We can only see the individual by seeing the group at the same time.

Psychodynamic group therapists avoid what they see as the artificial distinction between what is social and what is psychological. They believe that, in order to help the patient, one must always have in mind the 'total situation'.

> Foulkes wrote: *'Each individual – itself an artificial, though plausible, abstraction – is basically and centrally determined, inevitably, by the world in which he lives, by the community, the group, of which he forms a part'*[2] (p.10).

The concept of the *Matrix* is used to describe how we are embedded in relationships. The Matrix is a 'hypothetical web of communication'[3] (p.292) that connects us to other human beings. These connections include our biology, a shared language and culture, and our collective experiences of living. There are very few experiences that we have as individuals that have not been experienced by others, even if our *particular* experience is unique to us.

What is a psychological problem?

> *'Because we lack any real predators, the only major threat to humans is other humans. If we did not need other humans so much, it would make a lot of sense to avoid them'*[4] (p.214).

At the heart of our 'groupishness' is a paradox. We need relationships in order to thrive, yet this need makes us vulnerable to being hurt by others – especially by those people who are closest to us. Bion[5] (pp.168–9) referred to people as group animals at war with the group, including *that part of themselves* that needed the group. This is an important insight. He is suggesting that the conflict we experience is both interpersonal (with other people) and intrapersonal (within ourselves) at the same time. The psychodynamic approach views the managing of these contradictory aspects of our human-ness as the main challenge in achieving a full and satisfying life.

Difficulties often start in early childhood. If a child suffers neglect or intrusion, he may develop ways of psychologically protecting himself that avoid genuine intimacy or dependency on other people. One of the ways we manage conflict is to psychologically 'block things out' so that we are no longer connected to our experience. We still have traces of our feelings, but they are disconnected from the context that would allow them to make sense. Thus feelings – such as anxiety, depression or compulsion – are no longer meaningful to us. They appear simply as *symptoms*, and are felt by the patient as if they were 'things' to be got rid of rather than being part of himself. For patients with entrenched problems, removing one set of symptoms often results in another set of symptoms emerging to take their place.

A psychodynamic group therapist therefore does not focus on the presenting problem. Instead, she attempts to

CASE STUDY 1

Rebecca, a 42-year-old woman, came to group therapy with a diagnosis of obsessive–compulsive disorder (OCD). She felt that everything was unclean and constantly wanted to wash her hands. She lived alone and rarely mixed with other people for fear of catching their germs. Previous therapies had not relieved her of these problems. In the group she spoke about her father's parents being killed by the Nazis during the Holocaust and how, as a child, he told her never to trust people. As her therapy progressed, she expressed her regret at not having a closer relationship with her father and spoke about her sadness at not having children. After a year in therapy, she decided to take in a lodger and started to do an evening class. Her OCD symptoms remained, but she told the group, 'I've learnt that I can still do things when I really want to.'

explore the meaning of the patient's symptoms, especially in terms of his current and past relationships. Garland, in her article, 'Group-analysis: taking the non-problem seriously',[6] described how it is the experience of getting to know each other and 'play' that is transformative for patients in the group.

Group analytic concepts

Group analysis is the main psychodynamic approach to conducting therapeutic groups. It was established by S.H. Foulkes in the 1940s, and includes elements of psychoanalysis, Gestalt psychology, sociology and systems theory. It is an eclectic approach that continues to develop as practitioners incorporate new ideas such as attachment theory,[7] mentalization[8] and complexity theory[9] into group analytic thinking.

Group analysts use many of the concepts from individual psychodynamic theory to understand what is happening for patients in the group (see chapter 42 for more on psychodynamic approaches with individuals). In addition, there are a number of *group-specific* concepts[3] that are used to understand the processes that occur within groups.

These include:

- *Socialization.* This is the process by which group members develop a shared sense of belonging and the feeling of being at ease to talk openly in the group.
- *Free-floating communication.* The therapist encourages uncensored communication between group members in which the narrative of the group unfolds with spontaneous contributions from all group members.

- *Exchange.* Communication occurs and relationships develop through the process of exchange between group members (which is both conscious and unconscious).
- *Mirroring.* Group members are able to see aspects of themselves by *observing* others in the group. They also experience how they are *seen* by others. The multiple reflections in the group show different, and sometimes contradictory, aspects of the patient. Just as it takes two mirrors to see the back of one's head, a group is able to show aspects of the patient that are not easily seen in a dyadic relationship (such as rivalry, jealousy or voyeurism).
- *Resonance.* One of the reasons why we receive different mirroring experiences from group members is because the inner reactions to things that are said are different for each person. There are also whole group resonances that amplify the intensity of emotions and create a sense of shared experience within the group.
- *Location.* Sometimes a problem can appear to belong to one group member. The group therapist, however, is always thinking about the 'total situation'. For example, if a patient is anxious about the arrival of a new group member, we might wonder why this particular patient is expressing this feeling and whether it is shared by others in the group.
- *Condenser phenomena.* These occur when personal exchange and collective resonances lead to intense, shared emotional experiences in the group.

Not everything that happens in a group, however, is therapeutic. Nitsun described the destructive processes that can occur in groups which he referred to as 'the anti-group'.[10] A common anti-group phenomenon is *malignant mirroring*[11] in which two group members accuse each other of having the undesirable aspects of themselves that they have disowned.

Levels of communication in a group

Group analysts think about communication taking place, often simultaneously, at different levels within the group:

- *The current level* refers to the here and now of what is happening in the group. This communication is conscious and available to everyone in the group.
- *The transference level* refers to how communication reflects patients' formative relationships in the past, especially with parents and siblings.
- *The projective level* refers to aspects of the patient which are 'split off' and denied by the patient but which are then experienced as if these belonged to the therapist or other group members.
- *The primordial level* refers to our common biological and cultural inheritance as human beings. Deep and resonant conversations about fundamental aspects of our existence, such as birth and death, might be said to be at this level.

What is therapeutic about groups?

> Foulkes described the therapeutic task of groups as *'working towards an ever more articulate form of Communication'*[3] (p.169).

This means developing the capacity to talk about one's difficulties and to listen to others. This statement implies that underneath all difficulties lies our psychological disconnection from other people. As a consequence of this disconnection, we develop ways of thinking and behaving that prevent us from being able to learn from our experiences in relationships.

In other words, it is the act of communication that forms our relationships with others and develops our sense of self. It is by communicating our experiences that they are no longer expressed as psychological symptoms. Through communication we are reconnected to other people. We are able to make use of relationships with other people to test our perceptions of reality, rather than protecting ourselves from perceived attack by withdrawing from closeness to others.

Yalom identified 11 therapeutic factors in groups.[12] These are:

1. instillation of hope;
2. universality;
3. imparting information;
4. altruism;
5. the corrective recapitulation of the early family group;
6. development of socializing techniques;
7. imitative behaviour;
8. interpersonal learning;
9. group cohesiveness;
10. catharsis;
11. existential factors.

One striking aspect of these factors is how frequently they occur outside therapy. In other words, ordinary, everyday life is therapeutic – it gives pleasure and companionship, and we get to learn from our mistakes and come to terms with difficulties with the support from other people. Group therapy can be seen as a way of helping people reconnect to the normal, therapeutic processes of living by learning to share the troubles that are intrinsic to our lives.

REFLECTION

Can you remember a time when you felt upset or distressed in the past? What was it that allowed you to move on from this experience? What role did others play in helping you?

SERVICE USER'S PERSPECTIVE

Learning to accept and live with my own flawed humanity, including the ugly and vulnerable bits, was enormously liberating.

THE CRAFT OF CARING AS A GROUP THERAPIST

> *Care (verb): Old English carian, cearian 'be anxious, grieve; to feel concern or interest,' from Proto-Germanic *karo- 'lament,' hence 'grief, care' (cognates: Old High German charon 'to lament,' Old Saxon karon 'to care, to sorrow'), from Proto-Germanic *karo (cognates: Old Saxon kara 'sorrow;' Old High German chara 'wail, lament;' Gothic kara 'sorrow, trouble, care'.*[13]

Running a group is a complex activity. In many ways it is a *skill* like any other that can be taught. In some respects it is a very practical activity – a room has to be found, dates agreed, letters sent. There is also a body of literature to advise on how to intervene in a group. There are, however, so many new, unpredicted situations that the new group therapist often feels overwhelmed. She has to speculate about what is happening in the group and use her judgement to decide the best way of responding. In this respect, running a group is like a *craft*. The group practitioner develops her own style of intervening based on the setting, the client group and her personal preferences. It is not unusual for group therapists to respond in very different ways to the same situation, depending upon their perception of what is happening and their understanding of the craft of running a group.[14]

What underlies the different ways people conduct their groups is the idea that the most important quality of the group therapist is *the capacity to tolerate emotions*. Sitting in a room with a group of people who are in distress can be difficult. In other words, *care* is at the heart of developing one's craft as a group therapist. It is not, however, care as the term is commonly used today (i.e. feelings of concern or affection). In the old Germanic roots of the word, care is linked to the raw emotions of sorrow, wailing and lamenting. Group analytic psychotherapists are required to have their own therapy in order to develop the capacity to sit in a group without being overwhelmed by the intensity of their own and others' feelings. Emotional distress is difficult to bear – for patients, for staff and for society at large. It can be tempting to 'switch off', to do things mechanistically or by the book; in other words, to respond without care. Implicit in the following discussion is the belief that the most important aspect of being a group therapist is the ability to remain emotionally engaged with patients as they reflect upon themselves and attempt to make changes in their lives.

DYNAMIC ADMINISTRATION

Dynamic administration[15] refers to the practical tasks the therapist must do to set up and maintain her group. It is called *dynamic* administration because it has a significant impact on the therapeutic experience of group members.

When starting a group, the therapist is confronted with an endless list of questions: What sort of group shall I run? Who will be group participants? How many people should I have in the group? Where shall it take place? How long should each session last? Shall I have a co-therapist? How will I get referrals to the group? Answering these questions takes time. Group therapists use the analogy of a group developing in the mind of the therapist in the way a baby grows inside the mother. Value is placed on this preparation period and it is seen as crucial for avoiding many of the pitfalls that can beset therapy groups.

Different types of groups

There are a number of different types of groups, each of which has its advantages and disadvantages. Some of these types are:

- *Closed groups.* The membership of these groups is fixed at the beginning. Group members are expected to start and end the programme of group sessions together. This type of group is most suitable for short-term groups and where group cohesion is important.
- *Open groups.* These groups allow new members to join and leave at planned-for intervals throughout the year. This type of group is suitable for longer-term therapies because a group culture develops that is passed on to new members of the group. It is also a helpful model for service user and support groups.
- *Drop-in groups.* These are an extreme form of an open group, where there is no formal assessment prior to coming to the group, and no expectation that people will make a commitment for a set period.
- *Structured groups.* The content of the group is planned in advance by the group therapist. This type of group might start with a check-in and include some skills teaching by the therapist.
- *Unstructured groups.* The group does not have a formal programme. The focus of the group is the conversations between participants, who choose what issues they wish to bring to the group.
- *Homogeneous groups.* These groups focus on a particular problem (e.g. an anxiety management group) or highlight cohesiveness by group members having shared characteristics (e.g. a women-only group).

- *Heterogeneous groups.* These groups make use of multiple perspectives and life experiences to help group members explore their difficulties (e.g. having a mixed-age/gender group helps people explore what happens in their family relationships).
- *Single therapist.* A single therapist in the group is common for conducting long-term psychotherapy groups, and is logistically straightforward.
- *Co-therapist.* A co-therapist approach is common for groups that are part of a wider therapeutic system (e.g. inpatient settings). They are often used to give workers an experience of running groups with senior colleagues.

> ### REFLECTION
>
> What types of group are there for patients in your setting? If you were to set up a new group, what sort of group might you choose?

Groups that focus on specific 'problems' are likely to be short-term, structured and closed, whereas groups that focus upon reflection and exploration are likely to be longer-term, open and unstructured. In reality, many group therapists choose elements of different types of groups. For example, groups for people with a diagnosis of personality disorder are likely to have a mixture of structured and unstructured elements in a programme that lasts for a whole day or more per week. (See chapter 57 on therapeutic communities.)

The setting of the group

It is impossible to overestimate the importance of the setting for the successful running of a group. Group therapists talk about the *organizational container* that supports the functioning of the group. Consistency is an important element of this. Meeting in the same room, on the same day and at the same time each week, provides a sense of continuity and safety. The group therapy room should be a neutral space, with chairs that are the same for all participants, in a room that is light and warm but well-ventilated.

It is helpful to think that *it takes a group to run a group.* Time spent talking to the receptionists, clarifying arrangements with the service manager, speaking to cleaners and security staff, as well as knowing what other activities are going on in the building at the same time as the group, all ensure that the therapy extends to the patient's whole experience of coming to attend the group.

Assessment for groups

The group therapist needs to have a clear idea of who the group is for (and who it is not for) in order for it to have a recognized purpose and appropriate participants. Most groups therefore have some form of assessment of potential patients prior to their joining the group.[16] An assessment has three aspects:

1. *Understanding the patient.* Group therapists typically start by asking about the patient's personal history and finding out about his current circumstances. The therapist develops a *formulation* in order to understand the patient's 'problem' in terms of the dynamics of his relationships.[17]
2. *Deciding whether the group is suitable for the patient.* The criteria for joining will vary according to the type of group. Motivation is often a key indicator in assessment (e.g. does the patient have clear goals and *realistic* expectations of how the group might help?). The group therapist also has to consider the overall composition of the group. A teenage girl in a group of middle-aged men is likely to feel inhibited. It is usually better to delay a patient joining until there is a better mix of participants, rather than having an *isolate* in the group who is significantly different from the other group members.
3. *Preparation for the group.* The patient needs help to think about what it will be like for him in the group. It is important to discuss previous experiences of groups and to anticipate difficulties that may arise in the therapy group. For an open-ended group, the patient needs to discuss how he will know when to leave therapy and what help he might need to manage the process of ending.

Assessments vary from a single meeting (for shorter-term groups) to three or more sessions (for longer-term groups). Assessing a number of people at the same time can help the

therapist see whether the patient can use the group format, and it also helps the patient make an informed choice about joining the group. Although there can be pressure to carry out only a perfunctory assessment, this can lead to problems later on in the group (see chapters 13 and 14 for more on the importance of assessment).

> ### CASE STUDY 2
>
> Jed, a man in his 40s, was adopted as a child. He came asking for group therapy because he was depressed after the recent breakdown of a relationship. He had five children from three previous relationships, with whom he had no contact. When asked about his experience of being in groups, he replied that he had been the captain of a football team. He said that after an argument with the manager he led his team off the pitch, and the team never played together again. During the assessment he came across as charming and willing to talk openly about himself. The therapist put him in her group. After a few months Jed announced that he was going on an extended tour of South America. When the therapist said that she would not be able to keep his place open, he became very angry and refused to come back to the group.

> ### REFLECTION
>
> Could Jed's early departure (see case study 2) have been anticipated? What might the therapist have done differently in the assessment meetings? Would you have offered Jed a place in your group?

THE THERAPIST'S STANCE IN THE GROUP

> Group analysis is *'a form of psychotherapy by the group, of the group, including its conductor'*[18] *(p.3).*

Conducting a group can be a bewildering experience. There is so much happening that it can seem impossible to make sense of it all. It is helpful to hold in mind the idea that the agent of therapeutic change is the experience of being in a group and the relationships between the group members, rather than the actions of the therapist.

The group therapist is like the host of a party. It is her responsibility to make sure that the group takes place in a predictable and consistent way, and that everyone feels able to participate. The group therapist protects the boundary

of the group – making sure there are no interruptions, acknowledging group members who arrive late and following up on those who are absent.

When the group is working well, the therapist is likely to be an unobtrusive figure. She employs 'the rule of abstinence'.[19] She holds back from immediately reassuring or providing answers to group members. This is different from being a blank screen or emotionally distant. The group therapist pays attention to what is happening in the group without feeling that this needs to be actively directed or controlled by the therapist. The therapist holds in mind the task of promoting 'ever more articulate communication'.[2] (See chapter 3 for further discussion of developing and maintaining therapeutic relationships.)

REFLECTION

What term should you use for your role in the group? There are many different terms, such as leader, conductor, nurse-therapist, facilitator. Each of these terms has implicit messages about your role and authority. The term you use for group members can influence the expectations of the group. Are your group members patients, clients or service users? The terms you choose may be very important for some people.

Working through

Sometimes patients say everything about their difficulties as quickly as possible. There can be a sense of catharsis from expressing strong feelings, but this needs to be combined with an *understanding* of these feelings. A sense of *insight* often comes about slowly. Freud spoke about '*working through*'[20] – meaning that an emotional problem needs to be revisited over and over again and worked with in different ways before it is felt to be resolved. A group patient referred to this process as like baking a loaf of bread, where the dough must be kneaded over and over again before it is capable of rising. We can think of the patient's symptoms being made more pliable and flexible as they are worked with in different ways each time by the group.

Working with the transference

People often repeat the drama of their early family group in therapy. The therapist can be experienced by the patient as

CASE STUDY 3

Peter, a recovering alcoholic, says he is angry because his son was attacked by a gang of youths, and the police are doing nothing about it. He tells the therapist that he drank a bottle of cough medicine before coming to the group to 'take the hard edge off things'. The therapist wonders if he wants to take the hard edge off his anger in the group. He replies that it is not fair to let his anger out on other people. Peter says his father was a cruel man who beat him as a child. The therapist wonders if Peter expected a fatherly response from her today in the group. He replies that he doesn't know what a fatherly response is … Karen says she went for a walk with her foster father last week. He was imprisoned for sexually abusing children and she refused to have contact with him for many years. She says that, although she still hates what he did, she is grateful that he gave her a family life as a child. Rebecca cries. She says that she wishes her father was alive so that she could speak to him.

if she is an uncaring parent, or other group members can appear as if they are a favoured sibling. It is common for patients at times to feel criticized, excluded or rejected by the group. The therapist helps patients reflect upon what is happening and the meaning this has for each person in the group. Sticking with and exploring these difficult feelings (while not denying the validity of the experience for the patient *in that moment*) is an essential part of therapy.

In case study 3, the therapist makes a link between events outside the group (the assault on Peter's son) and what is happening inside the group (Peter's fear of getting angry). She mentions the transference to her as a father figure. This helps Peter link his past (violence from his father) to what he is feeling in the present (wanting to 'take the hard edge off things'). Other group members *resonate* with this discussion. Karen describes the possibility for change in a relationship with an abusive father. This helps connect Rebecca to her feelings of loss for a father who was never emotionally available to her. The therapist holds back from focusing on Peter's presenting problem (being an alcoholic who has drunk a bottle of cough medicine) and instead helps him explore the *meaning* of his actions. Through group discussion, themes emerge about physical/sexual abuse, trust of authority and coming to terms with the past. Peter begins to feel less isolated with his difficulties, and using substances to manage his anger seems less necessary.

The difference between an experience that is transformative and one that is distressing is often one of perception. A group with a strong sense of cohesion and safety is better able to challenge its individual members. A successful group is therefore one that has a high level of safety and a high level of challenge. It is this contradiction that can make the conducting of a therapy group initially so perplexing. The group therapist learns to listen to the group, and to tolerate not knowing for long periods before deciding how to act. Keats used the term *negative capability* to refer to when a person 'is capable of being in uncertainties, mysteries, doubts, without any irritable reaching after fact and reason'[21] (p.277). It is only by helping the group members to remain with *the uncertainties, mysteries and doubts* that they are able to develop new ways of seeing themselves and their difficulties.

SERVICE USER'S PERSPECTIVE

The greatest challenge that I encountered was finding a place for myself in the group … During the first months, I had dreams of being plunged into (and often rescued from) the depths of thrilling and scary waters! The process of finding a place for myself reminded me of previous experiences of joining groups, and opened up to me swathes of unexamined patterns in the way I relate to myself and others.

COMMON DIFFICULTIES IN GROUPS

Patients are often referred to a group because of difficult experiences in their past that have affected their ability to have trusting and intimate relationships. We therefore should not be surprised that difficulties occur in groups. The purpose of a therapy group is not to avoid difficulties, but for group members, with the help of the therapist, to work out their own solutions – and to gain the sense of satisfaction and togetherness that comes from having survived these moments.

Some of the common difficulties that occur in groups, and possible responses, are listed below.

The group that does not thrive

A group starts with low numbers and has a couple of early dropouts. This leads to an anxious group where participants are afraid to make an emotional commitment. The group staggers along as a collection of individuals without a sense of itself as a group. Existing patients can be hostile to new members and undermine attempts for the therapist to grow and develop the group. Zelaskowski calls this *the suboptimal group*.[22]

Response: Often it is better to delay a group rather than start with low numbers. Introducing new members can feel unsettling for a group, but that must be done sooner rather than later when numbers are very low. Supervision can help the therapist stick with the group and slowly build up a group culture.

Dropouts

Sometimes people abruptly leave group therapy. Such 'dropouts' can be a consequence of conflict and rivalry between group members. Patients can also have a 'flight into health', and leave the group prematurely, asserting that they no longer need therapy.

Response: It is helpful to discuss with patients what they might find difficult in the group during the assessment meetings. A group therapist learns to monitor group members who appear disengaged or dissatisfied, and encourages them to talk. Over time, group members spontaneously take over this role of checking out how each other are feeling.

Having only one 'patient' in the group

It is a strange that group members – having expended much time and effort to come to the group – often act as if they do not need to be there. Into this situation often steps one group member, who will mention a difficulty he is having. At this point the attention of everyone is focused solely upon him. Sometimes there is a succession of 'presentations' by patients who, one by one, speak without interruption. It is as if the group has decided that each person will take turns to have individual therapy in the group.

Response: A group is not therapeutic when there is no genuine exchange or sharing taking place. The group therapist might share her curiosity about the 'here and now' experience of being in the group rather than the content of the individual presentations. It is helpful to remind oneself that one's role is to promote a culture of curiosity and exploration, rather than to be the expert who solves the problems brought by patients to the group.

The difficult group member

Groups can have a person who is not liked by other members of the group. This person often talks more than other group members, offers advice, makes judgements and generally irritates people. The person is sometimes oblivious to the tension that is building up in the group and is in danger of being scapegoated.

Response: We might wonder what this person is expressing for the group as a whole. What *transference* drama might be being played out in the group? For example, is he unconsciously expecting to be rejected by the group? It can sometimes be helpful to find reasons to praise the difficult group member (e.g. for how active he is in the group). This paradoxical intervention can prevent him becoming isolated, and re-frame the difficulty as belonging to the group. There are occasions, however, when the group is not the right place for someone. The group member may need to be helped to leave the group in a way that does not feel humiliating.

Competition and conflict

Conflict can feel scary and evoke fears that it will get out of hand, especially for people who experienced violence or abuse as a child. Sometimes a pair of group members get caught up in a mutually hostile relationship that echoes their early family relationships (cf. malignant mirroring[11]).

Response: Competition and conflict are essential parts of life and are crucial to the development of healthy relationships. Sometimes, however, the therapist has to intervene forcefully to stop conflict from escalating, and help patients reflect upon what might be happening in the group. It is helpful to remember that strong feelings are likely to be fuelled by experiences in the patients' past (i.e. transference reaction). It is the re-working of these relational conflicts that often brings about change for members of the group.

Turning a blind eye

Steiner[23] describes this dynamic of ignoring what is in plain sight. It is common for things to be known about but unspoken in therapy groups. This can be subtly destructive, echoing the dynamic of family secrets for patients. Turning a blind eye can be linked to fears of shame and exposure, and lead to a pseudo-solution of 'don't ask, don't tell' being employed by the group.

Response: Transformative moments often come when someone takes the risk of saying something which feels silly or exposing. This can open up communication in a group that has become stuck.

It is a truism that we often learn more from our failures than we do from our successes. It is the responses to 'mistakes' that allow group members to develop new ways of seeing their problems, and create new ways of responding to difficulties in life. Rather than avoid problems in groups, we might instead follow the advice of Samuel Beckett, who

---

CASE STUDY 4

In a psychotherapy group of 7 women with a male therapist, the issue of gender was not mentioned. When the therapist pointed out that he was a man amongst female patients, he felt that he had said something salacious and felt ashamed. Several of the women said they had thought about this, and spoke of not knowing what went on in the minds of their fathers who didn't play with them as children. One group member spoke teasingly of wanting to sit on the therapist's knee, while another said she expected all men to be sexually abusive and wanted to keep far away from the therapist. Later they spoke about competition amongst women when in the presence of men and how this often went unspoken. The small comment from the therapist helped group members explore their relationships to men and acknowledge the rivalry between the women in the group.

---

wrote, 'Ever tried. Ever failed. No matter. Try Again. Fail again. Fail better'[24] (p.7).

REFLECTION

What difficult experiences have you had in groups? What did you learn from these experiences?

GROUPS FOR STAFF

Since the Francis Report,[25] there has been an increased appreciation of the *emotional labour*[26] that is needed by staff in order to provide *compassionate caring*[27] for patients. There is a recognition that the craft of caring is not just an individual act but one that is dependent upon good management and engaged relationships between colleagues.

Tasks in health settings can evoke anxious feelings that are linked to death, illness, and the physical and emotional intimacy that is involved in caring for people. Menzies Lyth[28] found that organizations develop defences in a way similar to how individuals protect themselves. Work procedures can be organized in a way that turns the act of caring into a series of disconnected tasks. Taken to the extreme, workers can become more concerned with completing tasks (and achieving organizational targets) than responding to the needs of the patient. Ballat and Campling[29] argue that health workers need to develop 'Intelligent Kindness' in order to be emotionally engaged and reflective practitioners.

There are different types of *reflective practice groups* that are designed to help staff to work better in their roles. These groups can be used to air difficulties and concerns, and to reflect upon how colleagues are working together. The purpose of these groups is to develop better communication in the team, to encourage reflection on practice, and to improve patient care. These types of staff groups are common in settings where workers have to work closely in emotionally intense environments (such as in therapeutic communities and some forensic settings). There is evidence that the use of such groups improves the quality of care for patients.[30]

In many ways it is more difficult to run a group for staff than it is to run a group for patients. Members of staff have to work together every day and there can be fears that airing difficulties will make things worse. It is helpful to remember that the purpose of a staff group is to improve the quality of care for patients and that this requires improving communication and working relationships within teams.[31]

DEVELOPING AS A GROUP THERAPIST

The group therapist can feel isolated if she is the only person who is running a group in her team. The group therapist also needs a group – one of like-minded colleagues – that will support her development. There are three ingredients necessary to be a thriving group therapist.

1. Supervision

Groups evoke feelings in the therapist that need reflection and digestion. It is helpful to have an outsider perspective on what is happening in the group. Being part of a *supervision group* offers the possibility of seeing one's group through multiple lenses. A supervision group can sometimes reflect the dynamic that is occurring in the therapy group. This helps the group therapist to see the group in a new light through exploring this *parallel process* in the supervision group.[32] (See chapter 10 on the importance of clinical supervision and chapter 11 on critical reflection.)

2. Training

There is no substitute for specialist training in groupwork. Training typically combines learning about theory, the experience of being in a group, and supervision of conducting a group. More advanced training requires trainees to be a patient in a long-term psychotherapy group. The main training in the psychodynamic approach to running therapeutic groups is provided by the Institute of Group Analysis (IGA). It provides a network of 1-year foundation courses, as well as postgraduate and Master's level training in group psychotherapy.

3. A network

It is enjoyable to meet other group therapists to share one's achievements and failures. Many people establish informal networks with people who are also interested in groups. The Group Analytic Society (GAS) is a formal membership network for group therapists. It provides workshops and events in the UK and Europe, and is a forum for people from different professional backgrounds who are interested in groups. The Group Analytic Society also publishes the *Journal of Group Analysis*.

CONCLUSION

The beginning group therapist often starts by wanting to know the rules of how to run a group. Over time, she develops a sense of her own authority that comes from experience. It is the capacity to learn from experience that is the hallmark of group therapy. The therapist asks group members to suspend existing preconceptions about themselves, their problems and the world around them, and to explore new ways of being with others.

Once one begins to think seriously about groups, one's stance on all aspects of therapeutic intervention is likely to change. The group therapist becomes curious about all types of groups in her work life. Is a psychiatric ward a group with a culture that is therapeutic? Is the community

mental health team really a team, or a fragmented series of individuals? The group approach entices us always to look at the *total situation*, whether or not we are running a group for patients.

Ultimately, the psychodynamic approach to groups is not about learning a specific model or technique, but about developing in oneself – and in one's team – a 'culture of enquiry',[33] in which one is able to ask fresh and challenging questions about the best way of engaging and assisting patients to make changes in their lives. Hopefully this chapter will have whetted your appetite to find out more about groups and to explore how group therapy might help patients.

SERVICE USER COMMENTARY

Steve Delaney

I had been in individual therapy for 7 years before joining a therapy group as part of my group analysis training. The psychological challenge of relinquishing individual attention in a group made me feel uncomfortable, and continues to be a source of frustration even now. I've had to go on a journey to be able to recognize the social animal within me.

Thirty years earlier I had another experience of joining a group during my psychiatric nurse training. My overwhelming memory is of being welcomed into a rich community

of hospital staff and patients. I became part of the team, a member of the community, and this experience remains one of the happiest of my life.

Both of these experiences reflect the rewards and the challenges of being part of a group. In a small way I have been able to recognize this social part of me through my experiences of sharing, learning and receiving from others in a therapy group.

Just like other patients' experiences expressed in this chapter, I still feel frustration at never quite getting to the end of something in a group. I have learnt though that I can complain, acknowledge the various parts of myself, and slowly feel safe with my and other people's frustrations. I have learnt that being with others in this way allows me to connect with my own humanity. I thought this was beautifully articulated in this chapter by the patient who writes that 'learning to accept and live with my own flawed humanity, including the ugly and vulnerable bits, was enormously liberating'.

References

1. Bridger H. Northfield revisited. In: Pines M (ed.). *Bion and group psychotherapy* (International Library of Group Analysis). London: Jessica Kingsley, 2000: 87–113.
2. Foulkes SH. *Introduction to group analytic psychotherapy.* London: Heinemann; 1948 [repr. Karnac Books, 1983].
3. Foulkes SH. *Therapeutic group analysis.* London: George Allen & Unwin, 1964 [repr. Karnac Books, 1984].
4. Christakis NA, Fowler JH. *Connected: the amazing power of social networks and how they shape our lives.* London: HarperPress, 2010.
5. Bion WR. *Experiences in groups, and other papers.* London: Tavistock, 1961.
6. Garland C. Group-analysis: taking the non-problem seriously. *Group Analysis* 1982; **15**(1): 4–14.
7. Marrone M. Attachment theory and group analysis. In: Brown D, Zinkin L (eds). *The psyche and the social world: developments in group-analytic theory.* London: Jessica Kingsley, 2000: 146–62.
8. Karterud S. Constructing and mentalizing the matrix. *Group Analysis* 2011; **44**(4): 357–73.
9. Stacey RD. *Complexity and group processes: a radically social understanding of individuals.* New York: Brunner-Routledge, 2003.
10. Nitsun M. *The anti-group: destructive forces in the group and their creative potential.* London: Taylor & Francis, 1996.
11. Zinkin L. Malignant mirroring. *Group Analysis* 1983; **16**(2): 113–26.
12. Yalom ID. *Theory and practice of group psychotherapy,* 4th edn. New York: Basic Books, 1995.
13. Online Etymology Dictionary. Available from: http://www.etymonline.com/ [Accessed 3rd July 2016].
14. Kennard D, Winter D. *A workbook of group-analytic interventions* (International Library of Group Analysis). London: Jessica Kingsley, 2000.
15. Behr H, Hearst L. *Group analytic psychotherapy in practice: meeting of minds.* Oxford: Wiley-Blackwell, 2008: 42–54.
16. Knowles J. How I assess for group psychotherapy. In: Mace C (ed.). *The art and science of assessment in psychotherapy.* London: Routledge, 2003: 78–89.
17. Mace C, Binyon S. Teaching psychodynamic formulation to psychiatric trainees: part 1: basics of formulation. *Advances in Psychiatric Treatment* 2005; **11**(6): 416–23.
18. Foulkes SH. *Group analytic psychotherapy: method and principles* (Maresfield Library). London: Gordon and Breach, 1975.
19. Young R. The analytic frame, abstinence and acting out. *Human Nature Review* 2005. Available from: http://human-nature.com/rmyoung/papers/pap110h.html [Accessed 3rd July 2016].
20. Freud S. Remembering, repeating and working-through (Further recommendations on the technique of psycho-analysis II). In: *Standard edition of the complete psychological works of Sigmund Freud.* London: Hogarth Press, 1956–74: vol. 12, 146–56.
21. Keats J. *The complete poetical works and letters of John Keats,* Cambridge edition. Boston and New York: Houghton, Mifflin and Company, 1899.
22. Zelaskowski P. The suboptimal group. *Group Analysis* 1998; **31**(4): 491–504.
23. Steiner J. Turning a blind eye: the cover up for Oedipus. *International Review of Psychoanalysis* 1985; **12**: 161–72.
24. Beckett S. *Worstward ho.* New York: Grove Press, 1983.
25. Francis R. *Report of the Mid Staffordshire NHS Foundation Trust Public Inquiry.* London: The Stationery Office, 2013. Available from: http://webarchive.nationalarchives.gov.uk/20150407084003/http://www.midstaffspublicinquiry.com/sites/default/files/report/Executive%20summary.pdf [Accessed 2nd July 2016].
26. Gray B. The emotional labour in nursing 1: exploring the concept. *Nursing Times* 2009; **105**(8): 26–9.
27. Cummings J, Bennett V. Compassion in practice – nursing, midwifery and care staff – our vision and strategy. 2012. Available from: http://www.england.nhs.uk/nursingvision/compassion [Accessed 2nd July 2016].
28. Menzies Lyth I. *Containing anxiety in institutions.* London: Free Association of Books, 1992.
29. Ballat J, Campling P. *Intelligent kindness: reforming the culture of healthcare.* London: Royal College of Psychiatrists, 2011.
30. Goodrich J. Supporting hospital staff to provide compassionate care: do Schwartz Center Rounds work in English hospitals? *Journal of the Royal Society of Medicine* 2012; **105**(3): 117–22.
31. Hartley P, Kennard D (eds). *Staff support groups in the helping professions: principles, practice and pitfalls.* Hove: Routledge, 2009.
32. Plant R, Smith M. Countertransference and parallel process in supervision groups. *Journal of the British Association for Psychoanalytic and Psychodynamic Supervision* 2009; 15–18.
33. Griffiths P, Hinshelwood RD. Enquiring into a culture of enquiry. In: Day L, Pringle P (eds). *Reflective enquiry into therapeutic institutions* (Cassell Hospital Monograph Series). London: Karnac Books, 2001: 29–44.

Further reading

Barnes B, Ernst S, Hyde K. *An introduction to groupwork.* Basingstoke: Palgrave Macmillan, 1999.
Behr H, Hearst L. *Group analytic psychotherapy in practice – meeting of minds.* London: Whurr, 2005.

Hartley P, Kennard D (eds). *Staff support groups in the helping professions: principles, practice and pitfalls.* London: Routledge, 2009.
Yalom ID. *Theory and practice of group psychotherapy,* 4th edn. New York: Basic Books, 1995.

Relevant web pages

GAS (Group Analytic Society). http://groupanalyticsociety.co.uk/
This is a membership network for people who are interested in the psychodynamic approach to groups. They run workshops and conferences in the UK and in Europe.

IGA (Institute of Group Analysis). http://www.groupanalysis.org/
The IGA provides a range of trainings in groupwork (from introductory to Master's level). Courses are available throughout the UK.

Journal of Group Analysis. http://gaq.sagepub.com
This is a peer-reviewed journal about the theory and practice of running groups. It is published by Sage on behalf of the GAS.

44 Mindfulness

MARY E. CAMPBELL AND LAURA BURKE

LEARNING OUTCOMES

- To be able to define mindfulness.

- To understand the practice of sitting meditation.

- To know some different ways in which mindfulness has been incorporated into clinical practice.

- To understand how mindfulness relates to the craft of caring.

- To understand the ways in which mindfulness practice has been found to be of benefit for nurses.

- To understand the ways in which mindfulness has been found to be of benefit to people experiencing mental health issues.

- To be able to give an example of how mindfulness has been introduced to individuals with a psychotic illness.

- To know about the areas of the brain that are affected by mindfulness practice.

SUMMARY OF KEY POINTS

- Mindfulness-based interventions are effective in promoting health, reducing physical and psychological distress and improving quality of life for people in diverse settings with a wide range of medical and psychiatric conditions.

- Mindfulness is the natural capacity to be present with our experience as it is unfolding.

- Mindfulness is strengthened over time through mindfulness practice.

- Mindfulness has been integrated into therapeutic work as mindful presence in therapy, mindfulness-informed therapy and mindfulness-based therapy.

- Mindfulness practice strengthens the ability to be present in relationship with others. Presence provides the ground for caring, empathy and compassion and enables one to see more clearly what is actually happening in the here and now, increasing the likelihood of a skilful response.

- For nurses, mindfulness-based stress reduction (MBSR) has been found to increase relaxation, self-awareness and self-care, decrease stress and risk of burnout, increase empathy and self-compassion and increase confidence in being able to establish a caring orientation.

- The various mindfulness-based therapies teach a way of paying attention to present-moment experience that has significant potential for reducing distress and enhancing health and well-being.

- Mindfulness practice has been shown to affect brain function and structure.

- It is necessary to establish an ongoing mindfulness practice before teaching it to others.

INTRODUCTION

This chapter will provide an introduction to mindfulness and its rapidly growing place within psychiatry and mental health. Mindfulness-based interventions are being integrated into the treatment of a wide range of medical and psychiatric conditions, including cancer, chronic pain, depression, anxiety, substance abuse, eating disorders and personality disorders. Mindfulness meditation practice and mindfulness-based interventions are recognized as effective approaches to manage stress, reduce physical and psychological distress, promote health and improve quality of life. For the clinician and care provider, mindfulness has been found to reduce stress, increase compassion and reduce the risk of burnout.

WHAT IS MINDFULNESS?

Mindfulness is *being present* with our experience as it is unfolding: experiencing *what* we are doing *while* we are doing it – open to whatever thoughts, sensations and emotions arise in the immediacy of the present moment. Mindfulness is characterized by non-judgemental attention, awareness and a synchronization of body and mind. The capacity to be present in our life is quite natural, something that we all experience from time to time. For most of us, the experience of *mindlessness* is more familiar – moving quickly from one thing to the next without paying attention, held captive by thoughts and opinions, likes and dislikes, memories of the past and plans for the future; all the while missing the experience of what is happening in the *here and now*.

The word mindfulness also refers to mindfulness meditation, the practice of cultivating mindfulness. While mindfulness is intrinsic and we are all mindful to varying degrees, through practice, this natural capacity is strengthened. Mindfulness is not an idea or concept that we can decide to enact, as in 'I am going to be mindful'. While it is helpful to set such an intention, mindfulness is a way of being that takes practice. The Tibetan Buddhist teacher Sakyong Mipham notes that, while there is general agreement on the importance of training and caring for the body through exercise and diet, there is little attention to training and caring for the mind. Mindfulness meditation practice is a way to develop the intrinsic strength, stability and clarity of the mind and the ability to be present.[1]

The present moment has a particular potency, a kind of magic – the power to simply *be* with whatever is going on: the magic of connecting with reality. Life unfolds in moments. Each moment has tremendous vividness and depth, and holds the resources to skilfully meet whatever is occurring in experience. As described by Jon Kabat-Zinn, founder of mindfulness-based stress reduction, paying attention to experience from moment to moment 'leads directly to new ways of seeing and being in your life because the present moment, whenever it is recognized and honoured, reveals a very special, indeed magical power: it is the only time that any of us ever has'[2] (p.29).

The teachings on mindfulness originate in Eastern contemplative traditions, particularly Buddhism. However, mindfulness does not belong to a particular religion or culture; it is universal. Within the contemplative traditions, mindfulness is understood to include an atmosphere or attitude of respect and caring for the mind. Mindfulness meditation practice is a way to deepen one's experience of being human, to care for the mind and to strengthen our innate human capacity for awareness, insight, compassion and skilful action.

MINDFULNESS PRACTICE

Mindfulness is 'paying attention in a particular way: on purpose in the present moment, and nonjudgmentally'[3] (p.4). The practice of mindfulness includes formal and informal approaches. Formal practice involves setting aside a time to practise, placing attention on a particular activity such as *breathing* or *walking*, being present to whatever thoughts, sensations or emotions arise, noticing when the mind wanders and gently returning to the object of attention. Informal practice involves bringing moment-to-moment non-judgemental awareness to ordinary daily activities such as eating, washing dishes, showering and brushing teeth. The aim of mindfulness practice is to bring gentle awareness to whatever arises in one's experience, without judging or trying to change it.

If you would like to try to practise mindfulness, the following instructions will get you started. The instruction presented here is a sitting meditation practice that includes both mindfulness and awareness. It is typically done in a seated position, either cross-legged on a firm cushion on the floor or in a straight-backed chair. When sitting in a chair, if possible, sit away from the back of the chair and place the feet firmly on the ground with the legs uncrossed.

- The posture is relaxed and alert, uplifted and dignified.
- Hands gently rest on the thighs, palms down.
- Eyes are open; the gaze is soft, directed slightly downward, resting on the floor, four to six feet in front of you.
- Mouth is slightly open and the jaw is relaxed.
- Begin by settling into the body, *feeling* your present moment experience – sense perceptions, bodily sensations, emotional tone. Bring kind attention to whatever you feel, moment to moment, without trying to change anything; just notice.
- Feel the movement of the body with the breath. Bring your awareness to the breathing. Actually *feel* the body breathing in the present and let your attention rest there.
- Thoughts will arise; the mind will wander. When you notice that you have been lost in thought, gently return to feeling the body breathing.
- It does not matter how often the mind wanders. When you notice, gently return to the breathing.
- Continue this practice for 10 minutes.

REFLECTION

- Practice mindfulness using these instructions.
- What was your experience?
- What did you notice?

When people begin to practise mindfulness, they are usually surprised to discover how *busy* the mind is: like a waterfall, one thought tumbling after the next. It may seem difficult to find the breath in the midst of all that mental activity. One may be inclined to try to push thoughts away in an effort to create a sense of relaxation, or to use the breath to separate from unwanted, distressing thoughts and feelings. Trying to push thoughts away or change one's experience serves only to set up an atmosphere of struggle and will ultimately increase distress.

> When people first sit down with themselves, I think it is common for them to experience a lot of self-directed aggression. So much comes up. It is important to not to have the expectation that it won't be there. It is important to find ways to be gentle. The magnitude of that self-directed aggression and that pushing from all sides to change and get better and not to be where you are is really huge. It can easily bleed into mindfulness practice – to sit down and be like 'Okay, now I've got to be peaceful, I've got to be calm.'
>
> *Laura Burke*

Mindfulness practice is *not* about struggle. Rather it is a way to extend kindness and accommodation to whatever is arising, even if it is uncomfortable. This involves feeling the busy mind, the sense of restlessness one may experience in attempting to be still and the unwanted or distressing thoughts and emotions. The practice is to simply feel all of it without judging or trying to change anything.

Mindfulness practice includes precision and gentleness: the precision of noticing what is happening, the waterfall of thought; the gentleness of bringing kind attention and being non-judgemental, not rejecting the busy mind. Over time, recognizing and releasing thoughts, gently returning to the feeling of the body breathing, the waterfall of thoughts does settle, becoming more like a river and eventually a lake, as the mind gradually relaxes into itself.

Dropping the struggle of trying to have things be other than they are gives rise to a sense of relaxation and ease. Mindfulness does not eliminate thoughts and emotions. Thoughts are seen *as thoughts* and the ability to recognize thoughts *as thoughts* frees one from the distorted sense of reality thoughts can create. One is able to step back and be less identified with thoughts and emotions. In this way, it becomes possible to experience a state of mind that includes, but is not conditioned by, thought.

MINDFULNESS AND MENTAL HEALTH

It probably comes as no surprise that a practice which helps one recognize thoughts as thoughts, and strengthens innate human capacities for awareness, insight, compassion and skilful action, has found its way into mental health. Mindfulness has been integrated into therapeutic work in various ways: mindful presence in therapy, mindfulness-informed therapy and mindfulness-based therapy.[4] In mindful *presence*, the clinician or caregiver who practises mindfulness cultivates a more mindful presence that serves to strengthen the therapeutic relationship. (More information on developing and maintaining therapeutic relationships can be found in chapter 3.)

Mindfulness-*informed* therapy is informed by insight and understanding derived from mindfulness practice and Buddhist psychology, while mindfulness-*based* therapy incorporates traditional mindfulness practices into the treatment itself. These categories are not mutually exclusive.

Mindfulness itself is *not* therapy; it is an unconditional way of *being*. From a contemplative perspective, human beings have basic sanity or intrinsic health.[5] Mindfulness practice is a way to develop unconditional friendliness toward oneself and, through that, connect with intrinsic healthiness.

Mindfulness is characterized by a kind, caring attention. When we care about something, we very naturally become interested and pay attention. This is why it is so important to enter the practice with gentleness, simply *feeling* one's present-moment experience, whatever that may be, and extending kind attention to whatever arises, as one might do for a loved one or a dear friend.

Mindfulness is a *not* a relaxation technique. Relaxation techniques attempt to control the physical symptoms of stress and anxiety. In bringing attention to whatever is happening in the present moment, mindfulness practice *may* initially increase discomfort by reducing distraction. The relaxation that develops through mindfulness does so over time, as a result of dropping attempts to control or manipulate one's experience and developing friendliness toward oneself based on genuine self-acceptance.

> For the consumer, there is so much shame in being given a psychiatric label. It's often a traumatic experience. Mindfulness can help loosen the fixation on the naturally drawn conclusion that one's life is over, a conclusion often propagated by the psychiatric system. Mindfulness mediates the focus on change, change without validation, without the acceptance piece, without the being with what is. To experience a transformative recovery-oriented process, one has to be able to be in the moment with what is. This is where the non-striving and non-judgemental aspects of mindfulness are very helpful and can serve to support and improve recovery.
>
> *Laura Burke*

Mindful presence and the craft of caring

Mindful presence refers to the way in which a personal mindfulness practice enhances the clinician's or caregiver's capacity to be present and to bring a more mindful presence to their work, strengthening the therapeutic relationship, the most potent predictor of a positive treatment outcome. A practice that enhances the ability to be present and cultivates compassion has enormous potential to improve care.

Psychiatric mental health nursing is an interpersonal process grounded in a professional caring relationship for the purpose of promoting health and forward movement of the person in the direction of creative and productive, personal and community living.[6] Nurses attend to the concerns of individual patients and families in particular situations, focusing on the *human response* to actual or potential health problems,[7] the experience of *illness* rather than the *disease process*.

Caring is central to nursing. Caring practices are shaped through engagement with others and learning together what is helpful. Effective caregiving requires more than skill and knowledge; it requires that the caregiver be in relationship with the person(s) receiving care in ways that foster mutuality, empowerment and growth.[8] This calls for presence, openness and self-awareness on the part of the nurse.

A fundamental aspect of presence is to simply be there, physically present for the other person. Once there, to be open and available with the fullness of one's being – willing to listen, willing to be there in the face of the uncertainty and distress associated with illness. It is not easy to be present in this way.

> Being present is really important. Being present with another human being draws them out. That sense of verbally and energetically feeling acknowledged – the way someone talks to you and listens.
>
> *Laura Burke*

To be present in relationship with others, one must first have the ability to be present with oneself. Mindfulness is a practice of being present with oneself. It brings greater self-awareness and strengthens the ability to be present in situations without getting caught up in thoughts or emotional reactions. This kind of presence provides the ground for caring and compassion. One can see more clearly what is actually happening in the here and now, increasing the likelihood of a skilful response.

REFLECTION

- Describe an experience of having someone offer you this kind of presence.

- Describe an experience when you were able to be present for another person in this way.

- In the clinical setting, what are the challenges to being present in this way?

- How might you work with these challenges?

The potential negative impact of stress, the risk of burnout and the need to attend to self-care are important issues for nurses. Mindfulness practice has demonstrated efficacy in reducing the risk of burnout in various health care disciplines including nursing.[9,10] Studies on the effects of mindfulness-based stress reduction (MBSR) with nurses have demonstrated the following positive outcomes: increased relaxation, self-awareness and self-care,[11] decreased symptoms of stress and burnout,[12–14] improvement in overall general health, increased empathy and self-compassion[13] and increased confidence in being able to establish a caring orientation.[12] Nurses identified the ability to be more fully present and less reactive in relationships as one of the benefits of mindfulness practice.[11] This has particular relevance to inpatient psychiatric treatment settings where the presence and availability of staff has been associated with a reduced incidence of aggression and violence.[15]

Mindfulness-informed therapy

Mindfulness-informed therapy is informed by insights derived from mindfulness practice and Buddhist psychology. *Morita therapy* and *the Windhorse Program for Recovery* are examples of treatment approaches informed by mindfulness practice and Buddhist psychology.

MORITA THERAPY

Morita therapy,[16] developed by Dr Shoma Morita, is a psychotherapy in which emotions such as anxiety and fear are understood as a natural phenomenon of the human psyche. Neurosis is understood to result from the secondary meanings attached to these emotional reactions rather than the emotions themselves.

Morita viewed his therapy as a combination of rest therapy and discipline therapy. The treatment occurs over 4 weeks: week 1 – bed rest; week 2 – light work period; week 3 – heavy work period; week 4 – training for practical living. The therapy directs one's attention receptively to what reality brings in each moment. For example, during the period of rest, the person is encouraged to accept whatever feelings and thoughts bubble into his or her awareness. In doing so, the person learns experientially that the waves of thought and emotion come and go. With successful treatment, the person learns to accept the internal fluctuations of thoughts and feelings and to ground his or her behaviour in reality and the purpose of the moment.

Morita therapy has been used to treat individuals with depression, anxiety disorders,[16] borderline personality disorder, alcohol dependence, childhood neurosis and schizophrenia.[17,18] It has also been applied to self-help activities and 'meaningful life therapy', an approach used with cancer patients.[17]

THE WINDHORSE PROGRAM FOR RECOVERY

The Windhorse Program for Recovery[19] provides individualized comprehensive home-based whole-person treatment for people experiencing extreme psychiatric distress. Developed by Edward Podvoll and colleagues,[20] the Windhorse Program draws from Buddhist psychology, particularly Vajrayana Buddhism as taught by the Tibetan meditation master Chögyam Trungpa. Windhorse is the energy of basic sanity or intrinsic health, a self-existing energy that can radiate tremendous strength and healthiness in one's life.

The Windhorse Program holds the view that significant recovery is possible for anyone experiencing psychosis. The mind, even when most disturbed, has what Podvoll calls 'islands of clarity'[20] (p.5) when there is a sudden shift in awareness that discriminates between dream and reality. Even in the wildest mind, moments of recovery are happening all the time and need encouragement and protection. Recovery depends on an atmosphere of simplicity, warmth and dignity. This is accomplished through creating a healing environment in the person's home.

A windhorse team has three primary components: a therapeutic household with live-in housemate(s), several therapists providing basic attendance, and individual psychotherapy provided by a principal therapist. The person spends several hours each day with housemate(s) sharing domestic activities. Basic attendance is provided in 3-hour shifts by a team of therapists who have trained in the practice of mindfulness awareness meditation.

Basic attendance is a way of being present that allows the other person to be present. It is paying attention to the entire situation and what the person needs to recover, doing whatever is called for – taking a walk, helping the person tidy his or her room, doing the laundry – all the while recognizing and appreciating the windows of opportunity provided by 'islands of clarity'. Basic attendance can occur in any setting – the kitchen, the laundromat, the grocery store. The activities become important practices for the person in relating calmly and accurately to his or her mind and developing stability of mind. For example, playing basketball becomes a way to bring the mind back to the present moment. The practice of basic attendance involves 'genuine nursing of the mind'[20] (p.264) and calls for a willingness to be open to learning from the person in care. It is being present in such a way that one's presence does not crowd, overpower or impose on the situation. Attending in this way supports the person and creates the necessary environment for recovery, an environment within which 'islands of clarity begin to gather and flourish'[20] (p.253).

REFLECTION

- How do you experience the mental health treatment settings in which you provide care?

- Consider the interpersonal and physical environment. In what ways do you notice the simplicity, warmth and dignity that is characteristic of a healing environment?

- Recall a recent interaction with a person experiencing an extreme state of mind.

- Were you able to notice 'islands of clarity' or moments of recovery?

- If so, describe that experience.

- If not, pay close attention the next time you have the opportunity.

Mindfulness-based therapy

Mindfulness-based therapy incorporates traditional mindfulness practices into the treatment itself. An expanding body of evidence supports mindfulness-based approaches in the treatment of a variety of psychiatric and physical problems.[21–24] Examples of these approaches include *mindfulness-based stress reduction* (MBSR),[2] *mindfulness-based cognitive therapy* (MBCT),[25] *dialectical behaviour therapy* (DBT)[26] and *acceptance and commitment therapy* (ACT).[27] Mindfulness approaches have also been adapted for people with anxiety disorders and post-traumatic stress disorder[28] and the treatment of psychosis.[29]

MINDFULNESS-BASED STRESS REDUCTION

MBSR[2] was developed by Jon Kabat-Zinn as a complement to medical treatment, to help people with chronic health problems work with the stress, pain and suffering associated with illness. MBSR is provided in a group format and includes education about stress and coping strategies in addition to mindfulness practice and awareness exercises. Formal and informal mindfulness practices are taught as a way to support awareness, insight, relaxation and behaviour change.

The formal mindfulness practices taught in MBSR include:

1. *the body scan* – mindfulness of body sensations while moving attention through the body in a sequential fashion, done lying down with eyes closed;
2. *sitting meditation* – attention is placed on the breath while sitting quietly in an upright, dignified and relaxed posture;
3. *walking meditation* – attention is placed on the physical sensation of walking;
4. *yoga* – mindfulness of body sensations during gentle movements, stretches and while holding a posture.

Informal mindfulness practice involves bringing moment-to-moment awareness to activities of daily living. For example, you can practise mindfulness while eating, brushing your teeth, doing laundry, working in the garden, walking the dog, doing the dishes or any of the many activities of daily life. The practice is to bring the fullness of attention to the activity at hand and when you notice that the mind has wandered (which it will), gently bring your attention back to the activity.

An example of an MBSR awareness exercise is the pleasant events calendar, in which participants are asked to bring awareness to one pleasant event each day while it is happening and later reflect on the event using a series of questions provided, for example, 'What mood, feelings, and thoughts accompanied this event at the time?'

Since its beginnings in 1979, over 20,000 people have completed MBSR training in the Stress Reduction Clinic at the University of Massachusetts. There are more than 250 MBSR programmes in a variety of settings around the world – hospitals, clinics, mental health settings, correctional facilities, schools, workplaces and corporate offices. MBSR has traditionally included participants with a wide range of health-related issues, rather than grouping participants according to diagnosis. It has also been used with specific populations, such as individuals with a diagnosis of cancer or a mental illness and groups of health care providers.

There is consistent evidence supporting the positive benefits of MBSR for a number of physical and psychological problems such as symptoms of anxiety and depression,[21,22,24] chronic pain,[22,24] fibromyalgia,[30] psoriasis,[31] multiple sclerosis[30] and cancer.[32] MBSR also improves general mental health and psychological functioning and is beneficial for healthy individuals and health care providers.[9]

MINDFULNESS-BASED COGNITIVE THERAPY

MBCT[25,33] is an adaptation of MBSR developed by Segal, Williams and Teasdale to prevent reoccurrence of major depression. Evidence supports the efficacy of MBCT in unipolar depression relapse prevention, residual depression and treatment-resistant depression.[21,22,34] Compared to maintenance antidepressant, the current treatment of choice, MBCT is equivalent in terms of relapse rate and superior in terms of quality of life and residual symptoms. MBCT is recommended in the UK National Institute for Health and Care Excellence (NICE) guidelines as an effective treatment for prevention of relapse.[35] The American Psychiatric Association's *Practice guideline for the treatment of patients with major depressive disorder* includes MBCT as a group intervention.[36] MBCT has also been found effective in bipolar disorder, generalized anxiety disorder, panic disorder and social phobia.[21,22]

MBCT combines mindfulness practice with traditional cognitive therapy strategies and education about depression. Individuals who have experienced an episode of major depression are at high risk of relapse and the risk increases with each episode. In previously depressed individuals, ordinary sad moods are likely to reactivate depressive thought content and ruminative thinking leading to a reoccurrence of depression. MBCT is a group intervention that provides training in how to disengage from depressive and ruminative thinking, reducing the risk of relapse for individuals with a prior history of major depression.

We all have a tendency to believe our thoughts. For those who have been depressed, the tendency to believe negative thoughts can be quite strong, particularly in moments of sadness. In mindfulness practice, one begins to see thoughts and emotions as mental events that come and go rather than some kind of truth or accurate reflection of reality. MBCT includes teaching on the role of pleasure and mastery activities in lifting one's mood and the development of an individualized relapse prevention action plan.

Mindfulness has also been associated with more fulfilling interpersonal relationships. Given the role of interpersonal factors in chronic depression, improved relationships may play an important role in relapse prevention. 'Relating mindfully',[37] the core construct identified in a qualitative study on MBCT, describes a change process that moves from increased understanding of self and other to a range of changes in relationships. In the words of one of the participants, 'mindfulness is a physicality first, then you're changing the relationship to thoughts and improving mental well-being, then these internal changes lead to eternal/relational changes'[37] (p.57).

MBCT introduces a mini-meditation, 'the 3-minute breathing space',[33] to provide a bridge between formal mindfulness practice and daily life. The 3-minute breathing space, a way to open to the present moment on the spot, is useful in working with challenging situations as they arise. This mini-meditation can be done with the eyes closed and has three steps: becoming aware, gathering and expanding. To do this practice, take an upright posture and bring awareness to your inner experience – thoughts, feelings and bodily sensations.

1. Ask the question 'What is my experience right now?' This is step 1, 'becoming aware', stepping out of automatic pilot and opening to the present moment.
2. 'Gathering' involves bringing your attention to the sensation of breathing, noticing each in-breath and out-breath as it occurs.
3. Next, expand awareness to include a sense of the body as a whole, including any sensations, allowing for a sense of spacious awareness.

Participants are asked to practise this mini-meditation three times per day, gradually using it as needed to work with challenging life situations.

REFLECTION

- Try the mini-meditation three times over the next day.
- Try it when feeling stressed.
- What was your experience?

DIALECTAL BEHAVIOUR THERAPY

DBT[26] is a cognitive behavioural treatment that was developed by Marsha Linehan to treat chronically suicidal individuals with borderline personality disorder (BPD). It was the first psychotherapy to incorporate mindfulness as a core component. DBT includes four sets of behavioural skills: mindfulness, distress tolerance, interpersonal effectiveness and emotional regulation. The central dialectic in DBT is the relationship between acceptance and change. DBT combines cognitive behavioural

interventions designed to help clients change thoughts, behaviour and emotions with mindfulness skills that are taught within the context of synthesizing acceptance and change. Mindfulness 'what' skills specify what one does when being mindful – observing, describing and participating. Mindfulness 'how' skills are how one does it – non-judgementally, one-mindfully and effectively. DBT does not prescribe specific mindfulness exercises or the frequency and duration of mindfulness practice. However, all team meetings and treatment groups begin with some form of mindfulness practice. Mindfulness has been found to be a strong predictor of the emotional well-being experienced by women diagnosed with BPD who are engaged in DBT.[38] Evidence now supports the use of DBT for substance abuse/dependence, eating disorders, post-traumatic stress disorder and depression.[39]

Mindfulness and psychosis

Mindfulness-based approaches such as MBSR have been successfully adapted for persons with psychosis and schizophrenia with positive results.[40–42] Adjustments to the standard approach include a therapeutic rather than class context, fewer participants per group, shorter periods of meditation practice (10 minutes) with less silence and more guidance during meditation periods. Guidance needs to include specific reference to the psychotic sensations (voices, thoughts and images) in a normalizing way, as sensations that arise and pass.

> I have found that shorter periods of meditation with more guidance works for me, particularly when I'm feeling like I'm more on the edge of something.
>
> *Laura Burke*

In one such mindfulness group programme for people with distressing psychosis, the following three-stage process of relating differently to psychosis emerged from participant descriptions: centring in awareness of psychosis; allowing voices, thoughts and images to come and go without reacting or struggle; and reclaiming power through acceptance of psychosis and the self.[41] In the words of several participants: 'It's like you have to unlearn your responses to these thoughts and feelings … not being tied to fighting with them and struggling with them'[41] (p.82). '[You are] aware of your breathing and that in turn makes you aware of your body and it relaxes'[41] (p.83). 'Voices can come and go as they please. Don't get distressed, just allow it to go away … you don't lose your mind to them'[41] (pp.83–4). 'You know this big thing that comes in with lots of bluster … You know it's just a load of hot air and bluster'[41] (p.84).

> One thing mindfulness can do is it can allow you to make friends with your mind again, especially after psychosis. It's like you're taught not to trust your mind which is not helpful, obviously. So it's really a process of making friends with it again.
>
> *Laura Burke*

Participants in an MBSR programme adapted for persons with a diagnosis of schizophrenia[42] reported that mindfulness practice helped them to recognize and stop negative thought patterns, become less withdrawn and isolated, feel more relaxed and less frustrated, accept the good and bad aspects of themselves and gain a better understanding of self and control of impulsive behaviour. For example, one participant described mindfulness as a way of grounding and a way to keep a sense of humour when things went wrong instead of becoming upset and unable to problem-solve effectively. There was no increase in psychotic symptoms reported by the participants or their primary clinicians.

> It's very painful sometimes to sit down with yourself when you're having a really chaotic or difficult time. When I actually sit down with it, I'm like 'Ugh'. I hate to practise sometimes, but I do it. It feels important not to have the expectation that it's going to be peaceful, that it's going to be anything other than what it is. In the long run, I feel like there's a flexibility and a resilience that builds. There's a sense of being able to work with anything that comes up so I don't get mired in it as much.
>
> I think one of the biggest parts of my recovery was creating a space where I could let go of expectation and let go of striving.
>
> *Laura Burke*

Singh and colleagues[43] introduced a simple mindfulness technique, 'meditation on the soles of the feet', to three men with psychotic illness whose aggressive behaviour had prevented successful placement in the community. All had been treated with various psychotropic medications and were currently taking medication. Prior attempts at behavioural treatment for physical and verbal aggression had not been effective. They had each been discharged to the community several times and were readmitted within weeks of discharge because of aggressive behaviour.

Meditation on the soles of the feet is a mindfulness technique that had been used successfully by a young man with mental illness and mild mental retardation to manage aggression.[44] In this technique, attention is directed from an emotionally charged thought or situation to a neutral part of the body, the soles of the feet. The participants received individual instruction in focusing on the soles of the feet while sitting, standing or walking slowly and while imagining a situation that had previously provoked an aggressive response. The participants were required to practise the mindfulness technique at least twice a day and when an incident occurred that might provoke aggressive behaviour. With this mindfulness practice, incidents of verbal and physical aggression decreased and all three were successfully placed in the community. During the 4 years of follow-up post-discharge, there was no evidence of physical aggression and verbal aggression was minimal.

Mindfulness and acute care

Mindfulness practices such as the body scan, sitting meditation and yoga are being introduced on inpatient psychiatric units for patients[45,46] and staff.[15] Early evidence indicates that these practices can be learned and practised by individuals experiencing acute psychiatric symptoms with positive results. In one small study,[45] participants in a weekly mindfulness group reported changes in the relationship to thought, increased ability to focus, a sense of peace and relaxation, a willingness to 'sit with' and observe difficult feelings and increased awareness of the present. Brady and colleagues[15] found that the reduction in stress levels and increase in intrapersonal presence experienced by acute care staff participating in a 4-week MBSR programme was associated with an increase in patient satisfaction and a decrease in patient safety events over the 3 months following the staff MBSR programme. Here we see the potential for mindfulness not only to benefit individual patients and staff members, but also to impact the treatment environment, contributing to a culture of safety.

MINDFULNESS AND THE BRAIN

There is now a growing body of evidence that mindfulness meditation has an impact on brain function and structure.[21,22,47] Changes in neurophysiology include brain regions implicated in the neurobiology of mood disorders, anxiety and pain, such as those associated with attention, awareness, self-referential thinking, emotional processing and regulation, executive behaviour control, cognitive function and pain response. Mindfulness is also associated with changes in anatomical structure in several brain regions.[48] For example, experienced meditators were found to have thickening in cortical regions associated with attention and sensory processing. The differences in prefrontal cortical thickness between meditators and non-meditators were most significant in older participants, suggesting that a regular meditation practice may offer protection from age-related neural degeneration.

TEACHING MINDFULNESS

The quality of teaching is an important factor associated with the positive outcomes in mindfulness-based interventions.[49] Mindfulness is a profoundly different approach to working with distressing thoughts and feelings in that it is a practice of being present with whatever is arising, without judging or trying to change things. To teach mindfulness, one must be able to embody the mindful approach that learners are being asked to adopt. This embodiment requires a personal mindfulness practice and a continual exploration of one's own experience through the lens of mindfulness.

SUMMARY

Mindfulness is a very natural, though underdeveloped capacity of mind that is strengthened through mindfulness practice. It is an unconditional way of being, a non-judgemental openness to present moment experience. The ability to be present with whatever is arising moment-to-moment provides a good foundation for caring relationships, beginning with oneself and extending to others. There is a rapidly growing body of evidence that supports mindfulness practices and mindfulness-based interventions as effective approaches to manage stress, reduce physical and psychological distress, and promote health and well-being in clinical and non-clinical populations. For the healthcare provider, mindfulness practice strengthens compassion, offers protection against burnout and has the potential to positively impact treatment environments. Current research is exploring the effects of mindfulness on brain function and structure with promising results. For those wishing to teach mindfulness, the importance of an ongoing personal mindfulness practice cannot be overemphasized.

References

1. Mipham S. *Turning the mind into an ally.* New York: Riverhead, 2003.
2. Kabat-Zinn J. *Full catastrophe living: using the wisdom of your body and mind to face stress, pain, and illness.* New York: Delacorte, 1990.
3. Kabat-Zinn J. *Wherever you go there you are: mindfulness meditation in everyday life.* New York: Hyperion, 1995.
4. Germer C. Mindfulness: what is it? What does it matter? In: Germer C, Siegel R, Fulton R (eds). *Mindfulness and psychotherapy.* New York: Guilford Press, 2005.
5. Trungpa C. *The sanity we are born with.* Boston, MA: Shambhala, 2005.
6. Peplau H. *Interpersonal relations in nursing: a conceptual frame of reference for psychodynamic nursing.* New York: GP Putnam's Sons, 1952.
7. American Nurses Association. *Nursing's social policy statement: the essence of the profession.* Kansas City: ANA, 2010.
8. Benner P. Caring as a way of knowing and not knowing. In: Philips S, Benner P (eds). *The crisis of care: affirming and restoring caring practices in the helping professions.* Washington, DC: Georgetown University Press, 1994.
9. Irving JA, Dobkin P, Park J. Cultivating mindfulness in health care professionals: a review of empirical studies of mindfulness-based stress reduction (MBSR). *Complementary Therapies in Clinical Practice* 2009; **15**: 61–6.
10. Goodman MJ, Schorling JB. Mindfulness course decreases burnout and improves well-being among healthcare providers. *International Journal of Psychiatry in Medicine* 2012; **43**(2): 119–28.
11. Cohen-Katz J, Wiley SD, Capuano T. The effects of mindfulness-based stress reduction on nurse stress and burnout, part III. *Holistic Nursing Practice* 2005; **19**(2): 78–86.
12. Pipe TB, Bortz J, Duek A, Pendergast D, et al. Nurse leader mindfulness meditation program for stress management. *Journal of Nursing Administration* 2009; **39**(3): 130–7.
13. Cohen-Katz J, Wiley SD, Capuano T. The effects of mindfulness-based stress reduction on nurse stress and burnout, part II. *Holistic Nursing Practice* 2005; **19**(1): 26–35.
14. Bazarko D, Cate R, Azocar F, Kreitzer MJ. The impact of an innovative mindfulness-based stress reduction program on the health and well-being of nurses employed in a corporate setting. *Journal of Workplace Behavioral Health* 2013; **28**: 107–33.
15. Brady S, O'Connor N, Burgermeister D, Hanson P. The impact of mindfulness meditation in promoting a culture of safety on an acute psychiatric unit. *Perspectives in Psychiatric Care* 2012; **48**: 129–37.
16. Morita S. *Morita therapy and the true nature of anxiety-based disorders (Shinkeishitsu).* Translated by Akihisa Kondo. Albany, NY: State University of NY Press, 1998.
17. Kitanishi K, Mori A. Morita therapy: 1919–1995. *Psychiatry and Clinical Neurosciences* 1995; **459**: 245–54.
18. He Y, Li C. Morita therapy for schizophrenia. *Cochrane Database of Systemic Reviews* 2007; **I**: CD006346.
19. Fortuna J. The Windhorse program of recovery. In: Warner R (ed.). *Alternatives to the hospital for acute psychiatric treatment.* Arlington, VA: American Psychiatric Publishing, 1995: 171–89.
20. Podvoll E. *Recovering sanity: a compassionate approach to understanding and treating psychosis.* Boston, MA: Shambhala, 2003.
21. Marchand W. Mindfulness meditation practices as adjunctive treatments for psychiatric disorders. *Psychiatric Clinics of North America* 2013; **36**: 141–52.
22. Marchand W. Mindfulness-based stress reduction, mindfulness-based cognitive therapy, and Zen meditation for depression, anxiety, pain and psychological distress. *Journal of Psychiatric Practice* 2012; **18**: 233–52.
23. Chiesa A, Malinowski P. Mindfulness-based approaches: are they all the same? *Journal of Clinical Psychology* 2011; **67**(4): 404–24.
24. Goyal M, Singh S, Sibinga E, Gould N, et al. Meditation programs for psychological stress and well-being: a systematic review and meta-analysis. *JAMA Internal Medicine* 2014; **174**(3), 357–68.
25. Segal ZV, Williams JMG, Teasdale JD. *Mindfulness-based cognitive therapy for depression,* 2nd edn. New York: Guilford Press, 2012.
26. Linehan M. *Cognitive behavioural treatment of borderline personality disorder.* New York: Guilford Press, 1993.

27. Hayes SC, Strosahl K, Wilson KG. *Acceptance and commitment therapy: the process and practice of mindful change*, 2nd edn. New York: Guilford Press, 2011.
28. Orsillo SM, Roemer L. *The mindful way through anxiety*. New York: Guilford Press, 2011.
29. Chadwick P. *Person-based cognitive therapy for distressing psychosis*. Chichester: John Wiley & Sons, 2006.
30. Chiesa A, Serreti A. A systemic review of neurobiological and clinical features of mindfulness meditations. *Psychological Medicine* 2010; **40**: 1239–52.
31. Kabat-Zinn J, Wheeler E, Light T. Influence of a mindfulness-based stress reduction intervention on rates of skin clearing in patients with moderate to severe psoriasis undergoing phototherapy (UVB) and photochemotherapy (PUVA). *Psychosomatic Medicine* 1998; **60**: 625–32.
32. Speca M, Carlson LE, Goodey E, Angen M. A randomized wait-list controlled clinical trial: the effect of a mindfulness-based stress reduction program on mood and symptoms of stress in cancer outpatients. *Psychosomatic Medicine* 2000; **62**: 613–22.
33. Williams M, Teasdale J, Segal Z, Kabat-Zinn J. *The mindful way through depression: freeing yourself from chronic unhappiness*. New York: Guilford Press, 2007.
34. Ma S, Teasdale J. Mindfulness-based cognitive therapy for depression: replication and exploration of differential relapse prevention effects. *Journal of Consulting and Clinical Psychology* 2004; **72**(1): 31–40.
35. National Institute for Health and Clinical Excellence. *Depression: the treatment and management of depression in adults (update)*. NICE, 2009.
36. Work Group on Major Depressive Disorder. *APA practice guideline for the treatment of patients with major depressive disorder*, 3rd edn. Arlington, VA: American Psychiatric Publishing, 2010.
37. Bihari JL, Mullan EG. Relating mindfully: a qualitative exploration of changes in relationships through mindfulness-based cognitive therapy. *Mindfulness* 2014; **5**(1): 46–59.
38. O'Toole SK, Diddy E, Kent M. Mindfulness and emotional well-being in women with borderline personality disorder. *Mindfulness* 2012; **3**: 117–23.
39. Linehan MM, Dimeff L, Koerner K, Miga EM. *Research on dialectical behavioral therapy: summary of the data to date*. Washington: Linehan Institute, 2014.
40. Chadwick P. Mindfulness for psychosis. *British Journal of Psychiatry* 2014; **204**: 333–4.
41. Abba N, Chadwick P, Stevenson C. Responding mindfully to distressing psychosis. *Psychotherapy Research* 2008; **18**(1): 77–87.
42. Davis L, Strasburger AM, Brown LF. Mindfulness: an intervention for anxiety in schizophrenia. *Journal of Psychosocial Nursing and Mental Health Services* 2007; **45**(11):23–9.
43. Singh NN, Lancioni GE, Winton ASW, et al. Individuals with mental illness can control their aggressive behaviour through mindfulness training. *Behaviour Modification* 2007; **31**(3): 313–28.
44. Singh NN, Wahler RG, Adkins AD, et al. Soles of the feet: a mindfulness-based self-control intervention for aggression by an individual with mild mental retardation and mental illness. *Research in Developmental Disabilities* 2003; **24**: 158–69.
45. York M. A qualitative study into the experience of individuals involved in a mindfulness group within an acute inpatient mental health unit. *Journal of Psychiatric and Mental Health Nursing* 2007; **14**: 603–8.
46. Knight M, Pultinas D, Collins S, Freeman DC, et al. Teaching mindfulness on an inpatient psychiatric unit. *Mindfulness* 2014; **5**: 259–67.
47. Fox KCR, Nijeboer S, Cixon ML, Floman JL, et al. Is meditation associated with altered brain structure? A systematic review and meta-analysis of morphometric neuroimaging in meditation practitioners. *Neuroscience and Biobehavioral Reviews* 2014; **43**: 48–73.
48. Lazar SW, Kerr CE, Wasserman RH, et al. Meditation experience is associated with increased cortical thickness. *Neuro Report* 2005; **18**(17): 1893–7.
49. Crane RS, Kuyken W, Williams MG, Hastings RP. Competence in teaching mindfulness-based courses: concepts, development and assessment. *Mindfulness* 2012; **3**: 76–84.

Further reading

Chozen-Bays J. *How to train a wild elephant & other adventures in mindfulness*. Boston, MA: Shambhala, 2011.
Germer C. *The mindful path to self-compassion: freeing yourself from destructive thoughts and emotions*. New York: Guilford Press, 2009.
Kabat-Zinn J. *Full catastrophe living (revised edition): using the wisdom of your body and mind to face stress, pain, and illness*. New York: Random House, 2013.
Smalley S, Winston D. *Fully present: the science, art, and practice of mindfulness*. Philadelphia, PA: Da Capo Press, 2010.
Williams M, Teasdale J, Segal Z, Kabat-Zinn J. *The mindful way through depression*. New York: Guilford Press, 2007.

Relevant web pages

Centre for Mindfulness in Medicine, Health Care and Society. http://www.umassmed.edu/cfm/index.aspx
The Linehan Institute (DBT). http://behavioraltech.org
Mindfulness-Based Cognitive Therapy. http://www.mbct.co.uk/
Windhorse Community Services. http://www.windhorsecommunityservices.com/
Windhorse Integrative Mental Health. http://www.windhorseimh.org/

Early intervention in psychosis

HENRIETTA MBEAH-BANKAS

LEARNING OUTCOMES

- To recognize what constitutes first episode psychosis (FEP) and its stages of development.
- To understand the principles of early intervention in psychosis (EIP).
- To be aware of evidence for the effectiveness of early intervention (EI) services.
- To demonstrate an understanding of the processes involved in identifying FEP and recommended treatment/support interventions.
- To recognize the complexities of working with EI service users and compounding factors.
- To demonstrate an understanding of factors that might limit the effectiveness of EI services.

SUMMARY OF KEY POINTS

- The onset of FEP can be at a critical time in an individual's life.
- Specialist EI services have been set up to provide targeted intervention and support for people who are deemed at risk of developing psychosis or have developed FEP.
- Nurses have a crucial role in identifying, providing interventions and coordinating the care of individuals requiring EI services.
- Services offered to people with suspected FEP or established FEP have to be sensitive and responsive to individual, family and community needs.

INTRODUCTION

This chapter will critically explore the concept of early intervention (EI), the effectiveness of the model and the nurse's role in delivering high fidelity care.

Any contact with health services about ill-health can increase anxiety for individuals. This anxiety is exacerbated when contact is with mental health services, at a time when an individual may be confused, in acute distress and worried about their health status and the implication of a developing or developed mental illness. It is imperative that the care they receive not only focuses on treatment of illness but is acceptable and collaborative in an environment that promotes hope and recovery. A number of considerations have to be made when providing care to individuals during their initial and continuing contact with mental health services, especially in specialized EI services.

Health professionals, particularly mental health nurses in EI services, are best placed to use their skills and expertise in supporting and providing care to individuals and the supportive systems around them, such as family, friends, schools and other community groups, during this crucial time.

EARLY INTERVENTION

Early intervention in psychosis (EIP) is not a recent idea; it dates back to Harry Stack Sullivan's work in the 1920s and has been established further with evolving evidence. The fundamental underlying principles are as follows:

- Intervening in early stages of psychosis can change the trajectory of illness and improve long-term prognosis.
- Early targeting of non-responders can reduce treatment resistance.
- Multi-faceted interventions promote psychological and social recovery and reduce treatment damage and carer burden.[1,2]

These principles are particularly important considering the time of onset – usually late adolescence to early adulthood. This is a high-risk period for developing mental disorders, with 7,500 young people developing an emerging psychosis each year in England.[3] About three-quarters of men and two-thirds of women experience their first episode by the age of 35; most are in their late teens and twenties.[4] Because of the typically young age of onset, psychosis can be particularly debilitating, with extensive overall implications for the individual and family. All aspects of life are affected: education, employment, relationships and social functioning, physical/mental well-being.[5] Interrupted or paused personal and social development can have life-long consequences and account for much of the disability experienced by people with chronic mental illness.[6]

The first 3 to 5 years following the development of psychosis are critical due to the rapid progress of symptoms and psychosocial deterioration, which require specialized, effective interventions.[7,8] Traditional mental health service provision has not been seen to address the specific needs of the 18–35 age group[9] during this 'critical period'. It has been shown that EI services produce better clinical outcomes and are cost-effective. Furthermore, provision of care under specialized EI services results in young people having better social and vocational outcomes and better engagement with services, with reduced hospital stays.[10]

EI can involve improving outcomes in established cases of psychosis by facilitating and consolidating recovery. It can also involve detecting hidden morbidity in the community or within mental health care by identifying untreated cases. Another aspect of EI is early detection (ED) to reduce the duration of untreated psychosis (DUP), or to prevent the emergence of psychosis in pre-psychotic and prodromal states.[9]

Despite a rapid expansion of EI services in many countries (Australia, Canada, Scandinavia and the United Kingdom (UK)), the presence of prodromal clinics and community awareness campaigns differ considerably.[11]

STAGES IN THE DEVELOPMENT OF PSYCHOSIS

Psychosis and schizophrenia are sometimes used interchangeably in the literature, but it is worth noting that the recommendations for treatment are not dissimilar.[12] Psychosis is a broad medical term used to explain symptoms evident in a number of mental disorders, of which schizophrenia is one. (See chapter 12 for further information on the classification of mental illness.)

Psychosis develops over time, usually with evidence of functional decline and other subtle behavioural changes. Nevertheless, a small proportion of people may experience acute psychosis, as a result of either stress or the use of mood-altering substances. Figure 45.1 outlines the developmental stages of psychosis.

Knowledge of the developmental stages of psychosis is important in assessment and targeted interventions. Special intervention programmes are targeted at individuals showing early signs and other related problem behaviours.[13]

Research findings suggest that there are three stages to developing psychosis: the prodrome, the first episode and the chronic phase of illness.[13,14] There is, however, further indication (as shown in Figure 45.1) that there is a premorbid phase before the prodrome.[15]

The prodrome is defined as the period in weeks from the time of first definite change in behavioural, psychological or emotional functioning to the onset of the first psychotic episode.[16]

Despite previous ethical concerns about interventions in the prodrome because of the clinical challenges it poses as a result of the non-specificity of symptoms,[17] there are ongoing studies that outline the benefits of interventions.[18–20]

There are a number of strategies required to address the needs of an individual experiencing an FEP. These include a multidisciplinary assessment of mental state, risk and other support needs, allocation of a keyworker/care coordinator

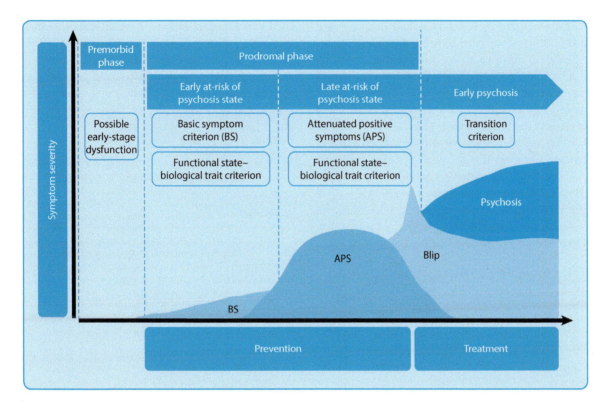

Figure 45.1 Stages in the development of psychosis.

and the use of atypical antipsychotics. It is also essential to ensure therapeutic engagement with the individual.[20]

The chronic stage of illness requires interventions relating to medication adherence, cognitive behavioural therapy (CBT), psycho-education and family intervention where indicated, vocational assessment and support and engagement of carers as partners in the care process. Furthermore, at this stage, assessment and management of comorbidity, especially substance misuse, is vital. Also indicated at this stage is regular, structured and documented

multidisciplinary review of the care plan, with user input into the needs assessment and the plan.

> ## REFLECTION
>
> Think about the three fundamental principles of EI, discussed earlier. What are the important factors to consider in ensuring that interventions are targeted for effectiveness?

ENGAGEMENT

Early engagement is the most important initial therapeutic goal in EI. A nurse's ability to assess and provide interventions to an individual is very much dependent on engaging the individual and the significant people in their lives (usually family and close friends). For some individuals, this could be with professionals in education, training and employment institutes. It could also involve professionals in housing projects or social care providers including foster carers. There are a number of factors that enhance engagement:

- flexibility in appointments offered – this includes timing, location (including the possibility of visiting the person's home) and the characteristics of professionals attending, as some individuals may have a preference, for example, for a particular gender due to previous experiences or cultural beliefs;

- addressing the needs that the person feels are important to them including issues relating to housing, finances, education, etc.;
- information-giving and rationale for planned actions – this should sometimes involve consideration of language and format, which may require the use of interpreters or information written in other languages.

A nurse may utilize various skills to engage a young person and their family. However, they may resist contact with EI services for a number of reasons, such as stigma, poor understanding of the young person's mental health needs and sometimes having had previous contact with services that are restrictive in provisions, such as the criminal justice system and emergency services.[20,21] Nevertheless, a dedicated EI service can influence long-term engagement by ensuring a considerate first contact with mental health services, while creating optimum hope and ensuring care delivery in a low-stigma environment. The nurse's skills and approaches are invaluable in achieving this. The skills that can be employed include active listening, negotiation skills and effective communication skills. This process of engagement is underpinned by the principles of assertive outreach (see chapter 37 for further details).[22] Nevertheless, the use of 'oneself' in connecting with others, to support care provision, is an art that is sometimes challenging to master.[23] (For more information on developing and maintaining therapeutic relationships, see chapter 3.)

Engagement efforts should not just be solely directed towards the affected individual, especially when there is an initial strong resistance. The effort can be focused on supporting other members of the family/professional network in maintaining the young person's well-being and providing them with information on individuals or services to contact in times of crisis.

> ## REFLECTION
>
> If you were a young person or a family member requiring access to an EI service, what efforts could the nurse or service make to engage you and your family?

KIP'S STORY

My name is Kip and I was sent to go and see this 'special service' about my mental health by my keyworker in CAMHS and probation officer. I first met the doctor and the nurse at my probation centre who told me that everyone was worried about me because I did not make sense when I talked to them. Also, I wasn't doing well in my college work and got angry with people easily. They asked me lots and lots of questions about myself, my family, what I get up to and many other things. I told them a lot about myself and even told them I 'smoked weed' and hung out with a 'bad crowd'. I also told them that I have been in a bit of trouble with the police a number of times for petty crime which was why I had a probation officer. I saw them a number of times and then was told that I don't need 'ongoing' support from their service. I was sent to the team a few other times and each time, someone met with me. I remember one time, I saw

another doctor at the college, who said she was a psychologist. All the people I saw were alright and always very friendly and didn't judge me, which is why I was happy to see them even though they kept sending me away. They were always 'cool' and professional; the nurse was really patient and called me to remind me about my appointment or made another one when I missed it. Then, I went on a 'binge' and felt 'proper mad' after taking a lot of different drugs and was sent to Accident and Emergency, then hospital. This time everything was different because the hospital doctor and the doctor from the EI team said I will need ongoing support. I had two community nurses; one was an EI keyworker and the other one was a specialist drugs worker who helped me with a lot of things: my housing, money and talking to my family to understand me better. My mum and sisters were happy with all the help.

> ## REFLECTION
>
> Kip was assessed a number of times and supported by different services. Even though services were concerned about his mental health, they could not clearly establish whether Kip was experiencing an FEP or a prodrome, or whether his presentation was due to excessive drug use.

- What factors do you feel contributed to him engaging in a number of assessments before an offer of support was made by the EI service?
- What do you feel will further help practitioners coming into contact with young people like Kip to identify an emerging mental health difficulty?

ASSESSMENT

Identifying whether a young person is experiencing an emerging or established FEP can be challenging and complex, as indicated by Kip's story. Young people can experience early symptoms of psychosis for up to 2 years before coming into contact with mental health services. This period preceding an evident psychosis is called the 'prodrome', 'at-risk mental states (ARMS)' or 'ultra high risk', with various indications including decline in function (sometimes apparent in a significant drop in grades at school or college), psychotic-like symptoms and sometimes somatic signs like those found in depression and anxiety. During this period it is extremely difficult to persuade a young person and their family to seek help, due to lack of awareness or sometimes the stigma associated with mental illness.[22] It also increases the risks posed to young people, including that of suicide and social isolation. A timely specialist assessment not only reduces the risk for young people and their families, but reduces the duration of untreated psychosis and consequently improves outcomes.

To ensure that a young person has received a comprehensive assessment of their needs, an EI team has to employ the full spectrum of skills of members of the multidisciplinary team.

There are a number of tools to aid assessment; some of the tools used have been developed locally by services, but there are others that are used in a number of EI services worldwide. Examples of such tools include the Positive And Negative Syndrome Scale (PANSS), the Brief Psychiatric

Rating Scale (BPRS) and the Strengths Assessment Tool. The various tools can only contribute one part of an overall view of a particular individual at a particular time. They should only be used as part of the overall assessment, with the nurse utilizing expertise within their team and other attributes. It has to be emphasized that the basis of good nursing practice is combining the 'art' and the 'science', which together become a 'craft of caring'.[23]

Assessment usually looks at the bio-psychosocial needs of the service user. Despite generic mental health services having the ability to conduct such assessments, it is evident in Kip's story that assessment of FEP or ARMS requires the use of specialist skills in early intervention or detection services. Furthermore, assessing risks posed by a young person suffering from an FEP can be difficult, as some areas of risk may be unknown. Risks usually relate to harm to self and/or others, vulnerability, and self-neglect. It is crucial to involve carers and family members in ensuring that information has been collected in relation to current and potential risk to support management.

THE EI NURSE'S ROLE IN ASSESSMENT

When assessing an individual, with contributions from the significant people in their lives, the aim should be to take a bio-psychosocial history of positive, negative, disorganized and general/affective symptoms.[24] In collecting this information, the domains to consider are severity, frequency and level of distress. The questions to ask in obtaining information in those domains include:

- How are you feeling generally in yourself?
- Have you noticed any changes in yourself, e.g. your mood, your thoughts, not enjoying things as much as you used to?
- How would you describe these changes?
- How long has it been going on for?
- Has it been worse recently?
- How much does it worry or upset you that you have experienced these changes?
- Have other people noticed a change? When did they notice the change?

During assessment, a nurse should avoid asking individuals closed questions, because a suggestible person may say 'yes' to questions and experiences they do not have. It has to be acknowledged that sometimes an individual may not be forthcoming with information and, rather than insisting that they give you answers, it is better to talk about other general things of interest to them but always assess any risks as soon as possible.

For the assessment of ARMS, training in using the various tools, such as the Comprehensive Assessment of At-Risk Mental States (CAARMS)[25] and the Structured Interview for Prodromal Symptoms (SIPS) including the companion

Scale of Prodromal Symptoms (SOPS),[26] is recommended to ensure accurate use.

In addition to collecting information to formulate an understanding of the experiences of the young person and their family, there are cases where issues of culture, religion and spirituality have to be considered to ensure sensitivity, accuracy of assessment, and appropriate formulation and treatment. (More information on assessment can be found in chapters 13 and 14.)

GOLA'S STORY

Gola is a 20-year-old who had stopped attending college and had become withdrawn, with periods of aggression to various family members. Prior to this period of decline, he was functioning at a very high level in the previous year. Despite evidence of significant decline in function, inability to comprehend simple conversations, withdrawal and aggression (which was out of character for him), his parents were adamant that it was a case of being possessed by the devil and hence would prefer to have input from the local religious leader. The nurse who was assessing Gola supported the family to seek religious interventions, but negotiated with the family to consider psychiatric treatment alongside. The practitioner, however, realizing the implications of the family pursuing religious treatment, had to find other means of engaging with the family's beliefs to support the initiation and maintenance of care provision in the EIS.

An issue of culture can thwart the assessment process and affect the information gathered and hence formulation and treatment. Nurses and other team members can take these steps to facilitate engagement and treatment of an individual and their family who have beliefs consistent with a specific culture:

• Listen to the young person's perception of the problem, and that of their family members.
• Explain the professionals' perception of the problem.
• Acknowledge similarities and differences in perceptions.
• Recommend options, with the involvement of the young person and their family.
• Negotiate treatment plans.[27]

Assessment is an ongoing process throughout the duration of a young person's care in an EI service. It establishes a service user's understanding of the illness and their aspirations early on, in order to inform the strategies that are used for engaging them in treatment and post-discharge from EIS.

> ## REFLECTION
>
> If you were a young person or a family member seeing a specialist mental health team with concerns about developing a psychosis, in addition to the questions you may be asked in assessment, what other things would you like the nurse or the team to consider when thinking about your care?

PHASE-SPECIFIC INTERVENTIONS

The broad aims and activities of EI services are prevention, detection, early intervention, improved treatment, relapse prevention and onward care-pathway connections. The nurse has a role in developing and delivering various interventions across these aims.

The nurse's role involves working with a group identified as being at ultra-high risk of developing psychosis. Additionally, the nurse's role in improving detection includes promoting public health education, and educating other professionals through social marketing strategies.[28] To support the improvement of detection, the nurse can have a role in setting up services that are accessible to help-seeking individuals, carers and other referrers.[6] Further to this, a nurse is also best placed to conduct a comprehensive assessment of a young person.

Once a FEP has been established, the nurse will provide other interventions, including psychological therapies, independently or with other therapists.

RECOVERY-FOCUSED INTERVENTIONS

There are a number of interventions with proven efficacy to aid recovery following a diagnosis of FEP. These interventions include medication/antipsychotic treatment, and psychological therapies – in particular, family intervention, and CBT for psychosis.[12] Psychosocial intervention skills are seen as essential for practitioners working in EIS.[29] Additional recommended interventions include access to a specialist training and employment worker and ensuring that the service user's physical health, including lifestyle choices, has been addressed.[12] In addressing the aim of reducing the duration of untreated psychosis, the nurse's role has evolved to include early detection of psychosis.

When a diagnosis of ARMS is established, the various recommended effective treatments are CBT for psychosis and support with returning to education and employment.[30] Depending on the stage of development, sometimes a young person may require a low dose of antipsychotic medication in addition to CBT for psychosis.[31]

Antipsychotic treatment

This involves the use of psychotropic medication and sometimes other forms of medication such as antidepressants or anxiolytics to manage comorbidities or to resolve adverse effects from the prescribed medication. To ensure adherence to both tablets and long-acting antipsychotic medication, the nurse has a role in providing further information to the service user. This is intended to address lack of knowledge, misperceptions and stigma related to the treatment of psychosis.[32] Further to this, the choice of antipsychotic treatment should result from a shared decision-making process wherein service users and clinicians have had open discussions about the advantages and disadvantages of the various options. The quality of the nurse–service user relationship/alliance is known to be associated with better medication adherence.[33] The nurse can support adherence by exploring the service user's beliefs and behaviour about medication. This can include:

• the service user's experience of medication taking;
• the service user's concerns – dependency, side effects, cultural beliefs;
• the cost of medication.

EXAMPLES OF ADHERENCE QUESTIONS

- Have you missed any medication in the last week?
- How many tablets do you have left today?
- What time do you take your tablets?
- Is it a problem taking it in the morning?
- Have you always been on this particular medication?

Chapters 47 and 48 provide more information on psychopharmacology and mental health.

JOYCE'S STORY

Joyce is a young woman who was admitted to hospital after becoming acutely ill and exhibiting psychotic symptoms. She was prescribed antipsychotic medication which both her parents and Joyce were not keen on, despite having received thorough explanation and information. Joyce subsequently stated she did not need the medication because she was well. Her parents, on the other hand, had been informed through hearsay that psychiatric medications can 'mess with your brain'. Following evidence and examples of how others have responded to medication as part of the interventions offered, Joyce's mother supported her adherence to treatment. Joyce was not able to consent to receiving antipsychotic treatment because of her poor mental state, but engaging with her parents became crucial for maintaining adherence.

REFLECTION

In addition to explanation, what would support you in deciding to adhere to prescribed medication if you or a family member were receiving treatment from an EI team?

Family support/intervention

The social networks of adolescents and young people experiencing an FEP can reduce significantly; however, during an FEP, many young people will stay in close contact with a number of family members.[34] The presence of psychosis can have a negative impact on family relationships which can be addressed using family intervention, a recommended evidence-based treatment in later psychosis.[12] Family intervention can be provided effectively with additional training;

however, a practitioner can use their existing skills in supporting other family members by establishing how their caring roles/caregiving experience impacts on their physical, social and mental well-being. It is very important to work with families, as they can contribute to information-gathering to support a young person, including providing information about risk and relapse. Due to the typical age of onset, family members – usually parents – may have a sense of loss about the young person not being able to fulfil their potential.[35] Family members or partners may also feel isolated and sometimes inadequate in their ability to support the individual, and may require support from others, including families in similar circumstances. Some of the questions that a nurse can ask to establish a carer's needs for support include:

- How are you feeling generally?
- How were you spending your time prior to your loved one becoming ill?
- What are you most worried about, with … becoming ill?
- Are you worried about your other children/siblings?
- What do you need support with at the moment?

Depending on the local or national policy operating in the nurse's area of work, the nurse should consider a formal assessment of needs for an identified carer. (Chapter 15 provides further information on conducting a family assessment.)

A MOTHER'S/CARER'S STORY

Jade is a mother of three adolescent children and her eldest, who is accessing an EI service, is always argumentative with other family members. During the assessment of Jade's daughter, it was clear that Jade was upset about her daughter becoming ill and the impact it had on the whole family, especially her. However, she remained positive and hopeful and was always very cheerful. As part of the EI care, her daughter's key nurse met with the family to ascertain what support they required, and they were all keen for their mother to be supported further as she had 'suffered the most'. The family was offered family intervention and, with support from the carers' centre, a comprehensive assessment was completed. This resulted in Jade accessing additional support and activities from the EI team and carers' centre. This included a range of support areas, welfare, health, leisure and respite. Jade felt the centre also gave her an opportunity to meet other carers and have time for herself. Additionally, there was some evidence and reports of improved relationships in the family unit.

Psycho-education

Relapse among individuals in contact with EI services tends to occur in the first 3 years after the initial onset of psychosis.[21] EI significantly reduces the risk of a second relapse, and psycho-education has been identified as an effective intervention in preventing relapse. Usually this is delivered by nurses and/or other members of the team and with the individual or, where possible and available, with family members. Topics that can be addressed include:

- optimum medication management;
- stress management strategies;
- psychotic disorders education;
- symptom management strategies;
- development and maintenance of effective social support;
- crisis resolution strategies;
- social living skills training for achieving personal goals;
- coping strategies;
- problem-solving education;
- communication skills;
- relapse prevention (early warning signs/action plan).[36]

SUBSTANCE MISUSE

Generally, substance misuse is more common in people with early psychosis than their non-psychotic counterparts. It is linked to poorer outcomes and a number of challenges in treatment.[37] This requires the EI nurse to have an understanding of the underlying reasons to be able to support the person, including sometimes involving specialist drugs and alcohol workers or services. Substance misuse needs to be addressed because it can exacerbate a psychotic illness, but it also has implications for an individual's psychological and social well-being. (For further information on substance misuse, see chapter 31.)

PHYSICAL HEALTH

Individuals with schizophrenia and psychosis die on average 15 to 20 years younger than the general population.[38,39] The reasons for this include the use of antipsychotic medications, lifestyles (poor dietary intake, sedentary lifestyles due to negative symptoms) and poor access to general health services and checks.[40] Poor physical health impacts negatively on self-esteem and mood, and therefore can exacerbate mental illness and affect well-being.

The Lester Positive Cardiometabolic Health Resource provides practitioners in any service, including EI, with a simple assessment and intervention framework. Following assessment, the EI nurse has to intervene by providing advice on diet and lifestyle and, if indicated, arrange consultation with the team doctor or the service user's GP.

Furthermore, there has been a lot of emphasis recently in the UK on achieving parity between mental and physical health.[41] To ensure that this is embedded in routine practice, there are various measures to monitor input by teams responsible for the care of individuals suffering from psychosis. To support the achievement of this parity, the nurse also has to address the needs of the individual as a whole, rather than separating their mental and physical health needs. (Chapters 69 and 70 provide further information about physical health care and health promotion respectively.)

MULTIDISCIPLINARY AND MULTI-AGENCY WORKING

Despite the nurse having a number of roles within an EI service, they have a number of resources to draw on to ensure that the care delivered is effective and meets the individual needs of the service user. EI services usually work well using a team-based approach. Also, since an individual nurse is not expected to be an expert or competent in providing all aspects of care, their skills in working with multidisciplinary and multi-agency teams are crucial.

A team-based approach to service delivery is recommended in EI services and this sometimes requires a willingness to share roles in meeting the needs of individual service users.[6,42] Chapter 37 has information on the care programme approach (CPA) and chapter 50 for collaborative care planning with service users and carers.

In addition to multidisciplinary team working, there are instances where multi-agency working between health and education, housing and children's services are required to address the needs of the service user, and the nurse has to be prepared to share roles with other professionals, teams and agencies.

AJ'S STORY

I am AJ, and my journey in EI started when I went out one day and felt that people were doing things to me. I wasn't entirely sure how they were doing it, but I always had a burning sensation anytime I was in a particular area of town. Well, at the time, I thought it was real until I started having other strange experiences, which was frightening. At this point, I knew something was wrong with my mental health, but my family thought it was spiritual. We sought help from the church pastor, but a conversation with a friend changed everything. I realized I needed help and went to my doctor who referred me to the EI team. They were very supportive and offered me a number of options. I was initially anxious about the medication but with a lot of explanation and reassurance from the doctor and my nurse, I agreed to have it. After a few weeks of treatment, I started feeling better in myself than I had done in a very long time, almost like my old self. I then started worrying that things could get bad again and it scared me. To help me cope with that fear, I started focusing on other things; mostly activities. It was at this point that I met with the training and employment advisor who encouraged me to go back to my course. I doubted myself because of everything that had

happened, but she gave me a lot of reassurance to go back. I enjoyed it so much and started finding myself again. My confidence continued to grow to the point where I was able to talk to other students about my experiences. I feel that my life has changed because of the help I got from the team. It is coming up to 3 years since my first contact with EIS. I still take my tablets and I am in full-time work. I was also very fortunate that my family were very supportive and information from the service helped them to support me.

I know that my story is a very positive one, but that is due to input from a range of professionals who were very skilled and seemed passionate about helping people in their care. I was particularly supported by my care coordinator, who was a nurse. I saw a lot more of her than others in my care team and developed a good working relationship with her. Everyone in the care team is crucial in providing you with some aspect of your care. I feel that EI services are great but the outcome of the intervention is dependent on so many factors. This includes accessing help early, complying with treatment offered and using a number of support systems, including a religious one in my case.

CONCLUSION

Early intervention in psychosis care has been developing extensively in the past two decades, with growing evidence on its effectiveness and outcomes in comparison to traditional mental health care. A number of interventions have been established to produce good outcomes for individuals and their families. The nurse has a role in working independently and with other members of the EI team to address the holistic needs of EI service users. This can be done using theory and research evidence, but awareness that nursing is not always a science and that sometimes the art of caring and our ability to use ourselves can become critical in our engagement with individuals and their families.

References

1. McGlashan T, Johannessen JO. Early detection and intervention in schizophrenia: rationale. *Schizophrenia Bulletin* 1996; **22**: 201–22.
2. McGorry PD, Edwards J, Mihalopoulos C, Harrigan SM, Jackson HJ. EPPIC: an evolving system of early detection and optimal management. *Schizophrenia Bulletin* 1996; **22**: 305–26.
3. Mental Health Network. *Early intervention in psychosis services.* Issue 219. Briefing. London: NHS Confederation, 2011.
4. Kirkbride JB, Fearon P, Morgan C, Dazzan P, Morgan K, Tarrant J, Lloyd T, Holloway J, Hutchinson G, Leff JP, Mallett RM, Harrison GL, Murray RM, Jones PB. Heterogeneity in incidence rates of schizophrenia and other psychotic syndromes: findings from the 3-center AeSOP study. *Archives of General Psychiatry* 2006; **63**(3): 250–8.
5. Yung AR, McGorry PD. The prodromal phase of first-episode psychosis: past and current conceptualizations. *Schizophrenia Bulletin* 1996; **22**(2): 353–70.
6. IRIS. IRIS guidelines update. IRIS Initiative Ltd., 2012. Available from: http://www.iris-initiative.org.uk/silo/files/iris-guidelines-update--september-2012.pdf [Accessed 7th September 2016].
7. Birchwood M, Todd P, Jackson C. Early intervention in psychosis: the critical period hypothesis. *British Journal of Psychiatry* 1998; **172**(33): 53–9.
8. McGorry PD, Killackey E, Yung AR. Early intervention in psychosis: concepts, evidence and future directions. *World Psychiatry* 2008; **7**(3): 148–56.
9. Singh SP. Early intervention in psychosis. *British Journal of Psychiatry* 2010; **196**(5): 343–5.

10. Singh SP. Outcome measures in early psychosis: relevance of duration of untreated psychosis. *British Journal of Psychiatry* 2007; **191**(50): 58–63.

11. Murphy BP, Brewer WJ. Early intervention in psychosis: strengths and limitations of services. *Advances in Psychiatric Treatment* 2011; **17**: 401–7.

12. NICE (National Institute for Health and Care Excellence). *Psychosis and schizophrenia in adults: prevention and management. Clinical guideline 178.* London: NICE, 2014.

13. Yung A, Phillips LJ, Yuen HP, Francey SM, McFarlane CA, Hallgren M, McGorry PD. Psychosis prediction: 12-month follow up of a high-risk ('prodromal') group. *Schizophrenia Research* 2003; **60**: 21–32.

14. Singh SP, Cooper JE, Fisher HL, Tarrant CJ, Lloyd T, Banjo J, Corfe S, Jones P. Determining the chronology and components of psychosis onset: the Nottingham Onset Schedule (NOS). *Schizophrenia Research* 2005; **80**:117–30.

15. Fusar-Poli P, Borgwardt S, Bechdolf A, Addington J, Riecher-Rössler A. The psychosis high-risk state. *JAMA Psychiatry* 2013; **70**(1):107–20.

16. Lappin JM, Dazzan P, Morgan K, Morgan C, Chitnis X, Suckling J, Fearon P, Jones PB, Leff J, Murray RM, McGuire PK. Duration of prodromal phase and severity of volumetric abnormalities in first-episode psychosis. *British Journal of Psychiatry* 2007; **191**(51): 123–7.

17. Harvey PD. Commentary: chickens and eggs; carts and horses: an outsider's perspective on the study of the early stages and potential prevention of psychosis and schizophrenia. *Schizophrenia Bulletin* 2003; **29**(4): 845–9.

18. Larson MK, Walker EF, Compton MT. Early signs, diagnosis and therapeutics of the prodromal phase of schizophrenia and related psychotic disorders. *Expert Review of Neurotherapeutics* 2010; **10**(8): 1347–59.

19. Morrison AP, French P, Walford L, Lewis SW, Kilcommons A, Green J, Parker S, Bentall RP. Cognitive therapy for the prevention of psychosis in people at ultra-high risk. *British Journal of Psychiatry* 2004; **185**(4): 291–7.

20. Singh SP, Fisher HL. Early intervention in psychosis: obstacles and opportunities. *Advances in Psychiatric Treatment* 2005; **11**: 71–8.

21. Rogers C. Principles of early intervention in the treatment of psychosis. *Nursing Times* 2006; **102**(5): 28–30.

22. DH. *Policy implementation guide.* London: DH, 2001.

23. Barker, P. In the need for nursing. In: Barker P (ed.). *Psychiatric and mental health nursing, the craft of caring.* Boca Raton, FL: Taylor and Francis Group, 2008: 2–3.

24. Loewy RL, Therman S, Manninen M, Huttunen MO, Cannon TD. Prodromal psychosis screening in adolescent psychiatry clinics. *Early Intervention in Psychiatry* 2011; **6**(1): 69–75.

25. Yung AR, Yuen HP, McGorry PD, Phillips LJ, Kelly D, Dell'Olio M, Francey SM, Cosgrave EM, Killackey E, Stanford C, Godfrey K, Buckby J. Mapping the onset of psychosis: the Comprehensive Assessment of At-Risk Mental States. *Australia and New Zealand Journal of Psychiatry* 2005; **39**(11–12): 964–71.

26. Miller TJ, McGlashan TH, Woods SW, Stein K, Driesen N, Corcoran CM, Hoffman R, Davidson L. Symptom assessment in schizophrenic prodromal states. *Psychiatric Quarterly* 1999; **70**(4): 273–87.

27. Berlin EA, Fowkes WC. A teaching framework for cross cultural health care: application in family practice. *Western Journal of Medicine* 1983; **139**: 834–8.

28. Marlowe K. Adults of working age. In: Bryne P, Rosen A (eds). *Early intervention in psychiatry: EI of nearly everything better in mental health.* Chichester: Wiley Blackwell, 2014: 92–102.

29. Craig T. A step too soon or a step too far? Early intervention in psychosis. *Journal of Mental Health* 2003; **12**(4): 335–9.

30. Brimblecombe N, Knapp M, Murguia S, Mbeah-Bankas H, Crane S, Harris A, Evans-Lacko S, Ardino V, Iemmi V, King D. The role of youth mental health services in the treatment of young people with serious mental illness: 2-year outcomes and economic implications. *Early Intervention in Psychiatry* 2015; **9**(6): doi:10.1111/eip.12261.

31. McGorry PD, Yung AR, Phillips LJ, Yuen HP, Francey S, Cosgrave EM, Germano D, Bravin J, McDonald T, Blair A, Adlard S, Jackson H. Randomized controlled trial of interventions designed to reduce the risk of progression to first episode psychosis in a clinical sample with subthreshold symptoms. *Archives of General Psychiatry* 2002; **59**: 921–8.

32. Das AD, Malik A, Haddad PM. A qualitative study of the attitudes of patients in an early intervention service towards antipsychotic long-acting injections. *Therapeutic Advances in Psychopharmacology* 2014; **4**(5): 179–85.

33. McCabe R, Healey PG, Priebe S, Lavelle M, Dodwell D, Laugharne R, Snell A, Bremner S. Shared understanding in psychiatrist–patient communication: association with treatment adherence in schizophrenia. *Patient Education and Counselling* 2013; **93**: 73–9.

34. Onwumere J, Bebbington P, Kuipers E. Family intervention in early psychosis: specificity and effectiveness. *Epidemiology and Psychiatric Sciences* 2011; **20**(2): 113–19.

35. Patterson P, Birchwood M, Cochrane R. Preventing the entrenchment of high expressed emotion in first episode psychosis: early developmental attachment pathways. *Australian and New Zealand Journal of Psychiatry* 2000; **34**: 191–7.

36. Johnson DL. Professional–family collaboration. *New Directions for Mental Health Services* 1987; **34**: 73–9.

37. Summers A, Goel C. Substance use in early intervention services for psychosis. *Advances in Dual Diagnosis* 2011; **4**(3): 115–24.

38. Thornicroft G. Physical health disparities and mental illness: the scandal of premature mortality. *British Journal of Psychiatry* 2011; **199**(6): 441–2.

39. Chang C-K, Hayes RD, Perera G, Broadbent MTM, Fernandes AC, Lee WE, Hotopf M, Stuart R. (2011) Life expectancy at birth for people with serious mental illness and other major disorders from a secondary mental health care case register in London. *PLoS ONE* 2011; **6**(5): e19590.

40. Shiers D, Campion J, Jones P, Taylor D. *Early intervention in psychosis; keeping the body in mind – 2014 update.* London: Royal College of General Practitioners and Royal College of Psychiatrists, 2014.

41. Royal College of Psychiatrists. *Whole-person care: from rhetoric to reality: achieving parity between mental and physical health.* Occasional paper OP88. London: Royal College of Psychiatrists, 2013.

42. Kane JM, Robinson DG, Schooler NR, Mueser KT, Penn DL, et al. Comprehensive versus usual community care for first-episode psychosis: 2-year outcomes from the NIMH RAISE early treatment program. *American Journal of Psychiatry* 2015; doi: 10.1176/appi.ajp.2015.15050632.

Further reading

Centre for Mental Health. *Investing in recovery: making the business case for effective interventions for people with schizophrenia and psychosis.* London: Rethink Mental Illness, 2014. Available from: https://www.centreformentalhealth.org.uk/investing-in-recovery [Accessed 21st June 2016].

Knapp M, McDaid D, Parsonage D (eds). *Mental health promotion and mental illness prevention: the economic case.* London: Department of Health, 2011. Available from: www.crisiscareconcordat.org.uk/wp-content/uploads/2014/11/Knapp_et_al__MHPP_The_Economic_Case.pdf [Accessed 21st June 2016].

Rethink Mental Illness and the IRIS Network. *Lost generation: why young people with psychosis are being left behind, and what needs to change.* London: Rethink Mental Illness, 2014. Available from: https://www.rethink.org/media/973932/LOST%20GENERATION%20-%20Rethink%20Mental%20Illness%20report.pdf [Accessed 21st June 2016].

Schizophrenia Commission. *The abandoned illness: a report by the Schizophrenia Commission.* London: Rethink Mental Illness, 2012. Available from: https://www.rethink.org/media/514093/TSC_main_report_14_nov.pdf [Accessed 21st June 2016].

Relevant web pages

IRIS. Early intervention in psychosis. http://www.iris-initiative.org.uk/

Mental Health Care. Early intervention services. http://www.mentalhealthcare.org.uk/early_intervention_services

MIND. http://www.mind.org.uk/

Orygen Youth Health. http://oyh.org.au/

Rethink Mental Illness. https://www.rethink.org/

Royal College of Psychiatrists. http://www.rcpsych.ac.uk/

Young and Well Cooperative Research Centre. http://www.youngandwellcrc.org.au/

46 Crisis assessment and resolution

JULIE TAYLOR, MRS M, MR M AND MISS M

LEARNING OUTCOMES

- To be able to articulate the core principles and function of a Crisis Resolution and Home Treatment service.
- To appreciate a service user perspective of an episode of mental health crisis.
- To appreciate a carer perspective of an episode of mental health crisis.
- To know how to apply principles of evidence-based practice to the field of mental health crisis.
- To be able to evaluate the effectiveness of a Crisis Resolution and Home Treatment model.

SUMMARY OF KEY POINTS

- Crisis services operate a 24-hour, 7-days-a-week multi-disciplinary mobile workforce, delivering intensive home treatment as close to home as possible, as an alternative to hospital admission.
- Crisis teams work closely with service users and their carers to achieve safe and effective partnerships.
- The evidence base for home treatment versus hospital admission includes the minimization of stigma and effects of institutionalization on the individual.

- Crisis mental health teams approach each case within a personalized recovery framework, taking into account the strengths/resources of the individual, and providing an opportunity to develop valuable life skills.
- Crisis practitioners intervene within a bio-psychosocial approach, viewing the person in a wider context than that of their medical diagnosis.
- The skill-set of crisis practitioners is allied closely to and is congruent with the '6 Cs' and the craft of caring.

INTRODUCTION

The word 'crisis' derives from the Greek word *krisis*, which means a 'turning point' or decision. Understanding that there are possibilities for new skills to be gained or for learning opportunities to take place during or following a period of crisis can be helpful when providing interventions. A phase of crisis can allow a fresh interpretation of difficult situations, which sits well with the notion of strengths-based personalized care. A mental health crisis may include:

- experiencing unusual thoughts or hearing voices, which can be very frightening or disturbing for both the service user and their family;
- feeling misunderstood or excluded from relatives, peer networks or communities, thus compounding the service user's sense of isolation or stigma;
- a significant disturbance in a person's usual degree of functioning, such as an inability to go to work or difficulty in attending to their own self-care needs or diet.

If this is a first episode of mental health crisis, the person's lack of previous experience may limit their repertoire of coping skills, leading to a sense of helplessness.

A mental health crisis is different for each individual person and cannot be defined within the bounds of the triggering event; it is more helpful to understand the emotional and psychological response to the event instead. A person experiencing a mental health crisis may need urgent help and this may be the point at which they enter the local mental health pathway.

CRISIS THEORY AND THE PERSON IN MENTAL HEALTH CRISIS

In the context of mental health, the word 'crisis' represents a failure to cope[1] and was first used in this context by Caplan in 1964.[2] Caplan suggested that a crisis is a brief non-illness response to stress. The experience of crisis is universal. People face crisis when they encounter an obstacle to important life goals. Caplan identified three components of crisis:

1. *Onset.* There is an immediate increase in tension as the individual realizes that the problem cannot be resolved quickly.
2. *Breakdown/disorganization.* Tension and anxiety quickly rise to intolerable levels and all of the person's coping strategies become exhausted. This is often the point at which the person's behaviour changes – they may stop meeting their responsibilities or cease caring for themselves.
3. *Resolution.* Because crises are often passing events, a resolution of some kind may occur; however, this resolution may be positive or negative. If the outcome is positive, then the person may have learned constructive ways of helping themselves in the future; alternatively, they may have developed ways of coping that are harmful.

Although crisis theory was built around the experiences of people who are normally psychologically healthy but are exposed to an extraordinary event, it has been successfully applied to people in mental health crisis. It is important to stress that mental health crisis is not a description of a specific event, but a subjective response to a set of circumstances which may lead to longer-term mental health difficulties, such as depression or adjustment disorder, if not resolved.

Mental health crisis and psychiatric emergencies are essentially different. A psychiatric emergency is when the person has gone beyond the breakdown phase and has adopted a maladaptive solution. A psychiatric emergency may require a more formal response if the maladaptive strategies involve risk to the person or to those around them, and these formal responses may include invoking mental health legislation or involving emergency services, as they often require immediate intervention.

The aim of crisis resolution is to help a person during the phase of breakdown or disorganization, when they may be amenable to learning or finding new ways of coping with their mental health difficulties.

DEVELOPMENT OF CRISIS SERVICES IN THE UK

The vast majority of mental health institutions were built as a result of the Lunatics Act 1845. They were large remote buildings that were viewed by the local populace with a significant degree of fear and stigmatisation. Many patients admitted to these 'asylums' were inappropriately placed (such as unmarried mothers or people with epilepsy) and received custodial-type care.

Advances in treatments in the 1950s and 1960s, such as the introduction of phenothiazine drugs and electroconvulsive therapy (ECT), enabled patients to be managed more effectively in the community. There was a peak of around 150,000 beds in 1955 which had reduced to around 22,300 by 2012;[3] between 1998 and 2012 alone,

there was a 39 per cent reduction in the number of beds.[4] This has been underpinned by a gradual programme of de-institutionalization, and a growing focus on services providing community-based care.

Based on the early pioneers, communities such as Dingleton in Scotland, Querido in Amsterdam and community-oriented developments in the USA,[5] the National Service Framework for Mental Health stipulated the development of 24-hour access and home treatment.[6] The NHS Plan in 2000 and further national policy[7] provided more detailed guidance for services to attain fidelity to the crisis model, including the size of home treatment caseloads, staffing ratios and funding requirements. The overall rationale for the development of Crisis Resolution and Home Treatment services across the UK includes:

- maintaining people within a familiar environment rather than removing them to a mental health facility; this maintains familial ties and relationships and people's integrity in the community setting;
- an overall reduction in reliance on inpatient settings, including the minimization of re-admissions to psychiatric facilities;
- improvement in context-driven coping strategies;
- congruence with user and carer preferences and feedback obtained via surveys and questionnaires;
- provision of a less stigmatizing alternative to inpatient care, which has an impact on prognosis and recovery;
- a more holistic approach to the service user's mental health within a social and cultural context.

However, it is clear that some people still require a period of hospital-based care, due to the presence of severe or critical risks or situational factors which impair the safe provision of intensive home-based treatment.

CORE FEATURES OF A CRHT

In 2000 the Department of Health set targets for mental health services in England to implement 335 crisis teams to treat 100,000 people by 2005,[8] with the aim of reducing the number and duration of psychiatric admissions by managing people who are in crisis in the least restrictive environment.

CRHT provides rapid response and assessment 24 hours a day, and offers intensive home-based treatment (the least restrictive environment) as an alternative to hospital admission. The core elements of CRHT are summarized as follows:

- providing a 24-hour mobile multidisciplinary workforce;
- targeting people who without CRHT intervention would be considered for admission to a mental health facility;
- responding rapidly to urgent requests for assessment, usually within a 0- to 4-hour timescale;

EVIDENCE BASE FOR CRHT IN THE UK

Following the introduction of crisis services from 2003 onwards, there was a considerable outpouring of research and evaluation of the changes introduced and the differences that they were making across the mental health pathway. There have been more than 30 research papers and other studies on CRHT, primarily with a focus on demonstrating whether or not they have made a difference to bed reduction and length of stay. Other outcomes that have been explored included the patient experience and

> **REFLECTION**
>
> Consider the bio-psychosocial factors which would determine hospital care versus home-based treatment.

During the emergence of Crisis Resolution and Home Treatment (CRHT) teams across the UK, a number of terms were used to describe their function. These include:

- home treatment teams;
- crisis assessment and treatment teams;
- rapid response service;
- crisis and home treatment teams;
- crisis resolution and home treatment teams;
- acute home treatment teams.

For the purposes of brevity, all crisis and home treatment services will be referred to as CRHT.

- having the capacity to provide at least daily visits (often more frequently) and to continue until the crisis is resolved;
- gatekeeping local acute inpatient beds;
- facilitating early discharge planning to reduce length of stay within a mental health facility;
- providing a range of psychosocial interventions which include medication management, practical advice or support, user and carer/family support, condition management and relapse prevention;
- joint working and appropriate referral on to other parts of the mental health pathway as indicated.

It has been acknowledged that there has been variation in the consistency of the provision of CRHT services, with a lack of fidelity to the recommended original model cited above. Many crisis services operate as an adjunct to community mental health teams and do not provide full 24-hour cover.

economic costs. More broad-based evaluations have considered not just the impact of the services on the pathway and beds provided across the UK, but also on matters such as the differences in structures and functions, and fidelity to the original model.

In summary, mental ill-health is the single largest cause of disability in the UK, contributing up to 22.8 per cent of the total burden.[9] The NHS has an annual expenditure of around £1.4 billion on adult mental health care,

£900 million of which is spent on hospital-based services. CRHT services account for £276 million each year.[10] Even though there were considerable guidance and targets regarding CRHT operations in England, more recent evaluations have pinpointed variations in the composition and practice of the teams. These evaluations have provided strong evidence that CRHT services in England and Wales have brought about a reduction in the number of admissions. However, considerable differences in the extent of bed usage and length of stay have been revealed, which may be underpinned by the variety in the composition and operation of crisis services.

A recent report from the Audit Commission in England undertook a review of resources used in adult mental health acute care pathways.[10] The Audit Commission identified a significant variation in admission rates after adjusting for age, sex and deprivation. One important issue that they addressed was the commitment to CRHT services, and they concluded that there was a variation in the effectiveness of CRHT teams in terms of gatekeeping. Published studies have considered the impact of CRHT, particularly upon admissions, but little or nothing has been written about the actual operation of these services and their cost-effectiveness.

There is mixed evidence regarding the effectiveness of CRHT services in reducing admissions and bed days in inpatient settings. There is some evidence that reductions in admissions do occur, accompanied by reductions in costs.[11] However, in 2011, Jacobs and Barrheno[12] concluded that there was 'no evidence' that crisis services have made any difference to admission rates in the UK. Several studies have demonstrated a reduction in informal admissions, but show an increase in compulsory admissions.[13]

More recent publications have identified a rise in completed suicides among service users who are under the care of CRHT services. The 2015 National Confidential Inquiry into Suicide and Homicide by People with Mental Illness stated that there were 1,333 suicides among mental health patients in England in 2011 – an increase from 1,175 in 2010. Suicides under CRHT are now three times greater than the number of deaths occurring in mental health inpatient settings in England, with an estimated 226 deaths in 2013.[14]

It is acknowledged within the literature that ongoing data collection, including randomized controlled trials and other further rigorous evaluation regarding the effectiveness of CRHT, is urgently required. Little evidence has thus far been gathered from carers and relatives regarding their experiences of mental health crisis services.

ACCESS AND ASSESSMENT

CASE STUDY 1

Mrs M is a 55-year-old married employed mother of an adult (Miss M). Mrs M was referred to the local crisis team in the context of a relapse of a transient psychotic episode. Mrs M presented with a range of acute clinical features, including elated mood, grossly disturbed sleep pattern and agitation with significant behavioural/functional changes.

SERVICE USER'S PERSPECTIVE

In a previous experience of a mental health crisis which resulted in admission to a psychiatric intensive care unit:

I woke up and didn't know where I was. The room was empty with a wooden bed in the middle of the floor. A stranger asked me if I would like some breakfast and I really had no idea who they were. This was a frightening time. Being taken out of my own environment and being in hospital was very scary and upsetting. Being able to stay in my own home with family around me, alongside knowing I had a team I could trust supporting me, reduced my anxiety and distress no end at this time.

CARER'S PERSPECTIVE

As a husband all you want to do is look after and protect your wife. When Mrs M was in hospital (the first time), I felt helpless and could see the fear in her eyes. Having restricted visiting times and leaving her in a bare room was heart-breaking. When she became unwell again, there was no question, we would do anything we could to keep her at home in her familiar, comfortable environment.

Mr M

One of the most important features of a fully functioning CRHT is to have clearly defined criteria for inclusion in the service, given the finite resources available. Only those people who would otherwise have been considered for admission are eligible for CRHT. If teams do not target the population correctly, then their capacity to provide safe and effective home treatment to people with severe mental health conditions or critical risks may be compromised.

The local CRHT service provides 24-hour telephonic access to triage to prioritize incoming demands. At the point of triage, an assessment by two clinicians can be arranged, usually within a 0- to 4-hour timescale. The assessment may take place in a variety of venues, such as GP surgeries, emergency departments, community settings or police suites, but it is preferable for this to be conducted in the person's home.

> ## REFLECTION
>
> Outline the reasons why an assessment in the person's home environment is preferable and why two clinicians are involved.

A prompt response to referrals alleviates distress, reassures carers and relatives and conveys the message that the situation is being taken seriously. This validates and improves engagement with the CRHT service.

A full bio-psychosocial assessment is completed, often involving relatives or carers. The assessment follows the principles of the Care Programme Approach (CPA), and covers a variety of topics related to social and physical health issues, previous risk events, current mental state, physical health, medicine reconciliation as well as a risk formulation. Please refer to chapter 37 for further information on the CPA and chapter 16 for more details on assessing the risk of suicide and self-harm.

> ## CARER'S PERSPECTIVE
>
> One of the most valuable aspects of the care we received as a family was having the same care team visit each day. Practically and understandably it was not possible to have the same person; however, it was possible to have three nurses who knew mum well. Our main nurse took the lead in meeting with the team and discussing our concerns. Following this, the home visits worked extremely well. The support of our main nurse was invaluable. We found having a plan extremely useful; it felt as though our nurse was there with us when we had plan A, B and C. Our experiences and concerns were always taken on board. For anyone working with a family in a crisis situation, making the family feel valued and included at this difficult time, I can say from my experience, is absolutely invaluable.
>
> *Miss M*

Many services no longer use a paper notes system and instead have electronic health care records available to practitioners, which reduces the necessity for service users

to be asked the same series of questions repeatedly and assessed on multiple occasions. As part of the assessment, people's strengths, resiliencies, competencies and resources are also identified. (Please refer to chapters 13, 14, and 15 for further information on assessment.)

The assessment is presented to the multidisciplinary team as soon as is practicable, to convey the formulation and propose a plan of care. This plan may require a timely medical review by a psychiatrist, the involvement of a pharmacist (Getting the Medicines Right 2),[15] social work input, or a mental health practitioner to provide structured home treatment and psychological interventions.

Working within a multidisciplinary framework allows a rich, multi-faceted approach to underpin people's care and treatment, and, for students, delivers a unique learning opportunity.

> ## REFLECTION
>
> What are the advantages and disadvantages of working within a full multidisciplinary team?

The input and contribution of significant others, family members or carers during the assessment process are invaluable. This provides an opportunity to attain corroborative information, to establish how robust the caring network is to be able to sustain the person in the home environment and also to share information and provide advice. Not all crisis assessments result in home-based treatment; a number of cases will be signposted to more appropriate services, such as non-statutory services, local planned care teams, drug and alcohol services or local authority agencies. A small number of referrals following assessment may require detention under the Mental Health Act or admission to hospital if home-based treatment is not deemed to be appropriate.

> ## CARER'S PERSPECTIVE
>
> Mum became unwell quite quickly. Initially, we contacted the GP who made a referral to the crisis team for assessment. Mum was unable to fully communicate with the team and was becoming quite distressed at being expected to do so. Initially, there was the assumption that mum would go into hospital, and we felt initially that our views about keeping mum at home were ignored. Our assessment with the psychiatrist was very positive. She was very interested in all of our views, wishes and concerns. We made a plan for mum to stay at home while it was practical to do so and felt very involved with the care. We understood that mum is the centre of the care and her needs must come first.
>
> *Miss M*

RISK ASSESSMENT

There are several definitions of the term 'risk', the majority of which associate the term with a negative consequence such as harm or dangerousness. However, there is a more contemporary definition offered by Morgan in 2004: 'the likelihood of an event happening with potentially harmful or beneficial outcomes for self and for others'[16] (p.18). In this context risk can be viewed as a potentially positive experience and that exposure to risk, if carefully managed, can promote the recovery process. More information on recovery and risk management is available in chapter 36.

SERVICE USER'S PERSPECTIVE

As I was able to stay at home during my episode of psychosis, it took away the unfamiliarity of a hospital environment. I could do simple things like sitting in my favourite chair, knowing where the bathroom is and going into the garden. This reduced my anxiety and also provided some comfort for my family.

By facilitating the development of more constructive coping strategies, CRHT is fundamentally opposed to the traditional, high-security, containment approaches to managing risk. Instead, CRHT favours what is known as positive risk taking, which has a significant influence upon the recovery pathway through the use of joint approaches to promoting independence and the development of contingency plans to manage future relapse periods.

Positive risk taking has been defined in the literature as 'the weighing up of potential benefits and harms of exercising one choice of action over another; the development of plans and actions that reflect the positive potentials and stated priorities of the service users; and using available resources and support to achieve the desired outcomes and to minimize the potential harmful outcomes'[16] (p.18).

INTENSIVE HOME-BASED TREATMENT

A CRHT has the capacity to provide twice-daily visits, if clinically indicated. The plan of care (including specific goal descriptions) is negotiated and developed in collaboration with the service user, carers and other agencies involved. See chapter 50 for further discussion on collaborative care planning with service users and carers. At times, CRHT can act as an augmentation service to local community-based teams, such as Early Intervention in Psychosis (EIP) (see chapter 45) or community mental health teams (providing out-of-hours cover, for example). The goals of the crisis service may include stabilization through effective regular

In any risk assessment process, CRHT services will consider the following factors:

- previous self-harm behaviours, including longitudinal risks;
- previous situations/triggers or precursors of harm to others;
- previous assessment and treatment plans and a description of the response by the service user;
- underlying causes and prognosis;
- mental state or impression;
- protective or mediating factors;
- incongruencies between observed and reported risk behaviours;
- vulnerability of others;
- available resources;
- external factors or hazards.

Suicide risk is one of the main concerns facing a CRHT team. One helpful model to assist staff who work in crisis services is that of Thomas Joiner.[17,18] Building on Shneidman's previous work,[19] Joiner proposes the following elements to guide practitioners in identifying suicide risk:

- a degree of *perturbation*, which is a high level of distress or turmoil and has been described as psych-ache;
- a perceived *burden* to others;
- lack of belonging or *connectedness*;
- an *acquired ability* for lethal action in which a person overcomes their fears to engage in risk-taking behaviour. Chapter 16 considers the assessment of suicide and self-harm.

REFLECTION

How might a person in mental health crisis think about the pathway to suicide?

(often daily) support, in the least restrictive environment. The CRHT team provides help for the user to cope with associated difficult social or domestic situations, while at the same time identifying and utilizing resiliency in the service user's personal repertoire or peer network.

The range of interventions can be varied, but it relies heavily on the degree of engagement and therapeutic alliance with the service user and their family. In the early phases of home-based treatment, a number of practitioners may visit the home, which service users often find very difficult to accommodate. In due course, a smaller number of staff provides continuity and clinical consistency, which improves the user's experience of the crisis pathway.

The range of psychosocial interventions provided by CRHT may include the following:

- ongoing risk assessment and risk management;
- practical help through liaison with local housing services or other agencies, or advice regarding debts or benefits;
- physical health monitoring providing electroconvulsive therapy and clozapine initiation in the community – this is becoming increasingly common in CRHT;
- medication management – a significant aspect of home-based treatment which includes the supervision of prescribed medications; the approach must be congruent with national standards (Getting the Medicines Right 2);[15]
- structured psychological interventions to address condition management and relapse prevention – WRAP planning may be a component of this;
- carer and family interventions and young carers' assessments – without consideration of the critical input of families during a mental health crisis, hospital admissions would probably increase;
- a range of psycho-education packages specifically related to particular mental health conditions, including treatment options and concordance issues.

The CRHT may provide a crisis respite placement as an alternative to hospital admission during the period of home-based treatment. This is usually for a fixed period, with ongoing support and intervention from the CRHT. Not all services across the UK have this facility, which reportedly service users find much less traumatic and less stigmatizing than traditional hospital based care.[20] (See chapter 56 for more information on assertive outreach.)

In terms of the practitioner skills required to provide intensive home-based treatment, a range of attributes and clinical skills are needed in order to provide high-quality, safe, effective, evidence-based care. These attributes may include being compassionate, respectful, empathic and confident with the ability to inject hope and work with a person's strengths. All these features are congruent within the '6 Cs'[21] (Compassion, Caring, Courage, Commitment, Competency and Communication) and have been well described by Barker.[22] These personal and professional attributes are central to the essence of nursing.

The necessary clinical skills include being able to work within professional boundaries; being able to take positive risks, be decisive and adaptable; and being aware of a range of mental health conditions and treatment options. These clinical skills can be viewed as secondary to the human/ personal interventions which mental health nurses provide at each contact, in order to potentiate growth through lived experience, which Barker describes as 'human helping'[23] (p.13). Chapter 3 focuses on developing and maintaining therapeutic relationships.

Working with people in crisis requires sensitivity, flexibility and creativity. The practitioner needs to remain aware of the issues of power, difference and dominance which have traditionally existed between those diagnosed with a mental health condition and professionals. Crisis workers must have a highly developed understanding of issues related to cultural and social difference. Consideration should be given to people's ethnicity, class, gender, sexual orientation and ability during an episode of home-based treatment. The service users and their families can expect to be treated with compassion, respect and dignity throughout their contact with the mental health pathway. Genuineness and empathy are the foundations of the craft of nursing, honed over a career's-worth of experience, or, as suggested by Barker, 'sharpened with every encounter'[23] (p.8).

CARER'S PERSPECTIVE

The home environment meant mum had us there and followed her normal routine as much as possible so we felt this reduced distress. During home-based treatment, we were also able to recognize very subtle changes which may indicate agitation and address this through our plan. I feel this is because me and Miss M knew Mrs M so well and could see these things quickly; however, in hospital these may not have been as quickly picked up. It was a challenging time, but less so than having Mrs M in hospital. We are a team, a unit, and being granted that trust and support from the health service to use our strengths and love I have no doubt shaped Mrs M's recovery.

Mr M

CARER'S PERSPECTIVE

Even when mum was in the depths of her psychosis, she could do these things almost on auto pilot and it was good to see some 'normality' at this time. The home environment meant mum had us there and followed her normal routine as much as possible so we felt this reduced distress. Mum had previously been on a psychiatric intensive care ward and her levels of anxiety and distress were very clearly elevated. However, this time in the home environment these levels were certainly nowhere near as bad. While living through this scary experience, anything to reduce levels of fear, such as a familiar environment, was very positive.

Miss M

As the crisis begins to resolve, CRHT teams engage in a collaborative approach with the user and carers to plan for discharge. During this exit planning phase, a variety of structured work needs to be completed, including crisis and contingency planning, underpinned by WRAP principles. There is often a short period of joint working with colleagues (if a transfer of care to another part of the mental health pathway has been identified) or signposting and referral on to non-statutory services, following agreement between the service user, carers and family alongside crisis service staff.

The discharge planning phase is an important component of intensive home treatment provided by CRHT teams. It is completed in the hope that the more effective the relapse prevention plan is, the less likely the person will require a future intervention from CRHT.

CONCLUSION

CRHT services are associated with the augmentation of community-based care for people suffering from acute mental health conditions for whom hospital admission is being considered. A fully functioning CRHT team, with high fidelity to the original model, has been identified as improving users' and carers' experience of crisis intervention and the prevention of future admission to hospital. The CRHT team attains this by maintaining the integrity of users and families in the community, which reduces the effects of institutionalization and stigma on a person's mental health care. However, CRHT requires a skilled multidisciplinary workforce with well-developed assessment and therapy skills in order to provide effective, evidence-based care to vulnerable people in the community.

Within CRHT services, despite the high volume of referrals and home-based treatment cases through the crisis pathway, a high degree of job satisfaction and a low incidence of burnout has been identified.[24] Rigorous clinical supervision and case management systems are required in order to reduce the negative impact on the workforce. Informal and formal mechanisms, such as debriefing and live supervision, also have a part to play in the longer-term effectiveness of crisis services.

There must be an acknowledgement that, without the invaluable contribution of carers, relatives and other significant others in the home treatment package, the viability and effectiveness of crisis services would suffer. Being invited into people's homes at the most difficult and stressful point in their lives is a huge privilege. Crisis staff are grateful for and remain impressed with the astonishing degree of care and resilience of service users and their families.

The practitioners will have a more strengths-based rather than problem-saturated perspective. The use of appreciative comments, and the provision of compliments where positive strategies are identified, amplifies the skills, resources and competencies of the service user.

SERVICE USER'S PERSPECTIVE

I am able to recall towards the end of my care with the crisis team. I felt very included in sessions when the crisis team visited. A small issue was going over old ground and having to repeat stories and past events which could be distressing. However, we were able to share this with the team and our views were taken on board.

SERVICE USER'S PERSPECTIVE

Being able to stay in my own home was really therapeutic. I felt more secure in my familiar environment rather than being removed to a hospital away from my family.

CARER'S PERSPECTIVE

Overall, we feel with the help and support from the crisis team we were able to provide the best care for Mrs M at the time of crisis. The familiar environment, including the whole family in decisions and being able to be involved with Mrs M's care as the people who know her the most was invaluable. We have no doubt this contributed to Mrs M's steady, successful recovery.

References

1. Minghella E. Home based emergency treatment. *Mental Health Practice* 1998; **2**: 10–14.
2. Caplan G. *An approach to community mental health.* London: Tavistock, 1964.
3. CAAPC (Commission on Acute Adult Psychiatric Care). *Improving acute inpatient psychiatric care for adults in England.* London: CAAPC, 2015.
4. King's Fund. *Mental health under pressure.* London: King's Fund, 2015.
5. Stein LL, Test MA. Alternative to mental hospital treatment. Conceptual model, treatment programme and clinical evaluation. *Archives of General Psychiatry* 1980; **27**: 392–7.
6. Department of Health. *National Service Framework: Mental Health.* London: Department of Health, 1999.
7. Department of Health. *The Mental Health Policy Implementation Guide.* London: HMSO, 2001.
8. Department of Health. *NHS Plan.* London: HMSO, 2000.

9. Department of Health. *No health without mental health.* London: HMSO, 2012.

10. Audit Commission. *Maximising resources in adult mental health.* London: Audit Commission, 2010.

11. McCrone P, Johnson S, Nolan F, Pilling S, Sandor A, Honet J, McKenzie N, White R, Bebbington P. Impact of a crisis resolution team on service costs in the UK. *Psychiatrist* 2009; **33**: 17–19.

12. Jacobs R, Barren, E. Impact of crisis resolution and home treatment teams on psychiatric admissions in England. *British Journal of Psychiatry* 2011; **199**: 71–6.

13. Carpenter RA, Falkenburg J, White TP, Tracy DK. Crisis teams: systematic review of their effectiveness in practice. *Psychiatric Bulletin* 2013; **37**: 232–7.

14. National Confidential Inquiry into Suicide and Homicide by People with Mental Illness. Annual Report July 2013.

15. Davies P, Taylor J. *Getting the medicines right 2.* London: National Mental Health Development Unit, 2010.

16. Morgan S. Positive risk-taking: an idea whose time has come. *Health Care Risk Report* 2004; **10**(10): 18–19.

17. Joiner T. *Why people die by suicide.* Cambridge, MA: Harvard University Press, 2005.

18. Joiner T. *Myths about suicide.* Cambridge, MA: Harvard University Press, 2010.

19. Shneidman E. Suicide thoughts and reflections 1960–1980. In: *Suicide and life threatening behaviours.* New York: Human Sciences Press, 1981: 195–364.

20. Hodge S, Buley N (eds). *Home Treatment Accreditation Scheme (HTAS). Standards for home treatment teams – second edition.* London: Royal College of Psychiatrists, 2015.

21. Commissioning Board Chief Nursing Officer and DH Chief Nursing Advisor. *Compassion in practice.* London: Department of Health, 2012.

22. Barker V, Taylor M, Kader I, Stewart K, Le Fevre M. Impact of CRHT services on user experience and admission to psychiatric hospital. *Psychiatric Bulletin* 2011; **35**: 106–10.

23. Barker P (ed.). *Psychiatric and mental health nursing. The craft of caring,* 2nd edn. Boca Raton: Hodder Arnold, 2009.

24. Nelson T, Johnson S, Beggington P. Satisfaction and burnout among staff of crisis resolution, assertive outreach and community mental health teams. A multicentre cross sectional survey. *Journal of Social Psychiatry and Psychological Epidemiology* 2009; **44**(7): 541–9.

Further reading

Appleby L, Sheehan A, Mahony J. *Mental health policy implementation guide: crisis resolution /home treatment teams.* London: Department of Health, 2001.

Crompton N, Daniel D. *Guidance statement on fidelity and best practice for crisis services.* London: Department of Health/Care Services Improvement Partnership, 2007.

Johnson S, Needle J, Thornicroft G. *Crisis resolution and home treatment in mental health.* Cambridge: Cambridge University Press, 2008.

Mental Health Crisis Care Concordat. *Improving outcomes for people experiencing mental health crisis.* London: Department of Health and Concordat Signatories, 2014.

Relevant web pages

CQC online. Thematic review of mental health crisis care. http://www.cqc.org.uk/content/thematic-review-mental-health-crisis-care

HelpGuide.org. Suicide prevention. http://www.helpguide.org/home-pages/suicide-prevention.htm

If U Care Share Foundation. www.ifucareshare.co.uk
This is a charity promoting emotional well-being in young people and supporting families affected by suicide.

MIND. www.mind.org.uk/crisis-care

47 Psychopharmacology and mental health

CARL HOLVEY AND NIKOLA NIKOLIĆ

LEARNING OUTCOMES

- To have an awareness of the underlying principles of the pharmacology of receptors and ligands.

- To describe how the pharmacology of mental illness and medicines used to treat mental illness affects the symptomology and side effects a service user may experience.

SUMMARY OF KEY POINTS

- The psychopharmacology and concepts behind medicines used to treat mental illness are important subjects, because of their role in the practical care of a service user.

- Clinicians need to know why adverse effects occur and why the management recommended should help at a cellular or chemical level.

- Physical health should be monitored while using medicines to treat illnesses.

- Clinicians must be aware of the theory behind the therapeutic efficacy of the medicines used to treat these conditions where it exists, as this enables them to change the treatment care plan in order to improve the service user's experience.

INTRODUCTION

Having an understanding of the underlying pharmacology of mental illnesses and the medicines used to treat them improves our ability to adjust and optimize the treatment given to a service user. This in turn enables monitoring and subsequent interventions they receive as a result.

CONCEPTS OF PHARMACOLOGY

The first concept to understand is that of receptor and ligands. Here, the idea of a 'lock and key' is useful. For a process in the cells in the body to change at a molecular level, a key (otherwise known as a ligand) needs to fit into a receptor (a lock) in order for that change to occur. The ligand may act at a receptor site, thus producing a variety of effects.

There are a number of types of ligand (key):

- *Agonist.* This is a ligand that activates the receptor (a key that opens the door). This activation initiates changes in cell functioning, e.g. dopamine agonists, levodopa at the dopamine receptor used in Parkinson's disease.

- *Antagonist.* This is a ligand that binds to the receptor, but does not initiate any changes in cell activity (a key that locks the door). For example, antipsychotics are dopamine antagonists. They stop the neurotransmitter dopamine from activating the dopamine receptor. This type of antagonism is non-competitive.
- *Partial agonist/antagonist:* This is a ligand that activates a receptor and produces activation/stops the activation at the receptor, but not as much as other ligands would (a key that opens the lock a little bit and by doing so stops another key from opening it fully), e.g. aripiprazole, an antipsychotic, is a partial dopamine and a specific serotonin subtype receptor agonist, while being an antagonist at a different serotonin subtype receptor.
- *Reversible competitive antagonist.* These ligands bind to the receptor without activating it, and in doing so they stop the agonist from binding to the same receptor, e.g. flumazenil, a benzodiazepine receptor antagonist which is used in benzodiazepine overdoses. This type of antagonism is reversible because the receptor can still be activated in the presence of the additional agonist, because the agonist is able to displace the antagonist.
- *Irreversible competitive antagonist.* Similar to a reversible competitive antagonist, but the additional agonist cannot activate the receptor because it is not able to displace it from the receptor, due to irreversibly formed bonds between the receptor and the antagonist, e.g. monoamine oxidase inhibitors (MAOIs) such as tranylcypromine, an antidepressant.

The most discussed ligands in psychiatry are neurochemicals (chemicals in the brain) that work at nerve endings. The gap between one nerve and another is known as the synapse. Neurochemicals released from one nerve pass through the synapse and act on the end of the next nerve cell to carry on the message (transmission). The main neurochemicals of interest to us, for the purposes of understanding the concepts of psychopharmacology, are dopamine (DA), noradrenaline (NA), and serotonin (5-HT).

Receptor concepts

A receptor is a site where a ligand has its effect. Most commonly in mental health, affected receptors that produce the therapeutic effect are proteins found at the end or beginning of nerve cells. Medicines used in mental health have their therapeutic effect by causing nerve cells to transmit electrical impulses either more or less frequently, depending on the medicine in question.

- Binding affinity describes how tightly a ligand attaches to the receptor and how strongly it affects the activity of the receptor with which it is associated. A ligand that binds tightly and has a strong effect at a receptor is said to have a 'high affinity' for the receptor.
- How a receptor causes changes to a nerve ending or cell depends on the type of receptor. A receptor can cause changes in how easily chemicals or molecules pass in or out of a cell (e.g. sodium/potassium pump), or it could initiate a change in activity of enzymes or chemicals within the cell (an intracellular message, e.g. G-coupled proteins).
- Some receptors may have a number of different versions of the same receptor, each with a slightly different role and distribution within the body, e.g. a DA receptor may have seven or more subtypes D_1, D_2, etc.

> ### REFLECTION
>
> - What other medicines do you know where the actual drug being given is the molecule that activates or inhibits a receptor from working?
> - Why do you think learning about the pharmacology of a medicine is important for safety?

NEUROBIOLOGICAL UNDERSTANDING OF MENTAL ILLNESS

This section describes some of the neurobiological ideas about how changes in the brain might be responsible for symptoms seen in mental illness. (See chapter 12 for a more in-depth review of symptomatology and the differentiation of illnesses.)

Depression

Medicines that affect 5-HT, NA and DA, such as tricyclic antidepressants (TCAs) and MAOIs, have been used since the 1960s to treat depression.

Evidence that low levels of NA, 5-HT and DA cause depression has been found by measuring their metabolites (the broken down molecules) in the brain. However, these results were not entirely convincing, because there are also environmental factors that cause depression. Depression is also linked to changes in hormones, such as cortisol, which affect levels of monoamines such as NA and 5-HT.

It has been hypothesized that 5-HT is the major neurotransmitter involved in the development of biological depression. 5-HT is produced in the brain from tryptophan, which is in turn produced from tyramine in the diet. 5-HT is stored in sacs or 'vesicles' at the nerve endings, ready for release into the synapse (the gap between nerve cells) once activated. When released into the synapse, 5-HT can activate the receptor on the preceding receptor, be transported back into the pre-synaptic nerve by a reuptake transporter enzyme and then be broken down and inactivated by monoamine oxidase (MAO) or put back into a vesicle for reuse.[1]

Selective serotonin reuptake inhibitors (SSRIs) work by stopping the 5-HT transporter enzyme from removing the 5-HT from the synapse (located from the mid-brain raphe to prefrontal cortex), extending the activity of 5-HT at the receptors. MAOIs work by stopping the breakdown of 5-HT in the nerve endings, hence increasing the availability of 5-HT to be put in vesicles ready for release on activation. TCAs block the uptake of amines by nerve terminals by competing with the binding site of the transport protein, having the most inhibitory effect on the NA and 5-HT reuptake and less so of DA.

Bipolar affective disorder (BPAD)

The neurobiology of BPAD is startlingly complex, and a variety of hypotheses have been generated. In recent times there is a growing belief that BPAD is a psychotic disorder and should primarily be treated as such.[2]

Gamma-aminobutyric acid (GABA) is the principal inhibitory neurotransmitter (neurochemical that stops rapid firing of nerves) in the brain. Medicines that are known to enhance the effect of GABA are known to have a positive effect on the symptoms of BPAD.

Glutamate is the principal excitatory neurotransmitter in the brain. Lithium is known to lower its levels in the brain, perhaps indicating a mechanism of action.

A communication pathway within the cell is also thought to be affected (phosphoinositide (PI) cycle), which causes inositol to be raised. An enzyme known as glycogen synthase kinase 3-beta (GSK3ß) is involved in the process of carrying the message from the DA receptor into the cell. It may be that there is a genetic malfunction in this enzyme in BPAD, and lithium may also lower its effect; however, a clinical effect of the GSK3ß enzyme abnormality is yet to be proven.

In line with guidance from the National Institute for Health and Care Excellence (NICE) and the British Association of Psychopharmacology (BAP), the focus of pharmacological treatment of BPAD is on mania and depression, and the most commonly used classes of medicines used are antipsychotics, mood stabilizers, antidepressants and benzodiazepines (BDZ).

In acute mania, it is essential to treat as quickly as possible. Medicines such as antidepressants are stopped, as these contribute to manic presentation. Note that other medicines may also induce mania, most commonly stimulants and non-psychotropic medicines such as corticosteroids (for example, prednisolone). Antipsychotics are the first-line treatment, as they have rapid anti-manic effects. When the symptoms are not as severe, lithium could be considered as an anti-manic, particularly in patients who have

previously responded well to it. In cases where sedation is required, BDZ are found to be effective in the short term, especially as these can be used orally and/or intramuscularly. There is growing evidence that the combination of an antipsychotic and a mood stabilizer is more effective than a mood stabilizer on its own. As in all other disorders, the choice of treatment should therefore always depend on the severity of the symptoms, side effects, previous treatment responses, prophylactic options for the future, comorbidities and patient preference.

Unlike in recurrent depression, also referred to as unipolar depression, bipolar depression is characterized by psychotic symptoms, diurnal mood variation, excessive sleepiness, and a greater number of episodes with shorter duration. The aim of the treatment of bipolar depression is first to optimize existing mood stabilizers, as often relapses occur due to non-compliance or sub-therapeutic doses, and only when this cannot be achieved are antidepressants added, with extreme caution. The antidepressant class of choice for the treatment of bipolar depression is SSRIs. SSRIs have clinical evidence supporting their use (in combination with an antipsychotic). TCAs are more likely to cause a switch from depression to mania, and are therefore the least preferred option of antidepressants used in bipolar depression. Any antidepressant should be used at the lowest effective dose, and stopped as soon as the depressive episode resolves.

Once acute episodes of BPAD are resolved, the goal of long-term treatment is future prevention of relapses. As per NICE guidelines, first-line treatment includes valproate, lithium and olanzapine. When monotherapy with any of these stops being effective, another monotherapy option should be commenced prior to using combination treatment (that is, a mood stabilizer and an antipsychotic). Alternatively, agents such as lamotrigine have been found to be particularly effective in BPAD with predominantly depressive episodes. Among the above-mentioned agents, evidence has found that lithium is effective in both manic and depressive episodes, and may be better at preventing mania; valproate is equally effective in mania and depression, and olanzapine is better at preventing mania than depression. Treatment in the post-acute phase of BPAD should last for at least 2 years, and in instances where there is a higher risk of relapse, it may need to be longer.

REFLECTION

We know very little for sure about how the biology of bipolar affective disorder results in symptomatic improvement. How will you decide which medicine is the most appropriate to treat a service user?

Schizophrenia/psychosis

Psychotic illnesses may be considered to be on a spectrum, and include schizophrenia, BPAD, delusional disorder and psychotic depression.

The DA hypothesis has been the basis of treatment research for schizophrenia for many years. Because the symptoms of schizophrenia are treated by DA blockade, this implies that the illness must be caused by an over-activity of DA.[3] Apart from environmental factors affecting the prognosis and time course of the development of psychotic illness, other pharmacological theories have been proposed: the glutamate hypothesis (involving abnormalities in glutamate transmission), the DA imbalance hypothesis (involving underactivity of dopamine in the frontal cortex) and abnormal 5-HT receptor genes.

Insomnia

Insomnia is a symptom of many mental health illnesses. Ensuring adequate treatment of any underlying comorbidity is important to prevent the need for additional treatment for insomnia. Rapid eye movement (REM) sleep is associated with the 'dream state' and is considered the beneficial element of sleep, while slow wave sleep is the deep sleep where the metabolic rate and steroid secretion are at their lowest.

BDZ and other hypnotics extend the total duration of REM sleep. However, due to tolerance, hangover and dependence effects, long-term administration is ill-advised.

Melatonin is a hormone released by the pineal and adrenal glands at night and is responsible in part for the circadian rhythm of the body. It mainly works on G-coupled receptors found in the brain and retina. The exact action of the melatonin receptor in the cells is unknown. Melatonin can be administered in oral form, and it is currently only licensed for short-term use as monotherapy for insomnia in people over the age of 55.

Anxiety

Anxiety presents as a mixture of psychological, physical and behavioural symptoms. It can generally be divided into: generalized anxiety disorder (GAD), panic disorder, social phobia, specific phobias, post-traumatic stress disorder (PTSD) and obsessive–compulsive disorder (OCD) (see chapter 12 for more on the classification of mental illness). Commonly, all anxiety disorders present clinically with the following features: fear or worry, sleep disturbance, concentration problems, dry mouth, sweating, palpitations,

gastrointestinal discomfort, restlessness, shortness of breath and avoidance behaviour. Additionally, each anxiety disorder has specific features – for example, a person with GAD experiences persistent, excessive and inappropriate anxiety on most days for at least 6 months; while a person with PTSD suffers intense fear or horror associated with exposure to an earlier traumatic event. To meet the diagnostic criteria, the above symptoms must be prolonged, cause significant distress and impair social or daily functioning. In two-thirds of the cases, patients with anxiety suffer with other disorders, and in many such instances treatment of the underlying disorder improves the anxiety.

The main guidelines for treatment of anxiety, provided by NICE and the BAP, advise that the first-line treatment should be psychological therapies, particularly cognitive behavioural therapy (CBT), which has the most evidence of effectiveness (see chapter 40 for more on CBT).

Treatment with medicines is reserved for moderate to severe anxiety, either as monotherapy or in conjunction with CBT. Most commonly, this includes antidepressants as the first-line treatment. Compared to depression, treatment of anxiety needs to continue for a longer time in order to produce results. SSRIs should be commenced at half the initial dose used in depression, as the symptoms tend to worsen in the initial weeks of treatment. TCAs, while effective for panic disorder, OCD and PTSD, have considerably more side effects than SSRIs (see the section on TCAs below). Venlafaxine has proved to be effective for all anxiety disorders but, like TCAs, the side effects associated with its use and discontinuation symptoms following withdrawal may be bothersome. Lastly, NICE recommends mirtazapine for use in PTSD. The minimum length of treatment with antidepressants is 6 months for GAD and panic disorder, and 12 months for PTSD, OCD and social phobia, although sufferers often continue with treatment beyond this length of time.

BDZ have been used in the treatment of anxiety for a long time. However, due to risks associated with developing dependence and tolerance, their use should be limited to the shortest possible time (2 to 4 weeks), at the lowest effective dose. They may be effective in severe and disabling anxiety disorders, but also at the start of treatment with SSRIs. Other pharmacological options include promethazine (a sedating antihistamine) for use as a short-term sedative, and pregabalin for use in GAD, while beta-blockers such as propranolol may be useful when anxiety is followed by physical symptoms such as palpitations, tremor, sweating and shortness of breath.

MEDICATION CLASSES

Benzodiazepines (BDZ)

BDZ belong to a group of medicines called anxiolytics. They are indicated for the short-term relief of severe anxiety.

They should not be prescribed on a long-term basis, and should not be prescribed for stress-related symptoms, unhappiness or minor physical issues, because that is inappropriate.

When prescribing BDZ, they should be prescribed at the lowest effective dose for the shortest amount of time possible, to avoid the risk of developing dependence. This is particularly an issue in patients who are likely to abuse other substances, or in disorders such as personality disorder.

BDZ relieve anxiety, cause sedation, relax muscles, stop seizures and may cause memory loss. These actions are caused by activation of GABA-mediated inhibition in the central nervous system.[4]

BDZ are usually taken by mouth, and are broken down by the liver. Despite being central depressants, they induce respiratory depression at higher doses. Their main side effects include drowsiness, impaired alertness, agitation and ataxia. Older people are especially sensitive to the effects of BDZ. Due to their centrally depressant activity, BDZ have even greater effects if given with alcohol, or other sedating medicines such as antihistamines. This should therefore be avoided.

Typical examples of BDZ include short-acting lorazepam and temazepam, and longer-acting nitrazepam and diazepam.

REFLECTION

What other strategies could you suggest to a service user to avoid the need to use medicines to help sleep?

Antipsychotic medicines

Antipsychotics, also known as neuroleptics, block DA receptors, and are licensed for use in psychoses. The therapeutic effect of antipsychotics in psychosis is due to DA blockade in mesolimbic/mesocortical pathways. DA is blocked in other parts of the brain, e.g. basal ganglia, causing side effects, such as movement disorders and endocrine side effects (hyperprolactinaemia).

Antipsychotics are broadly split into first generation (typical) and second generation (atypical). First generation antipsychotics are associated with causing hyperprolactinaemia and EPSE, while second generation antipsychotics have a greater propensity for metabolic side-effects. Antipsychotics are also associated with other side effects such as postural hypotension, dry mouth, constipation, increased appetite and weight gain.

First generation antipsychotics are: phenothiazines (e.g. chlorpromazine, pipotiazine, fluphenazine), butyrophenones (e.g. haloperidol,) thioxanthenes (e.g. flupentixol, zuclopenthixol) and benzamides (e.g. sulpiride).

Second generation antipsychotics differ from each other in their side-effect profiles; they are broadly as clinically effective as each other, with the exception of clozapine, which is superior at treating the symptoms of psychosis in comparison to all other antipsychotics. Side-effect profiles

can be explained by the activity at the receptors; for example, clozapine blocks DA, but also blocks serotonergic, adrenergic and muscarinic receptors. 5-HT receptor block may cause sedation and increased appetite leading to weight gain; adrenaline receptor block may cause changes in blood pressure and pulse, such as postural hypotension or tachycardia; and blockade of muscarinic receptors may cause dry mouth, urinary retention, constipation and drowsiness. Other important medicines in this group are olanzapine, risperidone, quetiapine, aripiprazole and paliperidone.

REFLECTION

- With the exception of clozapine, all antipsychotics are equally effective for schizophrenia. How would you choose the best treatment for a service user?

- What physical monitoring does a service user need when treatment is initiated?

- What things do you think a service user finds important when choosing treatment, as compared to what a professional thinks is important?

Antidepressants

Antidepressants are a group of medicines used to treat affective disorders, particularly moderate to severe depression associated with psychomotor and physiological changes. They should not be used in mild depression, as the treatment of choice in mild depression is psychological therapy (see chapter 40).

The main principle of action of antidepressants is the inhibition of the reuptake of norepinephrine (NE) and/or 5-HT, which in turn causes an increase of 5-HT available for the cells to use. Because this process of increase in 5-HT is quite gradual, most antidepressants take at least 2 to 3 weeks before they start exerting their benefits.[5] It is during this period that there is an increased risk of agitation, anxiety and suicidal ideation. All antidepressants are also known to cause hyponatremia, especially in the elderly population and possibly in patients with inappropriate secretion of antidiuretic hormone. Signs of hyponatremia include drowsiness, confusion and convulsions.

Antidepressants are split into SSRIs, TCAs and a third group that cannot easily be classified according to their mechanism of actions.

TCAs typically inhibit the reuptake of NE and/or 5-HT. They also block muscarinic, adrenergic and histaminergic receptors, causing side effects. They are well absorbed orally and have half-lives of 4 to 24 hours, apart from nortriptyline which has a long half-life of 24 to 96 hours. TCAs should be used with caution in the elderly, as they cause confusion, drowsiness, dry mouth, blurred vision, constipation and urinary retention, and in those patients who have cardiovascular disease. TCAs are particularly dangerous in overdose due to a high rate of fatality. Typically, dosulepin and amitriptyline are associated with the highest risk. TCAs should never be stopped abruptly because they may cause withdrawal symptoms, including chills, myalgia, sweating, headache, nausea and insomnia. The main side effects of TCAs in addition to those just described are postural hypotension, tachycardia and changes in electrocardiogram (ECG). Typical examples of TCAs are amitriptyline, clomipramine, lofepramine and nortriptyline.

SSRIs selectively inhibit the reuptake of 5-HT, increasing the amount of 5-HT available to activate the next nerve cell. They are well absorbed orally and have half-lives of 15 to 24 hours, fluoxetine having the longest (24 to 96 hours). Similarly to TCAs, sudden withdrawal of SSRIs may cause gastrointestinal disturbances, headache, anxiety, flu-like symptoms, electric shock sensation in the head, neck and spine, and sweating. Among the SSRIs, withdrawal effects are most commonly seen with paroxetine. Side effects SSRIs most commonly cause are nausea, vomiting, diarrhoea and constipation and they may also cause sexual dysfunction. SSRIs are now commonly used first-line antidepressants because, unlike TCAs, they are not associated with risks in cardiovascular disease and overdoses are less dangerous. Examples include sertraline, citalopram, fluoxetine and paroxetine.

The third group of commonly used antidepressants includes venlafaxine, mirtazapine and trazodone.

Venlafaxine inhibits the reuptake of both serotonin and norepinephrine in a non-selective manner. It is commonly referred to as a serotonin and norepinephrine reuptake inhibitor (SNRI). Venlafaxine has a very short half-life of 5 hours. Unlike TCAs, venlafaxine does not cause sedation or dry mouth, constipation or urinary retention. However, it is associated with a higher risk of withdrawal effects compared with other antidepressants, and can increase blood pressure at higher doses. Duloxetine is another example of an SNRI that is associated with an increase in blood pressure. Both venlafaxine and duloxetine are used in major depression, but are also licensed for use in GAD.

Mirtazapine and trazodone are sedative antidepressants. Mirtazapine increases the transmission of NA and 5-HT centrally by blocking α_2, 5-HT_2 and 5-HT_3 receptors, and has a half-life of 20 to 40 hours. Trazodone is a 5-HT uptake inhibitor which also blocks 5-HT_2 and H_1 receptors and has a half-life of 6 to 12 hours; it works similarly to mirtazapine but is in fact structurally related to TCAs. The side effects most often associated with mirtazapine are weight gain and sedation. Trazodone, unlike TCAs, does not have any cardiotoxic side effects, and in addition to being an antidepressant, it also has anxiolytic properties. Its main side effects are nausea and sedation.

REFLECTION

Given that it takes up to a month for antidepressants to exert their effects, what factors other than the efficacy do you think influence a service user's response to antidepressants?

Medicines for affective disorders

VALPROATE

Valproate exists in three forms: sodium valproate, semi-sodium valproate and valproic acid. The body breaks down both valproate and semi-sodium valproate to its active component, valproic acid, at the active site. For the purposes of understanding the basic concepts of how it works, all forms of valproate will simply be referred to as valproate.[6]

Valproate acts on the central nervous system, by potentiating the inhibitory action of GABA, somewhat similarly to BDZ, thereby reducing the symptoms of mania discussed earlier in the chapter. Its most common side effects are nausea and weight gain, and in some people it may cause lethargy, confusion, tremor and hair loss. Most of these side effects are dose-related; in other words, reducing the dose may improve the side effects.

One of the most important side effects of valproate is that it is teratogenic. This means that in women of child-bearing age, valproate may cause defects in the development of the fetus. As such, health care professionals must always ensure that this patient group receives counselling on effective contraception. When a pregnancy is planned, valproate can be changed to a suitable alternative (see chapter 50 for more on collaborative care planning with service users and carers).

PREGABALIN

Pregabalin is licensed for the treatment of GAD. However, NICE recommends that pregabalin is used for this indication only as an alternative to SSRIs and SNRIs (discussed above).[7] Pregabalin is an analogue of GABA, and as much as its name suggests that it works on GABA receptors, pregabalin in fact acts centrally on another type of receptor, called voltage-gated calcium channels, thus reducing neuronal excitability.[8]

The main side effects associated with the use of pregabalin are blurred vision, dizziness, nausea and sleepiness. Due to an increased risk of seizures on sudden withdrawal, pregabalin is always withdrawn gradually.

It is worth noting that some psychotropic medicines listed above are also used in physical health conditions – pregabalin and valproate for neuropathic pain and epilepsy, respectively. Amitriptyline (a TCA) is used for neuropathic pain and migraine prophylaxis, both as unlicensed indications, and duloxetine is also used for diabetic neuropathy and stress urinary incontinence.

LAMOTRIGINE

Lamotrigine has proven efficacy for the prophylaxis of bipolar depression only.[9] Lamotrigine selectively blocks N- and P-type calcium channels, and slows the opening of overactive calcium channels. Lamotrigine decreases the release of excitatory amino acid neurochemicals such as glutamate and aspartate, and may also have agonist effects on GABA. Lamotrigine may also decrease 5-HT reuptake, which contributes to its antidepressant effect.[10]

> ### REFLECTION
>
> Which would be the most appropriate treatment for a service user whose most problematic feature of their bipolar is mania, which results in repeated admission to hospital?

LITHIUM

Lithium is known to enhance 5-HT in the brain and the effect of GABA. Lithium may also inhibit an enzyme called inositol phosphatase in the intracellular messenger system or change G-coupled proteins and how they affect the messenger system within the nerve cells. The cellular processes listed above do not adequately explain the mechanism of action of lithium in the treatment of BPAD or unipolar depression.[11] The use of lithium for these conditions is based on its effectiveness in clinical trials. It is still the only medicine used to treat BPAD that has been shown to reduce the rate of suicide in this vulnerable group of patients.

Lithium is a salt (carbonate or citrate) which is almost completely removed from the body unchanged via the kidneys. If the dose is doubled, the blood serum level will double. The blood level range between therapeutic and toxic effect is small; hence there is a need for close blood monitoring. Patients should be empowered to reduce the likelihood of harm from their medicines by ensuring they know the importance of their physical health checks (using a patient help record paper or an appropriate app), and know the toxic effects, side effects and interactions related to their medicines.[12]

CARBAMAZEPINE

Carbamazepine is mainly used to treat bipolar disorder,[13] aggression and behavioural and psychological symptoms in depression. There is a paucity of evidence to support their use, and some clinicians believe the best thing you can do with carbamazepine is stop it and let the other medicines used to treat the illness work, due to the extensive interactions seen with this medicine. Carbamazepine exerts its effect through numerous pharmacological mechanisms: adenylate cyclases, phosphoinositol turnover and calcium influx into nerve cells through numerous mechanisms (including through inhibition of the N-methyl-D-aspartate (NMDA) receptor). Carbamazepine also decreases the release of glutamate, the excitatory neurochemical in the brain.[14]

SIDE EFFECTS

Extrapyramidal side effects (EPSEs)

EPSEs are the most common side effects associated with the use of first generation antipsychotics.[15] This is due to the blockade of DA in the basal ganglia of the brain. EPSEs are more likely to occur with those antipsychotics that have high potency.

EPSEs are divided into four types:

1. dystonias;
2. pseudo-parkinsonism;
3. akathisia;
4. tardive dyskinesia (TD).

Dystonias are uncontrolled muscle spasms that can occur in any group of muscles. Typical examples include eyes rolling upwards (oculogyric crisis) and side twisting of the neck and head (torticollis). Commonly, due to the spasms in the neck and the head, the patients may not be able to swallow or speak clearly. These spasms may be very painful and distressing.

Dystonias affect young males, and patients who have never had any neuroleptics, i.e. neuroleptic naïve. They appear within hours of treatment, and sometimes even minutes, especially in cases of intramuscular (IM) administration. Dystonias require immediate medical attention, and prescribing oral, IM or even intravenous (IV) antimuscarinics such as procyclidine provides effective treatment.

Pseudo-parkinsonism includes symptoms such as stiffness, tremor, bradykinesia, bradyphrenia and hypersalivation. Symptoms of bradykinesia could be mistaken for depression or negative symptoms of schizophrenia. Pseudo-parkinsonism affects elderly women and those patients with neurological damage, for example after a stroke. These are manifested days or weeks after initiating antipsychotic treatment or dose increases, and they respond best to reduction of the dose, or changing to an antipsychotic that is less likely to cause EPSEs, such as atypical, or short-term anticholinergics (for example, procyclidine), as they are commonly not needed for longer than 3 months.

Akathisia, a subjective feeling of inner restlessness with a desire to move constantly, is characterized by symptoms such as stomping feet when seated, crossing/uncrossing legs, rocking from foot to foot and pacing up and down. As such, it can be mistaken for psychotic agitation. Akathisia can occur within hours to weeks of commencing an antipsychotic or increasing its dose, but unlike in dystonias and pseudo-parkinsonism, anticholinergics are more likely to exacerbate the symptoms. The recommended treatment option is to change to an atypical antipsychotic, or reduce the dose. Alternatively, BDZ such as clonazepam, or lipophilic beta-blockers such as propranolol, may be effective.

Tardive dyskinesia (TD) includes a variety of abnormal movements, such as lip smacking, tongue protrusion, and pill rolling (that is, choreiform movements) and pelvic thrusting. These can often lead to difficulties in speaking, breathing, eating and swallowing, and are worse when under stress. TD affects elderly women, patients with affective disorders and those who have had EPSEs early on in the treatment. TD may take months or even years to manifest, and in up to 50 per cent of cases it is reversible. Anticholinergics are not used in TD, as good results are seen with antipsychotic dose reductions and changing to either clozapine or quetiapine, of which clozapine has the most evidence of efficacy.[16]

> ## REFLECTION
>
> What tools are available to help review the side effects of antipsychotics?

Metabolic side effects

Numerous psychotropics have metabolic effects on the body.[17] These effects include: weight gain, insulin resistance (type 2 diabetes) and hyperlipidaemia. Due to the combined possible genetic increase in risk of cardiometabolic disorders disease in those with serious mental illness and effects of antipsychotics, appropriate monitoring (of blood pressure, pulse, BMI, lipids and HBa1c) and physical health interventions are necessary.

Antipsychotics may affect brain-derived neurotrophic factor (BDNF). Diminished signalling of BDNF may be responsible for the increased feelings of hunger. Increased cortisol levels can occur during episodes of agitation and cause increased insulin resistance, but do not explain the prolonged weight gain that can occur with psychotropic medicines. Antipsychotics are known to increase the levels of leptin in the body, which may in turn affect the hypothalamus, increasing hunger and fat deposits, and thus are responsible for at least part of antipsychotic weight gain. D_2 antagonism may also increase craving and have an impact on increased food intake.

Antagonism of apha-1 and histamine-1 receptors may increase inactivity due to sedation and thus cause further weight gain.

> ## REFLECTION
>
> - What interventions are likely to be needed for a service user with metabolic syndrome?
> - How can the mental health clinician support service users to get the right physical monitoring and ensure they receive the right interventions for their physical health problems?

Cardiac side effects

Cardiac side effects of antipsychotics occur as a result of antagonism on adrenergic and cholinergic receptors.[18] Postsynaptic adrenergic receptor block results in postural hypotension, which may in turn cause reflex tachycardia. This is particularly common with clozapine, chlorpromazine, quetiapine and risperidone. Tachycardia, which is associated with clozapine, occurs as a result of clozapine's anticholinergic properties. ECG changes are also possible, and these may be prolongation of the Q-T and P-R intervals, as well as S-T depression and T-wave blunting. It is suggested that these ECG changes, and particularly the QTc prolongation with typical antipsychotics, are due to drug-induced arrhythmias.

An overdose with QTc-prolonging antipsychotics may lead to sudden cardiac death due to cardiotoxicity known as torsade de pointes. Cardiac side effects are dose-related, so it is essential to use the lowest possible dose of antipsychotic. Haloperidol is the typical antipsychotic associated with the greatest change in ECG, and therefore an ECG must be performed prior to its administration.

Note that antipsychotics are not the only medicines that cause ECG changes. Other psychotropics, such as citalopram, and TCAs are known to have a moderate effect too. Using combinations of antipsychotics, or doses above the maximum, increases this risk significantly. Some non-psychotropics are known to cause ECG changes too, namely antibiotics such as clarithromycin, erythromycin, medicines used for arrhythmias and others such as methadone.

However, the use of psychotropic medicines is just one of the risk factors. One must also consider other significant modifiable risk factors that pose a risk to the patient; these are smoking, obesity and impaired glucose.

Endocrine side effects

DA is the natural inhibitor of prolactin in the body. Thus, psychotropics that inhibit DA cause prolactin to rise. Hyperprolactinaemia is responsible for a number of sexual side effects: decreased libido, anorgasmia, galactorrhoea, amenorrhea, gynaecomastia, and erectile dysfunction in men. Long-term hyperprolactinaemia may also be linked to an increased risk of breast cancer and osteopenia.

Gastrointestinal (GI) side effects

The main GI side effects that are likely to occur as a result of psychotropic medicines described in this chapter include GI bleeds, constipation and transient GI disturbances.[19] These are most common at the start of the treatment.

GI bleeds are associated with the use of SSRIs. This is because a certain amount of 5-HT is needed by the platelets in order to promote platelet aggregation and clotting as a result of vascular injuries. By inhibiting the reuptake of 5-HT, SSRIs also inhibit the amount of 5-HT available for platelets, thus reducing the body's ability to form clots, resulting in an increased risk of bleeds. These bleeds may occur in the upper or lower GI tract. Concomitant use of medicines such as aspirin, and other non-steroidal anti-inflammatory drugs such as ibuprofen, will significantly add to the increased risk of bleeds.

Constipation is one of the most common side effects associated with clozapine. Unlike the transient GI disturbances such as nausea and diarrhoea that are seen at the initial stages of treatment with most medicines, clozapine-induced constipation persists throughout the treatment. It is imperative that patients with reduced gut motility are identified as soon as possible, because effective treatment or prophylaxis will reduce risk of death that may occur as a result of severe faecal impaction. Severe faecal impaction could lead to colon enlargement or even obstruction, leading to severe abdominal pain, high fever, vomiting blood, rectal bleeding or bloody stool. Constipation can be treated and prevented effectively by a high-fibre diet and the use of bulk-forming laxatives (such as ispaghula husk) and stimulants (for example, senna, bisacodyl).

SERVICE USER INVOLVEMENT

As seen in this chapter, the main concepts in psychopharmacology, and also those involved in understanding disease states, are very complex. Therefore it is essential to understand these in relation to what is important to service users. Service users receive information which explains both the way their medicines work, and also why they have a mental illness in the first place. A great deal of feedback from service users tells us that they often find this information overwhelming. In other cases, it is the carers who relay most of this information. It is imperative that the information we as health care professionals are able to provide is relevant information that service users and carers need and understand. It has also been found that some service users, and more frequently those who are involved in working with mental health services, have a special interest in psychiatry as a whole. They are particularly interested in how their medicines work, as they use their own knowledge to empower other service users to promote recovery and rehabilitation.

The questions most frequently asked by service users are:

- Why do I need this medicine? What is it for?
- What side effects will I get?
- How long do I have to take it for?
- When do I have to take it?
- What does it do?

See chapter 48 for more useful information on this topic.

> ### REFLECTION
>
> - You are asked by a service user how sertraline works: 'I know that it will improve my mood, but how exactly does that happen?'
>
> - Think about your own understanding of depression, and also about SSRIs. Now think what the service user is particularly interested in and attempt to address this. Always try to confirm their understanding by asking questions: 'How does that sound to you?' 'Would you like some more information?' Different people learn in different ways; therefore offer a patient information leaflet from the Choice and Medication website (see 'Relevant web pages').

CONCLUSION

Giving a medicine is the most common treatment intervention in the NHS and is becoming increasingly complex. As the ageing population increases, and the number of comorbidities each person has rises, issues related to medicines are becoming increasingly important. Nurses must have at least a basic understanding of the pharmacology of mental illness, as the medicines used to treat them will enable the practitioner to respond to the medicine treatment needs of the service user appropriately.

References

1. Vaishnav K, Nestler EJ. The molecular neurobiology of depression. *Nature* 2008; **455**: 894–902.
2. Kato T. Molecular neurobiology of bipolar disorder: a disease of 'mood-stabilizing neurons'? *Trends in Neurosciences* 2008; **31**(10): 495–503.
3. Ross CA, Margolis RL, Reading SAJ, Pletnikov M, Coyle JT. Neurobiology of schizophrenia. *Neurone* 2006; **52**(1): 139–53.
4. Bellantuono C, Reggi V, Tognoni G, Garattini S. Benzodiazepines: clinical pharmacology and therapeutic use. *Drugs* 1980; **19**: 195.
5. Willner P, Scheel-Krüger J, Belzung C. The neurobiology of depression and antidepressant action. *Neuroscience and Biobehioral Reviews* 2013; **37**(10) Part 1: 2331–71.
6. Perucca E. Pharmacological and therapeutic properties of valproate. a summary after 35 years of clinical experience. *CNS Drugs* 2002; **16**: 695–714.
7. Frampton JE. Pregabalin: a review of its use in adults with generalized anxiety disorder. *CNS Drugs* 2014; **28**(9): 835–54.
8. Calandre EP, Rico-Villademoros F, Slim M. Alpha2delta ligands, gabapentin, pregabalin and mirogabalin: a review of their clinical pharmacology and therapeutic use. *Expert Review of Neurotherapeutics* 2016; **16**(11): 1263–77.
9. Goldsmith DR, Wagstaff AJ, Ibbotson T, Perry CM. Spotlight on lamotrigine in bipolar disorder. *CNS Drugs* 2004; **18**(1): 63–7.
10. Xie X, Hagan RM. Cellular and molecular actions of lamotrigine: possible mechanisms of efficacy in bipolar disorder. *Neuropsychobiology* 1998; **38**(3): 119–30.
11. Malhi GS, Tanious M, Das P, Coulston CM, Berk M. Potential mechanisms of action of lithium in bipolar disorder. Current understanding. *CNS Drugs* 2013; **27**(2): 135–53.
12. Grandjean EM, Aubry JM. Lithium: updated human knowledge using an evidence-based approach: part III: clinical safety. *CNS Drugs* 2009; **23**(5): 397–418.
13. Post RM, Ketter TA, Uhde T, Ballenger JC. Thirty years of clinical experience with carbamazepine in the treatment of bipolar illness. *CNS Drugs* 2007; **21**(1): 47–71.
14. Albani F, Riva R, Baruzzi A. Carbamazepine clinical pharmacology: a review. *Pharmacopsychiatry* 1995; **28**(6): 235–44.
15. Holloman LC, Marder SR. Management of acute extrapyramidal effects induced by antipsychotic drugs. *American Journal of Health-System Pharmacy* 1997; **54**(21): 2461–77.
16. Klawans Jr HL. the pharmacology of tardive dyskinesias. *American Journal of Psychiatry* 1973; **130**(1): 82–6.
17. Bhuvaneswar CG, Baldessarini RJ, Harsh VL, Alpert JE. Adverse endocrine and metabolic effects of psychotropic drugs. *CNS Drugs* 2009; **23**(12): 1003–21.
18. Chong SA, Mahendran R. Cardiac effects of psychotropic drugs. *Annals of the Academy of Medicine, Singapore* 2001, **30**(6): 625–31.
19. Grover M, Drossman DA. Psychotropic agents in functional gastrointestinal disorders. *Current Opinion in Pharmacology* 2008; **8**(6): 715–23.

Further reading

Dale MM, Ritter JM, Fowler RJ, Rang HP (eds). *Rang and Dale's pharmacology*, 6th edn. London: Churchill Livingstone, 2008.

Katzung B, Masters S, Trevor A. *Basic and clinical pharmacology*, 11th edn. New York: McGraw-Hill, 2009.

McKay GA, Reid JL, Walters MR. *Lecture notes: clinical pharmacology and therapeutics*, 8th edn. Oxford: Wiley-Blackwell, 2011.

Stahl SM. *Stahl's essential psychopharmacology, neuroscientific basis and practical applications*, 4th edn. Cambridge and New York: Cambridge University Press, 2013.

Taylor D, Paton C, Kapur S. *The Maudsley prescribing guidelines in psychiatry*, 12th edn. Chichester: John Wiley & Sons, 2015.

Walker R, Whittlesea C (eds). *Clinical pharmacology and therapeutics*, 4th edn. London: Churchill Livingstone, 2007.

Relevant web pages

BNF (British National Formulary) Online. https://www.bnf.org/products/bnf-online/

Choice and Medication. http://www.choiceandmedication.org

Electronic Medicines Compendium. www.emc.medicines.org.uk
This website provides a full drug company-generated monograph about most medicines. It provides a range of information about medicines, ranging from some basic pharmacology to side effects and recommended monitoring, among other things.

MHRA (Medicines and Healthcare products Regulatory Agency). Medicines information: SPC & PILs. http://www.mhra.gov.uk/spc-pil/

NICE (National Institute for Health and Care Excellence) Clinical Knowledge Summaries. Mental health. http://cks.nice.org.uk/clinicalspeciality#?speciality=Mental health
These give practical tips on reviewing a wide range of medical problems faced by primary care practitioners that nurses may find useful when reviewing medicines with service users.

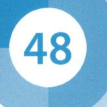

48 Medicines management and the mental health nurse

REBECCA M. BURGESS-DAWSON AND
STEVE HEMINGWAY

LEARNING OUTCOMES

- To understand the concept of medicines management.

- To be aware of the complex issues that need to be considered when assisting someone to manage their use of medicines.

- To appreciate the role of the mental health nurse in facilitating effective medicines management for service users.

SUMMARY OF KEY POINTS

- Medicines management is not simply administering medicines, or giving information, or making decisions about medicines, or ensuring the correct supplies are available – it is all of these complex activities and much more.

- Why and how medicines are prescribed for service users, how they get access to them and whether they choose to take them are key aspects of collaboration in care and treatment.

- Mental health nurses, whether directly involved in the prescribing of medicines or not, are well placed to engage with the service users for whom they are working to facilitate effective medicines management.

INTRODUCTION

This chapter is a practical examination of the mental health nurse's role in medicines management. Although the study of the medicines themselves is referred to as psychopharmacology and is discussed in chapter 47, this chapter concentrates instead on the practical use of those types of medicine in reality with service users, and some of the issues that can arise.

Medicines management refers to a wide variety of activities that encompass the choice, acquisition, use and review of medicines, so that they are used for optimal safety and efficacy. Figure 48.1 shows a simple cycle describing medicines management. In an ideal scenario, an individual would manage their own medicines when they knew they needed them, collaborating with health care professionals

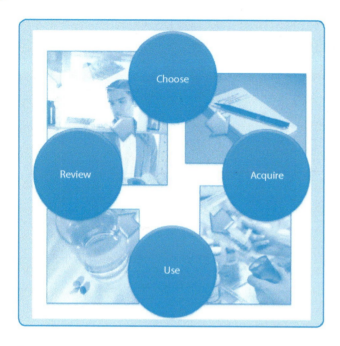

Figure 48.1 A representation of medicines management.

whenever necessary to choose, acquire, ingest, review and discontinue medicines as and when they were required, and these medicines would be as efficacious as possible without having other unwanted effects that were disabling.

In the real world, however, the relationship between an individual and health care is not so scientifically clinical – a myriad of factors exist that impact on all stages of the process, not least personal beliefs and relationships, social pressures, economic factors and availability of resources. Medicines management therefore must be a highly personalized arrangement for the individual considering the medicine, in order to make the best decisions possible at all stages. As the largest group of health care professionals working with those receiving services, mental health nurses are at the forefront of collaborating with service users and their carers to assist in this process. The chapter therefore looks closely at the overall process, examining key concepts such as adherence, concordance, capacity and choice. The legal and ethical considerations are also discussed, before an examination of the future role of nurses in medicines management is explored.

BACKGROUND

Medicines are a widely used treatment for mental illness and disorder. The vast majority of inpatient service users in mental health take medicines during their stay as part of their care.[1] Overall in England, prescriptions for mental health medicines rose between 1998 and 2010 by an average of 6.8 per cent each year.[2] This has led some to suggest that prescriptions for such medicines can be used to 'medicalize' emotional states that occur for other reasons,[3] although others equally point out that the increasing availability of medicines, coupled with a reduction in the social stigma towards accepting them, could also be factors.[4] However, the concept of taking prescribed psychoactive substances of any type to treat emotional distress can also be potentially contentious. Some suggest that medication should not be a first-line treatment for mental illness, although medicines may be used alongside other psychosocial interventions such as working with the whole family.[5–8] Others (sometimes referred to under the broad term 'antipsychiatry') challenge the biomedical model of treatment per se, and believe mental distress to be a result of social pressures upon an individual,[9] and that in some cases, administration of medicine in the long term, particularly by the use of long-acting injections,

could then be considered a method of exerting further social control.[10]

Every service user's experience of their illness is different, and therefore it must apply that their experience of using medicine is different, specific and individual to them. Medicines management issues exist not only personally for each service user, but also for wider society. Recent studies, for example, have shown a wide-ranging and marked increase in the prescription of antidepressant medicines in the world's richest nations.[11] The fact that they are more often prescribed has not been particularly contested – but the underlying reasons for this, such as whether depression is being diagnosed more frequently, or whether more antidepressants are being considered as treatment for depressive symptoms in today's society, are being intensely debated.[3,11,12] In any event, in the UK, with a national health care programme that has finite resources, medicines must be used judiciously; after all, the drugs bill is the second largest in the NHS after staffing costs.[13] In 2012 in England, new data showed that over 90 per cent of all prescriptions for all types of medicines dispensed were free of charge to the customer (most often because they were over 60 years old, or were prescribed for a child under the age of 16).[14]

THE ROLE OF THE NURSE

All nurses in the UK are required to meet their licensing body's standards for medicines management.[15] Although they previously concentrated on administration, where the nurses' role traditionally began and ended, the guidelines on competence in medicines management now cover a much broader area.

From the point of registration, the nurse is expected to have a wide variety of skills. See Box 48.1.

BOX 48.1: MEDICINES MANAGEMENT SKILLS FOR NURSES

People can trust the newly registered graduate nurse to:

- Correctly and safely undertake medicines calculations.
- Work within legal and ethical frameworks that underpin safe and effective medicines management.
- Work as part of a team to offer holistic care and a range of treatment options of which medicines may form a part.
- Ensure safe and effective practice in medicines management through comprehensive knowledge of medicines, their actions, risks and benefits.

- Safely order, receive, store and dispose of medicines (including controlled drugs) in any setting.
- Administer medicines safely and in a timely manner, including controlled drugs.
- Work in partnership with people receiving medical treatments and their carers.
- Use and evaluate up-to-date information on medicines management and work within national and local policy guidelines.
- Demonstrate understanding and knowledge to supply and administer via a patient group direction.

Source: NMC *Standards for pre-registration nursing education.*[15]

The Nursing and Midwifery Council's change of terminology from 'guidelines' to 'standards' for medicines management is in no way accidental – they describe what a registered nurse *must* do.[16] Despite being comprehensive, however, they cannot cover all situations and particular individual circumstances, so the broader values that are contained within the nurses' code of conduct also apply.[17] Mental health nurses are involved in assisting service users to choose, acquire and manage their medicines at all stages, and are often at the centre of medicines management activities.[18] Mental health nurses must therefore always consider their own attitudes, values and beliefs when working with service users, and this is certainly true in the use of medications. See Figure 48.2.

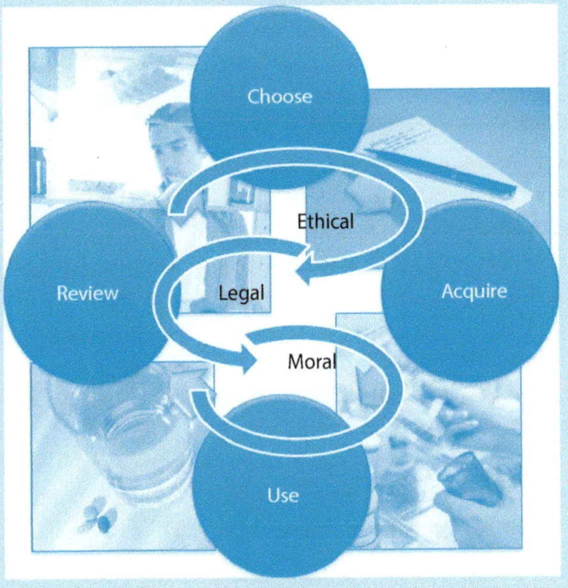

Overall, a central theme to the whole process is engagement with the service user to enable them to discuss their own rationale for potentially taking a medicine. Lack of adherence to a medication regimen, for example, can occur for practical or psychological reasons, or sometimes both combined.[19]

The nurse in such circumstances needs a sophisticated understanding of the psychopharmacology of the medicines prescribed, as well as how to practise medicines management interventions including administering, providing advice on the use of and assessing the outcomes of taking medication as prescribed. A 'stepped approach' to the education and training needs of mental health nurses involving a university and NHS Trust shows how such a pathway may follow pre- and postgraduate study.[20] See Figure 48.3.

Figure 48.2 Further considerations within the medicines management cycle.

REFLECTION

- Think about your experience of the mental health nurse undertaking medicines management activities. Are you comfortable with the thought that mental health nurses are investing so much time in medicines management activities?

- Do you think some of this time would be better spent on other interventions?

- Does the mental health nurse's role in medication serve to reinforce a biomedical model of disease and treatment?

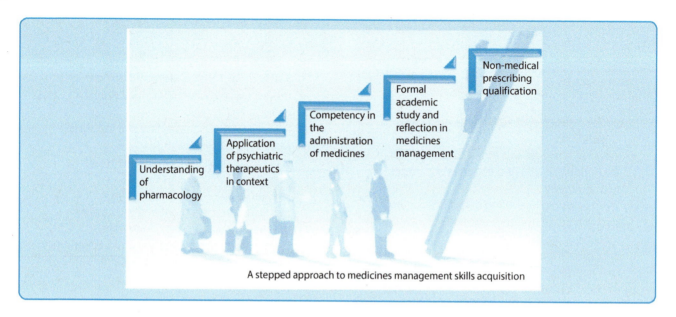

A stepped approach to medicines management skills acquisition

Figure 48.3 A 'stepped approach' to acquiring medicines management skills.

MEDICINES MANAGEMENT ACTIVITIES AND THE ROLE OF THE MENTAL HEALTH NURSE

Considering a prescription

Nurses are involved in negotiating with the service user at all stages of treatment, and the use of medications in an overall plan of care should therefore be no different. One of the key opportunities may present itself when a medicine is being suggested or considered for the first time. In the field of mental health care, a previously small number of potential treatments has increased considerably, particularly with the advent of atypical antipsychotics and newer hypnotics over the years. With a wider range of choice than ever before, specialist texts exist that examine the evidence to support the use of various mental health medicines.[21] Research into further novel preparations is also taking place, perhaps most notably into potential treatments for dementia.[22]

With such a variety of options to consider, it is more important now than ever that clinicians adopt the current clinical evidence in their decisions and advice given to service users. In the UK, the National Institute for Health and Care Excellence (NICE) has a wealth of researched guidance for clinicians to employ when treating a number of conditions.[23] In addition to this, there may be additional local guidelines to further outline the management of medicines within local population groups. Clinical Commissioning Groups, for instance, have a role in defining how best to utilize local health care resources.

However, the complex factors that arise from a very personal experience of mental distress,[24] coupled with a relatively rigid set of diagnostic criteria to provide formal diagnosis of mental ill-health or disorder,[25] can mean that it is difficult to treat an illness per se.

It is here that nurses must be especially mindful of ethical considerations, and their own bias. The pharmaceutical industry certainly has an effect on the promotion of medicines.[26] Strict governance on how and where it is permissible for industry representatives to engage with clinicians regarding a particular product has been further strengthened over time.[27] However, there is surely still the bias present when a clinician notes the efficacy of a particular product in an individual for whom they provide care – and then meets someone else with a similar presentation. Which product would they immediately think of?

Excepting a small number of cases where it is necessary to utilize legal powers to act in an individual's best interest when they are unable to do so themselves, everyone has the right to refuse treatment. Weighing up the risks and benefits can be difficult. Although rapid relief from distressing symptoms, and in some cases risk-taking behaviour, is of great benefit,[28] this must be considered alongside the potentially negative impact of the same treatments in the longer term. In the case of mental health medicines, possible iatrogenic onset of obesity and diabetes is of particular note.[29]

One of the key ethical dilemmas for mental health nurses in medicines management can be understanding how best to continue to engage and work with an individual who declines to take medication for their symptoms, sometimes despite the recommendation of the whole care team, including family and friends. At times such as these, the nurse's ability to empathize and truly appreciate the service user's point of view is often called upon, as the nurse can often find themselves directly engaging with both the service user and the wider care team as the service user's advocate.

When an individual does decide that medication is right for them, and consents to its prescription, the nurse is then equally well placed to discuss practical issues, such as in what formulation and at what time of day the medicine would be best taken to maximize efficacy, and what community or hospital pharmacy services should be utilized for support, advice and assistance in acquiring the medicines.

Initiating treatment

COMPLIANCE, CONCORDANCE OR ADHERENCE?

At its best, collaborating with a service user to choose and use a medication to enable them to feel well can additionally empower and inform that individual, which in its own right fosters well-being and fits within the craft of caring. However, the use of medication, perhaps unfortunately more than any other therapeutic intervention, can be perceived as coercive and even punitive.[30,31] It is crucial that this activity is approached in a facilitative and responsible manner. Successfully done, this collaboration not only increases service users' feelings of informed control, but also increases the likelihood that medicines will be taken correctly, increasing their efficacy.

It must be remembered that clinicians discussing treatment have in only the recent past been schooled in a relatively hierarchal culture, where it is the responsibility of clinicians to choose a treatment, as they were regarded as the most technically competent to do so. In this culture (of which some traditionalist practice may continue), 'collaboration' is sometimes seen as reduced to providing information about the selected medicinal product, and then checking agreement to take it.[32] This is fundamentally flawed – collaboration should utilize the service user's unique expertise to influence the discussion and eventual decision. However, it must also be remembered that sometimes the service user has for a long time received care in the same hierarchal culture, and may equally strongly hold the belief that choices about medicines are not theirs to make. This may be coupled with additional difficulties with engagement, social interaction, controlling emotions and thinking clearly and logically as the consequence of their illness.[33] It is clearly important to navigate this process well. Planning care in a collaborative way is discussed further in chapter 50 of this book.

ENGAGEMENT

One of the key skills that nurses can utilize in medicines management is engagement, via the therapeutic relationship they have with a service user, as discussed in chapter 3 and embedded in the craft of caring. Engagement is vital

SERVICE USER'S PERSPECTIVE: ENGAGEMENT

My own experience of inpatient and outpatient settings was different. In the hospital the nurses seemed distant and seemed to only emerge from their nurse station/office to administer 'scripts' and take people outside to smoke. If I asked them questions about my medicine, I was advised to take it up with the consultant psychiatrist if and when I saw him.

In contrast, as an outpatient, I saw my CPN regularly. (He was attached to my GP's Health Centre.) He was able and willing to answer questions about side effects and the pros and cons of different treatments. He also seemed able to influence the GP's prescribing and would seek out and take into account my own thoughts and feelings and treatment preferences.

Given the issues of control/coercion, doubts over efficacy, and the 'shooting in the dark' state of much psychiatric treatment, as well as suspicions about the way drugs are marketed to prescribers *and* the importance of 'therapeutic engagement', it seems right that the power in this setting is divided more equally among the doctor, the nurse and the service user.

Andrew Roe

in all humanistic interactions, and at least one large study has reflected the importance of engagement in medicines management activities.[34] Poor relationships, either with individual staff or indeed the inpatient environment or service generally, can greatly influence whether or not an individual continues to accept medicine.

Carers are often involved in assisting in lots of aspects of medicines management, from ensuring prescriptions are dispensed and collected, to assisting with self-administration in the community.[35] Department of Health literature therefore highlights not only the importance of collaborating with and involving carers wherever possible, but also the suggestion that they would benefit from specific training and knowledge around medicines, including side effects and storage requirements.[36]

CONSENT

It is *informed* consent that is important; the more complex the activity and the higher the risk, then the more difficult it is to achieve capacitous consent.[37] It is important for all those involved in medicines management to realize that there are risks associated with taking treatment, as well as those inherent in not. Overall, there has even been a move beyond 'adherence' to the concept of 'appropriate adherence', with the service user judging the overall value of a treatment for themselves[38] (p.283). This is a personalized evaluation of a treatment, but perhaps creates difficulties for carers and professionals who also wish to report on any benefits or difficulties they have subjectively noted. This can pose even greater difficulty in a scenario where the service user is unable to make decisions for themselves, whether this be an acute problem related to ill-health for which treatment is required, or a more permanent cognitive decline requiring longer-term compensatory care.

The Mental Capacity Act of 2010 has highlighted the significance of assisting people to make decisions when they are not able to act in their own best interest. Pivotally, the Act reinforces the fact that capacity can only be judged in relation to the decision at the time, and that capacity can be fluid – sometimes individuals are more able to make judgements at certain times or in specific situations.[39]

The Mental Health Act 1983 includes provision to legally enforce the use of medication when it is thought to be in an individual's best interest.[40] In mental health inpatient services, it is common for a detained patient's medication administration record to carry 'consent to treatment' legal papers, denoting whether an individual has given their full consent to receive treatment, or in rarer cases where a second opinion from a medical professional has been necessary to enforce that treatment. In the community, changes to mental health legislation in the UK have introduced community treatment orders (CTOs) in an attempt to offset the social and physical damage over time that can accompany discharge from hospital, non-adherence to medicines, deterioration in mental health and subsequent readmission to hospital.[41] Mental health nurses must therefore be able to work within the law but at the same time provide advocacy for those they care for. In situations where nurses are administering treatment against an individual's will, it is therefore necessary to consult an independent advocate for the service user, to ensure their legal rights are upheld.

Managing an active prescription

Assisting someone to manage their medication must involve strategies for making sure that supplies are always available. In modern health care, the use of different pharmaceutical manufacturers and brands to acquire generic medicines at best cost is now routine practice. Service users with paranoid thoughts about a change in the colour or shape of their oral medicines may need careful education, explanation and reassurance at these times. Some inpatient services are now advocating the use of patients' own medicines while in hospital. The primary benefit is one of safety, and to make the process of 'medicines reconciliation' easier; however, there can also be the added advantage of making

concordance easier when they return home, as the medicines themselves, their packaging and administration are all more familiar.

Engaging with the service user and making sure that medicines management activities are only one part of an overall package of care (as described in chapter 37, on the Care Programme Approach) can mean that the taking of medicine is a part of everyday life. Unwanted effects not immediately linked by the individual to their medicine regime can be quickly identified and managed more effectively if a holistic discussion about overall quality of life is initiated. Medicines reconciliation is also an important activity whenever an individual moves between teams or services, as this is a time of risk when information can be missed or misreported.[42]

Modern technology is able to provide some assistance when available, as clinical records can now be shared electronically between health care professionals. Electronic record keeping per se and e-prescribing are both now more widely available.[43] It must also be remembered that the same technology can be applied to informing and educating the service user and their carers. From the use of the internet to find information on various medicines to the use of text message reminders to an individual's phone, modern technology can improve adherence to treatment when used appropriately.[44–46]

It is not only the potential physiological side effects or practical issues with medicines management that can limit treatment and lead to a lack of adherence. Historically, it was considered that medicines used to treat mental illness should be taken for a lengthy period, if possible. Particularly in the case of antidepressants, there was cited evidence of a protective effect if medication were continued for a significant time after an individual felt wholly well.[47,48]

However, more recent literature, particularly in the case of psychosis and bipolar disorder, has questioned the benefit of long-term treatment with psychotropics and has called into question common recommendations that service users continue medicines as long as unwanted effects are not disabling.[49,50] Overall, non-adherence rates remain high in any event, and service users report distressing discontinuation syndromes from medicines.[51]

As when treatment is first discussed and initiated, it is certainly not the case that the mental health nurse's role should concentrate on promoting adherence; the engagement and subsequent therapeutic relationship (see chapter 3) between nurses and those they care for can often include not taking medicines, or managing the discontinuation of medicines those individuals no longer wish to take.[31]

Medication administration

Medicines management is a complex process, and the administration of medicine is equally complex in its own right. The Nursing and Midwifery Council concentrates on administration issues particularly in its standards for medicines management, underlining how pivotal a role this is for nurses in the whole process.[16] Nurses provide a particularly important opportunity to prevent errors, as in the administrative role they are often the 'last line of defence' before a service user takes their medicine. Traditionally at this time, they have been advised to follow the '5 rights' of medicines[52] administration; that is, to ensure that the right *patient, medicine, dose, time* and *route* are evident. However, this is a simple cognitive checking system, not a competency framework that incorporates all of the behaviours, cognitive skills and knowledge associated with the process. In inpatient medicines management, there can be a return to paternalistic nursing practices because of the organization of the environment.[53] Self-administration under the amount of nurse supervision that is necessary to ensure safety can be a possible way of tackling this.[54]

Overall, medication administration provides an ideal opportunity to engage with a service user about their treatment plan generally.[55] Having a quiet space to do this that affords dignity and privacy can be at odds with some more institutionalized methods of medication administration, but nurses should consider this as part of their practice. As part of previous work undertaken with local colleagues, the authors of this chapter were involved in the development of the Medicines with Respect (MwR) framework, in an attempt to map out the complex range of skills needed for the administration of medicines. These were found to include cognitive, psychomotor and humanistic skills,[56,57]

which, in early versions of the framework, were grouped into discrete stages of activity related to preparation, administration and housekeeping tasks. See Table 48.1 for some key examples of these stages.

It would be useful for the reader to search for the policies for the administration of medicines in the area where they practice. In particular, look for assessments of practice competence. To see an example of such a document, look at the MwR assessment of competence documents listed under 'Further reading' (South West Yorkshire Partnership NHS Foundation Trust).

In the absence of prescriptive authority, perhaps the greatest autonomy for the nurse in choosing medicines with a service user is in the case of *pro re nata* (PRN) or 'as and when required' medicines. This is particularly used in inpatient services when caring for those individuals in the acute or fluctuating phases of their illness, as the mental health nurse can utilize PRN medicine to treat those symptoms per se, or indeed to use other medicines as 'symptomatic relief' to make the service user feel more comfortable if they are in pain or physical discomfort.

There is evidence that PRN medicine is used for extremely complex presentations of agitation without clear rationale, and that, furthermore, medicines are often given in the early stages of admission to hospital, when the services user's underlying condition is as yet unknown, as is their potential response to medicines.[58] Perhaps particularly in the treatment of disturbed behaviour causing a potential for harm to the service user or people around them, or in cases of violence and aggression, it is important

Table 48.1 Skills in administration of medicine

The process of administration of medication		
Preparation	**Administration**	**Housekeeping**
Ensuring the environment is appropriate (clean, clear, well lit, free from distraction, etc.) Ensuring appropriate documentation (medicine cards, legal forms) are present Checking that all equipment necessary is available (and, if necessary, sterile, in date, etc.)	Correctly identifying the service user with multiple checks Ensuring consent, or legal capacity Checking physical health status (overall, and, for example in the case of injections, skin integrity) Identifying what is to be currently administered at this time, and by which route Offering time to the service user to discuss their prescribed medication Calculating the dose of medicine (check with another nurse or health care professional) Administering the medication using correct technique Checking as appropriate that the medication has been taken, and that there are no immediate adverse effects	Documenting the process Re-ordering and re-stocking medicines as appropriate Disposing of any waste, adhering to local policies and procedures Ensuring the environment is returned to its original state Ensuring that future administration of medication is planned for, and communicated to the service user

to note that the use of PRN medicine to relieve psychotic symptoms and/or provide a degree of sedation is part of a wide range of available options and therapeutic interventions. Overall, it is important that the nurse clearly records the clinical rationale for administration.[59]

Most often, it is appropriate to consider the use of PRN in these situations as a 'last resort', and certainly never as a substitute for humanistic interventions such as verbal de-escalation, behavioural interventions such as reduced stimulus environments, and good physiological care and management, such as attention to hunger, warmth or comfort needs.

REFLECTION

- After reading about the use of PRN medication, do you feel your own practice and that of those around you reflects competence, including engagement with the service user?

- Do you feel PRN medication is only used as a last resort to manage a service user's distress, or do you think that there are other factors?

CASE STUDY 1: THE USE OF PRN ON A PICU

G was prescribed an antipsychotic as part of her treatment in the psychiatric intensive care unit (PICU). Although G was already prescribed this type of medication on a regular basis, this was a different prescription, and had not so far proved effective in treating her symptoms.

G continued to be very distressed and agitated as a consequence of her delusional ideas. The team decided to try another antipsychotic, and use it as and when required (PRN).

The decision was made after a multidisciplinary meeting involving G's psychiatrist, primary nurse and the ward's specialist pharmacy team. G was also involved in this meeting, but it was felt that she lacked insight, so the nursing staff revisited conversations around medication almost on a daily basis as everyone was keen that G understood as much as possible about the treatment she was receiving and the reasons for it.

PRN medication was made part of G's overall plan of care at times when she became visibly agitated or distressed. Prior to this PRN medication being prescribed, G agreed to have her physical health quite closely monitored. The team was keen to do this, because the PRN medication plus her regular prescribed doses meant that

G was receiving a high overall daily amount of antipsychotic medication.

This monitoring included blood tests and electrocardiogram readings (ECGs) as well as more routine monitoring of pulse, blood pressure and respiratory rate, and was repeated often to track any potential changes from the normal range. G was also afforded dietary advice and monitoring of her weight.

As part of G's care plan, the PRN medicine was only administered when non-pharmacological techniques had been attempted without success. On a daily basis, G was allocated specific staff members to work with her. Over time, G responded positively to spending time in the relaxation room as a way of distracting her from distressing thoughts and also benefited from having somebody to talk through her delusional ideas with her as a way of rationalizing these thoughts. If these interventions were unsuccessful, nursing staff would then discuss the use of PRN medication on each occasion.

As G's insight improved, she was able to recognize for herself the times when she required additional medication and often approached staff herself to say that she felt she needed it.

Side effect management

It must be understood by those dealing with medicines management that *all* drugs have side effects. When new or novel preparations are licensed and added to formularies, it is often with the assurance that they are better than or 'superior to' what is currently available. Of course, when benzodiazepines first became widely available, they had many advantages over existing therapies – because the existing treatments were essentially limited to the effective but potentially very dangerous barbiturates.

However, the benzodiazepines themselves are not without unwanted effects, not least those of relatively rapid tolerance and reports of dependence, with often significant withdrawal symptoms and a necessarily prolonged withdrawal regimen.[60]

A similar picture emerged with the introduction of atypical antipsychotics. At first heralded as superior and therefore preferable to older medicines, modern trials have shown that they have different but equally significant side effect profiles – and that all licensed antipsychotics have a potential role in treatment.[61,62]

Therefore, the best way to manage the unwanted effects of medicines is to utilize the lowest therapeutic dose that provides relief from symptoms without unwanted effects that are disabling. On occasion, effects which can initially be thought of as 'unwanted' can be employed to therapeutic effect – for instance, an antidepressant or antipsychotic that has a particularly sedative effect could be taken at night by someone who suffers from insomnia, and thus avert the need for a separate hypnotic (with added side effects of its own). Discussion about the pros and cons of different treatments is a collaborative exercise, yet large proportions of service users still report not receiving information on side effects in a way that they could understand.[1]

The 'real world' efficacy of medications is much discussed. In this context, issues such as tolerability, side effect profile and safety are just as important as the baseline clinical effectiveness of the medicine per se. Recent history showed a prescribing preference for atypical antipsychotics – their lack of debilitating and lingering (sometimes permanent) unwanted effects, particularly tardive dyskinesia and movement disorders, made them perhaps more palatable to prescriber and service user. However, further wider-scale studies have shown that these medicines can also cause large degrees of sedation, weight gain and poor lipid control, leading to chronic conditions such as diabetes.[63]

Neither the nurse nor the service user can be expected to know all about each medicine's exact profile, and therefore the nurse's medicine management skills must include access to resources related to drug information, and knowledge of how to use them. The British National Formulary (BNF) is a well-known evidence-based resource, with the advent of electronic searchable versions assisting information gathering.[64] While service users are equally encouraged to perform their own research, they may require education regarding the reliability and validity of some sources, particularly those accessed via the internet.[65]

The nurse's relationship with the service user can facilitate asking about potentially sensitive side effects.

Sexual dysfunction, for example, is a common side effect of many medicines used in mental health care. It is in fact perhaps more common than the literature suggests, given that there is evidence that it is under-reported.[66] A nurse already involved in working with an individual may be best placed to have conversations of this nature, and should utilize their humanistic skills to approach such topics in the same manner as other potentially sensitive conversations, such as those related to the use of alcohol or other drugs.

Detecting any unwanted effects from medicines and implementing appropriate educational, intervention or preventative strategies with service users has multiple benefits.[67,68] Therefore, physical health monitoring strategies need to form a routine part of overall treatment plans for medicines management in order to identify these issues. These strategies can include the use of self-rating scales for specific treatments – for instance, those individuals prescribed an antipsychotic may be encouraged to complete a general scale for side effects, such as the Glasgow Antipsychotic Side Effect Scale (GASS)[69] or Liverpool University Neuroleptic Side Effect Rating Scale (LUNSERS), or an observer rated scale for a specific set of potential effects such as the Abnormal Involuntary Movement Scale (AIMS).[70] Overall, however, in cases where a more global physical health scale is used, such as the Health Improvement Profile (HIP),[71] this can afford the nurse an opportunity to have a much broader and more general discussion about health with an individual, and perhaps offer appropriate advice or assistance about contact with other types of health care. This can also promote the therapeutic relationship with the service user, rather than making the episode of care seem like a 'conveyor belt exercise'.[72]

Case study 2 gives an anonymized example of a case in which holistic assessment including rating scales has identified health needs for an individual which can be acted upon by referral to other health care professionals.

CASE STUDY 2: PHYSIOLOGICAL MONITORING IN MENTAL HEALTH SERVICES

Medicines management general health assessment
Background history
B is a 37-year-old male who has a diagnosis of paranoid schizophrenia dating back to 1998. Although B has had no past hospital admissions, he has a history of not adhering to prescribed oral medication for psychosis, and has been prescribed a long-acting antipsychotic injection in 2007 which he has adhered to ever since. The last time B experienced a relapse and psychotic symptoms was in 2008. B currently lives in supported accommodation with input from a community mental health nurse and a community care officer. B attends the treatment team in his local area every 2 weeks for his depot, and the team conduct an overall health check-up every 12 months.

Current medication		Flupentixol Decanoate 80 mg every 2 weeks	
Physiological observations			
Weight	109 kg	**BMI**	30.5
Height	189 cm	**Waist**	119 cm (less than 94 cm recommended for adult males)
BP	123/87		
Pulse	93 bpm	**Temperature**	36.3°C
Blood test results			
FBC	All measured within range	**Urea and electrolytes**	All measured within range
Calcium and albumin	All measured within range	**LFT**	All measured within range
Cholesterol	5.4	**TFT**	1.76 (Range 0.20–4)
Prolactin	599 (Range 0–400)	**Glucose**	4.5 (Range 2.5–7.8)
Additional items noted (as scored 'red' on the Health Improvement Profile (HIP))			
Teeth	no dental appointment attended in last 2 years		
Eyes	no eye examination attended in last 2 years		
Exercise	walks 'on occasion' (recommended < 30 minutes per day moderate exercise)		
Diet	<2 portions of fruit or vegetables per day, >3 portions of fat intake per day		
Further discussion			
B described his diet as 'mainly microwave meals and takeaways', stating he has no cooking skills.			
Other assessments:			
GASS (Glasgow Antipsychotic Side Effect Scale)	19 (Rated as 'mild side effects')		
Highest rated side effects: 'I feel sleepy during the day; My legs have felt restless and/or I couldn't sit still; I have had or people have noticed uncontrollable movements of my body or face.' B had had a recent change in his medication due to increased feelings of paranoia and feeling anxious when he left the house; he described these as lessening since the increase to his depot.			
Plan			
After discussion, with his agreement B was referred by the treatment team to a local voluntary agency which provides a practical educational cooking group specifically aimed at males, with a plan to then join their healthy lifestyle group. A referral was also made to another voluntary agency for B to be considered for their walking group. A copy of all the results of the treatment team's assessment was sent to B's GP and consultant psychiatrist. A comprehensive entry was made on the team's computerized clinical records system, so that the consultant could see the information when reviewing medication at B's next outpatient appointment. B's care plan is also regularly discussed with a specialist mental health pharmacist who attends the treatment team on a weekly basis. Finally, B was advised to attend a local optician, and was additionally given some support to search the NHS Choices website for a local dentist he might register with.			

Collaborating with a service user about their experiences of medicines does not just benefit the service user themselves. More knowledge is always required about the use of mental health medicines in the real world setting to improve the evidence base. Nurses should encourage colleagues and service users to join them in anonymously reporting new and/or unexpected effects from medicines. In the UK, this is done via the 'Yellow Card' scheme, which is available via a form at the back of the BNF and online (see 'Relevant web pages').

REFLECTION

- After reading about unwanted effects of mental health medicines, do you think the benefits of taking the medicine usually outweigh the risks?

- What specific skills and knowledge do you need in order to effectively support a service user to monitor and manage any unwanted effects from medicines?

Nurses as non-medical prescribers

In the last two decades, nurses with additional training in the UK have been given the opportunity to provide prescriptions.[73] The perceived benefits of mental health nurses prescribing are increased access to medicines, and more efficient use of the care team rather than relying wholly on the finite resources of the psychiatrist.[74] Adopting prescriptive authority has added accountability and responsibility for nurses, as they need the requisite skill, knowledge and governance arrangements to practise safely and competently.[75] A nurse prescriber in the UK can prescribe in two ways: 'supplementary' prescribing, where the nurse is restricted to prescribing medications from a clinical management plan as agreed with the supervising psychiatrist and the service user, and 'independent' prescribing, which is the ability to prescribe any medication within their specialist area of expertise.[73]

CASE STUDY 3: NON-MEDICAL PRESCRIBING IN OLDER PEOPLE'S SERVICES

D is 78 years of age and was referred to the memory service by his GP.

D's GP had completed a full set of cognitive screening blood tests and a baseline ECG before referring David to the older people's mental health service. A memory nurse visited D at home and completed specific clinical assessments which showed a mild to moderate memory deficit (from the Mini Mental State and Montreal Cognitive Assessments), no significant depression from the Geriatric Depression Scale and retained independence on the Bristol Activities of Daily Living Scale. Following this visit, D agreed to attend a cognitive screening brain scan, and a diagnostic appointment was booked with the nurse consultant in a memory clinic.

D's medical history included hypertension and hyperlipidaemia and he was prescribed Ramipril 5 mg, Simvastatin 20 mg and Aspirin 75 mg, all once daily. The CT brain scan had shown a moderate level of cortical atrophy and mild patchy ischaemia. The test results, history of onset and memory deficits described by D and his son (who also attended the appointment) resulted in the nurse consultant giving a diagnosis of Alzheimer's disease. The option of anti-dementia medication was discussed with D and agreed following discussion of the potential risks and benefits. D asked if such medication was safe to take with his other medicines and that it was not addictive in any way. It was agreed to prescribe Donepezil, initially at a dose of 5 mg once daily. Information on this medicine, possible side effects and the monitoring process from the memory service was provided.

D and his son also met with a member of staff from the local Alzheimer's society as part of the local dementia pathway, to receive information on education and support for people with dementia and their carers, including a benefits check and information on local social services provision.

An independent nurse prescription was issued by the nurse consultant and the memory nurse reviewed his progress by phone a month later before providing a further titrated nurse prescription for Donepezil 10 mg od. This was reviewed again by phone after a further month and the GP was then requested to issue a repeat prescription in line with a shared care protocol for this medication.

CONCLUSION

Overall, medicines management as it applies to mental health nurses encompasses a complex and diverse suite of skills. As can be seen in Figure 48.2, nurses consider ethical, legal and moral issues in all aspects of the medicines management cycle.

Mental health nurses are perhaps the best placed members of the health care team to create and develop genuine engagement with service users and their carers.

People can become emotive about the subject of medicines, and bring to discussions their own values, beliefs and attitudes, not only about the use of medicines generally, but also about the causation, nature and society's view of mental distress – if it should be treated, and if so, how.

Cooperation with a medication regimen can vary greatly, depending on how much an individual believes in the treatment. For instance, beliefs about mental illness or disorder that have spiritual or religious foundations may mean that the individual does not see medicine as a viable treatment option.[76] Mental health nurses need to reflect critically not only on the beliefs of the service user regarding medication, but also on their own viewpoint, both culturally and in terms of therapeutic optimism,[77] because this can affect their relationship and subsequent dialogue with the service user and their carers.[78]

See Figure 48.4 for the cycle of medicines management with some considerations described.

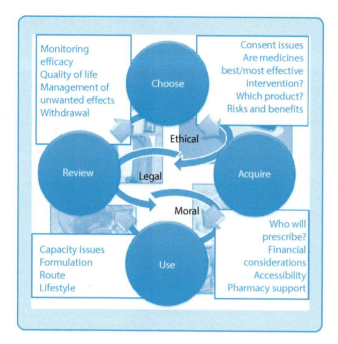

Figure 48.4 Some of the elements within medicines management.

More than ever before, the role of the mental health nurse is one of incredible diversity.[79] However, a theme that has remained constant is that of close collaboration with the service user to provide them with comfort and relief from distress. Mental health medicines, when used judiciously and sensitively, can help provide relief from at least a portion of that distress, and enable further engagement with the whole care team as part of a comprehensive treatment package.

Nurses must therefore use medicines management as part of a suite of skills of engagement and overall plans of care.

ACKNOWLEDGEMENTS

The authors wish to acknowledge the following individuals for their kind contribution of care studies:

Andrew Roe
Service User Representative
University of Huddersfield

Laura Ainslie
Senior Clinical Practitioner, Psychiatric Intensive Care Unit
South West Yorkshire Partnership NHS Foundation Trust

Richard Clibbens
Nurse Consultant, Memory Service
South West Yorkshire Partnership NHS Foundation Trust

Lindsay Holliday
Clinical Lead, Kirklees Treatment Team
South West Yorkshire Partnership NHS Foundation Trust

References

1. CQC (Care Quality Commission). *Supporting briefing note: issues highlighted by 2009 survey of mental health acute inpatient services*. London: CQC, 2009. Available from: http://www.nhssurveys.org/Filestore//documents/MH_Inpatient_Key_Findings.pdf [Accessed 12th October 2016].
2. Ilyas S, Moncrieff J. Trends in prescriptions and costs of drugs for mental disorders in England, 1998–2010. *British Journal of Psychiatry* 2012; **200**(5): 393–8.
3. Dowrick C, Frances A. Medicalising unhappiness: new classification of depression risks more patients being put on drug treatment from which they will not benefit. *BMJ* 2013; **347**: 7140.
4. Croghan TW, Tomlin M, Pescosolido BA, Schnittker J, Martin J, Lubell K, Swindle R. American attitudes toward and willingness to use psychiatric medications. *Journal of Nervous and Mental Disease* 2003; **191**(3): 166–74.
5. McMurrich S, Sylvia LG, Dupuy JM, Peckham AD, Peters AT, Deckersbach T, Perlis RH. Course, outcomes, and psychosocial interventions for first-episode mania. *Bipolar Disorders* 2012; **14**(8): 797–808.
6. Richter T, Meyer G, Möhler R, Köpke S. Psychosocial interventions for reducing antipsychotic medication in care home residents. *Cochrane Database of Systematic Reviews* 2012; **12**: CD008634.
7. Trawver K, Springer DW, Rubin A. *Psychosocial treatment of schizophrenia*. Hoboken: Wiley, 2011.
8. Gamble C, Hart C. The use of psychosocial interventions. *Nursing Times* 2003; **99**(9): 46–7.
9. Kotowicz Z. *RD Laing and the paths of anti-psychiatry*. New York: Routledge, 2005.
10. Patel MX, Taylor M, David AS. Antipsychotic long-acting injections: mind the gap. *British Journal of Psychiatry* 2009; **195**(52): S1–S4.
11. Reid I, Cameron I, MacGillivray S. Increased prescription of antidepressants shows correction of inadequate duration of treatment of depression. *BMJ* 2014; **348**: g228.
12. Moore M, Yuen HM, Dunn N, Mulle MA, Maskell J, Kendrick T. Explaining the rise in antidepressant prescribing: a descriptive study using the general practice research database. *BMJ* 2009; 339.
13. Bloor K, Maynard A. *Expenditure on the NHS during and after the Thatcher years: its growth and utilisation*. York: Centre for Health Economics, University of York, 1993.
14. Health and Social Care Information Centre. Prescriptions dispensed in the community, statistics for England – 2002–2012

[NS]. 2012. Available from: http://content.digital.nhs.uk/catalogue/pub11291/pres-disp-com-eng-2002-12-rep.pdf [Accessed 28th October 2016].

15. NMC (Nursing and Midwifery Council). *Standards for pre-registration nursing education*. London: NMC, 2010.

16. NMC (Nursing and Midwifery Council). *Standards for medicines management*. London: NMC, 2008.

17. Pattison S, Wainwright P. Is the 2008 NMC Code ethical? *Nursing Ethics* 2010; **17**(1): 9–18.

18. Hemingway S, Snowden A. Debating mental health nurses' role in medicines management. *British Journal of Nursing* 2012; **21**(20): 1219–23.

19. Haynes RB, Ackloo E, Sahota N, McDonald HP, Yao X. Interventions for enhancing medication adherence. *Cochrane Database of Systematic Reviews* 2008; 2(2): CD000011.

20. Hemingway S, Stephenson J, Allmark H. Student experiences of medicines management training and education. *British Journal of Nursing* 2011; **20**(5): 291.

21. Taylor D, Paton C, Kapur S. *The Maudsley prescribing guidelines in psychiatry*. Chichester: John Wiley & Sons, 2012.

22. Shabbir SH, Sanders AE. Clinical significance in dementia research: a review of the literature. *American Journal of Alzheimer's Disease and Other Dementias* 2014; **29**(6): 492–7.

23. NICE (National Institute for Health and Care Excellence). About NICE. 2014. Available from: http://www.nice.org.uk/aboutnice/ [Accessed 12th October 2016].

24. Bird V, Leamy M, Tew J, Le Boutillier C, Williams J, Slade M. Fit for purpose? Validation of a conceptual framework for personal recovery with current mental health consumers. *Australian and New Zealand Journal of Psychiatry* 2014; **48**(7): 644–53.

25. Kress V E, Hoffman RM, Eriksen K. Ethical dimensions of diagnosing: considerations for clinical mental health counselors. *Counseling and Values* 2010; **55**: 101–112.

26. Ashmore R, Carver N. The pharmaceutical industry and mental health nursing. *British Journal of Nursing* 2001; **10**(21): 1396–402.

27. Petryna A, Lakoff A, Kleinman A. *Global pharmaceuticals: ethics, markets, practices*. Durham, NC: Duke University Press, 2006.

28. Harris BA. A critical nursing perspective of pharmacological interventions for schizophrenia and the marginalization of person-centered alternatives. *Issues in Mental Health Nursing* 2012; **33**(2): 127–9.

29. Edward K-L, Rasmussen B, Munro I. Nursing care of clients treated with atypical antipsychotics who have a risk of developing metabolic instability and/or type 2 diabetes. *Archives of Psychiatric Nursing* 2010; **24**(1): 46–53.

30. Cutcliffe J, Happell B. Psychiatry, mental health nurses, and invisible power: exploring a perturbed relationship within contemporary mental health care. *International Journal of Mental Health Nursing* 2009; **18**(2): 116–25.

31. Barker P, Buchanan-Barker P. First, do no harm: confronting the myths of psychiatric drugs. *Nursing Ethics* 2012; **19**(4): 451–63.

32. Hamann J, Kruse J, Schmitz FS, Kissling W, Pajonk F-G. Patient participation in antipsychotic drug choice decisions. *Psychiatry Research* 2010; **178**(1): 63–7.

33. Stewart DC, Anthony GB, Chesson R. 'It's not my job. I'm the patient not the doctor': patient perspectives on medicines management in the treatment of schizophrenia. *Patient Education and Counseling* 2010; **78**(2): 212–17.

34. Day JC, Bentall RP, Roberts C, Randall F, Rogers A, Cattell D, Healy D, Rae P, Power C. Attitudes toward antipsychotic medication: the impact of clinical variables and relationships with health professionals. *Archives of General Psychiatry* 2005; **62**(7): 717–24.

35. Taylor J, Davies P. The medicines management needs of carers during an episode of mental health crisis. *Journal of Psychiatric and Mental Health Nursing* 2012; **19**(2): 190–2.

36. Worthington A, Rooney P. *The Triangle of Care; carers included: a guide to best practice in acute mental health care*. London: Princess Royal Trust for Carers and the National Mental Health Development Unit, 2010.

37. Ogston-Tuck S. *Introducing medicines management*. Harlow: Pearson Education, 2011.

38. Randall F, Wood P, Day J, Bentall R, Rogers A, Healy D. Enhancing appropriate adherence with neuroleptic medication. In: Morrison AP (ed.). *A casebook of cognitive therapy for psychosis*. Abingdon and New York: Routledge, 2014: 281–98.

39. Jones RM. *Mental Capacity Act manual*. London: Sweet & Maxwell, 2012.

40. Jones R, Cole M. *Mental Health Act manual*. London: Sweet & Maxwell, 2013.

41. Vaughan K, McConaghy N, Wolf C, Myhr C, Black T. Community treatment orders: relationship to clinical care, medication compliance, behavioural disturbance and readmission. *Australian and New Zealand Journal of Psychiatry* 2000; **34**(5): 801–8.

42. Brownlie K, Schneider C, Culliford R, Fox C, Boukouvalas A, Willan C, Maidment ID. Medication reconciliation by a pharmacy technician in a mental health assessment unit. *International Journal of Clinical Pharmacy* 2014; **36**(2): 303–9.

43. Rothbard AB, Noll E, Kuno E, Zubritsky C, Hurford MO, Holzer C, Hadley T. Implementing an e-prescribing system in outpatient mental health programs. *Administration and Policy in Mental Health and Mental Health Services Research* 2013; **40**(3): 168–78.

44. Diamond R. Psychopharmacology and medication adherence. In: McQuistion HL, Sowers WE, Ranz JM, Feldman JM (eds). *Handbook of community psychiatry*. New York: Springer, 2012: 329–38.

45. Bryant Howren M, Van Liew JR, Christensen AJ. Advances in patient adherence to medical treatment regimens: the emerging role of technology in adherence monitoring and management. *Social and Personality Psychology Compass* 2013; **7**(7): 427–43.

46. Koroneos G. *Adherence through education*. North Olmsted: Advanstar Communications, Inc, 2010.

47. Curtin F, Schulz P. Relapse prevention and antidepressants. *Lancet* 2003; **361**(9375): 2158–9.

48. Tylee A, Howard L, Anderson IM, Matthews K, Ferrier IN, Scott J, Tylee A. Evidence-based guidelines for treating depressive disorders with antidepressants: a revision of the 2000 British Association for Psychopharmacology guidelines. *Journal of Psychopharmacology* 2008; **22**(4): 343–96.

49. Fountoulakis K, Vieta E, Bouras C, Notaridis G, Giannakopoulos P, Kaprinis G. Long term lithium therapy: a neuroprotective or neurotoxic factor? A systematic review of existing data. *Annals of General Psychiatry* 2006; **5**(Suppl. 1): S329.

50. Moncrieff J. Questioning the 'neuroprotective' hypothesis: does drug treatment prevent brain damage in early psychosis or schizophrenia? *British Journal of Psychiatry* 2011; **198**(2): 85–7.

51. Salomon C, Hamilton B. Antipsychotic discontinuation syndromes: a narrative review of the evidence and its integration into Australian mental health nursing textbooks. *International Journal of Mental Health Nursing* 2014; **23**(1): 69–78.

52. Macdonald M. Patient safety: examining the adequacy of the 5 rights of medication administration. *Clinical Nurse Specialist* 2010; **24**(4): 196–201.

53. Murray A. The implementation of a self-administration of medication programmes within Older Persons Mental Health. *Journal of Psychiatric and Mental Health Nursing* 2011; **18**(2): 113–21.

54. Wright J, Emerson A, Stephens M, Lennan E. Hospital inpatient self-administration of medicine programmes: a critical literature review. *Pharmacy World and Science* 2006; **28**(3): 140–51.

55. Duxbury JA, Wright K, Bradley D, Barnes P. Administration of medication in the acute mental health ward: perspective of nurses and patients. *International Journal of Mental Health Nursing* 2010; **19**(1): 53–61.

56. Hemingway S, White J, Baxter H, Smith G, Turner J, McCann T. Implementing a competence framework for administering medication: reporting the experiences of mental health nurses and students. *Issues in Mental Health Nursing* 2012; **20**(10): 657–64.

57. Hemingway S, White J, Turner J, Dewhirst K, Smith G. The Medicine with Respect Project: a stakeholder focus group evaluation. *Nurse Education in Practice* 2012; **12**(6): 310–15.

58. Baker JA, Lovell K, Harris N. A best-evidence synthesis review of the administration of psychotropic pro re nata (PRN) medication in in-patient mental health settings. *Journal of Clinical Nursing* 2008; **17**(9): 1122–31.

59. Usher K, Lindsay D, Sellen J. Mental health nurses' PRN psychotropic medication administration practices. *Journal of Psychiatric and Mental Health Nursing* 2001; **8**(5): 383–90.

60. Bateman DN. Benzodiazepines. *Medicine* 2012; **40**(3): 111.

61. McKenna PJ, Mortimer AM. Current and future treatment modalities in schizophrenia: novel antipsychotic drugs and cognitive therapy. *Expert Review of Neurotherapeutics* 2014; **14**(1): 67–73.

62. Fervaha G, Agid O, Takeuchi H, Foussias G, Remington G. Effect of antipsychotic medication on overall life satisfaction among individuals with chronic schizophrenia: findings from the NIMH CATIE study. *European Neuropsychopharmacology* 2014; **24**(7): 1078–85.

63. Jarboe KS. Considering the impact on overall patient health when choosing antipsychotic therapy. *Journal of the American Psychiatric Nurses Association* 2007; **13**(5): S23–8.

64. Mizukami A. Useful medicines information sources. *Practice Nurse* 2006; **32**(5): 32.

65. Schwartz KL, Roe T, Northrup J, Meza J, Seifeldin R, Neale AV. Family medicine patients' use of the internet for health information: a MetroNet study. *Journal of the American Board of Family Medicine: JABFM* 2006; **19**(1): 39–45.

66. Reichenpfader U, Gartlehner G, Morgan LC, Greenblatt A, Nussbaumer B, Hansen RA, Van Noord M, Lux L, Gaynes BN. Sexual dysfunction associated with second-generation antidepressants in patients with major depressive disorder: results from a systematic review with network meta-analysis. *Drug Safety* 2014; **37**(1): 19–31.

67. Harris N. Treatment adherence. In: Harris N, Baker J, Gray R (eds). *Medicines management in mental health care.* Chichester: John Wiley & Sons, 2009: 114–33.

68. Nash M. Improving mental health service users' physical health through medication monitoring: a literature review. *Journal of Nursing Management* 2011; **19**(3): 360–5.

69. Waddell L, Taylor M. A new self-rating scale for detecting atypical or second-generation antipsychotic side effects. *Journal of Psychopharmacology* 2008; **22**(3): 238–43.

70. Factor SA, Lang AE, Weiner WJ. *Rating scales for movement disorders.* Malden, MA: Blackwell: 20–9.

71. White J, Gray R, Jones M. The development of the serious mental illness physical Health Improvement Profile. *Journal of Psychiatric and Mental Health Nursing* 2009; **16**(5): 493.

72. Phillips L, McCann E. The subjective experiences of people who regularly receive depot neuroleptic medication in the community. *Journal of Psychiatric and Mental Health Nursing* 2007; **14**(6): 578–86.

73. Hemingway S, Ely V. Prescribing by mental health nurses: the UK perspective. *Perspectives in Psychiatric Care* 2009; **45**(1): 24–45.

74. Snowden A. Integrating medicines management into mental health nursing in UK. *Archives of Psychiatric Nursing* 2010; **24**(3): 178–88.

75. Kwentoh M-L, Reilly J. Non-medical prescribing: the story so far. *Psychiatric Bulletin* 2009; **33**(1): 4–7.

76. Adewuya AO, Owoeye OA, Erinfolami AR, Coker AO, Ogun OC, Okewole AO, Dada MU, Eze CN, Bello-Mojeed MA, Akindipe TO, Olagunju AT, Etim E. Prevalence and correlates of poor medication adherence amongst psychiatric outpatients in southwestern Nigeria. *General Hospital Psychiatry* 2009; **31**(2): 167–74.

77. Procter N, Baker A, Grocke K, Ferguson M. Introduction to mental health and mental illness: human connectedness and the collaborative consumer narrative. In Procter N, Hamer HP, McGarry D, Wilson RL, Froggatt T (eds). *Mental health: a person-centred approach.* Cambridge: Cambridge University Press, 2013: chapter 1.

78. Caldwell TM, Jorm AF. Mental health nurses' beliefs about likely outcomes for people with schizophrenia or depression: a comparison with the public and other healthcare professionals. *Australian and New Zealand Journal of Mental Health Nursing* 2001; **10**(1): 42–54.

79. Hercelinskyj G, Cruickshank M, Brown P, Phillips B. Perceptions from the front line: professional identity in mental health nursing. *International Journal of Mental Health Nursing* 2014; **23**(1): 24–32.

Further reading

Harris N, Baker J, Gray R (eds). *Medicines management in mental health care.* Chichester: John Wiley & Sons, 2009.

Lehner T, Senthil G, Addington AM. Convergence of advances in genomics, team science, and repositories as drivers of progress in psychiatric genomics. *Biological Psychiatry* 2015; **77**(1): 6–14.

South West Yorkshire Partnership NHS Foundation Trust. Medicines with Respect: assessment of the administration of oral medicines. Available from: http://www.southwestyorkshire.nhs.uk/documents/783.pdf [Accessed 18th October 2016].

Relevant web pages

Medicines Complete. https://www.medicinescomplete.com/about/subscribe.htm

Register on this site to have access to the British National Formulary (often referred to as the BNF).

MHRA (Medicines and Healthcare products Regulatory Agency). Yellow Card. https://yellowcard.mhra.gov.uk/

MIND. Psychiatric drugs: an alphabetical list. http://mind.org.uk/information-support/drugs-and-treatments/medication-drugs-a-z/

NICE (National Institute for Health and Care Excellence). http://www.nice.org.uk/

This website provides clinical guidelines and pathways that follow the current best evidence for treatment.

Royal Pharmaceutical Society. Medicines optimisation. http://www.rpharms.com/what-we-re-working-on/medicines-optimisation.asp

Section 5

Services and support for those with mental health distress

What does it mean to be a carer for someone with a mental health problem?

GEORGINA WAKEFIELD AND GARY HICKEY

LEARNING OUTCOMES

- To realize the importance of giving carers sufficient information about the illness of the person for whom they care and options.

- To recognize that there are many factors and interventions, from a variety of professions and people, which contribute toward helping carers cope.

- To be aware that the attitudes and behaviours of professionals can impact significantly on the hopes of carers.

- To recognize that no two situations are exactly the same and that individual carers and service users will require their own unique, tailored support.

- To acknowledge the role of carers as part of the team and that they need support, education and information in order to carry out a vital role.

SUMMARY OF KEY POINTS

- Caring is a craft. Carers need help, support and information from professionals to help them overcome challenges and discover what factors will help them in their situation.

- The attitude and behaviour of professionals play a vital role in supporting and providing hope to carers.

- Professionals' provision of information to carers is particularly important. This information includes diagnosis and care and treatment options. This will enable carers to make informed choices and decisions.

- Professionals need to work in collaboration with carers. They need to listen to them and regard them as part of the care provision team.

INTRODUCTION

The aim of this chapter is to help readers gain a deeper insight into the impact having a son or daughter with a mental health problem has on the whole family of carers. This chapter is a personal story of our journey and the challenges that we, a family caring for our son, faced and the factors that have helped us cope. Although very much a personal perspective, I have collaborated with Gary Hickey in writing this chapter. He has helped me pull this information together, link it to some wider developments and structure it to fit with this book, while ensuring that it is my voice that you 'hear' on these pages.

It occurred to me recently that, if we lose a spouse, we are referred to as a widow or a widower. A child who loses a parent is referred to as an orphan. There is no name for a parent who loses a child, be it through death or a severe and enduring mental illness. Our son, Christian, was diagnosed with paranoid schizophrenia. We feel that we lost Christian around the age of 16 and the grieving process never really ends. Twenty-five years later, I have come to terms with the fact that there is nothing we can do to change this. Although I don't think I will ever come to terms with our loss, we, and Christian, have coped.

ME AND MY SON CHRISTIAN

Over the years we've had three very different sons: Christian before he became unwell; Christian when he was first given antipsychotic medication; and finally Christian as he is today. He has slowly recovered, but his cognitive functioning is very poor. He struggles to remember things, he has lost his spark, and he tends to be very quiet and finds it difficult to engage in conversations. But if he is having a good day, he is the happiest soul on this earth. He has dealt with his journey extremely well and has always shown his family the utmost respect. I have finally accepted the fact that there is only so much that we as parents can do, and that for our son there is no cure for schizophrenia. Having said that, we will never stop fighting his corner or indeed missing the son he was before this dreadful illness tore into all of our lives.

I've been on both sides of the fence. Although I am a carer for my son, I have suffered from severe anxiety/depression from the age of 18. I am now 66 years old. I have never been given a diagnosis but I would say after a lot of researching that I suffer from cyclothymia. I have taken medications from the age of 18. People often ask me why I have dedicated so much time to this subject of mental health and two words sum it up: injustice and respect. Having witnessed my son's suffering day in and day out for many years, I find it very hard to cope with the injustice that attaches itself to mental distress and in particular schizophrenia. As for 'respect', well, that is the very least that sufferers deserve.

I often use poetry because it can be quite difficult to talk about 'the mind'. I find that poetry captures lived experiences and the sometimes elusive language of personal reflection, thoughts, feelings and insights. In short, it is a unique way of communicating and it highlights emotional intensity very well.

This poem explains what it is like being on both sides of the fence and paints a picture of our family circumstances.

Both sides of the fence

Service User then Carer sometimes I think life could have been fairer
My label is Cyclothymia my son's? Paranoid Schizophrenia
His label promotes negative attitudes whilst the tabloids create the sensation
If you're wondering what's been the hardest? I'd say Carer … no hesitation
A helpless witness to your pain time and time and time again
Both sides of the fence entangled feelings so intense
A constant witness to your struggle your disordered thoughts are such a muddle
You believe we can hear your thoughts you're distressed and overwrought
I scream silently inside but tears must go uncried
I must not let you see how your suffering affects me
How are you today? not good I hear you say
My stomach starts to churn but I gloss things over now I've learned
Things will improve I say yeah I know mum 'one day'
A voice screams in my head I hide my fear and dread
Do you fancy a cup of tea? Distraction can help you see
I'll only throw it up so don't make me a cup
Both sides of the fence our combined feelings too intense
Where's the son we used to know has anyone seen him? Where did he go?
Now the TV is referring to you I try hard to explain it's not true
To you though it's so very real and hard to understand how you feel
I can see things mum you say why won't it just go away?
It's all part of the condition try hard to see it's not real
Take a Valium [sheer desperation] mum you don't know how I feel
Think of the starving children … Imagine being blind
I do mum but it makes no difference what the hell is wrong with my mind?
You don't ask much of this life despite all these painful years
I marvel at your tenacity despite such constant fears
Thrown into an endless battle a battle that's yet to be won
Always there for each other I'm your mother you're my son
Tangled by this web we're caught up in feelings so intense
A very confusing place to be on both sides of the fence

WHAT ARE THE CHALLENGES?

There are many challenges to being a carer for my son. In this section I give a personal account of the main ones that we faced:

- not knowing;
- maintaining hope;
- isolation;
- stigma.

Not knowing

In the UK, there have been various pieces of legislation and policy documents that have placed service users and communities at the heart of the design and delivery of services.[1–8] A distinction has been made between two approaches to involving service users and carers: consumerism and democratization.[9,10] Consumerism refers to service users or carers commenting and being consulted about decisions whereas democratization refers to their active engagement in partnership in decision making.[9,11]

But call it consumerism or call it democratization, a key requirement is the provision of information. It is only with this information that people are able to make informed choices and decisions. Indeed, the National Institute for Health and Care Excellence (NICE) 2014[12] clinical guideline about the treatment of psychosis and schizophrenia recommends that mental health professionals give family members and other carers written and verbal information about diagnosis and recovery, (see chapters 35 and 36 for more detail about recovery) the role of mental health teams and services and how to get help in a crisis. Our experience, however, was very different. We spent many years not knowing what was wrong and not being given the right information.

Christian had always been an outgoing lad. The illness came on very subtly and very slowly and it was hard to detect how much was raging hormones and normal teenage behaviour. I had this gut feeling that something far more sinister was going on. He started having problems concentrating at school. He became argumentative and stroppy at home, as teenagers do. He became increasingly reclusive and refused to sit at the dinner table. He'd take his food to his bedroom and insist on eating in there. One day he stood in the middle of the lawn in torrential rain for over an hour; his hair was stuck to his face, his clothes soaked through. He didn't seem to know what to do, where to go or even who he was. Remarkably, he had a couple of jobs after leaving school but struggled with his concentration. He started throwing clothes away that had patterns on them because he thought they interfered with his concentration. He would be scared that his friends would break in and harm us.

Getting help for Christian took 14 months and three appointments with his GP, who seemed to think that I was over-reacting. The first time I went to see him, he said, 'You will have to get him to come and see me.' I explained that

Christian didn't think there was anything wrong with him. The second appointment was just as bad. Luckily a friend came with me the third time and she asked the GP if he thought Christian was losing his mind. To my amazement, he said, 'I have no doubt that he is.' He finally agreed to send two social workers to our home a few days later. By now Christian weighed eight stone two pounds, and at six feet two inches tall, was little more than skin and bone.

Christian was eventually prescribed medication – intermuscular injections of Piportil every 4 weeks in his backside (which he hated). No one explained to us what it was for or what it was supposed to achieve. We thought he'd be his old self in a few weeks. No one told us what was wrong with him. The psychiatrist told us he had a 'thought pattern disorder'. He would talk gobbledegook (word salad). His words would be a jumble and nothing made any sense, but no one thought to explain thought disorder to us. The confusion this caused ('high expressed emotion', as practitioners refer to it) could have easily been avoided had someone explained things. Our son had changed from being an extremely articulate, witty and highly intelligent young man into someone who was unable to even follow a conversation. We needed to understand thought disorder, auditory hallucinations, visual hallucinations, thought block, thought disorder, etc. – so-called 'positive symptoms'. Chapter 28 describes these symptoms in more detail. We had no idea what 'CPN' (community psychiatric nurse) or 'ASW' (approved social worker) meant. To us it was like a foreign language.

We were not warned about the effects of the antipsychotic medication. We were not told about the inertia, total lack of interest and endless sleeping caused by the medication. Consequently, another son appeared, one who slept constantly and walked around like a zombie with lead boots on. I foolishly believed that he would just get up one day and the son we used to know would miraculously reappear. I would try to get him friends and part-time work, but I could not see that he was incapable of doing these things, all because we had no understanding and no idea what was wrong with him.

It was only when we applied for benefits almost 7 years into his illness, and a letter came through stating that 'Mr Christian John Wakefield' has paranoid schizophrenia, that we had a proper diagnosis. I remember dropping the letter. I was in a daze. The GP later said to me, 'Well, you did realize he had schizophrenia, didn't you?' I honestly didn't. No one had ever told us. Hindsight is a wonderful thing. Perhaps the GP and psychiatrist didn't tell us because of fears about the impact the diagnosis would have on us all. However, 'protecting' us in this way just delayed the inevitable. Being starved of valuable information meant the well-meaning things we were doing as family were sometimes making the situation worse. Chapter 12 has information on the classification of mental illness.

Christian now takes clozapine. His condition greatly improved after he was prescribed (See chapters 47 and 48 for information on psychopharmacology.) it. Sadly, this was prescribed 9 years into his illness. He might have been spared years of mental torture and us years of anxiety and heartache. This thought haunts me – would he have recovered to a far better level had I known about this drug? A loaded question, and one to which I will never know the answer. Again, this is a demonstration of the lack of information given to carers and service users far too often.

> ## REFLECTION
>
> What role does information play in empowering service users and carers? How else might you empower service users and carers to have a greater say in the decision making about their care?

Maintaining hope

Hope is very important to carers. We never expected Christian to be able to live independently or work part-time. Christian has lived in his own flat for over 10 years and he now manages 6 hours a week putting letters into envelopes in a hospital over the road from where we live. There was only one practitioner who had the confidence to predict that he would be able to do both of these things. Practitioners must understand that carers will look to them for guidance and hope, and to take hope away causes immense pain and life becomes even more difficult. Some practitioners can take away our hope and their words will go round and round our heads, whereas those that promote hope give us confidence and we feel far more able to cope with the caring role (see chapters 35 and 36 for for discussions on recovery).

We are well aware that things could be far worse. On our travels we have met many other carers; some of them have sons/daughters who have been in hospital for many years and it is likely that some of them will remain in care for the rest of their lives. Christian does have some quality of life and we live in hope that one day his cognitive functioning will improve as well as his symptoms.

> ## REFLECTION
>
> Reflecting on your own practice, what role do you think you play in giving service users and carers hope for their future? In what ways, if any, do you think you could do more?

Isolation

Christian relapsed aged 23 and the next 5 years were spent either in hospital or 24-hour care. He had no quality of life and mixing with friends and relatives became very difficult.

Christian's friends abandoned him very early on due to their lack of understanding. One of his friends actually said to me, 'Chris is in a mental hospital, isn't he?' When I replied, 'Yes', he said, 'It's very sad, but don't ask me to go to visit him, will you?'

We just existed. Relationships with other family members deteriorated big time. They had their own lives to live; normal lives, and mixing with us was like mixing oil with water. The illness consumes you. It infects you. You think: why my son? I do think that the younger people develop this condition, the poorer the prognosis. The older you are at its onset, the more you have to fall back on in recovery. Christian had no experience of the working world, relationships, driving a car, etc. Consequently, it's almost as if he hasn't evolved at the normal rate and is caught up in a sort of time warp. I would get frustrated with practitioners. I can vividly remember Christian's nurse saying, 'Mrs Wakefield, try going to college, you could do music or art.' I was thinking, 'How on earth do you think I could go to college and concentrate when my teenage son is losing his mind before my very eyes?'

Stigma

We know that there is still a lot of stigma around mental health[13,14] and that there is a particular public perception that people with schizophrenia are 'dangerous'.[15]

There is still much work that needs to be done in reducing the stigma associated with mental health. There were many experiences of the stigma faced by Christian and the family. Local residents smashed the security lights the night his new residential facility opened. A local headmistress called the police when she saw Christian sitting by the side of the local swimming pool trying to decide whether to get in or not. The police called him out of the pool and asked him, 'Why are you in there while there are children in there?' We were horrified. This incident caused him so much stress and he was prescribed even more medication which he has remained on to this day. His new neighbours wrote letters to the local paper stating that they did not want the mentally afflicted living near them because of the danger to their everyday lives. Injustice!

Out of all the conditions, schizophrenia seems to come off the worst. Lots of people react negatively to media headlines that use words like 'sicko', 'psycho', 'schizo', 'nutter' – sensationalism at its worst. I get so frustrated when I am asked, 'Is he violent?' Sometimes when asked, I reply, 'No. Are *you*?'

This poem, about stigma, is based on my favourite poem by Rudyard Kipling.

If

If you would try your best to combat stigma
That surrounds all those who suffer mental distress
Help people see it's not just an enigma
That can make us feel that we are even less

Less than human beings we're weirdos psychos
    schizos
We're just a waste of space we're crazy we're insane
If you could feel the depth of so much suffering
Or be witness to a loved one in such pain
If you can try to see that mental illness
Is just a tragic life event a twist of fate
If you can see the media just exploits us
Creating negativity promoting hate
If you can sense the evil behind the tabloids
Read between the lines and not be taken in
If you realize their motive is making money
The pain it causes to so many such a sin
If you'd been there to witness such tenacity
You'd been there too many times to watch them fall
Then pick themselves back up and that astounds you
Far too many times for you to just recall
If you could see just how much they've lost forever
Stolen from them in the blinking of an eye

You'd understand why so many take their own lives
The pain so intense it's easier to die
If you'd seen families torn apart beneath the weight
Of coping till they're sick of their hard lives
If you could walk a mile in carers' shoes
You'd question how these people can survive
If you can imagine how it feels to be excluded
Without someone there to lend a caring hand
If you'd spare the time to imagine what it feels like
Knowing so many people will never understand
If you should wonder why I've put these words
together
My son developed schizophrenia at 16
25 years on and he struggles on to deal with
What he's heard what he's felt and what he's seen
If you would pledge with me to combat stigma
Try to spread the truth wherever you may go
Till mental illness won't be seen as an enigma
You'd pave the way for better futures this I know

DISCOVERING HOW TO COPE

It is noted in chapter 15 that carers and family members take on the majority of care for people living in the community. It is vital that these people are adequately supported. There are now helpful guidelines for carers on how to cope[16] and how to get support.[17] Back then, though, there was much less support available. I see Christian's 'recovery' as due to a combination of so many things. He and we, his carers, have learned what to welcome and what to avoid. We have discovered, on our journey, what factors have helped us, as a family, cope. All of the following contribute toward the craft of caring:

- a compatible personal assistant;
- love and compassion;
- collaborative working partnerships;
- medication;
- talking therapy;
- some independent living;
- attention to diet and physical exercise;
- respite;
- family therapy;
- education for carers.

A compatible personal assistant

Employing a personal assistant (PA), through the government's personal budgets scheme, has, more than anything else, helped us all to cope. This personal budgets scheme is designed to provide funding for things that will improve quality of life. Christian was assessed by an occupational therapist for several weeks. His findings were that Christian was very lonely and isolated and that the best way forward was for Christian to employ a PA who could help him to socialize. We can say in all honesty that Christian has done more in the past few years than he did in the 17 years leading up to employing a PA. Having a PA is helping Christian to live both independently and safely. It also helps us because we are sharing the burden of caring, which makes life much easier to cope with.

His current PA, Denise, has made significant improvements to his life. He now enjoys going to shows (often, in London), shopping trips, breaks away and even holidays – something that he has not enjoyed since he was a boy. Caring can be exhausting but these days I feel free to do things that I wasn't able to do before. We still have daily contact and provide support and a safe, inviting place for him to come whenever he likes, but I am not constantly worrying like I used to. He has employed five PAs, but I feel that only one of them has been suitable. Denise had first-hand experience of mental health problems and it was very apparent from the start that, unlike his other PAs, she did not have to keep phoning me for advice on how to deal with problems that arose. Recovery is only possible if we can improve quality of life – relying on medication is only one small part of the jigsaw.

Love and compassion

Mental illness strips people of their precious self-esteem. We believe that love and solid family support is the biggest mover in recovery.

Our son's illness was handled as if we didn't really exist. Had he been suffering from a physical condition, we believe that we would have felt far more included. The government's mental health strategy[5] says that it seeks to

49

What does it mean to be a carer for someone with a mental health problem?

raise the profile of mental health and make it as important a priority as physical health. It also aims to promote good mental health through early intervention, particularly in childhood and the teenage years, and reduce the social inequalities that contribute to mental ill-health. It is high time that mental health was given exactly the same level of understanding and compassion as physical illnesses.

Pets have also played a role. We have a border terrier and a chihuahua. We've had five dogs during Christian's illness; whenever one got old, we bought another puppy. Alfie the border terrier is almost 9, and we have recently bought Lou Lou. Christian gets a lot of comfort from stroking the dogs.

Collaborative working partnerships

The World Health Organization is clear that the delivery of modern health care is dependent on professionals coming together as interdisciplinary teams.[18] In the UK, the Health and Social Care Act (2012)[6] and the National Collaboration for Integrated Care and Support (2013)[19] emphasize the need for professions to work collaboratively to provide integrated and safe patient care. There have been high-profile cases of inadequate collaborative working, for example the case of Baby P[20] and the scandal at Mid Staffordshire Foundation Trust, resulting in the Francis Report (2013).[21] Both reports highlighted how poor communication and team-working between professionals impacts negatively on patient care. A partnership between professionals and carers is also very important.[22] Chapter 50 outlines in more detail how to include service users and carers in collaborative care planning.

In recent years, we feel practitioners have listened to us, but more importantly heard us. Carers have a wealth of experience that should be tapped into and used. We need to work with professionals as partners in care, with both parties respecting each other for their individual but equally important expertise. Some professionals hide behind a smokescreen of patient confidentiality, even when the service user is happy for their carer to be involved in all aspects of their care. This is a major cause of 'high expressed emotion'. We have found that lack of understanding as to just how hard this is for families has been extremely difficult to cope with. The ongoing sadness never goes away; no matter where we are or what we are doing, Christian is in the back of our minds.

REFLECTION

What characterizes good partnership working between professionals and carers? Consider how you could improve how you work with carers.

Medication

Christian now takes 500 mg of clozapine daily; this drug is the gold standard for treatment-resistant schizophrenia (TRS). Within 12 weeks of it being prescribed, he moved from 24-hour to 12-hour care.

Christian still suffers from both auditory and visual hallucinations, his thoughts are often disordered, and he also gets thought broadcasting, which convinces him that people can actually hear what he is thinking. While watching TV, he often says that the people on TV know everything about him. This means that his confidence is often at an all-time low. Sometimes it can mean prompting him to do things, as he is often preoccupied with what goes on in his mind. Christian's mental health fluctuates regularly and dramatically throughout the day and this prevents him from doing everyday personal tasks; for example, sometimes he needs gently reminding about his washing and general hygiene routine, to get up and be motivated to face the day, to keep hospital appointments for blood tests and seeing his GP or consultant psychiatrist. However, this is not to the same degree as he used to before he was prescribed clozapine.

We stress that it has to be the right medication. Furthermore, this should be monitored and changed if there is little or no improvement.

Talking therapy

Christian was lucky enough to have 3 years of a psychodynamic therapy combined with art therapy which has given him an insight into his condition (see chapter 42 for information on psychodynamic approaches with individuals). Asking people to go through this journey without the benefit of talking therapy is like asking someone to climb a mountain without a compass, rope or light. The difference now is that when he experiences symptoms he knows that this is part of his condition. He knows that the things he is seeing are not real. And he knows that other people can't hear his thoughts – he just thinks they can sometimes. This has made things far less frightening for him.

Recently he came with us while I gave a talk to some student nurses. At the end of the session he read something about how he feels about his illness, and when his dad shed a tear, Chris suddenly walked out of the room. I apologized and went to find him. When I asked him what was wrong, he explained that 'When dad got upset, I thought everyone in the room hated me for having schizophrenia and then I realized that it was nonsense and that I was in "the other mind".'

Some independent living

There are two aspects to this: supported housing and part-time employment.

Christian has lived in his own flat for 10 years with support from his family and his PA. Staff are there from 9 am to 5 pm, Monday to Friday. He is one of the lucky ones; he has plenty of support. Some of the other young people who live there (eight altogether) are not so lucky and they rely heavily on staff, needing help with managing finances, keeping appointments cleaning, etc.

Chris also manages to work part-time (6 hours of paid employment per week), and this has provided structure, social inclusion and financial support too. If Chris needs to call me for reassurance, he is allowed to do so. He also has a 10-minute break and, because we live so close to his work, he comes over for a cup of tea.

Attention to diet and physical exercise

We encourage Chris to do as much walking as he can. He used to go swimming but, due to the incident outlined in the section on 'stigma', he refuses to go now. His current GP is very vigilant and keeps regular checks on his physical health. I am reminded by text message when he has an appointment and his GP also arranges, periodically, for a full blood count. Chapters 69 and 70 give details on physical health care and mental health promotion.

Respite

This is imperative for carers. As well as the personal budget Christian gets to employ his PA, we as carers are also given a budget for respite. We were assessed by Christian's social worker, who managed to get us an ongoing £800 per year, which pays for eight nights away in bed and breakfast. We never had a holiday for 20 years; now we usually take two nights at a time and come back feeling refreshed and far more able to care for our son.

Family therapy

Family therapy helped us to take a look at our own behaviour and address things accordingly. Christian and I especially were far too fused together. I put this down to me having suffered mental distress and I couldn't bear to think that my son was suffering in a similar way. I openly admit that I have 'over cared' and I have tried to make up for all of the things that have been taken away from Christian.

I often think that having suffered mental distress myself is both helpful and unhelpful in equal measure – helpful because I have been able to be very patient and because I understand (to a certain extent) what Chris has to cope with, but unhelpful because I have probably done far too much for him. Chapter 51 considers family involvement and support networks.

Education for carers

Hindsight is a wonderful thing and educating carers in the early years is what is needed. The section on 'not knowing' illustrated how much in the dark we were about Christian's condition and what options were available to us. We need a service that helps family members to understand, because I have seen so many families fall apart purely due to a total lack of understanding.

CONCLUSION

This chapter has been a personal account of my experience of caring for someone with a mental health problem. I have outlined the key challenges we faced: the need to maintain hope and the impact professionals can have on this; not knowing what was happening to my son and the lack of information we received from professionals; the isolation and lack of support; and the stigma that people with schizophrenia face.

The chapter has also detailed the things that have helped us cope with this situation: the key role played by a personal assistant with the right 'fit' for Christian; the importance of love and compassion from both family carers and professionals; and the need for good partnerships between carers and professionals. Talking therapy has also helped Christian. Getting the right medication can also be important, as can advice and guidance on diet and exercise. Carers can also receive support through education about mental health problems, respite and family therapy. That Christian is in work and lives in supported housing is both a consequence of these things and also a contributing factor to us coping with the situation.

I want to end this chapter by talking about the things that this journey has taught us. Although this is what you could say is a long, hard, rocky road, I believe we are all better human beings as a result of this journey.

I would say that for family members especially acceptance is the key, but the time it takes to come to terms with this situation will vary. We – Christian's dad and I – appreciate life. We have come into contact with many wonderful people; some are practitioners and some, like us, are informal carers. Knowing people who have walked the same path helps me to cope. Carers share an empathy that is almost tangible. It has taken us years to realize that all we can do is be here and support our son in any way that we can. We have finally accepted that this is a serious and chronic condition and we too have lives to live. None of us knows what life will throw at us and managing the situation takes time and patience and skill. Christian's strength helps no end and without this journey he would not be who he is today either; a kind, unassuming and compassionate young man.

I dedicate this poem to my son and to anyone who suffers from mental distress.

Proud

Our youngest son Christian John suffers from
  Schizophrenia
He suffers each day in silence with a kind and gentle
  demeanour

49

What does it mean to be a carer for someone with a mental health problem?

But look deeply beyond his label to the baby I held in
   my arms
To the happy mischievous four-year-old who
   captured the world with his charms
To the bright intelligent ten-year-old who excelled at
   school in his study
To the twelve-year-old football fanatic who'd come
   home exhausted and muddy
To the carefree handsome teenager who would greet
   me with a kiss
To the son I would lay down my life for but the man I
   was destined to miss
He waded through the torment hallucinations and
   angry voices
Robbed of the sweet years of youth and denied so
   many choices

Forced to deal with public ignorance and the pain
   that goes with stigma
He accepted that mental illness is still viewed as a
   kind of ENIGMA
Because my son was sent on a journey there were
   demons he had to face
Along with horrific memories he struggles each day
   to erase
A journey so long and relentless we can never
   measure his pain
So many times he would stumble and fall but rise to
   his feet yet again
Now he's quiet and unassuming but to me he stands
   out from the crowd
He's the son that he was always destined to be
And one word describes my feelings and that's PROUD

References

1. Department of Health. *Patient and public involvement in the new NHS*. London: Stationery Office, 1999.
2. Department of Health. *Commissioning a patient-led NHS*. London: Stationery Office, 2005.
3. Department of Health. *Independence, well-being and choice: our vision for the future of social care for adults in England*. London: Stationery Office, 2005.
4. Department of Health. *Our health, our care, our say: a new direction for community services*. London: Stationery Office, 2006.
5. Department of Health. *No health without mental health: a cross government mental health outcomes strategy for people of all ages*. London: Central Office of Communication, 2011.
6. Department of Health. *NHS Constitution for England*. Available from: https://www.gov.uk/government/uploads/system/uploads/attachment_data/file/480482/NHS_Constitution_WEB.pdf [Accessed 2nd December 2016].
7. *Health and Social Care Act*. 2012. London: Stationery Office, 2012.
8. Darzi A. *High quality care for all: NHS next stage review final report*. London: Department of Health, 2008.
9. Hickey G, Kipping C. Exploring the concept of user involvement in mental health through a participation continuum. *Journal of Clinical Nursing* 1998; **7**: 83–8.
10. Beresford P. User involvement in research: exploring the challenges. *Nursing Times Research* 2003; **8**(1): 35–46.
11. Collier R, Stickley T. From SUI to collaboration in mental health nurse education: developing a practical philosophy for change. *Journal of Mental Health Training, Education and Practice* 2010; **5**(4): 4–11.
12. National Collaborating Centre for Mental Health. *Psychosis and schizophrenia in adults; the NICE guidelines on treatment and management*. 2014. Available from: http://www.nice.org.uk/guidance/cg178/evidence/full-guideline-490503565 [Accessed 1st December 2016].
13. Thornicroft G. *Shunned: discrimination against people with mental illness*. New York: Oxford University Press, 2006.
14. Corrigan PW, Morris SB, Michaels PJ, Rafacz JD, Rusch N. Challenging the public stigma of mental illness: a metaanalysis of outcome studies. *Psychiatric Services* 2012; **63**(10): 963–3.
15. Denenny D, Bentley E, Schiffman J. Validation of a brief implicit association test of stigma: schizophrenia and dangerousness. *Journal of Mental Health* 2014; **23**(5), 246–50.
16. MIND. *How to cope as a carer*. Available from: https://www.mind.org.uk/media/859562/how-to-cope-as-a-carer-2014-.pdf [Accessed 1st December 2016].
17. Rethink Mental Illness. *Factsheet: Carer's assessment and support planning*, 2015. Available from: https://www.rethink.org/resources/c/carers-assessments-and-support-planning-factsheet [Accessed 1st December 2016].
18. WHO (World Health Organization). *Health workforce: nursing and midwifery*. Geneva: WHO, 2013.
19. National Collaboration for Integrated Care and Support. *Integrated care and support: our shared commitment*. Available from: https://www.gov.uk/government/publications/integrated-care [Accessed 1st December 2016].
20. Laming H. *The protection of children in England: a progress report*. London: Stationery Office, 2009.
21. *Report of the Mid Staffordshire NHS Foundation Trust Public Inquiry*. London: Stationery Office, 2013.
22. Gall SH, Eliott L, Atkinson JM, Johansen R. Mental health. Training nurses to support carers of relatives with schizophrenia. *British Journal of Nursing* 2001; **10**(4): 238–41.

Further reading

Schofield M. *January first: a child's descent into madness and her father's struggle to save her*. London: Hardy Grant Books, 2013.
Torrey ET. *Surviving schizophrenia, sixth edition: a family manual*. New York: Harper Perennial, 2013.
Wakefield G. *Schizophrenia: a mother's story*. Salisbury: Fivepin, 2002.
Wakefield G. *Addicts' language*. London: Chipmunka, 2003.
Wakefield G. *Surviving schizophrenia – through the maze and fighting back*. Salisbury: Fivepin, 2004.
Wakefield G. *Loving Christian: one family's journey through schizophrenia*. Monmouth: PCCS, 2010.

Relevant web pages

Georgina Wakefield. Spotlight on schizophrenia. www.georginawakefield.co.uk
Mind. www.mind.org.uk
Mental Health Care. www.mentalhealthcare.org.uk
Rethink Mental Illness. www.rethink.org
Schizophrenia.com. www.schizophrenia.com

50 Collaborative care planning with service users and carers

DOUGLAS HAMANDISHE AND DANIEL BARRETT

LEARNING OUTCOMES

- To understand the purpose of collaborative care planning.
- To know how to implement it into practice.
- To appreciate the importance of recovery.
- To be able to apply the principles of shared decision making.
- To be aware of challenges to collaborative care planning and how to overcome them.
- To understand how to involve the carer in the care planning process.

SUMMARY OF KEY POINTS

- Care planning should start from the point of view of the person[1] and focus on their individual needs, strengths, aspirations and personal goals.[2]
- The principles of shared decision making should underpin the care planning process.[3]
- The issue of who holds the power and control[4] is the key defining barrier to effective collaborative care planning.

INTRODUCTION

In keeping with the spirit of 'the craft of caring',[5] this chapter represents a collaborative effort between two people with varying experiences and varying ideas about the 'why, how and what?' of collaborative care planning. United by the principle that collaborative care planning is better for people than non-collaborative care planning, our process focused on agreeing a common set of topics we would both think and write about, and then comparing and reflecting on each other's point of view. The topics were as follows:

- What is the point in care planning?
- Process of collaborative care planning
- Recovery
- Shared decision making
- Barriers to effective collaborative care planning

Throughout our discussions, we found that we disagreed more than we agreed, so rather than straining for consensus, this chapter is written in two different voices, so that each is valued equally. Much of our disagreement can be summarized by the question: 'Who owns the care plan?'; is it a document for the individual receiving care, or a document for a nurse to deliver effective care for the individual? We have therefore included a final section to this chapter that is dedicated to answering that question.

WHAT IS THE POINT IN CARE PLANNING?

Douglas

Care planning has been an accepted part of mental health treatment for many years. It can be seen to have evolved from a loosely defined record of planned care for service users (produced exclusively by nurses following an initial assessment), to an ongoing and adaptive record of planned care written with and for the service user.

Across all disciplines of nursing, care plans have a bad historical reputation for a lack of service user involvement. Within mental health services the care plan was regarded as a once-only activity, serving more as a one-directional plan of the treatment applied to the recipient (the service user). Following a formal assessment, nurses would scurry away to a quiet room to write up the care plan, typically in paper format, which would end up confined to the relevant sections of the service user's clinical notes. Together with the service user's risk assessment and clinical progress notes, the care plan served as a prerequisite to facilitate the transfer of a service user to another ward or hospital, and was considered to be of little importance.[6]

Nurses were more concerned with identifying any potentially 'risky' behaviour traits that service users displayed to the nurses themselves or to others, resulting in an inpatient admission. Collaboration with service users was rarely sought and neither service users nor carers were routinely given a copy of the care plan, or the opportunity to discuss its content. In a study assessing user involvement in care planning, Lawson et al.[7] described user involvement in decision making regarding their needs, care planning and receipt of information as poor.

Care plans had relied on 'medical diagnoses' to encapsulate the perceived problems and paid little attention to challenges defined by service users or their carers. The diagnosis-focused, medically propelled care plans were riddled with jargon, medical terms and abbreviations that further alienated the service user. The language of the care plans has been described beautifully by a voluntary service user as being 'Impenetrable; a secret language used amongst so-called professionals to further alienate us service users and carers alike'.

Negative experiences such as this can become heightened when a service user is being treated under a section of the Mental Health Act. Under these circumstances, tensions commonly arise between the service user and the nurse, particularly when the service user is disputing the validity of the admission and its treatment regime.[8]

The care plan written in medical language by the nurse, based on their ideas of what the service user needs, failed to integrate the service user's own views and goals. This process eroded service users' confidence in drawing upon their own experiences, coping strategies, values and motivation to recover from mental illness. These conditions framed service users as passive recipients of care who had to rely on the expertise of nurses, rather than seeing themselves as being the source of their recovery.

Even with the best of intentions, the care plan will always fall short of meeting service users' expectations and needs for self-determination through making informed decisions about their care.[9] This is not because it fails to identify all the problems; rather it is because it fails to incorporate the service user's own goals to drive the treatment.

Fortunately, there are some signs that care plans are improving. In order to modernize the NHS, the Department of Health (DoH) has prioritized the goals of giving service users choice, promoting social inclusion, and ensuring that service users have control of their own lives and personal responsibility for their own well-being.[10] The DoH has also introduced the revised and updated Care Programme Approach (CPA),[11] which makes the point, with poignancy, that the care plan should promote recovery by giving weight to improving outcomes that mattered to the person.[12] However, in a study of 103 service users on the CPA, McDermott[13] found that service users were still not aware of their treatment plans, that the CPA process was difficult to understand and that little information was given to service users regarding their care. Interestingly, the study also revealed that service users felt their opinions, in both care planning and decision making, were valued less than the opinions of both professionals and carers.[14]

Changes to the ways in which health care is organized have challenged ideas about ownership of the care plan. Greater integration between mental health and other health care providers has brought about closer multidisciplinary team (MDT) involvement in care planning. This has been facilitated by electronic patient record systems (EPRS) such as Care Director, Cerner, RiO and Case Notes, which enable the contemporaneous recording and sharing of service user records across different locations.

Care plans have ceased to fall solely within the domain of the mental health nurse, overseen by the consultant. Collectively, with the involvement of the MDT imparting their own specialist knowledge and experience, the role of care plans and the ownership of them is now being debated, with each speciality citing nuances as to how best to implement the MDT recovery-focused approach. Notable differences include the frequency with which care plans are reviewed in the community compared with those being produced on inpatient wards, and variances in the format and quality of care plans produced for service users on CPA as opposed to those not on CPA.

Daniel

I had been under secondary mental health services for at least 3 years before I knew what a care plan was, let alone saw one. While that may seem like a terrible example of mental health practice, the essential conclusion I reached was that I had survived 3 years without seeing my care plan, so why did I now need not just to see it, but to be involved in its formulation? A national survey of people using community mental health services[15] showed that my experience was not an isolated one: 38 per cent of people either did not understand their care plan or simply did not know they had one. Therefore, my immediate answer to the question 'What is the point in care planning?' is that care plans exist to reassure mental health professionals that they are doing something of value and to feed the bureaucracy of the health and social care system.[15]

My initial feelings about care planning were only strengthened when I actually saw what was noted down in the care plan that had been written for me. The description bore no resemblance to the person I was, and only focused on my negative aspects: my problems, my symptoms, my needs. Within recovery-focused services, a care plan should be the driving force or action plan behind a person's recovery journey and focused on their individual needs, strengths, aspirations and personal goals.[2] Mine was somewhat lacking in everything but my needs.

What changed for me was that the same care coordinator who taught me what a care plan was is the same care coordinator who demonstrated to me that care planning can be a transformative experience, rather than a maintenance exercise, as long as it is about me and the things I want to achieve. The first principle of care and support planning, as defined by National Voices,[1] is that it 'Starts from the point of view of the individual', and as soon as my care coordinator did that, the care planning process became much easier for both of us. The fifth principle is that it 'Identifies manageable personal goals', and as soon as we did that, the care planning process actually achieved outcomes that were meaningful to me.

Progressively, the care plan became a document which enabled and supported me to self-manage my mental health problems as much as possible: an intention supported by the third National Institute for Health and Care Excellence (NICE) quality standard on service user experience in adult mental health.[16] Self-management offers people the opportunity to identify and build upon their own skills to manage their own mental health condition.

The idea of 'personal medicine' was first articulated by Deegan,[17] who was researching people's experiences of using psychiatric medication. However, participants also reported a variety of non-pharmaceutical strategies that served to improve mood, outlook, thought and behaviours, and defined 'personal medicine' as 'self-initiated, non-pharmaceutical self-care activities that served to decrease symptoms, avoid undesirable outcomes such as hospitalization, and improve mood, thoughts, behaviours, and overall sense of wellbeing' (p.4).

Deegan's research identified two main categories of personal medicine: activities that gave meaning and purpose to life, and specific self-care strategies. Research participants also reported that they did not generally disclose their personal medicine to clinicians, and clinicians did not routinely inquire about these strengths. Therefore self-management support can be viewed in two ways:[18]

- as a portfolio of techniques and tools that help people problem solve, set goals, identify triggers and warning signs and develop coping strategies;
- as a fundamental transformation of the person–professional relationship into a collaborative partnership.

If care plans are about offering people more than 'maintenance' and supporting them to 'build a life beyond illness', then ultimately the care plan must be about acknowledging the skills an individual has to self-manage their mental health problems, and how to enable the individual to learn new skills and build their confidence, all framed around the things they want to achieve.

REFLECTION

Consider the care planning process and ask yourself these two questions:

- What questions could I ask to establish the individual's point of view?
- How could I support the individual to identify meaningful goals?

THE PROCESS OF COLLABORATIVE CARE PLANNING

Douglas

Collaborative care planning requires MDT input, driven by the nursing process, which has four interrelated stages: assessment, planning, implementation and evaluation.[19] The success of this approach is primarily dependent on the cohesiveness of the MDT working together with service users, carers and other service providers in order to produce a coordinated, coherent and meaningful 'living' care plan for the service user across different demographic and clinical settings.[20] The aim of current collaborative care planning is for service users to work jointly with mental health and social care professionals to develop their care plan and agree a date to review it.[21] Copies of the care plan are then shared with the relevant people.

An analogy to illustrate the concept of 'collaboration' is that of a light, twin-engine propeller plane cruising at an altitude of 5,000 feet: one engine represents the expert service user, fuelled by lived experience; the other engine represents the professional, fuelled by clinical experience and academic qualifications. If either engine fails to work in tandem or fails totally, then the aircraft will instantaneously and dramatically deviate from a controlled flight in all three axes.[22] Conversely, smooth flying is maintained by embracing shared decisions, self-management and positive risk taking. Chapter 36 addresses the recovery approach and risk management in greater detail.

Collaboration is best approached from the perspective of two experts with different, and at times polar opposite, views regarding mental illness and recovery: the *expert service user*, clad in the armour of *lived experience* that draws upon knowledge, expertise, coping strategies and skills from the functional part of their lives; and the *expert clinician*, who utilizes personal and clinical experience as well as academic qualifications. They have two different points of view that are separate in conception and application, yet equal.

The recovery model aims to provide service users with the information, skills and access to resources they need to live their lives.[23] This way of working demands an equal balance of power in the relationship between professionals and service users and an emphasis on collaboration (including expertise and support from family, friends and community) and partnership. It represents a transfer of the authority to define and recognize recovery away from the professional to the individual.[2]

Therefore, collaboration can be seen as the silver thread woven *seamlessly* through each of the care planning processes (see Figure 50.1).

NICE guidance advises that, wherever possible, the service user should be able to write an advance directive in their own words which informs the professionals of their preferred choices/methods of treatment when they become unwell, thus significantly reducing the potential for situations where physical intervention may be required.

There are numerous challenges in MDT collaborative care planning that health care services are currently attempting to meet. These include:

- providing clarity on the implementation of recovery principles across the MDT;
- providing clarity concerning ownership, responsibility and accountability of the care plan, through a

conversation that is repeated many times over between the community care coordinator and the inpatient primary nurse/key nurse;
- encouraging greater carer involvement in collaborative care planning when consent has been given;
- reducing professional jargon and service-specific terminology to ensure the service user and carers engage in the care planning process;
- providing a suitable environment in which collaborative care planning can take place, which can be more of a challenge within busy inpatient settings than in the community;
- presenting the care plan in a format that best meets the needs of the service user or carer;
- upskilling the MDT with the training and support needed to be effective in integrating collaboration into the care plan process.

Daniel

It is difficult to be specific about the 'ideal' care planning process, as it is heavily reliant on the individual receiving care and their particular needs and strengths. What is clear, and often missed, is that genuine collaboration between a service user and mental health professional requires addressing the issue of who holds the power and control[4] and then relocating that power and control towards the service user. It requires service users to be acknowledged as the experts in their own circumstances, capable of making decisions, while professionals must move away from being fixers to being facilitators.[24]

Shared decision making offers a way to redress this power imbalance, by providing a way for service users and professionals to enter into a collaborative partnership when making decisions, and genuine collaboration between service user and professional must be underpinned by the principles of shared decision making:[3]

1. It involves at least two participants, the professional and the service user.
2. Both the professional and the service user take steps to participate in the process of decision making.
3. Information sharing is a prerequisite for shared decision making.
4. Both the professional and the service user take steps to build a consensus about the preferred treatment, weighted according to the specific characteristics and values of the service user.
5. A treatment decision is made and both parties agree to the decision.

The need to embed shared decision making in practice is widely acknowledged, and again reflected in the NICE guidelines on service user experience in mental health.[16] Furthermore, the White Paper *Equity and excellence: liberating the NHS*[25] announced the key principle of 'no decision

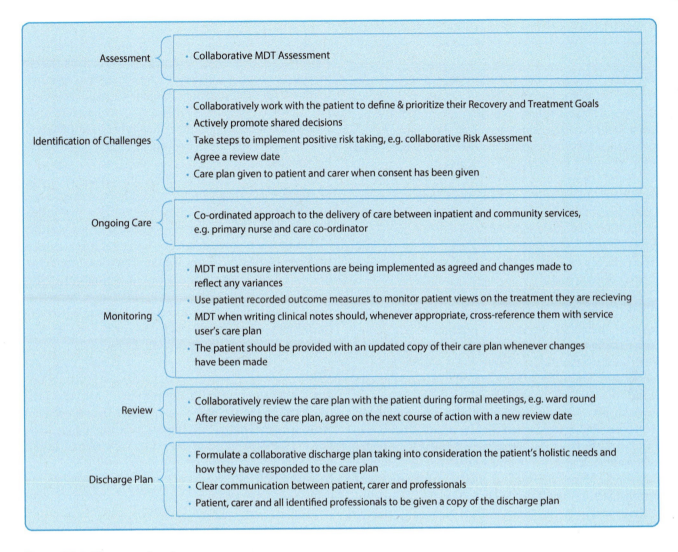

Assessment
- Collaborative MDT Assessment

Identification of Challenges
- Collaboratively work with the patient to define & prioritize their Recovery and Treatment Goals
- Actively promote shared decisions
- Take steps to implement positive risk taking, e.g. collaborative Risk Assessment
- Agree a review date
- Care plan given to patient and carer when consent has been given

Ongoing Care
- Co-ordinated approach to the delivery of care between inpatient and community services, e.g. primary nurse and care co-ordinator

Monitoring
- MDT must ensure interventions are being implemented as agreed and changes made to reflect any variances
- Use patient recorded outcome measures to monitor patient views on the treatment they are recieving
- MDT when writing clinical notes should, whenever appropriate, cross-reference them with service user's care plan
- The patient should be provided with an updated copy of their care plan whenever changes have been made

Review
- Collaboratively review the care plan with the patient during formal meetings, e.g. ward round
- After reviewing the care plan, agree on the next course of action with a new review date

Discharge Plan
- Formulate a collaborative discharge plan taking into consideration the patient's holistic needs and how they have responded to the care plan
- Clear communication between patient, carer and professionals
- Patient, carer and all identified professionals to be given a copy of the discharge plan

Figure 50.1 The care planning process.

about me, without me', while a report by the Care Quality Commission[26] stated that:

> *Plans should focus on individual needs and aspirations, involving service users at all stages so as to reflect their views and individual circumstances ... every effort should be made by providers to involve people in their own care, treatment and recovery. From a service user's position there should be 'no decision about me, without me' (p.9).*

However, it is recognized that there has been far more emphasis on strengthening professionals' skills to support shared decision making than there has been on developing the skills of people who use health services.[27] A greater emphasis on facilitative approaches to recovery that support the individual to engage in their own care and treatment is needed. Access to the right information can be a key stumbling block for service users trying to engage in shared decision making, and staff and services need to make more effort to provide people with enabling information, which supports them to make informed decisions about their care and treatment.

REFLECTION

Consider the care planning process and ask yourself these two questions:

- At what points could I meaningfully involve someone in their care plan?

- How can I embed shared decision making in practice?

RECOVERY

Douglas

'Recovery' improves the outcomes that matter to the person.[21] Recovery is deeply personal and affects all aspects of a person's life; it optimizes their strengths, skills, experience and knowledge, encapsulated by their hopes, beliefs and needs. Although clinical recovery is not its primary objective and for many people it remains a distant prospect, learning to harness these attributes helps the person to take back control of their lives and construct from themselves a new sense of self, meaning and purpose. Therein lays the conundrum that surrounds the 'recovery' debate within mental health: how to provide empirical evidence supporting its efficacy in improving health outcomes, aligned to a person's defined goal.

Every change made to clinical practice has its critics, and the process of defining a person's own recovery goals are not without its detractors. Criticisms of the recovery model include allegations that recovery goals are too wishy-washy, unachievable, vague and not easily defined, yet perhaps impossible to attain. On the surface, the root of their reservations may appear to be semantic; however, closer inspection reveals a disparity between traditional mental health practices, where the assessment process precipitates the formulation of treatment-orientated goals and interventions; and recovery-focused practices that result in the identification of two types of goal: treatment goals and personal recovery goals that are specific to the priorities of the individual.

Among the sceptics are service users who have become disillusioned with the traditional methods of care planning, and mistrust the new ones.

The aim of collaborative care planning is for care to be person-centred and individualized to meet the needs, preferences and strengths of the service user. However, providing personalized care is a complex task in the context of a political system that privileges equal access and standardized care. This has resulted in the use of 'buzzwords' such as 'hope', 'opportunity', 'control' and 'therapeutic alliance' in a way that fails to encompass the aim of the recovery model and can fail to engage service users in a meaningful way. If working in a recovery-focused way is about supporting people to find a fulfilling life beyond illness, then care plans need to focus on people's strengths, preferences, individual needs, aspirations and personal goals.[26]

Recovery goals should not be used as a euphemism to describe treatment goals;[5] instead, the professional must fully grasp the guiding principles of recovery before commencement of any goal-setting conversations with a service user. In doing so, the professional should approach the subject with a fresh, open mind-set, free from the old 'treatment'-focused practices. Professionals must be mindful to refrain from sounding commanding and judgemental. Instead, they should ask the service user how important each goal is; for example, 'How important is returning back to work for you? Is it very important, slightly important or unimportant?'

Nurses who struggle to make this transition should be supported through training, ideally co-delivered and co-produced with service users. The reality is that people with mental health problems can still set recovery goals.

From time to time, differences can emerge that cause a rift between the service user and the professional; for example, when a service user's goal is viewed as being unrealistic, unachievable or morally wrong. In these cases the professional should make every attempt to reach an agreement by engaging carers, family and friends (with consent). This subject is discussed in greater detail in chapter 35.

Daniel

There is no single definition of recovery; however, a central tenet of the recovery movement is that it does not claim to 'cure', but places emphasis on the unique journey experienced by those who live with mental health problems as they imagine and then build a life worth living, beyond the confines of illness.[28] Bill Anthony[29] has defined recovery as:

> *A deeply personal, unique process of changing one's attitudes, values, feelings, goals, skills and or roles. It is a way of living a satisfying, hopeful and contributing life even with the limitations caused by illness. Recovery involves the development of new meaning and purpose in one's life as one grows beyond the catastrophic effects of mental illness. (p.534)*

Therefore, what is clear is that recovery is not a defined action, intervention or outcome; it is an approach which reframes living with mental health problems as a personal and social challenge.[30] Within recovery-focused services, professionals facilitate this process through the central components of hope, control and opportunity.[4] It is these components which need to be reflected throughout the care planning process, by supporting people to manage their mental health problems and supporting them to access opportunities that offer them hope for the future. Linking the care planning process to more personalized plans, such as personal recovery plans,[31] can be a useful way of facilitating this process.

BARRIERS TO EFFECTIVE CARE PLANNING

Douglas

There are two mediums in which care plans are produced, stored and maintained: the traditional handwritten paper format, and the electronic version produced on the EPRS. Although they are outwardly different, they both have inherent shortcomings that prevent them from supporting the collaborative care planning process adequately.

Paper care plans are highly effective at promoting and evidencing collaboration between the service user and the professional; at the point of formulation, the document can be easily shared between both parties, and this enables dual entries to be recorded. However, the exclusive use of paper does in fact prevent the care plan from being a 'living document', since it does not lend itself to being reviewed and updated in its original form or when scanned/uploaded into EPRS. Any major additions or amendments will require an entirely new document to be produced and can result in several copies being in circulation. Service users can feel overloaded with care plans, with the result that the care plans can be perceived as a nuisance and discarded at the earliest opportunity (as commonly witnessed in ward environments where care plans are usually reviewed on a weekly basis).

Other notable deficits in using paper are issues regarding quality of print-outs, poor legibility caused by poor handwriting, and spelling and grammatical mistakes, all of which can result in important information being overlooked and not followed up. Therefore it can be said that paper care plans create a barrier to cohesive MDT involvement in helping a service user meet their defined goals.

However, electronic care plans are not without their own challenges; usually the only way a service user can access care plans while in hospital is to get them printed out by hospital staff, creating the same dependent relationship mentioned earlier in the chapter. It takes longer for the health care professional to transpose the care plan discussions onto the EPRS than writing them on paper. This has given rise to the use of smaller, hand-held devices, such as tablet and laptop computers, which have received mixed reviews from both health care professionals and service users.

REFLECTION

Consider the use of the electronic care planning process and ask yourself these two questions:

- How can health care professionals ensure service users can access and add their own comments to the electronic care plans?

- Is the time taken by health care professionals to input information into the system more beneficial to the service user or the health care system?

Daniel

While a failure to have the right tools and methods available can be an important barrier to effective collaborative care planning, my personal view is that a greater barrier, often overlooked, is an ineffective relationship between the service user and professional. Ineffective relationships between service user and professional can be characterized by an imbalance of power, control and information.[18]

SUPPORTING CARERS

Carers and families play an essential role in the lives of people who use mental health services and should be identified at the earliest opportunity; they should be encouraged to contribute to discussions relating to care and treatment. Carers are also entitled by law to have a Carer's Assessment and their own care needs reflected in a care plan.[32] Therefore services must ensure staff are trained in meeting their needs through 'Carer Awareness' training, underpinned by policies and protocols concerning confidentiality and sharing information. In paying greater attention to the views and concerns expressed by carers, staff must be sensitive to their feelings of guilt, fear, despair and anger, and take the necessary measures to ensure they are kept well informed and updated throughout the care episode.

Engaging carers, where consent is given, not only validates their role but also provides another pathway in getting to know the service user systemically, putting their needs and goals into context. In cases where a person has dementia or lacks capacity, the professional must act in their 'best interest', taking into consideration the Mental Capacity Act,[33] which aims to balance the needs and views of carers with that of the person with dementia.[33]

There is a lot of evidence that suggests that, within inpatient services, carers are still finding it difficult to be kept well informed of care planning, and decisions concerning discharge.[34] To explore the issue of consent further, it would be useful to read chapter 18. Box 50.1 lists opportunities to involve inpatient carers.

WHO OWNS THE CARE PLAN?

Douglas

Collaborative care plans aim both to synthesize the expertise of clinicians, service users and their families/carers, and to share responsibility for their design and delivery. This goal raises the complex question of 'Who owns the care plan?', reminding those responsible for delivering care that they cannot proceed with improving care planning until this question has been fully addressed.

Lack of clarity around ownership of and responsibility for the care plan can result in tensions and conflict between clinicians and service users. These tensions, when unchallenged, can result in a lack of effective coordination and delivery of the care plan and damage to the relationship between service users and professionals.

Currently, care plans can be regarded as property of the mental health services aiming to operationalize the care of service users. With this view, NHS Trusts have sought to audit the extent to which its departments are meeting their responsibilities to involve service users in jointly developing care plans with mental health and social care professionals, and whether service users have been provided with a copy, with an agreed review date.[16]

A number of recovery-inspired tools have been designed and implemented across the NHS including Wellness Recovery Action Packs (WRAP), crisis plans, and recovery and support plans. These tools all centre on goal setting and specify the actions needed to achieve them. They aim to bring structure, consistency and clarity to discussions that support shared decision making and self-management. Embedded in the recovery model, these plans aim to empower the service user through collaboration; the existence of standardized tools from which to then personalize each plan helps to support consistent care for all service users accessing the NHS, irrespective of their level of need, location, wealth, age, ethnicity, gender and so on.

Daniel

My thoughts on who should own the care plan can be perfectly summarized by the example given in Box 50.2. 'The reality of self-management'.

BOX 50.2: THE REALITY OF SELF-MANAGEMENT

Simon has a diagnosis of schizophrenia and lives independently in his flat. He hears voices and describes them as being rude, critical and abusive. He has trouble keeping track of thoughts and conversations and finds it hard to concentrate. As a result he has difficulty interacting with people in social settings and tends to withdraw, spending the majority of time on his own in his flat. Simon would like to gain more control over his life and has identified two recovery goals which are important to him: to give up smoking and to get a job. He receives support from his family and his care coordinator visits him every 2 weeks for an hour. Due to medication, Simon finds he needs to sleep for approx. 12 hours a day.

Reality

1. 1 hour visit from care coordinator x 26 weeks a year = 26 hours
2. 12 waking hours per day x 365 days a year = 4,380 hours
3. Percentage of time Simon receives support from his care coordinator over a year = 0.6%
4. Percentage of time Simon does not receive support over a year = 99.4%

Simon spends just a few hours a year in contact with health and social care services. The reality is Simon is self-managing his mental health condition 99.4% of the time.

Source: Rinaldi and Watkey[2] (p.30)

While the interactions which take place between service user and professional can be an important part of an individual's recovery, it must be viewed within the wider context of the individual's life and the life they would like to have (as described in chapter 35). The care plan must support a mental health professional to effectively provide the right care and treatment and make assessments of people's risk and vulnerabilities, but also acknowledge and value the day-to-day life of individuals living with mental health problems and the efforts they make to manage their problems.

The most effective way to do this is to develop a care plan that is owned by the individual, and support them to manage their mental health problems and live the life they want.

REFLECTION

- How much of a role does collaboration have in determining the ownership of the care plan?

- Examine your care plan template and ask a service user: if they could design its format, what would it look like? What would they leave out or include?

- Identify which enabling tools are used within your practice and ask service users if they find them more useful in encouraging self-management than the care plan.

- Identify a goal that is important for you and proceed in formulating your own care plan to achieve it. Then compare it with care plans produced for service users; pay particular attention to the language variations between the two.

BOX 50.3: TOP TIPS FOR COLLABORATIVE CARE PLANNING

1. Start from the point of view of the person.
2. Make enabling information available and accessible.
3. Build in time to consider the views of carers and others.
4. Take a collaborative approach, based on the principles of shared decision making.
5. Identify personal goals with the person.
6. Focus on supporting the person to self-manage and stay well.
7. Develop a care plan which is owned by the individual.
8. Agree next steps and a date for review and follow-up.

Adapted from National Voices, *Principles of care and support planning*[1]

CONCLUSION

Within this chapter we have essentially discussed three salient points. First, what is the point in care planning? Second, how do you develop a care plan collaboratively? Then lastly, who owns the care plan? While we may not have provided definitive answers, we do believe these are the most important questions for staff and service users to consider when engaged in the care planning process.

References

1. National Voices. *Principles of care and support planning: interactive pdf.* 2013. Available from: http://www.nationalvoices.org.uk/sites/default/files/public/publications/narrative-for-person-centred-coordinated-care.pdf [Accessed 7th September 2016].
2. Rinaldi M, Watkey F. Do our current approaches to care planning and the CPA enhance the experience and outcomes of a person's recovery? *Journal of Mental Health, Training, Education and Practice* 2014; **9**(1): 26–34.
3. Charles C, Gafni A, Whelan T. Shared decision-making in the medical encounter: what does it mean? (or it takes two to tango). *Social Science and Medicine* 1997; **44**(5): 681–92.
4. Repper J, Perkins R. *Social inclusion and recovery.* London: Balliere Tindall, 2003.
5. Barker P. *Psychiatric and mental health nursing: the craft of caring*, 2nd edn. London: CRC Press, 2003.
6. Hardcastle M, Kennard D, Grandison S, Fagin L (eds). *Experiences of mental health in-patient care – narratives from service users, carers and professionals.* Hove: Routledge, 2007.
7. Lawson M, Wolfson P, Strickland C. User involvement in care planning: the care programme approach (CPA) from the user's perspective. *Psychiatric Bulletin* 1999; **23**: 539–41.
8. Wyder M, Bland R, Crompton D. Personal recovery and involuntary mental health admissions: the importance of control, relationships and hope. *Health* 2013; **5**: 574–81. doi: 10.4236/health.2013.53A076.
9. Royal College of Psychiatrists/Social Care Institute for Excellence/Care Services Improvement Partnership. *A common purpose: recovery in future mental health services.* London: Social Care Institute for Excellence, 2007.
10. Roberts G, Hollins S. Recovery: our common purpose? *Advances in Psychiatric Treatment* 2007; **13**: 397–9.
11. Department of Health. *Making the CPA work for you. It is not about how you fit into services. It is about how services fit with you.* London: DH, 2008.

12. Department of Health. *Refocusing the Care Programme Approach: policy and positive practice guidance*. London: DH, 2008. Available from: http://webarchive.nationalarchives.gov.uk/20130107105354/; http://www.dh.gov.uk/en/Publicationsandstatistics/Publications/PublicationsPolicyAndGuidance/DH_083647 [Accessed 3rd December 2016].

13. McDermott G. The Care Programme Approach: a patient perspective. *Nursing Times Research* 1998; **3**(1): 47–63.

14. Anthony P, Crawford P. Service user involvement in care planning: the mental health nurse's perspective. *Journal of Psychiatric and Mental Health Nursing* 2000; **7**: 425–34.

15. Care Quality Commission. *Community mental health survey*. London: Care Quality Commission, 2012.

16. NICE (National Institute for Health and Care Excellence). *Service user experience in adult mental health: improving the experience of care for people using adult NHS mental health services. Clinical Guideline 136*. Manchester: NICE, 2011.

17. Deegan PE. The importance of personal medicine: a qualitative study of resilience. *Scandinavian Journal of Public Health* 2005; **33**: 1–7.

18. De Silva D. *Helping people help themselves: a review of the evidence considering whether it is worthwhile to support self-management*. London: Health Foundation, 2010.

19. Roper N, Logan W, Tierney A. *The Roper-Logan-Tierney model of nursing based on activities of living*. Edinburgh: Churchill Livingstone, 2008.

20. McHugh P, Byrne M. The teamworking challenges of care planning. *Irish Journal of Psychological Medicine* 2012; **29**(3): 29–33.

21. Adams N, Grieder DM. *Treatment planning for person centred-care: the road to mental health and addiction recovery*. Burlington, MA: Elsevier, 2005.

22. Turner T. Considering a twin. *Air Facts* 2012. Available from: http://airfactsjournal.com/2012/04/considering-a-twin/ [Accessed 27th June 2016].

23. Shepherd G, Boardman J, Slade M. *Making recovery a reality*. London: Sainsbury Centre for Mental Health, 2008.

24. Reape A, Wallace LM. *What is coproduction?* London: Health Foundation, 2010.

25. Department of Health. *Equity and excellence: liberating the NHS*. Norwich: The Stationery Office, 2010.

26. Care Quality Commission. *Monitoring the Mental Health Act in 2012/13*. London: Care Quality Commission, 2014.

27. Gigerenzer G, Muir Gray JA. *Better doctors, better patients, better decisions: envisioning health care 2020*. Cambridge, MA: MIT Press, 2011.

28. Smith-Merry J, Sturdy S, Freeman R. Recovering mental health in Scotland: 'recovery' from social movement to policy goal. *Knowledge and Policy in Health and Education Sectors*, 2010.

29. Anthony WA. Recovery from mental illness: the guiding vision of the mental health system in the 1990s. *Psychosocial Rehabilitation Journal* 1993; **16**(4): 11–23.

30. Alakeson V, Perkins R. *Recovery, personalisation and personal budgets*. London: Centre for Mental Health, 2012.

31. Perkins R, Rinaldi M. *Taking back control: a guide to planning your own recovery*. London: South West London & St George's Mental Health NHS Trust, 2007.

32. Department of Health. *National Service Framework for Mental Health. Modern standards and service models*. London: Department of Health, 1999.

33. The Princess Royal Trust for Carers. *The triangle of care: carers included: a guide to best practice in acute mental health care*. Andover: The Princess Royal Trust for Carers, 2010.

34. Royal College of Nursing. *Commitment to the care of people with dementia in hospital settings; how to guide*. London: RCN Publishing, 2013. Available from: www.rcn.org.uk/__data/assets/pdf_file/0011/480269/004235.pdf [Accessed 27th June 2016].

Further reading

NICE (2011) *Service User Experience in Adult Mental Health: Improving the Experience of Care for People Using Adult NHS Mental Health Services*. Manchester: NICE Clinical Guideline 136.

National Voices (2013) *Principles of care and support planning: interactive pdf*. See: HYPERLINK "http://www.nationalvoices.org.uk/read-our-guide" www.nationalvoices.org.uk/read-our-guide.

Rinaldi M. & Watkey F. (2014) Do our current approaches to care planning and the CPA enhances the experience and outcomes of a person's recovery? *Journal of Mental Health, Training, Education and Practice*.

Relevant web pages

http://www.cmft.nhs.uk/directorates/mentor/documents/Assessingplanningimplementingandevaluatingcare_001.pdf

http://www.mentalhealth.org.uk/help-information/mental-health-a-z/r/recovery/

http://mentalhealthrecovery.com/wrap-is/

http://www.rncentral.com/nursing-library/careplans/

http://www.rcgp.org.uk/clinical-and-research/our-programmes/collaborative-care-and-support-planning.aspx

51 Family involvement and support networks

MARTIN ATCHISON, JEANETTE PARTRIDGE AND
JO TWISS

LEARNING OUTCOMES

- To understand the experience of families who are in contact with mental health services.
- To understand the impact of confidentiality in mental health settings.
- To be able to work collaboratively with families.
- To know how to apply the Triangle of Care in clinical practice.
- To be aware of different ways in which families can be supported.

SUMMARY OF KEY POINTS

- Families can experience high stress levels when their relative has been diagnosed with a mental health problem.
- The ways in which family members respond to this are linked to the well-being of the service user.
- Supporting the family is a key part of the role of a psychiatric nurse/mental health nurse.
- Negotiating with the family and the service user to create the Triangle of Care is a process which embodies the ethos of the craft of caring.

INTRODUCTION

This chapter will explore the value of working in partnership with a service user's social network. The way in which we function is linked strongly to roles and relationships within our social networks. It is fundamental that the psychiatric/mental health nurse is capable of working in collaboration with, and providing support for, that social network.

Getting involved with the family can be more complex than working with an individual service user. Mental health services have traditionally been focused on working with individuals, despite the evidence that demonstrates the benefits of working with families. Whether on an inpatient unit or in the community, the psychiatric/mental health nurse is likely to be the professional who will have the most contact with the family, with the greatest opportunity to have a positive influence on the family's response to a relative being unwell.

This chapter will look at the experiences of families in contact with mental health services and some of the issues that families encounter, with emphasis on the use of confidentiality and the provision of accurate information to the family. The chapter will then examine some things that family members may find helpful, before exploring some principles that underpin *how* the psychiatric/mental health nurse can craft a relationship between the family, the service user and themselves that will create the conditions for everyone to thrive.

OUR FAMILIES

> ### REFLECTION
>
> Think about a time when a member of your family was unwell.
>
> - How did you feel?
> - What was the impact on relationships within your family?

This reflection is an exercise which has been used when training clinicians in family work from organizations across the world. The feedback has been consistent over time. Usually the illness being discussed is a physical health problem, and the experience of having someone in your family who is unwell creates a number of challenging feelings, such as stress, anxiety, worry, frustration and helplessness. The impact on family relationships can be that there are more arguments and family members can drift apart.

If the situation involves a mental health problem rather than a physical health problem, this can prove to be even more complex and challenging for families to manage. The family may not have an understanding of the diagnosis, what kinds of behaviour to expect, what to do that may be helpful, or any idea as to how long their loved one will be unwell. There can be an impact on the practicalities of family life, such as the working life of the family member, the financial pressures that can emerge, and the impact on the social life of the family.

There continues to be an uneven approach to families within services.[1] Too often, clinicians make statements which pathologize the family or describe them as dysfunctional.[2] 'If it wasn't for the family, the service user would be doing OK' is a comment that may sound familiar to you.

The above reflection will start to give some indication of what families in touch with mental health services will be experiencing. As a psychiatric/mental health nurse, you will be coming into contact with families at a time when they are at their most stressed, and you may be observing a skewed and a strained version of family life. If someone wanted to get a sense of your own family life, they would not get an accurate picture of this if they came round the day before you were moving house, or on Boxing Day after the in-laws have gone home. Putting yourself in the shoes of the family member and thinking about their experience is the first step to creating a positive relationship with the family. A broader understanding of the experience of families can be gained by reading chapter 49 of this book, written by a family member about her experiences.

> ### CARER'S PERSPECTIVE: GUILT AND BLAME
>
> It is all too common for a family member or carer to feel that they, in some way, have contributed to their relative's illness. They strive to find out why it has happened and can be overtaken by feelings of guilt. The most helpful comment from any professional is that they are not to blame and it is not their fault. When a carer hears this, they can begin their own recovery.

OUR FAMILIES AND THEIR CONTACT WITH SERVICES

> ### REFLECTION
>
> Think about a time when a member of your family was unwell.
>
> - What did services do well?
> - What could they have done differently?

This exercise is linked with the previous reflection, and has been used when training clinicians in family work, again with consistent feedback. A good experience of services can include such things as being listened to, having opinions taken into account, being given understandable information, and delivering an effective intervention to the person who is ill. Often, however, people report that services do not involve the family in decision making, do not listen to the family, and do not share information with the family in a timely and effective manner.

FAMILIES IN CONTACT WITH MENTAL HEALTH SERVICES

REFLECTION

- Have you heard the term 'high expressed emotion family' used in a clinical setting?
- What ideas about the family did this bring about?

Much has been written about the family being the source of mental health problems[3] and about the concept of 'expressed emotion'.[4] Expressed emotion is measured in terms of hostile comments, critical comments, and a sense of emotional over-involvement that the family exhibits. A link has been determined between communication in a family and the well-being of the service user. It has been shown that families viewed as having 'high expressed emotion' (HEE) – that is, those who make a lot of critical and hostile comments – tend to lead to poorer outcomes for service users.

These findings were valuable in the sense that they gave clinicians a focus to intervene with families and to explore how to readjust the patterns of communication within families. However, the label of 'high expressed emotion' is an easy one to apply to a family, but a difficult one to remove. The label may be something that you have heard in a negative context to describe what can be complex family situations.

If you are going to visit a service user and their family and you have heard them described as HEE, how will this impact on your ability to develop a positive relationship with the family? Will you be looking for the things that the family are coping well with? Or does this label lead you more towards looking for ways that the family are at fault?

It might be helpful to revisit the first reflection in this chapter, and think about our own families under stress.

Would your family have been given a label of HEE? How would this have influenced your family's relationships with services?

It may be more helpful to think about the family experiencing a *normal response to a stressful situation*. This is much more likely to lead to effective working relationships with families. As one family member put it: 'When mental illness comes through the door, communication goes out of the window'[5] (p.1).

CONFIDENTIALITY

Put a group of carers in a room and very soon the issue of confidentiality will come into the discussion. [6] *(p.12)*

REFLECTION

- What does the term confidentiality mean in the context of mental health care?
- What are some of the challenges of the issue of confidentiality?

Confidentiality is one of the key factors that influence how well a family becomes involved in the support of their relative.[7] Given the sensitive information that a psychiatric/mental health nurse has access to in discussion with service users, the process of whether and how to share this with the family can be a complex and challenging one. In situations where solutions to a complicated issue are not easy to find, the psychiatric/mental health nurse may find that a simple way to manage this confusion is to focus on working with the individual service user.[8]

The impact of confidentiality

From the service user's perspective, there may be worries about their family finding out about sensitive issues. Having their personal experiences or behaviours disclosed to their family can raise huge anxieties for service users, who may find discussions about sharing information with their family uncomfortable. The service user may find it difficult to talk with their family about their mental health, or may not want to worry their family by telling them about their traumatic experiences, and may find it beneficial to talk confidentially to a clinician. When discussions around sharing information take place, there may be some fantasizing about what, and how much, the family will get to find out. If family relationships are already strained, this can be a challenging issue.

From the family's perspective, without information about the mental health problem, it is difficult to know how best to support their relative. The family may have the best of intentions, but without knowledge of the service user's experience or diagnosis, or what is helpful to do, the family often have to guess what to do for the best. Family members develop their own (often quite different) models about the mental health problem, and the service user may experience a discrepancy in the kind of support they receive from others within the family.

From the psychiatric/mental health nurse's perspective, there is often a worry about breaking confidentiality. There may also be a concern that, by starting to

SERVICE USER'S PERSPECTIVE: IMPACT OF MENTAL HEALTH PROBLEMS ON FAMILY RELATIONSHIPS

When I was well, my relationship with my family was a very close and stable one with constant support, but when acute illness struck, this foundation was pulled apart. In illness, I lost all trust in family members as well as the professionals, as I felt they were all in it together, in removing me from the family home into a psychiatric ward. I really believed it was them who were unwell. I refused to allow my father to visit, made untrue accusations against him and also prevented my mother and sister from visiting me. When acutely unwell, I had harmful and abhorrent thoughts about my mother and gave a distorted view of family life.

CARER'S PERSPECTIVE: NOT KNOWING WHAT TO DO

It can be a real lottery to know how to support your relative. 'Will it work or won't it?' can be a common thought. In the absence of any information, or a difference of opinion about what to do, family members may decide to do nothing, rather than risking something else going wrong, worrying that intervening may lead to further arguments or a breakdown of communication between family members.

discuss family involvement, the nurse's relationship with the service user may be compromised. Without the routine involvement of the family, the psychiatric/mental health nurse is only getting a single view on family relationships – that of the service user. The family can give a different, more rounded view of family relationships, and also a wider view of the service user as an *individual*, as they will know the *person* much better than the professionals.

As can be seen, there are a wide range of factors in play that can make the management of confidentiality a challenging experience. The psychiatric/mental health nurse should be sensitive to all these factors, and the craft of caring consists of balancing these issues and creating a more resourceful partnership.

A useful exercise to encourage reflection on this subject is to ask everyone in your clinical team to read the Partners in Care leaflet on confidentiality,[9] and have a discussion with the team about how confidentiality is managed (see chapter 2 on ethics and mental health nursing and chapter 67 mental health, the law and human rights).

Sharing of information

Issues around confidentiality should not be used as a reason for not listening to carers, nor for not discussing fully with service users the need for carers to receive information so that they can continue to support them. Carers should be given sufficient information, in a way they can readily understand, to help them provide care effectively.[10] *(p.16)*

REFLECTION

How will the family having information about their relative's diagnosis and experience be helpful to the family, the service user and the clinician?

The main factor that determines whether the family are able to access important information is usually the clinician and how willing they are to get involved in potentially challenging situations related to confidentiality. Often, the psychiatric/mental health nurse is trying to manage these tensions without any previous training in how to share information with families proactively, safely and ethically. A simple starting point may be to ask the service user which information they *do not* want to be shared with the family, rather than ask whether information in a general sense can be shared. This will lead to better structured discussions.

It may also be useful for the psychiatric/mental health nurse to use different terminology. Confidentiality involves information that is intended to be kept secret.[11] If the process is described instead as the sharing of information, this has different connotations, and may lead the psychiatric/mental health nurse to have very different types of discussion with service users. Sutton[12] described this fluid process as *negotiated authorization*, that is, the psychiatric/mental health nurse negotiates with the service user and the family regarding what information can be shared.

It is vital that the psychiatric/mental health nurse does not make assumptions about what the family do or do not know. A good example of this is a family member who had a son with psychosis. She was very angry with services when she read an article in the newspaper about the link between psychosis and cannabis, as she was aware that her son was smoking cannabis, but had not done anything to intervene as he had said that it made him feel more relaxed. The clinicians involved in her son's care had assumed that she knew about the link between psychosis and cannabis use, and were bemused as to why she had not tried to stop him. This had led the team to develop views about the mother that were not particularly positive. Once the mother discovered this information (and following some heated discussion with her son's psychiatric/mental health nurse), she and the team started to have a consistent approach to cannabis use, and this led to a better long-term relationship between the service user, the mother and clinicians.

The vast majority of service users state that they want their relatives to be involved in their care,[13] yet family members still find it challenging at times to be as involved as they would like to be.[1] This may be partly due to clinicians making assumptions about confidentiality, thinking that service users will be reluctant or unwilling to share information.

SERVICE USER'S PERSPECTIVE: FAMILY SUPPORT

You lose touch with all your friends so the family step in and provide practical and emotional support as well as the professionals. It was especially important for me to have my family present during ward rounds to be informed of treatment, medication, for reassurance and an opportunity for everybody to ask questions. This sharing of information would reduce fear and confusion and keep all parties informed in achieving the same objective – keeping everyone well. My family's supportive role was my only contact with the outside world when under a section. Once home leave comes into play again, the family make sure the treatment carries on beyond the ward environment.

CARER'S PERSPECTIVE: FAMILY SUPPORT

Being given general information increases confidence to support your relative and helps a carer to cope with any criticism from others. When we had access to accurate information about my son's experience, I built a different relationship with him. I had thought that he would get back to how he was before, but with this information I was able to see a tremendous strength of character that he was demonstrating in coping with his experiences. This helped the family to cope better, and also helped us to know how best to support him.

Here are some key points for managing the sharing of information.

- It is vital that the family has some information about their relative's experience.
- Explore the reservations of the service user about information being shared.
- Discuss with colleagues about how to negotiate confidentiality. Confidentiality does not stop the clinician from listening to the family.
- Explain the issues of confidentiality to the family.
- Revisit the issue. Views will change over time.
- Do not make assumptions.

This quotation from a carer neatly outlines what carers need to know and what limits there may be on information being shared:

I need to know what you are trying to achieve for my son and how you are planning to do it. I need to understand the treatment that he is receiving so that I can play my part in his recovery programme. What I do not need to know are the personal details of what takes place between him and the professionals concerned.[9] *(p.1)*

SERVICES FOR CARERS

Carers' assessment

The entitlement of carers to have an assessment of their own needs and their own care plan came about in 1995[14] and was incorporated into the National Service Framework for Mental Health in 1999.[15] In terms of getting the family involved in the care of their relative, the carers assessment is a good starting point. The format for the assessment varies, but generally includes questions about how the mental health issue has had an impact on their life and what would help them to cope, and about accessing support for employment, training and leisure opportunities.

Carers' groups

Carers' groups fall into two broad categories: open support groups, and more educational, closed groups. The open support groups are for any carer to attend at any time, and include time for carers to discuss their experiences, have peer support and may have guest speakers. The educational groups tend to be time-limited, have a structured programme and endeavour to help the carers attending the group to develop coping skills, and to acquire information about mental health and the importance of looking after their own needs.

Speaking of attending a carers' group, a family member said: 'As soon as I walked through the door I knew

I was home. These were people who understood me. I did not have to hide anything. They have been my lifeline, supporting me to care for my relative better and protect my own wellbeing'[16] (p.131).

Carer support workers

Carer support workers were introduced into the workforce in 2002[10] following pioneering work by Making Space,[17] which introduced family support workers in 1991. Carers report that having a dedicated worker looking after their own needs is extremely helpful for their ability to cope with the demands of their role. They provide a range of services including signposting to other services, benefits advice, advocacy, counselling and provision of information about mental health issues.

> ## CARER'S PERSPECTIVE: CARER SUPPORT WORKERS
>
> To have access to a carer support worker can be like finding a long-lost friend! The listening ear and the offering of a carer's assessment means a carer can have *their* needs truly recognized and become a person in their own right again.

WORKING WITH FAMILIES

The Triangle of Care

The concept of the Triangle of Care[6] is crucial for the consistent involvement of families in mental health services. Traditionally, the relationship between the family, clinicians and service user has been viewed as a linear one, as shown in Figure 51.1.

From Figure 51.1, it can be seen that the only relationship between the clinician and the family is through the filter of the service user. Given the stress that the family may be experiencing and the possibility of tension between family members, this can mean that the clinician only sees part of the picture. If these relationships are triangulated, however, it is easy to see how this

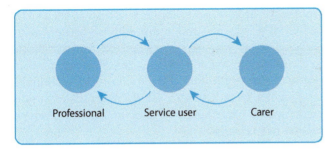

Figure 51.1 Traditional view of relationships.

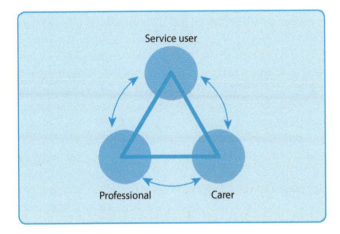

Figure 51.2 The Triangle of Care.

can make for more powerful and effective team working (Figure 51.2).

The Triangle of Care[18] was introduced in 2010 and was initially directed for families in contact with acute services. It was subsequently adapted for use across all fields of mental health care in 2013. The six key elements of the document are as follows:

1. Carers and the essential role they play are identified at first contact or as soon as possible thereafter.
2. Staff are 'carer aware' and trained in carer engagement strategies.
3. Policy and protocols regarding confidentiality and sharing information are in place.
4. Defined post(s) responsible for carers are in place.
5. A carer introduction to the service and staff is available, with a relevant range of information across the care pathway.
6. A range of carer support services is available.

Services wishing to examine their level of support for and contact with family members would do well to complete the self-assessment audit at the back of the document.[18] This will provide a benchmark for how well they are doing in achieving the six key elements, but will also provide guidance on how to start improving the involvement of families. Carers Trust[19] continues to broaden the scope of the concept of the Triangle of Care into other areas.

CREATING THE TRIANGLE OF CARE

As a newly appointed carers' support worker in 1991, I soon came to realize that in the quest to close the large institutions, the formal planning of community alternatives hadn't taken account of the needs of the very people who would be required to support the former patients in the home. In fact, the term 'carer' did not pass 'spell check' at that time! Information about mental health services was sparse, public knowledge and support were very poor and many clinicians had little practical advice to offer, probably because the training and experience up to that point had been based in institutions.

Having worked in education before retiring to be a carer and carers' support worker, it was not difficult to appreciate the insecurity that carers were experiencing. More education and training were needed! 'What do we need to know to carry out our responsibilities? What will make things better and what should we avoid doing? Where do we find this knowledge and support?'

Over 10 years in the role of a carers' support worker, listening to countless carers, I realized there was much duplication in their experiences. Carers commonly described a 'hitch' in the journey, sometimes with serious consequences. 'If only things could have gone differently!' These 'hitches' were then clustered together to form the six key elements of the Triangle of Care, each with a rationale and links with examples of best practice.

In creating the Triangle of Care, the psychiatric/mental health nurse will be required to focus on the spirit of the craft of caring. They may need to shift positions at times to respond to particular issues, regularly considering the family's views while continuing to respect the wishes of the service user, using all their personal skills to maintain the balance of the Triangle of Care.

Alan Worthington, author of 'The Triangle of Care'[18]

Engaging families

So far in the chapter there has been discussion of the importance of the routine involvement of the family in mental health care, and some discussion about what some of the barriers to this might be.

In terms of engaging families consistently, the following principles should act as a guide to the psychiatric/mental health nurse. They are taken from the principles of behavioural family therapy (BFT),[20] to which we shall return later in the chapter.

THE APPROACH TO THE FAMILY IS POSITIVE

From the first point of contact with the family, it is important to start off the relationship in a positive way and to view the family as partners in care and an additional resource to help you do your job. Chapter 50 looks at collaborative care planning with service users and carers.

THE EXPERTISE AND SKILL OF THE FAMILY IS RECOGNIZED

The family will be doing some things really well, and will have started to build up some expertise in terms of what helps and what is not helpful. Identifying these skills can help you to get to know the family and the environment in which the service user is living. For the family to hear that they are doing positive things can be extremely rewarding, and it can lessen the feelings of guilt that so many families experience.

THE ACTIONS OF THE FAMILY ARE SEEN AS THEIR BEST EFFORTS TO MANAGE THE SITUATION WITHIN THE LIMITS OF THEIR RESOURCES

There may well be things that the family are doing which may not appear to be helpful or positive. When exposed to these, it can be easy to develop a view of the family which is negative, or for the clinical team to extrapolate these incidents so that the kind of blaming statements mentioned earlier in the chapter start to become more commonplace. If the psychiatric/mental health nurse can use this principle to reframe some of these behaviours, this is much more likely to lead to positive relationships with families. The issue of cannabis use mentioned earlier is an example of how this could be applied. In this case, the mother was acting in a way that she thought was for the best, but once she became aware of the link between cannabis and psychosis, she was able to act in a more effective way.

DISTINGUISH BETWEEN THE ACTIONS OF THE FAMILY AND THEIR INTENTIONS

Again, the family may be doing things which do not seem to be helpful, but try and take some time to think about what lies behind some of these actions. Often some unhelpful behaviour can become established through the best of intentions. For example, a father, may shout at his son, who has psychosis, for failing to get out of bed in the morning. The son may tell his psychiatric/mental health nurse about this and subsequently the clinical team may start to develop critical views of the family. However, the father's intentions

are positive; he is desperate for his son to get out of bed, to be well, to go to work, and to mix with his friends again. Shouting at his son may have been effective previously, so the father continues to try it, as he is unaware of other strategies that might work. Taking a step back and thinking about the intentions of the family, rather than focusing on the actions of the family in isolation, can help to foster positive relationships.

EVERY FAMILY HAS ITS OWN CULTURE

Each family, regardless of whether any of its members have a mental health problem, has its own way of life. What is normal in one family may seem odd in another. It is vital to keep an open mind when coming into contact with a family. The family's culture may be difficult to discern amidst the stress and tension that they are experiencing, so it is important not to assume anything about the family during early contact with them.

With these principles in mind, the psychiatric/mental health nurse can start to get a sense of what the family's experience has been from a positive and realistic perspective, and can start to give the family a sense of hope that things can improve. This should be a routine approach to *all* families (see chapter 35 on what does the recovery approach really mean?).

Siblings

Much has been written about siblings and their involvement with services.[21-23] They can often be on the fringes of contact with services but may have a closer relationship with the service user than parents do. Parents may want to protect siblings from the difficulties the family are experiencing, but siblings may have useful information or viewpoints about the service user, and may have worries about their own mental health. It is vital that the psychiatric/mental health nurse takes time to involve siblings.

Working across different cultures

The need for the psychiatric/mental health nurse to be aware of cultural norms is especially important when working with families. The family may have a spiritual understanding of mental health, which needs to be taken into account. They may be using spiritual or faith practices which may well provide a great deal of solace for the service user. Other issues to consider include gender roles and traditional hierarchies in families, and communication styles in different cultures.[24]

SHARING INFORMATION WITH FAMILIES

As has been discussed previously, it is crucial that families have access to information about their loved one's experience. This can help the family to enhance their

understanding and empathy towards their loved one, and may start to help the family to fine-tune the support that they offer. This information can be provided in a general format, based on diagnosis, which does not breach confidentiality when given to a family. Some excellent leaflets explaining different diagnoses have been developed through the Partners in Care campaign.[25]

Most families will embark on a mission to access some general information about the diagnosis. Other families may need more guidance and support, either to access appropriate information, or to shape it to make it relevant and specific to their own situation.

The sharing of information with families is something that is important to assess, and is something that *most* families will need and find helpful, to a greater or lesser extent.

FAMILY INTERVENTIONS

Family intervention is identified as a core intervention for the treatment of a range of mental health problems. The National Institute for Health and Care Excellence (NICE) guideline for schizophrenia states: 'Offer family intervention to all families of people with psychosis or schizophrenia who live with or are in close contact with the service user. This can be started either during the acute phase or later, including in inpatient settings'[26] (p.10).

These interventions have been shown to reduce relapse rates and costs of care.[27] The additional benefits may be that family members are less at risk of being referred to mental health services themselves, and the clinician has additional resources available, i.e. working as a team with the family.

The model of Behavioural Family Therapy (BFT) is one of the models of family interventions that fit with the NICE guidelines. The key parts of the model include the following, though the way in which they are delivered depends on the information gained during the assessment process:

- *Individual assessment*. Each person taking part in the family work will have an assessment. This is to find out their understanding of the diagnosis and experience of the service user, which can differ greatly between family members. Each person is also asked to set personal goals for themselves, which can help each family member to focus on their own lives, rather than being consumed by their caring responsibilities.
- *Information sharing*. As discussed above, this is an important part of working with families. The family worker will already have a sense of what the family members know and understand through the individual assessments, and sessions are tailored to filling any gaps in knowledge or clearing up misunderstandings. This is not necessarily about the worker *educating* the family, but rather trying to get the family to understand each other's point of view and develop empathy for the service user.
- *Staying well plans*. Families are often aware of changes in the service user's well-being before the service user is, and will have a more rounded view of how the service user relapses compared to the clinician's perspective. Developing staying well plans with families (including the service user) is much more likely to lead to an effective plan than those developed with the service user alone.
- *Communication skills*. The family worker will guide the family to communicate in a more positive and clear way

that is much less likely to lead to stress. Families report finding these skills really useful, as it gives them something specific and positive they can do which has an immediate impact.[28]
- *Problem solving*. The family are shown a structured method of problem solving that they are asked to use. This enables the family to work together to achieve goals in a way that encourages all family members to be involved, and again gives the family a process to manage their own problems, rather than rely on clinicians to do so.[28]
- *Family meetings*. The family are asked to have a meeting themselves between the sessions with the family workers. The meeting is focused and structured, and gives the family time to focus on moving forward by discussing how the above skills and information are being utilized in the family. Family members will also discuss how to help each other achieve their goals.

The application of this kind of family work could be said to fit perfectly with concept of the *craft of caring*,[29] blending the *science* (a structured, evidence-based intervention with families) with the *art* of how to apply the model in different and potentially complex family situations. It is helpful for the psychiatric/mental health nurse to be familiar with the structure of the model in order to provide a focus for the time spent with families, but at the same time it is important to be mindful that every family is different, and the model needs to be crafted to suit each family.

CARER'S PERSPECTIVE: BEHAVIOURAL FAMILY THERAPY

The whole model of BFT brings to the fore the efforts families have made to adapt to the traumatic role of becoming a carer. The simplicity of the techniques does not make it an onerous task to apply to daily life, and equips each family member involved in the process with practical communication and problem-solving skills that have such a positive impact on the whole family.

CONCLUSION

This chapter has explored the impact on family life when someone becomes unwell, which is a situation that many of us have experienced ourselves. The impact of a mental health problem can prove to be even more challenging for families. Normalizing a family's response to a stressful situation, rather than pathologizing or blaming them, is a key factor in developing relationships with families. Confidentiality, and how its principles are applied, are also major influences on how families can access appropriate support.

A final message. Working in collaboration with families will save you time and effort in the long term. If all three points of the Triangle of Care – the family, the service user and the professional – can work together, positive changes can be brought about more effectively.

References

1. Chandler R, Bradstreet S, Hayward M, eds. *Voicing caregiver experiences: wellbeing and recovery narratives for caregivers*. Sussex Partnership NHS Foundation Trust and Scottish Recovery Network, 2013.
2. Leggatt M. Meeting the challenges. In: Froggatt D, Fadden G, Johnson DL, Leggatt M, Shankar R (eds). *Families as partners in mental health care. A guidebook for implementing family work*. Toronto: World Fellowship for Schizophrenia and Allied Disorders, 2007: 22–37.
3. Laing RD, Esterson A. *Sanity, madness and the family*. London: Penguin Books, 1964.
4. Vaughn C, Leff J. The measurement of expressed emotion in the families of psychiatric patients. *British Journal of Social and Clinical Psychology* 1976; **15**: 157–65.
5. Wyatt J. Jenni's story. 2003. Available from: Meriden Family Programme, Carers; Stories, http://www.meridenfamilyprogramme.com/family-work/carers [Accessed 5th August 2016].
6. Worthington A, Rooney P, Hannan R. *The Triangle of Care. Carers included: a guide to best practice in mental health care in England*, 2nd edn. London: Carers Trust, 2013.
7. Department of Health. *Briefing paper: sharing mental health information with carers: pointers to good practice for service providers*. London: SDO, 2006.
8. Fadden G. Involving and training professionals in family work. In: Froggatt D, Fadden G, Johnson DL, Leggatt M, Shankar R (eds). *Families as partners in mental health care. A guidebook for implementing family work*. Toronto: World Fellowship for Schizophrenia and Allied Disorders, 2007: 38–49.
9. Allison S, Fadden G, Hart D, Launer M, Siddle J. *Carers and confidentiality in mental health. Issues involved in information sharing. Partners in care*, 2nd edn. London: Royal College of Psychiatrists, Princess Royal Trust for Carers, 2010.
10. Department of Health. *Developing services for carers and families of people with mental illness*. London: Department of Health, 2002.
11. *Oxford dictionaries*. Available from: http://www.oxforddictionaries.com [Accessed 18th July 2016].
12. Sutton A. Confidence and confidentiality: carers, service users, service providers and service provision. Presented at Working with Families: Developing Partnerships. Meriden Family Programme Conference, Stratford upon Avon, 2007.
13. Cohen AN, Drapalski AL, Glynn SM, Medoff D, Fang LJ, Dixon LB. Preferences for family involvement in care among consumers with serious mental illness. *Psychiatric Services* 2013; **64**(3): 257–63.
14. Carers (Recognition and Services) Act 1995. Available from: http://www.legislation.gov.uk/ukpga/1995/12/enacted [Accessed 5th August 2016].
15. Department of Health. *National service framework for mental health*. London: HMSO, 1999.
16. Dowson E. Hearing the music and remembering to dance. In: Chandler R, Bradstreet S, Hayward M (eds). *Voicing caregiver experiences: wellbeing and recovery narratives for caregivers*. Sussex Partnership NHS Foundation Trust and Scottish Recovery Network, 2013: 121–36.
17. Making Space. Available from: www.makingspace.co.uk [Accessed 18th July 2016].
18. Carers Trust Professionals. Triangle of Care for mental health. Available from: http://professionals.carers.org/health/articles/triangle-of-care,6802,PR.html [Accessed 18th July 2016].
19. Carers Trust. www.carers.org [Accessed 18th July 2016].
20. Falloon I, Fadden G, Mueser K, Gingerich S, Rappaport S, McGill C, Graham-Hole V, Gair F. *Family work manual*. Birmingham: Meriden Family Programme, 2007.
21. Smith J, Fadden G, Taylor L. The needs of siblings in first-episode psychosis. In: French P, Smith J, Shiers D, Reed M, Rayne M (eds). *Promoting recovery in early psychosis: a practice manual*. Oxford: Wiley Blackwell, 2010: 235–44.
22. Sin J, Moone N, Harris P. Siblings of individuals with first-episode psychosis: understanding their experiences and needs. *Journal of Psychosocial Nursing and Mental Health Services* 2008; **46**(6): 33–40.
23. Smith J, Fadden G, O'Shea M. Interventions with siblings. In: Lobban F, Barrowclough C (eds). *A casebook of family interventions for psychosis*. Chichester: Wiley and Sons, 2009: 185–210.
24. Atchison M, Conneely P (producers). *Working with families across cultures* (DVD). Birmingham and Solihull Mental Health Foundation NHS Trust, National Institute for Mental Health in England and Birmingham City University, 2009.
25. Royal College of Psychiatrists. *Partners in Care campaign*. London: Royal College of Psychiatrists, Princess Royal Trust for Carers, 2004.
26. NICE (National Institute for Health and Care Excellence). *Psychosis and schizophrenia in adults: treatment and management*. London: NICE, 2014.
27. Pharoah F, Mari JJ, Rathbone J, Wong W. Family intervention for schizophrenia. *Cochrane Database of Systematic Reviews* 2010; **12**: CD000088.
28. Campbell AS. How was it for you? Families' experience of receiving behavioural family therapy. *Journal of Psychiatric and Mental Health Nursing* 2004; **11**: 261–7.
29. Barker P. The nature of nursing. In: Barker P (ed.). *Psychiatric and mental health nursing. The craft of caring*, 2nd edn. Boca Raton: Hodder Arnold, 2009: 3–11.

Further reading

Chandler R, Bradstreet S, Hayward M (eds). *Voicing caregiver experiences: wellbeing and recovery narratives for caregivers*. Sussex Partnership NHS Foundation Trust and Scottish Recovery Network, 2013.

Froggatt D, Fadden G, Johnson DL, Leggatt M, Shankar R (eds). *Families as partners in mental health care. A guidebook for implementing family work*. World Fellowship for Schizophrenia and Allied Disorders, 2007.

Worthington A, Rooney P, Hannan R. *The Triangle of Care. Carers included: a guide to best practice in mental health care in England*, 2nd edn. London: Carers Trust, 2013.

Relevant web pages

Carers Trust Professionals. Triangle of Care for mental health. http://professionals.carers.org/health/articles/triangle-of-care,6802,PR.html

Meriden Family Programme. http://www.meridenfamily programme.com/

MIND. How to cope as a carer. http://www.mind.org.uk/information-support/helping-someone-else/carers-friends-and-family-how-to-cope/

Rethink Mental Illness. Carers, family and friends. http://www.rethink.org/carers-family-friends

Royal College of Psychiatrists. Mental health information for all. http://www.rcpsych.ac.uk/mentalhealthinfo.aspx

52 The liaison psychiatric service

KATE CHARTRES, RIKKE ALBERT, SARAH EALES
AND ANGELA WARREN

LEARNING OUTCOMES

- To have an understanding of the origins of psychiatric liaison services.
- To be aware of the types of service models, and the advantages and disadvantages of different models of provision.
- To have an understanding of the competencies required by liaison mental health nurses.
- To appreciate liaison teams' emphasis on teaching and training.
- To have an understanding of the types of assessment completed by liaison nurses.
- To have an increased understanding of working with self-harm.
- To appreciate the multi-faceted role of the liaison nurse.

SUMMARY OF KEY POINTS

- Liaison psychiatry has existed worldwide at varying levels since at least the 1990s.
- There are a number of different types of service models, each with its own benefits and drawbacks.
- Liaison mental health nursing has a highly varied but very specialist set of requirements.
- Psychiatric liaison services benefit general hospital staff by providing a large amount of education and training, both formally and informally.

- A liaison nurse may work in different clinical settings, such as emergency department and ward settings; in all settings, assessment of the presenting problem will be required.
- Self-harm is one of the most common causes for attendance at emergency departments, and the liaison mental health nurse will be involved in supporting service users after self-harm.

INTRODUCTION

Mental health has historically been cast as the poor relation to general medicine in terms of service provision, particularly in the UK. Liaison psychiatry and the idea of treating body and mind together has existed at varying levels within acute hospitals the world over since the late 1990s, and perhaps earlier in some areas.

Specialist liaison psychiatry services are accessible to medical staff so that they can request assessment and advice for clients for whom there is a clear clinical need for treatment and support in terms of their mental health. However, there is a growing body of evidence to suggest that the mental health needs of patients within acute general hospitals have largely been unmet.

More than 60 years ago, *The work of nurses in hospital wards*[1] highlighted difficulties in meeting the needs of patients, due to a focus on delivering specific tasks in relation to care, which led to the needs of the patient on an emotional level not being specifically addressed. Psychiatric liaison nurses (PLNs), also referred to as liaison mental health nurses (LMHNs), work from a holistic viewpoint, taking into account the whole person and their clinical presentation from a multi-faceted perspective. They are particularly interested in the whole experience of living with a condition, or a number of conditions, from the individual's perspective. LMHNs will also ensure that the patient occupies a central role in formulating care plans and identifying bespoke interventions.[2]

In mental health, the 'parity of esteem' agenda,[3-6] which has gathered momentum since the previous edition of this book was published, has brought attention to the health outcomes of those with enduring mental illness. On average, those with enduring mental illness die around 14 to 32 years earlier than the wider population[7] and the lack of access to mental health care within the general hospital,[8] in particular within emergency departments, has meant that liaison mental health has seen an unprecedented growth in recent years. It is a really exciting time in the field of contemporary liaison psychiatry, particularly in the UK where large psychiatric liaison teams are being commissioned around the country. The requirement for these teams to operate on a 24/7 basis has led to them being largely nursing-led. However, despite the inherent need for expert nursing knowledge in light of this development, in contrast to our US counterparts who have liaison consultation nurses educated to Master's level, very few liaison nurses in the UK have received postgraduate training in the field. There is only one university offering a module in liaison mental health nursing. This, coupled with the need for large numbers of new liaison nurses, has led to services struggling to find appropriately skilled nurses and therefore having to cultivate innovative new ways of developing the skill sets of new starters. In a sense, services have been looking at how best to 'grow your own' LMHNs, and thus band 5 nurses have begun to take on roles that were historically the reserve of more experienced band 6 and band 7 practitioners. In such cases, competency frameworks have been developed and utilized, along with the provision of opportunities to shadow other specialist nurses (such as stroke specialists or chronic obstructive pulmonary disease (COPD) specialists).

> ### REFLECTION
>
> - Consider the extent to which you tend to work in a holistic way with people, taking into account their physical, emotional, psychological, spiritual and social needs.
>
> - What is your knowledge of physical health? For example, to what extent are you aware of the psychological impact of living with a long-term medical condition?

The need for liaison psychiatry services is emphasized by the fact that people presenting to the general hospital have a greater likelihood of experiencing psychological difficulties than those within the wider population.[9] Psychiatric liaison services benefit general hospital staff by providing a large amount of education and training, both formally and informally, which serves to maximize the quality of the care they provide, reduce stigma and generally improve the overall experience for the patient.[10,11] See Box 52.1.

There is now comprehensive evidence to suggest that, if left untreated, depressive and anxiety disorders delay the progress of patients presenting with a long-term medical condition and increase the frequency of inpatient admissions and presentations to emergency departments. The prevalence is estimated at 30 per cent for comorbidity, but in some studies much higher prevalence has been noted. Among 56 COPD patients, the prevalence of anxiety was as high as 52 per cent, and depression 43 per cent.[15] For those with diabetes, depression co-exists around twice as frequently compared with those without the condition.[16] Depression is generally the most common psychological disorder that can occur after a stroke, and it is estimated that this affects around one-third of patients.[17] In people with heart failure it is estimated that between 11 and 35 per cent will have comorbid depression. Unsurprisingly, this has a marked influence on outcomes, including increased mortality.[18]

There is no question that, left untreated, mental health problems co-existing with long-term medical conditions correlate with negative outcomes. This is due in part to a reduction of positive engagement with care packages. When working with long-term conditions, the effective

> ### REFLECTION
>
> Does anyone you know have a long-term medical condition? Have you noticed any signs or symptoms of depression or anxiety? Have you detected any links between the management of the condition and the person's mood and anxiety levels?

BOX 52.1: PEOPLE WITH MENTAL HEALTH PROBLEMS ATTENDING THE GENERAL HOSPITAL

- Older people occupy two-thirds of all general hospital beds.[12]
- In 2002, *Between two stools*[13] found that a quarter of all referrals to older persons' psychiatry came from general hospitals.
- The *Counting the cost* report on dementia[14] found that 77 per cent of carers were unhappy with the quality of care provided for dementia patients on general wards, and over a third had made a complaint. The main reason given was a lack of understanding and recognition of dementia.
- The overall prevalence of mental health problems for older people in acute hospitals is estimated at 60 per cent. These include dementia, depression, anxiety, alcohol dependence and schizophrenia.[9]
- It is widely thought that around 5 per cent of all emergency department attendances are related to mental health.
- Long-term conditions account for 70 per cent of all expenditure in general hospitals. People suffering from long-term conditions are believed to be two to three times more likely to have a comorbid mental health condition.[9]
- It is estimated that mental health comorbidity, including medically unexplained symptoms, cost the British economy around 13.5 billion a year.[9]

management of depression and anxiety can be delivered by employing relatively simple techniques, including brief cognitive behavioural therapy (CBT) based work, psycho-education and mindfulness (chapter 44) breathing and grounding techniques. (Chapter 40 provides further information on CBT.)

BRIEF HISTORY

It is generally accepted that the symbiotic relationship between mental and physical health was not conceptualized until the early twentieth century. In 1926, Pratt wrote that 'psychiatry may prove to be the liaison agent, the integrator that unifies, clarifies and resolves all available medical knowledge'[19] (p.897). The delivery of psychiatric liaison services is a relatively new development in comparison to other areas of mental health. It was first conceptualized in the USA and then in the UK, and is now a burgeoning worldwide phenomenon. In more recent times, Australia in particular seemed to be leading the way in terms of moving from a consultation approach towards full integration.[20]

Progress really intensified during the 1950s and 1960s, when collaborative relationships began to develop between physicians and psychiatrists as psychiatric wards were incorporated on site within the general hospital.[21] As more specialist nurse positions became available, nurses then began to follow their psychiatrist colleagues into the acute hospital, a process accelerated by the need for supply to be able to meet demand. During the 1960s, nurse education made the transition into universities in the USA and, alongside the academic and professional kudos this afforded, generic training was developed which meant that nurses were well versed in working within the general hospital. The emergent bio-psychosocial approach to care led to a number of nurses who demonstrated clinical competency in neurobiological knowledge being professionally acknowledged and accepted by their physician colleagues, and graduate programmes in consultation–liaison nursing were developed at Master's level.[10,11,21]

The evolution of the psychiatric liaison service was very different in the UK, however. According to Morriss and Mayou,[22] the early demand for liaison psychiatry services was attributable to the decriminalization of suicide in 1961, after which there was an expectation by the Ministry of Health that anyone who had made an attempt to take their own life would be reviewed by a psychiatrist before being allowed to leave hospital. Nurses were gradually recruited into positions that would lend support to this directive and the workload that it subsequently created.[23,24] However, at this stage they did not have the long-standing relationships with the general hospital that their US counterparts had established; rather, relationships had to be forged on a day-to-day basis. Without clinical specialist status or the opportunity to develop academically, the liaison nurse role was largely misunderstood as simply that of a risk assessor – unlike today when the role is recognized as that of a highly skilled and multi-faceted practitioner who demonstrates the craft of caring. Unsurprisingly, the reduction in bed numbers during the late 1980s and 1990s and the limited provision of community mental health care services increased the importance of having appropriately skilled mental health nurses available to assess those patients presenting to the general hospital following an episode of self-harm or with other mental health emergencies.

MODELS OF SERVICE PROVISION

As mentioned earlier, the movement towards ensuring adequate liaison psychiatry services in the UK has gathered momentum over the last 10 years. This has included a recommendation in 2008 by the Royal College of Psychiatrists[25] for raising the standards in the provision of liaison psychiatry for older people in acute hospitals. This was quickly followed by another paper, *Managing urgent mental health needs in the acute trust*,[26] which recommended provision of liaison psychiatry for other mental health conditions rather than solely concentrating attention on the service needs of dementia sufferers. In 2009, *No health without mental health*[27] reprised the recommendations for liaison teams from the 2008 Royal College of Psychiatrists report and linked adequate mental health care to physical health care, stating that 25 per cent of acute patients have a mental health need and that treatment of mental health problems improves physical health outcomes (more information on physical health can be found in chapter 69). Later in 2009, the NHS Next Stage Review recommended an alignment of mental health services with physical health care, and in the same year *New horizons*[28] supported the need for liaison psychiatric services. After a change of UK government, this was rapidly replaced by the current *No health without mental health* strategy.[29] At that time the Department of Health also supported work on developing a template for liaison mental health services. In 2011, the economic evaluation of the Birmingham Rapid Assessment Interface and Discharge (RAID) model was published, which stated that, for every pound spent on the service, investment showed a four-fold return (so for every pound spent, £4 was saved), improved health outcomes and a reduction in length of stay, readmissions and costs associated with medically unexplained symptoms.[30] The principles of the RAID include providing a service to adults of all ages; being available 24 hours a day, 7 days a week; and ensuring follow-up clinics to enable earlier discharge.[9]

Guidance for models of liaison psychiatry, commissioned by the Strategic Clinical Network for mental health, dementia and neurological conditions, was published in a February 2014 document entitled *Developing models for liaison psychiatry services*,[31] and identified four models of provision which are detailed in Table 52.1. The number of staff required to fulfil the model requirements grow in size according to the number of beds in an acute hospital, based on 500 beds and doubling for 1,000, and so on. However, there are very few services that stick rigidly to the numbers suggested by Aitken et al.[31]

According to Aitken et al.,[31] the Core model is based around a service that provides limited hours of cover (that is, not 24 hours), and senior nurses (band 6 or above) and consultant psychiatry cover.

1. The Core 24 model (Service C in Table 52.1) is currently gathering momentum as the UK government has

pledged affinity and stated that 50 per cent of emergency departments should have 24/7 front-of-house cover by 2020.[3] However, there is much concern among specialists within the field: if too much investment is focused providing a rapid response to the emergency department, and if, alongside this, investment is not given to allow teams to in-reach to the wider hospital, many of the savings realized from the Birmingham RAID model will not be demonstrated.[9,31]

2. Enhanced 24 (Service D in Table 52.1) is a 24/7 service which is able to offer outpatient work in the short term. This is useful for managing the psychological impact of long-term conditions, working with problematic self-harm and providing short-term support to people who do not easily fit into the pathway elsewhere. Many services are also enhancing their team with peer support. A peer support worker is someone who draws on their own experiences of emotional distress and use of mental health services in order to inspire, model and inform others in similar situations and support them in finding their own path to recovery, through developing innovative personal relapse prevention and care plans with the person presenting to the liaison service.

3. The Comprehensive service (Service E in Table 52.1) differs from the Enhanced by also providing very specialist interventions for complex cases.

The benefits of a liaison psychiatry service are well documented and some of these benefits are listed in Box 52.2.

Finally, the UK Department of Health has clearly set the national agenda for at least 50 per cent of all acute hospitals to have a service that is on a par with Core 24 by 2020, and to make services more accessible and reduce waiting times.[3] In support of this, the government has committed £30 million of initial investment in the last 6 months. The future is bright for liaison psychiatry and for liaison nurses.

At a recent national UK conference,[32] liaison nurses expressed enthusiasm for developing a variety of initiatives, including a UK network with regional and national groups and an evidence-based national website dedicated to the field of liaison mental health nursing. Those involved were also keen to set up a nursing conference dedicated entirely to the field.

REFLECTION

What is happening in liaison nursing in your area? Is there a website dedicated to the field? Are you aware of an annual conference?

Liaison mental health services within the UK can opt in to a national quality improvement programme that sets out quality standards for service provision.[33,34]

Table 52.1 Models of liaison psychiatry[31]

Types of liaison service	Team composition	Benefits	Drawbacks
A: Services providing 9–5 service or extended hours	Senior liaison nurses (band 6/7/8) and some psychiatry cover	Provides comprehensive bio-psychosocial assessment of need Builds strong relationships with acute colleagues Liaison nurses have specialist skills that tend to be associated with those people presenting under the age of 65, in terms of assessing for risk of self-harm/functional disorders (those for which after examination there is difficulty finding a medical problem) or older people's assessment skills (in terms of assessing for organic disorders and those associated with cognitive decline). Although on both sides there is often overlap, these services are often separated from each other, with dedicated clinicians providing older persons' services and dedicated clinicians assessing individuals post self-harm	Teams are relatively small and are under pressure in terms of delivering to all those in need Little or no out-of-hours response
B: Adults of all ages, 24-hour services where the focus is on an urgent and emergency response	Senior liaison nurses (band 6/7/8) Psychiatry cover x 2 (one for adults and one for older adults)	Provides comprehensive bio-psychosocial assessment of need Builds strong relationships with acute colleagues Liaison nurse work generically offering an ageless service where the specialism is around liaison mental health nursing and assessment/psycho-education and training for colleagues in acute care	Teams have less time to in-reach to inpatient wards to support the treatment of the mental health component of a medical illness or a long-term condition Very few services offer support to children and young people Some nurses report a loss of specialism in terms of working with older people and organic disorders

(Continued)

Table 52.1 (Continued)

Types of liaison service	Team composition	Benefits	Drawbacks
C: Ageless 24-hour liaison services where the focus is on urgent and emergency response	Senior liaison nurses (band 6/7/8) Dedicated input for children and young people, sometimes co-located, but more often a children's crisis service not based in the hospital will provide in-reach to the emergency department or the paediatric ward Psychiatry cover x 2 (one for adults and one for older adults) Scaffolding provided by child and adolescent psychiatry Recent input from band 5 nurses as a training opportunity and support workers and peer support in some areas	As service B All ages receive a service	Reduced opportunities to proactively in reach to inpatient wards to support in the treatment of the psychological impact of a medical illness or long-term condition Some nurses report a loss of specialism in terms of working with older people and organic disorders
D: Ageless 24-hour liaison services that provide an enhanced service including pro-active brief intervention treatment within acute hospitals	As model C but with increased numbers	As service C Teams have more capacity, so are able to provide brief psychological therapy to inpatients on acute hospital wards, which can impact positively on their length of stay	Clinical staff miss the opportunity to follow people up at home, particularly where they do not easily fit into another treatment pathway but would benefit from input
E: Ageless 24-hour liaison services that provide an enhanced service including pro-active brief intervention treatment within acute hospitals and follow-up in outpatient clinics post discharge	As model D but with increased numbers	As all other models, but with the added benefit of following people up to reduce re-attendance and admission	

BOX 52.2: BENEFITS OF THE LIAISON PSYCHIATRY SERVICE

- Provides comprehensive bio-psychosocial assessment of need.
- Staff are able to work in collaboration with one another to deliver integrated and less restrictive care.
- Provides brief psychological interventions to inpatients and, where commissioned, outpatients.
- Staff are able to understand and respect the roles and responsibilities of other professions and work together to provide the highest quality care.

- Staff are able to support the diagnosis of comorbidities and cooperatively engage in multidisciplinary treatment and care planning.
- Provides opportunities to engage in cross-boundary interprofessional training and education.
- Promotes communication, shared decision making and information sharing.

EDUCATION IN LIAISON MENTAL HEALTH

There are two core aspects of education in liaison mental health nursing. These are 1) the educational requirements of liaison mental health nurses themselves, and 2) their requirement as educators in relation to patients' mental health needs. Liaison psychiatrists also have their own competence and training programme in order to gain recognition as specialists in liaison psychiatry.

They are also expected to be independent practitioners who can operate both independently and within psychiatric liaison multidisciplinary teams. They are also required to be able to work as members of multidisciplinary clinical teams within the acute hospital and primary care setting. In theses settings, the clinical team is not mental-health-specific and LMHNs are joining these teams to ensure the patient/s has a more integrated health care service. For example, LMHNs operate within the emergency department, on acute hospital wards, in paediatric and maternity settings and in primary care services.

COMPETENCIES FOR LMHNs

A clear set of competencies can assist in understanding the specific role requirements, when undertaking a self-assessment of skills and knowledge. This listing can also help when developing a personal and/or team professional development programme. Nurses are not unfamiliar with the concept of competence because the measure of competence forms a key aspect of pre-registration education.[35] Competence has been defined as 'the expertise, clinical and technical knowledge to deliver effective care and treatments based on research and evidence'[36] (p.13).

Liaison mental health nursing has a highly varied but very specialist set of requirements. Liaison mental health nursing in the UK first began to focus on competencies in 2004, when work by the London Liaison Mental Health Special Interest Group sought to articulate the education, knowledge and skills required of LMHNs. This group produced a competency document which was revised and updated in 2014, reflecting the more varied grades at which LMHNs operate and thus incorporating a greater number of core competencies. Irrespective of grade, there are some core competencies:

1. Competency for providing liaison mental health nursing assessment and consultation
2. Competency for the assessment of risk including self-harm
3. Competency for providing nursing assessment and advice of patient's capacity
4. Competency in identifying and considering ethical issues
5. Competency for providing nursing advice on legal issues
6. Competency for interventions used in liaison mental health nursing
7. Competency for the admission and discharge of patients
8. Competency for Liaison Mental Health Nurses maintaining accurate records, documentation and report writing
9. Competency for providing nursing advice on the management and care of patients with complex psychosocial and/or challenging presentations
10. Competency for providing nursing advice on medication
11. Competency for Liaison Mental Health Nurses in working with people with specific physical illnesses
12. Competency for education, training, and supervision
13. Competency for evaluating Liaison Mental Health Nursing provision[37]

The level of competence would be expected to vary, depending on the grade of the LMHN.

The health care arenas that might employ LMHNs vary greatly, and so nurses may also be expected to have competence in regard to assessment, formulation and treatment of particular health issues and/or age groups. These competencies include:

1. Competency for Liaison Mental Health Nurses in working with older adults
2. Competency for Liaison Mental Health Nurses working with people with a substance misuse problem
3. Competency for Liaison Mental Health Nurses in working with people with specific psychosomatic disorders
4. Competency for Liaison Mental Health Nurses in working with people with learning disabilities
5. Competency for Liaison Mental Health Nurses in working with mothers and babies
6. Competency for Liaison Mental Health Nurses in working with children & young people[37]

Within a large multidisciplinary liaison team, utilizing the Core 24 model or the RAID model,[38] practitioners often develop areas of specialist interest, developing high levels of knowledge and skill in specific areas of clinical practice and forging strong links with the specialist health care team. This is in addition to working across the range of presentations and using the core competences outlined above. LMHNs may also be employed within one of the specific settings outlined above in a role that is intended to support one specific client group.

In order to achieve the core competencies, or skills to work with those having specific health issues, LMHNs may undertake formalized training or education in specific treatment approaches or clinical diagnosis. However, much of the education undertaken by LMHNs involves identifying and shadowing already competent practitioners from a variety of professional backgrounds, and also through discussion of individual cases within multi-professional meetings and clinical supervision (chapter 10). Therefore finding the right clinical supervisor is key to the development of LMHNs. LMHNs may also seek support from their non-mental-health colleagues who are specialists in their own field of health care. This leads to a better understanding of the physical health diagnosis and treatment options available to those referred for specific mental health issues or psychological distress.

A variety of models have been proposed to articulate the role of LMHNs and their colleagues.[39] Key to all of these role descriptions is that education of non-specialist health care colleagues is vital to the liaison remit. Evidence for the cost-saving benefit of one of the key models of liaison service, RAID, rests upon the impact that LMH practitioners can have without offering direct consultation to individual patients.[38] LMHNs need to be able to support health care teams in a variety of settings to better understand psychological distress and mental health needs, and to support nurses in particular, but also the wider health care team, in

understanding how to offer better and safer care and environments for those who have mental health needs but are not in hospital for the sole purpose of having that need met. Examples of specific education include:

1. supporting maternity services to understand how to identify emerging psychotic presentations which are often quick to develop after the birth of the baby, and require intensive and immediate specialist mental health intervention to protect the mother and the child;[40]
2. helping gastrointestinal services to understand the clinical diagnosis of an eating disorder and how their acute hospital intervention fits into the long-term care of a person with an eating disorder;[41]
3. supporting emergency department staff to understand the reason for self-harming behaviour, the clinical diagnosis associated with this behaviour and, from a service user perspective, how best to support those with a first presentation or repeat attendances;[42]
4. supporting clinical staff across services to provide better environments and care for those with medically unexplained symptoms, dementia and learning disabilities (support with communication strategies is often key to this educational work).[8,43]

> **REFLECTION**
>
> Can you identify situations where those offering specialist physical health care have required support to understand the mental health needs of those for whom they are caring? How have you sought to address these needs?

Education of clinical colleagues can take many forms. The busy nature of acute physical health care environments and the priority given to it, the most effective approaches are those that can be woven into the natural flow of a team or ward routine. These approaches include ensuring feedback is offered on all liaison mental health assessments, and that the diagnosis is clearly explained and the necessary interventions clearly outlined. By using a specific and real case example, individual staff and teams can learn. Working with approaches to implement in the future as appropriate. It is also possible to give brief teaching sessions that fit into education sessions already offered by the ward or team for their development, such as break-time seminars. Many teams have benefited from introducing the role of liaison psychiatry/liaison mental health, and key principles in caring for those with mental health issues, in induction programmes for all new staff. LMHNs also work nationally to develop e-learning packages that are accessible across the NHS and can be undertaken when time is available to the clinicians. Liaison mental health practitioners are also involved in developing accessible video resources to help clinicians, patients and carers understand the role of liaison mental health care.[44] The Northumberland Tyne and Wear Foundation NHS Trust has just developed its first training week for new starters, which includes training in assessment and management of risk, working with veterans, dealing with organic disorders and working with medically unexplained symptoms. This training week focused on utilizing case studies to demonstrate effective ways of working, and this will be delivered regularly throughout the year so that any new staff receive the training as part of their induction. Teams who typically see many people with mental health needs or who wish to develop their skills in this area can also be offered 1- or 2-day courses, normally based on clinical case studies and/or simulation. Written material can also be a means of supporting non-specialist colleagues in understanding the mental health needs of patients. When considering the development of formalized training, it is important to ensure that service user perspectives are integrated into the teaching package.[33]

LIAISON MENTAL HEALTH INTERVENTIONS

Assessment

Assessment in LMHN is a core function of the nurse. A liaison nurse may work in different clinical settings such as emergency departments, and ward settings; in all settings, assessment of the presenting problem will be required. The assessment should cover the patient's mental state, but also their level of engagement in care and treatment, challenges in behaviour, and risk. A bio-psychosocial approach to this assessment is needed in liaison work. This reflects the fact that patients are likely to be in hospital due to a physical condition. (Chapters 13, 14 and 15 contain further information on assessment and chapter 69 addresses physical health care.)

Although assessment forms part of clarifying the presentation of the patient, if it is done well and supportively it can also be an effective therapeutic intervention.[45] Giving someone an opportunity to tell their story and giving them the space to think through their situation are important aspects of supporting a person through a crisis or difficult situation.[46,47] The liaison nurse can help the person look at their strengths and coping strategies. This reflects the recovery approach utilized in mental health care.[48] If the person is too unwell at the time of assessment, they may not be able to engage fully in the process. If so, the liaison nurse can still use the recovery approach to help the person in the short term by ensuring they are safe and supportively cared for.[49]

REFLECTION

Think of a time when you supported a person to focus on their problem-solving skills and strengths. What did you do, and how did you share this work with others?

If a person is well known, it may be more appropriate to refer to their history, but it is also important to take into account any changes in the person's circumstances, as these changes may be a factor in their presentation to the emergency department or admission to the ward.

Over the years, a number of assessment tools have been developed, covering different areas of risk. Some are intended to predict risk, whereas others are aimed at helping the clinician structure the risk assessment.[50] Research shows that risk assessment based solely on a tool is unlikely to fully identify the risk the person may pose to themselves or others.[51] Risk assessment tools may help in the process of indicating areas of need, but for the most accurate risk assessment, a formulation – that is, interpretation of the information from the assessment alongside a clear management plan – is needed.[51] Understanding risk factors and indicators is useful when developing a care plan with the service user.[52] Positive risk taking in care planning is an important part of the recovery process, even when a person is in a mental health crisis,[48,53] (chapter 36) and is reflective of the craft of caring.

Assessments tools for specific conditions have been developed (see Table 52.2). Staff should be aware of the potential cultural bias that any tool may have. An example of cultural bias would be a cognitive tool which relies on the service user being familiar with the Roman alphabet or able to recognize English-sounding names. If the service user is not as familiar with either of those areas as a native speaker would be, the assessment may not reflect their cognition accurately. Work is being done to develop and understand the role of culture in cognition,[54] as well as developing screening tools that are more culturally sensitive, such as the Bangla Adaptation of Mini Mental State Examination (BAMSE).[55] Using collateral information for people who know the person well may help mitigate the bias.

The involvement of a service user's carer or social system is important in all fields of mental health. Understanding what the person is normally like, including their areas of strength, is important when trying to understand what that person's needs are.[56] The social system is the support a person may have in their life, such as family, friends and colleagues, but it can also include health professionals.[47] The people within the social system are likely to know the person best. The challenges of involving carers or the social system, at a time when the patient may be distressed and unwell, are well documented.[57–60] Conflict can arise when attempts are made to balance the service user's right to confidentiality with the needs of carers.[58–60]

Table 52.2 Mental health conditions and assessment tools to help in their identification and treatment

Condition	Tool
Dementia	Addenbrooke's Cognitive Examination – Revised (ACE-R), Montreal Orientation Cognitive Assessment (MoCA), Frontal Assessment Battery (FAB)
Psychosis	Health of the Nation Outcome Scales (HoNOS)
Mood disorder	Patient Health Questionnaire 9 (PHQ9)
Anxiety	Generalized Anxiety Disorder 7 (GAD7)
Alcohol misuse	Alcohol Use Disorder Identification Test – consumption questions (AUDIT-C), Clinical Institute for Withdrawal Assessment (CIWA)
Post-natal depression	Edinburgh Post-natal Depression Scale
Eating disorder	Body Mass Index (BMI), Management of Really Sick Patients with Anorexia Nervosa (MARSIPAN) for advice on treatment
Medically unexplained symptoms	European Quality of Life – 5 dimensions (EQ-5D-5L)
Delirium	Confusion Assessment Method (CAM)
Other	
Risk	Historical Clinical Risk – 20 (HCR20)

Source: Trigwell et al.[58]

Carers describe a sense of trauma and distress when caring for someone during a mental health crisis.[59,61] Staff are often faced with the challenge of trying to engage a service user during a crisis, who may ask for carers not to be involved. Understanding this challenge when supporting the person and their carers is important when deciding on effective personalized support.

> **REFLECTION**
>
> What are the challenges of involving carers and social systems when a person is in a crisis? Think of a time when you worked with both the person in crisis and their carers/social system. What were the challenges and how did you address them?

The mental state of the person in a crisis, whether in the emergency department or on a ward, may have an impact on their mental capacity. Being clear about the person's willingness to stay to be assessed is an important aspect of care.[62–64] If the person is in mental distress or is unwilling to stay, acute colleagues alongside the mental health liaison team have a duty to assess the person's capacity to make decisions in the person's best interest.[65] Please refer to local guidelines in managing lack of capacity.

The completion of any assessment should result in a clear management plan to support the person.[51] If done well, the voice of the person in crisis should be included although on rare occasions this may be difficult to do if the person is very unwell. Without the person's involvement the plan is less likely to support their needs. See chapters 13, 14 and 15 for further details on assessment.

Working with self-harm

Self-harm (SH) is one of the most common causes for attendance at emergency departments.[66] Over the years, the response to SH has improved, in part due to the increase in liaison services functioning within emergency departments and the 2004 guidelines from the National Institute for Health and Care Excellence (NICE).[62] Service users, on the other hand, still describe a sense of stigma, or a worry that they will face stigma, when attending emergency departments for help. This interplay between actual experiences of stigma and worries about being stigmatized is complex, and nurses will have to be aware of this when supporting people who have self-harmed. The NICE guidelines describe the best practice for managing self-harm (in the short and long term).[62,63] Anyone who attends the emergency department following SH should have a psychosocial assessment, including a full risk assessment. The guidelines focus on the joint approach of physical and mental health services in providing care for the person who has self-harmed.[62,63,66] Chapter 22 contains further information on SH.

The role of a liaison team in an emergency department or ward setting is not just to provide a psychosocial assessment of needs,[62,63] but also to support colleagues in acute care in understanding the emotional reasons for self-harming. Role modelling best practice and communication can help increase empathy in acute colleagues, which in turn may help to reduce the feelings of stigma which service users describe. The quality of the care therefore depends on joint working by the emergency department, wards and the psychiatric liaison.[62,63,66]

Self-harming behaviour is prevalent across all ages, but is more common in younger age groups (11 to 25 years).[67] Self-harm which leads to completed suicide is a particular concern for men in the middle age group (25 to 44 years), which has seen an increase in the last 10 years.[68] The assessment should clarify whether the self-harm is a way of managing emotional distress or an attempt to die. Service users themselves may not always be sure why they have self-harmed. The nurse also needs to be mindful that people who self-harm, whether once or regularly, are at risk of having thoughts of dying and completing suicide.[62] As such, each self-harm presentation should be assessed fully to establish the motivation for the behaviour and whether there are any changes in the usual reasons for harming or the type of self-harm used.

The reason for self-harming varies from person to person, but regular self-harming has the effect of reinforcing negative feelings, which may lead to the continuation of self-harm.[69,70] The psychological response to self-harm may initially be a sense of relief; however, this often turns into feelings of low self-worth. Understanding this dynamic in regular self-harming is important when supporting the person. If this vicious circle is not considered, the person who self-harms is likely to continue self-harming because the underlying feelings are being reinforced. Repeated self-harming may also indicate specific unmet needs, for example relating to current or past trauma, bullying or depression.[69] The role of the liaison nurse during assessment is to help the person understand their possible psychological responses and look at ways of breaking the cycle.

THE CLINICAL ROLE OF THE LIAISON NURSE

A nurse in a liaison team is part of a wider multidisciplinary team. Assessment and formulation form an important aspect of the nurse's role. The unique perspective which the liaison nurse will have within the liaison multidisciplinary team is a greater understanding of the challenges that acute nursing staff may face in managing a patient in distress 24 hours a day. The mental health nursing role is focused on the relationship with the patient, and on supporting the nursing care of the patient. It can be argued this is no different to other professional roles in health care, but the nursing role is unique in that this is the one profession which involves caring for the person for lengthy periods of time. (See chapter 3 for further detail on developing and maintaining therapeutic relationships.)

One area where liaison nurses can use their specific mental health nursing skills is in helping acute colleagues develop a personalized care plan for the patient and translate it into something the ward staff will be able to use. The emphasis should be on the care plan helping the person engage in their care and treatment. This will fit in with the role of liaison teams in minimizing the stigma of mental health problems, and increase tolerance towards patients who have mental health problems.[28,62,63,66] (Chapter 50 provides more information on collaborative care planning.)

Supporting acute colleagues in caring for a person who may have behaviour that challenges is another important role for the liaison nurse. Role modelling the use of ABC (antecedent, behaviour and consequence) can help the ward understand why the person's behaviour may be challenging and how to offer supportive interventions to prevent the behaviour from occurring. For this to work well, a clear understanding of the strengths and limitations of the acute staff is needed, as without this any personalized care plans are unlikely to work. This, alongside understanding the systemic issues and staff's response to anxiety when dealing with a person in distress, will help the liaison nurse support both acute colleagues and the person in distress.[71]

The life expectancy for a person with a mental illness is between 12 and 32 years shorter than the average person.[7,72] Supporting the person who may otherwise struggle to engage in their care and treatment for a physical condition is a hugely important part of the liaison nurse's role. Understanding the difficulties which the person with mental health problems may have in an acute setting, and advocating for them, will help in bridging this gap in life expectancy (see case study 1 for an example).

The clinical role of the liaison nurse can also involve providing short-term interventions such as education/teaching for the patient/carers and acute colleagues; brief interventions such as advice on alcohol, drugs and anxiety management; and psychological interventions such as CBT, among others.[37]

CASE STUDY 1

Sasha is a 27-year-old female who has been admitted multiple times for complications from endocarditis. She was using illicit substances and the ward suspected she was funding her drug-taking habit through prostitution.

She was referred to the liaison team on her seventh admission, as the team described feeling 'nihilistic' about her care. They felt stuck, as she would discharge herself before being fully treated and then would be admitted again in a worse physical state. She was described as being difficult. Sasha would use drugs on the ward and would disappear for a few hours at a time. She would refuse her intravenous antibiotics and physical tests. Other patients would complain about Sasha and ostracize her in the shared hospital bay. During her admission, following complications from her endocarditis, she had a stroke which left her unable to speak. The liaison nurse approached Sasha's referral in the following way.

Assessment

- Discussion was held with key members of the ward team to clarify concerns and conflict. The ward staff were offered the chance to debrief on their interaction with her and were supported in exploring and reflecting on their views on her presentation. The ward manager and consultant were champions of Sasha, and this was nurtured.
- Assessment of Sasha's mental state was difficult because she was wary of any engagement. The PLN used the approach of finding a common goal as a way of engaging rather than focusing on assessing her mental state. The common goal was for Sasha to be in a single room. She was initially assessed as having personality difficulties but was very guarded, so a clear mental state was not possible initially.
- A capacity assessment showed that initially she was not able to consent to care and treatment following the stroke. She was put on a Deprivation of Liberty Safeguard

(DoLS). Joint work between the PLN and the speech and language team identified her communication needs.

Personalized care plan

- Daily attendance on the ward was aimed at building a relationship – both with Sasha, but also with the ward, so that the ward clinical team felt they were supported by the mental health team.
- An ABC assessment of behaviour, around her response to requests for her to have care and treatment, was to be carried out.
- Sasha was given a single room. As a way to reassure staff, she was asked to take a drug test to check she was not using illicit substances. She agreed that if the drug test was positive she would return to a shared bay.
- Her replacement medication for her opiate use was to be increased.
- Ward staff were to give a 5-minute 'warning' call before asking to carry out intervention such as intravenous medication. Staff were given a suggested script of phrases that Sasha had said were less likely to make her decline care and treatment.
- A registered mental health nurse would help her engage in her care and treatment on a one-on-one basis. The intensive care helped orientate her and stopped her from wandering out of hospital, as following the stroke she was confused.

Outcome

- Sasha started taking her intravenous antibiotics – not all doses, but more than she had been accepting before.
- She agreed to an ECG and other scans.
- Daily drug testing increased staff's trust in Sasha, and reduced their anxiety about her behaviour, as she tested negative on most days.
- There was an increase in her engagement with acute colleagues in care and treatment.

SERVICE USER'S PERSPECTIVE

From a patient's perspective, I do not separate myself out into distinct parts. I am complex, with my mind, body and spirit interacting and having influence and effect on each other. I present with a set of symptoms, but against a backdrop of a life; a history and a context which may include pre-existing conditions. I live with a mental health condition that can affect every part of me. When a professional insists on taking blood or inserting a cannula into my right arm, I will resist and be deemed uncompliant. The reality is that I am hiding the pain and the shame of years of self-harm and the ugly scars that disfigure me.

Attending the emergency department for self-harm is a fearful experience; being in a busy waiting room, feeling vulnerable, being spoken to with disdain. I was there with all the thoughts and anguish of the precipitating event, at the same time my body going into shock. Experiences ranged from being 'treated' in silence and sent home with no follow-up, to seeing a LMHN who treated me as a person, with a name – whose sole focus was not on the deliberate self-harm, but on the reasons, my thoughts and emotions and what I wanted to happen next.

The 'kind' LMHN listened to me, gave me time and asked me what I wanted to happen next. It wasn't realistic to expect a nurse in a busy emergency department to do that, but I needed someone who would be 'with me' and enable me to identify what would help and formulate a plan, a way forward.

At first all I wanted was to be asked if I was cold; if I'd had a hot drink or eaten that day. I wanted the same treatment afforded to someone who had had a heart attack or an asthma attack, but I always felt I didn't deserve it.

The 'not so good' experiences indicated the need for education, the type that addresses not only the cognitive but also the affective domain of learning.

Frequent presentations for self-harm at the emergency department can lead to staff feeling anger and frustration towards the patient, but maybe also towards themselves for not 'making the patient better' – merely patching them up, sending them away, until the next time. To be deemed an attention seeker and time waster never contributed to easing my distress or providing hope and reassurance. There were too many assumptions and little understanding. The assessment was merely a form-filling exercise. Did they know why it had happened on this particular day? Was it an attempt on my life or a way of seeking some relief from emotional turmoil that seemed too great to bear? Was it the same as last time or had it become more severe, more concerning? Were the questions that were important to me the ones that they were actually asking?

Sometimes I couldn't speak for myself – my kind friend, who was more like a parent than mine ever were; she knew me. I wanted her to speak for me at times. I wanted the nurse to listen to her – to hear my voice through someone who knew.

However, not my next of kin – I wanted them to respect my request not to contact her. It wouldn't help; just cause further distress. They didn't know the history, the abuse, but I couldn't articulate that; by saying no, I was being 'difficult'.

CONCLUSION

Liaison mental health care has developed significantly in the UK in the last decade, bolstered by increasing concern that mental health needs should be treated on an equal footing with physical health care needs.[73–75] It is anticipated that this focus will reduce the significant difference in life expectancy and morbidity for those people who have mental health needs in comparison to the general population. Liaison mental health nursing is an integral part of evidence-based liaison psychiatric care within acute hospitals, and also in the community. Liaison mental health nurses require a wide set of competencies in order to support individual patients and their carers with their mental health needs, and also to support their non-mental-health colleagues in delivering effective, holistic care.

References

1. Goddard H. *The work of nurses in hospital wards.* London: Nuffield Provincial Hospitals Trust, 1954.
2. Merritt MK, Procter N. Conceptualising the functional role of mental health consultation–liaison nurse in multi-morbidity, using Peplau's nursing theory. *Contemporary Nurse* 2010; **34**(2): 158–66.
3. Department of Health. *The government's mandate to NHS England 2016–17.* London: DH, 2016.
4. Department of Health. *The mandate. A mandate from the government to NHS England: April 2015 to March 2016.* London: DH, 2015.
5. Department of Health. *The mandate. A mandate from the government to NHS England: April 2014 to March 2015.* London: DH, 2014.
6. Health and Social Care Act 2012. Available from: http://www.legislation.gov.uk/ukpga/2012/7/contents/enacted/data.htm [Accessed 24th August 2016].
7. Colton C, Manderscheid RW. Congruencies in increased mortality rates, years of potential life lost, and causes of death among public mental health clients in eight states. *Preventing Chronic Disease* 2006; **3**(2): A42.

8. Royal College of Psychiatrists. *CR183 Liaison psychiatry for every acute hospital. Integrated mental and physical health care.* London: Royal College of Psychiatrists, 2013.

9. Parsonage M, Fossey M, Tutty C. *Liaison psychiatry in the modern NHS.* London: Centre for Mental Health, Mental Health Network NHS Confederation, 2012.

10. Robinson L. Psychiatric consultation liaison nursing and psychiatric nursing doctoring: similarities and differences. *Archives of Psychiatric Nursing* 1987; **1**(2): 73–80.

11. Egan-Morriss E, Morriss R, House A. The role of the nurse in consultation liaison psychiatry. In: Benjamin S, House A, Jenkins P (eds). *Liaison psychiatry: defining needs and planning services.* London UK: Gaskell, 1994: 34–44.

12. Singh I, Ramakrishna S, Williamson K. The Rapid Assessment Interface and Discharge service and its implications for patients with dementia. *Clinical Interventions in Aging* 2013; **8**: 1101–8.

13. Holmes J, Bentley K, Camerson I. *Between two stools: psychiatric services for older people in general hospitals. Report of a UK survey.* Leeds: University of Leeds, 2002.

14. Alzheimer's Society. *Counting the cost. Caring for people with dementia on hospital wards.* London: Alzheimer's Society, 2009. Available from: https://www.alzheimers.org.uk/site/scripts/download_info.php?fileID=787 [Accessed 9th June 2016].

15. Yohannes AM, Alexopoulos GS. Depression and anxiety in patients with COPD. *European Respiratory Review* 2014; **23**(133): 345–9.

16. Holt R, de Groot M, Golden SH. Diabetes and depression. *Current Diabetes Reports* 2014; **14**(6): 491.

17. Rashid N. Post-stroke depression and expressed emotion. *Brain Injury* 2013; **27**(2): 223–38.

18. Nair N. Commonality between depression and heart failure. *American Journal of Cardiology* 2012; **109**(5): 768.

19. Lipsitt DR. Consultation–liaison psychiatry and psychosomatic medicine: the company they keep. *Psychosomatic Medicine* 2001; **63**(6): 896–909.

20. Smith G. From consultation–liaison psychiatry to integrated care for multiple and complex needs. *Australian and New Zealand Journal of Psychiatry* 2009; **43**(1): 1–12.

21. Lipowski Z. Review of consultation psychiatry and psychosomatic medicine. *Psychosomatic Medicine* 1967; **29**: 1–3.

22. Morriss R, Mayou R. International overview of consultation–liaison psychiatry. In: Guthrie E, Creed F (eds). *Seminars in liaison psychiatry.* London: Gaskell, 1996: 1–20.

23. Tunmore R. Encouraging collaboration. *Nursing Times* 1994; **90**(20): 66–7.

24. Tunmore R. Liaison psychiatric nursing in oncology. *Nursing Times* 1989; **85**(33): 54–6.

25. Royal College of Psychiatrists. *Inpatient care for older people within mental health services.* London: Royal College of Psychiatrists Centre for Quality Improvement, 2008.

26. AOMRC (Academy of Medical Royal Colleges). *Managing urgent mental health needs in the acute trust.* London: AOMRC, 2008.

27. AOMRC (Academy of Medical Royal Colleges). *No health without mental health. ALERT report.* London: AOMRC, 2009.

28. HM Government. *New horizons: a shared vision for mental health.* London: HM Government, 2009.

29. HM Government. *No health without mental health: a cross-government mental health strategy for people of all ages.* London: HM Government, 2011.

30. Parsonage M, Fossey M. *Economic evaluation of a liaison psychiatry service.* London: Centre for Mental Health, 2011.

31. Aitken P, Robens S, Emmens T. *Developing models for liaison psychiatry services – guidance.* Strategic Clinical Network for Mental Health, Dementia and Neurological Conditions South West, 2014.

32. Eales S, Chartres K. The needs of senior nurses and their teams in liaison psychiatry. *Psychiatric Liaison Accreditation Committee (PLAN) Annual Forum 2016: improving mental healthcare in general hospitals.* Available from: http://www.rcpsych.ac.uk/workinpsychiatry/qualityimprovement/ccqiprojects/liaisonpsychiatry/plan/newsandevents.aspx [Accessed 9th June 2016].

33. Royal College of Psychiatrists. *Quality standards for liaison services*, 4th edn. London: Royal College of Psychiatrists, 2014. [Accessed 9th June 2016].

34. Palmer L, Gill P, Dupin M. The psychiatric liaison accreditation network – an innovative project to improve quality in UK liaison psychiatry services. *Journal of Psychosomatic Research* 2010; **69**(6): 619–21.

35. NMC (Nursing and Midwifery Council). *Standards for pre-registration nursing education.* London: NMC, 2010. Available from: https://www.nmc.org.uk/standards/additional-standards/standards-for-pre-registration-nursing-education [Accessed 9th June 2016].

36. Department of Health. *Compassion in practice. Nursing, midwifery and care staff: our vision and strategy.* London: DH, 2012.

37. Eales S, Wilson N, Waghorn, J. *Competence framework for liaison mental health nursing.* London: Liaison Mental Health Nursing Special Interest Group, 2014. Unpublished. Available from: http://www.rcpsych.ac.uk/workinpsychiatry/qualityimprovement/ccqiprojects/liaisonpsychiatry/plan/membersarea/resources.aspx [Accessed 9th June 2016].

38. Tadros G, Salama RA, Kingston P, Mustafa N, Johnson E, Pannell R, Hashmi M. Impact of an integrated rapid response psychiatric liaison team on quality improvement and cost savings: the Birmingham RAID model. *Psychiatrist* 2013; **37**(1): 4–10.

39. Regel S, Roberts D (eds). *Mental health liaison. A handbook for nurses and health professionals.* Edinburgh: Balliere Tindall, 2002.

40. Royal College of Psychiatrists. *CR197: Perinatal mental health services: recommendations for the provision of services for childbearing women.* London: Royal College of Psychiatrists, 2015. Available from: http://www.rcpsych.ac.uk/usefulresources/publications/collegereports/cr/cr197.aspx [Accessed 9th June 2016].

41. Chelvanayagam S, Newell C. Differentiating between eating disorders and gastrointestinal problems. *Gastrointestinal Nursing* 2015; **13**(7): 56–62.

42. Palmer L, Blackwell H, Strevens P. *Service users' experiences of emergency services following self-harm. Better services for people who self-harm. National Quality Improvement Programme.* London: Royal College of Psychiatrists Centre for Quality Improvement, 2007.

43. GAIN (Guidelines and Audit Implementation Network). *Caring for people with a learning disability in general hospital settings.* Belfast: GAIN, 2010.

44. Central and North West London NHS Foundation Trust. Liaison psychiatry service. 2014. Available from: https://vimeo.com/98629035 [Accessed 9th June 2016].

45. Eales S. Service users' experience of liaison mental health care. PhD thesis, City University, London, 2013.

46. Kaplan D. Observations on crisis theory and practice. *Social Casework* 1968; **49**(3): 151–5.

47. Johnson S, Needle J, Bindman P, Thornicroft G (eds). *Crisis resolution and home treatment in mental health.* Cambridge: Cambridge University Press, 2008.

48. Slade M. *Personal recovery and mental illness: a guide for mental health practitioners.* Cambridge: Cambridge University Press, 2009.

49. Roberts G, Boardman J. Becoming a recovery orientated practitioner. *Advances in Psychiatric Treatment* 2014; **20**: 37–47.

50. Corbett E. *An organisation-wide document for clinical risk assessment and management.* London: NHS Litigation Authority, 2012.

51. Rahman MS, Gupta S, While D, Rodway C, Ibrahim S, Bickley H, Flynn S, Windfuhr K, Shaw J, Kapur N, Appleby L. Quality risk

assessment prior to suicide and homicide: a pilot study. 2013. Available from: http://research.bmh.manchester.ac.uk/cmhs/research/centreforsuicideprevention/nci/reports/ [Accessed 10th August 2016].

52. Department of Health. *Best practice in managing risk.* London: HMSO, 2007. Available from: http://webarchive.national-archives.gov.uk/+/www.dh.gov.uk/prod_consum_dh/groups/dh_digitalassets/@dh/@en/documents/digitalasset/dh_076512.pdf [Accessed 9th June 2016].

53. Boardman J, Roberts G. *Briefing: risk, safety & recovery.* London: Centre for Mental Health & Mental Health Network, 2014.

54. Mesudi A, Magid K, Hussain D. How do people become W.E.I.R.D? Migration reveals the cultural transmission mechanisms underlying variation in psychological processes. *PLoSOne* 2016; **11**(1).

55. Kabir Z, Herltiz A. The Bangla Adaptation of Mini Mental State Examination (BAMSE): an instrument to assess cognitive functioning in illiterate and literate individuals. *International Journal of Geriatric Psychiatry* 2000; **15**: 441–50.

56. Trigwell T, Kustow J, Santhouse A, Gopinath R, Aitken P, Reid S, Wilson N, Martin K. *Framework for Routine Outcome Measurements in Liaison Psychiatry (FROM-LP).* London: Royal College of Psychiatrists, 2015.

57. Wooff D, Schneider J, Carpenter J, Brandon T. Correlates of stress in carers. *Journal of Mental Health* 2003; **12**(1): 29–40.

58. Wynaden D, Orb A. Impact of patient confidentiality on carers of people who have mental disorder. *International Journal of Mental Health Nursing* 2005; **14**(30): 166–71.

59. Rapaport J, Bellringer S, Pinfold V, Huxley P. Carers and confidentiality in mental health care: considering the role of the carer's assessment: a study of service users, carers' and practitioners' views. *Health and Social Care in the Community* 2006; **14**(4): 357–65.

60. Gray B, Robinson C, Seddon D, Roberts A. 'Confidentiality smokescreen' and carers for people with mental health problems: the perspective of professionals. *Health and Social Care in the Community* 2008; **16**(14): 378–87.

61. Albert R, Simpson A. Double deprivation: a phenomenological study into the experience of being a carer during a mental health crisis. *Journal of Advanced Nursing* 2015; **71**(12): 2753–62.

62. NICE (National Institute for Health and Care Excellence). *Selfharm in over 8s: short term management and prevention of reoccurrence.* London: NICE, 2004.

63. NICE (National Institute for Health and Care Excellence). *Selfharm in over 8s: short term management and prevention of reoccurrence.* London: NICE, 2011.

64. 'Better Services for People who Selfharm' Project Group (eds). *Better services for people who selfharm – quality standards for health care professionals.* London: Royal College of Psychiatry, 2006.

65. Department for Constitutional Affairs. *Mental Capacity Act 2005: Code of Practice.* London: TSO, 2007.

66. Better Services for People who Selfharm Project Group (eds). *Better services for people who selfharm – quality standards for health care professionals,* 1st edn. London: Royal College of Psychiatry, 2006.

67. Rethink. Coping in a crisis. 2016. Available from: https://www.rethink.org/diagnosis-treatment/symptoms/self-harm [Accessed 10th August 2016].

68. NCISH (National Confidential Inquiry into Suicide and Homicide). *National Confidential Inquiry into Suicide and Homicide by People with Mental Illness, annual report.* Manchester: University of Manchester, 2015.

69. Arkins B, Tyrrell M, Herlily E, Crowley B, Lynch R. Assessing the reasons for deliberate self harm in young people. *Mental Health Practice* 2013; **16**(7): 28–32.

70. Gratz K, Dixon-Gordon K, Chapman A, Tull M. Exploring the association of deliberate self harm with emotional relief using a novel implicit association test. *Personality Disorder: Theory, Research and Treatment* 2016; **7**(1): 91–102.

71. Menzies IEP. *Social systems as a defence against anxiety.* London: Tavistock Institute of Human Relations, 1970.

72. Chesney E, Goodwin G, Fazel S. Risks of all causes and suicide mortality in mental disorder: a meta-review. *World Psychiatry* 2014; **3**: 153–60.

73. The Mental Health Taskforce. The Five Year Foward View for Mental Health. NHS England 2016. Available from https://www.england.nhs.uk/ourwork/futurenhs/nhs-five-year-forward-view-web-version/ [Accessed 5th December 2016].

74. NHS England. Implementing The Five Year Forward View for Mental Health. NHS England 2016. Available from: https://www.england.nhs.uk/mentalhealth/taskforce/imp/ [Accessed 5th December 2016].

75. NHS England, NCCMH and NICE. Achieving Better Access to 24/7 Urgent and Emergency Care - Part 2: Implementing for the evidence-based treatment pathway for urgent and emergency liaison mental health service for adults and older adults - Guidance. NHS England 2016.

Relevant web pages

https://www.england.nhs.uk/ourwork/futurenhs/nhs-five-year-forward-view-web-version/ [Accessed 5th December 2016].

The Mental Health Task Force. The Five Year Forward View for Mental Helath. NHS England 2016.

https:www.england.nhs.uk/mentalhealth/taskforce/imp/ [Accessed 5th December 2016].

NHS England. Implementing the Five Year Forward View for Mental Health. NHS England 2016.

53 The acute care setting

ANGELA SIMPSON, ROB ALLISON AND
RUTH LAMBLEY

LEARNING OUTCOMES

- To understand the purpose of acute psychiatric admission wards and the role of nurses within them.
- To recognize that interpersonal relationships underpin the role of mental health nurses working in acute psychiatric admission settings.
- To appreciate the power dynamic and tensions implicit in the provision of nursing care against a backdrop of informal or compulsory containment and treatment.
- To understand the therapeutic value of alternative forms of acute psychiatric care located outside hospital settings.

SUMMARY OF KEY POINTS

- People admitted to acute mental health services identify supportive relationships as essential for recovery.
- Interpersonal and therapeutic relationships are central to enable mental health nursing to develop a therapeutic milieu.
- Mental health nurses ought to consider models of care, such as the Tidal Model, to address the inherent power imbalance within services and emphasize empowering relationships.
- Alternative models of care exist, but there is little evidence of philosophical differences from approaches to care provided by traditional services.

INTRODUCTION

This chapter discusses the role of the nurse working in acute inpatient psychiatric settings. It begins by exploring the purpose of acute psychiatric admission wards and the tensions implicit in the provision of nursing care against a backdrop of psychiatric treatment and/or containment. The interpersonal focus of nursing work is highlighted as *the* essential therapeutic approach required when supporting people in acute distress.

The craft of caring is identified as involving the maintenance of a structured therapeutic environment while at the same time developing concerned, helpful, yet professional relationships. The experiences of people who use acute inpatient mental health services are explored. Close attention is paid to aspects of care provision reported as being either helpful or unhelpful while in recovery from acute crisis. Finally, the chapter considers the difficulties associated with providing acute psychiatric care in hospital settings and explores alternatives to hospital-based acute inpatient psychiatric care.

It is important to remember that, although this chapter focuses on the role of nurses in acute inpatient psychiatric units, nurses are members of a much broader multi-professional team, which commonly includes psychiatrists, social workers, occupational therapists and members of community mental health teams or agencies. Acute inpatient care is multi-professionally focused and it is essential to adopt a team approach to providing timely medical, nursing and social support.

THE PURPOSE OF ACUTE PSYCHIATRIC ADMISSION WARDS

Acute inpatient admission wards provide short-term admission to hospital for the purposes of psychiatric assessment, treatment and care. Acute inpatient care is distinguished from other forms of psychiatric support in that the person in crisis urgently requires admission to hospital where intensive 24-hour support can be provided. This also allows the person's changing condition to be closely observed. On admission to hospital, the person is usually highly distressed and requires a more intensive form of support than is usually available in community settings.

The aim of admitting someone to hospital in acute crisis is to assess the person's condition while also providing the human support and care environment necessary to establish emotional stability. In hospital, the person should be encouraged to become part of a collaborative helping process. Individual care needs are identified and constructive helping relationships developed. On discharge, responsibility for the individual's ongoing care is usually transferred to a mental health worker based in the community.

Over the last three decades mental health services have undergone radical restructuring as care provided for people with mental health needs shifted from institutions into community settings.[1] Community care is now a well-established feature of most Western mental health care, and the community teams responsible for providing treatment interventions to people experiencing psychic distress have become increasingly specialist in their approach. In line with the modernization of mental health services, clinicians aim to practise collaboratively. This means wherever possible providing care that is sensitive to the individual's

experience and in particular identifying what the person in distress finds most helpful for them when emotionally distressed. This individualized approach also emphasizes the need for nurses to work closely with the wider family and/or other supporters and, where possible, to involve them in a collaborative decision-making process.

As a consequence of the introduction of community care, the number of hospital beds available for acute inpatient psychiatric care has reduced.[2] Except in the most severe cases, admission to hospital for acute psychiatric care now only takes place once community-based interventions such as crisis intervention (chapter 46), early intervention or assertive outreach (chapter 56) (or local adaptations of these approaches) have first been attempted. Although mental health services have prioritized the provision of alternative forms of community-based care, research continues to indicate that demand for acute inpatient psychiatric care remains strong. In Australia, the UK and the USA, bed occupancy rates have remained high.[3-5] Given this context, it is perhaps unsurprising that the dependency of patients admitted to hospital has increased, with people in acute distress often admitted with multiple and complex care needs.[6,7] These combined factors make acute psychiatric admission care extraordinarily challenging to deliver. In particular, the uncertain and quickly changing ward environment means that it can be difficult to establish therapeutic rapport with patients,[8] while the fast-paced environment can also work against the establishment of structured one-to-one care as well as a supportive milieu/ schedule of organized therapeutic activities.[9,10]

THE ACUTE PSYCHIATRIC CARE ENVIRONMENT

Despite the shift into the community, acute inpatient psychiatric care remains for the most part hospital-based. At the point of acute admission, people present as profoundly emotionally destabilized. Most commonly the person is in a condition in which they themselves and/or other people may consider them to be at risk. Admission to hospital is usually organized as an emergency response to a crisis, which may include suicidal ideas, self-harm or profound self-neglect.

In some cases, distress can also present itself in a range of actions/interactions that can lead the individual, health professionals and family members to become seriously concerned for a person's welfare. In highly charged emotional situations such as this, the person in crisis may or may not feel as though they would benefit from the provision of space away from their natural environment in a hospital setting. Where a person is deemed to be a serious risk to themselves or other people and at the same time unwilling to countenance mental health support, care can be imposed against a person's will. Thus the acute psychiatric care environment is complex and in some ways unlike any other clinical area. Pilgrim[11] has defined acute mental health services as being 'accessed by or imposed upon people who are deemed to be in immediate need of containment to assess their needs, or to intervene when they are acting in a very distressed, disturbing or perplexing way' (p.85).

REFLECTION

Nurses working in acute psychiatric admission units are part of a multi-professional team that is able to detain and enforce psychiatric treatment against a person's will. How do you think this dynamic impacts on the care environment and the ability of the nurse to form helping relationships?

Some people are resistant to the idea of acute admission to hospital and at the same time can also appear to be seemingly unaware of the risks that their immediate condition and/or situation may present to themselves or other people. In these circumstances, people who do not consent to admission to hospital can be compulsorily admitted to or held in hospital for the purposes of psychiatric assessment and/or treatment.[12,13] Also, people who initially consent to admission to hospital can be detained while in hospital if they are deemed to be at risk to themselves or other people and/or if they refuse treatment or withdraw their consent to treatment. It is important to recognize that the multi-professional team responsible for providing respite from the person's natural environment and/or a place of safety also has the authority to detain and treat people against their will. This ever-present power dynamic profoundly influences how nurses and other health care professionals react to people in distress, as well as how service users perceive them and the services that they provide. It also frames the backdrop against which nurses must strive to forge supportive helping relationships. More information about freedom and consent in mental health practice is provided in chapter 18.

REFLECTION

Can care environments in which people can be detained and forced to accept treatments against their will ever be considered to be genuinely caring?

THERAPEUTIC RELATIONSHIPS AND THE PERSON IN ACUTE DISTRESS

It has long been acknowledged in psychiatric nursing literature that the development of therapeutic interpersonal (nurse–patient) relationships should underpin the work of mental health nurses, and this is also the case in acute inpatient settings. This relationship, first espoused by Peplau,[14] describes how nurses should aim to work closely with people on an individualized basis to nurture helping and concerned relationships, which are both caring and professional. Peplau[14] first described the importance of ensuring that all patients feel that they have the attention of nurses in ward environments and that nurses respond empathically. Assuming that a therapeutic relationship develops well, it should become the primary nursing intervention offered and be strong enough to sustain the person encountering emotional difficulties. However, if the relationship fails to develop, the likelihood is that the service user may feel cut adrift from the helping 'agency', isolated and alone.

The multiple and sometimes startling presentations of acute distress can lead nurses to stand back and observe the person as opposed to relating to them and getting to know them individually. It is well established[15] that behaviour that is 'acted out' is unlikely to be understood by either the nurse or the person in emotional crisis. Peplau[15] reminds nurses that they need to take every available opportunity to relate to the person in distress and also that they should be curious, particularly about how the experience of emotional crisis impacts on the person's ability to live everyday life. This illustrates the need for mental health nurses to use every available opportunity to come to better know and understand the person. It also underscores the view that the primary role of psychiatric/mental health nurses is interpersonal.[14,16]

Nurses are the mainstay providers of care in acute inpatient settings. They are in very close proximity to patients throughout the 24-hour period and this allows them the opportunity to get to know people in distress on an individual basis. An attentive and understanding nurse is able to relate to the person in distress, firstly by being a concerned and supportive presence during the most acute phase, and secondly, as things begins to settle, by creating a relationship with the person in which they begin to feel supported enough to share their experiences.

Developing and maintaining therapeutic relationships is challenging and purposeful work, and no more so than in cases where the person is felt to require hospitalization. The experience of acute psychiatric distress commonly affects a person's ability to function. For example, the person may experience episodes of feeling profoundly overstimulated, with boundless energy and no desire to rest, eat or sleep, or, on the other hand, might completely withdraw, lacking the motivation to communicate even the most basic messages or perform the simplest of day-to-day tasks. At both ends of this spectrum and in between, the experience of acute distress seriously impacts on the person's ability to live everyday life and can sometimes impair judgement and decision making. Chapter 3 discusses the importance of the development of therapeutic relationships in more detail.

THERAPEUTIC MILIEU

The atmosphere and social surroundings within any care environment are known as the milieu. Careful development of the milieu provides the social conditions in which it becomes possible for people in the ward surroundings to support and help each other.[17] Where a supportive milieu is created, the person in distress is able to share experiences with others in similar situations and, in so doing, help both themselves and others. Adopting an interpersonal approach to nursing work and developing the milieu requires nurses to structure care and ward activities in a purposeful way. For example, while in its initial stages of the admission, the interpersonal relationship may be developed by a nurse being a concerned and interested presence, and as the episode of crisis begins to settle, structured activities such as ring-fenced time for one-to-one discussion and structured group activities will help to promote a milieu that is both helpful and purposeful.

Developing an interpersonal focus to caring and promoting a structured and purposeful milieu is challenging in the context of contemporary acute psychiatric care. Since the introduction of community care, acute inpatient care has been characterized by a corresponding increase in perceived dependency at the point of admission to hospital.[6] This means that, on admission, people typically present with multiple and more complex needs and that typically the person's actions may be correspondingly chaotic or unfathomable. Alongside this, hospital stays have become shorter in duration and the documentation and risk assessment demands made on staff have considerably increased.[10] Unless carefully managed, these combined 'real world' factors can work against the formation of strong nurse–patient relationships and/or the creation of therapeutic ward environments. These can also be the circumstances in which the bio-medical approach to treating people for mental illness prevails. The bio-medical model assumes that biological factors underpin psychiatric conditions, tending to minimize or exclude psychological, environmental and social factors. It is the dominant treatment model that health professionals use to diagnose and treat. In the context of acute psychiatry, if the bio-medical approach dominates, then the primary focus of care becomes drug treatments rather than interpersonal.

SERVICE USER'S PERSPECTIVE

The big things that stood out to me when I was admitted to an acute psychiatric ward were nurses being too busy to really be able to talk when I felt I needed it, and a perception that they spent more time on paperwork than actually caring and building relationships. Also there was a lack of access to psychological therapy, either as an adjunct to prescribed medications or instead of it. For me it took three long inpatient admissions over 3 years before I was offered anything meaningful in psychological terms. When I first got ill, I would have preferred psychological/talking therapies to antipsychotic medication, and I suspect I'm not the only one to feel that!

I am a bit cynical now about 'patient choice' because it seems to me it is mentioned in circumstances where there are no real choices, i.e. choosing between two very similar medications, when what you really want is less, or no, medication. In my experience, the student nurses were often more therapeutic in their approach than the qualified nurses. I don't know if that's because they had more time to spend building relationships, or because they had been schooled in different ways of working with people.

Recognizing these tensions in the therapeutic environment, Barker[16] developed the Tidal Model, an approach to *being with* people in distress that respects the lived experience of the person and which also acknowledges that the experience of psychiatric distress is meaningful to the individual. It therefore differs considerably from other approaches, which assume that psycho- or organic pathology underpins mental health problems. The Tidal Model was developed through research, which took the form of detailed conversations with key stakeholders, including service users and health professionals. The topic of the discussions was 'What are psychiatric nurses needed for?' The Tidal Model is now internationally recognized as an empowering, recovery-focused approach to working with people in distress. It stresses the interpersonal nature of the nurse's role and is concerned with developing a therapeutic environment supportive of people learning through the experience of distress. The main areas of focus are:

- to collaborate with individuals and families to plan and deliver care;
- to empower the person in distress by putting their narrative at the centre of care planning and the wider therapeutic care environment;
- to identify strengths within the person that can be used to resolve problems;
- to promote mental health and well-being.

Barker[18] described the craft of caring as 'doing something quite ordinary, in highly extraordinary settings and circumstances' (p.2). He observed that psychiatric/mental health nurses are often required to make relationships and extend care to people who may have been abandoned by everyone else and be difficult to care for or about. He notes that, against the backdrop of these contextual challenges, ordinary acts of human kindness can be transformed into the extraordinary discipline of human caring.

> ### REFLECTION
>
> If nurses stand back from people in acute distress and observe them, as opposed to relate *with* them, what impact might this have on the developing nurse–patient relationship?

SERVICE USERS' PERSPECTIVES ON ACUTE INPATIENT PSYCHIATRIC CARE

Service users have long expressed their dissatisfaction with acute inpatient psychiatric care. Reports on acute-patient provision,[1,8] service-user-led/focused research[19] and service user commentary[20] all point to deeply etched problems with the predominant hospital-based approach to providing inpatient care for people in acute crisis. In particular, there are repeated reported concerns about the inaccessibility of nurses and other staff to form therapeutic relationships, the lack of therapeutic structure, a lack of involvement in treatment decisions and poor quality information, as well as poor ward and hospital-based facilities.[21]

Of these, the inability of staff to spend time with service users to forge therapeutic relationships based on trust and empathy stands out as the primary service user concern.[6,21] While nurses are acknowledged as being the occupational group that do spend the most time with the person in acute crisis,[22] there is a clear indication that more time spent in structured one-to-one involvement or other therapeutically focused activity would be viewed as beneficial from the service user perspective.[21] In particular, service users emphasize the need for relationships that develop over time, which include the development of trust, reassurance and individual understanding.[19] It is important to understand that, without this, the relationships between nurses, other mental health professionals and services users appear to collapse into an atmosphere of distrust and coercion[23] in which the common service user experience is one of having little, if any, control over personal circumstances, as well as an abiding sense of powerlessness. In these situations the primary role of staff as experienced by service users was described as being 'prescribing medications and rule adherence only.[21]

> ### REFLECTION
>
> How should nurses work to structure the care environment in order to strengthen the milieu?

> ### SERVICE USER'S PERSPECTIVE
>
> Reflecting on my admission to hospital, and after I had been able to discuss my problems in some detail with a psychologist, I felt that nurses were working in a very medical model way. I don't know why the nurses on the ward don't follow a Hearing Voices type approach, where they could talk in detail to me about my experience of hearing voices. In fact I wondered if the Hearing Voices approach might actually have scared them – assuming it would somehow make me more distressed? I also wondered how I would feel talking to nurses about some of the things I did talk through with my psychologist, such as suicidal thoughts and self-harm. I suspect the psychologist might tolerate 'risk' in different ways and also I realize now that I might be afraid of saying something like that to a nurse because it might delay my discharge.

> ### REFLECTION
>
> What steps should nurses take to minimize service users' sense of powerlessness and lack of involvement in decision making?

It is important to understand that these are not new observations; they have been a constant feature of literature relating to inpatient mental health care and more so over the last two decades and beyond. Despite this knowledge, little, if any, progress has been made in terms of improving the situation. The Sainsbury Centre for Mental Health[24] described acute inpatient environments as non-therapeutic, while MIND[13] reported that they have the capacity to make service users feel worse rather than better. Over the years there has been little reported progress in therapeutic terms. This is set against increased awareness of the scale of the problems that people using acute mental health services encounter. In an era in which modernizing health services to meet the needs of consumers has characterized the provision of health services more generally, acute psychiatric care continues to stand out as unprogressive and out of touch with the needs of the people using the service.

ALTERNATIVES TO ACUTE INPATIENT PSYCHIATRIC ADMISSION

As previously outlined, there is long-standing documented evidence that service users are unhappy with and critical of the treatment and care routinely delivered in acute inpatient psychiatric units and that many professional staff share these concerns.[23,25] Pilgrim[26] reminds us that service users commonly report that they do not receive individualized care and describe inpatient care as overcrowded holding areas only. Service user perspectives, and an increasing disenfranchisement from the dominant bio-medical approach to treatment by health professionals, support the need to develop alternative forms of community-based support for people – even in the most acute phases of distress. However, such approaches can only be considered genuine alternatives where they address the fundamental concerns of people using the service. This means acknowledging that service users want and need approaches that are focused on providing helping relationships that are tolerant of distress, as opposed to seeking either to medically treat it or to contain it. They would also value the prospect of learning from the episode of distress through being allowed to experience it, as opposed to being medically sedated and/or treated.

Alternative forms of acute inpatient care provision outside hospitals are important because, unlike hospitals, it becomes possible to 'normalize' both the environment and care setting, making it immediately less clinical, coercive and paternalistic. This approach appears to fit well with the introduction of recovery models (see chapters 35 and 36) which emphasize the need for care approaches rooted in interpersonal support, empowerment, choice and hope.[27] Where care for acute distress is located outside hospital, it engenders the prospect of a different type of atmosphere in which there is less emphasis on medication and containment and greater promotion of individual responsibility, peer support and the maintenance of routine everyday living. Where these services are located in the community, this also has the added benefit of enabling the person in distress to retain contact with friends, relatives and other supporters.[28]

> ### REFLECTION
>
> What elements of the acute inpatient care environment contribute to it being viewed as non-therapeutic?

As previously stated, the development of interpersonal relationships is the correct focus for mental health nurses working in acute mental health settings.[14,16] However, it is important to understand that this focus can and does become lost within the wider culture of hospital-based psychiatry. Although emphasis should be given to investing in relationships with patients, this can be challenging for practitioners to achieve. Menzies Lyth[29] first identified the struggle experienced by nursing staff in trying to manage their own anxieties in relation to caring for patients, observing that nursing staff often coped by emotionally distancing themselves from patients, focusing instead on physical tasks.

Recognizing that the wider culture of hospital-based psychiatry has the potential to dominate and dilute, if not negate, the potential for therapeutic relationships, a number of interesting projects have been developed which investigated alternative forms of care for people experiencing acute distress outside hospital settings. Of these, perhaps the most notable is Soteria House, developed by Mosher in the USA.[30] The aim was to determine whether people experiencing acute psychosis could be 'treated' successfully outside hospital with limited or no psychiatric medication.

Mosher[31] hypothesized that, in contrast to hospital interventions (predominantly medication) or a rehabilitation model (the development of basic living skills), therapeutic change would manifest within normal interactive processes, occurring when people within a supportive and tolerant environment came into contact with each other. Thus, close interpersonal relationships between the staff and residents (patients were called residents) were developed as a specific means of understanding 'unusual' thinking, ideas or behaviours. Residents often expressed unusual ideas but staff did not intervene (other than to prevent harm). To foster this approach, lay people were employed in the belief that, without preconceived professional theories and models, they had the potential to share the personal meanings underpinning the distress.

The process of 'being with' was fundamental to the development of the Soteria philosophy, as was the creation of an environment that did not abuse power or foster dependency. This could be achieved because of the underpinning therapeutic approach outside the hospital environment. The approach developed by Mosher suggested that it may be possible for some people to experience and recover from acute mental health problems without recourse to hospitalization or medication-focused treatment regimes.

Unsurprisingly, the Soteria project courted criticism from the traditional psychiatric community. Mosher's[31] account of this asserts that the therapeutic approach and results of Soteria challenged the prevailing approach to psychiatric treatment in traditional services, and, in particular, the suggestion that minimal if any medication was needed for the treatment and recovery of acute psychosis-related issues.

Research into alternatives to standard inpatient acute hospital wards continues. This includes a systematic review of the Soteria paradigm, evaluating the empirical evidence of the North American version of Soteria and a later Swiss version.[32] This was followed by a systematic review of residential alternatives to hospital-based acute inpatient care in the UK.[33] Johnson et al.[34] identified 131 so-called alternative services in England. However, in 109 of these, little identifiable difference was found in terms of the therapeutic approach between the alternative and standard services. This means that, although the services were located away from traditional hospital settings, the philosophy of care did not appear to be significantly different and that a relationship-centred approach was not necessarily adopted. Despite this, people using the services reported that they found alternative services to be less coercive and suggested that it was possible to build safer relationships within those environments. Alternative services were also cheaper to run and resulted in a shorter length of stay.[34]

In keeping with the interpersonal focus of mental health nursing underscored throughout this chapter, it has been suggested that in contemporary UK 'alternative' services, it seemed to be the therapeutic relationship that influenced patient perceptions regarding the quality of services provided.[35] However, these services are not necessarily being purposefully designed to achieve this objective, nor are they explicitly aimed at offering crisis support without recourse to containment and/or psychiatric medication (assuming that the person in crisis is able to respond responsibly in these circumstances). It would seem that publicly funded mental health facilities continue to be reluctant to offer *genuine* alternative approaches to acute inpatient mental health care, despite continued government rhetoric about developing person-centred mental health services and a concern with promoting choice and the least restrictive environment possible.[36] Government policy in the UK[36] continues to espouse that people with mental health problems should be fully involved in the design and delivery of services and have the greatest possible choice and control over treatment and care options. On the ground, however, while student nurses may witness changes in the physical care environment, they would be wise to question the extent to which new services are explicitly designed to allow interpersonal relationships to develop. Furthermore, they should explore whether the environment fosters a therapeutic milieu and question whether approaches to care that are respectful and tolerant of the lived experience of distress can be actively delivered.

CONCLUSION

This chapter has discussed the role of the nurse working in acute inpatient psychiatric settings. The interpersonal focus of nursing work has been highlighted as the essential professional focus, alongside the development of a therapeutic milieu. Service users have identified that there is a need for mental health services that are focused on building supportive relationships. The Tidal Model[16] is a model of care derived from conversations with service users and other key stakeholders. It is focused on recovery and empowerment and has become internationally recognized. Here, the philosophical underpinnings of the care emphasize empowering relationships in the least restrictive possible environment. It also promotes choice and supports the development of individual meaning(s) within the episode of crisis. While non-hospital-based residential alternatives to acute inpatient care are beginning to emerge, they are not necessarily structured to allow therapeutic relationships to happen or for a supportive milieu to be developed. As yet, these new services cannot be acknowledged as offering anything substantial or different, other than the environment in which they are located.

References

1. SCMH (Sainsbury Centre for Mental Health). *Beyond the Water Towers: the unfinished revolution in mental health service 1985–2005*. London: SCMH, 2005.
2. Lintern S. Mental health sector hit by bed shortage. *Health Services Journal* 2013; 10 October. Available from: www.hsj.co.uk/news/exclusive-mental-health-sector-hit-by-beds-shortage/5064061.article#.U4boXygQh5g [Accessed 1st June 2016].
3. Blader JC. Acute in-patient care for psychiatric disorders in United States, 1996 through 2007. *Archives of General Psychiatry* 2011; **68**(12): 1276–83.
4. AIHW (Australian Institute of Health and Welfare). *Australia hospital statistics 2011–12, health services series no. 50, cat. no. HSE 134*. Canberra: AIHW, 2013.
5. Thompson A, Shaw M, Harrison G, Davidson H, Gunnell D, Verne J. *British Journal of Psychiatry* 2004; **185**: 334–41.
6. Cleary M. The realities of mental health nursing in acute inpatient environments. *International Journal of Mental Health Nursing* 2004; **13**: 53–60.
7. Keown P, Tacchi M, Niemiec S, Hughes J. Changes to mental health care for working age adults. Impact on crisis teams and assertive outreach teams. *Psychiatric Bulletin* 2007; **31**: 288–92.
8. Healthcare Commission. *The pathway to recovery: a review of NHS acute inpatient care*. 2008. Available from: http://webarchive.nationalarchives.gov.uk/20110515082446/http://cqc.org.uk/_db/_documents/The_pathway_to_recovery_200807251020.pdf [Accessed 1st June 2016].
9. Bee PE, Richards DA, Loftus SJ, Baker JA, Bailey L, Lovell K, Woods P, Cox D. Mapping nursing activity in acute inpatient mental health settings. *Journal of Mental Health* 2006; **15**: 217–82.
10. Shattell M. The disappearance of one-to-ones in acute psychiatric care. *Issues in Mental Health Nursing* 2007; **28**: 229–30.
11. Pilgrim D. *Key concepts in mental health*. London: Sage, 2014.
12. Mental Health Act 1983 & 2007. Available from: http://www.legislation.gov.uk/ukpga/1983/20/contents and http://www.legislation.gov.uk/ukpga/2007/12/contents [Accessed 1st June 2016].

13. MIND. The MIND guide to the Mental Health Act 1983. 2012. Available from: http://www.mind.org.uk/media/7505/the-mind-guide-to-the-mental-health-act-1983-2012.pdf [Accessed 1st June 2016].

14. Peplau H. *Interpersonal relations in nursing*. New York: GP Putnam and Sons, 1952.

15. Peplau H. Interpersonal relations model: theoretical constructs, principles and general applications. In: Reynolds W, Cormack D (eds). *Psychiatric and mental health nursing: theory and practice*. London: Chapman Hall, 1990: 87–132.

16. Barker P. The Tidal Model: developing an empowering patient centred approach to recovery within psychiatric and mental health nursing. *Journal of Psychiatric and Mental Health Nursing* 2001; **8**(3): 233–40.

17. Altschul AT. *Patient nurse interaction*. Edinburgh: Churchill Livingston, 1972.

18. Barker P. *Psychiatric and mental health nursing: the craft of caring*, 2nd edn. London: Hodder Arnold, 2009.

19. Hopkins JE, LoeB SJ, Fick DM. Beyond satisfaction, what service users expect of inpatient mental health care: a literature review. *Journal of Psychiatric and Mental Health Nursing* 2009; **16**: 927–37.

20. MIND. Ward Watch: MIND's campaign to improve hospital conditions for mental health patients: report summary. 2004. Available from: http://socialwelfare.bl.uk/subject-areas/services-client-groups/adults-mental-health/mind/144546ward_watch_summary.pdf [Accessed 1st June 2016].

21. Walsh J, Boyle J. Improving acute psychiatric services according to in-patient experiences. A user-led piece of research as a means of empowerment. *Issues in Mental Health Nursing* 2009; **30**: 31–8.

22. Jackson S., Stevenson C. The gift of time from the friendly professional. *Nursing Standard* 1998; **12**(51): 31–3.

23. Shattell M, Andes M, Thomas S. How patients and nurses experience the acute care psychiatric environment. *Nursing Inquiry* 2008; **15**(3): 242–50.

24. SCMH (Sainsbury Centre for Mental Health). *Acute problems: a survey of quality of care in acute psychiatric wards*. London: SCMH, 1998.

25. Tansella M. Alternatives to standard acute in-patient care for people with mental disorders: from systematic description to evaluative research. *British Journal of Psychiatry* 2010; **197**: s1–s3.

26. Pilgrim D. *Protest and co-operation: the voice of mental health service users in* Beyond the Water Tower: *the unfinished revolution in mental health service 1985–2005*. London: Sainsbury Centre for Mental Health, 2005.

27. Pilgrim D, McCranie A. *Recovery and mental health: a critical sociological account*. Basingstoke: Palgrave Macmillan, 2013.

28. Warner R, Wolleson C. Cedar House: a non coercive hospital alternative in Boulder, Colorado. In: Warner R (ed.). *Alternatives to the hospital for acute psychiatric treatment*. Arlington, VA: American Psychiatric Press, 1995: 3–7.

29. Menzies Lyth I. Social systems as a defense against anxiety: an empirical study of the nursing service of a general hospital. *Human Relations* 1960; **13**: 95–121.

30. Mosher LR. Soteria and other alternatives to acute psychiatric hospitalization: a personal and professional view. *Journal of Nervous Mental Disorder* 1999; **187**: 142–9.

31. Mosher LR, Hendrix V, Fort DC. *Soteria: through madness to deliverance*. Bloomington, IN: Xlibris, 2004.

32. Calton, T, Ferriter M, Huband N, Spandler H. A systematic review of the Soteria paradigm for the treatment of people diagnosed with schizophrenia. *Schizophrenia Bulletin* 2008; **34**(1): 181–92.

33. Brynmore L-E, Slade M, Jagielska D, Johnson S. Residential alternatives to acute psychiatric hospital admission: systematic review. *British Journal of Psychiatry* 2009; **195**: 109–17.

34. Johnson S, Gilburt H, Lloyd-Evans B, Osborn DPJ, Boardman J, Leese M, Shepherd G, Thornicroft G, Slade M. In-patient and residential alternatives to standard acute psychiatric wards in England. *British Journal of Psychiatry* 2009; **194**: 456–63.

35. Johnson S, Brymor L-E, Howard L, Osborn DPJ, Slade M. Where next with residential alternatives to admission? *British Journal of Psychiatry* 2010; **197**: s52–s54.

36. Department of Health and Others. No health without mental health: implementation guide. 2012. Available from: https://www.gov.uk/government/uploads/system/uploads/attachment_data/file/216870/No-Health-Without-Mental-Health-Implementation-Framework-Report-accessible-version.pdf [Accessed 1st June 2016].

Further reading

Hughes R, Hayward M, Finlay WML. 2009. Patients' perceptions of the impact of involuntary inpatient care on self, relationships and recovery. *Journal of Mental Health* 2009; **18**: 152–60.

Lloyd-Evans B, Johnson S, Morant N, Gilburt H, Osborn DP, Jagielska D, Skinner R, Leese M, Shepherd G, Slade M. Alternatives to standard acute in-patient care in England: differences in content of care and staff-patient contact. *British Journal of Psychiatry – Supplementum* 2010; **53**: s46–51.

NICE (National Institute for Health and Care Excellence). *Quality standard for service user experience in adult mental health* (NICE Guideline). Available from: http://www.nice.org.uk/guidance/qs14 [Accessed 25th July 2016].

Sweeney A, Nolan F, Morant N, Fox Z, Lloyd-Evans B, Osborn D, Burgess E, Gilburt H, Mccabe R, Johnson S. A mixed-methods study exploring therapeutic relationships and their association with service user satisfaction in acute psychiatric wards and crisis residential alternatives. *Health Services and Delivery Research* 2014; **2**.

Relevant web pages

Hearing Voices Network. http://www.hearing-voices.org/

Mosher LM. Soteria Project. http://www.moshersoteria.com/bio-of-loren-mosher-soteria/

Theoretical foundations of nursing. http://nursingtheories.weebly.com/hildegard-e-peplau.html

Tidal Model. http://www.tidal-model.com/

54 The psychiatric intensive care unit

CHRISTOPHER DZIKITI AND REBECCA LINGARD

LEARNING OUTCOMES

- To be familiar with services and resources available in a modern psychiatric intensive care unit (PICU) that promote the concept of the craft of caring.

- To know how to apply the concept of the craft of caring in a PICU setting.

- To understand the functions of a specialist multidisciplinary team (MDT) in a PICU setting.

- To understand nursing within a multidisciplinary team.

- To be aware of alternative resources to seclusion, restraint and rapid tranquilization.

SUMMARY OF KEY POINTS

- PICUs are usually small wards (8 to 15 beds) with higher levels of nursing, and are built on an open plan to promote easy observation, are often locked, and at times (but not always) have facilities for seclusion.

- PICU care is for patients who are in an acutely disturbed phase of a serious mental disorder which is associated with loss of capacity for self-control, with a corresponding increase in risk, which does not allow their safe, therapeutic management and treatment in a less acute or a less secure mental health ward.[1]

- In PICUs, seclusion, physical restraint and rapid tranquilization are common methods of managing violence and aggression, and these are considered to be a very restrictive way of caring for patients which does not fully promote the craft of caring.

INTRODUCTION

Since the writings of Rachlin in 1973,[2] the world of psychiatric intensive care units (PICUs) has continued to advance, bringing new initiatives and many challenges along the way. PICUs contain the most acutely ill of all psychiatric inpatients.[3] The treatment of acutely disturbed patients can be challenging and inherently stressful, but it remains a ubiquitous requirement of psychiatrist practice. Aggression is common on a PICU and the target is often likely to be a member of staff (63 per cent) or a fellow patient (36 per cent).[4] Over the years PICUs have been based on seclusion, physical restraint and reliance on antipsychotic drugs, especially for behaviour management. However, these methods have the potential to cause considerable harm in inexperienced hands.[3] Donat[5] argues that reliance on these methods is tied to a variety of untoward outcomes that detract from the quality of care in psychiatric services. PICUs are criticized for poor environments, high levels of coercion and the lack of an evidence base from controlled trials or post-occupancy evaluations.[6] As a result, Donat[5] argues that alternatives to this line of treatment should be seriously considered; for example, psychological treatment which promotes the idea of the craft of caring. Modern-day PICUs have seen the introduction of more advanced resources and a recognition that science alone will not meet the needs of patients. Barker's concept of the 'craft of caring', where the basis of good nursing practice is considered to be a combination of both art and science, is increasingly becoming a cornerstone of PICUs. The concept of 'craft' encourages nurses to adopt a holistic approach to the practice of psychiatric and mental health nursing, rather than risk being trapped by technologically limiting approaches to 'treatment'.[7] Despite whether or not patients are being treated on a PICU, the Mental Welfare Commission in Scotland concluded that everyone with a mental illness, learning disability or other mental disorder should be treated in a certain way (Box 54.1).

Applying the concept of the 'craft of caring' in a PICU setting can appear to be challenging, but the benefits are evident, as many clinicians are more proactive and creative. Reducing or eliminating the use of restrictive interventions in inpatient facilities is seen as a priority by many regulatory agencies.[9] Psychological treatments need to be and can be an essential part of comprehensive mental health nursing, and there have been a number of influential reviews of their effectiveness. Cognitive behavioural therapy (CBT) is not just an effective treatment for anxiety, obsessive–compulsive disorder (OCD) and depression, but also for the management of hallucinations and delusions and in chronic mental illness.[10] Many resources available for patients in PICUs will be discussed in this chapter. Specialist multidisciplinary teams (MDT), especially nursing, lay the foundations for promoting the craft of caring which improves patients' experiences in PICUs.

CASE STUDY 1

Throughout this chapter, we will reflect on our own experience of caring for a patient on a PICU. Patient X was a 23-year old-woman with a history of several self-harming incidents. She displayed some psychotic symptoms, such as hearing voices that told her she was worthless, to self-harm by banging her head on walls and to physically assault other people. Both patients and staff were assaulted on many occasions, including some serious untoward incidents (SUIs). Most of these attacks were impulsive and hence unpredictable. This resulted in frequent staff attendance to the Accident and Emergency department following the physical assaults.

SPECIALIST MULTIDISCIPLINARY TEAMS

Over the years, the definition and composition of MDTs in PICUs has evolved, and these teams now provide a more structured and well-documented system of care.

This has given specialist MDT members (Box 54.2) a platform to express the craft of caring from one human being to another. At present we talk as if medicine or science generates healing, but these are only contemporary metaphors for the effects of nature or God, as suggested by Barker and Buchanan-Barker.[11]

BOX 54.1: TREATING PATIENTS AS PEOPLE

- Patients have the right to be treated with dignity and respect at all times.
- Patients have the right to treatment that's allowed by law and fully meets professional standards and guidelines.
- Patients have the right to live free from abuse, neglect or discrimination.
- Each patient must receive the care and treatment that best meet his or her needs.
- Each patient should be enabled to lead as fulfilling a life as possible.

Source: Adapted from NHS Quality Improvement Scotland.[8]

BOX 54.2: MULTIDISCIPLINARY TEAM MEMBERS

- Patients and carers
- Mental health nurses (qualified and non-qualified registrants)
- Consultant psychiatrists (in most PICUs they are the responsible clinicians)
- Clinical psychologists
- Junior doctors
- Pharmacists
- Occupational therapists
- Social workers

Despite all the science and technology, the MDT in a PICU is the most important resource that is instrumental to patients' recovery, especially when patients are considered as core members. MDT members require special skills to work successfully with aggressive and violent patients.[12] Whyte[13] surveyed all levels of security including prisons, and low-, medium- and high-secure units, and discovered a list of six core skills required when working with such patients in a PICU (Box 54.3).

However, MDT effectiveness cannot be assumed or guaranteed unless it is designed. In order 'to fully embrace a MDT multidisciplinary approach within these teams requires developing and implementing an ethos of shared vision with the teamwork philosophy at its core'[2] (p.326). This in return forms a strong foundation for an effective MDT. Examples of common team roles and responsibilities are described by Beer et al.[2] in Box 54.4.

It is essential for MDTs to be composed of staff with the necessary skills, knowledge and experience to ensure high-quality diagnosis, treatment and care in PICUs. Furthermore, Bowers[14] points out that PICU staff need to build enough expertise and knowledge of psychotic symptoms and cognitive deficits, so that these can be recognized and accommodated during daily life on a PICU ward. Bowers[14] clearly identifies PICU MDT members as not just ordinary clinicians but specialists in behavioural engineering. This means that PICU staff need to become experts in behavioural assessment, being able to utilize structured interviews, rating scales and structured real-time records with sequential analysis.[14] This is also supported by Barker and Buchanan-Barker,[10] who describe Edward Podvoll's writings in 1991. Podvoll discovered that a deeper set of clinical skills need to be cultivated to do basic nursing properly, ranging from what is immediately relevant to being with someone during the process of recovery, such as taking walks, to something approaching more traditional psychotherapy. (See chapter 3 for more information on developing a therapeutic relationship.)

Curtis et al.[15] looked at how to improve the quality of ward rounds, particularly reliability and patient experience. The study highlighted the role of nurses and other MDT members in contributing to an effective ward round. One of the outcomes of the MDT discussion was the creation of a checklist with key tasks that the team wanted to accomplish (Box 54.5), which was used as a measure of the key tasks carried out, including information presented for nursing during the ward round.[15] If PICUs are to become a centre of excellence for the craft of caring, MDTs in PICUs will need to continue to be rigorous, disciplined, constant, absolutely consistent behavioural responders to patients.[14]

BOX 54.4: EXAMPLES OF COMMON TEAM ROLES/ RESPONSIBILITIES

- Input into decision making
- Communicating information
- Promoting the unit's philosophy
- Induction of new team members
- Development of others
- Supporting relatives/carers
- Admission protocols
- Care and treatment planning
- Risk assessment
- Progress reviews
- Emergency management of disturbed behaviour
- Participation in referral assessments should be a common responsibility (each discipline will bring its own perspective completing a referral assessment, thus enabling a more thorough, rounded and complete assessment)

BOX 54.5: CHECKLIST KEY TASKS – NURSING CHECKLIST

- Mental state and behaviours (any changes in mental state presentation)
- Medication compliance and side effects
- Psychiatric observation level and rationale
- Urine drug screen/pregnancy test
- Social issues (accommodation/benefits)
- Sleep/diet/toilet
- Risk incidents (risk assessments and risk management)
- Legal and criminal issues (pending court cases)
- Patient and family views (user and carer involvement)
- Physical observations (vital signs)

Source: Adapted from Curtis et al.[15]

BOX 54.3: SIX CORE SKILLS FOR WORKING WITH AGGRESSIVE AND VIOLENT PATIENTS

- Basic interpersonal skills (tolerance, understanding)
- Humanity (empathy, warmth, non-judgemental attitude)
- Knowledge base (mental disorders, criminology, offending behaviour)
- Communication skills
- Personal qualities
- Teamwork skills

Source: Based on Whyte[13] (p.32).

NURSING WITHIN A MULTIDISCIPLINARY TEAM

Historically, the medical profession has traditionally dominated the care of mentally unwell individuals.[13] In modern PICUs, this concept has been challenged in order to have an effective MDT that incorporates different health care professionals. One difference between nurses and other MDT members is that nurses are able to forge long-standing relationships with patients, often spending much longer periods working with them, and thereby developing the trust essential to effective mental health care.[16] Nurses are ever-present on PICUs and in other inpatient services, and hence their contribution to MDT working as a resource is as important as that of a doctor, psychologist, occupational therapist or pharmacist. As part of an MDT, nurses practise the art of caring as they (most of the time) provide the human experience for patients. It is impossible to overemphasize the value of the patient–nurse relationship. At the focal point of mental health nursing care are the one-to-one personal relationships that nurses develop with patients. This is achieved through a combination of excellent communication skills, and knowledge of the patient and their presenting symptoms, together with an ability to observe behaviour, and an attempt to understand the underlying emotions and feelings (affect) and thinking (cognitions) that have produced any challenging behaviour.[16] Dooher[16] further suggests that there is a range of well-documented activities for nurses that are associated with developing a therapeutic rapport and a plan of care interventions which meet individual patients' specific needs (see Box 54.6).

If mental health care is to continue moving away from a medical approach, nurses will need to continue applying themselves more in MDT working by focusing on the most important item in their toolbox: the therapeutic relationships they build with patients, which form the foundation of the craft of caring. (See chapter 50 for more information on collaborative care planning.) This means that mental health nurses need to continue to develop their skills and knowledge set to provide evidence-based psychological therapies, better nursing assessments and health promotion activities that form the basis of care plans to meet the complex demands of individual patients in PICUs.[16] This in turn will position nurses as key drivers in practising the craft of caring in modern-day PICUs, as they implement more recovery-focused nursing interventions.

BOX 54.6: WORK ACTIVITIES FOR NURSES

- Listening to patients and interpreting their needs and concerns in an honest, non-judgemental and open manner, which respects the rights of individuals and groups, while actively engaging with patients in the provision of holistic, needs-led care that takes account of physical, psychological, emotional, social and spiritual needs
- Assessing and talking to patients, offering explanation and reassurance about treatment they are receiving
- Responding to distressed patients and attempting to understand the source of their distress in a non-threatening manner
- Participating in group and/or one-to-one therapy sessions, both as an individual and with other health professionals
- Devising plans of care that anticipate risks, and promote the safety, health and well-being of patients
- Applying the 'de-escalation' approach to help patients manage their emotions and behaviour
- Caring for patients who are acutely unwell or who have a long-standing or enduring mental health problem

Source: Adapted from Dooher.[16]

CASE STUDY 1 (CONTINUED)

We acknowledged that patient X was probably the most challenging patient in our 10-year experience of working on a PICU. While we were attempting to ensure safety for patient X and other patients, we encountered some ethical dilemmas: (a) the excessive use of segregation for the protection of others; (b) the ethics of using rapid tranquilisation when clinically beneficial; and (c) the use of physical restraint without consent. Patients experience tremendous loss when they are admitted onto PICUs. We recognized that our duty of care was to the patients and not to inflict pain or cause any harm. Some of the management techniques we used with patient X resulted in differences of opinion in the MDT, which made us reflect and question our own values and whether they reflected the true ethos of the craft of caring. Despite differences of opinion about clinical interventions, the MDT remained focused on better outcomes for patient X.

REFLECTION

Please reflect on your own values and how they influence your response to patients in distress.

TRAUMA-INFORMED SERVICES

Many of the patients who come through PICU services have extensive trauma histories, which have the potential to impact their recovery. Often patients can experience re-traumatization or triggers that will affect their emotional safety and mental state. It is therefore important that PICUs work towards becoming 'trauma-informed services' with an MDT skilled enough to care for patients' trauma-related needs. The focus on the craft of caring becomes even more important here, as human nurturing is vital for patients experiencing trauma. Blanch et al.[17] make an important distinction between providing trauma-specific interventions and being a trauma-informed service. Blanch et al.[17] state that 'trauma-informed practices provide a new paradigm for organising services and supports that recognizes the central role that trauma plays in people's lives and shifts the focus from what is wrong with you, to what happened to you?' (p.6). PICU services can make simple fundamental changes to their operational approach and ethos that can ensure that trauma-informed practices are embedded in day-to-day practice. The US National Center on Domestic Violence, Trauma and Mental Health published a series of tip sheets in 2011 to offer advice and support on how to create such services.[18] The basic principle of creating a safe and welcoming environment is key, and this includes considering how we choose our language to welcome our patients into our service.

SENSORY ROOMS

Sensory rooms are not a new phenomenon; they have been around since the 1970s. Sensory rooms first emerged in the Netherlands and were designed for people who experienced learning difficulties. The use of sensory rooms was first developed by Jan Hulsegge and Ad Verheul, two Dutch therapists working at the De Hartenberg Institute in Holland. The intention of a sensory room is to create an environment in which an individual can stimulate any of their five senses in a safe and non-threatening environment. The provision of safe and comfortable surroundings for people in distress creates an ideal opportunity to explore safe therapeutic relationships between patients and clinicians, and to begin to understand the basis of distress.

The beauty of using sensory rooms as an intervention is that they can be moulded to suit the environment and resources available in individual services. Sensory rooms can be as big or small, or as simple or complicated, as a service provider wishes. Over the last four decades, the use of sensory rooms has evolved into other care settings, and other innovative ideas are in development. Coldwell et al.[19] discuss the concept of 'caring and comfort rooms' in the context of reducing seclusion and restraint practices. The authors consider the importance of having a comfortable room, and debunk the idea of the usual uncomfortable 'time out' room. In their study they emphasize the importance of well-designed, comfortable rooms that include soft furnishings, soft lighting, music and soothing colours, all of which have the aim of 'reducing unsettled patients' level of stress'[19] (p.1).

Smith and Jones[20] looked at the application of sensory rooms specifically on a PICU. The research was conducted on a male PICU in East London and aimed to establish a link between sensory rooms and a reduction in seclusion rates. The quantitative data collated did not show any significant correlation between the implementation of a sensory room and the reduction in the use of seclusion practices. However, the qualitative part of the study indicated that there was a staff perception that the introduction of a sensory room reduced the use of seclusion. Additional findings were also of value. The study suggests that both patients and staff have found that sensory rooms are a positive therapeutic intervention which can improve communication and patients' overall experience of the PICU.[20] Most importantly, this study recommends that other PICU and psychiatric inpatient settings consider the use of sensory rooms as valid therapeutic interventions.

> ### CASE STUDY 1 (CONTINUED)
>
> We were privileged to have a sensory room on our PICU. The patients were involved in the planning, including choosing the equipment and colours of paint. The sensory room was a patient-informed project and became one of the alternatives for managing patient X. Due to the risk presented to other patients, patient X was nursed separately from other patients, including mealtimes. While it was accepted that such a solitary life was not helping her mental state, we assessed it to be high risk to bring her out of this situation in the absence of any identifiable clinical improvement. However, we had a duty of care not only to patient X, but also to the other 10 patients. Seclusion was not an option due to the high risk of self-harm. However, there was considerable anxiety among the staff about using physical

restraint for prolonged periods. We initially had to use the sensory room with four members of staff to ensure safety for the patient and staff. The sensory room created a stimulating and yet calming atmosphere for patient X. We realized that this was a more suitable and less restrictive alternative to physical restraint and rapid tranquilization. We can confidently say that we observed the craft of caring at its best.

REFLECTION

Please consider the possible thoughts and feelings experienced by both the patient and staff as they worked through the process described in case study 1.

RESTRICTIVE PRACTICES

The concept of restrictive practices has attracted greater scrutiny in recent years, and the scrutiny of care delivery within psychiatry has focused on the use of restrictive practices. Restrictive practices include physical restraint, the use of seclusion, enforcement of medication (under the use of the Mental Health Act), segregation and the use of banned items policies, which restrict items that patients are allowed to have in their immediate possession.

Restraint

There is a national drive to reduce the number of episodes of physical restraint and seclusion in psychiatric services. In April 2014 the Department of Health published guidance entitled 'Positive and proactive care: reducing the need for restrictive interventions'.[21] The authors were keen to acknowledge that vast numbers of staff in health care settings are committed to providing care in a safe, sensitive, dignified and respectful way. The paper also acknowledged the extreme and challenging situations that many staff face, and aimed to focus on the support and training that such clinicians need. This guidance was issued in response to previously published reports.

BOX 54.7: KEY ACTIONS FOR IMPROVING CARE

- People should not be deliberately restrained in a way that affects airways, breathing or circulation, 'such as face down restraint on any surface'[22] (p.26).
- Restrictive interventions should always represent the least restrictive option, and should not include the deliberate application of pain.[22]
- Seclusion should only be used for those patients formally detained under the Mental Health Act 1983.[22] In addition, the paper highlights the importance of services involving families and carers in the review process of all aspects of care and support.

In 2013, MIND released an important document that looked into the practice of physical restraint, which followed the much-publicized public outcry at the unacceptable treatment of people at Winterbourne View Hospital. MIND's 'Mental health crisis in care: physical restraint in crisis'[22] pointed out that physical restraint and restrictive interventions have not always been used as a last resort in health and social care settings.

MIND's 'Crisis in care' paper[22] highlighted the huge variation in the number of physical restraints between Trusts, ranging from 38 incidents in one Trust to 3,000 in another. However, caution should be taken in interpreting these statistics at face value. There are many factors that could account for the variation, not just differences in the ethical and moral stance of organizations. For example, there are many NHS Trusts which have forensic services within their remit, or Trusts that do not provide PICU services, which arguably deal with the most severe and enduring mental health presentations in acute settings. Additionally, there may be a variation in restraint figures based on the geographical location of the Trust. 'Positive and proactive care'[21] considers the importance of providing a framework 'within which adult health and social care services can develop a culture where restrictive interventions are only ever used as a last resort and only then for the shortest possible time' (p.1). See Box 54.7.

Seclusion

Seclusion, as defined by the Mental Health Code of Practice, is the 'supervised confinement and isolation of a patient, away from other patients, in an area from which the patient is prevented from leaving'[23] (p.300). The only clinical indication for the use of seclusion is to contain immediate and severely disturbed behaviour, and when there is an immediate threat to the safety of others. There are serious ethical considerations involved in the use of seclusion, and it should only be used as a last resort when all other clinical and therapeutic interventions, such as de-escalation and medication, have failed. Seclusion falls under the definition of medical treatment within the scope of the Mental Health Act (section 145). However, it should never be part of a planned intervention, and should not be used as a way of managing self-harming behaviour. The most important element of a clinician's practice with regard to seclusion is that, once commenced, the clinician should begin immediately to work with the patient on a care plan that would support them to leave seclusion safely and quickly and return to the ward's communal areas. The emphasis of practice should be on continued engagement and support to ensure that seclusion only occurs for the shortest time possible.

There is a great appetite for services to consider their environment, and how best to support someone who is agitated and at risk of potential seclusion. Current concepts that are popular include sensory rooms, de-escalation areas and comfort rooms. A systematic review conducted by Gaskin et al.[24] identified a wide range of therapeutic interventions that may assist in reducing the use of violence (and restraint). Although no causal relationship was established, the authors concluded that effective alternatives to seclusion are available and that this controversial practice could safely be reduced or even abandoned. The study also summarized key factors in the success of reducing seclusion rates. These included clinical leadership, the integration of new staff with positive attitudes, improved treatment plans, increased staff to patient ratios, and a good quality emergency response team, trained to support those experiencing distress and disturbed behaviour. In addition, the authors acknowledged that interventions would be particular to each service, and could also include good pharmacological interventions (chapters 47 and 48), patient involvement (the use of advance directives (chapter 37) on the interventions preferred at times of distress and agitation) and changes to the therapeutic environment. Chapter 25 has further information on caring for the person who is extremely distressed and disturbed.

Rapid tranquilization

Rapid tranquilization is defined by the National Institute for Health and Care Excellence (NICE)[25] as the 'use of medication to calm/lightly sedate the patient and reduce the risk to self and others' (p.17). The aim of using any medication in an emergency situation is not to render a patient incapable of activity, participating in groups or attending to any activities of daily living, but simply to reduce levels of distress, aggression or agitation that may impair normal routine and functioning, and interfere with overall recovery. In essence, 'the aim of rapid tranquilisation is to achieve a state of calm sufficient to minimise the risk posed to the patient or to others'[25] (p.202). When using rapid tranquilization, there are important practice implications that a treating team must consider, including ready access to medical emergency equipment, and access to a doctor. Macpherson et al.[26] have argued

that rapid tranquilization and physical interventions such as restraint and seclusion are management strategies, not primary treatment techniques. Antipsychotics are normally used in rapid tranquilization and can bring about rapid improvement in symptoms of psychosis and mania, to a greater extent than benzodiazepines.[27] However, akathisia, a side effect of antipsychotics, has been associated with suicidality and physical assault,[28] and the presence of this and other extra-pyramidal side effects means that the use of antipsychotics in behaviour control has a negative impact on the concept of the craft of caring, unless it is carefully balanced against the risks of side effects.

CASE STUDY 1 (CONTINUED)

It was a great achievement that our PICU no longer relied on seclusion, restraint and rapid tranquilization as part of providing care and treatment to patient X. There were certainly times when the use of these interventions seemed justified, but with patient X we learnt that these interventions still need to be seriously considered and should not be used as the first line of managing someone who is highly distressed.

Clinicians need to promote less frequent use of these restrictive practices as a major resource for PICU intervention, and promote alternative approaches. Initiatives such as sensory rooms and engagement in occupational therapy activities were good examples that we utilized in supporting patient X.

We are not advocating that seclusion, physical restraint and rapid tranquilization should be banned. These interventions have been and will always be part of PICUs, and they do serve a purpose in minimizing risk to patients and staff. The safe use of these interventions, together with psychological interventions and other initiatives (sensory rooms, occupational therapy groups/activities), will undoubtedly promote the creation of an environment that demonstrates the principles of the craft of caring.

REFLECTION

Think about situations that you have encountered where coercive interventions were used and consider, given the circumstances, what other options might have been used.

GROUPS AND ACTIVITIES

Have you ever imagined being locked up in a place where you cannot leave unless someone gives you permission to do so? Most patients in PICU wards are detained under the Mental Health Act and require section 17 leave to access the outside world. Groups and activities become a valuable resource on a PICU for reducing boredom for patients. Recreational activities are seen as therapeutic diversional interventions that include engaging in creative work, hobbies and special interests,[29] and these also improve clinical outcomes and patients' experiences. Furthermore, therapeutic activities not only enhance an individual's development but can also assist in the management of challenging behaviour and maintenance of a safe environment.[13] In the view of PICU patients,[30] activities keep patients occupied, give them outlets for creativity, and reduce agitation. Patients can be seen to benefit from structure and routine. In modern-day PICUs, there are many resources to keep patients engaged. A good example is Marion Janner's initiative, 'Star Wards'. This consists of 75 practical, mainly low-cost and easy-to-implement ideas which are increasingly acting as a catalyst to promote change through inspiring, collecting and disseminating best practice in inpatient care, from acute admission to high-secure units, to improve patients' experiences and clinical outcomes. A good example of the Star Wards initiative is Ward Buddy. Even though Ward Buddy is not a group activity, it is an activity that is available to accompany patients through various experiences of ward life, from arriving on the ward to the rediscovery of hope, among other themes. The Ward Buddy is filled with experiences of recovery and mini-snippets of ward life that have been kindly offered and beautifully illustrated by people who have had stays on mental health wards. Reports from the Star Wards initiative have indicated that violence has decreased on wards that have embraced the scheme,

and also indicate that one area for improvement is that of patient involvement.[31]

In a PICU in Blackpool, Antonysamy[32] discovered that outdoor activities had not been explored much. This could partly reflect a 'risk-averse' approach by clinicians, which can be found in most PICUs in UK. Like a pressure cooker, the patients' anger and frustration build up and unfortunately staff and other patients may be placed at risk as they may lash out at them.[32] Physical activity has the potential to improve the quality of life of people with severe mental health problems, such as schizophrenia and bipolar disorder, through improvements in physical and mental health.[33] Clinicians should always remember that people with these conditions have greater physical health needs (chapter 69) than the general population, as they are more likely to be inactive and have high rates of obesity, confounded by the side effects of antipsychotic medication. Consequently, patients in mental health services are at high risk of chronic medical conditions (cardiovascular disease, diabetes and obesity) associated with lack of activity, especially outdoor activity.[34] There is enough evidence to suggest that, for people with severe mental health problems, participating in physical activity may lead to improvements in quality of life.[33] Alexandratos et al.[35] reviewed 16 studies which included a physical activity intervention for people with severe mental illness and found that physical activities contributed to improved quality of life through social interaction, meaningful use of time, purposeful activity and empowerment. Another innovative activity for patients in PICUs is the use of pet therapy on Rosebank female PICU in East London (case study 2). The craft of caring can be practised once specialist MDTs start being creative and challenging the perceived normal cultures of PICUs.

CASE STUDY 2: PET THERAPY – ROSEBANK FEMALE PSYCHIATRIC INTENSIVE CARE UNIT, EAST LONDON NHS FOUNDATION TRUST

Pets have been used in medical settings for more than 150 years. However, it was only in the late 1970s that researchers began to uncover the scientific rationale for animal/human bonds.

One of the earliest studies, published in 1980, discussed the benefits of animal companionship for the health and well-being of adults and children. The study confirmed that 'social affiliation and companionship have important health effects'[36] (p.310). Specifically, the findings of the study suggested that social variables such as pet ownership could increase the survival rate of patients suffering with cardiovascular disease.

Furthermore, the study alluded to the transferability of using pets with people suffering from enduring mental illness.

Hardiman[37] reviewed research that focused on interactions between animals and individuals with a range of mental health issues. Simply put, Hardiman[37] states that contact and interactions with our 'animal friends' lower stress hormones, and increase hormones that affect levels of happiness, bonding, energy and elation. In the UK, 'Pets as Therapy' is a charity which has supported the use of animals in health and social care settings since 1983. The aim of the charity is to support volunteers and their cats or dogs to participate in therapeutic visits to health care settings.

One service that implemented the use of 'Pets as Therapy' is Rosebank ward in the East End of London. Rosebank ward is an 11-bedded female psychiatric intensive care unit, looking after vulnerable women who are detained under the Mental Health Act, and who often experience high levels of distress in the context of an enduring mental illness.

The service recently experienced a young dog spending a day with them. Leo, a young Cavachon (a cross between a Cavalier King Charles Spaniel and a Bichon Frise), was accompanied by his owner who has been assessed (along with Leo) as being suitable for a 'Pets as Therapy' provider. The visit was well planned and coordinated, with patients and staff alike well informed ahead of time. In addition, a protocol was developed that could be used by staff as guidance, and to offer structure and support during the visits. Prior to the visit, the staff also worked with patients to consider the goals of the visit, and to consider the therapeutic benefits. In summation, staff and patients deemed the visit a success, with 67 per cent of patients reporting a positive interaction.

CONCLUSION

In this chapter we looked at the resources available in PICUs. The chapter highlights the need for mental health professionals to continue to be innovative, which in turn improves patients' experiences in PICUs. The MDT remains the most significant aspect of a patient's journey while receiving treatment in a PICU. There is scope for clinicians to apply the concept of the craft of caring in PICUs. Total reliance on seclusion, physical restraint and rapid tranquilization appears to promote a restrictive practice which is being challenged by patient groups, families, professionals and the wider community. Trauma-informed services that employ initiatives such as sensory rooms and pet therapy are clearly spearheading positive changes in PICUs. This is the art of psychiatry; science continues to be crucial, but it is no longer the only foundation of PICUs and clinical interventions.

SERVICE USER COMMENTARY

Jo Thompson

The psychiatric intensive care unit (PICU) is without question one of the most challenging environments in which to be a patient. I was 19 years old when I spent approximately 5 months on a PICU. I was the only female on the unit, surrounded by seven highly distressed and angry men. I spent my first 3 weeks so medicated that I could hardly stand up. I was against my will, taking medication to which I had not consented. I was terrified, angry, hopeless and at times overwhelmingly bored. Like many others, I spent my time attempting to ligature from ligature-proof pipes, trying to sharpen plastic forks into self-harm devices and many other creative forbidden activities. Sometimes I did these things to try and regain some control and autonomy, sometimes it was out of sheer frustration and anger at the infantilizing nature of the PICU regime, and at other times to harm myself or others.

The main strength of this chapter is the appeal for a trauma-informed approach to containment and care. From the narrative above, it isn't difficult to see that a stay on a PICU can in itself be traumatic. This chapter promotes positive ways to ensure a more compassionate service is delivered. However, as a service user, it is difficult for me to imagine that a PICU can incorporate the principles of the craft of caring. The use of forced medication, seclusion and restraint are not obviously compatible with the 'craft of caring' ideal. Nevertheless, this chapter perfectly illustrates how this ideal can begin to be realized in even the most challenging of environments. Simple things, such as acknowledging that we as service users have often had very traumatic experiences that have contributed to our current states of distress, rather than using a purely medicalized approach to care, can be de-escalating in and of itself. The endorsement of the use of sensory rooms also feels like a positive move away from the abusive practice of restraint and seclusion, although I would also recommend a space within PICUs for anger and rage to be expressed in an appropriate way.

I am also encouraged to see the emphasis placed on the importance of the nurse–client relationship in the role of de-escalation and crisis prevention. In my experience, the relationship with key nurses on the PICU could mean the difference between a potentially re-traumatizing haloperidol injection and a positive opportunity to try new ways of coping. Being able to talk with a range of professionals was also important in my own recovery, and I fully support the recommendations for a diverse and organized MDT structure.

I am also pleased to see the issues of boredom highlighted by this chapter. Boredom was a real problem for me on the PICU. Unfortunately, the reality was that groups, when they happened, were usually poor in quality. Walking and other exercise groups are important not just for physical health needs, but, as explained in this chapter, they are also crucial to reduce the effects of antipsychotic medications, whether sedation or akathisia.

In conclusion, I feel that this chapter is a major step in the right direction towards a greater emphasis on care rather than mere containment for service users who need the kind of treatment a PICU can provide. Getting this balance right for PICUs will remain an ongoing challenge for nursing staff

and the MDT. However, the move towards providing a more sensitive service seems positive for staff in terms of job satisfaction and an increased awareness of their own emotional well-being. Ultimately, it is a crucial change for service users who, for too long, have been treated as prisoners without appropriate care in these types of units.

Jo Thompson, MSc, BSc (Hons), is a survivor researcher.

References

1. National Association of Psychiatric Intensive Care Units. *National minimum standards for psychiatric intensive care in general adult services.* East Kilbride: National Association of Psychiatric Intensive Care Units, 2014.
2. Beer MD, Pereira SM, Paton C. *Psychiatric intensive care*, 2nd edn. Cambridge: Cambridge University Press, 2008.
3. Pereira SM, Beer MD, Paton C. Good practice issues in psychiatric intensive care units. Findings from a national survey. *Psychiatric Bulletin* 1999; **23**: 397–400.
4. Cohen D P, Akhtar MS, Siddiqui A, Shelley C, Larkin C, Kinsella A, O'Callaghan E, Lane A. Aggressive incidents on a psychiatric intensive care unit. *Psychiatric Bulletin* 2008; **32**: 455–8.
5. Donat DC. Special section on seclusion and restraint: encouraging alternatives to seclusion, restraint and reliance on prn drugs in a public hospital. *Psychiatric Services* 2005; **56**(9): 1105–8.
6. Vaaler AE. Effects of a psychiatric intensive care unit in an acute psychiatric ward. PhD thesis, Faculty of Medicine Department of Neuroscience, Norwegian University of Science and Technology, 2007. Available from: http://www.diva-portal.org/smash/get/diva2:121844/FULLTEXT01.pdf [Accessed 4th July 2016].
7. Barker P. *Psychiatric and mental health nursing: the craft of caring*, 2nd edn. London: Edward Arnold, 2009.
8. NHS Quality Improvement Scotland. *The Healthcare Quality Strategy for NHS Scotland.* Scottish Government. Crown Copyright. 2010. Available from: http://www.scotland.gov.uk/Resource/Doc/311667/0098354.pdf [Accessed 8th July 2016].
9. Steinert T, Eisele F, Goeser U, Tschoeke S, Uhlmann C, Schmid P. Successful interventions on an organisational level to reduce violence and coercive interventions in in-patients with adjustment disorders and personality disorders. *Clinical Practice in Epidemiology and Mental Health* 2008; **4**: 27.
10. Turkington D, Kingdon D, Rathod S. Outcomes of an effectiveness trial of cognitive–behavioural intervention by mental health nurses in schizophrenia. *British Journal of Psychiatry* 2006; **189**: 36–40.
11. Barker P, Buchanan-Barker P. Caring as craft. *Nursing Standard* 2004; **19**(9): 1718.
12. Dawson P, Kingsley M, Pereira S. Violent patients within psychiatric intensive care units: treatment approaches, resistance and the impact upon staff. *Journal of Psychiatric Intensive Care* 2005; **1**(1): 45–53.
13. Whyte L. Working with a MDT team in secure psychiatric environments. *Journal of Psychosocial Nursing* 2001; **39**(9): 26–34i.
14. Bowers, L. Commentary – PICU possibilities. *Journal of Psychiatric Intensive Care* 2013; **9**(2): 68–71.
15. Curtis P, Sethi F, Ahmed F. Creating a high quality consultant led psychiatric intensive care unit multidisciplinary team ward round. *Journal of Psychiatric Intensive Care* 2013; **10**(1): 13–22.
16. Dooher J. *Fundamental aspects of mental health nursing.* London: Quay Books Division, MA Healthcare Ltd, 2008.
17. Blanch A, Filson B, Penney D, with contributions from Cave C. *Engaging women in trauma informed peer support: a guidebook.* National Association of State Mental Health Program Direction, 2012. Available from: http://www.nasmhpd.org/sites/default/files/PeerEngagementGuide_Color_REVISED_10_2012.pdf [Accessed 31st August 2016].
18. National Center on Domestic Violence, Trauma & Mental Health. Creating trauma informed services: tipsheet series. 2013. Available from: www.nationalcenterdvtraumamh.org [Accessed 21st June 2014].
19. Coldwell CM, Cummings KS, Grandfield SA. Caring with comfort rooms – reducing seclusion and restraint use in psychiatric facilities. *Journal of Psychosocial Nursing* 2010; **48**(6): 26–30.
20. Smith S, Jones J. Use of a sensory room on an intensive care unit. *Journal of Psychosocial Nursing & Mental Health Services* 2014; **52**(5): 22–30.
21. Department of Health. Social Care, Local Government & Care Partnership Directorate Policy. Positive and proactive care: reducing the need for restrictive interventions. 2014. Available from https://www.gov.uk/government/uploads/system/uploads/attachment_data/file/300291/JRA_DoH_Guidance_on_RH_Summary_web_accessible.pdf [Accessed 31st August 2016].
22. MIND. Mental health crisis in care: physical restraint in crisis. 2013. Available from https://www.mind.org.uk/media/197120/physical_restraint_final_web_version.pdf [Accessed 31st August 2016].
23. Department of Health. *Code of Practice: Mental Health Act 1983.* London: Department of Health, 2015.
24. Gaskin C, Elsom S, Happell, B. Interventions for reducing the use of seclusion in psychiatric facilities: review of the literature. *British Journal of Psychiatry* 2007; **191**(10): 298–303.
25. NICE (National Institute for Health and Care Excellence). Violence: the short term management of disturbed/violent behaviour in psychiatric in-patient settings and emergency departments. 2005. Available from: www.rcpsych.ac.uk/PDF/NICE%20Guideline%202005.pdf [Accessed 8th July 2016].
26. Macpherson R, Dix R, Morgan S. Revisiting: guidelines for the management of acutely disturbed psychiatric patients. *Advances in Psychiatric Treatment* 2005; **11**: 404–15.
27. Agid O, Kapur S, Arenovich T. Delayed onset hypothesis of antipsychotic action: a hypothesis tested and rejected. *Archives of General Psychiatry* 2003; **60**: 1228–35.
28. Crowner M, Dougon R, Convit A. Akathisia and violence. *Psychopharmacology* 1990; **26**: 115–18.
29. Department of Health. *Mental health policy implementation guide: national minimum standards for general adult services in psychiatric intensive care units (PICU) and low secure environments.* London: Department of Health, 2002.
30. O'Brien L, Cole R. Mental health nursing practice in acute psychiatric close-observation areas. *International Journal of Mental Health Nursing* 2004; **13**: 89–99.
31. Janner M. Creating Star Wards. *A Life in the Day* 2007; **11**(1): 6–8.
32. Antonysamy A. How can we reduce violence and aggression in psychiatric inpatient units? *BMJ Quality Improvement Reports.* British Medical Journal Publishing Group, 2013. Available from: http://qir.bmj.com/content/2/1/u201366.w834.full.pdf+html [Accessed 8th July 2016].
33. Mental Health Foundation. Let's get physical: the impact of physical activity on wellbeing, Mental Health Awareness Week 2013. 2013. Available from: http://www.bhfactive.org.uk/userfiles/Documents/lets-get-physical-report.pdf [Accessed 31st August 2016].

34. Davidson S, Judd F, Jolley D, Hocking B, Thompson S, Hyland B. Cardiovascular risk factors for people with mental illness. *Australian and New Zealand Journal of Psychiatry* 2001; **35**(2): 196–202.
35. Alexandratos K, Barnett F, Thomas Y. The impact of exercise on the mental health and quality of life of people with severe mental illness: a critical review. *British Journal of Occupational Therapy* 2012; **75**(2): 48–60.

36. Friedman E, Katcher AH, Lynch JL, Thomas SA. Animal companions & one year survival of patients after discharge from coronary care unit. *Public Health Reports* 1980; **95**(4): 307–12.
37. Hardiman D. Animal assisted therapy in mental health. *SCAS Journal* 2010; Autumn: 14–17.

Further reading

Barker P. *Psychiatric and mental health nursing: the craft of caring*, 2nd edn. London: Edward Arnold, 2009.
Barker P, Buchanan-Barker P. Caring as craft. *Nursing Standard* 2004; **19**(9): 1718.

Beer MD, Pereira SM, Paton C. *Psychiatric intensive care*, 2nd edn. Cambridge: Cambridge University Press, 2008.
Dix R. A nurse led psychiatric intensive care unit. *Psychiatric Bulletin* 1995; **19**(5): 258–87.

Relevant web pages

NAPICU (National Association of Psychiatric Intensive Care and Low Secure Units). www.napicu.org.uk

Snoezelen Multi-Sensory Environments. www.snoezeleninfo.com
Star Wards. www.starwards.org.uk

55 Mental health nursing in community care

DENIS RYAN AND JANE ALEXANDER

LEARNING OUTCOMES

- To understand the evolving need for community mental health services.
- To understand the challenges of working with persons suffering from severe and enduring mental illness.
- To be aware of health promotion and illness prevention roles.
- To be aware of the service user movement.

SUMMARY OF KEY POINTS

- In order to understand contemporary mental health nursing services internationally, it is important to be aware of the evolution of community mental health services from institutional care.
- The World Health Organization has identified the centrality of community mental health nurses (CMHNs) in health service development.
- CMHNs play a vital role in the care of those with severe and enduring mental illness.
- CMHN roles in health promotion and illness prevention have tended to be underemphasized, but this is beginning to change.

- The therapeutic relationship is a cornerstone of person-centred care.
- It is vital that CMHNs provide evidence-based interventions.
- CMHNs have a role in the promotion of individual as well as organizational recovery-orientated approaches.
- Conflicts and frictions naturally exist between the demands of organizational roles and growing service user and peer support worker involvement.

INTRODUCTION

The craft of caring demands a person-centred approach.[1] Since at least the middle of the twentieth century, there has been an increasing shift from institutionally based care towards 'community' care models in what are loosely referred to as 'western' countries or more developed economies. However, the World Health Organization (WHO)[2] has reported that there is a significant disparity in the resources provided to deal with mental health, between low- to middle-income countries on the one hand, and high-income countries on the other. The WHO[2] reported that almost half of the world's population lives in an environment where one psychiatrist serves the needs of 200,000 or more people, with even fewer personnel who are capable of delivering psychosocial interventions.

Within this context, a person-centred approach towards mental health nursing in the community is largely restricted to services available in higher-income countries, and it is a phenomenon which has evolved in a relatively short period within these countries. Later in this chapter, the development of mental health services and the place of community mental health nursing in these high-income countries will be traced. The shift from institutional care, which commenced following the Second World War, will be mapped, alongside discussion of how this shift changed the role of nurses. These developments were strongly linked with the increasing professionalization of nursing, which has led to ambiguity for CMHNs, who may be unclear on the boundaries of their role when working in interdisciplinary teams, and for those in other disciplines, who may be unsure of the distinctive contribution of CMHNs.[3] Some

authors have argued that the professional identity of community mental health nursing is poorly articulated, with CMHNs assuming roles more traditionally associated with other disciplines.[4] In assuming roles associated with 'talk therapies', it is arguable that they are positioning themselves to meet the needs of mental health service users (MHSUs) more appropriately,[5] but perhaps in doing so they have forged an identity for themselves which is inconsistent with more 'mainstream' nursing identities.

This chapter concentrates on the role of mental health nurses and developments in the craft of caring within this context. We are conscious that the luxury of such services is not freely available to large portions of the international community. Therefore, as indicated, this chapter examines the socio-cultural environment in which mental health nurses work within higher-income countries, and we recognize this as a limitation of international service provision.

THE EVOLVING NEED FOR COMMUNITY MENTAL HEALTH SERVICES

In many countries in the developed world, 'community care' is an evolving concept. Until the middle of the twentieth century, most mental health care for serious and enduring mental illnesses was provided within institutional settings, where the concept of rehabilitation was largely linked with work in the institutional laundry, kitchen, farm or gardens, and later in occupational or industrial therapy units where the facilities were designed to simulate real-life work settings.[6]

By the 1950s, there were a number of socioeconomic and political developments that made the evolution of alternative systems of mental health care possible. These included the development of phenothiazine medications, as well as other pharmacological initiatives. Additionally, increases in the costs of institutional care and the overcrowding of asylums occurred, coinciding with the evolution of the consumer movement. Essentially, deinstitutionalization efforts from the 1950s to the end of the twentieth century were part of a growing mental health reform movement that revolved around the broad concept of 'recovery', with an increased emphasis on a person-centred approach.

By the beginning of the current century, within an environment that increasingly emphasized the importance of 'evidence-based practice', some sought to identify the evidence that underpins the concept of 'recovery', which might include the ability to engage in work, study, engage in leisure pursuits in normative settings, as well as the ability to maintain normal relationships.[7] It has been argued that this reorientation of services promotes greater social inclusion.[2] One of the most influential figures in the consumer movement and the founder of the Wellness and Recovery Action Planning movement, Mary Ellen Copeland,[8] argued that recovery is based upon 'hope', 'personal responsibility', 'education', 'self advocacy' and 'support' – thus emphasizing personal responsibility and personal involvement in one's own health and well-being.

While the focus on the individual is important in emphasizing people's human rights, and in the development of indicators that might measure treatment outcomes, there is also a danger that this focus may not accommodate the wider ecological context in which recovery occurs,[5] thus placing the onus on service users to collaborate with other individuals and social systems to support recovery.

While individuals have limited control over their macro environment, or matters such as poverty, victimization, physical or sexual abuse and exploitation, they normally have greater control over their micro environment, and can influence their own well-being where they have the ability to understand, accept, manage or cope with their own levels of functioning. However, well-being is also influenced by people's own views of their situation, their perceptions of their health status, their self-esteem, cognitive processes, knowledge and insight[9] These have all been identified as determinants of health, or indeed layers of influence.[10, 11]

Community mental health services have tended to distinguish themselves from institutionally based care models by their greater emphasis on a 'recovery' orientation.[12] Chapters 35 and 36 of this book provide comprehensive definitions of the concept of recovery, as well as a view of what recovery-orientated services might look like. Chapter 35 highlights the individual experience of recovery, and in particular suggests that recovery may be a 'journey' which is experienced very differently at different points of the recovery process itself. Chapter 36 highlights the need for services which claim to be recovery-orientated to be characterized by a collaborative approach which values and places the voice of the service user at its centre. Services should be concerned with individual recovery, as well as systemic approaches to the factors that influence health. This demands a service ethos which is explicitly aware of the socio-political environment in which they operate, and proactively promotes inclusive practice and involvement among service users and providers alike. However, there may well be a distinction between the rhetoric of organizations which claim to be recovery-orientated and the actual experience of service users. For example, one recent Irish study reported that service users had little involvement in determining or influencing their treatment options, despite the policy commitment in Ireland to service user involvement.[13] Chapter 36 clearly outlines the fact that recovery-orientated services are rooted in an ethos of respect and mutuality as well as individuality. It points out that recovery-orientated services require organizational commitment and, for many traditional services, transformative change that promotes citizenship. However, according to some authors, service users' attempts to influence service planning and delivery challenge the general ethos of health service structures and power alignments, and while ostensibly service providers may argue that they are committed to service user involvement, the rhetoric is not always matched by the reality.[14] Service users tend to emphasize the social model of disability, favouring a holistic understanding of mental illness and distress that encompasses personal, spiritual, cultural and broader social and interpersonal concerns.

In at least one study, recovery was identified by consumers as constituting 'psychological' recovery from the consequences of the illness,[15] aligning the concept of recovery with the restoration of mental well-being (and this is certainly reflected in the reports in chapter 35 from service users at different stages of their recovery trajectory). This is an interesting conceptualization, in that it is perhaps less holistic than might be expected. The same

authors also identified four key processes associated with 'recovery', namely: (i) finding hope; (ii) re-establishment of identity; (iii) finding meaning in life; and (iv) taking responsibility for recovery. These key processes have been more recently echoed by other authors, who added 'empowerment', 'achieving a sense of agency' and 'coping',[5] which again certainly seem consistent with the types of sentiment expressed by service users in chapter 35.

While MHSUs may have limited control over the macro environment, including the community mental health services they receive, their efforts to influence the delivery of these services increases the pressure on CMHNs to provide recovery-orientated, collaborative and holistic care. (More on collaborative care planning can be found in chapter 50.) In order to fulfil the ethos of a 'recovery orientation', the macro and micro contexts of MHSUs' lives must be bridged, and thus CMHNs are positioned at the interface between the system of care and the MHSU. The macro and micro environments of service users (in which the CMHN operates) are interlinked. Practitioners have ethical and legal responsibilities to ensure that care provision structures take account of these layers of interconnectedness. Failure to be conscious (at least) of the wider socio-economic and political context in which practitioners and MHSUs operate (that is, the macro environment) may negate efforts to improve the health and well-being of individual MHSUs (that is, the micro environment), which, as previously stated, demands a socio-politically aware ethos on the part of health service providers. Consequently, it may be a challenge for CMHNs to align the general rhetoric of a 'recovery ethos' with the reality of all that this approach entails.

THE ROLE OF CMHNs IN PROMOTING OR SUPPORTING RECOVERY FOR INDIVIDUAL CLIENTS AND CLIENT GROUPS

The evolving role of CMHNs

Community mental health nursing has evolved over the past 60 odd years, and in many countries CMHNs are seen as pivotal to the delivery of mental health services. A number of reviews in the UK since 2006 have concluded that mental health nurses are a key resource in the effective delivery of a modern health service. However, all of these reports also highlighted the need for mental health nurses to embrace the recovery approach, to improve their skills in the delivery of psychological therapies, to promote physical health, and to focus on working with people with severe mental health problems.[16] This view of the multifaceted role of mental health nursing, and of community-based nurses specifically, is shared by service users, who regard the role as being concerned with the delivery of both practical and social support, as well as more formal psychological therapies,[17] which reflects developments in the craft of caring within services.

Others point out that the many different roles played by mental health nurses include those of clinicians, case managers, clinical nurse specialists and nurse practitioners in mental health care settings.[18] Mental health nurses are involved in the delivery of psychosocial interventions, and are mandated to work using a recovery-based ethos, in both primary care and residential-based services. They engage in direct client work and in medication management, and they support carers and advocacy groups. At the beginning of this century, the WHO recognized the central role played by CMHNs in multidisciplinary teams in the management of mental illness.[19] Others argue that health promotion is an important aspect of nursing generally, but somewhat under-recognized in the case of mental health care.[20] However, some authors comment that mental health nurses, especially those in community or primary care settings, are ideally placed to fulfil illness prevention and health promotion roles.[21] (More on medication management and the mental health nurse can be found in chapter 48.)

There is little doubt that mental health service reform has had a major international impact in the last half-century or more. CMHNs have been at the forefront of service provision and have widened service availability to include groups which had not received mental health care in the past. The professional cohort of CMHNs could not have come into existence had it not been for efforts to implement the policy of reducing reliance on inpatient services. Arguably, therefore, the introduction of community care precipitated the distinctive grade of CMHNs, and the relationship that CMHNs developed with other professionals – principally medical practitioners – facilitated their professional evolution. Their initial alignment with psychiatrists supported opportunities for professional development, while later GPs enabled greater autonomy for CMHNs in primary care. This professional closeness has also led to tensions and arguments, as a result of which CMHNs need to ensure that their roles are distinctive in order to ensure professional survival and development.[22]

While CMHNs appear to have adapted to enormous changes in community mental health provision, they arguably enjoy less autonomy because of an increase in multidisciplinary teamwork. Additionally, the service user and consumerist movement has gathered momentum, influencing changes that reflect the expressed needs of service users. The employment of peer support workers (PSWs) within community mental health services now impels CMHNs to modify their roles further and to develop new ways of working. According to Godin,[22] the survival of CMHNs is in question, and his warning has arguably come into sharp focus in the light of the increased involvement of service users in community mental health care and in mental health services overall. Carr[23] sums up the situation:

Analysis of the current situation suggests that such participation is challenging the very fabric of the institutions in which it is taking place, exposing problems with the political, strategic and structural elements of established non-user organizations. On many levels traditional power relations are being unsettled. The conceptual clash between citizenship and consumerism is being exposed as participation becomes more widespread and sites of resistance are revealed. (p.266)

Working with persons with serious and enduring mental illness

One of the key areas where community mental health nursing is seen as important is in the care of those with serious and enduring mental health problems. Working with such MHSUs is challenging, but efforts have been made to identify the core contributions of CMHNs in the care of such people. For example, it has been proposed that there are five areas that characterize the contribution of CMHNs, namely: development of therapeutic relationships; relapse prevention; enhancement of social function; stimulation of medication adherence; and support of family members.[24] Likewise, it has been argued that these nurses are ideally placed to address policy trends towards more integrated care, as well as health providers' concerns about the high incidence of physical disorders among MHSUs, because of their training, which draws on five sciences, namely medical science, neuroscience, psychiatry, relationship science and psychotherapy.[25]

SERVICE USER'S PERSPECTIVE: MOVING FROM HOSPITAL TO COMMUNITY CARE

The MHSU agreed to the discharge care plan as a condition of discharge, but did not view the process positively, as illustrated by the following statement on the transition from hospital to the community.

I came out of hospital 2 weeks ago and now they sent me a care plan; it made me a bit annoyed and made me feel like I was still a patient because 'Mental Health Trust' was printed across the top. Anyway I got out of hospital because I said it was OK for a nurse to visit me. Before I went into hospital I was thinking bad things, like kill yourself like this or with that. When I was in hospital there were so many different people working there so you can have a different person talking to you each time and I thought they were checking me out and then talking to each other about me even though they were friendly. Then sometimes they didn't speak to me but just talked between themselves and then said about diagnosis and stuff.

R.T.

More recently it has been reported that the work of CMHNs (at least in terms of first-episode psychosis) tends to be 'behind the scenes' and arguably somewhat invisible.[26] This invisibility perhaps reflects the institutional origins of psychiatric nursing, which were largely within medicalized models of care. When nurses moved to community care settings, this invisibility continued in many ways. Others have noted that CMHNs' invisibility may have been a pragmatic approach to professional survival. CMHNs have continually adapted and reinvented themselves to remain relevant in a dynamic policy context.[5] They arguably shifted from traditional nursing roles to become counsellors, therapists and befrienders to service users, and in that sense assumed roles more commonly associated with other professional groups.

The work of many CMHNs tends to focus almost exclusively on those with serious and enduring mental illness and also tends to draw on two treatment modalities, namely assertive community treatment and clinical case management.[27] This was consistent with the origins of CMHNs, since their original work mainly focused on post-discharge care of those who had been hospitalized, and thus their expertise evolved in relation to those with serious and enduring mental illnesses. Likewise, policy shifts in health care provision internationally have continually advocated the provision of care in the least restrictive environment, and also in community settings wherever possible, even for those with serious and enduring mental illnesses.

However, it may be wise for CMHNs and policy makers to reflect on the future needs of the population rather than remaining focused on the traditions and earlier incarnations of community mental health nursing. With an increasingly ageing population, it has been estimated that significant demand for appropriate mental health care for older persons will be needed in the future,[28] and perhaps this will require greater attention from CMHNs if they are to remain a responsive and relevant element of the health care workforce.

HEALTH PROMOTION AND ILLNESS PREVENTION ROLES

Utilizing a sizeable part of a workforce to support the rehabilitative and recovery needs of persons who have already been diagnosed with serious mental disorders is a necessary and worthy aspect of health service provision. Within the context of the craft of caring, it is vital to support people to maximize their potential and achieve optimal levels of functioning. However, arguably from a systemic perspective it is somewhat like locking the stable door after the horse has bolted.

One of the distinguishing characteristics of the professional ideology of nursing is that it is committed to a holistic view of the person, and it has been recognized that 'nurses have also led the health care profession in recognizing that health is a state of physical and mental wellness and that it is impossible to separate the former from the latter'[21] (p.105). Both health promotion and illness prevention are essential aspects of any health professional's role, even though they are frequently not attended to sufficiently.[29]

Mental health promotion 'is concerned with achieving positive mental health and well-being in the general population as well as addressing the needs of those at risk from, or experiencing, mental health problems'[30] (p.131). This implies a focus on the wider population as well as the individual at risk, and if a health-promoting ethos is to be form part of the role of community mental health nursing, then a culture shift in the education, practice and research of practitioners is necessary.

Mental health promotion should happen at a range of different levels (that is, at an individual, community and population level) and ideally there should be evidence of coherence between the levels at which mental health promotion occurs and the different 'settings' in which mental health is promoted. Within an overall population context, there will always be a need to pay particular attention to subsets of the population or take a targeted population approach (for groups that might be considered 'at risk'), with an emphasis on prevention. (For more on mental health promotion, see chapter 70.)

At its core, mental health promotion seeks to empower people, groups and communities through facilitating, teaching and supporting them to maximize their mental health.[29] Community and arguably individual empowerment can involve 'political' action, which might include facilitation of community-level interventions, activism, policy formulation and development, as well as a focus on individuals. CMHNs are arguably ideally placed to fulfil these types of roles at both the individual and the community level.

At an individual level, the Institute of Medicine has argued that practitioners' work should be focused on 'efforts to enhance individuals' abilities to achieve developmentally appropriate tasks (developmental competence) with a positive sense of self-esteem, mastery, wellbeing and social inclusion and to strengthen their ability to cope with adversity'[31] (p.67). In that sense, mental health promotion is for everyone, but surely those best positioned to provide leadership in relation to mental health promotion within community-based health teams would be those who have long subscribed to holistic views of humanity and have expertise in mental health – namely, CMHNs.

The effective improvement of the health of the population through health promotion requires many organizations and health care disciplines to work together. CMHNs are also well placed to participate in educational programmes for community groups and the public, and to endorse recovery, mental health promotion, social inclusion and vocational integration with other professionals. Through their work with MHSUs, their families and carers, they can provide links to organizations that engage in mental health promotion activities to enhance and sustain mental health.

REFLECTION

How can CMHNs engage in health promotion activities at a population level and demonstrate a distinctive contribution in this field?

CMHNs AND THE SERVICE USER MOVEMENT

Background

The participation of the public in the design and implementation of health care was designated as 'a right and duty' in the Alma Ata Declaration in 1978.[32] It was argued that incorporating varieties of views, experiences and expertise into the decision-making process promotes acceptance of policies and increases the responsibilities of the public for implementation.[33] Currently, the involvement of service users in mental health policy, planning and legislation is an intrinsic aspect of the new WHO Mental Health Action Plan.[34] Although individual choice may not be directly linked to systemic decision making, the collective impact of individual choices could change health policy.

Service user involvement in the planning and provision of services has grown, particularly in countries where mental health services have moved from institutions to the community,[35] but some perceive that the consumerist movement is driven by service providers. Their interest is to conserve budgets and promote efficiency, while offering customers or consumers a choice. Conversely, democratic approaches stem from service user organizations, whose main aim is to empower users to voice their concerns.[36]

However, a report by the WHO in 2010 on European systems of MHSU involvement stated that the Netherlands and the UK are the only countries that have passed laws associated with their participation in health care strategies.[37] Other European countries have adopted community systems with mechanisms to address MHSUs' rights and complaints. The findings of the report were based on the collection of baseline data in 42 countries in the European zone. The results revealed a paucity of evidence on systematic, significant MHSU or carer participation in ensuring the quality of mental health services. However, a recent qualitative study revealed that multidisciplinary mental health guidelines have incorporated MHSUs' views to some degree in the Netherlands.[38]

Constructions of the term 'service user'

At the level of care provision, the effective input of service users in influencing the direction and types of mental health services they receive is termed 'user involvement'. Specific developments in mental health services are also influenced by a consumer-focused movement that is based on receptiveness to service users' requirements, and by demands for shared decision making in treatment planning.

The language used to describe those who use mental health services is important in the avoidance of further social exclusion. A consumerist stance is challenged on the grounds that referring to service users as consumers, rather than as equal citizens with the right to mental health provision, further marginalizes them, so that they are perceived as impaired, dependent and uninvolved in normal society.[39] This position finds other supporters, who challenge the consumerist perspective by urging mental health nurses to promote more meaningful user involvement by identifying and giving voice to the positive resources and potentials of service users.[40] Others emphasize the role of nurses in facilitating true service user involvement, which may be attained with a shift in the use of the rhetoric associated with the phrase, by allowing service users to choose their own words to describe their relationships with services.[41]

These criticisms may have arisen because there appears to be no clear definition of service user involvement in mental health. An exploration of the literature shows that there are many variations in the interpretations of the term 'service user' by users, professionals and organizations. The different terms that are used – including client, patient, consumer, customer, expert by experience, survivor and service user – underscore the relationship between those who use and those who provide services. McLaughlin[42] has argued that, although the term 'service user' is in common parlance in health care, the term cannot incorporate the complicated facets of the relationship between service providers and recipients of care. One definition that is used in a number of service user involvement and primary care framework documents[43,44] says that:

> Service user involvement is simply a process by which people are enabled to become actively and genuinely involved in defining the issues of concern to them, in making decisions about factors that affect their lives, in formulating polices, in planning, developing and delivering services and in taking action to achieve change.[43]

However, the UK document[44] also identifies associated meanings intrinsic to the above definition, including leadership, peer support and co-production. All of these domains require the equal input of MHSUs with peer supporters in the planning and delivery of care, with the lived experiences of service users as a key reference point. Clearly, a problem with power relations is undermining service users' efforts to effect change.[23] Carr also thought that this problem stems from differing constructions of the meaning of service user involvement. She maintained that there is a disparity between the interpretations of involvement among health services, whose construction of the concept originates from a consumerist orientation, and those of service users. Mental health services have tended to view their participation as a means of engendering increased social inclusion and as a channel for the development of communication with other service users.

Power relations

There is evidence that certain groups – such as black and ethnic minority groups, as well as people from lower socio-economic groups and those with communication difficulties – are still failing to have their voices heard.[45,46] In that context it is hardly surprising that criticisms have arisen about a perceived divergence between the rhetoric and reality of service user involvement, as well as its intent. As far back as 1993, Beresford and Croft warned that increased MHSU involvement may not necessarily make service users more empowered, or health services more person-centred.[47] They identified other purposes behind the cloak of empowerment, which they referred to as 'incorporation', meaning that people are pulled into agreements by services that restrict and redirect their abilities to effect change. They used the term 'legitimation' to refer to the tendency to promote user involvement as a means of presenting an outward show of consensus so that service user involvement becomes an exercise in public relations, which conceals the lack of true participation.[47]

Reports from the Joseph Rowntree Foundation in 2003[48] and 2010[49] on the views of users about their involvement in the direction of services identified key difficulties relating to funding, tokenism and superficiality. Moreover, service users' experiential knowledge of mental illness was not taken seriously and was regarded as less worthwhile than that of professionals, though service users perceived that their own understanding was the most important means of exerting more impact on mental health services. The negation of their experiential knowledge and their unsuccessful attempts to have an equal say in service provision were disempowering and alienating experiences for MHSUs. Additionally, certain people experienced even more exclusion, including black and minority ethnic groups, older people and those with communication problems. Those interviewed stressed the crucial role of networking among service users, individually and in user-led forums, as these interactions served as a means of improving their quality of life and enabled them to continue trying to exert a strong voice.

Moves have been made to promote MHSU involvement in Ireland in various public bodies, such as the Mental Health Commission. These developments indirectly point to a philosophical and socio-political shift from a lack of attention to individual choice for people suffering from mental illness towards egalitarianism. While acknowledging the radicalism of these developments, in common with other researchers, McEvoy et al.[50] found that tokenistic structures exist for MHSU involvement and that people are insufficiently supported in their efforts to participate in health services forums. They argued that rebalanced systems are needed, in which MHSUs' experiences can be listened to, as they have much to contribute to mental health service provision by sharing experiential knowledge. In the UK the Community Health Survey, involving 13,500 participants, identified certain positive results but also highlighted the need for progress in many other areas covered in the questionnaire.[51] These included communication and information, reviews of care, involvement in decision making, and provision of understanding and support for other problematic areas besides mental health issues.

These reports on service user involvement from the UK and Ireland suggest that service users might be helped to express their views if they were accompanied to these decision-making forums by CMHNs – a suggestion which supports the view that nurses could promote meaningful participation on behalf of the people they serve.[40] However, advocating for MHSUs at these forums might be challenging for nurses, as they may find their loyalties divided between MHSUs and their employers.

This overview of the current situation suggests that moves to address the expressed needs of MHSUs have occurred, but developments are still partial and inconsistent. A statement by the WHO delineates empowerment and discusses the demands of this requirement, concluding that without the alignment of individual, service and social levels, empowerment activities will be ineffective, while stigma and discrimination will continue.[37]

Ideally, the work of the CMHN should take into account the priorities of MHSUs by providing truly client-centred care, which, as previously discussed, embodies the recovery-orientated focus of health care structures – which is not always consistently applied in practice. Chapter 3 of this book highlights the centrality of the relationship between service users and mental health professionals, especially nurses. Even though ways to restructure care, and new ways of working with MHSUs, those close to them and PSWs, need to be introduced in order to empower service users to take more control over their own mental health, the centrality of the therapeutic alliance with clients needs to be maintained.

The increasing orientation towards recovery-based community services and methods of shared decision making were pioneered by CMHNs, who carved out a place for themselves in the communities they served. Now, they face further challenges in preserving their relationships with MHSUs in the current context of health care. In chapter 3 of this book, Stenhouse and Muirhead correctly argue that the relationship between client and nurse needs to be 'grounded in equality, reciprocity and level playing fields' and in essence should involve a 'co-journeying' process or a partnership approach. This may be a challenge, as the increase in the statutory functions of the CMHN role forces an acknowledgement of the power differential that underpins their relationships with MHSUs. Issues of power and indeed power imbalances are obvious when working with involuntary service users. Indeed, the role of mental health nurses in the containment and involuntary detention of service users has been a long-standing function associated with hospital-based services in

particular. However, the capacity to set control functions in motion for voluntary service users is a more recent development and may not be as openly acknowledged by CMHNs in their work with MHSUs, but it has equally tangible consequences for service users. In order to preserve their relationships with MHSUs, the time is ripe to implement dialogues with service users that incorporate issues related to the dual therapeutic and containment functions of the CMHN's role. Although such issues may be difficult to address, they potentially impact on the meaningful empowered engagement of MHSUs in determining their care trajectories. In the case of CMHNs, recognition of a more empowered client group and the altered relationships associated with this development will demand further reflections on what is meant by the craft of caring in the community mental health setting.

> ## REFLECTION
>
> What should the 'ideal' relationship be between CMHNs and service users?

THE CHANGING ROLE OF THE CMHN AND MHSUs

> ## SERVICE USER'S PERSPECTIVE: MEDICATION MANAGEMENT AND SUPPORTING ADVOCACY
>
> *A traditional role of CMHNs has been medication management. In common with many MHSUs, this commentator was worried about the side effects of medication, as illustrated by this statement.*
>
> The drugs are making me fat, they did before, and most days I spend all afternoon sleeping. The community nurse told me that I could ask for my medication to be reviewed to see if I was on too much and she is going with me when I see the psychiatrist and she is making me an appointment with a dietician.
>
> *J.B.*

Policy changes in mental health may challenge the adjustment of CMHNs to new ways of working with clients who are becoming radicalized within service user networks and even further in working with PSWs. Further challenges are being faced; for example, in a submission to the Department of Health, the *Royal College of Nursing*[52] strongly argued that community treatment orders, incorporated in the Mental Health Act 2007, had the potential to damage the essential therapeutic relationships between clients and CMHNs. In the past, the risk of harming the therapeutic relationship was ameliorated, as legal controls were implemented by psychiatrists, GPs and social workers,

but now CMHNs may experience the full impact on their relationships with MHSUs in taking direct responsibility for these measures.[53] Chapter 3 notes that empathy, authenticity and congruence are the main qualities or attributes of effective interpersonal nursing and are essential to a therapeutic relationship. However, the same chapter also notes that friction may also be a natural feature of the relationship between client and nurse or health professional.

Nowhere is this friction perhaps more evident than in the fundamental contradiction that exists in mental health care, and arguably more so in community mental health care than in any other nursing or caring context. There is a basic conflict within mental health care, whereby services and practitioners present themselves as caring and co-journeying and in partnership with service users, when simultaneously detention and treatment can be enforced against the person's will. This power on the part of service providers directly challenges concepts of equity, as well as service user empowerment and involvement. This dichotomy is evident in the findings of a qualitative interview study of people on legally enforced community treatment orders, who were regarded as a risk to themselves or others, and professionals who provide care. Professionals reported that they were kind to MHSUs, and ethical in their practices, while using empathy with the MHSUs' experiences to reduce the impact of the coercive nature of the situation. However, most service user participants perceived the experience as a moral judgement and as a punitive measure for wrongdoing. Further, they perceived a lack of trust on the part of professionals and that their perceived failings had to be corrected by the imposition of care that mitigated their full involvement in recovery.[54] These developments in the role of CMHNs suggest that they may be being redirected into containment rather than a therapeutic function within

mental health services, with an increase in the input of PSWs, who may occupy aspects of the CMHN's hard-won therapeutic role.

SERVICE USER'S PERSPECTIVE: THE INCREASING EMPHASIS ON A PERSON-CENTRED APPROACH TO RECOVERY

This statement illustrates the development of the therapeutic relationship as a basis for recovery.

What I like about her [the CMHN] is that she listens to me and she sees that I didn't just have a breakdown out of nowhere. We looked back at the warning signs of it building up to help me if, please God it doesn't, ever happen again. I think I might have to stay on tablets even though I don't like taking them because they keep me steady when things go wrong. We have talked about what

she calls 'a recovery plan' so that maybe I can get back to where I was before or be even better. Next time she comes my Mum and my sister are coming round. I am glad she is going to be there because they had so much to put up with because of all the stuff I did when I was high and maybe she will help them understand more about what happened and what I need to do now.

A.C.

PEER SUPPORT WORKERS

SERVICE USER'S PERSPECTIVE: SUPPORT FROM OTHER MHSUS

The importance of the shared experiences of mental illness is illustrated by the following statement.

The other people in the ward were the ones who helped me. We were all in the same boat. My friend comes to see me nearly every day and if she doesn't come she phones me, she has been in hospital herself so she knows what it's like and she has the same thing as me, but she tries to make me feel better by talking about her and what she does to stop herself getting down. Sometimes that gets on my nerves but she does know what it's like.

R.M.

The employment of mental health workers with experiential knowledge of mental illness is regarded as one of the most pervasive means of reorienting mental health services to focus on the aims of service users. In a review of the literature, Simpson and House concluded that users of mental health services can be employed by mental health services without great problems.[55] These workers had a positive impact on trainees and elicited criticism of services that would not have been expressed by service users in another context. The Royal College of Psychiatrists also asserts that the inclusion of these workers could radically reorient mental health services.[56] Peer specialists could be employed to work in teams and elsewhere in health services, and the report pointed to examples from the UK and the USA where services became focused on the needs of service users as a result of these innovations. In North America, calls for the extensive involvement of PSWs

within all mental health services stemmed from the recovery movement and from research on these services. There is also a call for financial backing for consumer-led programmes that may lack a strong evidence base but are preferred by recipients of services.[57]

An Australian study highlighted important characteristics of effective consumer-led services where PSWs were involved. One of the main positive factors reported by service users was the perceived credibility of the PSW based on the fact that the PSW had personal experience of mental illness. They also reported improvement in the discharge experience and in continuity of care, with respondents reporting better community support, which they saw as being related to the efforts of the PSW. There was increased trust in the PSWs because they appreciated what service users were experiencing and used non-medical terms.[58] An analysis of two state-wide projects in Vermont and Minnesota, in which PSWs taught MHSUs self-management skills, identified significant changes in self-management attitudes and skills of 76 per cent of participants.[59] A review of the literature[60] on the employment of PSWs in mental health services concluded:

Clearly there has been exponential growth in the employment of peer support workers (PSWs) in the US, Australia and New Zealand over the past decade and more recently this expansion has spread to the UK. The focus of all recent mental health policy upon Recovery focused practice appears to be a key driver for these initiatives. (p.392)

According to the authors, controlled research trials indicated that PSWs do not have any effect on the mental health outcomes of service users. However, when a broader group of studies was considered, the beneficial effects of PSWs became apparent. It was evident that PSWs are more capable than professionals of instilling hope and confidence in the potential for recovery, and promoting self-esteem, better self-management and a decrease in social inclusion. The study concludes that these outcomes are parallel factors in recovery identified by people with experiences of mental illness.[60]

However, in a recent qualitative comparative study, several areas of concern were identified in relation to the employment of PSWs. The findings indicated that lived experiences, though valuable, needed to be augmented by interpersonal skills, dedication and resilience. Peer supporters experienced difficulties in expressing concerns about certain attitudes of professionals towards service users. Managerial support for PSWs who required debriefing was inconsistent, and stigmatizing attitudes and a lack of support from staff were also

apparent.[61] Although the study provided an understanding of the experiences of PSWs, their effectiveness in improving MHSUs' outcomes could not be ascertained. The authors concluded that a randomized controlled trial measuring peer support versus usual care was required.

According to the Joseph Rowntree Foundation,[49] PSWs are trusted by users and they can help to manage and strengthen connections between staff and users. Nevertheless, the authors found that PSWs could also be obstructive and, in some boroughs, workers were inconsistent in their support for service users or, if they worked for a voluntary organization, were torn between the role of employee and that of PSW. Service users delineated three distinct approaches by services to their involvement: services could be open to communication; superficially open, but in essence unwilling; or not open.

CONCLUSION

An examination of the rise in service user involvement in mental health services indicates that this is exerting pressure on existing services to rebalance structures in order to provide more choice, representation and voice to the people who use these services. These developments challenge the future direction of CMHNs: on the one hand professionals are urged to adopt more inclusive practices, while on the other hand mental health policies are also increasing the containment functions of CMHNs' roles in the community. Further challenges are presented by the negotiation of complex boundaries between service users' wishes, the input of PSWs, and institutional and social pressures to meet the

fundamental duty of safeguarding the MHSU and the public from harm. Perhaps CMHNs will continue to need to refine their own view of their roles, and identify and engage in relationships that are empathic, genuine, congruent, client-focused and respectful. Equally, they probably need to develop typologies of discourse with clients which avoid further stigmatization through the use of language that marginalizes individuals or inadvertently impedes clients' rights to fully empowered and equitable citizenship. All of these developments require CMHNs to continue to reflect on their evolving roles for those requiring collaborative and empowering services now and in the future.

References

1. Barker P. *Psychiatric and mental health nursing: the craft of caring*, 2nd edn. Boca Raton: Hodder Arnold, 2008.
2. WHO (World Health Organization). *Mental health action plan 2013–2020*. Geneva: WHO, 2013.
3. Cunningham G, Slevin E. Community psychiatric nursing's focus on effectiveness. *Journal of Psychiatric and Mental Health Nursing* 2005; **12**(1): 14–22.
4. Barker P, Buchanan-Barker P. Still invisible after all these years: mental health nursing on the margins. *Journal of Psychiatric and Mental Health Nursing* 2005; **12**(2): 252–6.
5. Crawford P, Brown B, Majomic P. Professional identity in community mental health nursing: a thematic analysis. *International Journal of Nursing Studies* 2008; **45**: 1055–63.
6. Killaspy H. Contemporary mental health rehabilitation. *East Asian Archives of Psychiatry* 2014; **24**(3): 89–94.
7. Liberman RP, Kopelowicz A. Recovery from schizophrenia: a challenge for the 21st century. *International Review of Psychiatry* 2002; **14**(4): 245–55.
8. Copeland ME. Wellness Recovery Action Plan. Available from: http://www.mentalhealthrecovery.com [Accessed 4th July 2016].
9. Ryan D, Mannix McNamara P, Deasy C. *Health promotion in Ireland: principles, practice and research*. Dublin: Gill and MacMillan, 2006.
10. Perese EF. Stigma, poverty, and victimization: roadblocks to recovery for individuals with severe mental illness. *Journal of the American Psychiatric Nurses Association* 2007; **13**(5): 285–95.
11. Dahlgren G, Whitehead M. *Policies and strategies to promote social equity in health*. Stockholm: Institute for Future Studies, 1991.
12. Gale J, Marshal-Lucette S. Community mental health nurses' perspectives of recovery-oriented practice. *Journal of Psychiatric and Mental Health Nursing* 2012; **19**(4): 348–53.
13. King A. Service user involvement in methadone maintenance programmes: the philosophy, the ideal and the reality. *Drugs: Education, Prevention and Policy* 2011; **18**: 276–84.
14. Van Hout MC, McElrath K. Service user involvement in drug treatment programmes: barriers to implementation and potential benefits for client recovery. *Drugs: Education, Prevention and Policy* 2012; **19**(6): 474–83.
15. Andresen R, Oades L, Caputi P. The experience of recovery from schizophrenia: towards an empirically validated stage model. *Australian & New Zealand Journal of Psychiatry* 2003; **37**(5): 586–94.
16. Higgins A, Callaghan P, deVries J, Keogh B, Morrissey J, Nash M, Ryan D, Gjibles H, Carter T. Evaluation of mental health recovery and wellness recovery action planning education in Ireland: a mixed methods pre–postevaluation. *Journal of Advanced Nursing* 2012; **68**(11): 2418–28.
17. Bee P, Playle J, Lovell K, Barnes P, Gray R, Keeley P. Service user views and expectations of UK-registered mental health nurses: a systematic review of empirical research. *International Journal of Nursing Studies* 2008; **45**: 442–57.
18. Hercelinskyj G, Cruickshank M, Brown P, Phillips B. Perceptions from the front line: professional identity in mental health nursing. *International Journal of Mental Health Nursing* 2014; **23**(1): 24–32.

19. WHO (World Health Organization). *The world health report: 2001: mental health: new understanding, new hope*. Geneva: WHO, 2001.

20. Verhaeghe N, Maeseneer J, Maes L, Heeringen C, Annemans L. Health promotion in mental health care: perceptions from patients and mental health nurses. *Journal of Clinical Nursing* 2013; **22**(11–12): 1569–78.

21. Calloway S. Mental health promotion: is nursing dropping the ball? *Journal of Professional Nursing* 2007; **23**(2): 105–9.

22. Godin P. The development of community psychiatric nursing: a professional project? *Journal of Advanced Nursing* 2008; **23**(5): 925–34.

23. Carr S. Participation, power, conflict and change: Theorizing dynamics of service user participation in the social care system of England and Wales. *Critical Social Policy* 2007; **27**(2): 268–76.

24. Dusseldorp LV, Goossens P and Achterberg TV. Mental health nursing and first episode psychosis. *Issues in Mental Health Nursing* 2011; **32**: 2–19.

25. Delaney KR. Psychiatric mental health nursing: why 2011 brings a pivotal moment. *Journal of Nursing Education and Practice* 2011; **1**(1): 42.

26. Moe C, Kvig EI, Brinchmann B, Brinchmann BS. Working behind the scenes: an ethical view of mental health nursing and first-episode psychosis. *Nursing Ethics* 2012; **20**(5): 517–27.

27. Wallace T, O'Connell S, Frisch S. Community psychiatric practice – what do nurses do when they take to the streets? An analysis of psychiatric and mental health nursing interventions in the community. *Community Mental Health Journal* 2005; **41**(4): 481–96.

28. Thompson P, Lang L, Annells M. A systematic review of the effectiveness of in-home community nurse led interventions for the mental health of older persons. *Journal of Clinical Nursing* 2008; **17**(11): 1419–27.

29. Ryan D, Deasy C. Mental health and mental health promotion. In: Morrisey J, Keogh B, Doyle L (eds). *Psychiatric mental health nursing: an Irish perspective*. Dublin: Gill and Macmillan, 2008.

30. Wand T. Real mental health promotion requires a reorientation of nursing education, practice and research. *Journal of Psychiatric and Mental Health Nursing* 2011; **18**(2): 131–8.

31. National Research Council and Institute of Medicine. *Preventing mental, emotional, and behavioral disorders among young people: progress and possibilities*. Washington, DC: National Academies Press, 2009.

32. WHO (World Health Organization). *Declaration of Alma-Ata*. Copenhagen: WHO Regional Office for Europe, 1978. Available from: http://www.euro.who.int/en/publications/policy-documents/declaration-of-alma-ata,-1978 [Accessed 5th August 2016].

33. WHO (World Health Organization). The world health report 2006. Available from: www.who.int/whr/2006/whr06_en.pdf [Accessed 4th July 2016].

34. WHO (World Health Organization). Development of a global health action plan. 2012. Available from: http://www.who.int/mental_health/mhgap/consultation_global_mh_action_plan_2013_2020/en/ [Accessed 5th August 2016].

35. Thornicroft G, Tansella M. Growing recognition of the importance of service user involvement in mental health service planning. *Epidemiologia e Psichiatria Sociale* 2005; **14**(1): 1–3.

36. Heikkila M, Julkunen I. *Obstacles to an increased user involvement in social services. A commissioned background document*. Stakes, Finland: Group of Specialists in Social Services (CS-US), 2003.

37. WHO (World Health Organization). *User empowerment in mental health: a statement by the WHO Regional Office for Europe*. Copenhagen: WHO, 2010.

38. Van der Ham A, Shields L, van der Horst R, Broerse J, van Tulder M. Facilitators and barriers to service user involvement in mental health guidelines: lessons from the Netherlands. *Administration and Policy in Mental Health* 2014; **41**(6): 712–23.

39. Lewis L. Politics of recognition: what can a human rights perspective contribute to understanding users' experiences of involvement in mental health services? *Social Policy and Society* 2009; **8**(2): 257–74.

40. Roberts M. Service user involvement and the restrictive sense of psychiatric categories: the challenge facing mental health nurses. *Journal of Psychiatric and Mental Health Nursing* 2009; **17**(4): 289–94.

41. Hui A, Stickley T. Mental health policy and mental health service user perspectives on involvement: a discourse analysis. *Journal of Advanced Nursing* 2007; **59**(4): 416–26.

42. McLaughlin H. What's in a name: 'client', 'patient', 'customer', 'consumer', 'expert by experience', 'service user' – what's next? *British Journal of Social Work* 2009; **39**(6): 1101–17.

43. Health Service Executive. Service user involvement and primary care: framework document. 2011. Available from: http://lenus.ie/hse/bitstream/10147/305219/1/ServiceUserInvolvement.pdf [Accessed 5th August 2016].

44. NSUN (National Survivor User Network). Summary of work. 2014. Available from: www.nsun.org.uk/about-us/our-work/2014-summary-of-work/ [Accessed 4th July 2016].

45. Rutter D, Manley C, Weaver T, Crawford M, Fulop N. Patients or partners? Case studies of user involvement in the planning and delivery of adult mental health services in London. *Social Science & Medicine* 2004; **58**(10): 1973–84.

46. Beresford P. Making service user involvement work: supporting service user networking and knowledge. Joseph Rowntree Foundation, 2006. Available from: https://www.jrf.org.uk/report/making-user-involvement-work-supporting-service-user-networking-and-knowledge [Accessed 5th August 2016].

47. Beresford P, Croft S. *Citizen involvement: a practical guide for change*. London: Macmillan, 1993.

48. Joseph Rowntree Foundation. Social service users' own definitions of quality outcomes. 2003. Available from: https://www.jrf.org.uk/report/social-service-users-own-definitions-quality-outcomes [Accessed 5th August 2016].

49. Scherer S, Sexton S. *Involving users in commissioning local services*. York: Joseph Rowntree Foundation, 2010. Available from: https://www.jrf.org.uk/sites/default/files/jrf/migrated/files/user-involvement-service-commissioning-full.pdf [Accessed 5th August 2016].

50. McEvoy R, Keenaghan C, Murray A. Service user involvement in the Irish health service. A review of the evidence. 2008. Available from: https://www.hse.ie/eng/services/publications/Your_Service,_Your_Say_Consumer_Affairs/Reports/LiteratureReview.pdf [Accessed 5th August 2016].

51. CQC (Care Quality Commission). Guidance for providers on meeting the fundamental standards and on CQC's enforcement powers. 2014. Available from: http://www.cqc.org.uk/sites/default/files/20140725_fundamental_standards_and_enforcement_consultation_final.pdf [Accessed 5th August 2016].

52. RCN (Royal College of Nursing). Congress Agenda Item 19. Community mental health nursing. 2011. Available from: https://www2.rcn.org.uk/newsevents/congress/congress_2011/congress_2011_agenda [Accessed 5th August 2016].

53. Legislation.Gov.uk. Mental Health Act 2007. Available from: www.legislation.gov.uk/ukpga/2007/12/contents [Accessed 4th July 2015].

54. Lawn S. Integrating service user participation in mental health care: what will it take? *International Journal of Integrated Care* 2015; **15**: e0004.

55. Simpson E, House A. Involving users in the delivery and evaluation of mental health services: systematic review. *British Medical Journal* 2002; **325**(7375): 1265.

56. Royal College of Psychiatrists. Mental health and social inclusion. 2009. Available from: http://www.rcpsych.ac.uk/pdf/

social%20inclusion%20position%20statement09.pdf [Accessed 5th August 2016].

57. Drake R, Latimer E. Lessons learned in North American community mental health from 1960–2010. *World Psychiatry* 2012; **11**(1): 47–51.

58. Lawn S, Smith A, Hunter K. Australian example of consumer driven and operated service. *Journal of Mental Health* 2006; **17**(5): 498–508.

59. Cook J, Copeland ME, Corey L, Buffington E, Joikas J, Curtis L, Grey D, Nichols W. Developing the evidence base for peer led services: changes among participants following Wellness Recovery Action Planning (WRAP) education in two state wide initiatives. *Psychiatric Rehabilitation Journal* 2010; **34**(2): 113–20.

60. Repper J, Carter T. A review of the literature on peer support in mental health services. *Journal of Mental Health* 2011; **20**(4): 392–411.

61. Davidson L, Chinman M, Sells D, Rowe M. Peer support among adults with serious mental illness: a report from the field. *Front Psychiatry* 2014; **5**: 178.

Further reading

Hudson B. Policy paradox and political neglect in community health services. *British Journal of Community Nursing* 2014; **19**(9): 428–31.

Kidd S, Kenny A, McKinstry C. Creating transformational change in community mental health services. *International Journal of Qualitative Methods* 2014; **13**: 522–3.

Shera W, Ramon S. Challenges in the implementation of recovery-oriented mental health policies and services. *International Journal of Mental Health* 2013; **42**(2): 17–42.

Yates I, Holmes G, Priest H. Recovery, place and community mental health services. *Journal of Mental Health* 2012; **21**(2): 104–13.

Relevant web pages

ImROC (Implementing Recovery through Organisational Change). Peer support workers in mental health recovery – benefits and costs. http://www.imroc.org/peer-support-workers-in-mental-health-recovery-benefits-and-costs/

Mental Health Commission (Ireland). http://www.mhcirl.ie

MIND. Seeking help for a mental health problem. http://www.mind.org.uk/information-support/guides-to-support-and-services/seeking-help-for-a-mental-health-problem/#.V59eA1c4n_U

Wellness Recovery Action Plan. http://mentalhealthrecovery.com

56 Assertive outreach

PAUL VEITCH, LISA STRONG AND
NICOLA ARMSTRONG

LEARNING OUTCOMES

- To have a critical understanding of the evidence base for the development of assertive outreach services for people experiencing mental health difficulties.

- To be able to describe the key components of such a service and understand how some elements can be adopted in other mental health teams.

- To demonstrate an affiliation with people who use services by appreciating how challenging services can be to utilize and navigate.

SUMMARY OF KEY POINTS

- It is important to consider what it is like to experience mental health difficulties, and how socially disabling such experiences can be.

- An accumulation of mental health difficulties, substance misuse, social disadvantage and stigma impact on help-seeking behaviours, at least partly because of how services are organized.

- Certain groups may experience specific challenges when encountering mental health services, and we should be able to understand the features of these groups that make them vulnerable.

- Community mental health workers should consider how to maintain their links to people in their caseload who are admitted to hospital.

INTRODUCTION

This chapter offers the reader an introduction to a particular type of community-orientated mental health service. This is a service model designed for people who experience considerable difficulty in tolerating or accepting care and treatment from a traditionally organized mental health service – that is, a service that has a tendency to be passive and expect people who use such services to be help-seeking. Do not bypass this chapter because you do not have a local assertive outreach team. There has been much to learn for all mental health workers as these services have developed over time. Think of assertive outreach as being a way of determining the approach you will take toward some people in your care who are struggling within a less flexible service.

We will describe how these services first emerged and how research and clinical experience have modified the approach in practice, and we will describe some of the challenges in adopting this approach. We will illustrate how key elements of assertive outreach working may be applied in everyday clinical practice for community mental health workers and nurses in particular, even those not working in a specialist assertive outreach team. Multidisciplinary working is always considered a key tenet of assertive outreach, but nurses are often the bulk of the workforce. A focus of this chapter is on thinking about how nurses shape their clinical practice and sometimes adapt their craft of care into novel ways of working.

We go on to look at how some people, deemed to be in need of services, can be peculiarly disadvantaged because of their circumstances or choices, and how services might be organized to overcome such issues. The chapter condenses the learning about designing and providing such services into some key learning points.

We draw on our own experience of assertive outreach services in the UK, but take an international perspective. Throughout the chapter, Nicola Armstrong has added challenges to our thinking and has given us insights from a service user perspective and experience of working within a specialist assertive outreach service in the north of England.

BACKGROUND

Assertive outreach is a service model and a way of thinking about, designing, organising and delivering community mental health services. Assertive outreach teams are multidisciplinary and sometimes multi-agency. They offer suitably intensive and yet flexible mental health care and treatment to individuals and their caregivers. The approach aims to benefit people with long-term mental health difficulties, typically psychoses, and invariably with complications of secondary morbidity, such as substance misuse.

The complex make-up of such teams, their intensity, their hours of operation and their team-working philosophy are such because they are not just aimed at people with severe psychiatric illness – they are aimed at those people who utilize the most mental health resources, the most disenfranchised and the most socially isolated. The people who are referred to assertive outreach teams are referred because they are disabled but also because they find accepting the help of a mental health service deeply dissatisfying and have often become adept at avoiding the attentions of such services. They are often deemed 'difficult to engage' inasmuch as they have struggled to maintain regular and helpful contact with less intensive community teams or have simply refused such contact.

An assertive outreach team is designed to make active and persisting efforts to improve relationships with the people who use the service. The most important aim of such an approach is not to accept as inevitable that people do not wish to use services, and to ensure that the service is agreeable and helpful. The prevention of repeated and harmful relapses and associated disability, which can occur after periods of poor cooperation with treatment and care, is also targeted. Such teams by nature are rehabilitative; they try to help restore the functioning of the person.

The approach is also known as 'assertive community treatment' and has been enshrined in public and independent sector mental health provision throughout the Western world, including the UK and elsewhere in Europe, the USA, Canada, New Zealand and Australia. In the UK, interest in the assertive outreach approach was prompted by serious crimes committed by people who disengaged from traditionally organized mental health services.

At least a third of people needing acute psychiatric wards will, at any one time, have a diagnosis of schizophrenia or psychosis. The individuals in hospital will be experiencing a significant crisis in their lives, often associated with an exacerbation of their psychotic illness or risk-related situation. In the UK, inpatient treatment of psychosis accounts for more than half of all secondary care mental health spending.[1] Such services are required because of the cost to independence caused by hospitalization, but also the cost to the public purse.

EVIDENCE BASE

The way in which we measure the success of any service approach is a complex area. The assertive outreach approach has been extensively evaluated since its beginnings in the USA over 30 years ago.[2,3] Early studies[4,5] have indicated that the approach, with its emphasis on counselling support, life skills training, family, medication and education, led to significant reductions in hospital admissions and improvements in quality of life for people who experience severe mental illness living in the community. Such studies led to the commissioning of assertive outreach teams across the USA, Australia and Europe. Two systematic reviews concluded that assertive outreach was an effective model in comparison to mainstream services.[3,6] These findings have directly influenced policy and guidelines in the UK.

Early optimism waned when studies showed that the approach had less impact on bed days than previously thought.[7] The UK700 study[8] and the REACT study[9] found that the approach made no difference at all to standard care.[10,11] In 2003, the Pan-London Assertive Outreach Project found that fidelity to the formal assertive outreach model varied greatly, and that characteristics of teams had little influence on outcome.[12–14]

The ability of an assertive outreach approach to aid engagement and improve satisfaction with services, however, was upheld in these studies, leading to new ways of thinking about the model and exploration of the value of each component of the approach. Recent studies have detected a positive impact of assertive outreach teams on numbers of hospital admissions, although findings may be related to an overall reduction in UK inpatient beds.[15,16]

Attempts to measure fidelity to the original model were popular in the 1990s, as it was widely held that the individual components of care were important, yet assertive outreach teams were not formed and did not all function in the same way.[17,18] The potential for teams to drift away from the original model was believed to undermine the efficacy of assertive outreach, and so the most salient characteristics by which services could be measured were defined. The Index of Fidelity Assertive Community Treatment (IFACT) and the Dartmouth Assertive Community Treatment Scale (DACT)[17,18] were widely used in service planning, addressing the structure and composition of the team, its organizational boundaries and the nature of the work.

UNDERSTANDING THE ASSERTIVE OUTREACH APPROACH IN PRACTICE

Here we consider the core elements of an assertive outreach approach that are essential in a specialist assertive outreach team, and may be incorporated within other service types.

Academic and clinical opinion is moving away from supporting stand-alone, specialized assertive outreach teams, and in the UK the number of specialist teams has diminished sharply.[19,20] However, studies continue to show that such teams are effective at engaging with individuals whom other services have failed to engage.[21–23]

The Flexible Assertive Community Treatment (FACT) model,[24] which originated in the Netherlands, integrates the supportive and coordinated elements of an assertive outreach approach within standard community mental health teams, providing two tiers of care. Core elements of the original assertive outreach approach – such as shared caseloads, whole-team working, daily meetings and planning – are protected.

Assertive outreach teams have up to 12 people per 'case manager'. Smaller caseloads allow workers time to design and provide high-intensity interventions and to coordinate the necessary multi-agency involvement. A team would typically have a caseload of around 90 and serve a population of approximately 250,000, but the configuration of a service is dependent on multiple factors, such as geography, demography and epidemiology, as well as the ways in which both health and social care services are organized locally.

A team leader who also carries an active clinical caseload is regarded as advantageous with regard to 'leading from the front', reinforcing the 'team approach' and demonstrating the values of the service. A team approach means that each person receiving care should be known to all members of the professional team. It provides an opportunity to share clinical contacts and to offer a variety of personalities to the person receiving support, which can improve engagement by offering choice and multiple perspectives. This aspect is also important in the maintenance of a 'healthy team', as individual staff are able to adjust their own level of input if needed without impacting on patient care. This can also offset the emotional challenges faced by staff as they provide intense support.

Regular team meetings have numerous benefits. The needs of those with complex mental health difficulties are prone to change; underlying degrees of 'stress vulnerability' without robust protective factors means difficulties can escalate rapidly into crisis. Progress and crisis need to be reviewed in a timely manner. The forum of a clinical team meeting also provides opportunities for staff to reflect on care plans and to receive and provide peer support.

It is widely acknowledged that consistent, compassionate relationships are essential in the delivery of effective care and support for people with severe mental illness.[25] Well-resourced, multidisciplinary teams ensure a bio-psychosocial approach which allows in-depth case discussion, intensive contacts and effective risk management plans. The sharing of up-to-date information enables clinicians to approach service users in a personalized and knowledgeable manner, which is especially crucial during times of crisis.[26]

Substance misuse specialists embedded within teams allow for an appropriate skill mix and supervision (see chapter 10) of other members.[27] Integrated models of care (as opposed to specialist substance use services working alongside mental health services) are more effective.[28]

The majority of people using assertive outreach services will be chronically unemployed and often sub-optimally educated. Vocational specialists can help to ensure that the issue of a meaningful occupation is addressed and acknowledged as a key component of recovery.[29] (See chapters 35 and 36 for further information on recovery.) Having a purpose and structure to one's day is particularly essential when living with mental illness. Meaningful occupation does not necessarily mean paid employment, however, and informal vocational and group activities are often the catalyst for huge progress in self-esteem and may lead to more formal training or employment.[30]

The entry criteria for an assertive outreach team usually include people who have a diagnosis of psychosis and a significant risk history, and whom previous services have struggled to engage (meaning people who have not kept appointments, have struggled to take medications or participate in therapeutic sessions and have been lost to follow-up or need frequent hospital admission).

The maintenance of a 'low intake' is important in order to maintain a stable service. New referrals require a significant investment of time and emotional energy from clinical staff as they begin the process of engagement and resolution of what are often very trying or poor social circumstances. Everyone in the team needs to get to know every person using the service, and so rapid influx of new patients can jeopardize the quality of engagement and team functioning.

A person with limited networking ability (including poor prior experience) may struggle to negotiate their needs appropriately. Avoiding unnecessary referrals to other professionals or agencies that might result in frustration for the individual is an important consideration. Facilitating and supporting the individual to learn how to achieve success in such encounters is considered important.

Community services taking an active role during discharge planning helps to facilitate the transition from hospital to home, as important aspects of the aftercare plan are shared across teams, allowing consideration of safety issues, roles and responsibilities. It also helps to ensure that shared expectations between the service user and worker are explored, maximizing collaborative working and building upon existing or new relationships.

Time-unlimited services were accepted as an original feature of assertive outreach teams, but are now more controversial. Initial evidence from the USA supported a time-unlimited service for those people with complex needs; however, recent studies indicates that episodic care can be effective.[31] From a 'recovery' perspective, some people find the prospect of lifelong service involvement disheartening and unhelpful. Others may desire a life without services but struggle to achieve this due to isolation in their community and social exclusion. Some view mental health services as essential for their long-term well-being and oppose the notion of total discharge from services.

People have a right to disengage from services; however, staff have a duty to ensure that, when this occurs, the decision has been an informed one. A 'no dropout' policy helps to ensure that disengagement motivated by paranoia/distrust, hopelessness, substance misuse and apathy is followed up, as these factors often herald the onset of a relapse in mental health.

The concept that people within an assertive outreach team were 'difficult to engage' was, in my experience, mostly misguided, and in fact people were more disenchanted about services and unclear how a mental health service could meet their needs. There is a need to be innovative and creative in order to understand services users' 'whole needs'.

Nicola Armstrong

Assertively seeking to improve engagement in order to prevent individuals from dropping out of services requires creativity, perseverance and persistence. Traditional approaches to engagement, such as sending appointment letters and invitations to attend a clinic, are likely to be ineffective, as the nature of complex difficulties often creates barriers to the organization and motivation required to attend an appointment. Instead, workers will be required to discover what is likely to incentivize and motivate an individual in order to achieve face-to-face contact. An assertive outreach worker will probably see most of their clinical contacts through home visiting, but meetings in public places, such as coffee shops, supermarkets or even car parks, may be necessary. The degree to which meaningful gains can be made from such (inevitably compromised) encounters is a question for the clinical team meeting to determine.

People's experiences suggest and support the concept that sometimes people in a position of power can't actually be trusted. For a number of people, this at some point in their life has been a reality. Did they have the opportunity to talk to someone then? Do mental health workers support the message that it is safe for people who have been exposed to previous trauma, from those whom they may have once trusted, to talk about how that might influence future therapeutic alliances? I still don't think services are fully understanding of the impact of trauma and abuse and there is so much more we can do.

Nicola Armstrong

REFLECTION

How do you establish 'trust' with service users? What aspects of your language and behaviour might you need to consider in order to combat negative assumptions about your position?

Mental health nurses frequently find themselves in a dilemma regarding the management of risk (see chapter 36). Working therapeutically and safely with service users can be challenging, but challenges occur in all mental health care services (see chapter 3). Effective teams are more likely to be able to manage unusual, risky or complex situations, and maintaining a culture of 'positive risk taking' is an approach more easily applied within a specially organized and focused arena. A multidisciplinary approach to assessment and shared decision making can help workers to manage their own anxiety by taking a comprehensive approach to risk management.

The challenges for services are about supporting the possibility of recovery, in whatever way the individual understands it, and some element of risk taking has to be supported to enable people to move forward and learn more about themselves. A 'clinical' culture can be one of trying to manage symptoms, pre-crisis and post-crisis interventions and trying to avoid or support hospital admission. A service is failing people where there is little or no real discussion about supporting positive risk taking and co-produced decisions and understanding.

People using an assertive outreach service may see 'harmful' ways of coping (such as substance misuse – see chapter 31) as their protective factors, as opposed to risk factors. Their experience might be that, at least for a period, their own way of coping may prevent things becoming worse and actually keep them safe. Few would have the opportunity to have essential open and transparent conversations with staff about their understanding of risk and safety, and what these things mean to them. As mental health workers, we should not make judgements about some people's lifestyle choices.

Nicola Armstrong

REFLECTION

Consider your own preferred ways of 'coping'. How might these be viewed in the context of 'risk'? What protective factors do you have that prevent maladaptive ways of coping from becoming 'risky'?

An assertive outreach approach anticipates and responds to periods of increased need, ensuring a high-intensity service when required. In order to do this, clinicians must have a full awareness of 'early warning signs' and 'relapse signatures', offering numerous daily contacts if needed. Working with the support system around an individual helps to incorporate multiple perspectives, which enriches both assessment and treatment. Integrating an assertive outreach approach with family interventions is essential in order for mental health services to be effective.[32] (See also chapter 15 on family assessment and chapter 51 on family involvement and support networks.)

Service users and their carers/family/friends should be seen as an essential part of 'the team' and, wherever possible, should have an understanding of the formulation and be meaningfully involved in its development, with agreed achievable goals (see chapter 15). Tricky and difficult conversations need to happen more often, as they are crucial to encourage understanding of the consequences of poor decision making.

While working as a user development worker within assertive outreach, it was apparent to me that relationships with staff were mostly very positive and our evaluation found that people who used the service preferred the more personable and informal approach that we adopted. Most people were happy to see team members other than their named key nurse, which was a surprise to us as a staff group, and people also liked the flexibility of evening and weekend staff availability. However, most were unaware of what was in their care plan and what goals, if any, there were in these plans. This suggested that people were not meaningfully involved in decisions and plans.

Nicola Armstrong

SPECIAL ISSUES FOR ASSERTIVE OUTREACH

Therapeutic alliance

Assertive outreach emphasizes the establishment of working relationships between clients and staff to achieve agreed goals. Therefore, effective engagement towards therapeutic alliance is of primary concern, both with the team and with other services.[20,26,33] Up to 30 per cent of people with mental health problems drop out of contact with mental health services, which significantly impacts upon continuity and quality of care, and so an assertive outreach team aims to sustain and improve long-term engagement.[34]

A qualitative study that explored patient engagement and disengagement found that concepts such as time and commitment of staff, social support that did not focus on medication, and a partnership model of the therapeutic relationship were inherently important in facilitating positive engagement.[21] A desire for autonomy, a lack of active participation/poor therapeutic relationships and loss of control due to medication and its effects were found to be significant causes of disengagement.

Being medicated challenges people's ability to process information in a way that makes sense to them. Within an assertive outreach team, there were also assumptions made around why people had stopped taking their medication. Most staff thought it was in relation to weight gain or that people just didn't want to take it and objected to any emphasis on medication. The feedback I received from people using the service was that an important reason for poor concordance was that it regularly caused sexual dysfunction. I learned that we need to collect more qualitative data and feedback from those who have lived experiences without jumping to our own conclusions. (See chapters 47 and 48 for further information on psychopharmacology and medication management).

Nicola Armstrong

Difficulties in sustaining relationships with services do not mean that people do not want help (see chapter 3 for further information). Apparent lack of motivation for treatment amidst acute distress and difficult social circumstances can lead to frustration and negative perceptions of people who are often considered 'hard to engage' (see chapter 39 for information on motivational interviewing). Knowing when to press for face-to-face contact, and when not to see the person in order to preserve a longer-term therapeutic relationship, involves nuanced decision making and is an important topic for discussion at team meetings.

Mutual respect should also work both ways and huge assumptions about staff can be made by service users about their perceived lack of understanding. There is a belief and misconception that staff have perfect lives, without having had lived experience themselves, or someone close to them. Appropriate disclosures could help dispel the assumptions that we can all make about one another. It may actually assist with engagement and help in reducing stigma. We could also regurgitate a list of values and principles, but the key is to demonstrate this in how we engage and work with people. You develop a skill of being able to know who is genuine and who is not.

Nicola Armstrong

REFLECTION

How do you feel about sharing your own experiences with service users? What might inform a decision to disclose personal information?

Mental health legislation

The issue of safety and its management can threaten to rupture the therapeutic alliance, and can create tension within teams, as thresholds for risk vary between individual clinicians. In England and Wales, in cases where risk is deemed unmanageable in a community setting, the Mental Health Act 2007[35] provides the authority to admit someone to hospital against their will. Similar legal systems are in place throughout the developed world. The stigma, loss of liberty and trauma of enforced treatment can have psychological effects that may last much longer than the actual admission. The use of coercive measures may be necessary when the potential benefits of treatment outweigh the cost to the therapeutic relationship and the service user's autonomy. The manner in which such legislation is implemented often determines the cost to the relationship, as evidence shows that coercion is less likely to be perceived negatively when people are treated fairly and with respect.[36] Considerable effort must be made on behalf of the clinician to ensure that supportive, open and honest conversations take place prior to and after a compulsory admission to promote partnership and collaboration. Post-admission reflections can be used to develop Wellness Recovery Action Plans.[37] Many countries also allow for some form of compulsion to accept treatment in the community, and assertive outreach teams are likely to work with people who experience such measures.

Working collaboratively towards independence – a socially inclusive, recovery-orientated approach

The term 'recovery' has historically been associated with the treatment of symptoms and the concept of cure. However, for many people with psychotic symptoms, cure is at best partial and often intermittent.[1] Recovery might be best understood as a process of learning to manage experiences and gaining a sense of control so that life can become meaningful and rewarding.[38] The role of the nurse is to hold on to hope for those whom they support during difficult times. This is a recovery skill and an aspect of the craft of caring for the nurse working in assertive outreach.

The road to recovery can be long and fraught with setbacks. Someone experiencing severe mental illness will often endure debilitating social, psychological and physical constraints that compromise their ability to meet their basic needs. When physiological and safety needs are neglected through poor diet and lack of adequate housing, the acquisition of positive relationships and mental well-being may be placed well beyond reach.[39]

There are still issues of stigma in our society and people using assertive outreach services are some of the most disadvantaged and do face terrible discrimination. In my opinion, people using assertive outreach were isolated and any friendships made were with other mental health service users. Such isolation made people grossly vulnerable to exploitation by others.

Nicola Armstrong

Social marginalization can be combated by socially inclusive services that adopt the aim of supporting personal recovery, embedding recovery principles of hope, agency and opportunity at all levels of an organization; that give primacy to outcomes that are valued by the people using the service; and that emphasize co-production and partnerships between all provider and commissioning agencies.[1]

The opportunity to have meaningful and open discussions about our past and present experiences and how these may affect us is significantly important. Making sense of it can help us move forward. How do we cope? What are our strengths? How do we recognize our difficulties and triggers? How can we learn from crisis in our lives? There are so many crucial issues that we could make sense of and learn about together in a genuinely meaningful and co-produced way, that may also include carers, family and friends.

Nicola Armstrong

Services that adopt an assertive outreach approach can help the service user re-establish confidence in their ability to influence their own position in society, reducing chaos and risk and, crucially, exposing them to non-judgemental, warm relationships with workers. The challenge may be to extend these relationships beyond mental health services, reconnecting individuals to family and initiating friendships when previous experience may have tarnished expectations. Stigma and social exclusion, particularly in relation to substance misuse, may perpetuate isolation and rejection.[40]

The high cost of inpatient care in the UK and the fact that such care accounts for over 50 per cent of spending on psychosis confirms the importance of relapse prevention interventions.[1] The expansion of co-production, drawing on the lived experience of service users, developing peer support roles, and making use of local community resources (education services, faith groups, hobby and leisure activities, friends and family), is a key element of the recovery approach.

Services that are difficult to engage

It may seem odd, in a chapter describing specialist services that are designed to address the needs of those who struggle to work well with routine services, to be thinking about services themselves as 'difficult to engage with'. However, we repeatedly come across examples of people who may be (comparatively mildly) disenfranchised who struggle to engage with such services. It can be helpful to consider how services may be difficult to engage with, rather than assuming that an individual possesses qualities that uniquely alienate him or her from helping services. The following are examples of how such services prevent seamless access to appropriate health and social care support.

PRIMARY HEALTH CARE

The gateway to most health services in the UK and many countries is through the provision of locally based multidisciplinary, general health care teams. The major focus on ensuring good quality care for those who experience common mental health problems has led to greatly improved access to locally provided, effective care. However, the primary care of people experiencing severe mental illness has not received such a focus, and there is a growing awareness of the toll of physical health problems (see chapters 69 and 70) in this group.[41] The ability to recognize that one is mentally unwell or the ability to self-manage a chronic condition (such as diabetes) may be impaired by psychosis. A mistrust of those who represent any form of institutional authority is likely to be more common in a group with disproportionately adverse experiences in childhood. We should also consider the range of skills necessary in negotiating an appointment system and consultations with busy general practitioners. Supporting a person through the process and helping them learn techniques to manage a consultation is a valuable use of an assertive outreach worker's time.

PEOPLE WHO ARE HOMELESS

People who are homeless are not a homogeneous group; however, they do have an unusually high degree of illness burden and a complex interplay between health, social and substance use difficulties. Mobility across the organizational geographical boundaries that are the usual routes to services is common in this group (for example, not having a permanent address). Homelessness itself carries a stigma, and shame is a common shared characteristic of people who become homeless and can cause reluctance to seek help, particularly where a poor or rejecting experience has been encountered previously. There are widespread prejudices held about homeless persons, and these include preconceived ideas about ulterior motives for seeking help. Disgust is not uncommonly encountered, and health care professionals may be concerned about dealing with complex multi-morbidity.

People I talked with in assertive outreach teams often reported poor care, poor support and poor attitudes from staff working in A&E and other hospital departments. Stigma is often greatly increased if someone is homeless and has mental health difficulties. I heard one staff member say 'We can't help you if you keeping harming yourself', as though judging the service user for something they didn't understand.

Gaining adequate housing for those who have substance abuse issues was often a challenge, and people would often get housed in inappropriate areas, which actually hindered their well-being and recovery.

Service users are often a target for bullying, and sometimes their community witnesses police/ambulance involvement in taking them to be detained in hospital. We need to understand the impact of this humiliating situation; can this be done in a more dignified way? Service users then have to return to those neighbours, street and estate, and try to rebuild sometimes damaged relationships.

Nicola Armstrong

HOSPITAL WARDS

People using assertive outreach teams have often had multiple compulsory hospital admissions, and hospital care can be seen as almost inevitable given the multiple complexities and challenges facing clinicians who are attempting to intervene and support individuals. However, the experience of long admissions, often as a detained patient and potentially having been exposed to coercive treatments, makes hospital care a significant concern for this group of people. Hospitals can be seen as places to dread and re-enact previous traumatizing experiences, places that individuals can feel resentful towards and vulnerable within. Alternatively, they can be places of asylum and places to avoid the loneliness and challenge of everyday life and poverty, in which case it is possible to develop dependency. The fact that the care team changes once a person enters hospital presents a significant challenge; the need to maintain regular contact with the person during a hospital stay is one of the most important learning points from assertive outreach for other community mental health workers.

> ### CASE STUDY 1
>
> Charlie has done well in his school studies and arrives at his new university full of hope and optimism for his future. He leaves his parents hundreds of miles away, but they fully support Charlie's new life. Within weeks, however, Charlie is missing lectures, he is not having meals or socializing with his peers and his flatmates complain that he is awake at night. One night, maintenance staff were called following a power cut caused by interference with the supply in Charlie's flat. The domestic housemaids are saying that Charlie's flat is in disarray. Charlie is not answering calls from his lecturers or from his parents. In this case we can see a number of concerning events, and we can see that a range of people have concerns about Charlie's welfare, but who should do what and in what event does this become an emergency (and for whom)?

Individual service users may not have thought about how they see themselves; sometimes things that affect you are so close that you don't see them, and issues that other people may find unacceptable can become the norm for you as a service user. These are important issues to discuss where possible. Trying to understand core beliefs about yourself and others, your responses, feelings and coping strategies, and sharing this information with those who support you, is crucial to effective wellness and recovery plans.

Nicola Armstrong

ESSENTIAL ATTRIBUTES FOR AN ASSERTIVE OUTREACH NURSE

In this section, we consider the skills and attributes necessary for a nurse who is working in a way that is associated with the assertive outreach approach. Some of these skills may be useful in any areas of nursing, or even in other disciplines. They are described here in order to capture the essence of what attributes should characterize a nurse practising within an assertive outreach team or using assertive outreach principles.

It is important to be *responsive* to need. Learning to be a thoughtful and reflective practitioner (see chapter 11) is part of nurse education and is distilled into practices such as clinical supervision. In talking about responsiveness being a key attribute, we make a significant distinction between becoming overly reactive to need, and ensuring an individual or team is enabled to be responsive. Recognizing patterns of coping or problem solving in an individual or family (or perhaps a care system, such as a residential care facility) helps the nurse plan effectively how to respond to a related challenge in future. This means learning about what works for this individual person in the context of, for example, a social crisis. Being an *innovative* and responsive nurse in an assertive outreach team often means becoming a good problem solver. Understanding how a patient has found him- or herself in a social crisis can be achieved through good knowledge of the individual patient, multi-agency skills, and networking ability in order to resolve such situations, and also to help the person receiving the service learn to utilize their own problem-solving skills.

Working *collaboratively* has attracted a shared meaning that is not always true to its origins. It has become a truism, rather than something we do to become more effective at our practice. In this context, 'collaboration' means being able to understand how the individual sees themselves and how they are perceived by significant others, working empathically and identifying how they might benefit from appropriate and thoughtful intervention. (See chapter 50 for further information on collaborative care planning.)

Anticipating the difficulties that an individual may encounter will always be more productive than intervening in a crisis. Knowing the person means relating well to the individual and their loved ones or carers. It means being able to make an accurate prediction of their responses to social stressors. Getting to know an individual is the most basic element of a therapeutic relationship, and it is achieved by spending time with the person during periods when one is invited to do so, taking advantage of privileged information – both privileged by the person in personal divulgences or by an institution (that is, in clinical records) – and taking care to respect that information.

Managing to *maintain* relationships over time is a key element in assertive outreach working. Therapeutic relationships are always subject to significant power differences, and these can be brought into sharp relief during episodes where risk is being considered, and especially where hospitalization (compulsory or otherwise) is considered necessary. Working through the experience of helping someone at an extremely challenging time in their life, even if aspects of the experience are negative, allows both parties to reflect on what went well and what was meaningful or potentially misconstrued, offering an opportunity for open dialogue.

Being a *team worker* is another positive attribute for the assertive outreach nurse. Teams are not only professional groupings, such as the formal assertive outreach team, but the coalescing of many small networks that are needed during different phases or periods of care. It is important to collaborate with, communicate with and utilize these networks for the benefit of the person using the service.

On the subject of the essential attributes for an assertive outreach worker, I would say that certain attitudes and values are key. We must treat people with respect and kindness, avoid jumping to conclusions and making assumptions or judgements about lifestyle choices, and keep an open mind about what might be possible to achieve. Wherever possible we should meaningfully involve people in decisions about their care, treatment and plan and have a shared understanding of problems (even if we don't agree). Have open and honest conversations (even about the difficult issues) to support greater understanding between all parties (where appropriate including family, friends, carers). Don't make promises you can't keep. Have insight into your own mental health; insist on meaningful supervision and reflection time. You need to look after your own well-being. No one is perfect or an expert in everything and at times people and situations will have a powerful impact on you.

Nicola Armstrong

REFLECTION

- What helps you to remain compassionate? Can you think of situations when compassion has been jeopardized by struggles with your own well-being?

- Sometimes we need to seek support from our line managers. How would you ensure you have access to the right support and supervision?

CONCLUSION

Assertive outreach is an approach aimed at tailoring mental health care to the needs of socially excluded individuals who have struggled to engage with treatment services that are provided in a less intensive and flexible manner. It has an evidence base stretching back to the early 1990s, and has been subject to considerable international interest, not least because huge amounts of financial resources have been dedicated to the provision of such services. Assertive outreach approaches have a good international track record of maintaining contact with people who otherwise may have dropped out of care, of preventing homelessness and of reducing the reliance on bed-based services (in some countries). There is moderately good evidence to suggest that assertive outreach services can help reduce symptom burden and improve the quality of life of those using services. However, assertive outreach as a model shows less impressive results when we consider how it helps people make appropriate social adjustments, and how it helps reduce the numbers of people being given prison sentences, being unemployed and abusing illicit substances or alcohol. The interest in developing such services has declined in the UK, but it has increased in other European countries.[42]

References

1. Knapp M, Andrew A, McDaid D, Valentina L, McCrone P, Park A-L, Parsonage M, Boardman J, Shepherd G. Investing in recovery: making the business case for effective interventions for people with schizophrenia and psychosis. 2014. *LSE Research Online*. Available from: http://eprints.lse.ac.uk/56773/ [Accessed 30th August 2016.].

2. Stein LI, Santos AB. *Assertive community treatment of persons with severe mental illness*. New York: W.W. Norton, 1998.

3. Marshall M, Lockwood A. Assertive community treatment for people with severe mental disorders. *Cochrane Database of Systematic Reviews* 2011; **4**: CD001089. DOI: 10.1002/14651858.CD001089.pub2.

4. Stein L, Test A. Alternative to mental hospital treatment. 1. Conceptual model, treatment program, and clinical evaluation. *Archives of General Psychiatry* 1980; **37**: 392–7.

5. Hout J, Reynolds I, Charbonneau-Powis M, Weekes P, Briggs J. Psychiatric hospital versus community treatment: the results of a randomised trial. *Australian and New Zealand Journal of Psychiatry* 1983; **17**: 160–7.

6. Marshall M, Gray A, Lockwood A, Green R. Case management for people with severe mental disorders. *Cochrane Database of Systematic Reviews* 2011; **4**: CD000050. DOI: 10.1002/14651858.CD000050.pub2.

7. Thornicroft G, Wykes T, Holloway F, Johnson S, Smzukler G. From efficacy to effectiveness in community mental health services; PRISM psychosis study 10. *British Journal of Psychiatry* 1998; **173**: 423–7.

8. Burns T, Firn M, Catty J, Healey A, Henderson J, Watt H, Wright C. Home treatment for mental health problems: a systematic review. *Health Technology Assessment* 2001; **5**(15): 1–139.

9. Killaspy H, Johnson S, Bebbington P, Blizard R, Johnson S, Nolan F, Pilling S, King M. The REACT study: randomized evaluation of assertive community treatment in north London. *British Medical Journal* 2006; **332**: 815–20.

10. Thornicroft G, Tansella M. Components of a modern mental health service: a pragmatic balance of community and hospital care: overview of systematic evidence. *British Journal of Psychiatry* 2004; **185**: 283–90.

11. Harvey C, Killaspy H, Martino S, White S, Priebe S, Wright C, Johnson S. A comparison of the implementation of assertive community treatment in Melbourne, Australia and London, England. *Epidemiology and Psychiatric Sciences* 2011; **20**: 151–61.

12. Billings J, Johnson S, Bebbington P, Greaves A, Priebe S, Muijen M, Ryrie I,Watts J, White I, Wright C. Assertive outreach teams in London: models of Operation Pan-London Assertive Outreach Study, part 2. *British Journal of Psychiatry* 2003; **183**: 139–47.

13. Priebe S, Fakhoury W, Watts J, Bebbington P, Burns T, Johnson S, Muijen M, Ryrie I, White I, Wright C. Assertive outreach teams in London: models of Operation Pan-London Assertive Outreach Study, part 3. *British Journal of Psychiatry* 2003; **183**: 148–54.

14. Wright C, Burns T, James P, Billings J, Johnson S, Muijen M, Priebe S, Ryrie I, Watts J, White I. Assertive outreach teams in London: models of Operation Pan-London Assertive Outreach Study, part 1. *British Journal of Psychiatry* 2003; **183**: 132–8.

15. Hamilton I, Lloyd C, Bland JM, Savage A. The impact of assertive outreach teams on hospital admissions for psychosis: a time series analysis. *Journal of Psychiatric and Mental Health Nursing* 2015; **22**: 484–90.

16. NHS England. Bed availability and occupancy data – overnight. 2014. Available from: http://www.england.nhs.uk/statistics/statistical-work-areas/bed-availabily-and-occupancy/bed-data-overnight/ [Accessed 30th August 2016].

17. McGrew JH, Bond G, Dietzen L, Salyers M. Measuring the fidelity of implementation of a mental health program model. *Journal of Consulting and Clinical Psychology* 1994; **62**(4): 670–8.

18. Teague GB, Bond GR, Drake RE. Program fidelity in assertive community treatment: development and use of a measure. *American Journal of Orthopsychiatry* 1998; **68**(2): 216–32.

19. Firn M. Assertive outreach: has the tide turned against the approach? *Mental Health Practice* 2007; **10**(7): 24–7.

20. Williams C, Macpherson R, Firn M, Wharne S (eds). *Assertive outreach in mental healthcare: current perspectives*. Chichester: Wiley-Blackwell, 2011.

21. Priebe S, Watts J, Chase M, Matanov A. Processes of disengagement and engagement in assertive outreach patients: qualitative study. *British Journal of Psychiatry* 2005; **187**: 438–43.

22. Killaspy H, Kingett S, Bebbington P, Blizard R, Johnson S, Nolan F, Pilling S, King M. Randomised evaluation of assertive community treatment: 3 year outcomes. *British Journal of Psychiatry* 2009; **195**: 81–2.

23. Brugha TS, Taub N, Smith J, Morgan T, Hill T, Meltzer H, Wright C, Burns T, Priebe S, Evans J, Fryers T. Predicting outcome of assertive outreach teams across England. *Social Psychiatry & Psychiatric Epidemiology* 2012; **42**: 125–30.

24. Van Veldhuizen JR. FACT: a Dutch version of ACT. *Community Mental Health Journal* 2007; **43** (4): 421–33.

25. Fosha D, Siegal D, Solomon M. *The healing power of emotion: affective neuroscience, development & clinical practice*. New York: Norton, 2009.

26. Molodynski A, Burns T. What does research tell us about assertive community treatment? In: Williams C, Macpherson R, Firn M, Wharne S (eds). *Assertive outreach in mental healthcare: current perspectives*. Chichester: Wiley-Blackwell, 2011: 1–14.

27. Barrowclough C, Meier P, Beardmore R, Emsley R. Predicting therapeutic alliance in clients with psychosis and substance misuse. *Journal of Nervous and Mental Disease* 2010; **198**(5): 373–7.

28. Cleary M, Hunt GE, Matheson S, Walter G. Psychosocial treatments for people with co-occurring severe mental illness and substance misuse: systematic review. *Journal of Advanced Nursing* 2009; **65**(2): 238–58.

29. Burns T, Catty J, White S, Becker T, Koletsi M, Fioritti A, Rossler W, Tomov T, Busschbach J, Wiersma D, Lauber C. The impact of supported employment and working on clinical and social functioning: results of an international study of individual placement and support. *Schizophrenia Bulletin* 2009; **35**(5): 949–58.

30. Tew J, Ramon S, Slade M, Bird V, Melton J, Le Boutillier C. Social factors and recovery from mental health difficulties: a review of the evidence. *British Journal of Social Work* 2012; **42** (3): 443–60.

31. Firn M, Hindhaugh K, Hubbeling D, Davies G, Jones B, White S. A dismantling study of assertive outreach services: comparing activity and outcomes following replacement with the FACT model. *Social Psychiatry & Psychiatric Epidemiology* 2012; **48**: 997–1003.

32. Burbach F, Carter J, Carter J, Carter, M. Assertive outreach and family work. In: Velleman R, Davis E (eds). *Changing outcomes in psychosis: collaborative cases from practitioners, users and carers*. Chichester: Wiley, 2007: 80–347.

33. Ardito RB, Rabellino D. Therapeutic alliance and outcome of psychotherapy: historical excursus, measurements, and prospects for research. Review article. *Frontiers in Psychology* 2011; **2**: 270.

34. Steer H, Onyett S. Multi-professional working in assertive outreach teams. In: Williams C, Macpherson R, Firn M, Wharne S (eds). *Assertive outreach in mental healthcare: current perspectives*. Chichester: Wiley-Blackwell, 2011: 15–38.

35. Department of Health. *The Mental Health Act*. London: DH, 2007.

36. Larsen IB, Terkelsen TB. Coercion in a locked psychiatric ward: perspectives of patients and staff. *Nursing Ethics* 2014; **21**(4): 426–36.

37. Copeland ME. *Wellness Recovery Action Plan.* London: Peach Press, 2011.

38. Repper J, Perkins R. *Social inclusion and recovery: a model for mental health practice.* London: Bailliere Tindall, 2003.

39. Maslow A. A theory of human motivation. *Psychological Review* 1943; **50**: 381.

40. Boardman J, Currie A, Killaspy H, Mezey G (eds). *Social inclusion and mental health.* London: Royal College of Psychiatrists, 2010.

41. Thornicroft G. Physical health disparities and mental illness: the scandal of premature mortality. *British Journal of Psychiatry* 2011; **199**: 441–2.

42. Wharne S. Whatever happened to assertive outreach? *Health Service Journal* 2013. Available from: https://www.hsj.co.uk/comment/whatever-happened-to-assertive-outreach/5064403.article [Accessed 30th August 2016].

Further reading

Holloway F, Kalidindi S, Killaspy H, Roberts G. *Enabling recovery: the principles and practice of rehabilitation psychiatry*, 2nd edn. London: Royal College of Psychiatrists, 2015.

Relevant web pages

Flexible Assertive Community Treatment Model. https://www.eaof.org

National Forum for Assertive Outreach. http://www.nfao.org/

RETHINK https://www.rethink.org/
    This is a UK-based federation.

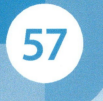

57 Therapeutic communities

SIMON CLARKE, GARY WINSHIP,
JENELLE CLARKE AND NICK MANNING

LEARNING OUTCOMES

- To understand some of the core principles underlying therapeutic communities (TCs).

- To be aware of the historic roots behind TCs in terms of providing an alternative therapeutic modality to conventional biological psychiatry, including the role of nurses in developing the core approach.

- Demonstrate an understanding of how TCs may support recovery from severe mental health difficulties through the personal account of a former TC member.

- To understand TCs in relation to recovery approaches in mental health.

- To appreciate the continuing relevance of TCs to the NHS, mental health nursing and current mental health services.

SUMMARY OF KEY POINTS

- TCs are planned social environments that involve both staff and service users in the therapeutic process.

- Despite considerable diversity across service setting, TCs share a common ethos and philosophy.

- Core values and principles underlying TCs include: attachment, containment, communication, respect, interdependence, relationships, participation, process, balance and responsibility.

- TCs in their current format emerged from post-Second World War therapeutic experiments with traumatized war veterans at three hospitals across the UK, and then during the radical critique of psychiatry in the 1960s and 1970s.

- TC principles became, to a lesser or greater extent, part of the fabric of organized health care, especially in terms of social psychiatric attempts to reform community mental health care.

- Despite a relative decline in the latter decades of the twentieth century and first decade of the twenty-first century, TCs are still at the forefront of developing alternative psychiatric practices in mainstream health care.

INTRODUCTION

This chapter provides an introduction to therapeutic communities (TCs). The chapter begins with a brief illustration of the core principles underlying TCs, before exploring the development of TCs in their historical context. The narrative is also interspersed with a service user's account of his experiences of being in a TC. With its emphasis from the start on social inclusion and user involvement, it is argued that TC methods continue to promise radically and politically informed mental health practice, compensating for the anti-therapeutic tendencies inherent in modern psychiatry. This relationship is further highlighted in the chapter through a discussion of TCs' version of 'recovery' compared to mainstream psychiatric care, and by illustrating TCs' unique craft of caring.

WHAT IS A THERAPEUTIC COMMUNITY? CORE PRINCIPLES AND STANDARDS

TCs are planned social environments that utilize the whole community – both staff and service users – in the therapeutic process.[1] Although TCs were formed largely within hospital institutions, they have evolved into many different types of organizations in a variety of settings. TCs focus on a range of issues including personality disorders, eating disorders, alcoholism, gambling addiction, psychosis, drug addiction and a range of other personal and mental health-related issues.[2] Despite the diversity of TCs across various sectors, they all share a common ethos and philosophy.[3] The mechanisms and principles of TCs are rooted in sociology/anthropology. Beginning with Rapoport, four main principles can be identified: democratization, permissiveness, reality confrontation and communalism.[4] More recently, Haigh updated Rapoport's principles with 'quintessential features': attachment, containment, communication, inclusion and agency.[5] These qualities were further refined in 2014 as attachment, containment, communication, respect, interdependence, relationships, participation, process, balance and responsibility (see Table 57.1).[2]

Whilst the core values do emphasize the individual's role in the TC, they clearly outline that the process of personal change is a social, rather than individual, pursuit.[6] Both the community and the individual share a responsibility to one another in order for the TC to function as a therapeutic mechanism of transformation.[2]

Table 57.1 Therapeutic community core values

Attachment	Healthy attachment is a developmental requirement for all human beings, and should be seen as a basic human right.
Containment	A safe and supportive environment is required for an individual to develop, to grow, or to change.
Respect	People need to feel respected and valued by others to be healthy. Everybody is unique and nobody should be defined or described by their problems alone.
Communication	All behaviour has meaning and represents communication which deserves understanding.
Interdependence	Personal well-being arises from one's ability to develop relationships which recognize mutual need.
Relationships	Understanding how you relate to others and how others relate to you leads to better intimate, family, social and working relationships.
Participation	Ability to influence one's environment and relationships is necessary for personal well-being. Being involved in decision making is required for shared participation, responsibility and ownership.
Process	There is not always a right answer and it is often useful for individuals, groups and larger organizations to reflect rather than act immediately.
Balance	Positive and negative experiences are necessary for healthy development of individuals, groups and the community.
Responsibility	Each individual has responsibility to the group, and the group in turn has collective responsibility to all individuals in it.

HISTORY OF THERAPEUTIC COMMUNITIES

A new concept of cooperative psychiatric therapy – the third revolution, as Rapoport eventually called it[4] – emerged against the backdrop of profound social change during the Second World War.[1] Three UK psychiatric hospitals were involved: Northfield in Birmingham, Mill Hill in London and the 312th Military Hospital in Stafford. These wartime experiments generated ideas of social participation. 'Talking therapy' and 'patient empowerment' came into sharp focus and formed the basis of social psychiatry. At the time of these early experiments, however, psychiatry was mostly characterized by the use of drugs such as sodium amytal, alongside deep insulin therapy, continuous narcosis and electroconvulsive therapy (ECT). Many soldier patients were unable to return to active service and those who returned to 'Civvy Street' had problems with unemployment and social disability. There was also a steady trickle of suicides.

A general sense of dissatisfaction with conventional biological treatments in psychiatry abounded, and there was an impetus to develop some of the new talking therapies expounded by Freud and his colleagues. At Northfield Army Hospital in Birmingham, Wilfred Bion, a psychiatrist and trainee psychoanalyst, took charge of a rehabilitation ward of soldiers with his colleague John Rickman. Group meetings were established on a daily basis and discussions held in which the analysis of conflict 'in the here and now' was examined. Bion took to strolling around the ward, having discussions with patients in the corridors and kitchen. This innovative approach brought about modest improvements and some reports even suggested that the ward became the cleanest and most disciplined unit in the hospital. The Northfield experiment continued when Bion and Rickman were replaced by Michael Foulkes. It was his junior colleague Tom Main who coined the term 'therapeutic community' as a way of describing the method in which all elements of life in the hospital community could be seen as therapeutically intentioned.[1,3,5–7]

As the same time as the experiments at Northfield, a young, newly qualified nurse called Hildegard Peplau began her work with soldier patients in the 312th Military Hospital in Staffordshire. Peplau had just graduated from Bennington College in the United States in 1943, with a BA in Interpersonal Psychology. At the 312th she began to put into practice what she had learned from her prior experiences at Chestnut Lodge, a hospital which at that time was well on its way to defining milieu therapy, and gaining a considerable reputation as one of the most radical treatment environments yet seen in psychiatry. The psychoanalytic work of Harry Stack Sullivan, among others, had been particularly influential at Chestnut Lodge and had shaped Peplau's early expectations and capacities. At the 312th, the shell-shocked soldier patients under Peplau's care were both depressed and anxious. She took it on herself to implement formal and informal group therapy sessions with soldier casualties, facilitating discussions over breakfast and in other everyday social situations, taking the opportunity to engage her patients in normalizing activities as part of a community programme. At the same time in London, Mill Hill was the site for evacuated patients and staff from the Maudsley Hospital. Here, a young medical psychiatrist called Maxwell Jones was experimenting with groups too. It is here that our other mental health nurse protagonist, Annie Altschul, enters the frame. Altschul later developed a renowned theory of nursing systems, a theory that seemed to be well fitted to therapeutic community practice.[1,8–11]

REFLECTION

How do you think these formative experiences influenced the careers of Annie Altschul and Hildegard Peplau?

In ways not dissimilar to the cooperative efforts of therapy at Northfield and the 312th, Jones found mutual learning to be beneficial in the treatment of shell-shocked soldiers at Mill Hill. Jones's approach differed from Northfield and the 312th insofar as he was not, ostensibly, working psychoanalytically, although Jones was far from analytically illiterate, having been under the guiding influence of Aubrey Lewis, his mentor and lead physician at the Maudsley.

The Department of Health and Labour was satisfied by the outcome of the rehabilitation of the prisoners of war and asked Jones to repeat the treatment with 100 homeless men suffering with concurrent mental infirmity. This formed the basis of the Belmont Social Rehabilitation unit in Sutton, which was established in 1947, later to become known as the Henderson Hospital. Belmont, and later Henderson, gradually deepened the use of democratic ideas, and the emphasis on these social democratic aspects of therapy culminated in a seminal book, *Social psychiatry*, published in 1952 by Jones and colleagues. Thus, the democratization and the urge towards egalitarianism emerged in their earliest articulated form from the Henderson Hospital during these years. The role of staff, such as Eileen Skellern, who went on to be an important figure in the mental health nursing profession, has often been underestimated and may have had far greater influence on the development of therapeutic democracy than is usually credited.[9,12–14]

Between 1962 and 1969, Jones returned to work in the UK as chief superintendent at Dingleton Hospital in Scotland. By then, TCs following the Mill Hill lineage rather than the more analytic TCs following the hierarchical approaches of Northfield (i.e. the Cassel Hospital and the Charles Hood Unit at the Maudsley) had forged a reputation synonymous with radical social psychiatry. Thus, the urge for a more liberated psychiatry blended with the aims and values of

SERVICE USER'S PERSPECTIVE

This community value of responsibility was reflected in the therapeutic community values of involvement, democratization and empowerment. Thus, community members were expected to take an active role in serving in the various community functions, to vote on issues such as electing the new leadership team, to be available to new members if necessary and to contribute to the day-to-day running of the community. As a community staffed entirely by volunteers, this ethos was the glue that held the community together in a web of mutual accountability. It was also the basis by which many of us acquired the valuable life skills of managing projects, organizing events and learning to put other people's needs first.

SERVICE USER'S PERSPECTIVE

The value of taking responsibility could have a dark side, in which people could be dismissed as 'not taking responsibility' for themselves when they genuinely did not have the skills or capacity to do so. Sometimes people found it impossible to accept this value and quickly left the community. For me, it was the basis by which I began recovering agency and empowerment, a sense of myself as the seat of action. As a psychiatric patient, the loss of agency is common: you quickly become a passive recipient of the system, learning very quickly that 'it's not your fault – it's your illness'. Of course, there were times when this explanation would be applicable. However, there were also times when I used my mental health problems as an excuse to avoid doing things that were difficult or challenging. Even though I had spent many years resisting it, the label became a core part of my identity. When I first told someone in the community I was bipolar, they shrugged and said, 'Aren't we all, mate?' Another member of the community remarked, 'I'm not – I take responsibility for my mood swings.' This form of 'reality confrontation' may seem harsh to an outsider but it really helped challenge me to become more active in my recovery.

the TC movement; George McDonald Bell had established Dingleton Hospital as the first 'open door' hospital in 1948, followed shortly by T. P. Rees at Warlingham Park Hospital in the early 1950s. David Clark likewise opened all but two of the locked psychiatric wards at Fulbourn, describing this as an 'experiment in freedom', which naturally paved the way towards the concept of patient self-government.[1,10,12,13,15]

The concept of a 'therapeutic community' became synonymous with the idea of progressive psychiatry between the late 1960s and mid- to late 1970s. The challenge for the organized second generation of TCs was to maintain the radical edge of progress towards egalitarianism arising out of the creative chaos of a fermenting ideology, while balancing the need for authoritative professional governance via standardization and statutory responsibilities. This challenge could be characterized as a difficulty of applying the concept of a flattened hierarchy to systems where a more traditional, or vertical, hierarchy was preferred. Although during the 1970s TCs became peripherally associated with the counterculture movement through the anti-psychiatry work of David Cooper and Ronnie Laing, who established Kingsley Hall as a therapeutic community, and later the Arbours Crisis Centre, many of the cornerstone principles of TC practice were adopted by an ever-increasing number of psychiatric

hospitals which saw *social psychiatry* as a progressive alternative psychiatric orthodoxy.[1,3,5,10,12]

The acceptance of the TC ideology in the very hierarchical establishment of the NHS seemed somewhat at odds with its radical anti-establishment roots. Anti-psychiatry itself became a dominant culture and there was fresh impetus to close the old asylums and reintegrate the mentally ill in the community under an agenda of social inclusion. TCs, which had been a sturdy haven for the interface of psychoanalysis, sociology and psychiatry, had produced a set of treatment ideologies which became embedded, to greater or lesser degrees, in all psychiatric treatments. But this 'established' place for TCs in the network of NHS provision was found to be precariously tallied to winds of political whim; when the idea of social therapy came under fire from new advances in pharmacology and behaviourism, the social method of TCs went out of favour. During the 1980s, the closure of the old hospital asylums, where many TCs had been rooted, saw many renowned TCs close. This drift away towards the anti-social inclinations of behaviour therapy and new biological theories saw further threats to the social type of approaches expounded by the TC method.[1,6,10,16–18]

REFLECTION

What do you understand to be the key ingredients that linked TC practice with social psychiatry from the 1960s onwards?

THERAPEUTIC COMMUNITIES AND THE RECOVERY MOVEMENT

In recent years we have seen the emergence of a new approach to the principles of mental health in what has been called 'recovery'.[19] This approach seeks to diminish the role of the expert and proposes that education, rather than therapy, is central to the process of recovery.[20] However, this 'New Recovery'[21] approach – coined for the purpose of debate here – is a specific addition to other well-established traditions in recovery. For example, New Recovery can be compared and contrasted with the progress of the TC movement that, over the last 60 years, has also been committed to changing the role of expert, user-involvement and theoretical co-construction.[22] Of course, TCs did not invent recovery, but there is a good case to be made that TCs have evolved some exacting methods of socially inclusive cooperative therapy that are the vanguard of achievements in the progress towards efficacious humanitarian intervention in the field of mental health.[23]

In the New Recovery movement, (see chapters 35 and 36) the concept of self-help and self-organization replaces the role of professionals.[20] The TC approach, on the other hand, while being committed to cooperative efforts that seek to engage with the concept hierarchy in order to diminish it, can be seen as rooted in approaches that are inclined to collectivist ideologies.[23] While the recovery approach has been strong on the rhetoric of service user involvement, TCs have developed the means to put principles into action in the deployment of formal democratic structures and quality checks, including service audit and review.[22]

Perhaps the most significant difference between the New Recovery approach and the way in which TCs operate might be considered in terms of what we think of as 'soft' versus 'tough' recovery. New Recovery begins with a pre-supposition of client cooperation.[20] Whilst TCs and New Recovery entirely agree that peer support is essential in building resilience in recovery, TCs begin with the notion that social inclusion is not a given. Social isolation lies at the root of many mental health problems and there are any number of steps which precede a client being able to be engaged with peers. TCs are therefore particularly well placed to help clients work through resistance and engage with conflict in a way that seems remote in the approach of New Recovery.

> ### REFLECTION
>
> What are the similarities to and differences from TCs compared to other approaches in modern mental health care in the UK?

THERAPEUTIC PROCESS IN THERAPEUTIC COMMUNITIES

This willingness and capacity to engage in the dynamics of conflict would be characteristics of a 'tough recovery' particular to TCs. TCs can sometimes get the reputation of being harsh and challenging places to be, and clients can initially find the experience hard and unsettling. Here is a brief illustrative extract from some field study notes drawn from in-depth observations of therapeutic community processes.[24] In this brief extract from J Clarke's research,[25] the client, Anna, who was new to the TC where she was residing, was talking about an experience of being in a community group where another client had been distressed:

> *And then we sit in a meeting and we're asking her all these questions and like, I don't know, I kind of wanted to say just leave her the fuck alone, she can't think straight. Like what you doing? You're asking people these really important questions when they're clearly not in a place where they can answer it. And I don't know, there's something really about it, struck me as quite cruel in a way. Um, but within 10 minutes, she was sat in the bay of the window with her headphones on, still upset but contained and able to be safe. And I just thought, God, this is really weird. Because all through the meeting*

> *I was just thinking, what the hell? And then you're like oh, I don't really get it but it does seem to work somehow. Um, and that was really strange … I really connected with [her] um right from the off. And I think it was that sense of nobody can help me. I think that's what I got from her, the fact that … she couldn't imagine there would be anyway that anybody could ever help …*

Perhaps Anna, in the vignette above, might have initially felt that the approach of the staff was rather haranguing the distressed client. However, within a short period of time Anna has witnessed that compassion can come in many forms and sometimes people may need a different approach at different times. In this case, for example, compassion has been tough rather than tender, but it appears to afford benefits to clients that may not have been possible through other forms of care. Chapter 43 has more detail on psychodynamic approaches to working in groups.

The reputation of TCs as rather tough places might point to one of the distinctive therapeutic imperatives of TC recovery approaches, which is the idea of 'reality confrontation', a phrase coined by Rapoport[4] based on his observation of work at the later Henderson. In the early 1980s, places like Phoenix House and Alpha House, Promis in Canterbury, and several other TC-minded services for addiction and eating disorder recovery, set up by Griffith Edwards in the 1960s along the lines of the DayTop Recovery Milieu therapy model in the USA, very much had the reputation of being tough places.[26] 'Tough love' was a catchphrase for recovery TCs and milieus. Some of the approaches would seem out of place today, such as 'mirror therapy', which involved a client sitting in front of a mirror for several hours taking a good look at themselves, or marathon large groups, for example, spending between 8 and 24 hours in the same room. Many clients, when faced with the choice of going to a TC or going to prison, would choose the latter.

Reality confrontation has never been a soft option. Today, the quintessential elements of TCs[5] such as containment and agency are the preferred descriptors for TC practice. However, the idea of reality confrontation in TCs

has never been entirely dispensed with. Reality confrontation is an interesting notion of course, and one that could be explored further. The clue is in the word 'confrontation'. One might also trace this harder edge back to the roots of TC in the army experiments at Mill Hill, Northfield and Staffordshire, where discipline and boundaries were extant.[7] There were also elements of the 1960s encounter group culture, where emotional confrontation was the order of the day.[6]

> ## REFLECTION
>
> What do you think of reality confrontation as a therapeutic technique and how does it compare with other psychotherapeutic approaches?

THERAPEUTIC COMMUNITIES AND THE CRAFT OF CARING

Reality confrontation as a therapeutic endeavour suggests that, somehow, the client needs reality. It might seem like a pejorative notion; the public image of TCs as a 'tough recovery choice' has perhaps not played out well over time, and there could be some clearer articulation of the way in which reality confrontation is a staged process. However, New Recovery and TCs would seem to overlap in their shared interest in ensuring that engaging in the real world is an outcome of recovery. While New Recovery is ambitious about clients developing an aptitude for work and civic membership, TCs are equally ambitious about developing clients' ability to consider how their attitudes and behaviour impact upon other people.[21]

TCs have therefore pioneered a version of the craft of caring that is somewhat unique in comparison to other psychiatric health care approaches.[21] However, this 'tough love' approach is also counterbalanced by innovative strategies to engage all clients in the process of caring for one another that go beyond merely 'telling it how it is'. This next excerpt from J Clarke's[24] research illustrates this process more clearly in terms of how reality confrontation and intrinsic care can work together in terms of confronting suicidality in clients:

Last night's Crisis Text was from Abby who is slumped very low in her chair, her head just poking up. Her fringe nearly covers her eyes and when they don't, her hand does. Abby says she was feeling very low over the weekend and is tired of her thoughts as they are 'not budging'. She continues to work on them but feels they are not getting better. She wanted to overdose over the weekend but only had antibiotics on her, 'which would just make me throw up again' (so not worth it?). However she did not self-harm, even though she really wanted to, and she says the texts she got from the clients were very

helpful – especially Brian's. Brian had told her that she would be letting not only herself down but others too if she self-harmed, meaning that he and the others would be disappointed if she did. Abby said this was a helpful reminder and she worries about when she goes and knows that no one will tell her that she'll be 'letting people down'.

As this scene shows, another client member confronted Abby with the consequences of her actions to other people: that other members in the community cared her for and her self-harm affected the whole group. Yet this idea was brought home to Abby in a way that was both confrontational *and* caring. While TCs might have a reputation for reality as a confrontation, it should also be stressed that reality for clients in TC recovery is not always an immediate big dose of reality; rather, it is more usual that reality is staggered. The model of reality confrontation in TCs is more like Winnicott's[27] idea that good enough maturational environments are characterized by reality in small doses. In TCs, new clients have much less responsibility than the more senior members who have been in treatment longer.

Therefore, despite their reputation for toughness and sometimes brutal honesty, TCs have also pioneered the use of peer support in often novel and creative ways. The participation of all community members in every aspect of the therapeutic programme is not just an afterthought or optional add-on, either in terms of cost–benefit (as we may find in some aspects of New Recovery) or as a top-down imperative of 'patient involvement' (such as is often found in the NHS). Rather, client members learning to care for each other is an intrinsic part of the TC model from The Retreat York and the post-war Northfield Park experiments. As this final excerpt from J Clarke's[24] research shows, this process can mean that clients become especially attuned to one another's needs:

> *It is nearly 9 pm and I join some of the clients in the lounge. Julie, who is sitting with Anna on the sofa, is sobbing. Julie is explaining that she wants to leave the unit but her mum will not come get her. Erica is colouring but clearly listening to the conversation. I (...) Julie says that the only time her mum really seemed 'bothered' about her is when she jumped off the roof. For the first time I am very concerned. Will Julie try something drastic to prove to her mother that she should be worried about her? Erica asks Julie about her urges and Julie says she does not feel safe and that is why she is in the lounge. Margaret (nurse) then comes in and joins the conversation. Talk revolves around*

> *Julie's eating disorder. Anna at times pats Julie's leg, and tells her she will get to the point where she can picture life without the disorder. She reminds Julie that the eating disorder is not her friend and does not help or protect her – it will kill her. Julie is crying and loudly sniffing. After a while the conversation moves on but every now and again someone will either gently pat Julie's shoulder or quickly check in with her.*

REFLECTION

How do you think reality confrontation and care are balanced in the TC approach? How does it compare with peer support initiatives?

CONCLUSION

The history of TC and milieu therapy movements usually features accounts of the key male psychiatrist figureheads, such as Harry Stack Sullivan, Dexter Bullard, Maxwell Jones, Michael Foulkes, Wilfred Bion, Tom Main and Ronnie Laing, among others. Suffice it to say, reports specific to nursing practice in the history of the TC tradition have been limited to a handful of accounts. In reappraising the history of TCs, we can glimpse the influence of some of the most eminent founders of mental health nursing in the evolution of TCs. Mental health nursing and TC practice emerge concurrently with the progressive traditions of user involvement and social psychiatry. So what place is there for TC practice today?

Although the recent era of modernized health care has resulted in the closure of some of the pioneering early communities,[17] TCs continue to thrive in a number of service settings including mental health in the NHS, independent/voluntary communities, prisons, children's homes and day centres, learning disabled communities, and faith communities.[28] Personality disorder (PD) remains a challenging condition for most mainstream psychiatric services, yet TCs have emerged as a particularly well-adapted treatment modality for the difficulties encountered in this client group.[29] The evidence for TCs in PD is generally positive,[30] albeit limited,[31] although the first major randomized clinical trial for TCs in PD is currently underway.[32]

We know at present that acute psychiatric inpatient units are particularly difficult environments, which stretch the resources of even the most capable individuals. The *Audit of violence*[33] drew attention to the wide array of problems encountered by staff, including the unsafe atmosphere of acute wards, compounded by inadequate staffing, with large numbers of vacancies and inexperienced leadership. The

report characterized treatments as coercive, and identified chronic staff demoralization, with 78 per cent of nurses, 41 per cent of clinical staff and 36 per cent of service users reporting that they had been personally attacked, threatened or made to feel unsafe.[33] *Acute care*[34] also noted high levels of boredom and inactivity among patients. In the aftermath of the Bennett Inquiry,[35] and more recently the problems identified in the Francis Report on Mid-Staffordshire NHS Foundation Trust,[36] it is timely to review some of the theoretical underpinnings of ward management by mental health nurses.

SERVICE USER'S PERSPECTIVE

Over time, I became an established and senior member of the community. In many ways, responsibility is learned through a process of helping other people. This 'living learning' approach provided me with many of the skills that I had lost through my recurrent bouts of mental distress. Through involvement with the community's various programmes, I began to learn how to support others in their therapeutic journeys. I eventually decided to retrain as a mental health professional and qualified as a clinical psychologist in 2009. I now work as a practitioner in a multidisciplinary team in the NHS.

There is some emerging evidence that TC group-based therapy, emerging from the traditions of TC and user involvement, is effective in producing a safe milieu.[18] There is also some persuasive evidence, albeit limited, that democratic administration and collective rule-setting in the milieu might have a positive impact on reducing levels of aggression, violence, seclusion and staff sickness and increasing staff morale.[37] It is perhaps through principles of TC practice that the transformative potential of mental health nursing practice might counter anti-therapeutic milieus.[16] A revitalized agenda for psychosocial mental health nursing might also produce more active service user engagement, a renewed focus on compassionate but reflective health care delivery and an increased emphasis on recovery and relational self-determination. All these aspirations are familiar givens in TC practice.

> **REFLECTION**
>
> What role do you think there is for TC philosophy and practice in the future?

References

1. Kennard D. *Introduction to therapeutic communities.* London: Jessica Kingsley, 1998.
2. Royal College of Psychiatrists. *Service standards for therapeutic communities 8th edition.* London: Royal College of Psychiatrists, 2014.
3. Campling P. Therapeutic communities. *Advances in Psychiatric Treatment* 2001; **7**: 365–72.
4. Rapoport RN. *The community as doctor.* London: Tavistock, 1960.
5. Haigh R. The quintessence of a therapeutic community. In: Campling P, Haigh R (eds). *Therapeutic communities: past, present and future.* London: Jessica Kingsley, 1999: 246–57.
6. Hinshelwood RD. The therapeutic community in a changing cultural and political climate. *International Journal of Therapeutic Communities* 1989; **10**(1): 63–9.
7. Harrison T. *Advancing on a different front: Bion, Rickman & Foulkes and the Northfield Experiment.* London: Jessica Kingsley, 2000.
8. Callaway B. *Hildegard Peplau: psychiatric nurse of the century.* New York: Springer, 2002.
9. Jones M. *Social psychiatry in practice.* London: Tavistock, 1968.
10. Main, T. The concept of the therapeutic community: variations and vicissitudes. In: Pines M (ed.). *The evolution of group analysis.* London: Routledge and Kegan Paul: 1983, 197–217.
11. Peplau HE. *Interpersonal relations in nursing.* New York: G.P. Putnam's Sons, 1952.
12. Manning N. *The therapeutic community movement: charisma and routinization.* London: Routledge, 1989.
13. Whitley SA. Community study. In: Warren F, Dolan B (eds). *Perspectives on Henderson Hospital.* Sutton: Henderson Hospital, 2001.
14. Clarke DH. *Administrative therapy.* London: Tavistock, 1964.
15. Winship G. Karl Mannheim and the 'third way': the democratic origins of the term 'group analysis'. *Group Analysis* 2003; **36**(1): 37–51.
16. Ballatt J, Campling P. *Intelligent kindness: reforming the culture of healthcare.* London: Royal College of Psychiatrists, 2011.
17. Haigh R. The trouble with modernisation: we need better relationships, not policies and procedures. *Mental Health Review Journal* 2005; **10**(3): 3–7.
18. Tucker S. *A therapeutic community approach to care in the community: dialogue and dwelling.* London: Jessica Kingsley, 2000.
19. Slade M. *Personal recovery & mental illness: a guide for mental health profession.* Cambridge: Cambridge University Press, 2009.
20. Repper J, Perkins R. *Social inclusion & recovery.* London: Balliere Tindall, 2003.
21. Winship G. A meta-recovery framework: positioning the 'New Recovery' movement and other recovery approaches. Paper presented at the Royal College of Psychiatrist's Community of Communities Annual Forum, Brunei Gallery SOAS, London, 2014.
22. Winship G. Democracy in practice in 14 UK psychotherapeutic communities. *Therapeutic Communities* 2004; **25**(4): 275–90.
23. Winship G. Marcuse, Fromm & the Frankfurt School – reflecting on the history of ideas in therapeutic communities. *International Journal of Therapeutic Communities* 2013; **34**(2/3): 60–70.
24. Clarke JM. The role of everyday interaction rituals within therapeutic communities. In: Middleton H. Jordan M (eds). *Mental health uncertainty and inevitability: rejuvenating the relationship between social science and psychiatry.* London: Palgrave, 2017.
25. Clarke JM. Where the change is: everyday interaction rituals of therapeutic communities. Unpublished Doctoral Thesis, University of Nottingham, 2015.
26. Winship G. A brief history of addictions treatment in the UK. *Austin Journal of Drug Abuse and Addiction* 2014; **1**(1): 1–7.
27. Winnicott DAW. *Maturational processes and the facilitating environment.* London: Hogarth Press, 1965.
28. Royal College of Psychiatrists. *Community of Communities Annual Report 2013–2014.* London: Royal College of Psychiatrists, 2014.
29. Winship G, Hardy S. Perspectives on the prevalence and treatment of personality disorder. *Journal of Psychiatric and Mental Health Nursing* 2007; **14**(2): 148–54.
30. Lees J, Manning N. A culture of enquiry – research evidence and the therapeutic community. *Psychiatric Quarterly* 2004; **75**(3): 279–94.
31. Gask L, Evans M. Personality disorder. *British Medical Journal* 2013; **347**: f5276.
32. Pearce S. Trials of therapeutic communities in personality disorder are under way. *British Medical Journal* 2013; **347**: f6036.
33. Royal College of Psychiatrists. *Audit of violence.* London: Healthcare Commission, 2007.
34. Sainsbury Centre for Mental Health. *Acute care 2004 report.* London: Sainsbury Centre, 2005.
35. The Bennett Inquiry. *Independent inquiry into the death of David Bennett.* Cambridge: Cambridgeshire, 2003.
36. Francis R. *Report of the Mid Staffordshire NHS Foundation Trust Public Inquiry: executive summary.* London: Stationery Office, 2013.
37. Mistral W, Hall A, McKee P. Using therapeutic community principles to improve the functioning of a high care psychiatric ward in the UK. *International Journal of Mental Health Nursing* 2002; **11**(1): 10–17.

Further reading

Campling P. Therapeutic communities. *Advances in Psychiatric Treatment* 2001; **7**: 365–72.

Haigh R. The quintessence of a therapeutic community. In: Campling P, Haigh R (eds). *Therapeutic communities: past, present and future.* London: Jessica Kingsley, 1999, 246–57.

Manning N. *The therapeutic community movement: charisma and routinization*. London: Routledge, 1989.

Relevant web pages

Community of Communities Project at the Royal College of Psychiatrists. http://www.rcpsych.ac.uk/workinpsychiatry/qualityimprovement/qualityandaccreditation/therapeutic communities/communityofcommunities.aspx
This is the quality improvement and accreditation programme for TCs.

Royal College of Psychiatrists. *Service standards for therapeutic communities 8th edition*. London: Royal College of Psychiatrists, 2014.

Consortium for Therapeutic Communities (TCTC). http://www.therapeuticcommunities.org
This organization represents TCs across the UK.

Services for children and young people

STEVEN PRYJMACHUK AND HANNAH WELSBY

LEARNING OUTCOMES

- To understand the ways in which mental health services for children and young people are organized.
- To identify the types of problem with which children and young people are referred to mental health services.
- To weigh up the evidence base for children's mental health services and the interventions used within these services.
- To reflect on the skills required to care for children and young people with mental health problems.
- To understand what using mental health services is like from a young person's perspective.

SUMMARY OF KEY POINTS

- Mental health problems in children and young people are relatively common and can have wide-ranging and long-lasting effects on the child or young person, and on the people close to them.
- In the UK, services for children and young people tend to be organized using a four-tier approach based on level of need.
- The craft of caring for children and young people with mental health problems requires a range of

child-centred interpersonal and communication skills as well as knowledge of the evidence base.

- The evidence base in children and young people's mental health is concerned with organizational effectiveness (how good service provision is) as well as intervention effectiveness (how good individual treatments are).

INTRODUCTION

Mental health problems and mental illness in children and young people can only really be conceptualized if we are aware of what the determinants of a mentally healthy child or young person are. These determinants are wide and varied but can be broadly categorized as originating within *the child or young person*, within *the family context*, or within

the community. Determinants of good mental health originating from within the child or young person include good communication skills; a capacity to enter into and sustain personal relationships; an ability to play, learn and attain; high self-esteem; and a developed sense of right and wrong.[1,2] Family determinants are largely related to the extent that parents or carers are interested in, or involved with, their children – through affection, supervision, appropriate discipline, and support for the child or young person's education, for example – and through the attendant absence of discord in parental relationships, whether these are parent–parent or parent–child relationships.[2] Community-related determinants include good housing and a high standard of living, a supportive network, and schools that provide both academic and non-academic opportunities.[2]

When faced with significant life challenges – the death of a close relative, a new school or job, or a relationship break-up, for example – children and young people, like most of us, are less able to cope if they have deficits in any or all of these determinants. Without the personal, family or community resources to deal with normal life stresses, a child or young person's mental health can be threatened. Where this threat results in emotions or behaviours that are distressing to the child or young person or to their family, the child or young person might be said to have a *mental health problem*. When these emotions or behaviours persist and are severe enough to interfere with the child or young person's or family's everyday lives, the child or young person might be said to have *severe mental health problems*, or even a *mental disorder* or a *mental illness*.

At any one time, around one in five children and young people in the UK will experience mild-to-moderate mental health problems, with around 1 in 10 having more serious problems that might be called mental illness or mental disorder.[2–5] In addition:

- Mental health problems in children and young people can have wide-ranging effects on educational attainment, social and family relationships, criminality and life chances.[2]
- Fifty per cent of mental illness in adult life starts before the age of 15, and 75 per cent by the age of 18.[5]
- Socio-economic disadvantage, parental mental illness, parental criminality and emotional and sexual abuse can all have a significant impact on children's and young people's mental health.[2]
- Looked-after children (children in care) are at greater risk, with as many as 50 per cent having mental health problems.[4]
- Self-harm rates among young people in the UK are the highest in Europe, affecting at least 1 in 15 young people.[6]
- Children with a physical or learning disability and children with serious and long-term physical illnesses are all at greater risk of developing mental health problems.[2,4]

REFLECTION

Do any of the statistics above surprise you? Given that 20 per cent of children and young people potentially require help, do you think the current provision of mental health services for children and young people is adequate?

ORGANIZATION OF SERVICES FOR CHILDREN AND YOUNG PEOPLE

Services for children and young people – in the Western world at least – have been organized around two conceptual models.[2] Both are hierarchical in that they are made up of discrete levels, with the levels at the top being reserved for the smaller population of children and young people with severe mental health problems and the levels at the bottom being reserved for the wider, general, 'universal' population of children and young people.

The first model (see Table 58.1) is more common in Australia and the USA than in the UK and focuses on the

Table 58.1 Service organization by level of intervention

Type	Level	Details
Preventative	Universal	Includes all children and young people Enhances resilience in children and young people Screening not required Avoids stigmatization
	Selective	Selects children and young people at risk Involves screening
Management	Indicated	Selects children and young people displaying mild symptoms Involves screening
	Treatment	Targets children and young people with a *diagnosed* condition

Source: Adapted, with the permission of Cambridge University Press, from Lowry-Webster et al.[7]

type of intervention available. In this model, services are organized according to the population at which the intervention is targeted. Two of the intervention levels (universal and selective) are what might be called 'preventative' interventions because they are designed to promote mental health or prevent mental ill-heath developing in one of two populations: (i) the population of children and young people as a whole; and (ii) the population of those who might be deemed 'at risk'.

The other two intervention levels might be termed 'management' interventions because they are designed to manage mild-to-moderate mental health problems (indicated) or the more severe mental health problems (treatment).

The second model (see Table 58.2) focuses on the level of need and is essentially the model on which UK mental health services for children and young people – colloquially known as 'CAMHS' (an abbreviation for 'child and adolescent mental health services') – are predicated.

This 'tier' model emanated from a 1995 publication[1] by the now defunct NHS Health Advisory Service (a forerunner of the Care Quality Commission). It remains the current organizational model for CAMHS throughout the UK, though it is not without criticism and may soon face changes in England at least.[8] The tiers are designed to operate in such a way that children and young people are dealt with in the lowest appropriate and least restrictive tier (and, some would also argue, the least stigmatizing tier) in the first instance, with referral to higher tiers based on a lack of progress or poor outcomes at that tier, or on insufficient expertise and resources being available.

Tier 1 services

Tier 1 services are concerned with *promoting mental health*, *preventing mental ill-health* and *early intervention*. As a consequence, most Tier 1 services operate in general community (universal) settings rather than in formal, health-related settings. Those working in Tier 1 services tend not

Table 58.2 Service organization by level of need

Tier	Level of need	Services	Service locale	Professionals involved
1	At risk of mental health problems Mild mental health problems	Screening Advice Mental health promotion and prevention Self-help Early intervention Referral to formal CAMHS (Tier 2)	Primary care Schools Community premises, e.g. youth centres, church premises, voluntary sector premises	GPs Health visitors School staff Youth workers Police officers
Formal CAMHS start at Tier 2				
2	Moderately severe mental health problems	Advice and training to Tier 1 professionals Assessment/outreach Early intervention Self-management support	Primary care Community mental health settings Psychology services Outpatient psychiatry	Child mental health professionals (usually singularly), e.g. psychologists, mental health nurses, psychiatrists Mental health liaison workers/primary mental health workers
3	Severe and complex mental health problems (i.e. mental disorders)	Specialist assessment and treatment services largely outside institutional settings	Community mental health settings Outpatient psychiatry Possibly day patient units	Multidisciplinary child mental health team
4	Very severe and/or persistent mental health problems (i.e. persistent mental disorders)	Specialist assessment and treatment services largely within institutional settings	Day patient units Local, regional and specialist (e.g. eating disorder, intensive care) inpatient units Specialized outpatient teams (e.g. self-harm teams)	Multidisciplinary and highly specialized child mental health team, often including an expanded range of professionals (e.g. occupational, creative, family and psychological therapists)

to be mental health specialists; indeed, anyone who works with children and young people – a teacher, youth worker, school nurse, GP, etc. – could be described as a Tier 1 professional. If they work as planned, Tier 1 services can provide children and young people with appropriate support in an ordinary, non-stigmatizing environment, possibly preventing referral to higher tiers or even inpatient admission. This is not always the case, however, as Hannah's story shows.

TIER 1 SERVICES – HANNAH'S STORY

The involvement that I had with Tier 1 services in the beginning wasn't very effective. I felt at the time my problems were being brushed aside and ignored. It wasn't until I was self-harming and suicidal at the age of 14 that I felt people were actually beginning to listen to me. Recently I went through my very first notes at CAMHS which stated I had told a school nurse at the age of 11 that I was struggling and that this was ignored. I strongly believe that if that nurse had listened to what I was telling her, my mental health wouldn't have deteriorated to the point it did. It took 3 years before people began to listen.

I told my head of year at school first, with the help of a friend. The teacher was helpful most of the time. However, on one occasion she grabbed my arm, and forced up my sleeve in order to see the cuts on my arm. This was quite unhelpful to say the least. The first GP that I saw was a junior doctor. She was lovely but was unprepared and out of her depth to be dealing with mental health problems. She offered to support me as best she could. However, on one occasion, I went to see her for the regular appointment and she prescribed about nine boxes of paracetamol. I was struggling a lot at this point and this almost became my first suicide attempt. At 14, emotions and an unhelpful friendship led to a suicide pact. This involved three major overdoses taken in school. School could no longer control the situation. I didn't understand what was happening during the course of those 3 years. I did not feel and still don't feel like my needs were met. If I was listened to, I do not think that things would have got to the point that they did. I lost trust in the people who were supposed to protect me.

Tier 2 services

Tier 2 services are the first formal level of CAMHS provision – the first tier at which mental health specialists are actively involved. One of the principal roles of Tier 2 specialists is to *provide advice and guidance for Tier 1 professionals.* Indeed, some CAMHS providers employ *mental health liaison workers* or *primary mental health workers* whose role is to act as a Tier 1/Tier 2 'go-between', providing training and advice for Tier 1 professionals and acting as gatekeepers to formal CAMHS by assessing children and young people about whom Tier 1 professionals may have concerns.[9] The outcome of these assessments may be that the child or young person is, indeed, referred to a Tier 2 specialist, but it may also be that the liaison/primary mental health worker feels the child or young person can be helped within Tier 1, as long as the Tier 1 professionals involved have the support and guidance of Tier 2 specialists.

A formal referral to a Tier 2 specialist usually means that the child/young person and their family are seen by a single mental health specialist, such as a child psychiatrist, child psychologist or nurse specializing in children's mental health, most often for *assessment.* Should intervention be required, it is usually one that is relatively short and which can be conducted in a primary care or community setting or on an outpatient basis. Should more complex or intensive interventions be required, or should the Tier 2 professional have concerns about the safety of the child or young person or those close to them, a referral can be made to Tier 3, which is often part of the same service.

Tier 3 services

The defining feature of Tier 3 services is that they are *multidisciplinary.* While more than one mental health specialist will work with the child/young person and their family, the locale of the service tends to remain community- or outpatient-oriented. Occasionally, day services may be available whereby the child or young person attends the service for one or more whole days, perhaps receiving schooling in the morning from specialist education staff and therapeutic work from specialist mental health staff in the afternoon. Again, a lack of progress or continuing concerns about risk at this tier would warrant a referral to a higher tier, Tier 4.

Tier 4 services

Tier 4 services are the very specialized mental health services. They are usually, but not necessarily, *inpatient services* and may include day services, home-based service and outreach services.[10,11] These services may be local, general inpatient services for children and young people or they may be more specialized regional or national services – specialized eating disorder, self-harm, forensic or psychiatric intensive care services, for example. Because the needs of children and young people in these units are complex and the therapies intensive, staff–patient ratios tend to be relatively high and an extended team of mental health specialists is usually available that may include – in addition to psychiatrists, mental health nurses and psychologists – occupational therapists, creative therapists (such as play, art and drama therapists), psychotherapists, family therapists and support workers. Education professionals such as teachers and educational psychologists are also available in order to ensure that there is as little disruption to the child/young person's schooling as possible. This is especially important given that the length of stay for a child/young person in Tier 4 services tends to be months rather than days or weeks.[12]

TIER 4 SERVICES – HANNAH'S STORY

I spent 4½ months in an inpatient service. This was my first experience of a Tier 4 service. I was not told much about the unit or what would happen to me. I had no time to prepare myself or to ask questions. Tier 4 services were difficult to cope with at times because of staffing levels and ineffective communication which meant it wasn't possible to facilitate vital 1:1 sessions with a staff member or information wasn't passed on. The pressures that the nurses were under clearly affected service users in a negative way, though some staff tried their best and always tried to keep us busy. For me, the group activities and walks were the most important part of ward life.

In retrospect, I feel that the admission to this service was the break that I needed from my family and school. It gave me the chance to find new ways of coping and build myself back up so that I was able to go back to a 'normal' life. One of the most important things that helped me during my stay was a self-harm group. I finally felt like I was understood. It was a controlled and supportive environment. Another helpful aspect was my key nurse. She understood the difficulties that I have with attachments and helped me to create a formulation. The onsite college gave me the opportunity to continue with my education and gave me a place to escape to from the ward. Once I moved on to the day service, the college supported me through the transition into my own school. I feel that the day service, however, was the most useful aspect of my therapy. I was given freedom whilst still receiving the same level (if not better) quality of care. I finally felt like I was understood and was now able to verbalize my emotions in an appropriate way. The day service gave me the right pathways to be able to speak at conferences and training courses and to contribute to research.

TYPES OF PROBLEM REFERRED TO CAMHS

Children and young people are referred to CAMHS for a variety of problems (see Figure 58.1). It is beyond the scope of this chapter to offer anything more than a cursory examination of these problems, and more detailed information can be found in the resources listed at the end of this chapter (McDougall,[13] Dogra and Leighton,[14] and chapters 9 and 10 in Pryjmachuk[15] in particular). Since many childhood problems are similar to those experienced in adulthood, the chapters in this book on anxiety (chapter 20), depression (chapter 21), self-harm (chapter 22), eating disorders (chapter 30) and early interventions in psychosis (chapter 45) may also be useful, though it should be borne in mind that additional skills and safeguards are often needed when working with children and young people rather than adults. It is, however, worth mentioning a few terms that you may be unfamiliar with, and worth pointing out those problems that are peculiar to children and young people or for which the incidence is much greater or much smaller in children and young people than in adults.

Emotional and behavioural problems are the most common reason for referral to CAMHS.[4] Behavioural problems such as *conduct disorder* and *attention-deficit hyperactivity disorder* (ADHD) are much more common in children (boys in particular) than in adults, though some believe that conduct disorder manifests as anti-social personality disorder in adulthood[16] (more detail about personality disorders can be found in chapter 27). Most of the emotional problems children and young people present with are also common in adults (indeed, in adults, the term 'common mental health problems' is frequently use to describe them).[17] *School refusal*, however, is a particular anxiety-based condition that can, by definition, only affect those legally obliged to attend school – children and young people, in other words. (This opens up interesting questions over the validity of a psychiatric condition that ceases to exist the minute a young person hits school-leaving age.) School refusal is sometimes known as 'school phobia' but its more common label reflects that fact that the condition is more about a fear of separation from

Emotional problems

- **Anxiety problems**: non-specific (generalized) anxiety; phobias; obsessive–compulsive disorder (OCD); social anxiety; separation anxiety; school refusal; post-traumatic stress disorder (PTSD); somatoform disorders
- **Depression** including 'dysthymia' (which is mild-to-moderate depression of a long-term nature)
- **Self-harm** (including suicidal ideation), e.g. self-cutting, self-burning and self-poisoning
- **Attachment problems**: insecure-avoidant attachment; insecure-ambivalent attachment

Behavioural problems

- **Conduct issues**: conduct disorder (CD); oppositional defiant disorder (ODD); fire-setting
- **Attention-deficit hyperactivity disorder** (ADHD); hyperkinesis (hyperactivity)

Developmental problems

- **Speech and language problems**
- **Disorders of bladder and bowel control**: enuresis (bed-wetting); encopresis (soiling)

Eating problems

- **Anorexia nervosa**
- **Bulimia nervosa**
- ? childhood obesity

Psychosis

- **Schizophrenia**
- Drug-induced psychosis

Figure 58.1 Types of problems referred to children and young people's mental health services.

home or a parent (i.e. separation anxiety) than about a real fear of school. *Somatoform* conditions are conditions where stress or anxiety seems to elicit persistent physical symptoms such as headache or nausea. They are also seen in adults, another name for these disorders being 'medically unexplained symptoms' which perhaps give you more insight into their nature. *Self-harm* is a particular concern, especially in older children and young adults.[6] *Psychosis* before the teenage years is rare,[18] and thus most referrals to CAMHS tend to be in the upper age range (15 to 18 years) and, in almost all cases, are first-episode referrals. Despite its relative rarity, psychosis accounts for around a quarter of Tier 4 admissions;[19] other common reasons for Tier 4 admission are severe eating disorders and serious self-harm.

THE ROLE OF NURSES IN CAMHS

Nurses are the largest occupational group working in formal CAMHS, accounting for around 25 per cent of the workforce[20] and they are designated, along with child psychiatrists and child psychologists, as one of the key professionals that define a mental health service for children and young people.[1,21] Consequently, nurses can play a key role in CAMHS at all tiers, though some specialist therapies (such as family therapy, interpersonal therapy or cognitive behaviour therapy) may require additional post-registration and/or postgraduate training. Interestingly, not all nurses who specialize in CAMHS are mental health nurses – a minority are children's nurses or have some other qualification, such as health visiting – and this opens up the (controversial) question of whether you need to be a mental health nurse to work in children's mental health. Nonetheless, even though the figures show that more mental health nurses work in CAMHS than non-mental health nurses, it is rare to find anything more than a cursory exposure to children and young people's mental health in most pre-registration mental health and children's nursing curricula, and few students have the opportunity for a placement in this area.

REFLECTION

- The craft of caring for children and young people with mental health problems requires that nurses have particular communication and interpersonal skills. Nurses may have to be – as well as therapist – any or all of parent, teacher, arbiter, disciplinarian and confidant.

- What do you think are the important characteristics of a nurse working in children and young people's mental health? What skills do you think they need? Why wasn't 'friend' on the list of roles above? (Hint: think about boundaries.)

- Once you have thought about this, compare your views with Hannah's perspective on nurses.

HANNAH'S PERSPECTIVE ON NURSES

A good mental health nurse must always keep in mind why they went into the job, especially in the midst of the hardest situations. This is vital as any health care professional who loses sight of their purpose in that role will have their judgement and the quality of care given affected. A mental health nurse should not be patronizing or authoritarian and should be able to approach a service user as they would any other human. This means that they should talk about daily issues and laugh with their patient but should also keep strong boundaries.

My nurse-therapist talks to me about some of her experiences whilst keeping these boundaries in place. I don't feel like I am going to a mental health service but see it as a calm and supportive environment. Bad mental health nurses allow their judgement to become clouded. Any health professional should not let personal issues or other work issues be taken into any appointment. From my own experiences, I know that the thing that helped me bond the most with my nurse-therapist, doctor and other professionals was being able to have a down-to-earth conversation with another human being.

THE CRAFT OF CARING: SKILLS REQUIRED BY NURSES WORKING WITH CHILDREN AND YOUNG PEOPLE

As with adults, the care of children and young people with mental health problems is predicated on *effective communication and interpersonal skills* (see chapter 3). Some of these skills are discussed in Section 2 of this book and in other core mental health texts,[15,22] but it is worth highlighting a few aspects that apply specifically to children and young people. Firstly, children and families tend to prioritize the ability of health care practitioners to *listen* and their *accessibility, approachability* and *child-centredness* over whether they have mental health expertise or not.[2,23,24] Secondly, since children and young people frequently have different views from adults about what matters in their care and since peers may be more important than parents, it is important that the child or young person's views are taken seriously. Thirdly, while *safeguarding* is paramount, safeguarding has to work within the constraints of building *trust* – the nurse must always be upfront with the child or young person if a safeguarding issue arises, and not make promises that they cannot keep, or report issues to other agencies without the child or young person being fully prepared and supported. Finally, a positive or strengths-based approach is less stigmatizing than one that focuses on problems and deficits;

protective factors as well as risks should be explored during the assessment and caring processes.

Risk assessment can be a particular challenge. While it is a core aspect of the craft of caring, it does require great care when working with children and young people, since an over-zealous risk assessment can lead to children and young people feeling controlled, mistrustful, stigmatized and avoidant of services, rather than protected or cared for.[6,25] Risk assessment is not always easy but it can be enhanced by asking the child and his or her family direct questions and exploring a wide variety of individual, family, community and environmental risk and protective factors[2] (e.g. relating to academic success/failure, relationships, substance misuse, poverty, homelessness, parental criminality or parental mental illness). (For more on risk assessment in general, see chapters 16 and 17.)

THE EVIDENCE BASE IN CHILDREN'S AND YOUNG PEOPLE'S MENTAL HEALTH

The craft of caring for children and young people with mental health problems requires knowledge as well as skills, and knowledge of the *evidence base* in particular. The evidence base in children's and young people's mental health can be considered from two related perspectives:

- the evidence that CAMHS provision, as organized, is effective;
- the evidence that individual interventions delivered within CAMHS are effective.

In other words, we can ask how good *services* for children and young people are (to some extent how good those running them are at caring), and how good *individual treatments* are.

Organizational effectiveness

Regarding organizational effectiveness, in 1999 the Audit Commission (a government body that oversees how public money is spent) published a review focusing on the value-for-money of CAMHS in England and Wales.[20] It described services with long waiting lists that often restricted access, and concluded that there was poor investment in CAMHS, unacceptable regional variation and little inter-agency working (between health, social care, education and voluntary sector bodies, for example). Almost a decade later, another review – the 2008 English CAMHS Review[2] – noted that children and young people did not think services were particularly responsive, accessible or child-centred. Moreover, it reported that unacceptable regional variations and problems in accessing services remained, and that little evidence-based practice was evident. Similar problems were reported in Wales a year later.[26] Tier 4 CAMHS

were subjected to particular criticism around this time: the Children's Commissioner for England published a report[27] condemning the practice of placing young people with mental health problems in adult inpatient facilities, and the NHS commissioned research to explore alternatives to inpatient CAMHS.[28]

In 2011, the frustration of the government and of commissioners of services, about the fact that little had changed in more than a decade, led to the implementation, in England, of the Children and Young People's Improving Access to Psychological Therapies (IAPT) initiative. Unlike the earlier adult IAPT initiative (see chapter 40), the children and young people's IAPT initiative does not operate as a stand-alone service; instead, it is designed to transform and improve services through the (re)training of staff in evidence-based interventions and routine outcome measurements.[29] In early 2015, yet another critical review of CAMHS was published,[8] drawing similar conclusions about high levels of unmet need, difficulty in accessing services and the need to develop the CAMHS workforce.

Throughout these reviews and reports, CAMHS provision has been criticized for its lack of accessibility, poor inter-agency working, inappropriate care environments, limited staff capability and the delivery of interventions and therapies without reference to the evidence base. There are certainly indications that these limitations are being taken seriously by CAMHS professionals. The Royal College of Psychiatrists,[21] for example, recommends that services consider evidence-based systems of managing demand and capacity to improve accessibility, the most well-known being perhaps the Choice and Partnership Approach (CAPA),[30] a collaborative approach that puts the child/young person and their family at the centre of decision making (for more on collaborative care planning, see chapter 50). Regarding inter-agency working, there is evidence that the Tier 2 liaison/primary mental health workers are valued, especially by schools,[9,21] and there are many voluntary sector organizations (such as YoungMinds, the Place2Be and Barnardo's) which are more than willing to work in partnership with established CAMHS providers. Indeed, within the current English health care framework, there is no reason why these organizations cannot be CAMHS providers themselves and, increasingly, voluntary sector organizations can be found delivering services in partnership with the NHS, especially in Tier 1.

As you will shortly discover, it is clear that there is an established and growing evidence base in children's and young people's mental health. Why there is so little reference to the evidence base in contemporary CAMHS provision is a complex question that cannot be resolved in an introductory text like this. The CAMHS Review of 2008[2] speculated that busy professionals with little time may be one reason; other possibilities could be the lack of training and education opportunities available to health care professionals in their pre-qualifying courses, or it may simply be a result of entrenched attitudes ('this is the therapy I like and I have always used it and I am not going to change').

REFLECTION

If the craft of caring requires both knowledge (theory; science) and skills (practice; art) what do you think could be done to improve the craft of caring for children and young people with mental health problems? (Think about, for example, inter-agency working, the physical care environment, evidence-based interventions, child-centred attitudes and the accessibility of services.)

Effectiveness of individual therapies

In determining the evidence base for individual interventions in children's and young people's mental health, the principal sources of information available are the guidance produced by the English and Scottish clinical guidelines agencies – the National Institute of Health and Care Excellence (NICE)[31] and the Scottish Intercollegiate Guidelines Network (SIGN)[32] – and the work emanating from the CAMHS Evidence Based Practice Unit (CAMHS EBPU),[33] a joint Anna Freud Centre/University College London initiative. The discussion that follows is grounded on information from these sources, together with other relevant evidence, such as systematic reviews of the literature.

In looking at the evidence base in children's and young people's mental health, it is possible to group and discuss interventions in a variety of ways: by the conditions targeted (depression, anxiety, self-harm, etc.); by the level at which they operate (universal/selective/indicated/treatment; prevention versus management); by the theoretical or conceptual approaches employed (neurobiological, cognitive-behavioural, psychodynamic, etc.); or by the tiers in which they are used. Since all of the four countries of the UK currently operate the four-tier model, perhaps the most pragmatic approach is to consider the interventions first according to the arbitrary division between non-specialist and specialist services (i.e. Tier 1 versus Tiers 2 to 4), and then, when discussing specialist services, consider interventions by target condition or problem, because specialist interventions tend to be designed with a particular condition or problem in mind.

Tier 1 interventions

Given that the focus in Tier 1 is principally mental health promotion and prevention, the interventions operating solely in Tier 1 tend to be universal, whole-population interventions. Sometimes, however, while remaining preventative, interventions are selective in that they are targeted at a particular sub-population (e.g. children at risk of anxiety or young people at risk of self-harm).

Universal interventions are largely concerned with a child or young person's social and emotional well-being and most universal interventions are delivered within schools, because schools are the very place where whole populations of children and young people can be found. Specific public health guidelines from NICE[34–36] provide a framework for good practice in universal interventions. The NICE guidance for primary and secondary schools[34,35] recommends a whole-school approach to social and emotional well-being that involves children, parents, teachers and health staff (e.g. CAMHS staff, school nurses and health visitors) all working together. Interventions typically focus on integrating into the curriculum social and emotional skills development (e.g. problem solving, coping, conflict management, and understanding and managing feelings and relationships) to enhance social and emotional well-being, instil resilience and prevent bullying and aggression. Teachers and other school practitioners should also be able to identify and assess early signs of emotional distress so they can – perhaps with the support of a Tier 2 liaison/primary mental health worker – offer 'low-level' targeted interventions like group problem-solving and parenting.

Guidance for the early years (pre-school) suggests that interventions with this age group should be selective rather than universal,[36] targeting mainly 'vulnerable' children, i.e. those exposed to socio-economic disadvantage, parental mental illness or parental criminality. With these families, parents should be supported at home to develop *parenting skills*, though midwives and health visitors are more likely to undertake this work than mental health staff.

In terms of whether Tier 1 interventions work, the evidence is somewhat equivocal, with targeted interventions seeming to work better than universal interventions. For example, an England-wide evaluation of a national, universal 'social and emotional aspects of learning' (SEAL) programme[37] found that SEAL generally failed to meet its intended objectives; on the other hand, an evaluation of an earlier 'targeted mental health in schools' initiative[38] found some evidence that school-based targeted interventions worked well for behaviour problems in primary school children but not so well for emotional problems, or in older children. Regarding parent training, a recent Cochrane review found that group parenting programmes such as *Triple P* and *The Incredible Years* appear to be effective in preventing a range of behaviour problems in young children.[39]

> ## REFLECTION
>
> Look back at Figure 58.1. There is a question mark next to *childhood obesity* under 'eating problems'. While discussing Tier 1 interventions, it is worth thinking about preventative interventions to tackle childhood obesity. Would you consider childhood obesity to be a mental health disorder? What about if you were told obesity had severe, negative consequences on self-esteem?

Specialist CAMHS interventions

For each of the broad range of conditions outlined in Figure 58.1, available evidence-based interventions are summarized in Table 58.3, together with the tiers in which these interventions are typically delivered.

It is worth mentioning that *medication* appears on the list of evidence-based interventions far less than it would

Table 58.3 Interventions used to manage specific problems in CAMHS

Problem type	Interventions with some evidence of effectiveness	Relevant tiers
Emotional problems		
Anxiety problems	Many of the approaches used to treat anxiety in adults can be used with children and young people, though interventions should be made age-appropriate. For generalized anxiety disorders, specific phobias and OCD, *behavioural or CBT approaches* or *group CBT* appear to be the most effective;[40,41] *guided self-help* may also be useful for OCD.[42] Individual CBT may work for school refusal.[41] For PTSD, *trauma-focused CBT* has some evidence of effectiveness.[40] For medically unexplained symptoms – especially abdominal pain – there is evidence that *CBT* is effective.[40]	Tiers 2–3
Depression	NICE guidance[43] recommends *watchful waiting* in the first instance. Watchful waiting is a 'light-touch' intervention whereby individuals are monitored on a regular basis to see whether the condition or problem worsens.	Tier 1
	If intervention is required, the NICE guidance[43] suggests *group CBT*, *nondirective supportive therapy* or *guided self-help* in the first instance; if there is no response, a further, brief course of psychological therapy is recommended, perhaps with the use of the SSRI antidepressant fluoxetine (Prozac); if there is still no response, a more intensive course of psychological therapy is recommended, augmented if necessary with an SSRI such as fluoxetine, citalopram or sertraline. The CAMHS EBPU suggests there is some evidence of the effectiveness of *psychotherapy* and *family therapy* for depression.[40]	Tiers 2–3; Tier 4 usually only if there is serious self-harm as well as depression
Self-harm	Serious self-harm is a *medical emergency* and may require admission to Accident and Emergency.	

(Continued)

Table 58.3 *(continued)*

Problem type	Interventions with some evidence of effectiveness	Relevant tiers
	Regarding the longer-term management of self-harm, there is little evidence of any specific intervention being effective,[44] though NICE guidance[45] suggests that specific therapies should be tailored to the individual's needs and could include *CBT*, *psychodynamic* or *problem-solving* elements. Drug treatments, however, are not recommended. There is a small amount of evidence for *group therapy*[40,46] and, at the time of writing, a large trial of family therapy for self-harm is underway.[47]	Largely higher tiers (Tiers 2–4)

Behaviour problems

Problem type	Interventions with some evidence of effectiveness	Relevant tiers
Conduct disorders	*Parent training*, combined with individual problem-solving and social skills training in older children, and *multi-systemic therapy* (an intensive therapy that takes into account community and family factors such as home, friends and school as well as individual factors) are the most effective interventions.[40]	Tier 1 Tiers 2–3
ADHD	*Stimulant medication* such as methylphenidate (Ritalin), perhaps combined with parent training and individual therapy in 'multimodal treatment', is the most effective intervention,[40,48,49] although recent NICE guidance[50] recommends *parent training* in the first instance, with medication being reserved for those with more severe ADHD.	Tiers 2–3

Developmental problems

Problem type	Interventions with some evidence of effectiveness	Relevant tiers
Speech/ language problems	Referral to specialist speech and language therapists.	Tier 1
Enuresis and encopresis	Specific NICE guidelines for enuresis[51] suggest that an *alarm system* (a bed pad that sets off an alarm when urine connects electrical contacts) should be the first-line treatment for persistent enuresis; *desmopressin* (a synthetic hormone that regulates retention of water) may also be useful. There are no NICE guidelines on encopresis but a recent review[52] suggests that *behavioural techniques* (e.g. toileting coupled with a reward system) are the most effective.	Mostly Tier 1

Eating disorders

Problem type	Interventions with some evidence of effectiveness	Relevant tiers
	The CAMHS EBPU[40] and NICE guidance[53] recommends *family therapy* as the treatment of choice for anorexia nervosa; for bulimia nervosa, there is some evidence for an adapted form of *CBT* and, perhaps, an antidepressant. The NICE guidance suggests that anorexia nervosa should be managed in primary care whenever possible.	Tiers 2–4

Psychosis

Problem type	Interventions with some evidence of effectiveness	Relevant tiers
	Both NICE[19] and SIGN[54] recommend that young people with psychosis are dealt with by a specialist, multidisciplinary early intervention service or team. NICE, SIGN and the CAMHS EBPU[40] recommend *antipsychotic medication* as a first-line treatment for psychosis but the NICE guidance – which is specific to children and young people – adds that medication should be used in conjunction with *family interventions*. NICE guidance also suggests that *CBT* may have some value for psychosis, and that creative therapies (art, drama, music, etc.) may be useful for young people with negative symptoms.	Higher tiers, especially Tier 4

for adults with mental health problems. One reason for this is the controversy over using potent medications such as stimulants and antidepressants with children and young people when the long-term effects on physical and mental development may not be known. Chapters 47 and 48 has information on psychopharmacology.

HANNAH'S REFLECTIONS ON MENTAL HEALTH TREATMENTS

At the beginning of my treatment, especially in the inpatient unit, I was not asked my opinion on my care. Some of this was due to risk, but I know now that this is something that should happen throughout any treatments. I was not aware of care plans until halfway through my care and it wasn't until I was transitioning back into school that I was involved in this process. In the past 4 years, the services that I have been with have helped me to understand my difficulties better and helped me to think about suitable methods of coping. My care has been about me taking responsibility for my care and making my own decisions in order to aid my recovery. I have had both good and bad experiences with mental health professionals. Boundaries in my care have been important to me as I can become attached to professionals very quickly and perceived abandonment has been devastating. I have been caught in unhelpful power struggles with my care team due to various factors. In the past few years I have felt more able to understand the impact of my behaviour on myself, others and my care team whilst allowing myself to express how I feel, and to ask questions about my care.

REFLECTION

How do Hannah's reflections on her treatment map on to what is known about the evidence base? Are there things from her perspective – particularly about her own attitude and the qualities of the therapists – that seem to be more important than the actual therapy? How might Hannah's perspective influence the way in which you might help children and young people with mental health problems?

CONCLUSION

In reading this chapter, you will have learnt about the organization of CAMHS provision across the UK and about the four-tier model in particular. While exploring service organization, you will have become aware of some of the criticisms that have been aimed at CAMHS over the last decade or so, and of some of the attempts to redress these criticisms. In doing so, the notion of evidence-based practice arises, and you will have had an opportunity to look at the evidence for the effectiveness of CAMHS provision overall and for individual interventions used in CAMHS. The value of nursing skills in CAMHS provision should also have become apparent. Finally, through reflecting on Hannah's experiences, it is hoped that you will have become much more aware of the importance of what the child or young person has to say about their care and treatment, because without acknowledging this, you will not be able to deliver truly child-centred, compassionate, collaborative and effective care.

References

1. NHS Health Advisory Service. *Child and adolescent mental health services: together we stand*. London: HMSO, 1995.
2. CAMHS Review. *Children and young people in mind: the final report of the National CAMHS Review*. London: Department for Children, Schools and Families/Department of Health, 2008.
3. Meltzer H, Gatward G, Goodman R, Ford T. *Mental health of children and adolescents in Great Britain*. London: Stationery Office, 2000.
4. Green H, McGinnity A, Meltzer H, Ford T, Goodman R. *Mental health of children and adolescents in Great Britain, 2004*. Basingstoke: Palgrave Macmillan, 2005.
5. Murphy M, Fonagy P. *Mental health problems in children and young people. Our children deserve better: prevention pays, annual report of the Chief Medical Officer 2012*. London: Department of Health, 2013.
6. National Inquiry into Self-harm among Young People. *Truth hurts: report of the National Inquiry into Self-harm among Young People*. London: Mental Health Foundation, 2006.
7. Lowry-Webster HM, Barrett PM, Dadds MR. A universal prevention trial of anxiety and depressive symptomatology in childhood: preliminary data from an Australian study. *Behaviour Change* 2001; **18**(01): 36–50.
8. NHS England. Future in mind: promoting, protecting and improving our children and young people's mental health and wellbeing. London: NHS England, 2015. Available from: www.gov.uk/government/uploads/system/uploads/

attachment_data/file/414024/Childrens_Mental_Health.pdf [Accessed 1st June 2016].

9. Atkinson M, Lamont E, Wright B. *NFER review: the role of primary mental health workers in education.* Slough: National Foundation for Educational Research, 2010.

10. McDougall T, Worrall-Davies A, Hewson L, Richardson G, Cotgrove A. Tier 4 Child and Adolescent Mental Health Services (CAMHS) – inpatient care, day services and alternatives: an overview of Tier 4 CAMHS provision in the UK. *Child Adolescent Mental Health* 2008; **13**(4): 173–80.

11. Kurtz Z. *The evidence base to guide development of Tier 4 CAMHS.* London: Department of Health, 2009.

12. Health and Social Care Information Centre. Hospital episode statistics, admitted patient care, England – 2012–13: main specialties. 2013. Available from: www.hscic.gov.uk/catalogue/PUB12566/hosp-epis-stat-admi-main-spec-2012-13-tab.xlsx [Accessed 1st June 2016].

13. McDougall T (ed.). *Children and Young People's Mental Health: Essentials for Nurses and Other Professionals.* London: Routledge, 2016.

14. Dogra N, Leighton S (eds). *Nursing in child and adolescent mental health.* Maidenhead: Open University Press, 2009.

15. Pryjmachuk S (ed.). *Mental Health nursing: an evidence-based introduction.* London: Sage, 2011.

16. Hill J. Early identification of individuals at risk for antisocial personality disorder. *British Journal of Psychiatry* 2003; **182**(44): s11–s14.

17. NICE (National Institute for Health and Care Excellence). Common mental health disorders: Identification and pathways to care (CG123). 2011. Available from: http://guidance.nice.org.uk/CG123/NICEGuidance/pdf/English [Accessed 1st June 2016].

18. Nicolson R, Rapoport JL. Childhood-onset schizophrenia: rare but worth studying. *Biological Psychiatry* 1999; **46**(10): 1418–28.

19. NICE (National Institute for Health and Care Excellence). Psychosis and schizophrenia in children and young people: recognition and management (CG155). 2013. Available from: http://guidance.nice.org.uk/CG155/NICEGuidance/pdf/English [Accessed 1st June 2016].

20. Audit Commission. *Children in mind: child and adolescent mental health services.* London: Audit Commission, 1999.

21. Royal College of Psychiatrists. *Building and sustaining specialist CAMHS to improve outcomes for children and young people: update of guidance on workforce, capacity and functions of CAMHS in the UK.* London: Royal College of Psychiatrists, 2013.

22. Callaghan P, Playle J, Cooper L. *Mental health nursing skills.* Oxford: Oxford University Press, 2009.

23. Pryjmachuk S, Elvey R, Kirk S, Kendal S, Bower P, Catchpole R. Developing a model of mental health self-care support for children and young people through an integrated evaluation of available types of provision involving systematic review, meta-analysis and case study. *Health Services and Delivery Research* 2014; **2**(18).

24. Pryjmachuk S, Graham T, Haddad M, Tylee A. School nurses' perspectives on managing mental health problems in children and young people. *Journal of Clinical Nursing* 2012; **21**(5–6): 850–9.

25. YoungMinds. *Stigma: a review of the evidence.* London: YoungMinds, 2010.

26. Wales Audit Office. *Services for children and young people with emotional and mental health needs.* Cardiff: Auditor General for Wales, 2009.

27. Children's Commissioner for England. *Pushed into the shadows: young people's experiences of adult mental health facilities.* London: Office for the Children's Commissioner, 2007.

28. Shepperd S, Doll H, Gowers S, James A, Fazel M, Fitzpatrick R, Pollock J. Alternatives to inpatient mental health care for children and young people. *Cochrane Database of Systematic Reviews* 2009; 2.

29. IAPT. Children and young people's project. Available from: https://www.england.nhs.uk/mentalhealth/cyp/iapt/ [Accessed 5th December 2016].

30. National CAMHS Support Service, Mental Health Foundation. *Evaluation of the choice and partnership approach in child and adolescent mental health services in England.* London: Mental Health Foundation, 2009.

31. NICE (National Institute for Health and Care Excellence). 2014. Available from: http://www.nice.org.uk/ [Accessed 1st June 2016].

32. Scottish Intercollegiate Guidelines Network (SIGN). 2014. Available from: http://www.sign.ac.uk/ [Accessed 1st June 2016].

33. Anna Freud Centre. Evidence Based Practice Unit (EBPU). No date. Available from: http://www.annafreud.org/pages/ebpu-home.html [Accessed 1st June 2016].

34. NICE (National Institute for Health and Care Excellence). *Social and emotional wellbeing in primary education (PH12).* 2008. Available from: http://guidance.nice.org.uk/PH12/Guidance/pdf/English [Accessed 1st June 2016].

35. NICE (National Institute for Health and Care Excellence). *Social and emotional wellbeing in secondary education (PH20).* 2009. Available from: http://publications.nice.org.uk/social-and-emotional-wellbeing-in-secondary-education-ph20 [Accessed 1st June 2016].

36. NICE (National Institute for Health and Care Excellence). *Social and emotional wellbeing: early years (PH40).* 2012. Available from: http://guidance.nice.org.uk/PH40/Guidance/pdf/English [Accessed 1st June 2016].

37. Humphrey N, Lendrum A, Wigelsworth M. Making the most out of school-based prevention: lessons from the social and emotional aspects of learning (SEAL) programme. *Emotional and Behavioural Difficulties* 2013; **18**(3): 248–60.

38. Wolpert M, Humphrey N, Belsky J, Deighton J. Embedding mental health support in schools: learning from the Targeted Mental Health in Schools (TaMHS) national evaluation. *Emotional and Behavioural Difficulties* 2013; **18**(3): 270–83.

39. Furlong M, McGilloway S, Bywater T, Hutchings J, Smith S, Donnelly M. Behavioural and cognitive-behavioural group based parenting programmes for early-onset conduct problems in children aged 3 to 12 years. *Cochrane Database of Systematic Reviews* 2012; **2**: CD008225.

40. Wolpert M, Fuggle P, Cottrell D, Fonagy P, Phillips J, Pilling S, et al. *Drawing on the evidence: advice for mental health professionals working with children and adolescents,* 2nd edn. London: CAMHS Publications, 2006.

41. Silverman WK, Pina AA, Viswesvaran C. Evidence-based psychosocial treatments for phobic and anxiety disorders in children and adolescents. *Journal of Clinical Child and Adolescent Psychology* 2008; **37**(1): 105–30.

42. NICE (National Institute for Health and Care Excellence). *Obsessive-compulsive disorder: core interventions in the treatment of obsessive-compulsive disorder and body dysmorphic disorder.* 2005. Available from: http://publications.nice.org.uk/obsessive-compulsive-disorder-cg31 [Accessed 1st June 2016].

43. NICE (National Institute for Health and Care Excellence). *Depression in children and young people: identification and management in primary, community and secondary care (CG28) (update).* 2015. Available from: http://guidance.nice.org.uk/CG28/NICEGuidance/pdf/English [Accessed 1st June 2016].

44. Pryjmachuk S, Trainor G. Helping young people who self-harm: perspectives from England. *Journal of Child and Adolescent Psychiatric Nursing* 2010; **23**(2): 52–60.

45. NICE (National Institute for Health and Care Excellence). *Self-harm: longer-term management.* 2011. Available from: http://www.nice.org.uk/guidance/CG133/NICEGuidance [Accessed 1st June 2016].

46. Wood A, Trainor G, Rothwell J, Moore ANN, Harrington R. Randomized trial of group therapy for repeated deliberate self-harm in adolescents. *Journal of the American Academy of Child and Adolescent Psychiatry* 2001; **40**(11): 1246–53.

47. SHIFT Trial. Family therapy vs treatment as usual for young people seen after second or subsequent episodes of

self-harm. Available from: http://www.controlled-trials.com/ISRCTN59793150 [Accessed 1st June 2016].

48. MTA Co-operative Group. A 14-month randomized clinical trial of treatment strategies for attention-deficit/hyperactivity disorder. *Archives of General Psychiatry* 1999; **56**:1073–86.

49. Scottish Intercollegiate Guidelines Network. *SIGN 112: management of attention deficit and hyperkinetic disorders in children and young people: a national clinical guideline.* Edinburgh: SIGN, 2009.

50. NICE (National Institute for Health and Care Excellence). *Attention deficit hyperactivity disorder: diagnosis and management of ADHD in children, young people and adults (CG72).* 2013. Available from: http://publications.nice.org.uk/attention-deficit-hyperactivity-disorder-cg72 [Accessed 1st June 2016].

51. NICE (National Institute for Health and Care Excellence). *Nocturnal enuresis: the management of bedwetting in children and young people (CG111).* 2010. Available from: http://publications.nice.org.uk/nocturnal-enuresis-cg111 [Accessed 1st June 2016].

52. Matson JL, LoVullo SV. Encopresis, soiling and constipation in children and adults with developmental disability. *Research in Developmental Disabilities* 2009; **30**(4): 799–807.

53. National Institute for Clinical Excellence. *Eating disorders: core interventions in the treatment and management of anorexia nervosa, bulimia nervosa and related eating disorders (CG9).* 2004. Available from: http://publications.nice.org.uk/eating-disorders-cg9 [Accessed 1st June 2016].

54. Scottish Intercollegiate Guidelines Network. *SIGN 131: management of schizophrenia.* Edinburgh: SIGN, 2013.

Further reading

CAMHS Review. *Children and young people in mind: the final report of the National CAMHS Review.* London: Department for Children, Schools and Families/Department of Health, 2008. Available from: http://webarchive.nationalarchives.gov.uk/20081230004520/publications.dcsf.gov.uk/eorderingdownload/camhs-review.pdf [Accessed 1st June 2016].

Dogra N, Leighton S (eds). *Nursing in child and adolescent mental health.* Maidenhead: Open University Press, 2009.

McDougall T (ed.). *Children and Young People's Mental Health: Essentials for Nurses and Other Professionals.* London: Routledge, 2016.

Murphy M, Fonagy P. *Mental health problems in children and young people. Our children deserve better: prevention pays, annual report of the Chief Medical Officer 2012.* London: Department of Health, 2013. Available from: http://www.gov.uk/government/publications/chief-medical-officers-annual-report-2012-our-children-deserve-better-prevention-pays [Accessed 1st June 2016].

NHS England. *Future in mind: promoting, protecting and improving our children and young people's mental health and wellbeing.* London: NHS England, 2015. Available from: www.gov.uk/government/uploads/system/uploads/attachment_data/file/414024/Childrens_Mental_Health.pdf [Accessed 1st June 2016].

Pryjmachuk S (ed.). *Mental health nursing: an evidence-based introduction.* London: Sage, 2011: chapters 9 and 10.

Wolpert M, Fuggle P, Cottrell D, Fonagy P, Phillips J, Pilling S, et al. *Drawing on the evidence: advice for mental health professionals working with children and adolescents,* 2nd edn. London: CAMHS Publications, 2006.

Relevant web pages

Barnardos. www.barnardos.org.uk/what_we_do/our_projects/mental_health.htm

CAMHS Evidence Based Practice Unit. http://www.ucl.ac.uk/ebpu

MindEd. www.minded.org.uk
    This website provides free e-learning resources on children and young people's mental health.

National Institute for Health and Care Excellence. www.nice.org.uk

The Place2Be. www.theplace2be.org.uk

Scottish Intercollegiate Guidelines Network. www.sign.ac.uk

YoungMinds. www.youngminds.org.uk

59 Group treatments with adolescents

GEMMA TRAINOR, 'AIDEN' AND
REBECCA McPHILLIPS

LEARNING OUTCOMES

- To understand how group treatments developed historically.
- To be able to identify the goals of this approach with young people with a range of presenting mental health difficulties.
- To be able to reflect on the skills and competencies required of an effective group therapist.
- To have insight into the personal experiences of service users who have accessed the modality.
- To comprehend the importance of confidentiality and supervision.

SUMMARY OF KEY POINTS

- Group treatments have received considerable attention over recent years for a variety of mental health difficulties affecting young people. However, a lot of the literature is focused on other treatments, and in the adult population.
- Nursing staff are uniquely placed to carry out such interventions, and as group therapists they need to cultivate an open, safe, non-judgemental space to promote positive change and compassionate care.
- Groups are used to facilitate discussions, to provide support, to normalize disorders and to motivate group members.[1]
- Group therapy allows for larger numbers of young people to be treated in a shorter period of time.
- The peer group plays a pivotal role in adolescence, and therefore the group approach can be more attractive to its participants than conventional treatments.

INTRODUCTION

This chapter examines theoretical approaches to group therapy with adolescents who present with mental health difficulties. Just as individual therapies do not speak solely about a single therapy, likewise there are a variety of different group approaches. Mental health nurses and other health care professionals can often be group therapists, and group therapy can provide an integral component of holistic care for young people with complex difficulties.

The delivery of compassionate care in the group setting should promote active engagement of group members to effect positive change. There is compelling evidence for the benefits of Child and Adolescent Mental Health Services (CAMHS) being creative, responsive and nurturing to enable young people to develop their sense of themselves, sociability and the maturational tasks inherent in adolescence. This chapter does not include group work with younger children, as often this type of group therapy is especially focused on play and other techniques. Parent groups are also not discussed, as these are predominantly about education and teaching parenting skills. The practice of group therapy with the adolescent population is the focus of this chapter.

HISTORY AND DEVELOPMENT OF GROUP TREATMENTS WITH ADOLESCENTS

The use of group treatment with adults has an extensive history. However, it was Slavson[2] who first used activity group therapy, derived from group psychotherapy, to treat children in the 1930s. From this point on, group treatments for adolescents have developed and are frequently recognized as a particularly effective type of treatment for adolescents. It is recognized that adolescents are often more comfortable with their peers than with adults, and frequently spend time in peer groups.[3] Since Slavson's[2] introduction of group treatment with children in the 1930s, group treatment with adolescents has reflected the various psychological theories that have been influential throughout the latter half of the twentieth century and to date. In the 1940s Axline[4] introduced group therapy based on Rogerian non-directive principles, and later Ginott[5] developed group therapy that was based on psychoanalytic principles. Both of these group treatments were utilized with adolescents, who were encouraged to use talk, play or activity-based therapy.[6] When these types of group treatments were used with adolescents, it was frequently the case that only minimal rules regarding danger and destructiveness were set, resulting in uncontrolled and potentially distressing sessions.[6,7]

From the 1980s onwards, cognitively orientated strategies began to be employed in group treatment with adolescents. For example, Sarason and Sarason[8] used modelling and role playing in order to improve the cognitive and social skills of adolescents. They found that, when compared to a control group, the young people who had received group treatment were able to adapt better to problematic situations and present themselves more effectively, and after 1 year had fewer absences and behavioural referrals.[6,8] Cognitive behavioural therapy (CBT), (chapter 40) has also been used to treat adolescents in groups successfully. For example, Clarke et al.[9] found that group CBT was an effective intervention for adolescents with major depression when compared to the control group who were placed on a waiting list. Additionally, group cognitive treatments have been used to prevent depressive disorder in adolescents; Clarke et al.[9] utilized a 15-session cognitive group with the aim of preventing unipolar depressive episodes and found that this reduced the incidence of depression at 6- and 12-month follow-up.

Historically, group treatment protocols have been fairly long term.[10] However, with the emphasis of modern health care on cost-effectiveness and time efficiency, more recent group treatments for adolescents often include fewer sessions than their predecessors. Burlingame et al.[11] also suggest that group treatment itself has also grown beyond demonstrating general effectiveness and towards identifying effective treatments for particular disorders. One example of the ways in which group treatments for adolescents have developed can be seen in the work of Kruczek and Vitanza,[12] These authors adapted Dolan's[13] Ericksonian and solution-orientated interventions with adults to use with adolescent females with one confirmed instance of sexual abuse specifically. Ericksonian techniques enable clients to resolve dissociated trauma and transform dissociation into a resource for healing, and solution-orientated therapy aims to provide clients with functional behaviours and perceptions that replace those based on trauma.[13] Kruczek and Vitanza's[12] group treatment included six modules, which were designed as 'stand-alone' sessions, so that girls could join at any point during the series. This particular group treatment design is particularly applicable in today's health care climate. Art therapy was also integrated into Kruczek and Vitanza's[12] group treatment, and in recent years has been increasingly used as a group treatment for adolescents. Vick[14] suggested that benefits of group art therapy for adolescents include the opportunity for the group leader to point out shared visual and content themes in the group's art work, which in turn can facilitate relationships in the group setting. This is particularly useful in health care settings where clinicians work with clients for briefer periods of time.

Throughout this book there is an underlying theme of compassionate care and the craft of caring. More recently, compassion-focused therapy (CFT) groups have been added to the literature. CFT is a transdiagnostic approach, which has been developed to help people who struggle with issues relating to shame and self-criticism.[15,16] The aim of this treatment approach is to help people be more compassionate with themselves and other group members. It has been designed for working with young people experiencing eating disorder difficulties. Compassionate care is a central and significant concept within the nursing discipline, and nurses are uniquely placed to take a lead in running such groups. Group therapy should be considered in settings where many clients share common problems, such as self-harm or eating disorders. Chapter 43 has a more general discussion on psychodynamic approaches to working in groups.

The brief review of the history and development of group treatments with adolescents presented here has frequently focused on group treatments that have been shown to be effective in facilitating positive change. It is important to note, however, that some of the research on group treatments for adolescents points towards potential harmful effects. Dishion et al.[17] draw upon evidence which suggests that group treatments for adolescents can actually increase problematic behaviour, such as violence, substance misuse and later adult maladjustment, as interaction with peers may inadvertently reinforce problematic behaviour.

This chapter focuses on group psychotherapy; however, there are other types of therapeutic groups with young people that are beyond the scope of this chapter.

THE GOALS OF GROUP THERAPY

The group can provide a safe arena for members to become aware of their thoughts and feelings and learn from others about how to reach their individual potential. The group setting offers an opportunity for skills building and a forum for modelling behaviours and interpersonal communication with peers. It prevents isolation and encourages inclusive practice.

Not all young people benefit from this approach, and therefore therapists must use their best judgement in determining the appropriateness of group interventions for particular clients. The group offers the additional benefits of support, peer modelling, a sense of commonality and an environment where members can practise a variety of skills acquired from the other participants and the therapist.

Trust, self-identity and the ability to be independent are key factors in adolescent development. The main goal is that therapists are required to develop a trusting and confidential relationship for all the group members.

Ideally, the members decide themselves the specific goals of the group. According to Corey,[18] some of the more general goals shared by members of counselling group are:

- To learn to trust oneself and others.
- To achieve self-knowledge and develop a sense of one's unique identity.
- To recognize the commonality for the participant's needs and problems and develop a sense of universality.
- To increase self-acceptance, self-confidence, and self-respect in order to achieve a new view of oneself.
- To find alternative ways of dealing with normal developmental issues and of resolving certain conflicts.

- To increase self-direction, autonomy, and responsibility toward oneself and others.
- To become aware of one's choices and to make choices wisely.
- To make specific plans for changing certain behaviours and to commit oneself to follow through with these plans.
- To learn more effective social skills.
- To become more sensitive to the needs and feelings of others.
- To move away from merely meeting others' expectations and to learn to live by one's own expectations.
- To clarify one's values and decide whether and how to modify them.

The overarching goal of group therapy, for the therapist, is to facilitate an open, self-disclosing, warm, spontaneous group interaction. It is also to encourage positive mutual identification of shared experiences, in keeping with the craft of caring. Successful groups depend on the continued growth of cohesion, trust and frankness.[19]

REFLECTION

- In what ways might the therapist encourage participation from young people for whom trust is a significant issue?

- How would the therapist create a safe environment for group members?

CASE STUDY 1

Maria, aged 15, has significant difficulties with trusting adults due to a long-term history of emotional abuse from adult caregivers. She struggles to engage in individual sessions; however, she is popular with her peers and shares her feelings with them much more readily.

Through the group process Maria realizes that the other group members seem to trust the facilitators even though they are adults. Maria was able to ignore her previously held beliefs and used the group sessions to explore where her mistrust of adults may have stemmed from.

ISSUES IN THE USE OF GROUPS WITH ADOLESCENTS

Adolescence is a developmental phase during which a number of important tasks are worked through in order to achieve independent adult functioning. These include identity formation, psychosexual maturity, working towards financial independence and developing and maintaining healthy sustaining relationships.[20] The transition from dependent child to independent adult involves changing the balance of relationships with family and adolescent counterparts. Thus the peer group is an important arena for some of this work to take place. Adolescents can show ambivalence towards authority figures and it can be difficult for a lone clinician to forge such relationships with young people, which may mean that the 'group' can be an attractive influential therapeutic milieu. In a lot of settings it is an untapped resource. The peer group plays a pivotal role in adolescence, and therefore being with other young people may be a way to engage those who may otherwise drop out of conventional treatments.

Adolescence involves the negotiation of a variety of dilemmas and the key task for adolescents is to formulate a stable identity to carry them into the future.[21] The adolescent years can be extremely lonely and a young person can often perceive that no one can help. There are common struggles such as dependence versus independence, acceptance versus rejection, identity crisis, a search for security and peer group pressures to conform. They strive to be accepted by peers, and a form of experimenting takes place. It is a critical developmental phase for the expression of vulnerabilities for behavioural symptoms and syndromes, ranging from substance use to major mental illness.[22] Therefore a prime goal is to promote the necessary conditions within the group to support young people to tackle this developmental process. Nurses are often in the closest proximity to clients, and therefore in a uniquely special position to promote positive change for young people within the context of the craft of caring. The Rogerian or person-centred concept of the importance of the relationship, being genuine and unconditionally accepting of the young person, demonstrates an empathetic understanding of their needs and issues.[23] (More can be found on developing and maintaining the therapeutic relationship in

chapter 3.) Adolescence is a time of continually testing limits, of conflict and of establishing a new identity. The young individuals struggle to define who they are, where they are going and how they will get there. They often experience pressure from school, as well as their parents' and peer group demands which are often conflicting. The task therefore is to negotiate a stable self-concept, with a clear sense of goals, to be able to make informed decisions. In group therapy a great deal of time is devoted to the exploration and resolution of the dependence/independence conflicts that are so prevalent in adolescence. Group counselling is especially important for adolescents, as it provides a forum in which they can express and explore such issues with like-minded people.

A YOUNG PERSON'S PERSPECTIVE

I felt I was accepted by the group and they understood me more than other people who haven't been through what I had been through. They helped me find ways to cope by telling the group about what they did when they were in a bad place. Their suggestions were much more honest and I could connect with them. They didn't pretend it would always get better but instead talked about how you could manage things better. I have had all sorts of treatments since I have been to CAMHS but this one was best for me. I like coming and I got to see other young people move on with their lives.

REFLECTION

- What are the core conditions described by the Rogerian approach, that are required to promote an effective therapeutic relationship?

- What are the similarities to these and 'compassionate care' in nursing?

The importance of 'caring' in nursing is well known and is a central defining concept within the nursing discipline. The term 'nursing' is actually derived from the word 'nurturance', which by definition means 'caring'. Today we might define compassion as a sensitivity to the distress of self and others, with a commitment to try to do something about it. It is an important aspect of patient-centred care.[24] Group therapists are required to be mindful that caring is an intersubjective human process based on the belief that, as is the case with group treatment, people learn from one another how to be human by identifying with others.[25] A fundamental assertion of the group approach is that each person constructs an individual inner world which is continuously being reconstructed through interactions with others which determine their view of themselves.

COMPOSITION OF THE GROUP

There are usually about 4 to 8 adolescents in the group; however, it is sensible to recruit around 12 young people to allow for potential absences at any given time. The group may be a fixed short-term closed group, or an open, more long-term group, depending on the needs of the participants. There are normally two therapists, one of whom takes the lead, while the other co-facilitates. Ideally, a third independent professional will observe and evaluate the group. The group usually lasts for 30 to 90 minutes. Younger children tend to have a shorter session, due to issues of attention and engagement.[26]

Frequency varies depending on the needs of the potential members. A thorough assessment of group members is crucial. The assessment may vary based on the setting or presenting problems. Clinicians need to consider these factors and the influence they may have on group processes. Assessments should include standardized outcome measures and an interview with the young person and parents/carers by the therapists. The group aims and rules should be discussed at the initial meeting, as well as the young person's concerns and hopes for the treatment. Issues of confidentially are explained at the interview to the young person and carers/family. (More information on assessment can be found in chapters 13 and 14.)

Inclusion criteria

It is essential that a working alliance is forged with the group leaders. Therefore, there should be the right mix of young people either with the same or with a variety of mental health difficulties. Most groups tend to be diagnosis-specific, although some might be centred on the general themes and maturational growth of adolescence. The inclusion criteria will therefore depend on the purpose of the group. One key assumption is that each young person wants to participate in the process. Additionally, to embark on a group programme, it is extremely important that the members are well versed in the principles and aims of the group treatment.

Exclusion criteria

Some young people may not be suitable for group therapy; for example, due to being acutely psychotic. Young people who do not speak English or have severe learning difficulties may also be unable to use this medium. Those with severe psychopathology or who are acutely suicidal may require a different type of treatment.

The group members should be able to cope with feelings that are aroused within the group setting without responding to them impulsively, and in between sessions they need to be able to continue to function in their normal life.[27]

PLANNING THE GROUP INTERVENTION

The planning stages of group therapy are essential to successful delivery. First, the group facilitators need to make decisions about the type of group they wish to run; for example, young people aged 14 to 17 who repeatedly self-harm may be offered developmental group psychotherapy.[20] Effective group treatment requires that specific goals be determined at the outset. The goals can be varied but should be measurable. In the example of developmental group psychotherapy described above, the main goal of the treatment was to reduce self-harming behaviour. This was measured at the end of the course, as the group progressed; however, additional agreed goals can be added. Regular attendance is a vital factor for the group. As stated previously, careful selection and preparation help to make successful groups. All members should receive the same information and preparation. Prior to the group commencing, it is useful to send out a written statement of what is on offer, where it will take place and the date and time. Sometimes the therapist can offer a meeting with a previous group member to offer reassurance.

In order to ensure the group is helpful to its members, objective outcome measures chosen by therapists should be conducted pre- and post-interventions; for example, the Beck Depression Inventory – Youth, Second Edition[28] is an excellent tool for monitoring depressive symptomatology in young people.

A YOUNG PERSON'S PERSPECTIVE: BEGINNING GROUP

When my CAMHS worker mentioned coming to a group with other young people with the same problems as me, I said no 'cos I didn't like speaking in front of people. She asked me if I wanted to speak to a young person from the group so they could tell me about it. I agreed. The young person was really nice and had been to about three sessions. He said it could be fun and that everyone was really nice. He said he really looked forward to it and learning about how everyone was getting on. He convinced me into giving it a try and I am so glad he did. It was easier because I had met one of the members.

GROUP THERAPISTS

The group leader/facilitator/therapist should be able to identify potential conflicts that are likely to cause difficulties with group members; to construct a balanced group; and to establish ways in which to manage any issues. Those leading the group should be neither passive nor aggressive, but should be able to reflect on and observe what is going on in the group. They should model helpful group behaviour to its members, such as modelling respectful attention, and giving the young person appropriate empathy for what is being discussed by them.

Sometimes groups may operate with one leader, but it is usually better to have a co-therapist/leader. Group members can be challenging even for two therapists, and it allows for greater objectivity and clarity. It is essential that the group leaders work together, and they should meet before and after sessions. Good communication is key to effective treatment. The leaders are required to determine their roles and identify how to handle potential sabotaging of the group processes by the group members. Therapists need to be competent in the technique and to have additional skills suited to the particular population with which they are working. Group therapists can come from a variety of professional backgrounds, and specific guidelines for the training of group therapists have been developed by professional organizations such as the American Group Psychotherapy Association (AGPA) and the Association for Specialists in Groupwork (ASGW). These are provided only as models for consideration, as it is not always possible to get in-depth training in group work with adolescents. However, group therapists are required to be trained professionals in fields such as nursing, social work or occupational therapy. It is ideal to have therapists who have at least 3 years, post-qualifying experience in child and adolescent mental health. Lifelong learning is another aspect of competence, and clinicians are required to provide evidence of continued education.

A YOUNG PERSON'S PERSPECTIVE: WHAT MAKES A GOOD GROUP THERAPIST

There are many qualities needed to make a good and effective group therapist. It starts off with patience; if you become inpatient easily, this isn't the career for you. Patience will help you deal with the service users, whilst allowing them to have the time to have their say and allowing them to go at their own compatible pace. If not, they may feel rushed and like they aren't listened to. Good listening skills are important. This can tie in with being patient, because as a therapist you will need to pay attention to what the service users have to say, but with an intent to understand and not just to reply, for example, by nodding your head, or phrases like 'Mmm'.

Topics to be addressed in each session can be chosen in advance, by discussion in the previous session. This discussion should only last around 10 to 15 minutes. These topics can vary, depending on the type of group; it is always best to allow the group members to pick the topics, identifying things that bother or concern them; for example, recent news.

GROUP PROCESSES

Therapy is typically viewed in evolving stages. There are no hard and fast rules; however, generally the first, exploratory or initial stage occupies the first few sessions. This is characterized by rule setting, planning the direction, and changing the focus of the group from the therapists to the collective membership of the group.[29]

Ground rules in group therapy are usually agreed at the initial session with members and facilitators. The therapists

BOX 59.1: SAMPLE SET OF RULES FOR A GROUP

1. No smoking, drinking, or other substance abuse.
The reasons for this rule are obvious.

2. No displays of aggression, either verbal or physical.
The reasons for this rule are obvious.

3. No eating or drinking.
This can be extremely distracting and may detract from the concept of *working* in sessions.

4. No interrupting when someone else is talking.
Each member has equal rights and needs. It is unacceptable for one member to be demanding or destructive towards another member, and what each member contributes is valuable and worthwhile.

5. Confidentiality
This is particularly important. The rule is that it is each member's responsibility to maintain confidentiality outside of the session. The only time when this rule can be breached is when clients themselves or someone else is at risk. If the therapists are concerned that a child is at risk then they will have to tell social services.

encourage members to reach consensus on rules to ensure the group is safe.

The ground rules include a statement of mutual expectations, an agreement about what is acceptable and not acceptable and possibly what sanctions may be invoked if they are breached. Negotiating the ground rules is a demonstration of care for group processes.[30]

REFLECTION

- Look at the sample set of rules in Box 59.1. Are there any other common ground rules you would suggest?

- Which one of these rules would be viewed as the most important when planning to run a group programme?

THE INITIAL SESSION

To start initial sessions, therapists may use techniques known as ice-breakers, especially if the group is new or if there is a new member. This helps reduce the tension and awkwardness, as people are engaging in simple activities that make them feel more comfortable.

It is essential that therapists provide the conditions for members to feel mutually supported. The next stage or evolution is where members can explore and initiate new behaviours. Group members can develop new ways of thinking and acting as they begin to trust the process.

In this middle stage the group members are central to the process, and there is an emphasis on cohesiveness and, hopefully, a higher level of participation and communication. While the leaders initiate processes, the dynamic occurs when the members adapt and utilize them. The leaders can point out the dynamics in relation to the progress of the group.

In the latter stages of therapy there is a need for enhanced decision making by leaders and members. It involves transferring the learning from the group to life

A YOUNG PERSON'S PERSPECTIVE: ENDINGS

I attended the group most weeks and when the therapist mentioned moving on I would go quiet. I felt sad that I may not get to see the other group members. I spoke about it to my CAMHS worker who suggested I bring up my concerns in the group. She helped me think about life after the group and other endings I had faced in my life. One of the young people in the group said something which really helped me come to terms with things. She said that it is never a good time to end things so it is best to end in a good way. This really helped me think about how my life so far has been and about ending things and moving on. I was due to start college which is an end to my high school days and a beginning of a new experience. I wanted to be in my new school and I realized I could stay in contact with my friends from high school.

away from the group. Both initial and final stages are characterized by decision making. Endings, although unavoidable, can pose some difficulties for group members and therapists. Therapists need to announce potential ending early throughout the course. The group members may experience issues of loss and grief. This may result in a re-emergence of symptoms or withdrawal from the group, hence the need for preparation. The leaders need to facilitate this type of discussion and emphasize what a successful ending may look like. A good way to consolidate may be for members to discuss what they have learned and how they can apply this learning to life away from the group.

CONFIDENTIALITY

This is a central theme commonly brought up by group members. The group leaders need to be very clear to define confidentiality at the screening interviews, aside from the obvious legal limits to confidentiality such as disclosing threats to harm self or others, reports of abuse or the need to respond to court orders. The therapist should explain in detail why and when they would disclose certain other information. This denotes a level of respect for the young person's cognitive, social and emotional level of functioning.[31] Young people may be concerned if everything they say is shared with parents/guardians, and therefore agreements of confidentiality are also agreed with the young people and their parents/carers. A more difficult task is ensuring that all group members adhere to issues of confidentiality outside the group setting. The therapist should remind young people regularly about the consequences of violation of confidentiality; for example, termination of group treatment. Agreement about how group members should react if they meet each other outside so as not to compromise the members' confidentiality should be obtained at the outset. With the proliferation of virtual relationships on the internet, there is also a need to ensure the anonymity of group members and again outline the consequences of not doing so. The young people are encouraged to understand and be empathetic about how such breaches can seriously affect trust in the group process.

Therapist nurses should be consistently reminded about when, where and how to share information. How much detail of client participation and progress in the group setting will be shared is agreed at the outset with the young person and their parents/carers. The group member, even if classed as a minor, should always be empowered to make choices about his or her behaviour during the group, including how much and what information to share;[32] for example, deciding on which disclosures can be made to parents/carers, teachers or others.

As is the case in all therapies, there are legally mandated limits to confidentiality. Although clinicians do not necessarily have to get permission from the young person before disclosing confidential information, it is good practice to tell them what information you will be disclosing, why you need to do that and to whom you will be disclosing it. When considering confidentiality with teenagers, therapists are often faced with issues regarding age limits for certain activities, such as drinking. In order to avoid censoring information or compromising discussions, therapists can develop mutual agreements with relevant family/carers. Of course, the parents/carers may want to know, and in that instance the young person would have to know in advance what information would be shared.

RECORD KEEPING

One of the central dilemmas is whether to keep records separately or for the group as a whole. Keeping individual records does not really capture the subtleties or dynamics that occur collectively. No reference to other group members can be involved in individual recordings. For individual recordings, the following are commonly included: date of attendance, diagnostic impression, treatment goals and progress towards achieving those goals. Another inclusion could be significant feedback received by the group member from another member of the group.[33]

EVALUATION

For any group treatment, sessions are required to be purposeful and relevant, and to have well-structured areas of objectives to achieve positive outcomes for its participants. The needs of the group membership need to be clear, and the objectives realistic and achievable. Most group therapists use evaluation tools to measure whether the objectives are met.

REFLECTION

- What may be the objectives of group treatment?
- What type of evaluation tools could be used in group therapy?

SUPERVISION

Obtaining effective supervision is essential for group therapists. Supervision can be both informal and formal. Pre- and post-group treatment sessions are a form of supervision. Supervision can give therapists a chance to stand back and reflect, to learn from difficult situations and to get support. (See chapter 11 for further reading on critical reflection.) Supervision is a very important part of taking care of oneself and staying open to new learning. It helps group therapists by recognizing growth and change and promoting self-development. A lack of supervision can lead to therapists becoming defensive, overwhelmed and deflated, which can contribute to 'burnout'. (Further information on clinical supervision can be found in chapter 10.)

The group observer can support post-group supervision, and there are a variety of ways in which to conduct supervision. There is no tangible product and very little evidence whereby we can rigorously assess the effectiveness of supervision.

It is well recognized that the role of the group observer is valuable and an integral part of the group process.

CONCLUSION

This chapter has addressed group psychotherapy with adolescents, placing specific emphasis on the role of the group therapist in conducting such groups. The goals of treatment are to provide adolescents with the skills necessary to promote recovery. It is difficult to describe actual groups, as they can take on a life of their own, and each group is a unique experience for therapists and members. Adolescence is a major development stage for identity construction, social belonging and regulation of emotions. Group therapy, as an adjunct to other therapies, can be extremely attractive and effective in normalizing these experiences.

Integrating group treatment with individual and family work is both rewarding and challenging. This chapter has also outlined the basic elements of group processes, and deals with some ethical and professional issues particular to group work with adolescents. However, its richness is in the personal testimonies of the young people themselves.

References

1. Kronenberger WG, Meyer RG. *The child clinician's handbook*, 2nd edn. New York: Allyn & Bacon, 2001.
2. Slavson SR. *An introduction to group therapy*. New York: International Universities Press, 1943.
3. Arunson S, Kahn GB. Group interventions for treatment of trauma in adolescents. In: Buckle B, Spitz H (eds). *Group intervention for treatment of psychological trauma*. New York: American Group Psychotherapy Association, 2004: 89–115.
4. Axline VM. *Play therapy*. New York: Ballantine Books, 1947.
5. Ginott HG. *Group psychotherapy with children: the theory and practice of play therapy*. New York: McGraw-Hill, 1961.
6. Callias M. Group treatments. In: Rutter M, Hersov L (eds). *Child and adolescent psychiatry: modern approaches*. Oxford: Blackwell Scientific, 1987: 871–87.
7. Kraft IA. Child and adolescent group psychotherapy. In: Kaplan HI, Sadock BJ (eds). *Comprehensive group psychotherapy*. Baltimore, MD: Williams and Wilkins, 1971: 534–65.
8. Sarason IG, Sarason BR. Teaching cognitive and social skills to high school students. *Journal of Consulting and Clinical Psychology* 1981; **49**: 908–18.
9. Clarke, GN, Hawkins W, Murphy M, Sheeber LB, Lewinsohn LB, Seeley JR. Targeted prevention of unipolar depressive disorder in an at-risk sample of high school adolescents: a randomized trial of a group cognitive intervention. *Journal of the American Academy of Child and Adolescent Psychiatry* 1995; **34**(3): 312–21.
10. Donahue WT, Elliot AN. Treatment of the sexually abused child: a review. *Journal of Clinical Child Psychology* 1992; **21**: 218–28.
11. Burlingame GM, Fuhriman A, Moiser J. The differential effectiveness of group psychotherapy: a meta-analytic perspective. *Group Dynamics: Theory, Research and Practice* 2003; **7**(1): 3–12.
12. Kruczek T, Vitanza S. Treatment effects with an adolescent abuse survivor's group. *Child Abuse and Neglect* 1999; **23**(5): 477–85.
13. Dolan YM. *Resolving sexual abuse: solution-focused therapy and Eriksonian hypnosis for adult survivors*. New York: WW Norton and Company, 1991.
14. Vick RM. Utilizing pre-structured art elements in brief group art therapy with adolescents. *Art Therapy: Journal of the American Art Therapy Association* 1999; **16**(2): 68–77.
15. Gilbert P. Introducing compassion-focused therapy. *Advances in Psychiatric Treatment* 2009; **15**(3): 199–208.
16. Gilbert P, Irons C. Focused therapies and compassionate mind training for shame and self-attacking. In: Gilbert P (ed.). *Compassion: conceptualisations, research and use in psychotherapy*. London: Routledge, 2005: 263–325.

17. Dishion TJ, McCord J, Poulin F. When interventions harm: peer groups and problem behavior. *American Psychologist* 1999; **54**(9): 755–64.
18. Corey G. *Theory and practice of group counseling*, 4th edn. Pacific Grove, CA: Brooks/Cole, 1995.
19. Davies M. Dramatherapy and psychodrama. In: Gennings S (ed.). *Dramatherapy in theory and practice.* Beckenham: Croom Helm, 1987.
20. Wood A, Trainor G. *A manual of developmental group psychotherapy.* In press.
21. Moretti MM, Holland R. The journey of adolescence: transition in self within the context of attachment relationships. In: Johnson SM, Wiffen VE (eds). *Attachment process in couple and family therapy.* New York: Guilford, 2003: 234–57.
22. Walker EF, Romer D. Conclusions. In: Romer D, Walker EF (eds). *Adolescent psychopathology and the developing brain: integrating brain and prevention science.* New York: Oxford University Press, 2007: 463–74.
23. Rogers C. *On becoming a person.* Boston: Houghton Mifflin, 1961.
24. King AC. Group therapy for adolescent depressive disorder: a comparison of social skills and therapy support.

25. Watson HJ, Allen K, Fursland A, Byrne SM, Nathan PM. Does enhanced cognitive behaviour therapy for eating disorders improve quality of life? *European Eating Disorders Review* 2012; **20**(5): 393–9.
26. Kolvin I, MacMillan A, Wrate R. Psychotherapy is effective. *Journal of the Royal Society of Medicine* 1988; **81**(5): 261–6.
27. Aveline M, Dryden W. *Group therapy in Britain.* Milton Keynes: Open University Press, 1993.
28. Beck JS, Beck AT, Jolly J. *Manual for the Beck Youth Interventions of Emotional and Social Adjustment*, 2nd edn. San Antonio, TX: Psychological Corporation, 2005.
29. Lewis C, Beck A. Experiencing level in the process of group development. *Group* 1983; **7**(2): 18–26.
30. Doel M. *Using group work.* London: Routledge, 2006.
31. Koocher GP, Keith-Spiegel PC. *Children, ethics and the law: professional issues and cases.* Lincoln: University of Nebraska Press, 1990.
32. Brabender V. The ethical group psychotherapist. *International Journal of Group Psychotherapy* 2006; **56**(4): 395–414.
33. Brabender VA, Fallon AE, Smolar AI. *Essentials of group therapy.* Hoboken, NJ: Wiley, 2004.

Further reading

Cole-King A, Gilbert P. Compassionate care: the theory and the reality. *Journal of Holistic Healthcare* 2011; **8**(3): 29–37.
Corey G. *Case approach to counselling and psychotherapy*, 3rd edn. Pacific Grove, LA: Brooks/Cole, 1991.
Dies RR. Current practice in the training of group psychotherapists. *International Journal of Group Psychotherapy* 1980; **30**: 169–86.

Lakin M, Lieberman M, Whitaker D. Issues in the training of group psychotherapists. *International Journal of Group Psychotherapy* 1969; **19**: 307–25.
Yalum I. *The theory and practice of group psychotherapy.* New York: Basic Books, 1983.

Relevant web pages

FPSA (The Foundation for Professionals in Services to Adolescents). http://www.foundationpsa.org.uk/. FPSA is a charity that works with, cares for and cares about adolescents and produces briefings and advice e.g. FPSA Briefing Paper No 6 (G. Trainor) 'Developmental Group Psychotherapy (DGP): A review of randomised controlled trials (RCT) in different international contexts and prospects for future utilisation'. http://www.foundationpsa.org.uk/cms/upload_area/documents//006_Briefing_Paper_Gemma_Trainor.pdf [Accessed 25 January 2017]

MindEd. https://www.minded.org.uk A free educational resource on children and young people's mental health for all adults. [Accessed 25 January 2017]

NICE. https://www.nice.org.uk/guidance/cg28 Depression in children and young people: identification and management.

Clinical guideline [CG28] Published date: September 2005 Last updated: March 2015. [Accessed 25 January 2017]

Royal College of Psychiatrists. http://www.rcpsych.ac.uk/workinpsychiatry/faculties/childandadolescent/generalinformation.aspx Information for children and adolescents and publications for parents, carers and professionals. [Accessed 25 January 2017]

Young Minds. http://www.youngminds.org.uk/Access to publications and resources for children, parents and professionals. Including 'Future In Mind Taskforce Report'. http://www.youngminds.org.uk/news/blog/2548_future_in_mind_taskforce_report_main_recommendations?gclid=COWMj6ux3dECFYm4GwodpzYLqQ [Accessed 25 January 2017]

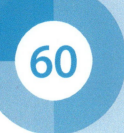

60

Services for individuals with both a learning disability and a mental health disorder

CHRIS KNIFTON, RICHARD POSTANCE AND DOROTHY HEMEL

LEARNING OUTCOMES

- To understand the term, condition, and concept of 'learning disability' as used in contemporary health and social care practice.

- To understand the different use of the term 'dual diagnosis' in learning disability services when compared with traditional mental health services in the UK.

- To be aware of a range of evidence-based mental health assessment/screening tools suitable for people with a learning disability.

- To be aware of a range of mental health disorders/conditions commonly associated with learning disability.

- To be aware of the use of mental health evidence-based interventions with people with a learning disability.

- To understand the extent and suitability of current service provision.

- To be able to reflect on the role of the mental health nurse in supporting people with learning disabilities, to engage with generic mental health services where necessary, and the need to challenge discriminatory attitudes and beliefs.

- To be able to reflect on the interconnectedness of the art and science of nursing practice in this area and the craft of caring for people with a learning disability.

SUMMARY OF KEY POINTS

- People with a learning disability are at a higher risk of having mental health problems than those within the general population.

- There are various forms/causes of learning disability, with different levels of severity ranging from mild to profound.

- People with a mild or moderate learning disability and a mental health disorder (dual diagnosis), where appropriate, should be accessing mainstream mental health services.

- The term 'dual diagnosis' may be used differently in learning disability and mental health services.

- A number of mental health screening and assessment tools have been developed specifically for use with people with a learning disability.

665

- Access to psychosocial interventions should not exclude people with a learning disability.
- Mental health services have a legal requirement to make reasonable adjustments for people with learning disabilities accessing their services.

- The 'Green Light Toolkit' provides practical assistance to help mental health services support people with a learning disability.

INTRODUCTION

This chapter aims to provide an understanding that people with learning disabilities and mental health problems should be able to access generic mental health services, particularly where this learning disability is mild to moderate. This supports the need to equip mental health nurses with a basic understanding of these two superimposed conditions of mental health and learning disability, often termed 'dual diagnosis' within learning disability services.

The Department of Health (DH)[1] has defined learning disability as:

- *impaired intelligence:* a significantly reduced ability to understand new or complex information and to learn new skills;
- *impaired social functioning:* a reduced ability to cope independently;
- *onset of disability before adulthood* which has a lasting effect on development.

The 'degree' of disability is frequently used within this client group; this is largely based on the Wechsler Adult Intelligence Scale – Revised (WAIS-R), a form of intelligence quotient (IQ) test, and provides four categories of severity of learning disability (LD). This is depicted as *mild LD* (score 50–69); *moderate LD* (score 35–50); *severe LD* (score 20–35); and *profound LD* (score 0–20). Approximately 1.2 million people in England have a mild or moderate learning disability, and 210,000 with a severe or profound learning disability, with 1.5 million in total across the UK.[1] In Scotland, this number is estimated at 120,000.[2] Currently affecting 2 per cent of the population,[3] this number is set to rise as improvements in health and social care are made across the UK. Emerson

and Hatton[4] suggest that improved life expectancy will result in a 37 per cent increase in people over 65 years with a learning disability by 2021. This is an increasingly important area for mental health services; despite the persistence of misguided and outdated beliefs that people with learning disabilities are not susceptible to mental disorders, high rates of mental health problems have been reported in people with learning disabilities, ranging from 10 to 50 per cent.[5] Crucially, the full range of psychiatric disorders remain common in people with learning disabilities,[1] with prevalence rates higher than those of the general population.[6,7]

This chapter considers the need for a greater understanding of learning disability for mental health nurses, given the potentially increasing use of generic or mainstream mental health services required by this client group. To help you navigate through the chapter, it has been subdivided into four parts. We begin by exploring the term 'learning disability'. The second section introduces the concept of 'dual diagnosis' from a learning disability perspective, and then discusses diagnosis, assessment and screening for mental health problems, before then considering common mental health disorders and the possible manifestations or atypical signs/symptoms observed in this client group. Interventions suitable for people with a learning disability are discussed in the third part followed by an overview of current service provision in the final part to support anti-discriminatory practice, attitudes, values and, importantly, the *craft of caring*.

Service user experiences are presented throughout the chapter, both directly within the form of text boxes, and also by the joint and inclusive writing of this chapter with the service user representative.

WHAT IS A LEARNING DISABILITY?

For centuries a wide variety of terms have been used to describe this condition. Some of these are noted in Box 60.1. Many of these terms are now considered inappropriate but may still be used in some countries, cited in reading text/source material, used within classification systems, or even noted in service user medical notes/records.

The term 'idiocy' was commonly used during the nineteenth and early twentieth centuries.[8] During the nineteenth century, conceptualization of the condition

underwent many significant changes, including an observance of its separation from insanity/mental health disorders.[9] In the UK, the term most commonly used in current practice since its adoption in 1992 is *learning disability*, replacing the terms 'mental handicap' and 'mental retardation'. Importantly, this not the same as 'learning difficulty', a term used mostly within the education system, and indicating sensory impairments, physical disabilities, behavioural problems or specific learning problems, such as dyslexia, dyscalculia or dyspraxia.

BOX 60.1: TERMS COMMONLY USED OVER TIME

Amentia	Learning disability
Developmental disability	Mental handicap
Feeble-minded	Mental retardation
Idiot	Mental sub-normality
Imbecile	Moral defective
Intellectual disability	Moron
Intellectual impairment	Oligophrenia

SERVICE USER'S PERSPECTIVE

On one particular occasion I remember supporting a number of service users with a mild to moderate learning disability at a local MENCAP advocacy meeting. As part of a group activity to give a voice to people with a learning disability, they were asked about terminology used by health and social care professions and their views on this. The majority of the group preferred the term 'learning difficulty', rather than 'learning disability' or 'mentally handicapped'.

Although this term may have different connotations for service providers, it was important that we heard the voice of the service users themselves and how labels are perceived.

CARER'S PERSPECTIVE

As a sibling I get very cross with all these terms. My younger sister is mentally handicapped. It doesn't matter to me what the professionals call it. She needs help washing, dressing, feeding and cannot do simple tasks. Nor can she speak. And she is 26. That makes her mentally handicapped. To say she has a learning disability appears to me to disregard the support she actually needs and minimizes the amount of support and time I need to give her as her carer. The people at the health centre and at the day centre, however, do not like me using this term.

REFLECTION

- Consider these two experiences. Why do you think their views are so different?
- As originally noted by Barker and Whitehill,[10] the value of care is defined by those who receive it. Now, take a moment to consider how the use of terminology can thus impact on your craft of caring.

It is important to note that there is not yet one agreed term, nationally or internationally. The current ICD-10 manual,[11] with which most mental health nurses will be familiar, for example, still uses the term 'mental retardation'.

Learning disability remains an umbrella term covering a wide range of separate conditions. However, it is important to note that in 40 to 80 per cent of learning disability cases, the causes or specific condition may not be known.[12]

Due to the overtly medical orientation of such classifications (see chapter 12 for more on the classification of mental illness), there is a growing encouragement to focus on the individual needs of people, rather than these groupings,[3] as the quotation from a carer below clearly shows.

CARER'S PERSPECTIVE

As a mother of a son with learning disabilities I want to tell staff to look at the person and not just the label of the condition, or degree/severity of disability. Looking at the person makes you see his uniqueness and his personal qualities. His 'label' won't tell you this.

The craft of caring is so much more than understanding the scientific knowledge of medically orientated classifications. Behind any label there is a person, and the craft of caring needs to involve a person-centred agenda.

In addition, people with learning disabilities tend to have significantly more health problems (comorbidity) than those in the general population (see Box 60.2), although often this may be overlooked. It is important to understand that what may be thought of as mental health symptoms may in fact be due to a physical comorbidity. By considering the 'whole' of the person, physical health remains an important consideration.

Finally, people with learning disabilities may also have autism, or be on the 'autistic spectrum', a term used to include *autism*, *Asperger's syndrome* and *atypical autism*.

Autism is usually classified as a neurodevelopmental disorder, and in children, may be classified as a pervasive

Communication problems 50–90%
Physical disability 40%
Sensory impairments 33%
Epilepsy 20%

Source: Adapted from Bhaumik and Branford.[13]

developmental disorder. It usually includes a typical 'triad of symptoms':

- difficulties with social interaction;
- stereotypical behaviours;
- difficulties in communication.

Diagnosis of autism in adults with learning disabilities is based largely on a comprehensive assessment, direct observation of core autism signs, and often the use of the Autism Diagnostic Observation Schedule – Generic (ADOS-G)[14] and the Autism Diagnostic Interview – Revised (ADI-R).[15] However, it is important to note that many people in the general population may also be on the autistic spectrum, and so, autism should not always be associated with a learning disability or an impaired intelligence.

Learning disability can thus be taken as an umbrella term that includes a wide variety of forms, types and levels of ability. The craft of caring for people with this long-term condition needs to include not only a clear and knowledge-able understanding of the patho-physiology presented, but also the psychosocial effect and the total experience for the person, and often their carer. Given the potential for dual diagnosis, the vulnerability of this client group and the eroding of emotional resilience cannot be underestimated. As noted by Barker and Whitehill,[10] 'If we are to develop a craft of care in psychiatric nursing, then we need to know what the experience of mental ill health means to the person who is "in" that experience' (p.21).

DUAL DIAGNOSIS – LEARNING DISABILITY *WITH* A CO-EXISTING MENTAL HEALTH DISORDER

Often the starting point in accessing mental health services for people with a learning disability is having a suspected or actual 'dual diagnosis'. The term 'dual diagnosis', however, can be misleading. For many mental health nurses, the term is commonly associated with co-existing substance misuse and mental health problems.[16] When applied to learning disability, the term has a very different meaning, and is instead used to indicate that a person has a learning disability *and* a diagnosed mental health disorder. Some forms of learning disability may also carry an increased risk. Examples are listed in Table 60.1.

Table 60.1 Forms of learning disability associated with mental health disorders

Fragile X syndrome	Anxiety disorders[17,18]
Phenylketonuria (PKU)	Anxiety disorders[18]
Down's syndrome	Dementia[19,20]
	Depression[21,22]
Turner syndrome	Depression[18]
Foetal alcohol syndrome	Mood disorders[18]
Rubinstein–Taybi syndrome	Mood disorders[18]
Prader–Willi syndrome	Mood disorders[18]
	Cycloid psychosis[23]

CASE STUDY 1

Sally is 41 and has Down's syndrome and attended a day centre. Over the course of the last year, her behaviour has begun to deteriorate. She has difficulty washing and dressing without assistance, and will sometimes refuse support with personal care. She appears withdrawn, more forgetful and, over the last year, has started to put on weight. She has also begun to talk to what her carers call her 'imaginary friend'. This is a new behaviour that coincided with the above symptomology.

Dementia, particularly Alzheimer's disease, is common in people with Down's syndrome, and usually starts at a much earlier age than noted in the general population. Symptoms can include hallucinations. A presumption was made that Sally had dementia, and arrangements were made for her to move to a dementia registered care provider. However, a series of assessments and screening showed this not to be the case. A *physical health check*, including blood screening, revealed an underactive thyroid gland, and mental *health screening* highlighted both negative and positive signs of schizophrenia.

REFLECTION

Consider case study 1, and how evidence-based 'generalizations' and diagnostic overshadowing may result in inappropriate care management. The craft of nursing is the ability to *skilfully* apply the knowledge or science of evidence-based practice in a way that relates to the individual, understanding their personal circumstances, and seeing beyond (or through) any obvious descriptors or labels.

There are resources available to support dual diagnosis with this client group. The Diagnostic Criteria for Psychiatric Disorders for Use with Adults with Learning Disabilities (DC-LD)[18] is one such example. It is a diagnostic classification system for adults with moderate to profound learning disabilities, based on the ICD-10 classification.[24] In addition, the authors of this system state that it may be used in conjunction with both the ICD-10 and DSM-IV in a complementary way, when working with adults with mild learning disabilities. This is an important point, given any potential increase in demand from mainstream mental health services, particularly by people with mild learning disabilities. Following the recent change to the newly published DSM-5,[25] and proposals for the soon-to-be ICD-11, it will be interesting to consider the accuracy of its current application, and thus this remains a potential area for further research and understanding.

REFLECTION

Do you think the current DSM-5 is sensitive to the needs of people with learning disabilities? If you have access to a copy of the DSM-5 and the DC-LD, compare the two. What are the subtle or not-so-subtle differences? Based on the above, would you consider the act of providing supporting evidence to make a diagnosis to be a science, an art or a craft? Go back to chapter 19, on what it means to have a diagnosis of mental illness. Now take a few minutes to really consider the person who is 'in' that experience. Now also add a cognitive impairment to that experience too. The craft of caring is to really understand this. Although diagnostic criteria and classifications are important, your actions should reflect that you are genuinely interested in the *person*, rather than the classification.

Assessment

An accurate diagnosis is based on a comprehensive assessment. It will involve understanding and a creative response to cognitive deficits and communication problems. It will also involve working with family members or carers, who may play a crucial role when using informant-based tools, a key blend between person-centred and relationship-centred agendas (see chapter 3). Assessment includes a large number of factors, many of which are discussed in much greater detail in other chapters in this book. Physical health screening, mental health screening, client interview, observation, as well as specific assessments for specific disorders, are all pertinent. However, it is always important to remember that the true craft of caring requires a serious attempt at a genuine understanding of the person and their world view.

Assessing mental health in people with a learning disability is not easy. Chapters 13, 14 and 15 have information on assessment. A number of 'screening tools' have been developed to support this process.

For many screening tools, a 'threshold score' is provided. This usually indicates that, if a score is met or exceeded, further detailed psychiatric assessment may be warranted within that specific category/area. As such, screening tools are useful in providing a global mental health overview of presenting signs and symptoms, and remain an important first step in assessment. However, they do not provide a definitive diagnosis but rather prompt the need for a more detailed mental health assessment of a particular aspect. The craft in using such tools with the required level of caring, sensitivity, attention to detail and respect is not to be underestimated.

CASE STUDY 2

Simon has a mild learning disability and during the 1990s lived in a local authority home. Simon accessed local facilities and undertook part-time work in a factory; he was supported in the home by carers. In the late 1990s Simon was admitted to a local treatment and assessment facility as a result of the breakdown of the placement. His 'bed' (placement) was closed at the local authority home, preventing his return. Following a stroke, Simon spent a further 3 months rehabilitating in an acute hospital before being placed in an independent sector home. Simon states that he enjoys living here and expresses a desire to stay at the home that he has now lived in for nearly 10 years. He is aware that discussions have taken place regarding his future and whether he would benefit from a move into supported living.

A number of screening tools have been designed to be used specifically for/with people with learning disabilities. Many of these tools are described as 'informant-based tools', meaning they are usually completed with the help of a family member or carer who knows the person well. For the assessment to be valid and reliable, many tools will actually state the length of time the person needs to have known the person, thus ensuring the information is accurate and up to date and reducing the risk of diagnostic overshadowing. A number of tools will actually specify this period as a minimum of 6 months.

Both screening and interview formats help clinicians gather information to assess for dual diagnosis, often providing a 'global mental health assessment'. This can be used to highlight specific areas that could warrant more

BOX 60.3: SCREENING TOOLS AND INTERVIEW SCHEDULES

Screening tools

- Assessment of Dual Diagnosis (ADD) (Matson and Bamburg 1998)[26] (compatible with DSM-IV)[27]
- Diagnostic Assessment for the Severely Handicapped – II (DASH-II) (Matson 1995)[28]
- Learning Disability version of the Cardinal Needs Schedule (LDCNS) (Raghavan et al. 2004)[29]
- Mini Psychiatric Assessment Schedule for Adults with Developmental Disabilities (Mini PAS-ADD) (Prosser et al. 1996)[30]
- Psychiatric Assessment Schedule for Adults with Developmental Disorders Checklist (PAS-ADD Checklist) (Moss et al. 1998)[31]
- Reiss Screen for Maladaptive Behaviour (Reiss 1994)[32]

Interview schedules

- KGV (Manchester) Scale (Krawiecka et al. 1977)[33]
- Psychiatric Assessment Schedule for Adults with Developmental Disabilities Interview (PAS-ADD Interview) (Moss et al. 1996)[34]

detailed investigation. Thus, it is also useful to consider how common mental health disorders may manifest in people with learning disabilities, and how this may or may not differ from the general population. Examples of assessment tools and interview schedules can be seen in Box 60.3.

CARER'S PERSPECTIVE

I had to call the consultant to my home to see my son. His behaviour seemed to be worsening and he was 'hiding' under blankets. I knew this wasn't his normal behaviour and was getting increasingly concerned. To me he seemed depressed. A joint home visit I remember was carried out by his consultant and a nurse to assess his depressive symptoms.

Following a series of screening questions, the consultant finally asked: 'Adam, can you hear voices?'

Adam replied: 'Yes.'

The consultant then informed me, 'I think he is having a psychotic episode as he is hearing voices.'

I then had to ask if I could rephrase the question to my son, and instead asked Adam: 'Whose voices can you hear?'

Adam replied: 'Doctor and Mummy.'

My son wasn't hearing voices; he was merely answering the question asked of him.

Type, incidence and manifestation of common mental health disorders in people with a learning disability

DIAGNOSTIC OVERSHADOWING

An important consideration when diagnosing mental health disorders in people with a learning disability is the possibility of diagnostic overshadowing. This is a common concept in mental health that describes an occasion when the physical health (chapter 69) needs of a service user are falsely attributed to the service user's mental health condition, leading to unmet physical health needs.[35] This can also be considered with reference to learning disability, where signs and symptoms of mental health problems become falsely attributed to learning disability traits/behaviours or vice versa. In addition, any presenting mental health problems experienced by someone with a learning disability then become seen as less salient and significant.[36]

REFLECTION

As a health care professional, why is it important for you to consider a service user's history when conducting an interview/assessment?

Incidences of common forms of mental health disorder experienced by people with learning disabilities are often higher than in the general population. In this client group, dementia has the highest incidence, affecting over 50 per cent of people with Down's syndrome aged over 60.[37] Anxiety disorders, particularly generalized anxiety disorder, are also more common in people with a learning disability,[38] with some studies suggesting this accounts for 28 per cent of all occurring mental health disorders.[39] Personality disorders account for 10–13 per cent,[40] depression 3–8 per cent,[41] cyclical behaviour and mood changes 4 per cent,[42] and finally schizophrenia, with a prevalence rate of 3 per cent,[40] three times higher than that of the general population.[43] Some of these are discussed in more detail below.

DEMENTIA (see also chapter 33)

People with learning disabilities have a higher risk, perhaps three to four times more, of developing dementia when compared to the general population,[44] with a significantly higher risk for people with Down's syndrome.[45] In addition, typically in people with Down's syndrome, prevalence rates have been seen to increase between the ages of 40 and 60, possibly in excess of 50 per cent for those aged 60 and over.[46] It is also important to note that the age of dementia onset is still usually much earlier in people with Down's syndrome than in the general population, with the mean age at diagnosis of 55 years[45].

Perhaps the biggest reason why people with Down's syndrome are more likely to develop dementia, usually Alzheimer's disease, is due to the formation of amyloid plaques. Amyloid is a protein that forms neural plaques, characteristic of Alzheimer's disease, in the brain. The gene coding for the corresponding amyloid precursor protein (APP) that gives rise to these amyloid plaques is located on chromosome 21. Down's syndrome is associated with chromosome 21 and usually involves a trisomy or extra copy, thus accounting for the subsequent over-expression of amyloid protein.

Some localities may have access to the services of an Admiral Nurse. Admiral Nurses work through the charity Dementia UK and are specialist dementia nurses who give expert practical, clinical and emotional support to families and carers living with dementia to help them cope. At the time of writing, there are currently only 180 Admiral Nurses in the UK, although this number is set to increase and, depending on the complexity of cases and their eligibility criteria, may be a useful contact.

Possible scales for screening include the Dementia Questionnaire for People with Learning Disabilities (DLD) (previously known as DMR);[47] the Dementia Scale for Down's Syndrome (DSS);[48] Dementia Screening for Individuals with Intellectual Disabilities (DSQIID);[49,] and the Adaptive Behaviour Dementia Questionnaire (ABDQ).[50]

ANXIETY DISORDERS (see also chapter 20)

Despite anxiety disorders being the most common psychiatric disorder in the general population, little is known of its incidence in people with a learning disability.[51] It is believed to have a higher incidence rate in people with learning disabilities than the general population, with a recent study suggesting that the rate in people with learning disabilities is 3.8 per cent.[52] One important consideration is that some behaviours may require elevated degrees of reassurance, which, for staff not familiar with this client group, may easily become labelled as demanding or attention seeking. Loss of temper, and catastrophic reactions to what may be considered as minor concerns by the person with learning disabilities, may be typical, and should not therefore be dismissed.

Possible scales for screening include the Zung Anxiety Rating Scale: Adults Mental Handicap Version;[53] and the Glasgow Anxiety Scale.[54]

AFFECTIVE DISORDERS (see also chapters 21 and 26)

Affective disorders, such as depression and bipolar disorder, may be prevalent in up to 6.6 per cent of learning disability cases.[52] Detection of these disorders is difficult, as often atypical signs, such as tearfulness, excessive sleepiness and overeating, may get overlooked.[55,56] Also it is important to note that people with a learning disability may not always be able to express their emotions and feelings in words. Consequently, there is an increasing reliance on the observance of depressive-type or defined behaviours as offering a more promising approach to detection.[19] Although useful, an important limitation is that minor degrees of depression are less likely to be recognized.[57] These inherent difficulties in the detection of affective symptoms need careful consideration.

Possible scales for screening include the Affective Rating Scale;[58] the Beck Depression Inventory;[59] the Hamilton Depression Scale – Mental Handicap Version;[60] the Mental Retardation Depression Scale;[61] the Self-Report Depression Questionnaire (SRDQ);[62] and the Glasgow Depression Scale Carer Supplement (GDS-CS).[63]

SCHIZOPHRENIA AND 'PSYCHOTIC EPISODE' (see also chapters 24 and 28)

The prevalence of schizophrenia in people with learning disabilities is possibly three times higher than in the general population.[43] Deb et al.[20] reported a prevalence of 1.3–3.7 per cent. It also has an earlier average onset of 22.5 years, compared to 26.6 years in the general population.[64] As noted in earlier chapters, the symptoms of schizophrenia are usually split into 'positive' and 'negative' but there are additional important considerations to make within this client group. These are discussed below.

Positive symptoms. The content of hallucinations and delusions may reflect the limited experiences of people with a learning disability and thus are likely to be less complex.[65] Grandiose delusions, for example, are not uncommon, often incorporating a belief that they are someone of great importance. Examples include a client with grandiose delusions who believes they are the charge nurse on a busy learning disability ward; this may be compared to grandiose delusions in the general population which may include being a film star or someone linked to the royal family. It is also important to bear in mind that the developmental or cognitive level of the person should also be considered, so that an 'imaginary friend' may not necessarily be considered a delusion belief. Communication difficulties or a limited vocabulary may also affect the interpretation of what the person says; as such it is important to guard against diagnostic overshadowing, and a skilled interviewer is also important, as discussed above.

Negative symptoms. It may be difficult to distinguish the negative symptoms of schizophrenia from apathy and lack of engagement in a person with learning disabilities. Although often less dramatic than positive symptoms, negative symptoms are usually more persistent. It may be more difficult to observe these symptoms in people with severe and profound learning disabilities, and consequently 'withdrawal from daily life' must be considered in the context of the person's usual responses. Reduced attempts at communication including eye contact, slower movements and refusal to eat food previously enjoyed, or showing reduced pleasure in dressing/personal grooming may be examples. Care and attention need to be taken to avoid confusing negative symptoms of schizophrenia with symptoms of depression.

Sometimes people with a learning disability may not demonstrate the full criteria range for schizophrenia under ICD-10.[11] In such cases, a diagnosis of 'psychotic episode' may sometimes be made.[3] However, the diagnosis of schizophrenia is progressively difficult to apply as the severity of learning disability increases. Thus, in practice, diagnosis of schizophrenia may rarely be used in people with severe learning disability.

Although not specifically designed for use in learning disability, the Hallucinations Rating Scale[66] or the Psychotic Symptom Rating Scales (PSYRATS)[67] may be considered as scales for screening. Alternatively, questions from the PAS-ADD[31] (as discussed above) could be considered.

PERSONALITY DISORDERS (see also chapter 27)

There are clear difficulties in understanding the prevalence rates of personality disorders in people with learning disabilities. Some studies estimate this as 22 per cent,[68,69] but state that the range may be as great as 1 per cent to 92 per cent, demonstrating the complexity of diagnosing personality disorder within the learning disability population. The Royal College of Psychiatrists[18] in the DC-LD suggest that personality disorder should not be diagnosed in people with a learning disability under the age of 21 years, and that a diagnosis should be avoided in people with severe and profound learning disabilities.

A possible scale for screening is the Standardized Assessment of Personality (SAP).[70]

INTERVENTIONS

It is important to note that people with learning disabilities with a dual diagnosis have a right to the 'full range' of mental health interventions that are available to the general population. Creativity and some level of adaptation will be required, based on their level of ability, including communication skills. In addition, all interventions must continue the journey of togetherness between the nurse and the person requiring support, sometimes referred to as collaborative caring. It is only through this that the right conditions for growth, development and recovery can begin. It is only in this sense that our interventions, our practice, can be crafted.

Psychosocial interventions

Non-physical and non-pharmacological interventions fall under the umbrella term of 'psychosocial interventions' and are often recommended as first-line treatment/management before medication or other physical interventions are considered. (See Section 4 of this book for a more detailed discussion of models of therapeutic practice in this area.) Rush and Frances[71] in particular list seven types of psychosocial intervention that can be used with people with a learning disability:

- cognitive behaviour therapy (CBT);
- counselling;
- classical behaviour therapy;
- applied behavioural analysis;
- psychotherapy;
- environment management;
- education (client/family).

For many years, there was a 'therapeutic disdain' or assumption that people with learning disabilities were unable to benefit from or take part in psychological interventions.[72] In particular, psychological interventions were not considered beneficial because the person was wrongly believed to be lacking the cognitive and communication skills to benefit from sessions.[3,73] The first published case of using psychotherapy in this client group, in the 1980s, involved a man with an IQ of 59.[74] There are, however, a number of challenges in using psychotherapy with this client group, including a clear lack of services and therapists experienced in working with people with learning disabilities.[75] The recent Improving Access to Psychological Therapies (IAPT) Programme in Primary Care[76] reminded providers that services must also be accessible to people with learning disabilities, and subsequently additional Department of Health guidance[77] on reasonable adjustments has been produced. Their applicability to people with a learning disability continues to be a topic of discussion.[78] This needs to be favourably considered in light of the growing evidence that people with learning disabilities can make good use of psychosocial interventions where these therapies are appropriately adapted.[79–82]

Drawing on the suitability of CBT as an example, Hatton[83] argues this may often require assessment of communication skills, cognitive aptitude, capacity to identify emotions and capacity to understand the CBT model. The important consideration here is how these areas can be creatively managed, although an element of realism must still remain[83] (see chapter 40 for more discussion of the use of CBT). Here, the craft of mental health nurses is to consider what reasonable adjustments they could make based on the abilities of the person with learning disabilities, while also adhering to the validity and integrity of the proposed intervention. If, despite such reasonable adjustments, the person would not be able to engage suitably, then the intervention may be ineffective.

Pharmacological and physical interventions

MEDICATION (see also chapters 47 and 48)

People with a learning disability are equally at risk of developing 'metabolic syndrome' when taking antipsychotic medication. Although it remains unclear if having a learning disability increases the risk, it is important to note the link between weight gain and metabolic syndrome. It has been estimated that between 4 and 20 per cent of people with a learning disability are on antipsychotic medication.[84] Reasons for psychotropic drug use include the treatment of mental health disorders, behavioural problems and stereotypical behaviours that may affect activities of daily living. It is also unclear if people with a learning disability are at any greater risk to adverse drug effects then the general population, although there is increasing evidence that people with organic impairments are more likely to develop tardive dyskinesia than the general population.[85]

ELECTROCONVULSIVE THERAPY (ECT) (see also chapter 62)

There is little available evidence on the use of ECT with people with learning disabilities, although a few early studies[86,87] have discussed its use, efficacy and safety. Overall it has been argued to be just as safe and effective as its use in the general population. However, it is important to consider the issues of informed consent and capacity and how this may need to be additionally considered in people with cognitive impairments.

SUPPORTING SERVICE DEVELOPMENT

One of the first attempts to seriously consider the mental health needs of people with learning disabilities can be found in the Department of Health Mansell Report.[88] There were a number of key recommendations in this report which included the need to develop individualized care packages, small-scale and community-based services and local specialist services. Although the main focus appeared to be on people with challenging behaviour, the report did highlight the mental health needs of this group and thus the policy context was born. This followed the move from institutional care for many people with a learning disability to community-based services, and placed a greater emphasis on primary care services to assess and treat common mental health problems or to provide a gateway to secondary mainstream or specialist services.

Specialist services for people with learning disabilities generally include community learning disability teams (CLDTs), outreach teams, and inpatient learning disability services. CLDTs and outreach teams may, among other roles, be involved in the assessment and treatment of mental health problems in people with a learning disability living in their own homes, or in formal care settings, and may include supported living and residential care. Inpatient learning disability settings admit people with a range of complex behaviours, including mental health disorders, for assessment, treatment and/or management, often when community placements break down, despite the support of the CLDTs. There are no nationally agreed criteria on who should use specialist in-services and who should use mainstream mental health services, although government policy is clear that people with a learning disability should use mainstream/generic services wherever possible.

Given the growing move to mainstream services, concern has been voiced as to whether mainstream services are able to adequately support people with learning disabilities. Consequently, in 2004, the 'Green Light Toolkit'[89]

Table 60.2 The three audits used within the audit tool, used by the 'Green Light Toolkit 2013'[91]

1. Basic Audit	Physical health; eligibility and access; secure settings; safeguarding; assessment; equalities; personalization; staff attitudes and values; accessible information
2. Better Audit	Research; health and care records and care plans; local plans; how specialist services relate to local provision; skilled workforce; people needing personal care; user involvement in governance of service; psychological therapies; working together
3. Best Audit	Advocacy; commissioning; buildings and environments; leadership; family and friends; employment support; checking services; monitoring; challenging behaviour

was published. This document acted as a self-audit framework for all mental health services in assessing their suitability for people with a learning disability and a mental health problem, supporting efforts, where possible, to improve services. Some years later, a second report, *Reasonably adjusted?*,[90] was commissioned to report on what had been put in place. Although the report highlighted some good practice examples, few had comprehensively and systematically audited their practice or redesigned aspects of their service to ensure fair access and effective interventions for people with learning disabilities. A result of this has been the publication of 'Green Light Toolkit 2013',[91] which provides practical assistance to help mental health services develop their practice to better support people with learning disabilities. This includes a new audit framework and a database of reasonable adjustments.

This new audit tool consists of three audits, *Basic Audit*, *Better Audit* and *Best Audit*, depending on the level of complexity involved. These are shown in Table 60.2. Although the audit tools can be used in a number of ways, the National Development Team for Inclusion (NDTi) recommends using the Basic Audit to generate the first service action plan and achieve progress before moving on to potentially more challenging objectives in subsequent audits. In addition, a traffic light system, with a description of each element, is incorporated, allowing for progress to be monitored, hence its name: 'Green Light Toolkit'.

It is important that mental health services understand that they have a legal requirement under the Equality Act 2010 and the NHS and Social Care Act 2008 to make reasonable adjustments for 'people with learning disabilities' accessing their services. This legal requirement, or duty, is an 'anticipatory' one, meaning adjustments or changes need to be considered in advance, rather than waiting until people with a learning disability are actually using the service. This point is clearly endorsed in the much-publicized Winterbourne View Hospital Report[92] in the recommendation that all local services should build an understanding of the reasonable adjustments needed so that people with a learning disability with mental health problems can access and make use of local generic/mainstream mental health services. This supports the need to increase joint planning and reciprocal arrangements between commissioning groups, in both learning disability and mental health services. The implementation of this legal obligation serves to focus the minds of health and social care professionals on the needs of people with a learning disability and their carers.

At the time of writing, the National Institute for Health and Clinical Excellence (NICE) has recently published new guidance specifically on the mental health needs of people with a learning disability. The publication of this new guidance, will have a large impact on future service provision and, potentially, the role and competency of mental health nurses in developing the craft of caring, as access to mainstream generic services continues to grow.

CONCLUSION

Within this chapter a number of factors relating to the assessment and diagnosis of people with a learning disability have been identified. While an array of tools are available to assist in these processes, the craft of caring lies within the implementation of the processes. Time must be taken to consider the individual needs of the person presenting for assessment. For example, could there be underlying sensory impairments that affect the person's ability to participate in the process, or does information need to be made available in a more accessible format? The term 'craft' denotes a degree of skill within the practitioner, and this chapter encourages practitioners to reflect on their

own interpersonal skills and how they may be developed to facilitate interaction with people with a learning disability, sharing their journey, and creating the right conditions for growth, development and recovery. In a care sector that is measured on the achievement of outcomes, when working with people with a learning disability it is clear that a focus on the craft of caring is more important now than ever before to improve the outcomes for people with a learning disability and their families. This is particularly important when recognizing that the mental health needs of people with learning disabilities is a growing area for mental health nursing, particularly for people with mild or moderate learning disabilities, for whom access to generic services needs to be first considered.

However, it should always be at the forefront of every mental health nurse's mind that the nature of nursing in this area is more than just the knowledge or aesthetics of learning disability practice, but rather the blending together of these agendas to form a true craft of caring. This craft can be seen in a number of ways: the way we undertake our assessments, select appropriate therapeutic interventions and develop our services, with a careful attention to detail, sensitivity and respect for the person we are caring for. Nursing is, after all, a human service. Here the mental health nurse needs to understand the person with learning disabilities through both a person-centred *and* a relationship-centred agenda. This can involve understanding the individual experiences of the person, as well as starting the journey of togetherness between the person, their carer and the nurse. It is only through undertaking such a journey 'with' the person that the true conditions for growth, development and recovery can be fostered, and we can then begin to understand the experience of their mental health with them. After all, we must never forget that the true focus of nursing, whether in mental health, learning disability or a combination of the two, is ultimately the 'craft of caring'.

ACKNOWLEDGEMENTS

The authors would like to acknowledge the contribution of other service users and carers who helped with the reflection points and case studies throughout this chapter but who wished to remain anonymous.

References

1. Department of Health. *Valuing people: a new strategy for learning disability for the 21st century.* London: Stationery Office, 2001.
2. Scottish Executive Health Department. *The same as you? A review of services for people with learning disabilities.* Edinburgh: Stationery Office, 2000.
3. Royal College of Nursing. *Mental health nursing of adults with learning disabilities.* RCN guidance. London: RCN, 2010.
4. Emerson E, Hatton C. *Estimating future needs/demands for support for adults with learning disabilities in England.* Lancaster: Institute for Health Research, 2004.
5. Hardy S, Holt G. Assessment of mental health problems. In: Holt G, Hardy S, Bouras N (eds). *Mental health in learning disabilities. A reader.* Brighton: Estia Centre/Pavilion, 2005: 19–26.
6. Borthwick-Duffy SA. Epidemiology and prevalence of psychopathology in people with mental retardation. *Journal of Consulting and Clinical Psychology* 1994; **62**: 17–27.
7. Day K, Jancar J. Mental and physical health and ageing in mental handicap; a review. *Journal of Intellectual Disability Research* 1994; **38**: 241–56.
8. Miller E. Mental retardation. Clinical section – part I. In: Berrios G, Porter R (eds). *A history of clinical psychiatry. The origin and history of psychiatric disorders.* London: Athlone Press, 1995: 212–24.
9. Berrios GE (1995) Mental retardation. Clinical section – part II. In: Berrios G, Porter R (eds). *A history of clinical psychiatry. The origin and history of psychiatric disorders.* London: Athlone Press, 1995: 225–38.
10. Barker P, Whitehill I. The craft of care: towards collaborative caring in psychiatric nursing. In: Tilley S (ed.). *The mental health nurse: views of practice and education.* Oxford: Blackwell Science, 1997.
11. WHO (World Health Organization). *The ICD-10 classification of mental and behavioural disorders.* Geneva: WHO, 1992.
12. Wymbrandt J, Ludman MD. *Genetic disorders and birth defects.* New York: Facts on File, 2000.
13. Bhaumik S, Branford D. *The Frith prescribing guidelines for adults with intellectual disabilities.* Leicestershire Partnership NHS Trust: HealthComm UK, 2008.
14. Lord C, Risi S, Lambrecht L, et al. The Autism Diagnostic Observation Schedule – Generic: a standard measure of social and communication deficits associated with the spectrum of autism. *Journal of Autism and Developmental Disorders* 2000; **30**: 205–23.
15. Lord C, Pickles A, McLennan J et al. Diagnosing autism: analyses of data from the Autism Diagnostic Interview. *Journal of Autism and Developmental Disorders* 1997; **27**: 501–17.

16. Ryrie I, McGowan J. Staff perceptions of substance use among acute psychiatric inpatients. *Journal of Mental Health Nursing* 1998; **5**: 137–42.
17. Bregman JD, Leckman JF, Ort SI. Fragile x syndrome; genetic predisposition to psychopathology. *Journal of Autism and Developmental Disorders* 1998; **18**: 343–54.
18. Royal College of Psychiatrists. *DC-LD Diagnostic criteria for psychiatric disorders for use with adults with a learning disabilities/mental retardation.* London: Gaskell, 2001.
19. Cooper SA, Collacott RA. Depression in adults with learning disabilities: a critical review. *Irish Journal of Psychological Medicine* 1996; **13**: 105–13.
20. Deb S, Mathew T, Holt G, Bouras N. *Practice guidelines for the assessment and diagnosis of mental health problems in adults with intellectual disability.* Brighton: Pavilion Publishing, 2001.
21. Khan S, Osinowo T, Pary R. Down syndrome and major depressive disorder: a review. *Mental Health Aspects of Developmental Disabilities* 2002; **5**(2); 46–52.
22. Cooper SA, Cllacott RA. Clinical features and diagnostic criteria of depression in Down's syndrome. *British Journal of Psychiatry* 1994; **165**: 399–403.
23. Verhoeven WMA, Curfs LMG, Tuinier S. Prader-Willi syndrome and cycloid psychosis. *Journal of Intellectual Disability Research* 1998; **42**: 455–62.
24. Cooper SA, Melville C, Einfield S. Psychiatric diagnosis, intellectual disabilities and diagnostic criteria for psychiatric disorders for use with adults with learning disabilities/mental retardation (DC-LD). *Journal of Intellectual Disability Research* 2003; **47**(1): 3–1.
25. American Psychiatric Association. *Diagnostic and statistical manual of mental disorders. Fifth edition. DSM–5.* Washington: APA, 2013.
26. Matson JL, Bamburg JW. Reliability of the assessment of dual diagnosis (ADD). *Research in Developmental Disabilities* 1998; **19**(1): 89–9.
27. American Psychiatric Association. *Diagnostic and statistical manual of mental disorders. Fourth edition. DSM-IV.* Washington: APA, 1994.
28. Matson JL. *The diagnostic assessment for the severely handicapped II.* Baton Rouge: Scientific Publishers, 1995.
29. Raghavan R, Marshall M, Lockwood A, Duggan, L. Assessing the needs of people with learning disabilities and mental illness: development of the Learning Disability version of the Cardinal Needs Schedule. *Journal of Intellectual Disability Research* 2004; **48**(1): 25–36.

30. Prosser H, Moss S, Costello H, et al. *The Mini PAS-ADD: an assessment schedule for the detection of mental health problems in adults with developmental disabilities.* Manchester: Hester Adrian Research Centre, 1996.

31. Moss S, Prosser H, Costello H, et al. *Reliability and validity of the PAS-ADD Checklist for detecting psychiatric symptoms in people with learning disability. Social Psychiatry and Psychiatric Epidemiology* 1998; **32**: 344–54.

32. Reiss S. *The Reiss screen for maladaptive behaviour test manual*, 2nd edn. Worthington OH: IDS Publishing, 1994.

33. Krawiecka M, Goldberg D, Vaughan M. A standardised psychiatric assessment scale for rating chronic psychotic patients. *Acta Psychiatrica Scandinavica* 1977; **55**: 299–308.

34. Moss S, Goldberg D, Patel P, et al. *The psychiatric assessment schedule for adults with a developmental disability: PASS-ADD.* Manchester: Hester Adrian Research Centre, 1996.

35. Nash M. Diagnostic overshadowing: a potential barrier to physical health for mental health service users. *Mental Health Practice* 2013; **17**(4): 22–6.

36. Mason J, Scior K. 'Diagnostic overshadowing' amongst clinicians working with people with intellectual disabilities in the UK. *Journal of Applied Research in Intellectual Disabilities* 2004; **17**: 85–90.

37. Cooper SA. High prevalence of dementia among people with learning disabilities not attributable to Down's syndrome. *Psychological Medicine* 1997; **27**: 609–16.

38. Raghavan R. Anxiety disorders in people with learning disabilities: a review of the literature. *Journal of Learning Disabilities for Nursing, Health and Social Care* 1997; 2(1): 3–9.

39. Day K. Psychiatric disorders in the middle aged and elderly mentally handicapped. *British Journal of Psychiatry* 1985; **147**: 660–7.

40. Weissman MM. The epidemiology of personality disorders: an update. *Journal of Personality Disorders* 1993 (Suppl): 44–62.

41. Clarke DJ. Functional psychoses in people with mental retardation. In: Bouras N (ed.). *Psychiatric and behavioural disorders in developmental disabilities.* Cambridge: Cambridge University Press, 1999: 188–99.

42. Deb S, Hunter D. Psychopathology of people with mental handicap and epilepsy. II. Psychiatric illness. *British Journal of Psychiatry* 1991; **159**: 826–30.

43. O'Hara J, Sperlinger A. *Adults with learning disabilities: a practical approach for health professionals.* Chichester: Wiley, 1997.

44. Sinai A, Chan T, Strydom A. The epidemiology of dementia in people with intellectual disabilities. In: Watchman K (ed). *Intellectual disability and dementia. Research into practice.* London: Jessica Kingsley, 2013: 24–33.

45. British Psychological Society. *Dementia and people with intellectual disabilities. Guidance on the assessment, diagnosis, interventions and support of people with intellectual disabilities who develop dementia.* Leicester: BPS, 2015.

46. Strydom A, Shooshtari S, Lee L, et al. Dementia in older adults with intellectual disabilities – epidemiology, presentation and diagnosis. *Journal of Policy and Practice in Intellectual Disabilities* 2010; 7(2): 96–110.

47. Evenhuis HM, Kengen MMF, Eurlings HAL. *Dementia questionnaire for people with learning disabilities (DLD). UK adaptation.* San Antonio: Harcourt Assessment, 2007.

48. Gedye A. *Dementia Scale for Down's syndrome – manual.* Vancouver: Geyde Research & Consulting, 1995.

49. Deb S, Hare M, Prior L, Bhaumik S. The dementia screening questionnaire for individuals with intellectual disabilities. *British Journal of Psychiatry* 2007; **190**: 440–4.

50. Prasher VP, Holder R, Asim F. The Adaptive Behaviour Dementia Questionnaire (ABDQ): screening questionnaire for dementia in Alzheimer's disease in adults with Down Syndrome. *Research in Developmental Disabilities* 2004; **25**: 385–97.

51. Ollendick TH, Ollendick DG. Anxiety disorders. In: Matson J, Barrett RP (eds). *Psychopathology in the mentally retarded.* New York: Grune and Stratton, 1982: 77–120.

52. Cooper SA, Smiley E, Morrison J, Williamson A, Allan L. Mental ill-health in adults with intellectual disabilities: prevalence and associated factors. *British Journal of Psychiatry* 2007; **190**: 27–35.

53. Lindsay WR, Michie AM. Adaption of the Zung self rating anxiety scale for people with a mental handicap. *Journal of Mental Deficiency Research* 1998; **32**: 485–90.

54. Epsie CA, Mindham J. Glasgow Anxiety Scale for people with intellectual disability (GAS-ID): development and psychometric properties of a new measure for use with people with mild intellectual disability. *Journal of Intellectual Disability Research* 2003; **47**(1): 22–30.

55. O'Brien G, Whitehouse A. A psychiatric study of deviant eating behaviour among mentally handicapped adults. *British Journal of Psychiatry* 1990; **157**: 281–4.

56. Meins W. Symptoms of major depression in mentally retarded adults. *Journal of Intellectual Disability Research* 1995; **39**: 41–5.

57. O'Brien G. Dual diagnosis in offenders with intellectual disability: setting research priorities: a review of research findings concerning psychiatric disorder (excluding personality disorder) among offenders with intellectual disability. *Journal of Intellectual Disability Research* 2002; **46**(S1): 21–30.

58. Wieseler NA, Campbell GJ, Sonis W. Ongoing use of an affective rating scale in the treatment of a mentally retarded individual with rapid-cycling bipolar affective disorder. *Research in Developmental Disabilities* 1988; **9**: 47–53.

59. Beck AT, Ward CH, Mendelson M, Mock J, Erbaugh J. An inventory for measuring depression. *Archives of General Psychiatry* 1961; **4**: 561–71.

60. Sireling L. Depression in mentally handicapped patients: diagnostic and neuroendocrine evaluation. *British Journal of Psychiatry* 1986; **149**: 274–8.

61. Meins W. A new depression scale designed for use with adults with mental retardation. *Journal of Intellectual Disability Research* 1996; **40**: 220–6.

62. Reynolds WK, Baker JA. Assessment of depression in persons with mental retardation. *American Journal of Mental Retardation* 1988; **93**: 93–103.

63. Cuthill FM, Espie CA, Cooper SA. Development and psychometric properties of the Glasgow Depression Scale for people with a learning disability. *British Journal of Psychiatry* 2003; **182**: 347–53.

64. Meadows G, Turner T, Campbell L, Lewis S, Rouley M, Murray R. Assessing schizophrenia in adults with mental retardation: a comparative study. *British Journal of Psychiatry* 1991; **158**: 103–5.

65. Došen A, Day K. Epidemiology, etiology, and presentation of mental illness and behaviour in persons with mental retardation. In: Došen A and Day K (eds) *Treating mental illness and behaviour disorders in children and adults with mental retardation.* Washington: American Psychiatric Press, 2001: 3–24.

66. Haddock G. *The hallucinations rating scale.* Brighton: Pavilion Publishing, 1994.

67. Haddock G, McCarron J, Tarrier N, Faragher EB. Scales to measure dimensions of hallucinations and delusions. The Psychotic Symptom Rating Scales (PSYRATS). *Psychological Medicine* 1999; **29**(4): 879–89.

68. Reid AH, Ballinger BR. Personality disorder in mental handicap. *Psychological Medicine* 1987; **17**: 983–7.

69. Alexandra R, Cooray S. Diagnosis of personality disorders in learning disability. *British Journal of Psychiatry* 2003; **182**(44): 28–31.

70. Mann AH, Jenkins R, Cutting JC, Cowen PJ. The development of a standardized measure of abnormal personality. *Psychological Medicine* 1981; **11**: 839–47.

71. Rush A, Frances A. Treatment of psychiatric and behavioural problems in mental retardation. *American Journal on Mental Retardation* 2000; **105**(3): 159–226.

72. Bender M. The unoffered chair: the history of therapeutic disdain towards people with learning disability. *Clinical Psychology Forum* 1993; **54**: 7–12.

73. Beail N. What works for people with mental retardation? Critical commentary on cognitive-behavioural and psychodynamic psychotherapy research. *Mental Retardation* 2003; **41**(6): 468–72.

74. Symington N. The psychotherapy of a subnormal patient. *British Journal of Medical Psychology* 1981; **54**: 187–99.

75. Arthur AR. The emotional lives of people with learning disability. *British Journal of Learning Disabilities* 2003; **31**: 25–30.

76. Department of Health. *Improving Access to Psychological Therapies (IAPT): best practice guidance commissioning toolkit.* London: DH, 2008.

77. Department of Health. *Improving Access to Psychological Therapies (IAPT): learning disabilities positive practice.* London: DH, 2009.

78. Dodd K, Joyce T, Nixon J, Jennison J, Heneage C. Improving access to psychological therapies (IAPT): are they applicable to people with intellectual disabilities? *Advances in Mental Health and Intellectual Disabilities* 2011; **5**(2): 29–34.

79. Dagnan D, Chadwick P. Cognitive behaviour therapy for people with learning disabilities: assessment and intervention. In: Stenfert Kroese BS, Dagnan D, Loumides K (eds). *Cognitive behaviour therapy for people with learning disabilities.* London: Routledge, 1997: 110–23.

80. Haddock G, Lobban F, Hatton C, Carson R. Cognitive-behaviour therapy for people with psychosis and mild intellectual disabilities: a case series. *Clinical Psychology & Psychotherapy* 2004; **11**: 282–98.

81. Lindsay WR, Howells L, Pitcaithly D. Cognitive therapy for depression with individuals with intellectual disabilities. *British Journal of Medical Psychology* 1993; **66**: 135–41.

82. Lindsay WR, Neilson C, Lawrenson H. Cognitive-behaviour therapy for anxiety in people with learning disabilities. In: Stenfert Kroese B, Dagnan D, Loumides K (eds). *Cognitive-behaviour therapy for people with learning disabilities.* London: Routledge, 1997: 124–40.

83. Hatton C. Psychosocial interventions for adults with intellectual disabilities and mental health problems. *Journal of Mental Health* 2002; **11**: 357–73.

84. Deb S, Fraser W. The use of psychotropic medication in people with a learning disability. Towards rational prescribing. *Human Psychopharmacology* 1994; **9**: 219–72.

85. Clarke DJ. Treatment of schizophrenia. In: Došen A, Day K (eds). *Treating mental illness and behaviour disorders in children and adults with mental retardation.* Washington: American Psychiatric Press, 2001: 183–200.

86. Cutjar P, Wilson D. The use of ECT in intellectual disability. *Journal of Intellectual Disability Research* 1999; **43**(5): 421–7.

87. Kessler RJ. Electroconvulsive therapy for affective disorders in persons with mental retardation. *Psychiatric Quarterly* 2004; **75**(1): 99–104.

88. Department of Health. *Services for people with learning disabilities and challenging behaviour or mental health needs.* London: HMSO, 1992.

89. Foundation for People with Learning Disabilities et al. *Green Light: how good are your mental health services for people with learning disabilities? A service improvement toolkit.* London: Turning Point, 2004.

90. NDTi (National Development Team for Inclusion). *Reasonably adjusted? Mental health services and support for people with autism and people with learning disabilities.* 2012. Available from: http://mentalhealthpartnerships.com/resource/reasonably-adjusted-mental-health-services-and-support-for-people-with-autism-and-people-with-learning-disabilities/ [Accessed 9th August 2016].

91. NDTi (National Development Team for Inclusion). *Green Light Toolkit. A guide to auditing and improving your mental health service so that it is effective in supporting people with autism and people with learning disabilities.* 2013. Available from: http://www.ndti.org.uk/uploads/files/Green_Light_Toolkit_2013_final_word_doc_revised.pdf [Accessed 9th August 2016].

92. Department of Health. DH Review: Winterbourne View Hospital Interim Report. Department of Health, 2012.

Further reading

General mental health in LD

Holt G, Hardy S, Bouras N. *Mental health in learning disabilities. A reader.* Brighton: Estia Centre/Pavilion, 2005.

Priest H, Gibbs M. *Mental health care for people with learning disabilities.* London: Churchill Livingstone, 2004.

Raghavan R, Patel P. *Learning disabilities and mental health.* Oxford: Blackwell Publishing, 2005.

Diagnosis of mental health problems in LD

Deb S, Mathew T, Holt G, Bouras N. *Practice guidelines for the assessment and diagnosis of mental health problems in adults with intellectual disability.* Brighton: Pavilion Publishing, 2001.

Royal College of Psychiatrists. *DC-LD: the diagnostic criteria for psychiatric disorders for use with adults with learning disabilities.* London: RCP, 2001.

WHO (World Health Organization). *ICD-10 guide for mental retardation.* Geneva: WHO, 1996. Available from: http://www.who.int/mental_health/media/en/69.pdf [Accessed 16th August 2016].

Improving services

Hardy S, Kramer R, Holt G, Woodward P, Chaplin E. *Supporting complex needs: a practical guide for support staff working with people with a learning disability who have mental health needs.* London: Turning Point, 2006.

NDTi (National Development Team for Inclusion). *Green Light Toolkit. A guide to auditing and improving your mental health services so that it is effective in supporting people with autism and people with learning disabilities.* 2013. Available from: http://www.ndti.org.uk/uploads/files/Green_Light_Toolkit_2013_final_word_doc_revised.pdf [Accessed 9th August 2016].

Royal College of Nursing. *Mental health nursing of adults with learning disabilities. RCN guidance.* London: RCN, 2010.

Interventions

Bhaumik S, Branford D. *The Frith prescribing guideline for adults with intellectual disability. Second edition.* Aberdeen: Healthcomm UK, 2008.

Department of Health. *Improving Access to Psychological Therapies (IAPT): learning disabilities positive practice.* London: DH, 2009.

Stenfert Kroese B, Dagnan D, Loumides K. *Cognitive-behaviour therapy for people with learning disabilities.* London: Routledge, 1997.

Depression and LD

Townsley R, Goodwin J. *All about feeling down* (accessible booklet). London: Foundation For People with Learning Disabilities, 2003.

Dementia and LD

British Psychological Society. *Dementia and people with learning disabilities. Guidance on the assessment, diagnosis, interventions and support of people with intellectual disabilities who develop dementia.* Leicester: BPS, 2015.

Dodd K, Turk V, Christmas M. *Down's Syndrome and dementia – a resource for carers and support staff*. Birmingham: BILD, 2009.

Kerr D. *Understanding learning disability and dementia. Developing effective interventions*. London: Jessica Kingsley, 2007.

Watchman K. *Intellectual disability and dementia. Research into practice*. London: Jessica Kingsley, 2014.

Watchman K, Kerr D, Wilkinson H. *Supporting Derek*. York: Joseph Rowntree Foundation, 2010.

Autism

NICE (National Institute for Health and Care Excellence). *Autism diagnosis in children and young people: recognition, referral, diagnosis of children and young people on the autistic spectrum.*

Relevant web pages

General

British Institute of Learning Disabilities. www.bild.org.uk/

Down's Syndrome Association. www.downs-syndrome.org.uk

Forster M, Wilkie B, Strydom A, Edwards C, Hall I. Accessible information about mental health medication. Elfrida Society. http://www.elfrida.com/publications.html

Intellectual Disability and Health. www.intellectualdisability.info/

MENCAP. Resources for health care professionals. www.mencap.org.uk/about-learning-disability/information-professionals/health

National Association for the Dually Diagnosed. *Diagnostic manual – intellectual disability (DM-ID): a clinical guide for the diagnosis of mental disorders in persons with intellectual disabilities*. http://www.dmid.org/clin-about.htm

NICE (National Institute for Health and Care Excellence). Learning Disabilities: identifying and managing mental health problems quality standard (QS142) https://www.nice.org.uk/guidance/qs142

NICE clinical guideline 128. 2011. Available from: www.nice.org.uk/guidance/cg128 [Accessed 16th August 2016] (NB: this guideline is due to be reviewed; please see website for updated version if necessary).

NICE (National Institute for Health and Care Excellence). *Autism: recognition, referral, diagnosis and management of adults on the autistic spectrum. NICE clinical guideline 142*. Available from: www.nice.org.uk/guidance/cg142?unlid=5627139520166155426 [Accessed 16th August 2016].

Royal College of Psychiatrists and Gaskell Publishing. Books beyond words. http://www.rcpsych.ac.uk/usefulresources/publications/booksbeyondwords.aspx

Services

National Development Team for Inclusion. Learning disability. www.ndti.org.uk/who-were-concerned-with/learning-disability/

Royal College of Psychiatrists. Learning disability and mental health. http://www.rcpsych.ac.uk/healthadvice/partnersincarecampaign/learningdisabilityleaflet.aspx

Dementia and LD

Admiral Nurses. www.dementiauk.org

Alzheimer's Society. www.alzheimers.org.uk

Bereavement and grief counselling

HUGH PALMER

LEARNING OUTCOMES

- To be able to describe current models of grief.
- To be aware of the mental health problems that result from bereavement.
- To understand the impact of bereavement upon people with existing mental health problems.
- To be able to consider interventions, including counselling, for people experiencing bereavement and loss.

SUMMARY OF KEY POINTS

- Bereavement and grief are not illnesses – they are a normal part of the human experience.
- Bereavement can sometimes become complicated and lead to mental health difficulties, and bereavement can be more problematic for people with existing mental health problems.
- There are different approaches to bereavement, and more recent models have moved away from the idea of 'moving on' to the concept of maintaining a bond with the deceased person.
- Most people who are bereaved do not necessarily need or benefit from counselling.

- Providing support to those who are bereaved requires basic counselling skills along with an appreciation of the process of grief.

If you listen long enough and are open and nonjudgmental you will hear at least one story from each person about something 'weird' and unexplainable that connects them with the one who died. It's there. They may not choose to disclose it for fear of ridicule.

(Mother, aged 33, cited in Sormanti and August[1] (pp.467–8))

INTRODUCTION

This chapter is intended to introduce the reader to the topic of grief and bereavement work, with the recognition that bereavement can sometimes be a source of mental health difficulties and that people experiencing mental health problems will also experience bereavement too. It is now recognized that there can be value in limited interventions made by health care practitioners (including mental health practitioners) in better outcomes for the bereaved.

In the chapter, we will explore models of grief and bereavement, beginning with earlier approaches arising from Freud's writing on melancholia, and moving on to cover attachment and more recent moves toward the idea of continuing bonds[2] and 're-membering'.[3] Following this, we will begin to think about bereavement and mental health, identify problems that arise as a result of bereavement, and consider issues related to bereavement in people who have existing mental health problems. A section on interventions will consider approaches to working with the bereaved, and the chapter will conclude with a general discussion. This chapter is very much concerned with the craft of caring; even though this concept is not discussed in great detail here, the topic of grief and bereavement, especially with recent moves away from pathologizing some aspects of grief, marks this as a subject that encourages a holistic approach.

WHAT DO THE TERMS 'BEREAVEMENT' AND 'GRIEF' MEAN?

Before exploring models of bereavement, it is worth understanding what the concepts of grief and bereavement entail. The English word *bereavement* comes from an ancient Germanic root word meaning 'to deprive of, take away, seize, rob', and the word *grief* stems from Middle English version of the Old French *grief*, from *grever*, 'to burden', which itself stems from the Latin *gravare*, 'to cause grief, make heavy'. Another word frequently used in this context is *mourn*, from the Old English *murnan*, 'to mourn, bemoan, long after'.

Modern use of the term bereavement is associated with the loss of a loved one, usually of a person or animal, normally through death. The response to this loss is typically grief, which can include a sense of sorrow, burden and heaviness, and mourning the loss is associated with feelings of longing for the person.

All of us will have experienced loss of one sort or another, but how we respond to the loss is, in part, associated with our attachment to that which is lost. Our strongest attachments are usually to other people, especially family and close friends.

REFLECTION

Spend a few moments thinking about something that you lost and did not find; perhaps a key or a favourite object. Write down your answers to the following questions:

- What was your immediate reaction when you realized you had lost the item?
- What words might describe your feelings at this time?
- After your initial reaction, what were your following responses?
- What other responses are you aware of having in the days and weeks following the loss?

Often our immediate reaction to a loss is panic; perhaps even thinking that it cannot be true, that there must be some mistake. This is sometimes followed by searching for the lost object, eventually realizing that the object may never be found, perhaps feeling angry or sad about the loss and, in time, accepting that the object is gone. Depending on what the object was, we might replace it with something else, but of course, if it had sentimental value, that emotional aspect of the item can never be replaced.

Many approaches to grief and bereavement identify similar processes to those discussed above in describing responses to the loss of a loved person, and as the chapter progresses you will be able to relate your own experiences to the theoretical ideas and consider how you might use them in practice.

MODELS OF GRIEF AND BEREAVEMENT

Bereavement affects all of us, and up until recently, grief often was treated as if it was an illness, with models drawing on Freud's[4] writing on mourning and melancholia, which conceptualized loss as a state that required a path to 'recovery', often identifying various stages of grief (for example, Worden's[5] four tasks of mourning or Kübler-Ross's[6] five stages of grief), before a resolution culminating in the redirection of emotional 'energy' elsewhere.

More recent bereavement theorists, particularly Klass et al.,[2] have challenged this approach, instead considering that bereaved people have a continuing bond with the deceased. Independently, some social constructionist, narrative therapists, notably White[7] and Hedtke and Winslade,[3] have also questioned traditional approaches to working with death and bereavement, instead exploring ways for the bereaved individual to maintain a relationship with the dead person. They keep open possibilities of staying in love with a dead partner and the possibility of being able to continue to maintain and shape the identity of that person. This is in stark contrast with help that is directed towards enabling the bereaved person to recognize their feelings of loss and sadness, to accept the reality of the death and emotionally to move on to a life without the deceased person.

Thinking about the concept of the craft of caring, it is evident that the experiences of bereaved people can be viewed through two different lenses; one that considers aspects of grief (particularly those experiences that might be perceived as denying the reality of the loss) as abnormal or even pathological; or one that views these experiences holistically, and considers them normal, even if no more than a means to continue the relationship or bond with the deceased person.

REFLECTION

Take a few minutes to consider your own views on bereavement and grief. Write down your answers to the following questions:

- Do you think it is best for a person to 'move on' and get on with their life when someone close to them has died? If so, when should this happen?

- Do you think that it is common for people to have unusual experiences, for example seeing or hearing a deceased person, when they are grieving? What explanations might there be for these experiences? What is your opinion?

FREUD AND ATTACHMENT-BASED MODELS OF GRIEF

In his seminal paper, 'Mourning and melancholy', Sigmund Freud[4] identified two forms of grief: *Trauer* (mourning) and *Melancholie* (melancholy). According to Freud, mourning is a normal reaction to the loss of a loved person, or to the loss of some abstraction (for example, 'home' or 'liberty'). He identified that this is a normal response to loss and should not be considered to be an illness, and, following a period of grieving, a person will overcome their sorrow and become free and unburdened.

In contrast to mourning, Freud suggested that, although melancholy derives from the same circumstances, it can present in more extreme and damaging ways, where the individual experiences profoundly painful dejection, loss of self-esteem, and loss of interest in the outside world. He suggests that, in melancholia, the loss suffered can be of a real person or an idealized entity and the person sometimes does not know what they have lost; therefore melancholy can be related to the unconscious loss of a love object. According to Freud, someone with melancholia is preoccupied by the loss of the idealized object and can become extremely self-destructive and have very impaired self-esteem.

Bowlby's[8] attachment theory was heavily influenced by Freud's writing about the relationship people have to idealized objects and real figures, and attachment theory in turn influenced later writers on bereavement, particularly William Worden and Colin Murray Parkes. Bowlby identified three stages of grief – shock and numbness, yearning and searching, despair and disorganization. Later, Parkes[9] added a fourth: reorganization. Bowlby agreed with Parkes and he also supported the idea of four stages that did not

necessarily follow sequentially, but might be experienced at different times. These stages are:

- *Shock and numbness.* In this phase, there is a sense that the loss is not real and is not easy to accept. There can be physical distress during this phase, which can result in physical symptoms.
- *Yearning and searching.* Here, the person is aware of the gap in their life left by the loss, with a loss of the imagined future that included the person. At this time, attempts to fill this void are made and the person may appear preoccupied with the deceased.
- *Despair and disorganization.* Here, the bereaved person is able to accept that life has changed and cannot go back to how it was or how the person hoped. Some of the emotions associated with this phase are hopelessness, despair and anger and questioning.
- *Re-organization and recovery.* In this phase the person begins to rebuild their life without their loved one and move on.

Elizabeth Kübler-Ross was strongly influenced by Bowlby and Parkes and her well-known model of grief appeared in her book *On death and dying*,[6] which outlines five stages of grief: denial, anger, bargaining, depression and acceptance. These stages are usually remembered by the acronym 'DABDA'. As with the previous model, these stages are not necessarily experienced in sequential order.

During the stage of denial, grieving people are unable or unwilling to accept the reality of the loss. They might feel as though they are experiencing a bad dream, that the loss is unreal, and they are waiting to 'wake up' as though from a dream, expecting that things will be normal.

Once accepting the reality of the loss, the person may begin to feel anger at the loss and the unfairness of it. They may become angry at the person who has been lost or towards other people – for example, friends, relatives or caregivers. The next phase, bargaining, is characterized by the person begging a higher power to undo the loss, perhaps saying that if the person is returned to them, they will change. The next stage is one of depression, where the person confronts the reality of the loss and their own helplessness to change it. Ultimately, according to Kübler-Ross, the person will enter a stage of acceptance when they will have processed their initial grief reactions, accept the loss and begin to move on and plan for a future without the loved one.

A similar model to these earlier approaches was proposed by Worden,[5] whose tasks of mourning followed a similar set of stages, although in the latest edition, instead of the idea of 'moving on', he incorporated the concept that the bereaved can find an enduring connection with the dead person.

- *Task I: To accept the reality of the loss.* When someone dies, there is often a sense of unbelief; that it cannot really have happened. This is sometimes referred to as denial, and part of this first task is to arrive at the realization, both intellectually and emotionally, that the person is dead and will not return. Rituals, such as funerals, are helpful to clients as they signify the reality of the death.
- *Task II: To process the pain of grief.* Sometimes clients will try to avoid the intense pain of losing a loved one. Society offers us lots of opportunities to distract ourselves, and it encourages this due to subtle messages about not showing distress and a general discomfort with grieving. However, processing the pain of loss and grief is necessary and can help stop individuals carrying the pain into their future where it may be more difficult to work through.
- *Task III: To adjust to a world without the deceased.* Losing a loved one requires the bereaved to make external, internal and spiritual adjustments. External adjustments might include having to take on roles previously undertaken by the dead person and having to undertake the normal tasks and activities of living in their absence. Internal adjustments are those changes that are required to create a new sense of identity without the person; 'Who am I now?' Spiritual adjustments are about the wider meaning of being bereaved and a changed relationship with the world, perhaps with a revision of spiritual beliefs.
- *Task IV: To find an enduring connection with the deceased in the midst of embarking on a new life.* In this task the clients may find themselves considering how to stay emotionally connected with the deceased without it preventing them moving on in their own life. It is not a forgetting of the deceased, but rather the client finding themselves reconnecting and enjoying their life while remembering the memories and thoughts of and feelings about the loved one.

Worden makes the point that there is no set time for these tasks to be completed, although it is likely that it would occur over months and years. He also acknowledges that, while it is essential to address these tasks to help adjust and assimilate to loss, any given individual may not experience loss or its intensity in the same way.

STROEBE AND SCHUT'S DUAL PROCESS MODEL

Stroebe and Schut's[10] model proposes that the bereaved tend to cope with stressors by oscillating between two types of coping processes that they describe as 'loss-orientation' and 'restoration-orientation'. Loss-orientation refers to how the bereaved cope with issues that are directly related to the loss (for example, feeling lonely or sad), and restoration-orientation refers to coping with issues related to the secondary changes brought about by the loss (for example, dealing with financial matters), and adapting to them.

Stroebe and Schut consider that loss-oriented coping behaviours, such as crying and talking about feelings, can help people to process their emotions. On the other hand, restoration-oriented coping behaviours, which might include developing new skills, such as managing finances, can help the bereaved person by distracting them, to an extent, from the focus on 'loss' as well as helping them to adapt to a different life.

This dual process model proposes that the bereaved oscillate between confronting their stressors and taking breaks from their stressors. Stroebe and Schut recognize that the focus will shift between these dual processes, and that there will be times when individuals may be more focused on coping with the loss itself, while at other times they may be more focused on adapting to an altered life.

CONTINUING BONDS

There has been a recent move towards thinking about 'continuing bonds' with the deceased person rather than 'letting go',[2] and some social constructionist, narrative therapists (for example, Michael White[7] and Hedtke and Winslade[3]) offer therapeutic approaches intended to enable the bereaved individual to maintain a relationship with the dead person.

Klass et al.[2] used the expression 'continuing bonds' as an alternative to the familiar model of grief that requires the bereaved to 'let go' from the deceased. They argued that the bereaved maintain a link with the deceased, which leads to the construction of a new relationship. This relationship continues and changes over time, typically providing the bereaved with comfort and solace. According to Normand et al.,[11] ways in which the bereaved person can build a 'new' relationship with the deceased include talking to them, locating them (often in heaven), experiencing them in their dreams, visiting the grave, feeling the presence of the deceased, and participating in mourning rituals.

Fraley and Shaver[12] suggested that some forms of continuing bonds may be 'healthier' than others, and Epstein et al.,[13] in a study that conflates dreaming and yearning, found that those who looked for their deceased partner in a crowd would also tend to dream of them still being alive.

They concluded that:

> this may imply a conscious wish for the deceased to be alive again, a process reflected in, and occurring in parallel with, dreams of the deceased, and may constitute a lack of willingness to accept the death of their spouse.[13] (p.264)

It seems that incorporating the idea of continuing bonds within the traditional model still leaves considerable room to find pathology, especially if the overriding discourse is materialistic.

However, if we can accept the view that maintaining a relationship, rather than 'letting go', might be a helpful approach to working with the bereaved, instead of considering whether or not experiences of contact with the deceased person are imagined or real, simply considering them as a means to continue the bond with the deceased person may prove to be useful.

NARRATIVE THERAPY: 'SAYING HULLO AGAIN' AND 'RE-MEMBERING'

White,[7] in a brief article entitled 'Saying hullo again', offered an alternative to the predominant 'saying goodbye' metaphor characterized by 'letting go' in traditional approaches to bereavement and, following on from his work, Hedtke and Winslade[14] describe a focus of 're-membering': a process that redirects the focus of grieving toward maintaining an ongoing relationship with the dead person. Here the bereaved can seek comfort in keeping the deceased person's membership current in their own 'membership club' of life. They utilize the subjunctive as a means to open up new possibilities and new ways of understanding situations; in terms of bereavement, moving away from talking about the dead person in the past (she or he *was* a keen reader of *Hello!*) to ways of including the dead person in the present (she or he *would* enjoy this edition of *Hello!*).

Nell,[15] also inspired by White's paper, identified several strategies for saying hullo again, including writing letters to the deceased, visiting the grave and remembering them with others, but importantly also recognized the importance of using dreams as a means to say hullo again.

According to Nell:[15]

> Dreams of the deceased have an immense, yet mostly underutilized potential for assisting clients in dealing with their grief. Such dreams can powerfully instigate a saying hallo process in therapy which can be built upon by other methods in order to aid the client in reincorporating the lost relationship back into his or her life. Ignoring such dreams would be to unnecessarily deprive the client of a valuable connection with the deceased, and a powerful opportunity for healing. (p.8)

BEREAVEMENT AND MENTAL HEALTH

Mental health problems as a result of bereavement

Complicated grief refers to a description of the normal mourning process that leads to chronic or ongoing mourning (see Table 61.1). Psychoanalytically, mourning refers to the conscious and unconscious processes and behaviour related to the development of new ties, adapting to the loss (the internal process of redefining one's view of self and the world) and adaptation to the loss (the external process of relating to the world, people, one's roles, responsibilities and so on). It has been in this area of complicated mourning and pathological grief that numerous terms came into

existence to further clarify different factors of complicated mourning or pathological grief.

Complicated grief occurs in about 10 per cent of bereaved people, and results from the failure to transition from acute to integrated grief.[16] In these situations, acute grief is prolonged, in some cases even indefinitely. Individuals experiencing complicated grief generally are those who have difficulty accepting the death, and the intense separation and traumatic distress may last well beyond 6 months. Bereaved individuals with complicated grief find themselves in a repetitive loop of intense yearning and longing that becomes the major focus of their lives, along with sadness, frustration and anxiety. The person experiencing

Table 61.1 Complicated grief

A. Stressor	Loss of a significant other
B. Intrusion	1. Occurrence of distressing, intrusive images, ideas, memories, recurrent dreams, or nightmares; the mind is flooded with emotions without a sense of reduction in intensity. 2. Illusions or pseudohallucinations. The mind is 'haunted' by a sense of presence of the deceased without a sense of reduction in intensity.
C. Denial	1. Maladaptive reduction in or avoidance of contemplation in thought, communication or actions on some important topics related to the loss. 2. Having an implicit relationship for more than 6 months with the deceased as if alive; keeping the belongings of the deceased exactly or completely as before.
D. Failure to adapt	1. Inability to resume work or responsibilities at home beyond 1 month after the loss. 2. Barriers to forming new relationships beyond 13 months after the loss. 3. Exhaustion, excessive fatigue or somatic symptoms having a direct temporal relation to the loss event and persisting beyond 1 month after the loss.

complicated grief may perceive their grief as frightening, shameful and strange, and might believe that their life is over and that the intense pain they constantly endure will never cease.

Bereavement in mental health

A bereaved individual with a pre-existing psychiatric disorder is especially vulnerable to depression (chapter 21) and depression-related physical illnesses,[17] and a study by Macias et al.[18] found a correlation between the severity of grief and increased service contact by individuals with serious mental illness, who would often turn to their service providers when facing bereavement. They noted that, as the majority of individuals with serious mental illness are middle-aged and have aging parents, it seems imperative that mental health services are able to provide practical planning for bereavement as an essential service. The authors added that planning for this type of service should incorporate counselling, help with funeral arrangements and financial planning, and may include arranging for a move to supported housing.

Something to bear in mind is that the person's pre-existing mental health problems may overshadow a grief reaction, and consequently practitioners may be tempted to explain a change in symptoms as a change in the underlying mental health problem rather than considering that the person may actually be grieving. For this reason, it is important to be aware of baseline behaviour that would normally be expected for the person, and be alert for exacerbation of pre-existing mental illness. Sometimes previous unresolved losses may resurface during bereavement, particularly if the person is ambivalent about the relationship they had with the person who died. It is important that practitioners do not avoid discussions about the concepts of death, and maintain an awareness of the level of cognitive ability of the person that may influence their experience of loss.

Sense of 'presence' of the deceased

One particular aspect of grief that many bereaved people report is that of sensing the presence of a deceased person in some way. These experiences are not uncommon – between 30 and 50 per cent of bereaved people experience this, according to some studies (for example, Guggenheim and Guggenheim[19] or Marris[20]). Traditional grief literature typically describes these types of experience as 'wishful thinking' symptoms of grief (Parkes[9]) or even 'hallucinations', while popular literature attributes these experiences (chapter 28) to 'afterlife communication', 'afterlife encounters' or sometimes 'after death communication' (for example, Arcangel,[21] Newcomb,[22] and Guggenheim and Guggenheim[19]).

Surprisingly little research has been undertaken into this relatively common phenomenon; most research done so far focuses largely on recording the types of experience (for example, Guggenheim and Guggenheim,[19] Heathcote-James,[23] Arcangel,[21] and Newcomb[22]). While all of these authors speculate on the significance of these experiences in providing evidence for an afterlife, none of them explores in any depth the meanings that are made by the people who have had the experiences. One notable exception is a paper by Sormanti and August,[1] who have explored this type of phenomenon in terms of the effects upon the perceiver, and they identified that most parents in their study benefited from such experiences following the death of a child. According to Sormanti and August, bereaved parents use a range of strategies to handle their grief and to integrate both their experience of their child's death and the dead child into their lives. They identified that one of these strategies is the:

phenomenon of continuing connection between parents and their deceased children, which has received little attention in the literature. In intensive work with a large number of bereaved parents, the authors have heard numerous reports of what might be termed 'spiritual' encounters with their deceased children. The encounters have included visions, physical sensations, dreams, and a variety of other experiences that made the parents feel connected to the children and seemed to help them in dealing with their grief.[1] (p.461)

Prevalence of after death communication experiences

One of the earliest studies of these phenomena was reported by the sociologist Peter Marris[20] in his book on widowhood, in which he reported that 50 per cent of widows experienced the presence of their deceased spouse. More recently, Guggenheim and Guggenheim[18] estimated that at least 50 million Americans (40 per cent of the population) have had one or more after death communications. This is based upon their research, which largely has been a collection of more than 3,500 reports of after death communication sourced from their project which began in 1988. It is not clear, however, how they arrive at their estimate, as their study consists largely of people who self-reported afterlife contacts, so it is hard to understand how they measured their sample against the wider population.

In an earlier 1973 study, reported by Greenley,[24] 27 per cent of a sample of 1,467 Americans who were asked if they had ever felt they had contact with someone who had died replied that they had. In the UK, Rees[25] discovered that of a sample of widows in Wales, 47 per cent had experiences (sometimes repeatedly over several years) that convinced them that their dead spouses had been in contact with them, although it is worth noting that this study described these experiences as 'hallucinations' and discounted dreams of the deceased. It is worth noting that Rees[26] returned to this study nearly 30 years later, as he revised his opinion on the nature of the experiences, considering them to have important philosophical and psychological implications not only for individuals, but for society as a whole.

Rees's study was repeated in Canada by Dunn and Smith,[27] who also found that 50 per cent of widows and widowers reported experiences of contact with their deceased spouse. Many of these respondents reported that they thought that they were 'going crazy' and had not previously informed anyone of their experiences as they expected to be ridiculed.

All these studies undertaken in the West (even discounting Guggenheim and Guggenheim's estimate) indicate that between 30 and 50 per cent of bereaved spouses experience some sense of afterlife contact with their deceased partner, and it can be safely assumed that this is a common feature of bereavement. Costello and Kendrick,[28] in an ethnographic study that retrospectively explored the grief experiences of 12 older people whose partners had recently died in hospital, noted that in all but one case, the respondents reported having dreams about their partners.

While recognizing these experiences are normal, they have been located as 'hallucinations' but 'real to the people who experience them', and this perhaps sums up the attachment-based tradition that suggests people who report a sense of contact with the deceased could be considered to have not completed the mourning process. Stroebe et al.[29] went so far as to describe the traditional view of bereavement as the 'breaking bonds perspective', which holds that bonds with the deceased need to be broken for the healthy adjustment of the bereaved, and that any efforts to retain ties are abnormal and can lead to maladjustment.

REFLECTION

Take a few minutes to think about someone you know who has been bereaved, and what might have helped them in the process. Write down your answers to the following questions:

- What sort of skills do you think might be needed to support a bereaved client?

- What issues might you need to consider before considering offering interventions?

- How might you approach working with bereavement holistically?

INTERVENTIONS AND COUNSELLING

It is important to remember that most people who are bereaved do not necessarily need or benefit from counselling, and in fact, according to a literature review by Wimpenny,[30] interventions for some people experiencing normal grief may even be harmful. Intervening too early can impair the experiencing of emotional pain that is a normal, healthy response to loss, and is a necessary experience for the bereaved.

Nevertheless, both Wimpenny[30] and Arthur et al.[31] suggest that health, education and social care staff require a basic understanding and awareness of grief reactions in order to provide the confidence to provide the care that many say they lack.

To provide appropriate support to those who are bereaved requires basic counselling skills along with an appreciation of the process of grief, such as that proposed by Worden.[5]

While it is not the purpose of this chapter to explore specific counselling skills, any intervention with a bereaved person should be undertaken with the core conditions of warmth, empathy and genuineness outlined by Rogers.[32]

According to Worden,[5] the overall goal of grief counselling is to 'help the survivor adapt to the loss of a loved one and be able to adjust to a new reality without him or her' (p.84). He goes on to link the process of counselling with the four tasks of mourning.

It is important to bear in mind that, occasionally, medication might be required for depression or anxiety (chapter 20) associated with chronic grief (see chapter 48 for more on psychopharmacology in clinical practice), but usually medication is not beneficial in resolving the sadness associated with bereavement;[33] it is advisable that the grieving person experiences the pain of loss in order to move forward and recover.

Increasing the reality of the loss

At this point, it is important to help the bereaved person talk about their loss. This can be encouraged through asking questions about the death; for example, where it happened, how the person found out about the death; or talking about the funeral: who was there and what was said about the dead person. Rituals such as visiting the gravesite, or the place where ashes were scattered, can also be helpful in reinforcing the reality of the loss.

Careful and attentive listening can enable the bereaved person to talk and process the reality of the loss, especially as in most social and family situations the person may feel actively discouraged from being able to talk about their feelings.

One important tip is to avoid using euphemisms such as 'passed away' or 'resting in peace' when counselling a person who is bereaved. When talking to a bereaved person, using the terms 'dead' or 'died' are unambiguous and reinforce the reality of the loss.

Helping the client deal with both the emotional and behavioural pain

Often, people who are bereaved will want to avoid the pain they are experiencing and may even ask for medication to help them. However, it is really important to help the person accept and work through their pain, which may also include feelings of anger, guilt, anxiety, helplessness and loneliness. Sometimes a bereaved person will be angry – at the person who died, with themselves or towards other people, perhaps family members or professionals who cared for the person who died. Sometimes this anger will be directed at you. Letting the person know that these feelings are normal and providing a safe space for the person to ventilate them can be very healing. Gently encouraging the person to find counterexamples to the anger, perhaps feelings of forgiveness and acceptance, can be helpful, although this should be undertaken with care and sensitivity so as not to appear to be invalidating the person's feelings.

Helping the client overcome various impediments to readjustment after the loss

The focus of interventions here is on supporting the bereaved person to adapt to a loss by facilitating their ability to live without the deceased and to make decisions independently.

Worden[5] recommends that the counsellor uses a problem-solving approach that explores the specific problems the survivor faces, and the means by which they can be resolved. It is worth bearing in mind that the person who died may have fulfilled several roles in the life of the bereaved person – for example, friend, companion, sexual partner, financial organizer, cook or decision-maker. Depending on these roles, the bereaved partner might feel quite lost, and sometimes help in developing practical, financial or decision-making skills can be valuable. Sometimes advice regarding social activities will encourage the bereaved person to create networks that provide company and companionship. Issues regarding the loss of a sexual partner will need handling with sensitivity, especially as some bereaved people will not feel ready to engage in intimate relationships for a considerable time following the death of a partner, if at all.

Helping the person to find a way to maintain a bond with the deceased while feeling comfortable reinvesting in life

Utilizing the narrative therapy concept of 're-membering', described previously, can be tremendously helpful in enabling the bereaved person to maintain a bond with the deceased person, with the aim of keeping the voice of the dead person as a resource. Being able to talk freely about the dead person can bring renewed strength into a person's life. You might consider asking the person about their relationship with the deceased person, and what they would think about the client now. This type of conversation has the potential to raise a new sense of worth and suggest that memories of their deceased loved one may serve as a resource for the future.

Systemic approaches to counselling

From a more systemic, constructionist perspective, Gunzburg[34] offers a helpful process of affirmation, deconstruction and reconstruction during therapy or counselling for people who are grieving. This process includes defining the problem, exploring the context and exploring options for the future.

- *Defining the problem.* Here, the role of the therapist is to encourage clients to describe their emotions related to unresolved grief; therapists gain an understanding as to how clients construct their views of the context within which those emotions arose.

- *Exploring the context.* When clients relate their problem to loss, the role of the therapist is to affirm the client's view, highlight their strengths, and utilize creative resources to express unresolved grief. Alternately, some clients may relate their problem to a cause other than loss, often involving blaming and linear thinking. The role of the therapist is to deconstruct the client's view, offering another context in which to view the problem. Therapists then can affirm the client's changes and utilize creative resources to express unresolved grief.

- *Options for the future.* Therapists and clients mutually reconstruct a context which offers autonomy, increased options, freer emotional expression, creative and holistic thinking, and new direction towards a more rewarding life and agreeable relationship.

CONCLUSION

While this chapter is not intended to provide all the skills and knowledge that are necessary for formal grief counselling, it has provided an up-to-date overview of bereavement and grief counselling that will equip the reader with an awareness of the need for the bereaved to talk through their loss, and an ability to recognize that people experiencing mental health problems can experience bereavement too. An awareness of the value of limited interventions by mental health practitioners in appropriate situations can lead to better outcomes for the bereaved.

SERVICE USER COMMENTARY

I lost my mother in 2010, aged 77. Although it was at the end of a long illness, the passing of mum was a very traumatic time for me. I was already having an episode of depression; then losing mum escalated the deterioration of my mental state.

I consider this chapter to give a very comprehensive insight into the issues surrounding bereavement and grief and the connection with mental illness. It emphasizes that bereavement and grief are a normal part of the human experience, while highlighting that bereavement can be more problematic for those with existing mental health problems. Quite importantly, it states that recent approaches to bereavement have moved away from the idea of 'moving on' to the concept of maintaining a bond with the deceased person. I believe it is a matter of personal choice whether a person should 'move on' and get on with their life when someone close to them has died. My experiences of my deceased mother are often moments of reflection on the happy times we spent together, and also remembering her words of wisdom and encouragement.

Though I knew mum had gone, there was this void in my life which is very difficult to explain, but it left me with a very empty feeling of total loss. At this stage the rebuilding process began as I accepted that my life has to go on, with my focus being my wife, children and myself.

The chapter suggests that many people who are bereaved do not necessarily need or benefit from counselling. This I would agree with, as counselling sessions may not necessarily be the most effective way of dealing with such a great loss. However, support for the bereaved may require basic counselling skills and appreciation of the process of grief.

I would agree that a bereaved individual with a pre-existing disorder is more vulnerable to depression and depression-related physical illnesses. I feel it is particularly important to remember that a high percentage of individuals with serious mental illness are middle-aged and have ageing parents. I strongly believe that the bereaved should be supported to accept and work through their pain, which may include dealing with anger at the person who has died. Loneliness, anxiety and helplessness can also be a major challenge. Therefore I want to stress the importance of having an active, supportive network of family and friends to help with the grieving process.

For me, this chapter gives a good overview of bereavement and grief counselling, while acknowledging that it does not provide all the skills and knowledge necessary for formal grief counselling.

References

1. Sormanti M, August J. Parental bereavement: spiritual connections with deceased children. *American Journal of Orthopsychiatry* 1997; **67**(3): 460–9.
2. Klass D, Silverman P, Nickman S (eds). *Continuing bonds.* New York: Routledge, 1996.
3. Hedtke L, Winslade J. *Re-membering lives: conversations with the dying and the bereaved.* Amityville: Baywood Publishers, 2004.
4. Freud S. *Mourning and melancholia.* Standard Edition of the Complete Psychological Works of Sigmund Freud, vol. XIV (1914–1916): *On the history of the psycho-analytic movement, papers on metapsychology and other works.* London: Hogarth Press, Institute of Psycho-Analysis, 1957: 237–58.
5. Worden W. *Grief counselling and grief therapy: a handbook for the mental health practitioner*, 4th edn. New York: Springer, 2009.
6. Kübler-Ross E. *On death and dying.* London: Routledge, 1969.
7. White M. Saying hullo again. In: White M (ed). *Selected papers.* Adelaide: Dulwich Centre Publications, 1989: 17–29.
8. Bowlby J. *Attachment. Attachment and loss. Volume 1.* New York: Basic Books, 1969.

9. Parkes CM. *Bereavement: studies of grief in adult life*. London: Tavistock, 1972.

10. Stroebe MS, Schut H. The dual process model of coping with bereavement: rationale and description. *Death Studies* 1999; **23**(3): 197–224.

11. Normand C, Silverman P, Nickman S. Bereaved children's changing relationship with the deceased. In: Klass D, Silverman P, Nickman S (eds). *Continuing bonds*. New York: Routledge, 1996: 87–111.

12. Fraley RC, Shaver PR. Loss and bereavement: attachment theory and recent controversies concerning 'grief work' and the nature of detachment. In: Fraley RC, Shaver PR (eds). *Handbook of attachment theory and research*. New York: Guilford, 1999: 735–59.

13. Epstein R, Kalus C, Berger M. The continuing bond of the bereaved towards the deceased and adjustment to loss. *Mortality* 2006; **11**(3): 3.

14. Hedtke L, Winslade J. The use of the subjunctive in remembering conversations with those who are grieving. *Omega* 2005; **50**(3): 197–215.

15. Nell HW. The saying hallo metaphor as alternative approach to death-related counselling. Paper presented at 3rd Global Conference on Making Sense of Dying and death, Vienna, Austria, 2004. Available from: https://www.inter-disciplinary.net/ptb/mso/dd/dd3/nell%20paper.pdf [Accessed 25th July 2016].

16. Zisook S, Shear K. Grief and bereavement: what psychiatrists need to know. *World Psychiatry* 2009; **8**(2): 67–74.

17. Mazure C, Bruce M, Maciejewski P, Jacobs C. Adverse life events and cognitive-personality characteristics in the prediction of major depression and antidepressant response. *American Journal of Psychiatry* 2000; **157**(6): 896–903.

18. Macias C, Jones D, Harvey J, Barreira P, Harding C, Rodican C. Bereavement in the context of serious mental illness. *Psychiatric Services* 2004; **55**(4): 421–6.

19. Guggenheim B, Guggenheim J. *Hello from heaven!* New York: Bantam, 1997.

20. Marris P. *Widows and their families*. London: Routledge & Kegan Paul, 1958.

21. Arcangel D. *Afterlife encounters*. Charlottesville: Hampton Roads, 2005.

22. Newcomb J. *Angels watching over me*. London: Hay House, 2007.

23. Heathcote-James E. *After-death communication*. London: Metro Publishing, 2004.

24. Greenley AM. *The sociology of the paranormal: a reconnaissance*. London: Sage, 1975.

25. Rees WD. The hallucinations of widowhood. *British Medical Journal* 1971; **4**(5778): 37–41.

26. Rees WD. *Death and bereavement: the psychological, religious and cultural interfaces*, 2nd edn. London: Whurr, 2001.

27. Dunn E, Smith J. Ghosts: their appearance during bereavement. *Canadian Family Physician* 1977 (October):121–2.

28. Costello J, Kendrick K. Grief and older people: the making or breaking of emotional bonds following partner loss in later life. *Journal of Advanced Nursing* 2000; **32**(6): 1374–82.

29. Stroebe M, Gergen MM, Gergen KJ, Stroebe W. Broken hearts or broken bonds: love and death in historical perspective. *American Psychologist* 1992; **47**(10): 1205–12.

30. Wimpenny P. *Literature review on bereavement and bereavement care*. Aberdeen: Robert Gordon University, 2006.

31. Arthur A, Wilson E, James M, Stanton W, Seymour J. *Bereavement care services: a synthesis of the literature*. London: Department of Health, 2011.

32. Rogers CR. *On becoming a person: a therapist's view of psychotherapy*, 4th edn. London: Constable, 1967.

33. Warner J, Metcalfe C, King M. Evaluating the use of benzodiazepines following recent bereavement. *British Journal of Psychiatry* 2001, **178**: 36–41.

34. Gunzburg J. 'What works?' Therapeutic experience with grieving clients. *Journal of Family Therapy* 1994; **16**: 159–71.

Further reading

Wilson J. *Supporting people through loss and grief: an introduction for counsellors and other practitioners*. London: Jessica Kingsley, 2014.

Worden W. *Grief counselling and grief therapy: a handbook for the mental health practitioner*, 4th edn. New York: Springer, 2009.

Relevant web pages

These websites provide useful information on bereavement and resources for both professionals and clients.

Cruse Bereavement Care. http://www.cruse.org.uk/

NHS. Bereavement. http://www.nhs.uk/Livewell/bereavement/Pages/bereavement.aspx

Royal College of Psychiatrists. Bereavement. http://www.rcpsych.ac.uk/healthadvice/problemsdisorders/bereavement.aspx

62 The nurse's role in the administration of ECT

JOY BRAY AND JEANNETTE HARDING

LEARNING OUTCOMES

- To recognize that the decision to have electroconvulsive therapy (ECT) is an individual one, with the person's wishes being paramount.

- To be able to reflect on your own attitude towards ECT and record any changes.

- To be aware of the reasons for administering ECT and to be able to discuss alternatives.

- To understand the effects of ECT on memory and to be able to discuss this with service users and carers.

- To be aware of the current neurobiological theories about the effects of ECT.

- To understand the procedure for delivering ECT and for recovery.

- To recognize when the Mental Capacity Act and the Mental Health Act may be applied.

SUMMARY OF KEY POINTS

- ECT remains a controversial treatment; the decision to initiate this treatment is made collaboratively with the involvement of service users and carers.

- National/state guidelines and policies are available and provide information about which diagnosis will respond to ECT, how to work with adverse effects and guidance on the actual procedure.

- The therapeutic relationship developed with the service user is critical, as this will enable the service user to discuss fears and apprehensions around treatment and adverse effects, and allows the nurse to give information and discuss the procedure and adverse effects.

- Memory loss remains a potential adverse effect, and memory is continually assessed alongside strategies to stimulate memory.

- There are neurobiological findings about the effects of ECT which suggest reasons for its efficacy.

- There is now evidence for the therapeutic action of ECT and for adverse effects following ECT. It is important that any nurse has knowledge of this, to enable an honest, evidence-based discussion between nurse, service user and carer.

- Prior to working with service users receiving ECT, there is a need to examine your own attitudes towards the treatment as your role is to facilitate the individual to decide for themselves whether ECT is a suitable treatment that they want to have, and not to persuade them either way.

- The Mental Capacity Act and the Mental Health Act may be implemented if the patient is severely ill, in danger and refusing treatment.

- ECT is delivered in a custom-designed suite with a specialist ECT nurse in charge, and is delivered by an anaesthetist and psychiatrist, accompanied by a nurse known to the patient.

- While ECT is administered in specialized units under the care of a specialist ECT nurse, the process and procedure need to be understood by all to enable thorough preparation and aftercare. Adverse effects, such as memory loss, can be less distressing with informed aftercare, involvement of carers and the use of aids such as memory diaries.

- Following recovery, the patient is assessed by the multidisciplinary team to recognize improvement and ensure the fewest treatments needed are given.

INTRODUCTION

The prescribing and administration of electroconvulsive therapy (ECT) remains one of the most controversial areas in psychiatry. However, now it is good practice and indeed critical to discuss the treatment with a service user;* consideration of the service user's wishes now drives treatment, echoing the ethical stance taken throughout this book.

In order to help you discuss ECT with your service users, it is important to be able to answer their questions. We have asked service users, and in particular Jeannette, the second author of this chapter, what questions they would like to have answered and have structured the chapter around these questions.[1] The evidence base will be integrated throughout.

> ### REFLECTION
>
> Before you continue reading this chapter, think about your experiences and attitudes towards ECT. Write down your thoughts. After you finish reading the chapter, write down your thoughts again and compare with the original list.

Carrie Fisher, who played the part of Princess Leia in *Star Wars*, writes in her memoirs about ECT. She has a diagnosis of bipolar disorder and is a recovered alcoholic.[2] This extract may be useful to share with service users to initiate discussion about both the process and potential side effects.

> *Why did I feel I needed ECT? Well, it had been recommended by several psychiatrists over the years, to treat my depression. But I couldn't bring myself to consider it as it seemed too barbaric. My only exposure to it was Jack Nicolson in One Flew Over the Cuckoo's Nest, which wasn't exactly an enticing example. From the seizures to the biting down on a stick to the convulsions, it looked traumatic, dangerous and humiliating. I mean what do we know for certain about it? Aren't there a bunch of risks? What if something goes wrong and my brain blows up?*

> *But I'd been feeling overwhelmed and pretty defeated. I didn't necessarily feel like dying – but I'd been feeling a lot like not being alive. The second reason I decided to get ECT is that I was depressed. Profoundly depressed. Part of this could be attributed to my mood disorder, which was, no doubt, probably the source of the emotional intensity. That's what can take simple sadness and turn it into sadness squared. It's what revs up the motor of misery, guns the engine of an unpleasant experience, filling it with rocket fuel and blasting into a place in the stratosphere that is oh-so near to something like a suicidal tendency – a place where the wish to continue living in this painful place is all but completely absent.[2] (p.13)*

While Carrie is quite clear that ECT has helped her, she also writes about the side effect of memory loss in a typically humorous way.

> *Perhaps now is as good a time as any to share with you the message that currently greets all callers on my answering machine ... 'Hello and welcome to Carrie's voice mail. Due to recent electroconvulsive therapy, please pay close attention to the following options. Leave your name, number, and a brief history as to how Carrie knows you, and she'll get back to you if this jogs what's left of her memory. Thank you for calling and have a great day.'[2] (p.14)*

She has an attitude to her memory loss – frequently experienced as the most distressing side effect of ECT – which is helpful to her.

> *It's just that ECT has forced me to rediscover what amounts to the sum total of my life ... Some of my memories will never return. They are lost – along with the crippling feeling of defeat and hopelessness. Not a tremendous price to pay when you think about it. Totally worth it.[2] (p.11)*

This chapter is very much about respecting the decisions and wishes of the service user. The following, written by Marion Janner, provides a strong contrast to Carrie's beliefs and experiences.

---

* We have used the term 'service user' when it seems the person may have choices about treatment and 'patient' where they are designated as under professional care. This is not ideal; however, currently no term is.

ECT, or at least the concept of it, completely freaks me out. I run a project working with mental health wards (Star Wards) and we've produced masses of materials – the equivalent of probably thousands of pages on everything from ward rounds to therapy dogs but there isn't a single reference to ECT. Despite the unbearable emotional pain of my illness (Borderline Personality Disorder), and behaving in arguably a very ferocious way to myself with all the self-harming and suicidal compulsions, ECT was never, ever an option ... My profound aversion to it stems from many sources – a solid grounding at university of the 'medical imperialism' model

of psychiatry, the shattering experience of watching One Flew Over the Cuckoo's Nest *many years ago and the naked, unnatural brutality of the process, however sensitively and evidence basedly it is applied.[3]*

It is not unusual for service users to have this viewpoint, meaning that being realistic and honest, and taking these views seriously, are critical to allow sensitive care to be delivered.

We discussed questions that Jeannette wanted answered as she waited to see if her treatment team thought ECT was the best option for her, and this chapter has been structured around these questions.

SERVICE USER'S PERSPECTIVE: JEANNETTE'S STORY

About a year ago I was sent for some physical health checks on my heart by my psychiatrist. I had been taking amitriptyline 150 mg for severe depression over a period of 14 years. I always feared that a change of psychiatrist might mean that they would pressure me into trying a different anti-depressant. Over the years several had tried me on different ones and it had always ended badly for me, usually precipitating a lengthy bout of depression and a subsequent return to amitriptyline.

This time the ECG showed that my heart was being affected and there was no choice but to stop amitriptyline immediately. The withdrawal was nightmarish. Indeed, most nights were spent in what felt like a waking nightmare of hallucinations, and a desperate yearning for sleep as my eyes felt as if they had been 'pinned open'. Trials of different antidepressants and zopiclone at night followed, but I remain more than I have done for many years at the mercy of my returning very low mood and since the heart scare I also experience high levels of health anxiety.

I have lived with suicidal ideation on and off for almost all my adult life. The thoughts are transient and I am used to ignoring them and frankly telling them where to go. However, over a month ago now, I was unlocking the car ready to go shopping and suddenly started to listen to the thoughts rambling at speed through my mind. They went something like this:

I know I am going to die soon. Mum hasn't got much longer, and Jess (my cat) is old and probably has kidney disease and I will lose him. My life is not worth living without Mum and Jess. It is best I prepare to kill myself after they have gone. I need to plan my funeral. Can I discuss my funeral at the same time as I complete my will? I want a humanist funeral with Caribbean Blue *by Enya as my coffin comes in and* Sylvia *by Focus as my coffin leaves. I don't know whether to have my ashes scattered on Mum and Dad's grave or on Grandma's. I loved Grandma so much ...*

I couldn't stop them. They became both repetitive and relentless and the more they re-ran, my mood deteriorated. When I told my psychiatrist, she strongly suggested ECT. This has thrown up a whole load of other concerns and worries.

I didn't know I was that bad. I think a lot of what I am saying is true and I am being practical.

My memory is already terrible. With all the brain cells that ECT will 'knock off' it will make it worse, not better.

I have a phobia about anaesthetics. I am terrified of them.

I can't remember if it worked last time I had it.

What if it doesn't work? What then?

I will have to be admitted to hospital. I don't want that. I can't leave my cats!

The first step when working with service users is to familiarize yourself with the guidelines and policies of your local health institution and also national guidelines – be aware that some states and countries ban the use of ECT. National guidelines will also consider the culture within which ECT will be administered – for example, the Royal Australian and New Zealand College of Psychiatrists (RANZCP), in their *Guidelines for the administration of ECT*,[4] state that cultural factors need to be considered when planning ECT as among the New Zealand Maori the head is sacred and the patient and their family will need to be closely involved and consulted prior to any treatment. Other issues needing recognition and understanding are that refugee and immigrant populations may have been subjected to ECT involuntarily and without a diagnosable psychiatric disorder.[5] Throughout this chapter we follow the *ECT handbook* published by the Royal College of Psychiatrists[1] as it is contemporary with an excellent evidence base. However, it is Eurocentric and also advocates ECT; this needs to be understood and adjustments made to ensure a cultural fit within the service user's stated wishes.

JEANNETTE'S QUESTIONS

'Why are you thinking I need ECT? That really scares me.'

The National Institute for Health and Care Excellence (NICE) is clear that ECT should be considered for severe depression that is life-threatening, where a rapid response is needed or where other treatments have failed. ECT should not be used routinely in moderate depression, but can be considered if there has been no response to multiple drug treatments and psychological interventions.[6]

ECT can be prescribed for severe mania if associated with life-threatening physical exhaustion or treatment resistance. However, the treatment of choice for mania remains a mood-stabilizing drug alongside antipsychotic medication.[7] ECT can be prescribed for catatonia, a syndrome that may complicate both psychiatric and medical conditions. The treatment of choice is a benzodiazepine drug. Lorazepam is widely used, but ECT may be considered when treatment with Lorazepam is not effective.[7]

Although ECT is sometimes recommended for patients with schizophrenia who are drug-resistant, are catatonic, or have aggressive or suicidal behaviour, we do *not* advocate this use. However, ECT can be considered as a fourth-line option for treatment of schizophrenia if other treatments including clozapine have proved ineffective or intolerable because of side effects.[8]

Clearly, your responsibility as a nurse is to be aware of the patient's diagnosis and be prepared to discuss with them the reason that ECT has been proposed as the most suitable treatment option for them.

'Are you saying that there are no other treatment alternatives that will help?'

It is very easy to dismiss these concerns, as the treatment team will have thought about other treatment modalities in detail and will have a sound rationale for deciding upon ECT. However, your responsibility is to care for and support the patient during the whole process of deliberation and treatment, and you may need to discuss concerns repeatedly. When discussing issues, the symptoms of severe depression may interfere with cognitive processing – psychomotor retardation, delusions, etc. – and so a patient may ask repeatedly to cover the same material. In addition, we should initiate discussion with them regularly to ensure understanding.

It can be argued that there are suitable alternatives to the prescribing of ECT; these include intensive nursing care, cognitive behaviour therapy and psychotherapy, which seem to be rarely considered.

There are sufficient current guidelines delineating best practice, which all state that unless it is a life-threatening situation, ECT should not be given without fully informed consent, after the patient has been given full details of adverse effects.[9] When the patient has had full information and freely consents to the treatment, we would suggest that there is no dilemma, as we follow the patient's wishes, as in the case of Carrie Fisher. If the patient wants other treatment, your role is to be fully informed of these alternatives and to support the patient in their request.

Alternative therapies include repetitive transcranial magnetic stimulation, vagus nerve stimulation and deep brain stimulation, for which there is an emerging clinical evidence base.[10]

Repetitive transcranial magnetic stimulation (rTMS) is a non-invasive technique where a train of magnetic pulses stimulate (via an external wire coil) the superficial layers of the cerebral cortex. NICE is uncertain about its clinical efficacy and suggests that further comparative studies should be carried out.[11]

Vagus nerve stimulation (VNS) involves an implanted programmable neurostimulator being wrapped around the vagus nerve (the cervical portion of the left vagus nerve) to deliver small electrical stimuli. The device is battery-powered and is implanted subcutaneously in the upper left chest. VNS has been approved by the US Food and Drug Administration as an adjunct to treatment-resistant depression. In 2009 NICE concluded that current evidence to use VNS for treatment-resistant depression is inadequate and therefore it is not recommended.[12]

Deep brain stimulation (DBS) involves a battery-powered pulse-generating device which is implanted under the skin of the upper chest. This neurostimulator device delivers electrical stimuli to deep brain structures (subgenual anterior cingulate white matter tracts, the internal capsule/ventral striatum/nucleus accumbens region) via bilaterally implanted electrodes. There are no current NICE guidelines on the efficacy of DNS for treatment-resistant depression, though NICE guidelines are available on DNS for neurological conditions such as Parkinson's disease.

For a detailed presentation of these treatments, refer to the *ECT handbook*.[1]

'I've heard terrible things about ECT. Will it "kill off" lots of brain cells? Will it have long-term effects on my memory or functioning?'

ECT can cause cognitive impairment, though the severity, permanence and range of such deficits remain contentious.[13]

For many years, service users have felt that professionals have downplayed the severity of side effects. A woman who received ECT in the last 2 years provided the following account in response to a MIND survey:

> *The ECT affected my memory long term, has slowed down my thinking process and has damaged my ability to associate words and ideas. Because of this my speech is sometimes not as fluent as it was before I had ECT. I cannot recognize some of the faces of people I have known for some time. My confidence and self-esteem are very low and the ECT treatment has contributed to this.[14] (p.18)*

There is a clear difference between studies which have used methods to test memory objectively and those accessing the service user experience. The subjective findings describe much more persistent and severe memory deficits. Freeman[13] states that a small number of patients complain of severe memory impairment, cognitive changes and sometimes even personality change; he adds the caveat: 'There have been no such findings in carefully controlled follow-up studies' (p.77). This statement is contentious and will be discussed later.

BOX 62.1: TERMINOLOGY USED FOR DESCRIBING ECT'S ADVERSE EFFECTS ON MEMORY

- *Anterograde amnesia:* amnesia for the time after ECT.
- *Autobiographical memory:* one's store of knowledge of past experiences and learning, sometimes referred to as personal remote memories.
- *Retrograde amnesia:* amnesia for the time before ECT.
- *Working memory:* the ability to store and access information in daily life – often involves accessing both autobiographical memory and new memories that have been laid down after ECT.[11]

NICE guidelines[6] recognize that cognitive impairment does occur but state that the evidence from service users suggests that the cognitive impairment following ECT often outweighs what they see as the benefits. However, some people believe that depression itself can, and does, cause cognitive impairment.

Two systematic reviews considered memory and ECT. Semkovsa and McLoughlin[15] reviewed cognitive performance and ECT in patients with depression and found that:

- over 70 per cent of tests showed a significant decrease in cognitive performance 0 to 3 days after the last ECT;
- between 4 and 15 days post-ECT the test results improved;
- 15 days after the last treatment no negative effects on cognitive function were measurable;
- nearly 60 per cent of tests at 15 days following ECT showed improvements when compared to the tests carried out pre-ECT.

They concluded that processing speed, working memory, anterograde memory and some aspects of executive function improved beyond baseline level. This review included patients who had been given both bilateral and unilateral ECT.

Unilateral ECT has been thought to cause fewer cognitive deficits. A study[16] has tried to clarify the differing effects of unilateral and bilateral ECT, if any. The findings showed that bilateral ECT was associated with more deficits in verbal and episodic memory than unilateral ECT, and brief pulse ECT caused less impairment than sine wave ECT. They concluded that it was not possible to make a clear statement about retrograde amnesia and commented that this is remarkable considering the amount of research done.

Importantly, a systematic review[17] of autobiographical memory studies was conducted in 2008. The authors concluded that:

- Autobiographical memory impairment does occur as a result of ECT.
- Objective measures found memory loss to be relatively short term (less than 6 months post treatment).
- Subjective accounts reported amnesia to be more persistent (longer than 6 months post-ECT).
- ECT predominantly affects memory of prior personal events that occurred near the time of treatment (the 6 months before).
- Autobiographical memory loss is reduced by using brief pulse ECT rather than sine wave ECT.
- Unilateral ECT causes less memory loss than bilateral ECT.
- There is less autobiographical memory loss if the electrical current is titrated relative to the patient's own seizure threshold.[13]

These conclusions recognize the impact of memory loss on the patient.

When nursing service users after ECT, it is important to be aware of and note the following as indications of memory difficulty: not being able to hold on to recently acquired information; forgetting simple things; having to make lists to aid memory; not being able to recognize faces or put names to these; losing the thread of what they are saying; getting lost in supermarkets or other places with which they usually cope; and losing memory of holidays, birthdays and important life events.[13]

Clearly, patients and families should be informed of these effects. Usually the psychiatrist in charge of treatment will give this information. However, an important part of the nursing care is to be open for discussions about the nature of ECT and its side effects. The discussion and reiteration of information will need to be informed and not related to the nurse's personal views. Freeman[13] suggests that the following information should be given:

1. ECT does cause memory problems.
2. It is anticipated that difficulties with everyday memory, learning and retaining new information will be relatively short-lived (less than 6 months following treatment).
3. Because memory and cognitive abilities are affected by both ECT and depression, their everyday memory may actually function better a few weeks after the end of ECT.

In addition, Freeman recommends, that the person is told on a separate occasion about autobiographical memory loss, and that the effects of this can be longer-lasting and may continue for up to 6 months and beyond; some individuals complain of gaps in their memory which last much longer.

In order for the individual to weigh up the information, Freeman suggests presenting information about depression, stating that it has a marked effect on cognitive abilities, and that the longer the depression goes on, the more persistent these memory problems will become, so it is important that the depression is treated.

This seems straightforward; however, two well-known and respected academics and clinicians, Read and Bentall,[18] deliver a detailed (indeed forensic) investigation of current research on ECT. In this, they discuss the placebo effect, which they state has been widely ignored. Their concluding statements are so important that I quote directly from them. Referring to a prior study by Read, they state that:

Since the 2004 review there have been no findings that ECT is effective, but significant new findings confirming that the brain damage, in the form of memory dysfunction, is common, persistent and significant, and that it is related to ECT rather than depression.[18] (p.333)

This is a firm conclusion and differs from the more speculative conclusion in the *ECT handbook*.[1]

REFLECTION

What is your understanding of the alternatives to ECT? How would you describe and discuss these alternatives with a service user? How would you describe and discuss the adverse effects of ECT? Do you think it is your responsibility to have this knowledge?

'How safe is it? What if it makes me worse or doesn't work at all?'

The adverse effects of ECT are a concern for the individual being treated and for their family. Ways of preventing, minimizing and treating adverse effects need consideration. The mortality rate is a major concern. ECT is viewed as a low-risk procedure and the mortality rate is usually stated as similar to that of anaesthesia for minor surgical procedures.[9] Benbow and Waite cite an audit carried out in the USA, stating that between 1999 and 2010 there were no deaths directly related to ECT in any Veterans Affairs hospitals. This suggests ECT mortality is less than 1 death per 73,440 treatments.[9] Cardiovascular and pulmonary complications are the most frequent, and any patient presenting as high risk needs close, intensive monitoring during treatment.[9]

Read and Bentall[18] make the important point that patients having minor surgery cannot be directly compared, as their smoking habits and weight (either obesity or low weight) are not taken into account. In addition, the person having ECT has six to eight episodes of anaesthesia over a relatively short period. They describe an interesting study from 1980 where 183 patients were followed up 1 year post-ECT to ask about their attitude to ECT, and found that 12 were dead, which would give a mortality rate of 1 per 91.5 patients, which at the least brings into question the usual comparison of ECT with short-term anaesthesia. They continue to argue against accepted 'facts':

Few of those exposed to the risks of memory loss, and to the slight but significant risk of death, receive any benefit even in the short-term. There is no evidence at all that the treatment has any benefit for anyone beyond the duration of treatment, or that it prevents suicide.[18] (p.344)

This statement directly opposes cited literature and is of great interest, as the beneficial effect on suicidality is frequently the rationale for giving ECT. Benbow and Waite[9] discuss the rate of suicide post-ECT and cite Danish studies which found the suicide rate post-ECT was only marginally higher than that of all mental health patients at risk of suicide. They thought this was because patients with severe suicidal ideation are more likely to receive ECT, accounting for the higher figure. Many nurses will say they have seen a rapid improvement in mental state over a course of therapy; however, we do not have randomized control trials to underpin this anecdotal evidence, for example, comparing ECT with intense nursing care alongside therapy, and, as Read and Bentall[18] suggest, the placebo effect is rarely considered. Read and Bentall conclude: 'The continued use of ECT therefore represents a failure to introduce the ideals of evidence-based medicine into psychiatry'[18] (p.344). Their suggestion that ECT produces powerful placebo effects is largely ignored in clinical practice. It is of note that Dr Ted Kaptchuk, director of the Harvard University Program in Placebo Studies, is generating fascinating scientific findings concerning the power of the placebo effect.

'How does it work?'

Studies are constantly being published which shed light on the possible mechanisms involved.

Sheline et al.[19] have suggested that depression may be caused by an overactive brain. In the words of Schwartzbauer: 'There may be so much internal communication that the brain becomes preoccupied with itself, less able to process information coming in from the outside world'.[20] Sheline et al.[19] found that people with depression have heightened conductivity among brain networks involved in paying attention, monitoring internal and external cues, remembering the past and controlling emotion. They found these overactive networks converged at a point in the dorsal medial prefrontal cortex; this common point – the dorsal nexus – may 'hotwire' the brain not working together in a way that leads to depression. They speculate that it is this nexus affected by ECT. Because the dorsal nexus is a place where attention, memory and emotion all converge, its emergence as the area affected by ECT explains why it may work and also the side effects, including memory impairment.

Perrin et al.[21] carried out a study in Aberdeen, in which nine depressed patients had functional magnetic resonance imaging (fMRI) carried out pre- and post-ECT. After ECT, connectivity was reduced in the prefrontal cortex. This decrease in connectivity reflected improvements as reported by patients. This is a small study and findings cannot be generalized; however, these new areas of research present objective data which are fascinating.

Anderson and Fergusson[22] suggest that ECT is relatively under-researched, and review the neurobiological effects of ECT as currently understood. Common models of psychiatric disorder, and in particular mood, suggest that these are a result of disruptions of neural circuits (networks of neurons that mediate thought, feelings and behaviour). Key areas concerned with networks and mood disorder include

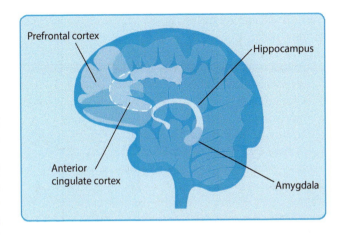

Figure 62.1 Areas of the brain currently considered to be involved with the development of mental ill health.

the hippocampus and amygdala, cingulate cortex and other areas of the prefrontal cortex (see Figure 62.1). There is evidence that ECT has important effects on the function and possibly the structure of neurons in these areas. Considering the effects on neurotransmitters, they conclude that ECT has a variety of actions on neurotransmitter systems involved in neuronal functioning that are likely to contribute to both the therapeutic and adverse effects. ECT has been shown to increase cell proliferation in some areas, such as the hippocampus, in common with other antidepressant treatments. It is suggested that neurogenesis and alterations in synaptic plasticity may be the mechanism underlying the antidepressant effect – this would influence the neuronal function and connectivity between brain areas relevant to mood and cognition.[22]

There are several current neurobiological theories about the effects of ECT: first, that ECT causes altered activity of monoamine neurotransmitter (antidepressant) systems; second, that it causes changes in the endocrine pathways, particularly the hypothalamo–pituitary–adrenal (HPA) axis (a growing body of evidence points to links between disturbances in the immune system and depression);[23] third, that it causes increased neurogenesis (plasticity); fourth, that it brings about changes in the immune system; and lastly, that it works via increased neuronal activity in the frontal and temporal lobes. It is thought that these effects interact with each other, so no single theory explains the effects in total.[24]

Epigenetics is a rapidly developing area of research – it refers to the processes that modify gene expression independent from the primary DNA (that is, life events which modify our DNA). There is increasing evidence for the role of epigenetic mechanisms in major depressive disorders. Early evidence arising from animal studies supports the notion of the impact of ECT on epigenetic mechanisms.[24]

The current lack of research into ECT is of concern. Two major areas that need to be addressed are the high rates of relapse following treatment and the adverse cognitive effects. Sienarert[25] summarizes the situation as seen by pro-ECT experts (of course, others may disagree with his last sentence):

> As of today there is no definitive unified theory on how ECT works, on how cognitive adverse effects are explained, and on how both are related. This is, however, not a sign of a failing science but of a continuously growing insight in the complex mechanism underlying the most effective and indispensable treatment in psychiatry. (p.85)

REFLECTION

- How would you summarize this discussion in order to inform a service user or carer?
- Do you think this discussion is an aspect of the nurse's role?

'Can you explain to me what happens during treatment?'

Any explanation of what happens during treatment needs to be grounded in a relationship where the person feels able to question decisions made by the treating team and knows that their preferences will be recognized and acted on (we know that at times ECT is administered when the person does not consent; this will be discussed later in the chapter). Barker and Buchannan[26] cite the Standards of Practice for Australian Mental Health Nurses 2010, Standard 3:

> the Mental Health Nurse develops a therapeutic relationship that is respectful of the individual's choices, experiences and circumstances.
> This involves building on strengths, holding hope and enhancing resilience to promote recovery – later defined as a subjective experience, defined by the individual.[26] (p.341)

On the subject of discussing ECT, nurses have said to me, 'I don't want to discuss the treatment; if the person knows about it they may refuse it.' This is precisely why the treatment needs discussion, to ensure we are 'respectful of the individual's choices, experiences and circumstances'. We must be aware that patients will have looked up and downloaded information about ECT from the internet and social media – our role is to discuss this information.

INFORMED CONSENT

The legal framework of the relevant state or country defines 'informed consent'. In this chapter we follow the legal

Any explanation of ECT should include information about anaesthesia, including the need for nil by mouth and venflon insertion; the placement of EEG (electro-encephalograph) equipment to monitor the seizure; the use of short-acting anaesthetic agents and muscle relaxants; and recovery time (see section on 'The nursing role and functions'). Following treatment, the person may experience headaches (reported after 22 per cent of episodes), muscular aches (9 per cent) or nausea (6 per cent).[27] These side effects can be treated post-ECT.

In addition, it is good practice for the individual and/or relatives to visit the ECT suite where the full process can be talked through in detail and equipment explained. As we reiterate throughout this chapter, in the UK consent can be withdrawn at any stage up to actual anaesthesia.

The Scottish ECT Accreditation Network (SEAN) reports on an excellent initiative, the development of a peer-led support group that supports service users, and it is hoped and anticipated that these groups may become standard practice. If so, an aspect of the support could be a discussion with a peer support worker prior to treatment, arguably the most powerful intervention.[27]

'How many do I have to have?'

The aim of ECT is the remission of symptoms. SEAN[27] states that the average (median) length of an episode of ECT treatment is eight sessions. However, if after six satisfactory treatments there is no clinical response, clinicians should consult the patient and reassess. A patient who has no response within 12 treatments is unlikely to respond. So we can conclude that the treatment length will be 6–12 sessions.[28]

In the UK and other European countries, ECT is given twice weekly; in the USA, three times weekly is common. For patients with marked cognitive adverse effects, having twice-weekly ECT changing to once-weekly should be considered, though this is less therapeutically effective.[28]

'Can you force me to have ECT?'

Throughout this chapter we are quite clear that we believe no person should be 'forced' to have ECT. It would benefit to consult other chapters in this book, such as chapter 2 on ethics and nursing and chapter 3 on developing and maintaining therapeutic relationships. If all other treatments have been thoroughly and exhaustively trialled and have failed, such as intensive nursing care, this case may alter. In the situation described above by Marion Janner, even then it should not be given. However, in exceptional circumstances, ECT may be administered under a legal framework.

framework of England and Wales. Professional guidelines exist for use in conjunction with the relevant mental health legislation, and these provide protection for both the patient and the professional.[29] ECT is unusual in that consent (chapter 18) obtained is for a course of treatment. As the person has a disorder sufficiently severe for ECT to be considered, this has implications for their capacity.

The first requirement is to explain the procedure, the rationale as to why ECT is being suggested now, any anticipated benefits and any potential adverse effects. Adverse effects will need to be presented clearly, particularly cognitive deficits, using the latest evidence and service user research. As obtaining consent involves assessment of capacity, it is suggested that a senior clinician does this, usually the person's consultant. Alternatives to ECT must be discussed and it should be made clear that refusal will not jeopardize the patient's continued treatment.

Obtaining valid consent is a process, not a one-off event, as the patient is given time to reflect on the information given to enable an informed decision.[30] Information can be absorbed in different ways, via written information, face-to-face interview, video, podcast, interactive DVD, etc. Useful information leaflets can be downloaded from several websites (see 'Relevant web pages').

Written consent is usually obtained using a standard form designed for use with ECT.

An assessment of capacity is an integral part of gaining consent, and this should be carried out by the most senior clinician in charge of treatment. If the person refuses, no coercion is to be used to gain consent, such as saying, 'If you don't consent, I won't be able to treat you.' Legally, any form of coercion invalidates the consent. However, in some circumstances, the patient may need to understand that a possible consequence of their refusal might be assessment for compulsory treatment.

The current legal test of capacity is: can the person:

- understand the information relevant to the decision in question?
- retain that information?
- weigh that information in the balance to arrive at a choice?
- communicate that decision (whether by talking, writing, using sign language, or any other means)?[29]

Robertson and Pryor[30] rightly suggest that service users are encouraged to speak with, or read accounts written by, people who have experienced amnesia (some can be found in the work of Pedler[14] and Rose et al.[31]). Encourage your patient to look online for discussion forums; these may be anti-ECT, which will provide a useful base for discussion. If the patient is not talking about it, it does not mean they are not actively using the internet, and so it is good to open a discussion about the variety of material published online; you can discuss the conflicting accounts in this chapter, including the conflicting academic work.

The capacity to consent and the person's expression of consent are dynamic, with the potential to change throughout the course of ECT. Vaughn McCall differentiates refusal and reluctance, suggesting that reluctance is often seen in the morning of treatment and can be a combination of issues, fear of anaesthesia or of the procedure and suchlike.[32] Where treatment is refused, the competent person should not proceed to ECT. The individual consents to a course of treatments, not each separately, and so it is critical that they understand *they can withdraw from treatment at any time.* The Mental Capacity Act 2005[33] is clear that, except in an emergency (where a person will be sectioned under the Mental Health Act), ECT may not be given to a person who has capacity to refuse consent to it, and may only be given to an incapacitated person where it does not conflict with any advance directive or decision of a deputy or of the Court of Protection.[29] If the incapacitated person has no friends or relatives to speak on their behalf, an independent mental capacity advocate (IMCA) must be involved.[29]

Where a patient cannot consent to ECT, the proper course of action is to use the Mental Health Act 1983, which was significantly amended in 2007, when Part IV, dealing with consent to treatment, was altered. ECT is now regulated by Section 58A of the amended Act. Under this Section, ECT cannot be given lawfully to a detained patient who has capacity and refuses the treatment. Practitioners need to be aware of the Mental Health Act *Code of Practice.*[34]

If ECT is necessary immediately to save life, it could be administered under emergency Section 62 (1A), but this does not give authority to complete a course. For adults detained under Sections 2 or 3, who have the capacity to consent to ECT, either the patient's responsible clinician or a second appointed doctor (SOAD) acting on behalf of the Care Quality Commission (CQC) must provide the consent form. For patients without capacity, a SOAD may authorize a course of ECT – the SOAD must speak to the patient and two other people involved in care, specifically a nurse and another person involved in care. The CQC expects that the care team will have checked that there is no conflict with a proxy decision maker or an advance decision to refuse treatment. If there is doubt that an advance decision refusing ECT is valid, then a ruling from the Court of Protection can be sought.[29]

However, these safeguards appear, at times, to be disregarded. Some of the survey respondents noted above said that they had consented 'under duress' or had felt 'coerced'. A number said they had been threatened with the use of the Mental Health Act if they did not comply.[14]

The roles of advocates and advance directives are central to the resolution of this issue.

Waite et al. provide a useful table, slightly adapted here (Table 62.1).[29]

In England the CQC produces an annual report on the monitoring of the Mental Health Act (see 'Relevant web pages'). This contains comments on the use of ECT under

Table 62.1 Assessment of patients over 18 years in England and Wales

Legal status	Capable of consenting?	Resisting or objecting?	Recommended action
Informal	Yes	No	Treat under normal rules of written consent
	Yes	Yes	Cannot treat with ECT
	No	No	It may be possible to treat under Section 5 of the Mental Capacity Act. Independent opinion (informal) advised
	No	Yes	Not appropriate to use the Mental Capacity Act. If ECT is to proceed, the patient may need to be detained under the Mental Health Act
Detained (where Part IV, which deals with consent to treatment, of the Mental Health Act applies)	Yes	No	Treat with written consent
	Yes	Yes	Cannot treat with ECT except to save life or prevent serious deterioration (Section 62)
	No	No	Treat if approved by SOAD from CQC
	No	Yes	Treat if approved by SOAD from CQC

Source: Waite et al.[29] (adapted).

the Mental Health Act. As mentioned previously, the CQC has a panel of psychiatrists (SOADs) who assess and approve treatment. In 2012/13 there were 1,281 completed SOAD visits. This represents approximately the number of people given ECT without their consent, demonstrating a real need for insightful, supportive nursing care[35] (p.56, fig.24).

THE NURSING ROLE AND FUNCTIONS

The nurse's role in ECT involves:

- preparation of the patient;
- care during the procedure – carried out by a specialist nurse;
- care following the procedure.

There is a need to individualize care through carrying out a comprehensive assessment, using standardized assessment tools where relevant, within the Tidal Model, a collaborative nursing framework.[36]

Each mental health service should possess relevant practice and procedure guidelines, framed within state/national directives from relevant professional bodies. ECT should take place in a purpose-built clinic within a hospital, with a waiting area, treatment clinic and *separate* lying recovery and sitting recovery areas.

ECT in the UK takes place in designated areas or, increasingly, in day surgery facilities. There should always be a nurse employed who is a specialist in ECT in charge of the whole process for outpatients, and responsible, while undergoing treatment, for inpatients. The nurse's role includes:

- spending time with patients and their carers in order to provide support and information;

- liaising with the prescribing teams and the ECT team;
- assisting in treatment sessions;
- updating protocols and policies;
- performing audit and risk assessment;
- training of staff and updating own skills and knowledge.[37]

The ECT nurse is responsible for care during treatment, alongside the escorting nurse and the nurse in charge of recovery. The escorting nurse should *always be a trained nurse* and, critically, should know the patient. Each patient should be individually escorted. The nurse should have:

- up-to-date training in life support and be competent in the practice;
- a good knowledge of the ECT process, especially the side effects and the nursing actions required;
- familiarity with the clinic and the emergency equipment.[38]

REFLECTION

- Think about a time you worked with a service user who had ECT.

- What was the experience like for that person?

> • Did you ask about side effects and wonder how you could help with these?
>
> • How well prepared and confident did you feel?
>
> • If it was a poor experience – for either yourself or the service user – what would have empowered you both and altered the experience?

Patient preparation

PSYCHOLOGICAL PREPARATION

This involves education of, and discussion with, the service user and family/carer. This should be repeated as often as requested. Video and written information should be offered that might be viewed or read afterwards. Time must be spent discussing the possibility of adverse effects with the service user, and encouraging them to read accounts of having ECT and to access online discussion forums. The patient's anxiety can be overwhelming and will need to be understood within the context of a potentially threatening procedure. Best practice suggests that preparation be carried out by the patient's primary nurse.[39]

Many clinics offer educational and orientation visits to relatives/carers prior to treatment.

Memory diaries can be employed as a way of helping the individual re-orientate themselves following treatment; these contain information which the patient finds meaningful and can contain current or old material. This work can be done collaboratively with the service user and their carers. The aim is for the person to have a source of material which will help prompt the memory. The patient may have an idea of what they would like in their diary: for example, photos, favourite pieces of writing, lists of favourite music and memories associated with these, a narrative/plan of their daily, weekly routines, and so on. The carers can put a recording on the person's phone or tablet computer to aid memory.

REFLECTION

• Reflect on what is important in your life, memories, relationships, the reassurance of daily routine.

• In light of this, consider what skills you will need to carry out patient preparation.

PHYSICAL PREPARATION

Tests need to be done to ensure physical fitness prior to a general anaesthetic; chest X-ray; electrocardiogram (ECG); baseline electroencephalogram (EEG); blood count and erythrocyte sedimentation rate (ESR). For an extensive list, refer to Walker et al.[40] (Cardiovascular complications are the major cause of death associated with ECT. Blood tests assess current health and consider any other relevant pathology.)

Ensure the patient understands that they are not to have solids or drinks containing milk for 6 hours before the general anaesthetic (to prevent regurgitation and inhalation of undigested food during the anaesthesia). They may drink clear fluids until 2 hours before treatment; chewing gum counts as clear fluids. A low-fat meal is advised the evening before. Patients prescribed cardiac and antihypertensive drugs may take these with sips of water only.[41]

On the day of treatment:

• Ensure that the patient has fasted.
• Property (such as rings and necklaces) should be deposited for safe keeping.
• Comfortable clothes should be worn, which can be readily opened at the front for monitoring equipment (such as ECG leads) to be positioned.
• Spectacles may be worn, but contact lenses should not.
• Hair must be clean and dry for optimal electrode contact, and hair ornaments removed.
• Nail varnish and make-up should be removed, to allow monitoring of changes in colour, which may indicate cardiovascular functioning.
• Take temperature, pulse, respiration rate and blood pressure to provide a baseline measure.
• Immediately prior to treatment, ask the patient to visit the toilet to empty their bladder.[41]

The escorting nurse may use a checklist to ensure preparation is complete. The key role is to act as the patient's advocate, offering support and reassurance, ensuring that their privacy and dignity are maintained, and relaying any anxieties, if expressed, to the core team. Some patients benefit from being accompanied by a relative/friend throughout treatment. If clinic staff consider that the patient will benefit, they may remain present throughout all treatment stages. *The patient may withdraw consent* at any time *before anaesthesia commences.*

Care following recovery

• The escorting nurse provides frequent reassurance and reorientation. The relative or friend may wish to take this role. Confusion may be an unwanted effect. The nurse can use material from the memory diary to help orientation. The presence of confusion is documented.
• Patients who are fully conscious, responsive to verbal commands and willing to move should be accompanied to a quiet area in the ECT suite and given refreshment.
• Ask if there are any unwanted effects such as headache, muscle aches or nausea (they may not always

say so spontaneously). Prescribed medication should be administered and checked for efficacy.

- Accompany the person back to their ward where they may well want to rest. The primary nurse will be responsible for monitoring their condition, including vital signs, for a reasonable interval (usually 4 hours) following their return.
- Night staff will continue to observe the person the night following treatment.
- The patient may want to discuss their experience of treatment, issues that were disturbing, and also what was

helpful; this information can be integrated into the care notes.

- Continued monitoring and discussion of side effects and adverse effects is important and may indicate a need to alter prescribed treatment (for example, an increased dosage of analgesia).
- An assessment of mental state between treatments is essential to monitor improvement or otherwise. Standardized assessment tools are used such as the Beck Depression Inventory. Memory will also need to be assessed; this is a responsibility of the whole multidisciplinary team.[42]

CONCLUSION

The administration of ECT continues to be a controversial and emotionally difficult area of nursing care. Poor practice in the area of administration has been evident in systematic audits carried out in the UK; it is important that nurses involved in the administration of ECT have specific training and are professionally accountable for their actions. The evidence base is now quite clear and states that all service users should be informed of adverse effects; this is very encouraging.

By involving independent advocates throughout the process, an individual will be able to give true informed consent.

Working collaboratively means that individuals who choose, and may request, ECT should be enabled throughout the process. However, it seems an anachronism that in the twenty-first century we are relying on an individual to choose their treatment rather than making the judgement from a recognized empirical evidence base.

Finally, there is considerable evidence showing that exposure to family and social disadvantages (particularly multiple) during childhood can predispose individuals to major depression in adulthood. This suggests a real need to consider preventative methods which may help this vulnerable population to lead mentally healthy lives.

References

1. Waite J, Easton A (eds). *The ECT handbook*, 3rd edn. College Report CR 176. London: Royal College of Psychiatrists, 2013.
2. Fisher C. *Wishful drinking*. London: Pocket Books, 2009.
3. Marion Janner, personal communication, 2014.
4. Royal Australian and New Zealand College of Psychiatrists. *Guidelines for the administration of ECT*. Clinical Memorandum #12. Royal Australian and New Zealand College of Psychiatrists, 1999.
5. SANE Australia. *Electroconvulsive therapy (ECT)*. Factsheet 24. Available from: https://www.sane.org/mental-health-and-illness/facts-and-guides/electroconvulsive-therapy-ect [Accessed 16th November 2016].
6. NICE (National Institute for Health and Care Excellence). *Depression: the treatment and management of depression in adults. Clinical Guideline CG90*. London: NICE, 2009.
7. Royal College of Psychiatrists' Special Committee on ECT and Related Treatments. Introduction: the role of ECT in contemporary psychiatry. In: Waite J, Easton A (eds). *The ECT handbook*, 3rd edn. London: Royal College of Psychiatrists, 2013: xii–xv.
8. Pompili M, Lester D, Dominici G, Longo L, Marconi G, Forte A, Serafini G, Amore M, Girardi P. Indications for electroconvulsive treatment in schizophrenia: a systematic review. *Schizophrenia Research* 2013; **146**(1–3): 1–9.
9. Benbow SM, Waite J. Non-cognitive adverse effects of ECT psychiatry. In: Waite J, Easton A (eds). *The ECT handbook*, 3rd edn. London: Royal College of Psychiatrists, 2013: 71–5.
10. Browne S, Christmas D, Steele D, Eljamel M S, and Matthews K. Other brain stimulation treatments. In: Waite J, Easton A (eds). *The ECT handbook*, 3rd edn. London: Royal College of Psychiatrists, 2013: 113–25.
11. NICE (National Institute for Health and Care Excellence). *Transcranial magnetic stimulation for severe depression* (Interventional Procedure Guidance IPG242). London: NICE, 2007.
12. NICE (National Institute for Health and Care Excellence). *Vagus nerve stimulation for treatment-resistant depression* (Interventional Procedure Guidance IPG 330). London: NICE, 2009.
13. Freeman CP. Cognitive adverse effects of ECT. In: Waite J, Easton A (eds). *The ECT handbook*, 3rd edn. London: Royal College of Psychiatrists, 2013: 76–86.
14. Pedler M. *Shock treatment, a survey of people's experiences of electro-convulsive therapy*. London: MIND, 2001.
15. Semkovska M, McLoughlin DM. Objective cognitive performance associated with electroconvulsive therapy for depression: a systematic review and meta-analysis. *Biological Psychiatry* 2010; **68**: 568–77.
16. Semkovska M, Keane D, Babalola O, McLouglin DM. Unilateral brief-pulse electroconvulsive therapy and cognition: effects of electrode placement, stimulus dosage and time. *Journal of Psychiatric Research* 2011; **45**: 770–80.
17. Fraser LM, O'Carroll R E, Ebmeier KP. The effect of electroconvulsive therapy on autobiographical memory: a systematic review. *Journal of ECT* 2008; **24**: 10–17.
18. Read J, Bentall R. The effectiveness of electroconvulsive therapy: a literature review. *Epidemiologia e Psichiatria Sociale* 2010; **19**(4): 333–47.
19. Sheline YI, Price JL, Yan Z, Mintum MA. Resting-state functional MRI in depression unmasks increased connectivity between networks via the dorsal nexus. *Proceedings of the National Academy of Sciences USA* 2010; **107**: 11020–5.
20. Norton E. Insight into a shocking therapy for depression. *Science* 2012; Available from: http://www.sciencemag.org/news/2012/03/insight-shocking-therapy-depression [Accessed 16th November 2016].

21. Perrin JS, Merz S, Bennett DM, Currie J, Steele DJ, Reid IC, Schwartzbauer C. Electroconvulsive therapy reduces frontal cortical connectivity in severe depressive disorder. *Proceedings of the National Academy of Sciences USA* 2012; **109**: 5464–8.

22. Anderson IM, Fergusson GM. Mechanism of action of ECT. In: Waite J, Easton A (eds). *The ECT handbook*, 3rd edn. London: Royal College of Psychiatrists, 2013: 1–7.

23. Guloksuz S, Rutten B, Arts B, van Os J, Kenis G. The immune system and electroconvulsive therapy for depression. *Journal of ECT* 2014; **30**(2): 132–7.

24. de Jong JOZ, Arts B, Boks M, Sienaert P, van den Hove, Kenis G, van Os J, Rutten B. Epigenetic effects of electroconvulsive seizures. *Journal of ECT* 2014; **30**(2): 152–9.

25. Sienaert P. Mechanisms of ECT: reviewing the science and dismissing the myths. *Journal of ECT* 2014; **30**(2): 85–6.

26. Barker P, Buchanan-Barker P. Myth of mental health nursing and the challenge of recovery. *International Journal of Mental Health Nursing* 2011; **20**: 337–44.

27. Scottish ECT Accreditation Network. *Annual report 2013*. Available from: http://www.sean.org.uk/AuditReport/SEAN-report-2013-web.pdf [Accessed 24 October 2016].

28. Dunne RA, McLoughlin DM. ECT prescribing and practice. In: Waite J, Easton A (eds). *The ECT handbook*, 3rd edn. London: Royal College of Psychiatrists, 2013: 28–44.

29. Waite J, Barnes R, Bennett DM, Lyons D, McLoughlin DM. Consent, capacity and the law. In: Waite J, Easton A (eds). *The ECT handbook*, 3rd edn. London: Royal College of Psychiatrists, 2013: 204–23.

30. Robertson H, Pryor R. Memory and cognitive effects of ECT: informing and assessing patients. *Advances in Psychiatric Treatment* 2006; **12**: 228–38.

31. Rose D, Fleischmann P, Wykes T. Consumers' views of electroconvulsive therapy: a qualitative analysis. *Journal of Mental Health* 2004; **13**(3): 285–93.

32. Vaughn McCall W. Refusal versus reluctance. *Journal of ECT* 2006; **22**(2): 89–90.

33. Department for Constitutional Affairs. *Mental Capacity Act 2005: Code of Practice*. London: Stationery Office, 2007.

34. Department of Health. *Code of Practice: Mental Health Act 1983*. London: Stationery Office, 2008.

35. CQC (Care Quality Commission). *Monitoring the Mental Health Act in 2012/13*. London: CQC, 2014.

36. Barker P, Buchanan-Barker P. *The Tidal Model*. Hove: Brunner-Routledge, 2004.

37. Cresswell J, Murphy G, Hodge S. *The ECT Accreditation Service (ECTAS): safeguards for the administration of ECT*, 10th edn. London: Royal College of Psychiatrists Centre for Quality Improvement, 2012.

38. Scottish ECT Accreditation Network. *SEAN Standards. Version v1.0*. Edinburgh: National Services Scotland, 2010.

39. Finch S. *Nurse guidance for ECT*. London: Royal College of Nursing, 2005.

40. Walker SC, Bowley CJ, Walker HAC. Anaesthesia for ECT. In: Waite J, Easton A (eds). *The ECT handbook*, 3rd edn. London: Royal College of Psychiatrists, 2013: 14–27.

41. RCN (Royal College of Nursing). *Perioperative fasting in adults and children*. London: RCN, 2005.

42. Cullen L, Finch S, Heaney E. Nursing guidelines for ECT. In: Waite J, Easton A (eds). *The ECT handbook*, 3rd edn. London: Royal College of Psychiatrists, 2013: 99–108.

Further reading

Andre L. *Doctors of deception: what they don't want you to know about shock treatment*. New Jersey: Rutgers University Press, 2009.
Difficult reading, you may not agree with the material presented but patients/carers will be reading evidence such as this and you need to be able to discuss this.

Bentall R. *Doctoring the mind*. London: Penguin, 2009.
Argues that we focus on the patients as individuals rather than concentrating only on the mechanics of the brain.

Cutcliffe J, Stevenson C. *Care of the suicidal person*. London: Elsevier, 2007.
Qualitative study, investigating how mental health nurses care for suicidal patients, draws on service user data, clinical application throughout.

Gilbert P. *The compassionate mind*. London: Constable & Robinson, 2010.
Reminds us to be compassionate to ourselves as carers/people, as well as to those we care for.

Lewis G. *Sunbathing in the rain: a cheerful book about depression*. Harper Collins, 2006.
A different way of thinking about depression.

Whitaker R. *Anatomy of an epidemic*. New York: Broadway Paperbacks, 2011.
Analysis and discussion about the rise in psychiatric diagnosis and medication.

Relevant web pages

Many countries have their own mental health charities, which provide excellent information and support such as:
Mind (UK). www.mind.org.uk
NAMI (National Alliance on Mental Illness) (USA). www.nami.org
SANE (Australia). www.sane.org
Search for a mental health charity in your area, as it will reflect the culture of the country you work in.

Brief Encounters. http://www.starwards.org.uk/brief-encounters-pub/
General nurses also work with patients having ECT, and this resource is specifically to help general nurses work with distressed patients who may have a mental health diagnosis.

CQC (Care Quality Commission). www.cqc.org.uk
NICE (National Institute for Health and Care Excellence). Guidance on the use of ECT. https://www.nice.org.uk/guidance/ta59

Bipolar UK. www.bipolaruk.org.uk
This website for individuals diagnosed with a bipolar disorder is also helpful for carers and professionals.

Royal College of Psychiatrists. www.rcpsych.ac.uk
The professional and educational organization for UK psychiatrists produces very good education leaflets that are clear and balanced.

Rethink. www.rethink.org/
This UK national mental health charity provides resources including a useful factsheet on ECT.

Star Wards. www.starwards.org.uk
This mental health charity works with mental health wards to improve everyone's outcomes: patients, staff, friends and family. The website provide lots of resources and ideas to access and implement on the ward.

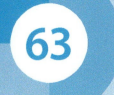

63

Services for people requiring secure forms of care

MICHAEL McKEOWN, FIONA EDGAR AND IAN CALLAGHAN

LEARNING OUTCOMES

- To be able to think critically about key issues in forensic mental health.

- To be aware of different approaches to care and treatment for this client group, and the key role of supportive relationships.

- To understand the role of risk as an organizing feature of all mental health care.

SUMMARY OF KEY POINTS

- The delivery of mental health care within secure, or forensic, settings remains a significant and substantial element of service provision.

- Aspects of compulsion and coercion are ever-present and unarguably influence the experience of care in these environments.

- The centrality of concerns over risk and its management in secure mental health services need not impede progressive models of care that hinge upon interpersonal and social relations.

- Recent developments in recovery-orientated forensic practice are welcome and demand critical appraisal.

- Forensic care thus presents opportunities for rewarding nursing careers, with scope for critical reflection upon the professional role.

- The focus upon nursing relationships allows for consideration of the meaningful translation of a *craft of caring* into these often inopportune environments.

INTRODUCTION

This chapter discusses nursing care in a multidisciplinary context in secure mental health settings; sometimes called forensic nursing. Of the three authors of this chapter, one of us was a nurse in secure environments and two of us have been detained therein, but we are all now active in research, teaching or practice development roles. Hopefully, our different perspectives on care in these settings will offer helpful insights born out of varied experiences. As such, the chapter combines personal viewpoints with a constructively critical account of available research.

Forensic services are typically defined in terms of their role in protecting the public from risk associated with mental disorder.[1] As such, a plethora of risk assessment and risk management processes have been devised.[2] Despite the obvious necessity for risk minimization, these systems have been criticized for their broader social impact and detrimental effect on therapeutic relations.[3] For many observers of nursing care in secure settings, however, the establishment, maintenance and eventual dissolution of therapeutic relationships is key (see chapter 3 for further information on therapeutic relationships).[4–7] Steve Burrow[8] and other early pioneers of the professionalization of forensic mental health nursing were at pains to point out how the quality of the therapeutic relationship could be constrained by the effects of the secure environment. A number of more recent studies demonstrate that service users in secure services particularly value relational aspects of care, and these can go a long way to mitigate deleterious intrusions of security into daily life.

An emphasis upon relationships connects with the *craft of caring* discussed in earlier editions of this book[9,10] and more recent prescriptions for organizing mental health care around recovery and involvement principles. For nurses concerned with practising a craft of caring, therefore, forensic settings represent interesting places that can potentiate or imperil nursing practice that seeks to emphasize the importance of relational skills. The means by which developments in the craft of caring can be articulated and made to work within the limitations of secure environments will have implications for progressive thinking across wider services that are becoming increasingly framed by compulsion and coercion. In services dominated by risk management goals, the art and craft of nurses involving service users in their own care can be mistrusted by risk-averse staff, but they can be a means by which people begin to assume responsibility for their own behaviour.[11] The various developments described in the chapter illustrate some of these tensions and highlight our contention that, if there is to be a recognizable craft of caring anywhere, then it must be operable within secure settings, regardless of the obvious constraints.

DEFINING TERMS

A number of terms have come in and out of fashion for describing users of forensic services. The appellation 'mentally disordered offenders' is widely used, suggesting a category of person located in the cross-over of interests of psychiatry and the law. Individuals who receive care in secure settings are usually compulsorily detained. As such, the descriptor 'service user', now widely applied within mainstream services, can appear something of a misnomer for people who have not chosen to 'use' the service. Indeed, many people in secure services prefer to be called patients, for that is how they perceive themselves. Nevertheless, we use the term service user within the chapter in preference to alternatives which variously have their own semantic shortcomings.

Similarly, the 'forensic' label is not universally approved of, but it has been adopted internationally and again indicates the nexus between mental health care and criminal legal systems. Forensic care is provided in a range of services; typically inpatient secure units designated at different levels of security, but there are also community forensic services. Secure hospital provision in the UK includes high, medium and low secure units, or smaller step-down facilities. Many of the low secure units are mainly constituted for non-forensic service users, focusing instead upon care of individuals presenting risk management issues that are beyond the scope of mainstream acute or rehabilitation units, but who have not necessarily come under the purview of the criminal justice system.

In the last two-and-a-half decades there has been growing international interest in the care of people in secure settings (for example, in Sweden,[4] New Zealand,[12] Australia,[13] Turkey,[14] Germany[15] and the USA[16]). This has included early deliberations about professional identity, definition and role.[8,17–32] Associated with this professionalization trajectory have been international efforts to define forensic nursing competencies and educational curricula[33–35] and attempts to inform generalist mental health nurse training with forensic ideas and practices.[36] Largely but not exclusively associated with North America, the 'forensic nursing' category can also include practitioners who support the victims of crime, or collect crime scene evidence.[37–41]

In this period a number of edited volumes presented ideas for optimizing practice in the care of individuals detained in secure environments.[42–44] To some extent, these books constituted a prescription for change, urging nurses and others working in forensic settings to take up the challenge of shaping more therapeutic environments. As such, these texts were influential and have aged well, so that, despite some advances in wider practice, they continue to offer a decent point of departure for describing effective practice or considering practical service developments. Latterly, the burgeoning momentum for reconsidering mental health care in terms of recovery has also impacted upon forensic services, presenting them with perhaps new challenges.[45–52] Turton and colleagues report that, despite the very different environment, key themes and principles of recovery translate readily and meaningfully into forensic care.[53]

> ### REFLECTION
>
> What are the practice implications of the fact that different people hold different points of view on the value of the 'forensic' terminology?

HISTORY AND CONTEXT

Peter Nolan has written a comprehensive history of forensic care in the UK, noting a distinct nursing role and the powerful influence of relationships on outcomes.[54] Critical commentators narrate a history of isolation – both geographically and from wider centres of professional expertise and knowledge[55] – culminating in the damning critique levelled by a series of official inquiries. These included two public inquiries in the 1990s at Ashworth Hospital in England. Variously, secure hospitals were criticized for poor standards of care and abuse, leading to something of a liberalization of the regime. Then a few years later security and managerial systems at Ashworth were seen to be failing to such a considerable extent that a national review of security was undertaken, and to some extent the pendulum swung back.[56] Wider criticisms of secure care include disquiet at the over-representation of various groups, notably ethnic minorities[57] and deaf people.[58]

The nature of these environments necessitates certain specialized interventions, largely focused upon the effective management of risk or addressing particular forms of behaviour. Nevertheless, much of the nursing care within secure settings is not so far removed from more mainstream practices, and many progressive developments from wider mental health services have been taken up, albeit sometimes in an adapted form. Arguably, the main difference for nurses working in the forensic context is a conspicuous concern with balancing the delivery of care and the maintenance of security. This imperative places forensic services in a somewhat unique position in society, with complicated relations to systems of governance and public consciousness.

Embedded in increasingly risk-conscious societies,[59] the mission of nursing care within secure or forensic settings has always been entangled with concerns over public safety, and has stood accused of exemplifying the extreme end of a psychiatric continuum of social control.[60–62] In part this is to do with social representation of those residing in secure hospitals as 'bad' rather than 'mad', 'monsters', or, on occasion, irredeemably 'evil'.[63–67] As such, practitioner staff must work hard at overcoming a sense of alienation from service users constructed as essentially different and 'other',[68] sometimes involving efforts to 'reclaim the humanity' of this client group.[69] Similarly, service users exiting forensic units have to renegotiate identity, and do so in a context of stigma.[70] Forensic nursing can undoubtedly be stressful work[71–74] and this is often understood in terms of working with quite difficult individuals in constraining environments,[75] but it can also be a highly interesting and fulfilling role.

Despite certain barriers to research implementation,[76] varied approaches to offender rehabilitation have been put into practice. Reflecting divergent histories, these have developed somewhat differently between prisons and mental health care systems. Latterly there have been efforts to learn lessons across this divide.[77] In the 1990s pioneers such as James McGuire attempted to draw upon and improve a steadily expanding evidence base of 'what works' in terms of offender rehabilitation.[78] Over the years a number of programmatic approaches have been adopted, including the recent Good Lives model.[79,80] Nursing and psychology leadership have been in the vanguard of implementing psychosocial approaches,[81] specialist care for women (chapter 65), recovery initiatives,[48,51] and trauma-informed care,[82,83] though sometimes the pace of change has been frustrating.[84]

REFLECTION

How has the history of forensic care shaped its development? What do you think are the main drivers now for the future development of secure mental health services?

There are issues concerning the degree to which care and treatment approaches developed and evaluated within non-forensic settings are applicable to the secure care environment. But, equally, it can be argued that many of these are highly relevant and should be implemented, if necessarily in an adapted form, and the evidence base can be built from there. Arguably, there are some initiatives and practices that have originated in secure care that are also applicable in more mainstream settings. Whether or not forensic nursing is indeed recognized as a distinct specialism in its own right, nurses in secure services have taken up approaches developed primarily in the mainstream – for instance, humanistic approaches to care,[85] including the Tidal Model.[86]

Access to formal psychotherapies and interventions can be haphazard in some secure settings, and it is often transacted away from the wards where service users spend most of their time. Relationships with staff, in and out of formally therapeutic contexts, are crucial in forming the opinions of service users of the value of institutional care and framing any recovery. Ward atmosphere and cultures are, hence, vitally important in this regard. Chandley and Rouski remark upon the experiences and therapeutic impacts of different professional staff groups, singling out ward-based nursing staff for particular attention.[52] These authors, one a nurse and one a service user, argue that the interpersonal qualities of ward-based nurses are paramount in establishing helpful relationships, influencing any sense of recovery and shaping positive identities. Despite the potential for conflict and strained relationships, wards can equally be sites for productive mutuality rather than an 'us and them' dynamic. This can involve skilled nursing support, without necessarily being highly reflexive; the nurses acting 'without being conscious of the extent of their skills or contemporary recovery ideas'[52] (p.89) (chapters 35 and 36) consider receovery.

REFLECTION

To what extent are ideas of best practice in mental health care different between forensic and mainstream services?

FIONA'S STORY: THE CENTRALITY OF RELATIONSHIPS

I began my journey in secure care as an adolescent. Following a suicide attempt in the children's home where I was living and a short spell on an adult ward, I was transferred to a regional secure unit and eventually a secure children's unit. Later, when I reached 16, I found myself pregnant, but having no support and because of my previous mental health issues, my son was taken from me. Following a period of homelessness, I met my future husband. He was 17 years older than me, and using and dealing drugs. Very soon, I became embroiled in a life of drugs and crime.

At 20, I had a daughter, was married by 21, and was imprisoned for robbery aged 23. When I came home, I discovered my daughter had been abused. My father-in-law committed suicide and we took in his elderly widow, suffering dementia. By the time I was 25, we had no money, no future and the care of his mother was getting to be too much. I think, by then, I thought I was better off in prison and so after a particularly bad argument I rushed out of the house and committed an armed robbery locally. Within days I was caught and remanded to prison to await sentencing.

Just 4 weeks after arriving, an officer came to my door and told me my husband had been found dead and my daughter had been taken into care. I broke down, not knowing when I'd be able to look after my kids and ashamed that it was someone else who told my now 6- and 8-year-old children their father was dead. Weeks after receiving an 8-year sentence I was found bleeding heavily in my cell, unconscious and almost dead. The Home Office ordered a hospital transfer and I eventually went to a high secure hospital. On arrival I was stripped and placed on observation. I was 7 stone 2 pounds on admission, but that wasn't to last. I was given heavy doses of clozapine and spent 2 years laying on a couch in the day room, eventually putting on 14½ stone in weight. Throughout, my relations with staff were distant. Thankfully, the criteria for holding women in high secure care changed so I was moved to a medium secure unit.

It was here that I met many excellent nursing staff and one in particular who supported me through most of my journey and coincidentally became my CPN when discharged. She was a wonderful person who employed amazing skills to get me back to normal and I have since written about her and the value of therapeutic relationships.[87]

Whilst still in hospital, I was instrumental in setting up user groups on the secure wards and became a board member for the Trust. I also joined a local charity which allowed me to do admin-type duties, but it wasn't enough for me to sit round a table debating the local mental health services but not making many changes. So, in 2010, I was encouraged to apply for a job as research assistant at the local university. It was a huge gamble. I had to come off benefits completely and be sure in my own mind that I was up to the job. Thankfully, other people had faith in me too and I was offered the job. I knew the lead researcher quite well and I admired his values and ethos around bringing people into the university to teach the health care professionals of tomorrow. The sort of projects I would be working on included evaluating involvement initiatives in secure settings and an appreciative inquiry study with inpatient teams.

It was very frightening for me to go through the airlock again and I wondered if it was an elaborate ruse to get me back in services. I needn't have worried, my colleague was right beside me all the time and I knew if it got too much I could simply ask to be let out. Many service users were unsure about talking to a bunch of academics but when they found out I was an ex-service user myself, that paved the way for some really good data collection and I was impressed by how much services had changed since I was in. Many good things were happening and I began to believe that this wasn't just tokenism; my view was as important as anyone else's, if not more so at times. It felt great to know that, although emotionally stressful for me, I was part of the changes, for real people at a real place.

I have since gone on to do a study about recovery in the same high security hospital that I was detained in, again pleased to see the progress which the system is making to include service users in their own care and make tangible changes to environments; something that was just not talked about whilst I was there. I am now assisting in implementing and evaluating a project to reduce physical restraint in acute inpatient wards.

User involvement becomes a different thing when you are out of hospital. More things need to be put in place for the support of researchers from a service user background. It's the little things that you won't know about, like how it feels to go back to services that have detained you, and it's hugely emotional. I would not have been able to do this job without supportive colleagues. My immediate supervisor, an ex-mental health nurse, has been there to answer

frantic emails sent at 3am when I questioned my ability or whether I was doing a good job. He knows when I need to get off the ward, if only for a minute, and has helped build my capacity so I now feel confident and capable. There's no point employing a service user just to say you have user involvement. We need support and someone to tell us we're doing OK even when we feel we're not. It's hard to reconcile yourself with the services that may have mistreated you but it is also the best thing about the job.

My life has gone on an upward trajectory and I feel the best I have ever felt. I have a sense of purpose and I'm not just talking about what should happen; I am making changes to people's future care. Not bad for someone who was written off, over-medicated and imprisoned by the system. I went into this as a research assistant but I have also found myself as a person.

Fiona's story pivots on her encounters with a nurse who demonstrated kindness and appeared to show an interest in her as a person in her own right. This meant attending to and talking about non-clinical things, like shared interests in music. Also important is continuity in valued relationships, though in this case the fact that Fiona's most valued staff relationship extended beyond her transition into the community occurred more by accident than design. The establishment of social ties with the community before discharge was also hugely beneficial, as was subsequent engagement in meaningful occupation. There is a

contrast drawn between negative experiences of a simple bio-psychiatry and more beneficial psychosocial support, and it is to these sorts of interventions that we now turn.

REFLECTION

What lessons are there from Fiona's story for organizing forensic care services? How does her story connect with the principle of putting relationships at the heart of care?

PSYCHOSOCIAL APPROACHES TO CARE

One of the more interesting innovations within secure settings has been the translation of so-called psychosocial interventions (PSI), largely developed for mainstream community settings, into the predominantly inpatient forensic environment.[88-96] These initiatives simultaneously attempt to improve engagement and support of family and friends of forensic service users, and also to treat the forensic setting and staff–service user relationships as a focus for psychosocial stress management. The panoply of psychosocial interventions includes systematic and individualized approaches to minimize stress, especially within close relationships, tailored approaches to cope with distressing psychotic experiences, including CBT (chapter 40) and self-management, and active measures to recognize and intervene in early signs of relapse. There is an emphasis on a range of family interventions, including but not exclusively family therapy, elements of which can also be applied to consideration of the particular psychosocial stressors at play within ward settings when family members are absent.

The support and involvement of family carers and friends of individuals under the care of secure services is a policy priority across forensic care[97] and is now a central feature of the setting of UK commissioning targets (see chapter 51). Family carers are well placed to contribute positively to their relatives' recovery, and they demonstrably have their own needs;[98-101] though many do not accept the label 'carer'.[102] Their experiences of contact with services are mixed,[98,103] with many feeling neglected by services, necessitating more empathic institutional responses.[104] Challenges for families can involve fear of violence, troubled family relationships or stress in their dealings with services, including having to negotiate security regimes.

Quite particular negative experiences can result from the actual index offence and relations with the judicial system and the police, or critical and sensational media coverage, which can in turn lead to ostracism or hostility from neighbours. Families can also be afflicted by profound worries for the safety of their relative detained in secure settings, with perceived threats from other dangerous service users or abusive staff, again stoked by media stereotyping. They can often experience difficulty and uncertainty concerning how best to deal with their relative's mental health problems and they can feel considerable guilt and self-blame. Perhaps because of these stresses and tensions, visiting times can become particularly fraught or stressful. Forensic carers often report disappointments in their previous contacts with psychiatric services, not least in terms of missed opportunities, despite their exhortations for help, for early interventions which may have prevented deteriorations in mental state contributing to the actual offence.[98,105,106]

Most recently, Absalom-Hornby and colleagues conducted a number of studies of PSI in secure settings.[96,107–110]

THE TURN TO RECOVERY

In recent times the development of an ethos of recovery in mental health care has been creatively extended into forensic services. This has been predicated upon efforts to involve service users more thoroughly in decision making about their own care and wider strategic thinking about service development. We were involved in a systematic evaluation of such initiatives within the Yorkshire and Humber region which have formed the basis of wider national developments, such as the My Shared Pathway approach to case management.[111] An indicative feature of the involvement practices in this context was the extent to which these were rendered meaningful by attention to the setting conditions under which they would have to take place.[11] An earlier study of user involvement in secure care drew somewhat pessimistic conclusions regarding the extent to which the environment and atmosphere of secure units militated against authentic and meaningful involvement.[112] We noted that efforts to alter aspects of space and place, and associated communicative relations, could foster an appreciation for the value of collaborative involvement on the part of staff and service users alike.

Practitioners associated with the more broadly cast Implementing Recovery through Organisational Change (ImROC) initiative have been developing ideas for guiding

Recognizing that geographical separation can adversely impact upon forensic services' capacity to deliver effective family support, the research team went on to study the potential benefit of interventions provided using digital technologies. The innovation of utilizing web cameras to conduct family therapy remotely was appreciated by families, who experienced a number of positive social, emotional and practical gains.

> ### REFLECTION
>
> To what extent do you feel that secure services could respond better to the needs of relatives and friends?

recovery practices within forensic settings, and numerous recovery-orientated practices are now at the cutting edge of innovation in mental health services.[113] High secure hospitals, for instance, have developed a range of participatory initiatives and championed meaningful occupation based upon the Recovery College model. There is also now a growing interest in innovatory peer-support practices.[114] The national roll-out of the My Shared Pathway approach has been supported by an extensive network of regional Recovery and Outcomes Groups that bring together large numbers of forensic staff and service users for regular strategic meetings that are beginning to have a real impact upon strategic planning and commissioning arrangements. In many ways, these developments are in advance of involvement practices in mainstream services, which arguably do not extend beyond the boundaries of individual Trusts and may have more limited impact.[115]

> ### REFLECTION
>
> How do you think ideas of recovery might be shaped by experiences leading up to detention in secure services and progress through such services?

IAN'S STORY: USER INVOLVEMENT AND SHARED DECISION MAKING

It was August 2007 and the end of a long period of desolation and hopelessness, culminating in crisis as an alternative to suicide, and after a brief spell in prison, I was admitted to a medium secure unit. I had no idea what to expect, except that during my assessment I'd been told the hospital had a swimming pool, which conjured up images of luxury – perhaps my crisis was to have a relaxing

ending. I should have known what to expect, of course, as not much before then I'd worked briefly in a secure unit. But the perspective from the inside is so completely different from that from the outside. I'd always tried to work compassionately and fairly, but always felt quite distant from the service users – constant awareness of boundaries and safeguarding issues seemed more of a barrier than the 5.2 metre fence.

My world had been inverted so catastrophically that the alien landscape of my past seemed as unreal as my present had become. I could not see a way out, no resolution of any of my many difficulties, and desperation soon kicked in. Care seemed a word unsuitable to describe my initial experiences. The ward was too busy, with an air of uneasiness and anticipation that things might go wrong at any minute. There was little explanation of what was going on and in my confused state I wasn't sure what I wanted to ask anyway. High turnover and use of unfamiliar bank or agency workers was also unsettling. I would have really benefited from a 'buddy', someone to take me under their wing and show me the ropes. I'm pleased we've encouraged this latterly, as part of the My Shared Pathway project.

Though I didn't realize it, people were caring for me. I wasn't an easy person to care for – always complaining, arguing and playing games on the staff. It may have been out of boredom, but more likely out of the pent-up anger and rage I seemed completely unaware of at first; I seemed to enjoy tripping staff up. I was both aware of and perpetuated a sense of 'them and us'. Of course, staff didn't have an easy job reconciling this person who used to be 'one of them' and was now someone on the 'other side'. At that time, however, I had a superb primary nurse, though I didn't necessarily appreciate her at the time.

So what was good about the ways she worked with me? Simple things really, but just what I needed. She listened to my rants and didn't judge me. She gently reflected what I said, bringing it back to the reality of my situation. Keeping and describing the therapeutic boundary (which I found in my desperation so frustrating), she encouraged me to meet with her even when I felt it was pointless. My hopelessness didn't seem to faze her and I came to realize retrospectively that she held the hope for me – something she would occasionally say and which of course I always rejected. Years later, when I've spoken about the importance to service users of good relational security and the need for clinical supervision and a reflective space for staff, I often think of how much this nurse must have needed it when working with me. It saddens me when visiting units as a member of a peer review team from the Quality Network for Forensic Mental Health Services that so often staff are unsupported in this way. As service users we much prefer our security

to be managed relationally rather than physically and procedurally – it's a challenge, but it can be done effectively.

It took me a couple of years to settle down, though I thought I never would, and with the encouragement again of staff who saw my improvement, I became more involved in the life of the unit and the world outside. As well as being supported to participate in hospital governance, I was pointed in the direction of a group of people trying to improve secure services and address some of the frustrating aspects of life in 'the system'. I came to realize that it wasn't just me that found the secure life difficult. Many others were saying the same thing: 'How long will I be here?', 'What do I have to do to get out?', 'Why do I not feel listened to?', 'Why do I feel I go backwards when I should be moving on?' Out of a collective sense of desperation, and building on great involvement projects taking place in the Yorkshire and Humber region, My Shared Pathway was born.

By this time, I was beginning to realize I was responsible for what had brought me into secure care, and I was the person needing to change to get out of it. I hadn't ever imagined it would be so difficult. As well as previous medical and psychological knowledge (but little application), I'd also had years of therapy. As my psychotherapist used to say, that had probably kept me alive (through many suicide attempts) but hadn't really addressed my personality difficulties or underlying problems. Through the trials and tribulations of psychological therapy in the secure unit, these started to be addressed. Again, it took staff encouragement, perseverance and sheer determination to get me to and through those sessions. I kicked and screamed (and occasionally others did so too in return) but, once more, staff dedication prevailed.

The My Shared Pathway work was timely. I'd progressed to having escorted community leave and sufficient trust between myself and my multidisciplinary team that they were happy for me to travel to meetings. Again, I didn't realize the lengths others went to in order to facilitate this. They believed in what I was doing as much as I did. I found the work inspirational and emancipatory – here was an opportunity to give something back and help bring about meaningful change. I quickly became involved in developing new processes and materials to support others in addressing their concerns – we insisted that the recovery paradigm could and should be adopted in secure services. Some staff seemed to intuitively 'get' this; others (particularly medics) seemed to struggle – 'Isn't it too risky?', 'Won't service users pull the wool over our eyes and pretend to be getting better?', 'Won't it all just be giving people false hope?'

We also realized that we needed to address some of the hard questions about what we needed to do (on both sides) to move on. We wanted to work out some outcomes to guide people on their journey, as well as making the therapeutic relationship more transparent. Again, it was challenging to some (both service users and staff) – seeing desired achievements in black and white can be both liberating and constraining, but we strongly felt this was the direction we needed to take. I continued to be supported by staff and my team at the hospital. Along the way, with encouragement, belief, persuasion and in particular the commitment of my social workers, I'd rebuilt some of the bridges I'd burned with my family and friends throughout my life before and during my time in hospital. This was opportune – one of the areas identified by the

service user focus groups as needing particular support was relationships, which became the focus of a challenging Pathway Resource Book.

As my 5-year stay in secure services came to a close, I started to live in an emotionally better place. There were still times of desolation, but the relationships built with certain staff were sustaining and supportive, helping me get back on track. I came to see the usefulness of the tiresome therapy. It took me over 2 years to 'engage' with the system in the conventional sense. What I and some others around me realized was that, even at my most distressed and distressing, I was indeed engaging – not constructively, but nevertheless engaging. I was communicating my very great distress; expressing the enormity of my internalized anger and rage; and trying to discover who, what and where I really was. Yes, I would have preferred to have done this elsewhere, but it may be that the only place safe enough for me to go through this process was in a medium secure unit.

Ian's story brings to life the importance of having a voice within decision making (see chapter 50) surrounding one's own care and how this can extend into becoming involved in processes of strategic consultation, participation and change. His role in national initiatives to support secure service developments demonstrates the growing influence of recovery and involvement philosophies.[116] As in Fiona's account, key relationships with practitioner staff were pivotal. Both narratives involve surviving suicidal impulses, and the value of supportive, relational interventions in this regard (see also chapter 16). We now turn to discuss

relational aspects of secure care in a context of increasing emphasis upon recovery goals.

REFLECTION

To what extent does Ian's story provoke critical thinking about service user involvement in secure care services? What might be your blueprint for how best to organize such involvement?

RISK MANAGEMENT AND RELATIONAL SECURITY

There is an apparent tension between progressive implementation of recovery and involvement strategies and the ever-present requirement for effective risk management. Yet there may not indeed be so much of a contradiction, as therapy is always a factor in maintaining security.[56] A case can be made for more systematically involving service users and relatives in risk management.[105,117] Furthermore, relational approaches to security can capitalize upon the centrality of relationships within progressive models of nursing care – though effective clinical supervision is a must.[118,119]

In community settings, carers remark on various ways in which they informally attend to risk, though they refer to this in terms that differ from those used by professionals.[120] Kennedy suggests a risk management framework that recognizes the potential contribution that supportive families might make.[121] Similarly, a model of community forensic care

has been proposed in Australia that identifies relatives as key partners in formulating and acting upon risk management plans.[122] In the Irish context, a recovery-oriented Integrated Care Pathway has been proposed, which has some similarities to the My Shared Pathway programme. The effect of this would be to reshape the traditional emphasis on security and open up opportunities for greater involvement of service users and carers in key decisions.[123] Implications for practice include enabling service users and their relatives to forge better alliances with care teams and to pinpoint and understand needs and risks as a basis for more thorough recovery.

On a note of caution, our research suggests that service users really appreciate opportunities for involvement or efforts to enhance their voice, such as independent advocacy, even if their actual wishes or demands are not immediately met. While this state of affairs undoubtedly reflects some of the complexities of balancing concern with risk management and expediting progress through the system, or factors beyond the control of practitioners, like limited availability of step-down accommodation, there must also be grounds for caution. What if the emancipatory, empowering appeal of involvement and recovery practices are merely illusory, and the real function is benignly to assist service users to adapt to the secure care system and its severe curtailment of liberties without too much fuss?[124] Service users in a high secure setting can view their recovery as primarily about compliance with an illness model of problems and needs and, first and foremost, agreeing to take medication as and when prescribed (chapters 47 and 48 have information on psychopharmacology).[125]

Despite some notable, even remarkable, stories of collaborative care framed in these terms, a minority of individuals never achieve this level of cooperation and actively resist the system; indeed, many present cooperators have previously been more recalcitrant, kicking against the system. In such circumstances, the very idea of recovery is extremely loaded and open to critical questioning.[126,127]

> **REFLECTION**
>
> How do you think that concerns over risk management might affect thinking regarding progressive developments in service design?

CONCLUSION

The last decade or so has seen a significant amount of innovation and development in secure mental health services and associated scholarly interest and research. That said, there is arguably a way to travel before the tensions between care and security are resolved to the extent that some of the practical impediments to ideal conceptualizations of services are removed. Undoubtedly, however, advances in thinking and practice around recovery and involvement have made a substantial impact upon these service settings that, not too many years earlier, were subject to some damning critique.

All of this is grounds for celebration, and for practitioners a future career in forensic services is now replete with the promise of stimulating and rewarding work. Nevertheless, despite the fact that for some residents of forensic institutions long-term or indefinite containment is most appropriate, the true test of further progress will be the extent to which thinking about recovery and involvement permeates risk assessment and management procedures. Perhaps only then might the current recalcitrants and refusers be persuaded to engage more meaningfully in cooperative relationships.

References

1. Buchanan A, Grounds A. Forensic psychiatry and public protection. *British Journal of Psychiatry* 2011; **198**: 420–3.
2. Doyle M, Dolan M. Understanding and managing risk. In: Soothill K, Rogers P, Dolan M (eds). *Handbook of forensic mental health*. Uffculme: Willan Publishing, 2008: 244–66.
3. Szmukler G, Rose N. Risk assessment in mental health care: values and costs. *Behavioral Sciences & the Law* 2013; **31**(1): 125–40.
4. Rask M, Levander S. Interventions in the nurse–patient relationship in forensic psychiatric nursing care: a Swedish survey. *Journal of Psychiatric and Mental Health Nursing* 2001; **8**(4): 323–33.
5. Rask M, Brunt D. Verbal and social interactions in Swedish forensic psychiatric nursing care as perceived by the patients and nurses. *International Journal of Mental Health Nursing* 2006; **15**: 100–10.
6. Rask M, Brunt D, Fridlund B. Validation of the verbal and social interaction questionnaire: nurses' focus in the nurse–patient relationship in forensic nursing care. *Journal of Psychiatric and Mental Health Nursing* 2008; **15**: 710–16.
7. Martin T, Street A. Exploring evidence of the therapeutic relationship in forensic psychiatric nursing. *Journal of Psychiatric and Mental Health Nursing* 2003; **10**: 543–51.
8. Burrow S. An outline of the forensic nursing role. *British Journal of Nursing* 1992; **2**: 899–900.
9. Barker P. The nature of nursing. In: Barker P (ed). *Psychiatric and mental health nursing: the craft of caring*, 2nd edn. London: Hodder Arnold, 2009: 3–11.
10. Barker P, Buchanan-Barker P. Getting personal: being human in mental health care. In: Barker P (ed). *Psychiatric and mental health nursing: the craft of caring*, 2nd edn. London: Hodder Arnold, 2009: 12–20.
11. McKeown M, Jones F, Wright K, Spandler H, Wright J, Fletcher H, Duxbury J, McVittie J, Simon, Turton W. It's the talk: a study of involvement practices in secure mental health services. *Health Expectations* 2014; DOI: 10.111/hex.12232.
12. Dhondea R. An ethnographic study of nurses in a forensic psychiatric setting: education and training implications. *Australian and New Zealand Journal of Mental Health Nursing* 1995; **4**(2): 77–82.
13. Doyle J. Forensic nursing: a review of the literature. *Australian Journal of Advanced Nursing* 2001; **18**(3): 32–9.
14. Gökdoğan M, Erkol Z. Forensic nursing in Bolu, Turkey: a survey. *Journal of Clinical Forensic Medicine* 2005; **12**(1): 14–17.
15. Lambe A, Gage-Lindner N. Pushing the limit: forensic nursing in Germany. *Journal of Forensic Nursing* 2007; **3**(3–4): 117–26.
16. Shelton D. Forensic nursing in secure environments. *Journal of Forensic Nursing* 2009; **5**(3): 131–42.
17. Topping-Morris B. An historical and personal view of forensic nursing services. In: Morrison P, Burnard P (eds). *Aspects of forensic psychiatric nursing*. Aldershot: Avebury, 1992: 2–44.
18. Tarbuck P. The therapeutic use of security: a model for forensic nursing. In: Thompson T, Mathias P (eds). *Lyttle's mental health and disorder*. Oxford: Bailliere Tindall, 1994: 552–70.
19. Lynch V. Advances in forensic nursing: new dimensions for the 21st century. *Journal of Psychosocial Nursing and Mental Health Services* 1996; **34**(10): 6–7.
20. Whyte L. Forensic nursing: a review of concepts and definitions. *Nursing Standard* 1997; **11**(23): 46–7.
21. Robinson D, Kettles A. The emerging profession of forensic nursing: myth or reality? *Psychiatric Care* 1998; **5**: 214–18.
22. Mason T. Forensic nursing: international origins and directions. *British Journal of Forensic Practice* 2000; **2**(4): 10–15.
23. Mason T. Forensic psychiatric nursing: a literature review and thematic analysis of role tensions. *Journal of Psychiatric and Mental Health Nursing* 2002; **9**(5): 511–20.

24. Saunders L. Forensic nursing. Formalising a new role or recognising existing practice? *Australian Nursing Journal* 2000; **8**(3): 49.

25. Martin T. Something special: forensic psychiatric nursing. *Journal of Psychiatric and Mental Health Nursing* 2001; **8**(1): 25–32.

26. Mercer D, Mason T, Richman J. Professional convergence in forensic practice. *Australian and New Zealand Journal of Mental Health Nursing* 2001; **10**(2): 105–15.

27. Sekula K, Holmes D, Zoucha R, DeSantis J, Olshansky E. Forensic psychiatric nursing. Discursive practices and the emergence of a specialty. *Journal of Psychosocial Nursing and Mental Health Services* 2001; **39**(9): 51–7.

28. Baxter V. Nurses' perceptions of their role and skills in a medium secure unit. *British Journal of Nursing* 2002; **11**(20): 1312–19.

29. Burgess A, Berger A, Boersma R. Forensic nursing: investigating the career potential in this emerging graduate specialty. *American Journal of Nursing* 2004; **104**(3): 58–64.

30. Clements P, Sekula L. Toward advancement and evolution of forensic nursing: the interface and interplay of research, theory, and practice. *Journal of Forensic Nursing* 2005; **1**(1): 35–6.

31. Bowring-Lossock E. The forensic mental health nurse – a literature review. *Journal of Psychiatric and Mental Health Nursing* 2006; **13**(6): 780–5.

32. Lynch V, with Duval J. *Forensic nursing.* St Louis, MO: Elsevier Mosby, 2006.

33. Kent-Wilkinson A, McKeown M, Mercer D, McCann G, Mason T. Practitioner training, future directions, and challenges for practice. In: Mercer D, Mason T, McKeown M, McCann G (eds). *Forensic mental health care: a case study approach.* Edinburgh: Churchill Livingstone, 2000: 349–57.

34. Mason T, Coyle D, Lovell A. Forensic psychiatric nursing: skills and competencies: II clinical aspects. *Journal of Psychiatric and Mental Health Nursing* 2008; **15**(2): 131–9.

35. Kent-Wilkinson A. Forensic nursing educational development: an integrated review of the literature. *Journal of Psychiatric and Mental Health Nursing* 2011; **18**(3): 236–46.

36. Freedberg P. Integrating forensic nursing into the undergraduate nursing curriculum: a solution for a disconnect. *Journal of Nursing Education* 2008; **47**(5): 201–8.

37. Lynch V. Clinical forensic nursing: a new perspective in the management of crime victims from trauma to trial. *Critical Care Nursing Clinics of North America* 1995; **7**(3): 489.

38. Rutty J. Does England need a new genesis of forensic nursing? *Forensic Science, Medicine, and Pathology* 2006; **2**(3): 149–55.

39. International Association of Forensic Nurses. *Forensic nursing: scope and standards of practice.* Silver Spring, MD: American Nurses Association, 2009.

40. Lyons T. Role of the forensic psychiatric nurse. *Journal of Forensic Nursing* 2009; **5**(1): 53–7.

41. Hammer R, Moynihan B, Pagliaro E. (eds). *Forensic nursing: a handbook for practice.* Sudbury, MA: Jones & Bartlett Publishers, 2011.

42. Robinson D, Kettles A (eds). *Forensic nursing and multidisciplinary care of the mentally disordered offender.* London: Jessica Kingsley, 1999.

43. Mercer D, Mason T, McKeown M, McCann G (eds). *Forensic mental health care: a case study approach.* Edinburgh: Churchill Livingstone, 2000.

44. Chaloner C, Coffey M (eds). *Forensic mental health nursing: current approaches.* Oxford: Blackwell Science, 2000.

45. Allen S. *Our stories: moving on, recovery and well-being.* London: South West London & St George's Mental Health Trust Forensic Services, 2010.

46. Pouncey C, Lukens J. Madness versus badness: the ethical tension between the recovery movement and forensic psychiatry. *Theoretical Medicine and Bioethics* 2010; **31**: 93–105.

47. Mezey G, Kavuma M, Turton P, Demetriou A, Wright C. Perceptions, experiences and meanings of recovery in forensic psychiatric patients. *Journal of Forensic Psychiatry and Psychology* 2010; **21**: 683–96.

48. Drennan G, Alred D. *Secure recovery: approaches to recovery in secure mental health settings.* London: Routledge, 2012.

49. Ferrito M, Vetere A, Adshead G, Moore E. Life after homicide: accounts of recovery and redemption of offender patients in a high secure hospital. *Journal of Forensic Psychiatry and Psychology* 2012; **23**: 322–44.

50. Livingston J, Nijdam-Jones A, Brink J. A tale of two cultures: examining patient-centred care in a forensic mental health hospital. *Journal of Forensic Psychiatry and Psychology* 2012; **23**: 345–60.

51. Ayres J, Fegan T, Noak J. The recovery orientation of patients and staff in a high secure hospital. *Mental Health Practice* 2014; **17**(7): 20–4.

52. Chandley M, Rouski M. Recovery, turning points and forensics: views from the ward in an English high secure facility. *Mental Health and Social Inclusion* 2014; **18**(2): 83–91.

53. Turton P, Demetriou A, Boland W, Gillard S, Kavuma M, Mezey G, Mountford V, Turner K, White S, Zadeh E, Wright C. One size fits all: or horses for courses? Recovery-based care in specialist mental health services. *Social Psychiatry and Psychiatric Epidemiology* 2011; **46**(2): 127–36.

54. Nolan P. The historical context. In: Wix S, Humphreys M (eds). *Multidisciplinary working in forensic mental health care.* Edinburgh: Churchill Livingstone, 2005: 1–18.

55. Mullen P. Forensic mental health. *British Journal of Psychiatry* 2000; **176:** 307–11.

56. Exworthy T, Gunn J. Taking another tilt at high secure hospitals: the Tilt report and its consequences for secure psychiatric services. *British Journal of Psychiatry* 2003; **182**: 469–71.

57. McKeown M, Stowell-Smith M. 'Big, black and dangerous'?: the vexed question of race in forensic care. In: Landsberg G, Smiley A (eds). *Forensic mental health: working with offenders with mental illness.* Kingston, NJ: Civic Research Institute, 2001: 23.1–23.8.

58. Mitchell T, Braham L. The psychological treatment needs of deaf mental health patients in high-secure settings: a review of the literature. *International Journal of Forensic Mental Health* 2011; **10**: 92–106.

59. Beck U. *Risk society, towards a new modernity.* London: Sage, 1992.

60. Mason T, Mercer D. Forensic psychiatric nursing: visions of social control. *Australian and New Zealand Journal of Mental Health Nursing* 1996; **5**(4): 153–62.

61. Holmes D. Police and pastoral power: governmentality and correctional forensic psychiatric nursing. *Nursing Inquiry* 2002; **9**(2): 84–92.

62. Holmes D. Governing the captives: forensic psychiatric nursing in corrections. *Perspectives in Psychiatric Care* 2005; **41**(1): 3–13.

63. Mercer D, Mason T, Richman J. Good & evil in the crusade of care. Social constructions of mental disorders. *Journal of Psychosocial Nursing and Mental Health Services* 1999; **37**(9): 13–17.

64. Richman J, Mercer D. The vignette revisited: evil and the forensic nurse. *Nurse Researcher* 2002; **9**(4): 70–82.

65. Bowers L. *Dangerous and severe personality disorder: response and role of the psychiatric team.* Abingdon: Taylor & Francis, 2002.

66. McKeown M, Stowell-Smith M. The comforts of evil: dangerous personalities in high security hospitals and the horror film. In: Mason T (ed). *Forensic psychiatry: influences of evil.* Totowa, NJ: Humana Press, 2006: 109–34.

67. Jacob J, Gagnon M, Holmes D. Nursing so-called monsters: on the importance of abjection and fear in forensic psychiatric nursing. *Journal of Forensic Nursing* 2009; **5**(3): 153–61.

68. Peternelj-Taylor C. Engaging the 'other'. *Journal of Forensic Nursing* 2005; **1**(4): 179–80.

69. Wright K, Haigh K, McKeown M. Reclaiming the humanity in personality disorder. *International Journal of Mental Health Nursing* 2007; **16**: 236–46.

70. Coffey M. Negotiating identity transition when leaving forensic hospitals. *Health* 2012; **16**: 489–506.

71. Coffey M, Coleman M. The relationship between support and stress in forensic community mental health nursing. *Journal of Advanced Nursing* 2001; **34** (3): 397–407.

72. Happell B, Pinikahana J, Martin T. Stress and burnout in forensic psychiatric nursing. *Stress and Health* 2003; **19**(2): 63–8.

73. Dickinson T, Wright K. Stress and burnout in forensic mental health nursing: a literature review. *British Journal of Nursing* 2008; **17**(2): 82–7.

74. Lauvrud C, Nonstad K, Palmstierna T. Occurrence of post traumatic stress symptoms and their relationship to professional quality of life (ProQoL) in nursing staff at a forensic psychiatric security unit: a cross-sectional study. *Health and Quality of Life Outcomes* 2009; **7**(31): 1–6.

75. Holmes C. Services for people requiring secure forms of care: a global problem. In: Barker P (ed). *Psychiatric and mental health nursing: the craft of caring*, 2nd edn. London: Hodder Arnold, 2009: 463–76.

76. Carrion M, Woods P, Norman I. Barriers to research utilisation among forensic mental health nurses. *International Journal of Nursing Studies* 2004; **41**(6): 613–19.

77. Howells K, Day A, Thomas-Peter B. Changing violent behaviour: forensic mental health and criminological models compared. *Journal of Forensic Psychiatry and Psychology* 2004; **15**(3): 391–406.

78. McGuire J. *What works: reducing reoffending: guidelines from research and practice*. Oxford: John Wiley & Sons, 1995.

79. Ward T. Good lives and the rehabilitation of offenders: promises and problems. *Aggression and Violent Behavior* 2002; **7**(5): 513–28.

80. Ward T, Mann R, Gannon T. The good lives model of offender rehabilitation: clinical implications. *Aggression and Violent Behavior* 2007; **12**(1): 87–107.

81. McCann G, McKeown M. Applying psychosocial interventions within a forensic environment. *Psychiatric Care* 1995; **2**(4): 133–6.

82. Aiyegbusi A, Tuck G. Caring amid victims and perpetrators: trauma and forensic mental health nursing. In: Gordon J, Kirtchuk G (eds). *Psychic assaults and frightened clinicians: countertransference in forensic settings*. London: Karnac Books, 2008: 11–26.

83. Miller N, Najavits L. Creating trauma-informed correctional care: a balance of goals and environment. *European Journal of Psychotraumatology* 2012; **3**: 10.3402/ejpt.v3i0.17246.

84. McKeown M. Psychosocial interventions at Ashworth: an occupational delusion. In: Pilgrim D (ed). *Inside Ashworth: professional accounts of institutional life*. Oxford: Radcliffe Publishing, 2007: 59–80.

85. Gillespie M, Flowers P. From the old to the new: is forensic mental health nursing in transition? *Journal of Forensic Nursing* 2009; **5**(4): 212–19.

86. Jacob J, Holmes D, Buus N. Humanism in forensic psychiatry: the use of the tidal nursing model. *Nursing Inquiry* 2008; **15**(3): 224–30.

87. Jones F. The naughty child. *Asylum: the Magazine for Democratic Psychiatry* 2013; **20**(2): 11–12.

88. Savage L, McKeown M. Towards a new model for practice in a HDU. *Psychiatric Care* 1997; **4**(4): 182–6.

89. McKeown M, McCann G. Psychosocial interventions. In: Chaloner C, Coffey M (eds). *Forensic mental health nursing: current approaches*. Oxford: Blackwell Science, 1999: 232–51.

90. MacInnes D. Interventions in forensic psychiatry: the caregiver's perspective. *British Journal of Nursing* 2000; **9**(15): 992–8.

91. McKeown M. Psychosocial interventions for a person with serious mental health problems, using street drugs, with a history of related offending. In: Landsberg G, Smiley A (eds). *Forensic mental health: working with offenders with mental illness*. Kingston, NJ: Civic Research Institute, 2001.

92. Baker J, O'Higgins H, Parkinson J, Tracey N. The construction and implementation of a psychosocial interventions care pathway within a low secure environment: a pilot study. *Journal of Psychiatric and Mental Health Nursing* 2002; **9**: 737–9.

93. Walker H. Using psychosocial interventions within a high security hospital. *Nursing Times* 2004; **100**(31): 36–9.

94. Isherwood T, Burns M, Rigby G. Psychosocial interventions in a medium secure unit for people with learning disabilities: a service development. *Mental Health and Learning Disabilities Research and Practice* 2004; **1**(1): 29–35.

95. Gleeson J, Nathan P, Bradley G. The need for the development and evaluation of preventative psychosocial forensic interventions in mainstream adult community mental health services. *Australasian Psychiatry* 2006; **14**(2): 180–5.

96. Absalom-Hornby V, Gooding P, Tarrier N. Family intervention using a web camera (e-FFI) within forensic health services: a case study and feasibility study. *British Journal of Forensic Practice* 2012; **14**(1): 60–71.

97. NIMHE (National Institute for Mental Health England). *Cases for change: forensic mental health services*. London: NIMHE, 2004.

98. McCann G, McKeown M, Porter I. Understanding the needs of relatives of patients within a special hospital for mentally disordered offenders: a basis for improved services. *Journal of Advanced Nursing* 1996; **23**: 346–52.

99. MacInnes D, Watson J. The differences in perceived burden between forensic and non-forensic caregivers of individuals suffering from schizophrenia. *Journal of Mental Health* 2002; **11**(4): 375–88.

100. Tsang H. Family needs and burdens of mentally ill offenders. *International Journal of Rehabilitation Research* 2002; **25**(1): 25–32.

101. Ferriter M, Huband N. Experiences of parents with a son or daughter suffering from schizophrenia. *Journal of Psychiatric and Mental Health Nursing* 2003; **10**: 552–60.

102. Ridley J, McKeown M, Machin K, Rosengard A, Little S, Briggs S, Jones F, Deypurkaystha M. *Exploring family carer involvement in forensic mental health services*. Edinburgh: Support in Mind Scotland, 2014.

103. Hughes J, Hughes C. Family and friends. In: Mercer D, Mason T, McKeown M, McCann G (eds). *Forensic mental health care: a case study approach*. Edinburgh: Churchill Livingstone, 2000: 19–24.

104. Rowe J. Great expectations: a systematic review of the literature on the role of family informal carers in severe mental illness, and their relationships and engagement with professionals. *Journal of Psychiatric and Mental Health Nursing* 2012; **19**: 70–82.

105. Nordstrom A, Kullgren G, Dahlgren L. Schizophrenia and violent crime: the experience of parents. *International Journal of Law and Psychiatry* 2006; **29**(1): 57–67.

106. MacInnes D, Beer D, Reynolds K, Kinane C. Carers of forensic mental health in-patients: what factors influence their satisfaction with services? *Journal of Mental Health* 2013; **22**: 528–35.

107. Absalom V, McGovern J, Gooding P, Tarrier N. An assessment of patient need for family intervention in forensic health services and staff skill in implementing family interventions. *Journal of Forensic Psychiatry and Psychology* 2010; **21**(3): 350–65.

108. Absalom-Hornby V, Gooding P, Tarrier N. Coping with schizophrenia in forensic health services: the needs of relatives. *Journal of Nervous and Mental Disease* 2011; **199**: 398–402.

109. Absalom-Hornby V, Gooding P, Tarrier N. Implementing family intervention within forensic health services: the perspectives of clinical staff. *Journal of Mental Health* 2011; **20**(4): 355–67.

110. Absalom-Hornby V, Hare D, Gooding P, Tarrier N. Attitudes of relatives and staff towards family intervention in forensic health services using Q methodology. *Journal of Psychiatric and Mental Health Nursing* 2012; **19**: 162–73.

111. Ayub R, Callaghan I, Haque Q, McCann G. Increasing patient involvement in care pathways. *Health Service Journal* 2013; June 3. Available from: http://www.hsj.co.uk/home/commissioning/increasing-patient-involvement-in-care-pathways/5058959.article [Accessed 31st August 2016].

112. Godin P, Davies J, Heyman B, Reynolds L, Simpson A, Floyd M. Opening communicative space: a Habermasian understanding of a user led participatory research project. *Forensic Psychiatry and Psychology* 2007; **18**: 452–69.

113. Drennan G, Wooldridge J, with Aiyegbusi A, Alred D, Ayres J, Barker R, Carr S, Eunson H, Lomas H, Moore E, Stanton D, Shepherd G. *Making recovery a reality in forensic settings*. London: ImROC/Centre for Mental Health/Mental Health Network, NHS Confederation, 2014.

114. Shaw C. *Peer support in secure services*. London: Together (for mental wellbeing), 2014.

115. McKeown M, Jones F, Wright K, Burns M, Wright J, Ayub R, Fletcher H, McVittie J, Turton W, Rawcliffe-Foo S, Browning G, McCann G. Open market: let patients in on commissioning. *Health Service Journal* 2013; November. Available from: http://www.hsj.co.uk/5064889.article [Accessed 2nd September 2016].

116. NSUN (National Survivor User Network) & WISH. *Unlocking service user involvement practice in forensic settings: research into the provision of service user involvement in secure settings*. London: NSUN/WISH, 2011.

117. McCann G, McKeown M. Risk and serious mental health issues. In: Harris N, Williams, S, Bradshaw T (eds). *Psychosocial interventions for people with schizophrenia: a practical guide for mental health workers*. Basingstoke: Palgrave Macmillan, 2002: 205–10.

118. Aiyegbusi A, Clarke-Moore J. *Therapeutic relationships with offenders: an introduction to the psychodynamics of forensic mental health nursing*. London: Jessica Kingsley, 2008.

119. Urheim R, Rypdal K, Palmstierna T, Mykletun A. Patient autonomy versus risk management: a case study of change in a high security forensic psychiatric ward. *International Journal of Forensic Mental Health* 2011; **10**(1): 41–51.

120. Ryan T. Exploring the risk management strategies of informal carers of mental health service users. *Journal of Mental Health* 2002; **11**: 17–25.

121. Kennedy H. Therapeutic uses of security: mapping forensic mental health services by stratifying risk. *Advances in Psychiatric Treatment* 2002; **8**: 433–43.

122. Kelly T, Simmons W, Gregory E. Risk assessment and management: a community forensic practice model. *International Journal of Mental Health Nursing* 2002; **11**(4): 206–13.

123. Gill P, McKenna P, O'Neill H, Thompson J, Timmons D. Pillars and pathways: foundations of recovery in Irish forensic mental health care. *British Journal of Forensic Practice* 2010; **12**(3): 29–36.

124. McKeown M, Poursanidou D, Able L, Newbigging K, Ridley J, Kiansumba M. Independent mental health advocacy: still cooling out the mark? *Mental Health Today* 2013; November/December: 20–1.

125. McKeown M, Jones F, Foy P, Paxton T, Blackmon M. Putting the past behind us: making sense of recovery in a high secure setting. *International Journal of Mental Health Nursing* 2016; **25**: 234–42.

126. Harper D, Speed E. Uncovering recovery: the resistable rise of recovery and resistance. *Studies in Social Justice* 2012; **6**(1): 9–25.

127. Pilgrim D, McCranie A. *Recovery and mental health: a critical sociological account*. Basingstoke: Palgrave Macmillan, 2013.

Further reading

Aiyegbusi A, Clarke-Moore J. *Therapeutic relationships with offenders: an introduction to the psychodynamics of forensic mental health nursing*. London: Jessica Kingsley, 2008.
This key book explores the often neglected relational and emotional features of forensic nursing. Close reading affords nurses the necessary knowledge for understanding their own reactions to working in these challenging environments and how to make the best use of their own relational skills. The book is part of a 'forensic focus' series which is also worth investigating.

Chaloner C, Coffey M (eds). *Forensic mental health nursing: current approaches*. Oxford: Blackwell Science, 2000.
An edited text that, despite being published some time ago, presents lucid accounts of key aspects of nursing in secure environments. Much of the content has dated well, not least because of the real-time lag between introducing progressive developments, such as psychosocial approaches and support for families, and their consistent uptake into routine practice.

Drennan G, Alred D. *Secure recovery: approaches to recovery in secure mental health settings*. London: Routledge, 2012.
A vanguard text, promoting adoption of recovery ethos and practices into forensic settings. Precisely what recovery means at different levels of secure care is open to debate and contestation. Nevertheless, introducing thinking about recovery as an organizing feature for secure services could be a defining progressive moment in their historical development.

Livingston J, Nijdam-Jones A, Brink J. A tale of two cultures: examining patient-centred care in a forensic mental health hospital. *Journal of Forensic Psychiatry and Psychology* 2012; **23**: 345–60.
An interesting study that makes the case for person-centred care in secure environments. As such, the actual practices focused on are congruent with other developments concerning recovery and service user involvement practices.

McKeown M, Jones F, Wright K, Spandler H, Wright J, Fletcher H, Duxbury J, McVittie J, Simon, Turton W. It's the talk: a study of involvement practices in secure mental health services. *Health Expectations* 2014; DOI: 10.111/hex.12232.
This paper presents an evaluation of some very interesting developments concerning involvement practices in one region of England, some of which, like the My Shared Pathway initiative featured in this chapter, are being rolled out across the country. The discussion poses critical questions about the pivotal nature of communication between practitioners and service users and the conditions which need to be achieved to optimize impact.

Mercer D, Mason T, McKeown M, McCann, G (eds). *Forensic mental health care: a case study approach*. Edinburgh: Churchill Livingstone, 2000.
Another fairly old edited collection, but notable for its case study approach – presenting numerous care and treatment interventions framed by real cases. The argument for more extensive implementation of such measures in forensic services remains valid. This book was also notable for presenting some of the first published first-person accounts from service users and carers within a practitioner-facing text.

Relevant web pages

International Association of Forensic Mental Health Services. http://iafmhs.org/

International Association of Forensic Nurses. http://www.forensicnurses.org/

Recovery and Outcomes. http://www.recoveryandoutcomes.org/

64 Services for older people with mental health problems

HELEN PUSEY AND JOHN KEADY

LEARNING OUTCOMES

- To understand the main models of mental health service provision for older people.
- To realize how ageism can impact on mental health service provision for older people.
- To be able to describe the influence of policy on the development of mental health services for older people.
- To be able to identify the key barriers to older people in primary care mental health services.
- To be aware of the barriers and benefits of memory assessment services for people with dementia.

SUMMARY OF KEY POINTS

- In response to numerous policy and legislative initiatives, mental health services for older people have undergone significant change and development in recent years to improve the quality of dementia care and access to other services.
- The concepts and resources attached to the notion of 'recovery' should be made applicable and available to people living with dementia.
- There remains a risk that the drive to improve care in dementia will potentially disadvantage those with functional mental health problems.
- The complex nature of mental health problems in old age require specialist nursing expertise and it is unclear how well current provision and configuration will meet this need.

INTRODUCTION

The craft of caring maps directly onto the provision of quality services for older people with mental health needs. Services based on mechanistic interventions cannot provide a comprehensive solution to the complex care needs of older people. The essence of the craft of caring lies in person-centred care and a rights-based holistic approach to the needs of the individual. While this approach has been at the core of developments to enhance care for older people for some time, the challenge to services is still apparent. Services need to facilitate mental health nurses to provide care that is not only scientifically coherent, but which embraces individual need and challenges stigma and discrimination. A service underpinned by the craft of caring is an empowering and liberating service.

In the UK, since the time of asylum-based care, mental health nurses and their attendant predecessors have played a pivotal role in the care and support of older people, i.e. those aged 65 years and older. However, while the need is great (for example, older people are more likely to experience higher levels of depression and suicidal ideation than any age group across the life span), it has long been recognized that older people with mental health problems do not receive the same level – or quality – of service as younger people.[1,2] While a sociological and theoretical explanation for such inequality is beyond the scope for this chapter, we will, however, explore mental health services for older people through three domains: first, primary care mental health services where the majority of common mental health problems are found; second, memory assessment and treatment services, usually associated with the diagnosis of dementia and its follow-up (we recommend that readers combine this with chapter 33 on the care of the person with dementia); and third, specialist service provision for older people. From the third domain we have selected three areas to examine in more detail (marked in Box 64.1 with an asterisk): (1) community mental health teams, (2) NHS inpatient service provision and (3) crisis intervention. Finally, in light of the recent UK-based equality legislation[3] that promotes heterogeneity and inclusion, the chapter will present a challenge by asking if it remains appropriate to have age-specific models of mental health service provision.

OUTLINE OF SERVICE PROVISION

Mental health services for older people, although subject to some regional and local variation, are generally configured around the models outlined below; these services may be open to all ages or delivered on an age-specific basis.

> ## BOX 64.1: EXAMPLES OF SPECIAL MENTAL HEALTH SERVICE PROVISION FOR OLDER PEOPLE
>
> *Primary care mental health services:* medical support delivered by general practitioners and talking based therapies delivered by psychological well-being practitioners or specialist mental health staff
>
> *Memory assessment and treatment services:* multidisciplinary team providing a range of assessment, treatment and support
>
> **Community mental health teams:* multidisciplinary team supporting people at home
>
> **NHS inpatient services:* multidisciplinary hospital-based care for a range of organic and functional disorders
>
> **Crisis intervention services:* home-based support for acute mental health problems
>
> *Liaison psychiatric services:* acute hospital-based service providing assessment and/or intervention in issues of comorbidity and deliberate self-harm
>
> *Assertive outreach:* teams to work specifically with those who need frequent and intensive support and find it more difficult to engage with services
>
> *Intermediate care:* often time-limited inpatient care for people with dementia who have complex physical and mental health needs
>
> *Specialist services:* these will vary but may include drug and alcohol services, forensic services, homeless services, public health activity, and services specifically for people with a diagnosis of personality disorder

BACKGROUND

We live in an ageing society. There are over 10 million people over the age of 65 in the UK. Over the next 30 years this figure is likely to double. Furthermore, the numbers of people aged over 80 is projected to reach 8 million during this time.[4] Currently, those over the age of 65 account for around one-third of all mental health service activity.[5] One in four older people has symptoms of depression (chapter 21) that would warrant intervention[6] and up to 50 per cent of mental health inpatient admissions are for those aged over 65.[7] These demographic and prevalence trends clearly demonstrate that there will be an increasing demand for mental health services for older people.

Traditionally, mental health services have been configured around a model of 'working age adults' (up to the age of 64) and services for 'older people' (from the age of 65 upwards). While the merits or otherwise of this division can be debated, from the end of the last century the development of mental health services for older people has been influenced by a series of policy guidance. Arguably, the first of these directives, the National Service Framework (NSF) for Mental Health,[8] was unhelpful for older people as the report specifically excluded older people, except those who had a diagnosis of a psychotic disorder, both from their general recommendations and from ring-fenced funding that arrived with the NHS Plan.[9] This funding was specifically available to develop assertive outreach and crisis intervention services. In the public, policy and professional mind, this exclusionary act also cemented the notion that older people were somehow 'set apart' from mainstream mental health service provision.

An example of this focus was apparent in the Audit Commission's report, *Forget me not: mental health services for older people*.[10] Conducted in 12 areas of England and Wales, this study used a range of instruments to measure practice in primary, secondary and tertiary care, including surveys of general practitioners, carers' individual case information and case file analysis. From this approach, three key aims of a mental health service for older people emerged, namely: (1) to maintain the mental health of older people and to help preserve their independence; (2) to support family carers as well as older people themselves; and (3) to provide intermittent or permanent residential care for those who are so disabled that it is the most practical and humane way of looking after them.[10] Building on these findings, UK government policy guidance for older people's mental health needs took shape under the National Service Framework for Older People (NSFOP)[11] which set out a 10-year programme of action and reform to deliver higher quality services for older people and contained eight standards: (1) rooting out age discrimination; (2) person-centred care; (3) intermediate care; (4) general hospital care; (5) stroke; (6) falls; (7) mental health in older people; and (8) the promotion of health and active life in older age. While each of these standards is important in its own right, standard 7 specifically addressed 'mental health in older people' with the overarching aim: 'to promote good mental health in older people and to treat and support those older people with depression and dementia'[11] (p.90).

Arguably, the diluted focus applied to both the range of mental health conditions as well as the location in the policy document,[11] resulted in restricted national impact and placed mental health services for older people on a back foot. In many ways, in England at least, the situation would not recover (for dementia services) until the publication of the *National Dementia Strategy* (NDS)[12] and its aim to 'ensure that significant improvements are made to dementia services across three key areas: improved awareness, earlier diagnosis and intervention, and a higher quality of care'. This aim of the NDS was articulated through 17 key objectives – an 18th objective was later added, relating to the use of antipsychotic medication[13] – and encouraged local services to deliver quality improvements to dementia services through innovation and partnership working within and between health, social care and third sector services. On the expiry of the NDS, the first Prime Minister's *Challenge on dementia*[14] further embraced this focus on service innovation by emphasizing that the first (of three) key areas of his report was dedicated to 'driving improvements in health and care' (the other two key areas were 'creating dementia friendly communities that understand how to help' and 'better research').

While dementia services are finding policy support and political backing, the same cannot be said for other mental health conditions of old age which are significantly lagging behind.[15]

> ## REFLECTION
>
> What characterizes a service that meets the needs of older people?

PRIMARY CARE MENTAL HEALTH SERVICES

In 2007 one of the most radical changes to mental health service delivery was launched. With an investment of over £400 million, the Improving Access to Psychological Therapies (IAPT) programme transformed the way in which mental health interventions are delivered in primary care. This initiative aimed to train around 6,000 people to deliver evidence-based psychological therapies, predominantly for depression and anxiety and based on a cognitive behavioural therapy (CBT) approach. There were two main drivers for this new policy direction; the first was the publication by National Institute for Health and Care Excellence (NICE) of a number of reports.[16–18] These reports presented evidence-based guidance, based on robust research supporting CBT-based interventions for depression and anxiety. They also indicated that a Stepped Care model would be the most appropriate mode of service delivery. The Stepped Care model moved away from the 'one size fits all' approach to interventions, and is predicated on the notion that

therapies should be offered in differing degrees of intensity depending on the individual needs of the patient. Built on a foundation of research evidence, these proposed changes to service delivery provided a vehicle for an economic argument, namely that improving access to psychological therapies would become self-sufficient. It was argued that enhanced access to therapies would result in improved outcomes for depression and anxiety. It was also proposed that these better outcomes would lead to reduced welfare benefit and medical costs for those who were unemployed as a result of their mental health problem. Furthermore, treasury revenue would be increased by the higher number of people able to work.[18]

It is this economic argument that illustrates why there have been so many obstacles for older people: older people are seen as unproductive members of society. From a financial perspective this policy was clearly designed for working age adults and at its launch older people were not directly considered. It appeared that yet again an important clinical initiative would bypass their needs. However, the development and subsequent launch of the Equality Act 2010[3] forced a re-think. The Equality Act states that services should be equally accessible and not discriminate on the grounds of age, and this provided a chance to redress the injustice. Alongside other groups deemed to be at risk of unequal access, such as Black and Minority Ethnic groups, an Older People Special Interest Group[19] was convened in an attempt to improve uptake. There was clearly work to do, with figures suggesting that only 5.2 per cent of people accessing the IAPT service were over the age of 64, despite making up 18 per cent of the population.

Alongside the economic motivations for IAPT there are numerous barriers that may be standing between older people and equal access to the service. Historically, there was a perception that older people were less likely to benefit from psychological therapies and this has led to therapeutic nihilism,[20] but there is now firm evidence that demonstrates they are just as likely to benefit as those under 65 in treatments for depression and anxiety.[21] However, many older people are likely to have complex comorbidity issues (such as complications from arthritis, diabetes and other long-term conditions), which raises an uncomfortable question about IAPT services not being able to meet assessed needs. For example, older people with depression often present with symptoms that do not neatly correspond to expectations, and there have been long-standing problems with practitioners from all professions being unable to distinguish between depression and physical health problems.[21]

Location of the service can also be an issue. Many IAPT services do not offer home visits due to pressures on resources; this may reduce the likelihood of some older people being able to attend appointments, given potential mobility issues or caring responsibilities. Furthermore, IAPT appointments are generally of a fixed length and duration. There can be very little flexibility in the length of appointment times. Older people may need longer appointment times or a higher number of sessions. This could be due to the need for a slower pace of work – perhaps the person had had a problem for decades rather than months, or perhaps they have memory or sensory impairments.

Many of the staff who were first recruited to work in IAPT teams had very little or no experience of working with older people. Not unsurprisingly given the objective of the IAPT programme, the initial preparation for Psychological Wellbeing Practitioners and High Intensity Therapists had very little, if any, content about the needs of older people. This has now been addressed by the publication of competencies that are required of graduating practitioners, and there is a roll-out of training for those already in post. However, despite this initiative, it may take a long time for the 'newcomer' to become embedded within the nature of the service. It could also be argued that 2 or 3 days of training is an insufficient amount of time to tackle a discrimination that is at a societal level alongside providing the necessary knowledge and skills.

> ### REFLECTION
>
> What is the impact of concurrent physical health problems on the provision of primary care mental health services for older people?

MEMORY ASSESSMENT AND TREATMENT SERVICES

The NHS Confederation[22] included the following definition of dementia in a recent report on improving hospital care for people with dementia: 'Dementia is a syndrome (a group of related symptoms) that is associated with an ongoing decline of the brain and its abilities. These include thinking, language, memory, understanding and judgement; the consequences are that people will be less able to care for themselves' (p.5).

The most commonly occurring dementia in both older and younger people is Alzheimer's disease,[23] although there are many different causes of dementia which vary in their presentation and progression. The greatest risk for the acquisition of dementia is age, with one in five people aged over 80 having a form of dementia.[23] Worldwide, 36 million people live with dementia, with these numbers projected to double every 20 years to 66 million by 2030 and 115 million by 2050.[24] In the UK, it is estimated that there are currently around 800,000 people with dementia and this number is forecast to rise to over 900,000 by 2021 and over 1.7 million by 2051.[23] Moreover, as no national epidemiological studies have been conducted in the UK, it is simply unknown how many younger people (i.e. aged under 65 years) have dementia, with recent estimates placing the figure at around 64,000 (or 8 per cent of all cases)[25] (p.19). However, compared to onset in older age, those diagnosed with young onset dementia are more likely to experience a more rapid progression through the 'stages' of dementia (mild–moderate–severe) and a significant shortening of the life span.[26] Unfortunately, access to specialist services and support for younger people with dementia across the UK is fragmented, with access to (any) specialist service provision dependent upon a postcode lottery rather than through a coordinated national plan of action.[27,28] Presently, in the UK, two-thirds of people with dementia currently live at home and one-third are resident in a care home.[23]

Tellingly, an Alzheimer's Disease International report[29] on the benefits of early diagnosis and intervention suggests that as many as 28 million of the world's 36 million people with dementia have yet to receive a diagnosis, and therefore 'do not have access to treatment, information, and care' (p.6). In the UK around half of all people living with dementia do not have a diagnosis.[30] This represents a personal and political predicament that the first Prime Minister's *Challenge on dementia*[14] sought to redress by setting ambitious and quantified targets for improving diagnostic rates across the country. underpinned by 'robust and affordable local plans' (p.6). This right to a diagnosis of dementia is not a recent phenomenon. For instance, at the end of the last century, Alzheimer Europe[31] compiled a seven-item 'Declaration of the needs and rights of people with dementia and their carers'. This Declaration called for: accurate and timely diagnosis; better information and public understanding about dementia; integrated health and social care provision; a right for the person to be involved in decisions about their own lives; people with dementia to have protection under the law; and people with dementia and their carers to have access to the best available health and social care services in the country in which they live.[31] The Declaration also noted that carers and family members were 'essential' in the domestic support of people living with dementia, and that carers also have a right to be consulted – and involved – in the provision of post-diagnostic care and development of services.

Traditionally, in England at least, a diagnosis of dementia was available through three main pathways:

Pathway 1: General practitioner (GP) in primary care.
  For the majority of the population, up until relatively recently, a diagnosis of dementia was usually made in primary care and performed by the person's GP.[32–34] In the 1990s especially, this led to a stream of research and supportive interventions that were aimed at helping GPs and primary care staff, such as practice nurses, to formulate and communicate a diagnosis of dementia in the surgery/health centre setting. Such research was usually in the form of conducting accessible and accurate cognitive and physical (blood tests, etc.) screening tools[35,36] and in the provision of diagnostic information about dementia to assist in decision making and follow-up care.[37–39] Here, the nursing role was conducted by a community mental health nurse whose role was largely confined to post-diagnostic care, such as home visits and/or setting up support groups for people with dementia/carers and, in some limited cases, to undertaking pre-diagnostic counselling.[40]
Pathway 2: Memory assessment and treatment service (also known as a 'memory clinic'). The first memory clinic was set up in the UK in 1983 with the aim of providing a complementary, and arguably more holistic, diagnostic service.[41] The number of memory clinics grew by 1995 to 22 and their service role was augmented by a developing research base to practice.[42] This research-driven role was consolidated when the

first licensed drug treatment for Alzheimer's disease (Tacrine) was piloted in the UK at the start of the 1990s and mushroomed when the licensing of new drugs to alleviate some of the symptoms of Alzheimer's disease were made available: donepezil (Aricept) was launched in 1997, rivastigmine (Exelon) in 1998 and galantamine (Reminyl) in 2000.[43,44] In many instances, memory clinics were set up specifically to ensure delivery of treatment with acetylcholinesterase inhibitors, and mental health nurses, who were usually employed as part of the multidisciplinary memory assessment and treatment service, found a new service role in performing medication monitoring.[45]

Pathway 3: Specialist regional/national neurological centres. In many ways, this pathway is self-explanatory. Such centres exist for the identification of rare and unusual dementias, such as 'non-fluent primary progressive aphasia',[46] and have a multidisciplinary staffing. An example of a recent specialist national memory assessment service, set up in 2012, is for Deaf people (British Sign Language users) that has been established at the Cognitive Disorders clinic at the National Hospital for Neurology and Neurosurgery in Queen Square, London, where Deaf people with presenting memory problems undergo full medical and neuropsychological assessment for dementia and other neurodegenerative disorders.[47]

The relationship between pathways 1 and 2 above was to change radically a few years ago with the publication of the NDS,[12] when the commissioning guidance that accompanied the NDS included the following statement:

NDS objective 2: Good-quality early diagnosis and intervention for all. All people with dementia have access to a pathway of care that delivers: a rapid and competent specialist assessment; an accurate diagnosis sensitively communicated to the person with dementia and their carers; and immediate treatment, care and support following diagnosis. The system needs to have the capacity to attend to all new cases of dementia in the area. (p.84)

This service reconfiguration stemmed directly from the NICE and the Social Care Institute for Excellence (SCIE) dementia clinical guideline[48] and the key recommendation that memory assessment services should act as a point of referral for a diagnosis of dementia and that there should be integrated working across all agencies. However, at a stroke, the diagnosis of dementia moved away from primary care to being a specialist activity provided by locally based memory assessment and treatment services, with providers challenged to develop (if they did not have one already) a 'rapid and competent specialist assessment'. Such a service reconfiguration also meant that the role of primary care changed so that it was now solely there to 'screen' for any potential signs of dementia in those patients who attended the surgery complaining of poor memory performance, for example, and refer them to memory assessment and treatment services. Hence, there has been a recent upsurge of information issued to primary care staff about the use and efficacy of various short cognitive screening tests, such as the Six Item Cognitive Impairment Test (6-CIT), as an evidence-based rationale for referral.[49]

This service reconfiguration has had far-reaching consequences, not only for those living with undiagnosed and then diagnosed dementia, but also, in the context of this chapter, for mental health nursing staff working at memory assessment and treatment services. This is because mental health nurses have a relatively long-standing role as members of multidisciplinary memory assessment and treatment services, although as Page[50] reminds us, up until the turn of the twenty-first century, the nursing role was mainly administrative and comprised blood taking and the conducting of clinical tasks at the behest of other professionals, such as the psychiatrist and the clinical psychologist.

However, as memory assessment and treatment services developed in the 2000s onwards, then so did the nursing role in such clinics. Page[50] draws upon his clinical experience at the Manchester Memory Clinic to outline the evolvement of a nurse-led memory clinic where the nurse has specific responsibility for the undertaking of suitability assessments; pre-treatment education; and assessments of compliance, tolerance and efficacy of pharmacological treatments (p.128). The importance of the mental health nursing role was also highlighted by Watts et al.,[51] with Keady et al.[52] demonstrating the role played by the memory clinic mental health nurse in integrating biographical assessments into both diagnostic and neuropsychological assessment/s. More recently, a pilot study conducted by Page et al.[53] suggests that after attendance at a diagnostic educational programme – mainly consisting of better understanding and applying neuropsychological assessment forms – nurses and allied health/social care professions (occupational therapists and social workers) can be trained to accurately diagnose 'uncomplicated' dementia alongside their (neuro)psychological and medical colleagues.

Such a proactive response to clinical practice begins to fit within the Chief Nursing Officer's review of mental health nursing in England, entitled *From values to action: the Chief Nursing Officer's review of mental health nursing*[54]. This report, similar to the mental health nursing review in Scotland,[55] promoted the adoption of the 'recovery approach' to all aspects of mental health care, including working with people with dementia and their families. Adapted from the *From values to action* report[54] (p.17), the recovery approach is based around a number of principles that stress the importance of working in partnership with service users (and/or carers) to identify realistic life goals

and enabling achievement; the value of social inclusion; and the need for professionals to be optimistic about the possibility of positive individual change.

It is not a huge conceptual leap to begin to link the principles of recovery to people with a recent diagnosis of dementia and the need to recover, for example, their self-esteem, self-belief and aspects of their memory performance. (We suggest readers consult chapter 35 for more on the recovery approach.) This service connection, therefore, further legitimizes nursing involvement in memory assessment services, although what that role is and how it should develop needs to be embedded within the Memory Services National Accreditation Programme.[56] Moreover, developing mental health nursing within the public health arena and with a focus on the prevention of dementia[57] would seem a logical extension of service roles and responsibilities.

SERVICE USER'S PERSPECTIVE

As a consequence of my diagnosis of AD in 2007, I am aware of certain priorities in coming to terms with my dementia.

I was a little unlucky to have a positive diagnosis, but very fortunate that I went to a Memory Clinic so early. I realize this has been crucial for my well-being; I have been able to do all the right things to slow down my AD.

As the community ages, the proportion of people with a dementia increases exponentially. Something must be done to correct this forecast; as I see it, the way forward is by routine screening of the older generation through primary care.

Physical health in the community is largely under control; the emphasis must be on mental health, with increased resources made available to put in place the screening routine. Raised awareness with the general public, along with the reduced stigma, this screening must be made a top priority for funding. In this regard, it should be noted that government resources allocated to mental health are approximately 10 per cent of those for cancer, even though far more patients are living with dementia. Because most people go to their GP every year or so, dementia nurses at the clinic should be enabled to refer those with a memory problem to a specialist unit.

On a final note, my part-time employment in mental health and my continuing search for dementia information gives me plenty to think about, and a consequent good feeling about life.

Mike Howorth, person living well with dementia

COMMUNITY MENTAL HEALTH TEAMS

The foundation stone of secondary care provision is the community mental health team. These are the multidisciplinary community teams providing specialist care for complex mental health problems in older people. In some areas they also provide support for primary care services, nursing and residential homes and acute hospitals. Although varying in make-up and exact remit, a set of core attributes has recently emerged as a gold standard by which teams could be measured. The members of the team should ideally be drawn from mental health nursing, psychiatry, social work, occupational therapy, psychology and support staff. The team should also have ready access to specialisms such as physiotherapy and dietetics. Referrals should be from a range of sources, including self-referrals as well as GPs, using single case files and joint documentation.[11,58,59]

Two surveys of composition and management arrangements in 2004 and 2009[60] found there had been a radical change in the role of unqualified support staff. In 2009, a quarter of teams had no access at all to support staff, but by 2009 they had become the second-largest grouping within teams. Psychologists appeared to remain on the fringes of the team, being the least likely profession to be line-managed within the community mental health team. However, concerns about this relative lack of access to psychology services[60] may be superseded by the advent of new ways of providing psychological therapies. Another worrying finding was that, despite integration with social care being a cornerstone of working age community mental health teams, nearly 70 per cent of teams were not mutually sharing records.

The NDS[12] called for an increase in community mental health service provision to enable additional support for care homes. It also suggested the further development of specialist liaison teams to support acute hospital staff. In a survey of 376 community mental health teams,[61] most (96 per cent) provided support for staff in non-specialist settings, with the majority providing formal support for care homes and a third providing formal support for acute hospital settings. The provision overall appears patchy, with a lack of time, staff and resources cited as preventing the level of service they perceived was required (chapter 55 has information on community care).

NHS INPATIENT PROVISION

Although there has been an increasing focus on the alternatives to hospital-based care, inpatient provision remains an essential feature of services for older people with mental health problems. When there is a need for care that exceeds the remit of community-based service or where there is a specific need to assess within a 24-hour setting, provision still draws on the hospital ward. This provision also extends to some longer-term care, but since changes to funding rules in 2007,[62] much of this care is now provided by independent nursing homes, with the NHS focused on those whose needs are too complex or challenging for the independent sector.

From the historical 'backwaters' of the asylums, inpatient care has progressed considerably, although there remains a concern that these wards are vulnerable to poor quality care.[63] This was highlighted by the Rowan Ward investigation[64] in 2003 that identified geographical isolation, low staffing levels, a lack of training and a lack of nursing leadership as risk factors. There remains some evidence to suggest that wards for older people are still the poor relation, and are less clean and more noisy and violent than average.[65,66]

Good practice guidelines indicate that wards should now be configured on a basis of diagnosis rather than just on geographical lines.[58] This means that wards can be separated into 'functional' or 'organic' provision. Here the 'functional' wards will provide care for those with diagnoses such as depression, psychosis (chapters 24 and 26) and personality disorder (chapter 27). The organic wards will accommodate those with dementia. Although it could be argued that this concentrates the skills and expertise of staff in the corresponding area, it will also potentially lead to a dilution of service provision. It seems likely that the group of people most at risk will be those who have a primary diagnosis of dementia. Where does this system acknowledge and address issues related to co-existing mental health problems such as dementia and depression or personality disorder? In addition, dementia can often be accompanied by psychotic experiences; does this separation mean these issues will receive less than optimum input?

CRISIS INTERVENTION

The changing nature of services, in part driven by financial pressures and in part reflecting a change in clinical models evidenced in the NSF for Mental Health,[8] has led to a decrease in the number of hospital beds available. Although crisis intervention models vary, the general aim is to encourage assessment and treatment at home as an alternative to hospital and facilitate timely discharge from inpatient units. However, a survey of 79 English NHS Trusts in 2006[67] found only 36 per cent were offering a full crisis resolution service to older people. On the one hand, this finding is unsurprising given that older people were initially excluded from the home treatment services developed under the guidance provided by the NSF for Mental Health.[8] On the other hand, the actual and perceived service need is even greater. For example, older people with mental health problems can quickly move from a situation of coping to one of not coping in the face of a minor illness or to a change in personal circumstances. It could be argued that this lack of alternative services leads to an unnecessary and potentially damaging hospital admission.[68]

This need is reiterated by the Mental Health Care Crisis Concordat,[69] designed to ensure people of all ages receive appropriate services when they experience a mental health crisis. This Concordat specifies that early intervention should be appropriate for people with dementia to ensure they are engaged with services.[69] However, it fails to identify the needs of older people in the Next Steps section, although other groups are afforded their own Action, Timetable, Lead and Outcome. Yet again, the service needs of older people are at risk of being overlooked and set outside the mainstream. Chapter 46 has more general information on crisis assessment and resolution.

> ### REFLECTION
>
> How can services best provide timely support for older people in crisis?

CONCLUSION

This chapter has outlined mental health service provision for older people and sought to capture the key issues and challenge for nurses. Services are undergoing considerable change and development in the wake of legislation and policy initiatives that are attempting to improve quality in dementia care and ensure equity of access for those with a range of mental health needs. As the pressure mounts to meet this ambition, there is a perception in some quarters that mental health services for older people risk becoming increasingly focused solely on dementia.[70] There are inherent challenges, or arguably advantages, to this potential development. The most obvious question is: what will be the quality of service for people over the age of 65 presenting for the first time with a functional mental health problem? Some working age teams are raising the age limit of referral, and others are combining services, but there is widespread concern that there is a lack of expertise and will within established community mental health teams to embrace

and deal effectively with the often more complex nature of functional mental problems in older people.[15] This situation is further complicated by the fact that in the UK social services operate with a 65 years cut-off point.[70] A survey of commissioners, with a 76 per cent response rate across the UK, found that of 11 types of service provision, 7 were either unavailable or did not provide equality of access to older people in more than a third of commissioning areas.[71] The greatest inequality was demonstrated in a lack of access to crisis resolution and home treatment services. However, merely measuring the number of older people accessing a particular service in no way indicates the 'true' equality of provision when it fails to take into account the quality of that service in terms of its ability specifically to meet the needs of older people. As we have seen, the craft of caring in service provision requires a person-centred approach, appropriately trained staff and older people taking a central role in the development and appraisal of quality.

ACKNOWLEDGEMENTS

We would like to express our thanks to Mike Howorth for his invaluable contribution in highlighting the experience of services from the perspective of someone living well with dementia.

References

1. Care Services Improvement Partnership. *Everybody's business: integrated mental health services for older adults: a service development guide.* London: Care Services Improvement Partnership, 2005.
2. Mental Health Foundation. *All things being equal.* London: Mental Health Foundation, 2009.
3. Great Britain. *Equality Act 2010.* Chapter 15. London: Stationery Office, 2010.
4. Office for National Statistics. *National population projections, 2012-based.* London Office for National Statistics, 2013.
5. Banerjee S, Chan J. Organization of old age psychiatric services. *Psychiatry* 2008; **7**(2): 49–54.

6. Godfrey M. *Literature and policy review on prevention and services. UK Inquiry into Mental Health and Well-Being in Later Life.* London: Age Concern/Mental Health Foundation, 2005.

7. Mental Health Act Commission, Care Services Improvement Partnership and Healthcare Commission. *Count me in: results of the 2006 national census of inpatients in mental health and learning disability services in England and Wales.* London: Commission for Healthcare Audit and Inspection, 2007.

8. Department of Health. *National Service Framework for Mental Health.* London: HMSO, 1999.

9. Department of Health. *NHS Plan: a plan for investment.* London: NHS, 2000.

10. Audit Commission. *Forget me not: mental health services for older people.* London: Audit Commission, 2000.

11. Department of Health. *National Service Framework for Older People: modern standards and service models.* London: HMSO, 2001.

12. Department of Health. *Living well with dementia: a national dementia strategy.* London: Department of Health, 2009.

13. Banerjee S. *The use of anti-psychotic medication for people with dementia: time for action.* London: Department of Health, 2009.

14. Department of Health. *Prime Minister's challenge on dementia: delivering major improvements in dementia care and research by 2015.* London: Department of Health, 2012.

15. Keady J, Watts S. *Mental health and later life: delivering an holistic model for practice.* London: Routledge, 2010.

16. NICE (National Institute for Health and Care Excellence). *Anxiety: management of anxiety (panic disorder, with and without agoraphobia, and generalised anxiety disorder) in adults in primary, secondary and community care. Clinical guideline 22.* London: NICE, 2004.

17. NICE (National Institute for Health and Care Excellence). *Depression: management of depression in primary and secondary care. Clinical guideline 23.* London: NICE, 2004.

18. Clark D. Implementing NICE guidelines for the psychological treatment of depression and anxiety disorders: the IAPT experience. *International Review of Psychiatry* 2011; **23**: 375–84.

19. Department of Health. *How to make IAPT more accessible for older people: a compendium.* London: Department of Health, 2013.

20. Burroughs H, Lovell K, Morley M, Baldwin R, Burns A, Chew-Graham C. 'Justifiable depression': how primary care professionals and patients view late-life depression. A qualitative study. *Family Practice* 2006; **23**(3): 369–77.

21. Rabins P. Barriers to diagnosis and treatment of depression in elderly patients. *American Journal of Psychiatry* 1996; **4**: 79–84.

22. The NHS Confederation. *Acute awareness: improving hospital care for people with dementia.* London: NHS Confederation, 2010.

23. Alzheimer's Society. *Dementia UK: 2014 edition.* London: Alzheimer's Society, 2014.

24. Alzheimer's Disease International. *World Alzheimer Report 2009.* London: Alzheimer's Disease International, 2009.

25. Alzheimer's Research Trust. *Dementia: The economic burden of dementia and associated research funding in the United Kingdom.* London: Alzheimer's Research Trust, 2010.

26. Thompson D. *Service and support requirements for people with younger onset dementia and their families, literature review.* Prepared for Alzheimer's Australia NSW 2011. Available from: https://www.sprc.unsw.edu.au/media/SPRCFile/2011_9_1Alzheimers_YOD_lit_rev_FINAL_DT_Oct11final.pdf [Accessed 23rd August 2016].

27. Alzheimer's Society. *Younger people with dementia: a guide to service development and provision.* London: Alzheimer's Society, 2005.

28. Roach P, Keady J, Bee P, Williams S. 'We can't keep going on like this': identifying family storylines in young onset dementia. *Ageing and Society* 2013. First View. doi:10.1017/S0144686X13000202.

29. Alzheimer's Disease International. *World Alzheimer report 2011: the benefits of early diagnosis and intervention.* London: Alzheimer's Disease International, 2011.

30. Alzheimer's Society. *Dementia 2012: a national challenge.* London: Alzheimer's Society, 2012.

31. Alzheimer Europe. Declaration of the needs and rights of people with dementia and their carers. *Alzheimer Europe Newsletter* 1999; **1**(January): 7.

32. Downs M, Turner S, Bryans M, Wilcock J, Keady J, Levin E, O'Carroll R, Howie K, Iliffe S. Effectiveness of educational interventions in improving detection and management of dementia in primary care: cluster randomised controlled study. *British Medical Journal* 2006; **332**: 692–6.

33. Ahmad S, Orrell M, Iliffe S, Gracie A. GPs; attitudes, awareness, and practice regarding early diagnosis of dementia. *British Journal of General Practice* 2010; **60**(578): e360–e365.

34. Thomas H. Attitudes of primary care team to diagnosing dementia. *Nursing Older People* 2010; **22**(3): 23–7.

35. Brayne C, Calloway P. The case identification of dementia in the community: a comparison of methods. *International Journal of Geriatric Psychiatry* 1990; **5**: 309–16.

36. Downs M. The role of general practice and the primary care team in dementia diagnosis and management. *International Journal of Geriatric Psychiatry* 1996; **11**: 937–42.

37. Cooper B, Bickel H, Schäufele M. The ability of general practitioners to detect dementia and cognitive impairment in their elderly patients: a study in Mannheim. *International Journal of Geriatric Psychiatry* 1992; **7**: 591–8.

38. Iliffe S, Eden A, Downs M, Rae C. The diagnosis and management of dementia in primary care: development, implementation and evaluation of a national training programme. *Aging and Mental Health* 1999; **3**(2): 129–35.

39. Turner S, Iliffe S, Downs M, Wilcock J, Bryans M, Levin E, Keady J, O'Carroll R. General practitioners' knowledge, confidence and attitudes in the diagnosis and management of dementia. *Age and Ageing* 2004; **33**(5): 461–7.

40. Clark C. The community mental health nurse role in sharing a diagnosis of dementia: practice approaches from an early intervention study. In: Keady J, Clarke CL, Adams T (eds). *Community mental health nursing and dementia care: practice perspectives.* Maidenhead: Open University Press, 2003: 134–47.

41. Philpot M, Levy R. A memory clinic for the early diagnosis of dementia. *International Journal of Geriatric Psychiatry* 1987; **2**: 195–200.

42. Wright N, Lindesay J. A survey of memory clinics in the British Isles. *International Journal of Geriatric Psychiatry* 1995; **10**: 379–85.

43. NICE (National Institute for Health and Care Excellence). *Alzheimer's disease – donepezil, rivastigmine and galantamine for the treatment of Alzheimer's disease TA19.* London: NICE, 2001.

44. NICE (National Institute for Health and Care Excellence). *Alzheimer's disease – donepezil, galantamine, rivastigmine (review) and memantine for the treatment of Alzheimer's disease (amended) TA111.* London: NICE, 2007.

45. Page S, Hope K, Bee P, Burns A. Nurses making a diagnosis of dementia – a potential change in practice? *International Journal of Geriatric Psychiatry* 2008; **23**: 27–33.

46. Snowden J, Neary D, Mann D. Frontotemporal dementia. *British Journal of Psychiatry* 2002; **180**: 140–3.

47. Young A, Keady J, Woll B, Marshall J, Atkinson J, Rogers K, Burns A, Geall R, Ferguson-Coleman E, Denmark T. *Overcoming obstacles to the early identification of dementia in the Deaf community.* London: Alzheimer's Society, 2013. Available from: http://www.alzheimers.org.uk/site/scripts/documents_info.php?documentID=1129 [Accessed 2nd June 2016].

48. NICE (National Institute for Health and Care Excellence)/SCIE (Social Care Institute for Excellence). *Dementia: supporting people with dementia and their carers in health and social care. NICE clinical practice guideline 42.* London: NICE, 2006.

49. Upadhyaya A, Rajagopal M, Gale T. The Six Item Cognitive Impairment Test (6-CIT) as a screening test for dementia: comparison with Mini-Mental State Examination (MMSE). *Current Aging Science* 2010; **3**(2): 138–42.

50. Page S. From screening to intervention: the community mental health nurse in a memory clinic setting. In: Keady J, Clarke CL, Adams T (eds). *Community mental health nursing and dementia care: practice perspectives.* Maidenhead: Open University Press, 2003: 120–33.

51. Watts S, Harkness L, Domone R, Shields G, Moss G, Bilsborough N. Memory services: psychological distress, co-morbidity and the need for flexible working – the reality of late life mental health care. In: Keady J, Watts S (eds). *Mental health and later life: delivering an holistic model for practice.* London: Routledge, 2010: 104–24.

52. Keady J, Williams S, Hughes-Roberts J. Emancipatory practice development through life-story work: changing care in a memory clinic in North Wales. *Practice Development in Health Care* 2005; **4**(4): 203–212.

53. Page S, Hope K, Maj C, Mathew J, Bee P. 'Doing things differently' – working towards distributed responsibility within memory assessment services. *International Journal of Geriatric Psychiatry* 2011; **27**: 280–5.

54. Department of Health. *From values to action: the Chief Nursing Officer's review of mental health nursing.* London: HMSO, 2006.

55. Scottish Executive. *Rights, relationships and recovery: the Report of the National Review of Mental Health Nursing in Scotland.* Edinburgh: Scottish Executive, 2006.

56. Memory Services National Accreditation Programme. Available from: http://www.rcpsych.ac.uk/workinpsychiatry/qualityimprovement/qualityandaccreditation/memoryservices/memoryservicesaccreditation.aspx [Accessed 2nd June 2016].

57. World Health Organization. *Dementia: a public health priority, 2012.* Available from: https://extranet.who.int/agefriendlyworld/wp-content/uploads/2014/06/WHO-Dementia-English.pdf [Accessed 23rd August 2016].

58. Royal College of Psychiatrists. *Raising the standard: specialist services for older people with mental illness.* London: Royal College of Psychiatry, 2006.

59. Abendstern M, Harrington V, Brand C, Tucker S, Wilberforce M, Challis D. Variations in structures, processes and outcomes of community mental health teams for older people: a systematic review of the literature. *Aging and Mental Health* 2011; **16**(7): 861–73.

60. Wilberforce M, Tucker S, Abendstern M, Brand C, Giebel CM, Challis D. Membership and management: structures of inter-professional working in community mental health teams for older people in England. *International Psychogeriatrics* 2013; **25**(9): 1485–92.

61. Tucker S, Wilberforce M, Brand C, Abendstern M, Challis D. All things to all people? The provision of outreach by community mental health teams for older people in England: findings from a national survey. *International Journal of Geriatric Psychiatry.* 2014; **29**: 489–96.

62. Social Care Policy and Innovation. *The National Framework for NHS Continuing Healthcare and NHS-Funded Nursing Care.* London: Department of Health, 2007.

63. Age Concern. *Improving services and support for older people with mental health problems.* London: Age Concern, 2007.

64. Commission for Health Improvement. *Investigations into matters arising from care on Rowan Ward, Manchester Mental Health and Social Care Trust.* London: Commission for Health Improvement, 2003.

65. Mental Health Act Commission. *In place of fear: eleventh biennial report, 2003–2005.* London: Mental Health Act Commission, 2006.

66. Healthcare Commission. *National audit of violence 2003–2005.* London: Healthcare Commission, 2006.

67. Cooper C, Regan C, Tandy AR, Johnson S, Livingston G. Acute mental health care for older people by crisis resolution teams in England. *International Journal of Geriatric Psychiatry* 2007; **22**: 263–5.

68. Kings Fund. *Making our health and care systems fit for an ageing population.* London: Kings Fund, 2014.

69. Department of Health. *Mental Health Crisis Care Concordat – improving outcomes for people experiencing mental health crisis.* London: Department of Health, 2014.

70. Sikdar S. Old age psychiatry risks turning into a dementia-only service (Correspondence). *Psychiatric Bulletin* 2013; **37**: 116.

71. Anderson D, Connelly P, Meier R, McCracken, C. Mental health service discrimination against older people. *Psychiatrist* 2013; **37**: 98–103.

Further reading

Brooker, D. *Person-centred dementia care: making services better.* London: Jessica Kingsley, 2007.

Department of Health. *No health without mental health: delivering better mental health outcomes for people of all ages.* London: HMSO, 2011.

Downs M, Bowers BJ. *Excellence in dementia care: research into practice.* Maidenhead: Open University Press, 2008.

James I. *Cognitive behavioural therapy with older people: interventions for those with and without dementia.* London: Jessica Kingsley, 2010.

Keady J, Clarke CL, Page S. *Partnerships in community mental health nursing and dementia care: practice perspectives.* Maidenhead: Open University Press, 2007.

Kitwood T. *Dementia reconsidered: the person comes first.* Buckingham: Open University Press, 1997.

Royal College of Psychiatrists Social Inclusion Scoping Group. *Mental health and social inclusion: making psychiatry and mental health services fit for the 21st century.* London: Royal College of Psychiatrists, 2009.

Relevant web pages

Alzheimer's Society. www.alzheimers.org.uk
Dementia Action Alliance. www.dementiaaction.org.uk
Dementia Engagement and Empowerment Project. http://dementiavoices.org.uk/

IAPT (Improving Access to Psychological Therapies) (Older People). http://www.iapt.nhs.uk/equalities/older-people
Social Care Institute for Excellence. www.scie.org.uk

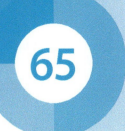

65 Working with women: compassionate and gendered care

ANN JACKSON AND JESSICA WORNER

LEARNING OUTCOMES

- To understand the place of 'compassion' in mental health nursing.
- To realize the role gender plays in violence and abuse and in mental health.
- To understand how policy has failed to address the mental health needs of women.
- To appreciate the role of peer support in mental health and the development of nursing practice.

SUMMARY OF KEY POINTS

- The concept of compassion is important to mental health nursing and the craft of caring.
- While compassion is poorly defined, there are sources that are useful for deeper understanding.
- Compassion is closely aligned to the concept of 'empathy' which has a long history of underpinning mental health nursing.
- Women's experience of violence and abuse is a gender issue.
- Policy addressing violence and abuse has been poorly implemented.

- Some mental health nurses may be survivors of violence and abuse.
- Peer Supporters mutually share experiences in their caring and compassionate relationships.
- Peer Supporters have an important role in supporting nurses to be compassionate.
- A deeper understanding of compassion requires a commitment to act to change women's experiences.

INTRODUCTION

We do not need to look too far in the current UK health policy and practice literature to find 'compassion' and 'compassionate care' littered through the various texts, either as an expected quality or as a workforce training issue.[1] As a nurse, it is impossible to deny that compassion is an attribute or an act that should be valued highly, but it is given an almost 'taken for granted' status that is, as yet, not evidenced or even well defined. Compassion has a currency that provides the nursing profession with both an opportunity and a challenge.

One of the challenges is its definition, and the ease with which nurses from across the different fields of nursing can identify with the intentions and motivations behind the limited policy language. Further, as it is used so prolifically, it must be said that it loses its real potential when given superficial treatment. A closer look at compassionate practice literature may help us to understand the potential of the concept, and the opportunity that is provided by the emphasis that current policy places on compassion. However, the authors of this chapter are not convinced that compassion is sufficiently well defined to be easily articulated and demonstrated in the specific area of mental health nursing and working with women. More specifically, we are concerned that women with mental health problems who have histories of experiencing violence and abuse are still not receiving high quality care that is both competent and compassionate.

This chapter will look at the response of mental health nursing to gendered violence, mental health nursing as a gendered profession, its application or not of compassion and the challenges and opportunities that exist to provide care and services that are both appropriate and lead to better experiences of care.

The advent of recovery and peer support, as shaped and led by people with lived experience, provides a final landing place for this discussion.

Throughout the chapter, we have referred to 'mental health nurses/nursing' in preference to 'psychiatric nurses/nursing'. This is the first author's personal and professional choice as a long-held view in favour of nursing with an emphasis on health, and a dislike for paternalism and patriarchy within traditional models of psychiatry. In support

of 'mental health nursing', Chambers[2] argues: 'there needs to be a movement away from pathology and medicine to health, lifestyle and health promotion embedded within a humanistic philosophy, grounded in hope and the principles of recovery' (p.36).

We also need to acknowledge that, while this chapter is exclusively about working with women and is written by women, we do not wish to diminish the important role that our male colleagues, in any guise, have in creating safe and therapeutic spaces for women.

Finally, we are conscious that to write, even briefly, about recovery and peer support for a professional nursing purpose runs a contradictory risk. We are keen to ground the ownership and leadership of both recovery approaches and peer support with service users. We write about peer support here to illustrate, and promote, the changing domain of the 'nurse–patient' relationship, where mental health nurses increasingly share – as equals – this 'helper' space with people with lived experience of mental health problems. Thus, we would not wish to compromise the role of Peer Supporter, which is 'authentically' different from that of a professional/nurse.[3]

We therefore write about it together – one author as a mental health nurse, the other as someone who has used mental health services and now works around peer support. As women, we share a common intention to further knowledge, understanding and mutual respect in our mental health work.

WHY COMPASSION?

We are reminded constantly about the need for compassion within services, or the lack of compassion of nurses (and other health professionals) across all areas of health care. Melanie Phillips, writing in the *Daily Mail*[4] about the findings of the Care Quality Commission's Dignity and Nutrition Inspection Report, provides a typically unpleasant narrative:

> *These horrifying revelations do not signify merely incompetence nor that perennial excuse, the effect of 'the cuts'. No, they illustrate instead something infinitely grimmer: the replacement of altruism by indifference and compassion by cruelty.*

However, it is true that many of the recent scandals within health care, addressed comprehensively by the failings in Mid Staffordshire NHS Trust, and the resultant inquiries and publication of the Francis Report, have raised similar concerns.[5] Numerous previous reports have also highlighted the 'grim' reality of poor, neglectful and at times abusive care.[6] At the same time, key reviews and reports heralded an ever-increasing emphasis on health care strategies to improve quality and the patient experience.[7, 8]

Compassion and compassionate practice are reflected in the recent new Nursing and Midwifery Council (NMC) Code of Practice,[9] the basis upon which all UK nurses are registered. From April 2016 it is proposed that a nursing revalidation process will require nurses to provide evidence that their practice reflects the four areas of the code: prioritize people, practise effectively, preserve safety and promote professionalism and trust.

The four statements in the Code that relate specifically to compassion or compassionate practice are:

1.1 treat people with kindness, respect and compassion
2.6 recognise when people are anxious or in distress and respond compassionately and politely
3.2 recognise and respond compassionately to the needs of those who are in the last few days and hours of life
11.2 make sure that everyone you delegate tasks to is adequately supervised and supported so they can provide safe and compassionate care[9] (pp.4,5,10)

Since these are the regulatory expectations of the nursing profession, we might assume that a clear definition of compassion exists to help nurses demonstrate it in their daily practice. However, this is yet to be crafted or evidenced; the UK Chief Nursing Officer's 2012 nursing strategy[9] suggests that care is given through relationships based on empathy, respect and dignity; it can also be described as intelligent kindness and is central to how people perceive their care. This is an undeveloped and superficial understanding of compassion, although it aptly identifies some key attributes, which will be discussed further later in the chapter.

Compassion within nursing attracts critique from a range of commentators. For example, Roy Lilley writes in his well-known blog:

> *Compassion is a word, I fear, in the NHS, we may use too lightly … compassion can't be learned or traded. To pretend it can be means the word has been hijacked, professionalised, sloganized and devalued. Compassion is a big word, defining, huge and must be used sparingly, not sprinkled across the pages of another report, destined to be another shelf-warmer.[10]*

Compassion, therefore, should not go without professional critique or be taken for granted; to wrongly assume that nurses 'just have it' is to understate its importance and potential. In addition to current developments to train and facilitate compassionate practice,[11] investment in the future nurse workforce will be required. This will need to have a genuine and thoughtful approach to its development. 'Top-down' policy approaches have been criticized as insufficiently likely to engage or 're-awaken' the practitioner to the values of compassion.[12] *The Shape of Caring*,[13] which is the policy basis for future nurse education in the UK, states: 'Placement and education providers must foster a culture and environment where learners feel that their views are respected, acknowledged and acted upon; where they are encouraged to ask questions and inspired to act with honesty, integrity and compassion' (p.48).

The attributes of empathy, respect and dignity are well established within all fields of nursing literature. The Royal College of Nursing in 2010 developed a set of Principles of Nursing Practice, the first of which laid the foundation for modern, person-centred nursing practice.[14] Principle of Nursing Practice A is stated fully as:

> *Nurses and nursing staff treat everyone in their care with dignity and humanity – they understand their individual needs, show compassion and sensitivity, and provide care in a way that respects all people equally. (p.35)*

In a paper by Goodrich and Cornwell,[15] the first author states that 'too often patients have reported that little or no attempt has been made to identify their individual needs in a way that is sensitive and compassionate'.

REFLECTION

If compassion is more than kindness, how can mental health nurses demonstrate this in their actions? How can we achieve a shared understanding of what is 'compassionate' in mental health nursing?

For our purposes, we prefer the definition of compassion as offered by Cole-King and Gilbert:[11] 'a sensitivity to the distress of *self and others* with a commitment to try *to do* something *about it* and prevent it' (p.30, emphasis added). They also note that the evidence for the effect of compassion is well established and no longer a 'woolly add-on' area in need of evidence.

Closely aligned to person-centred care, compassion, as an action, has the potential to allow nursing to be more critical and perhaps more political, as part of its application is to understand the needs of others more deeply, and this will include the broader social issues that impact on health. This is compatible with the aspirations of most professional health strategies, but particularly in mental health, where the social determinants of health and illness are well established.

Chambers and Ryder[16] outline six components of compassionate care as:

- empathy and sensitivity;
- dignity and respect;
- listening and responding;
- diversity and cultural competence;
- choice and priorities;
- empowerment and advocacy.

This empowerment and advocacy role for nurses is summarized in a sharp reminder by Cole-King and Gilbert:[11] 'Compassion is not synonymous with pity: it does not depict one person as being weak, inferior or lesser in comparison with another' (p.30).

Adding to the action element of compassion, Purtilo,[17] cited in Danielsen and Cawley,[18] describes three aspects of compassion as sympathetic understanding; a moral duty to carry out professional responsibility; and a 'readiness to go beyond the call of duty' (p.267).

Most importantly, Cole-King and Gilbert,[11] among others, raise the thorny issue of organizational compassion. This is an urgent issue, as observers fear the current austerity measures within UK health and social care systems are impacting negatively on the human resources required to give compassionate care, and will continue to do so. These human resources include not only the emotional labour and commitment of nurses but also nurses as a staffing resource. There is currently a contradiction in the overall policy approach to nurse staffing, where safe staffing[19] figures are routinely reported on internally and publicly, and for which providers are held to account. We have been warned recently that 'nurse shortages are life threatening'.[20]

It is a constant paradox that the very reason why nurses may have entered nursing – that is, to be caring and compassionate – has become an overall indicator for patient experience, and yet, the pressure of financial constraints is likely to have an immediate and long-lasting impact on the ability of individual nurses to deliver care that is truly compassionate.

EMPATHY IN MENTAL HEALTH NURSING – A SHORT WALK TO COMPASSION?

Compassionate care is expected by service users and patients across health settings. This is a highly relevant debate in mental health care, as the dilemmas and complexity of health, lifestyle choice and control are perhaps more acutely drawn in this area.

For us, we are interested in the extent to which mental health nursing demonstrates compassion towards women with mental health problems who have experienced violence and abuse. A compassionate approach should reflect a deeper understanding of the social context of women's experiences,[21] illustrated well by the question 'What has happened to this woman?' as opposed to 'What is wrong with this woman?'[22]

As an essential attribute within the definitions of compassion, 'empathy' has a long history in mental health nursing.[23] However, few authors have linked this to gender – either in relation to working with women, or to work as a female nurse.

As one of the few feminist nurse academics to write about this subject, in a book that dates from 1997, Ruth Gallop[23] says:

I still believe in the centrality of the interpersonal relationship but I believe that many of the defining qualities of that relationship are shaped by gender; the particular way empathy and/or caring develops in women, the role of the nurse/woman in the health care system, the social conditions of practice, and, more generally, the social condition of women in society. (p.29)

She goes on to contend that, as nursing is concerned with empathy, 'the nurse comes to know and understand the world of the other and to use that understanding constructively'[23] (p.34).

Gallop also highlights the importance of reflection and supervision as necessary in the development and enhancement of capacity. This chimes with the current focus on 'compassion training' – even though many people believe compassion cannot be taught – which is now becoming more accepted, and the authors of this chapter would agree that, in order to be consciously compassionate, a significant level of reflection and support is required. As we learn more about the complexity of compassion and self-compassion,[11] thoughtful reflection is necessary if we are to support and nurture this quality in nursing.

Gallop again offers us a straightforward way of understanding this when she writes:

acquiring insight into how one's own personal baggage informs the way one is in the world helps a person know when and where she/he ends and the other begins. But most importantly, by experiencing an increased understanding of self and the difficulties of the human condition, one is better positioned to hear and reflect upon the human condition of others (i.e. be empathic).[23] (p.35)

We are interested in the potential for compassion to underpin the work we do with women who have mental health problems and who have experienced violence and abuse, in whatever form this has occurred.

> ### REFLECTION
>
> What do mental health nurses need to know to understand the experience of others at a deep level? What kind of relationships do mental health nurses develop with women?

Gendered violence is a global issue; women across social and cultural groups are disproportionately victims of all forms of violence and abuse, and men are predominantly, though not exclusively, the perpetrators.[24] This is accepted as a gender inequality, where being female is a risk factor and being a victim of violence is linked to further social and health inequality.

There is a growing awareness of this issue and increasing action to 'end violence against women and girls' across UN states, alongside a developing understanding of the social dimensions which are directly affected by gendered violence. There is compelling evidence about the impact of gendered violence and abuse, in all its forms, on immediate and long-term health,[25] and there is a well-established causal link between 'psychiatric disorders' and domestic violence.[26] In addition, there is a significant economic and social cost,[27] which has provided a lever for campaigners to argue for both social and health policy to address issues of prevention, provision and protection.[28]

There have been several calls to UK policy and practice for health professionals to identify and respond meaningfully to women experiencing violence and abuse.[29–31]

Empathy in mental health nursing – a short walk to compassion?

65

Nurses are in a key position to provide important opportunities for women to talk openly and to receive practical support to help them make choices. In spite of the knowledge we have that the effects of child sexual abuse (chapter 29) and other forms of violence and abuse can be contributory factors to all mental health illnesses, there continues to be a lack of 'routine enquiry'.[31]

There has been little movement in this area of practice since the following statement from the NHS Confederation in 2008:[32]

> *There is a notable reluctance on the part of mental health professionals of all disciplines to routinely explore service users' experiences of abuse, and to directly affect their healing process if they are a known victim or survivor, particularly of child sexual abuse.*

It is disappointing that the main policy in this area is now over 12 years old and is yet to realize all of its intentions and aspirations for high quality gender-specific care. This is particularly the case in relation to the long-term effects of violence and abuse and the lack of services designed to meet the specific needs of survivors. Importantly, the social experiences of women, particularly as survivors of all forms of violence and abuse, were put at the centre of the attempt to understand women's mental health. In addition to being safe, the 3,000 women who participated in the study *Women's mental health: into the mainstream* wanted services to do four things: to promote empowerment, choice and self-determination; to place importance on the underlying causes and context of women's distress; to address issues relating to roles as mothers and the need for work and accommodation; and to value women's strengths and abilities and their potential for recovery.[21] It has been stated elsewhere that 'safe' and gender-specific services are difficult to achieve,[29,33] and current policy continues to emphasize the need to completely eradicate mixed-sex inpatient accommodation.

Ten years ago, the first author was involved in developing a set of principles to underpin mental health nursing, with a view to developing anti-oppressive and action-oriented practices, based on the rights of women and nursing values.[34] We believe that these principles are still a priority today and that the need to understand the experiences of women *and* to act in a way that is empowering and preventative is fundamental to the provision of care that is genuinely compassionate. The following principles are relevant to this discussion:

- Women need environments that are free from all forms of discrimination; nurses challenge discriminatory language and practices and draw attention to gender-blind policy.
- Women need relationships that are empowering; nurses, through their values and actions demonstrate and promote anti-oppressive practices.

- Women need access to staff who identify the signs of physical, sexual and emotional violence and abuse; nurses formally assess and act to prioritize the safety of women.

However noble the attempts to influence practice through good policy, it remains the case that there are areas within women's mental health that are inherently challenging and difficult. The second author is particularly concerned to hear, in both her everyday work and personal experiences, repeated accounts of women experiencing care that has been less than kind, caring, empathic and compassionate. Rather, women have continued to be 'blamed' for their experiences and then further re-abused within relationships with staff, who make little attempt to understand or validate their experiences. (For more information on developing and maintaining therapeutic relationships, see chapter 3.)

If we take self-harming behaviours (chapter 22) as an example, Sandy and Shaw's[35] study demonstrated that nurses continue to have negative attitudes, and use pejorative labels, such as 'manipulative' and 'attention seeking'. Sandy and Shaw state that, 'The use of these labels in this study indicates a serious misinterpretation of the motives underpinning service users' behaviour; which in essence relates to the communication of unbearable emotions'[35] (p.72).

Language is powerful here. For example, where nurses have been found to have negative views about women as either 'victim' or 'survivor', this may have an effect on their attitude towards caring[36] and will therefore compromise the acceptance that is a fundamental to a definition of compassion.[22] Table 65.1 presents some 'better ways of speaking'.[22]

Table 65.1 Better ways of speaking

Jargon and labels	Better ways of speaking
Attention seeking	She is trying to build relationships; she finds it hard to be alone with her thoughts and feelings
Borderline personality disorder	She is doing her best despite early experiences of deprivation and trauma
Manipulative	She doesn't believe that she is entitled to get her needs met if she is open about what she wants
Personality disordered	She is emotionally distressed, has low tolerance of frustration, and relies on coping strategies developed in situations of great deprivation

It has been suggested by some that the experience of nurses in the health care system parallels the dynamic of (not) 'being heard' that is experienced by women with the label of borderline personality disorder.[23] Clearly, if this means that nurses are unable to ask the right questions or hear the stories of those for whom they care, and there is continued deployment of labelling language and traditional psychiatric responses (that is, pathologizing of diagnoses), it is not surprising that some women will not disclose the true extent of their distress.

What might be happening to get in the way of nurses playing their part in tackling violence and abuse in their practice? It has been suggested that 'distress tolerance' is a facet of compassion skills. This has been described as an 'ability to bear difficult emotions both within ourselves and in others'[11] (p.31).

Spandler and Stickley[37] eloquently summarize the challenge this poses for nurses:

> *It may be difficult for professionals to develop compassionate relationships with clients and alleviate their suffering when they are struggling themselves – with their own suffering, heavy workloads, and inadequate supervision – when they do not have the resources to care. (p.562)*

It would be interesting to understand more fully the impact of mental health nurses' personal experiences and identity on practice in relation to gendered violence and abuse; how such practice issues impact on the workplace in which female nurses are situated; and the potential of nursing as a gendered profession to support global social change to improve the welfare, health and safety of all women.

It seems to the authors that there continues to be a disconnect between what is known about this area of need and risk and the amount of evidence and policy on the one hand, and the (apolitical) response of nursing to be fully engaged in this agenda on the other. There is evidence to suggest that NHS staff, including nurses, are themselves victims/survivors of violence and abuse and that this might be a factor in reluctance or sensitivity with regard either to addressing violence and abuse in their direct practice and contact with their patients/clients, or indeed to the lack of identification and activism around a gendered phenomenon.

As the largest professional health group, nurses are a key group to support successful implementation of practices which improve the experience of women attending health care in distress, with physical injuries and undetermined symptoms. Therefore, despite knowledge about incidence of violence, risk factors and vulnerable groups, there

continues to be variable practice. This is an acknowledged area of practice inconsistency, and while there have been suggestions and some evidence of NHS staff as victims of gendered violence themselves, the impact of this on individual practice is largely unexplored. This was recognized by a taskforce set up to tackle violence against women and girls,[38] and was addressed in one of the taskforce's 23 policy recommendations: 'NHS organisations should have health and well-being policies specifically for staff who are victims of domestic and sexual violence. A clear pathway should be implemented in every NHS-funded organisation so that staff and managers know where and how to access support'[8] (p.6). It is unclear to what extent this recommendation has been implemented within health services.

REFLECTION

Policy has indicated the kind of services that women with mental problems want. What do nurses need to do to ensure quality services for women? How do nurses hear the stories and validate the experience of women? How do they cope with their own experiences of violence and abuse?

Finally, Gallop[23] summarizes the important link between being female and being a nurse:

> *Nurses can learn most … from considering the role of interpersonal intimacy or caring, in the light of feminist or emancipatory goals such as choice, awareness, freedom to act intentionally and involvement in change. Nurses espouse valuing and attending to the subjective experience of the other, of understanding the 'lived experience' of the other. All of these values are completely compatible with feminist goals, which reflect the feminine relationship. (p.39)*

Even within the current policy driver for UK mental health, *The five year forward view for mental health* (2016), the three mentions of 'compassion' do not provide any narrative or descriptor of the care process, the quality of relationships, or the environment in which all the aspirations for 'recovery' can be achieved.[39] For more on recovery see chapters 35 and 36.

It would be reasonable to question the 'lens' through which current policy is being developed and services reconfigured; one might wonder about the future of women's services, and those related to gendered violence specifically, which depend on an appreciation of gendered causes and consequences.

Recovery and peer support – a different route to compassionate care?

65

RECOVERY AND PEER SUPPORT – A DIFFERENT ROUTE TO COMPASSIONATE CARE?

The relationships between compassion, hope-inspiring practices and achievement of recovery have been well articulated by Spandler and Stickley.[37] While that information is not going to be repeated here, they helpfully carve out the policy and literature base for an argument that supports compassionate practice at individual, relational and community levels.

The authors of this chapter are interested in another way to establish a relationship based on compassion – that of peer support. We are attracted to the description of peer support provided by Repper and Perkins:[40] 'a reciprocal relationship, based on mutuality and a shared journey; a way of sharing our personal story; a way of being in a relationship that empowers people to recover; a way of offering help and support as an equal; a way of teaching, learning and growing together and an attitude that values each person's experience' (p.77).

Mead and Hilton[41] describe this further:

> Peer Support programmes have been at the cutting edge of exploring new practices. They are grounded in the knowledge that neither person is the expert, that mutually supportive relationships provide necessary connections and that new contexts offer new ways of making meaning. (p.88)

The extensive and increasing range of peer support approaches are described fully by Stamou,[3] although we are interested in the developing ideas that support formal roles within mental health provision.

It is important that Peer Supporters lead the development of their own roles, and that innovation in this area honours the Peer Supporter as completely different from, but of at least equal value, to clinical and professional roles. It is not a step too far to suggest that peer support is a core role within workforce and service development. This should be constructed to achieve 'authentic peer support' – it is not about combining professional roles with an experience of mental health problems; it is, as Jessica has stated above, about 'sharing lived experience, hope and coping strategies to identify and achieve goals that lead to fulfilling and independent lives'. In addition, there is value in the Peer Supporter's independence, the fact that they are not part of the 'system', and have not been contaminated by 'professional' training.

So while the aspect of 'being with' the patient for a compassionate purpose is shared with nurses, the Peer Supporter has negotiated this space with the service user as a mutual foundation to their relationship. However, there are central parts to compassionate relationships that come very easily and naturally to a peer support relationship. While some of these are unique to peer support, other

SERVICE USER'S PERSPECTIVE: PEER SUPPORT

I am a woman with lived experience of mental distress myself, and I work closely with voluntary Peer Supporters who use their own experiences to support others on a mutual and reciprocal basis, based on equal peer relationships. Many people who have given and received peer support, whether informally through friendships made amongst people with similar experiences, or more formally through the provision of voluntary or paid Peer Supporters, will often speak of the importance of compassion within the peer support relationship. For women who have experienced trauma, who may self-harm and/or have been given psychiatric labels that are often experienced as stigmatizing, the complete acceptance and safety that comes with talking to someone who has been through, or is still going through, similar experiences can be lifesaving.

For those of us who have experienced 'care' that is not compassionate, this can reinforce a lack of self-compassion and in turn the severe distress arising from this. It also serves to reinforce a divide in which we come to expect less compassion from professionals who we assume will not understand us. Compassion within a peer support relationship, however, is mutual. By understanding and relating to another person as an equal, and using shared experiences to support them in a way that is compassionate to the other person, this can also help you develop compassion towards yourself, which may have been destroyed in the past. When I share parts of my own 'story' with Peer Supporters, I often talk about how I 'learnt to make friends with myself', after years of physical and mental self-destruction, and peer support has been a central part of that. When I have supported someone who has been through a similar experience to myself, it has made it difficult to continue to hate myself when I have provided compassion towards someone with whom I identify. Similarly, when I have received support from someone who has had similar experiences, I have felt safe – that they have really understood and they still value me as someone who should be here.

Jessica Worner

parts are not necessarily so. We believe that nurses could learn from these in their own practice, and this provides an opportunity that was not envisaged even a decade ago. As practice develops, we feel confident that Peer Supporters will be key partners in collaborative learning, reflection and supervision for nurses.

> **REFLECTION**
>
> How can mental health nurses be helped to reflect and be reflexive about their practice? Do you agree that Peer Supporters can educate and support nurses to be compassionate?

CONCLUSION

In this chapter we have aimed to outline the case for compassionate and gendered care. We are conscious that in our attempt to articulate what we believe and know to be right, our thoughts are not always underpinned by anything accepted as 'evidence'. As women who have a personal and professional interest in the experience of violence and abuse, it is a challenging area to write about. There is still much to be done across health, social and judicial services to transform responses to the specific needs of women. What, then, is the potential contribution of nurses as activists in local, national and global challenges to violence and abuse against women? One might ask what the role of nurses is in 'activism' – and maybe this is an unrealistic or undesirable objective, although it seems insufficient to leave social change to policy makers or indeed to the actions and protest of service users alone. As a professional nurse, the first author believes there is a relationship between nursing 'praxis' and the values inherent within professional codes, the 'craft of caring' and the motivation for social change. As a peer support leader, the second author believes that there is great value in social change emerging as part of the evolution of this new kind of worker, described earlier in the chapter. Together, we are committed to the idea that we can learn from each other – that in spite of the attempt to professionalize compassion, it is not the province of the professional helper only. That said, more needs to be done to provide a framework of what 'good compassion looks like', and it cannot be the case that expertise by experience alone provides the only basis for compassionate care.

Compassion offers an opportunity to re-think or re-author some of the basic tenets of mental health and nursing – we wonder whether it can move us away from 'empathy' as *the* key skill for practice. We believe that, if women are to be cared for, about and with, in a way that understands the social contexts of their experiences and the consequent impact, we must move beyond the rhetorical language of compassion within current policy. It is essential that all stakeholders in protecting and advancing women's safety and mental health work together to make the very most of diminishing health and voluntary sector resources. The putting of policy into practice for violence against women and girls has hitherto taken decades, and while we can look back to the past for the policy steer, we need to look to the future for its application, for considered actions that are meaningful and authentic. In other words, policy and practice should share the same territory of purpose and intent, and be connected by a genuine attempt to *make it different*.

This, for us, would unify those strands of compassion – the care that can be crafted, within a deep understanding of women's stories, with action that works to prevent and address the causes and consequences of women's inequality.

References

1. NHS England. *The five year forward view for mental health – a report from the Independent Mental Health Taskforce to the NHS in England.* 2016. Available from: https://www.england.nhs.uk/wp-content/uploads/2016/02/Mental-Health-Taskforce-FYFV-final.pdf [Accessed 20th October 2016].
2. Chambers M. The case for 'mental health' nurses. In: Cutcliffe J, Ward M (eds). *Key debates in psychiatric/mental health nursing.* Elsevier, 2006: chapter 2.
3. Stamou E. Reclaiming user leadership in peer support practice. *Journal of Mental Health Training, Education and Practice* 2014; **9**(3): 167–76.
4. Phillips M. The real reason our hospitals are a disgrace. *Daily Mail*, updated 17 October 2011. Available from: http://www.dailymail.co.uk/debate/article-2049906/How-feminism-nurses-grand-care.html [Accessed 20th October 2016].
5. Francis R. *Report of the Mid Staffordshire NHS Foundation Trust Public Inquiry.* 2013. Available at: https://www.gov.uk/government/publications/report-of-the-mid-staffordshire-nhs-foundation-trust-public-inquiry [Accessed 26th October 2016].
6. Department of Health. *Transforming care: a national response to Winterbourne View Hospital, final report.* 2012. Available from: https://www.gov.uk/government/uploads/system/uploads/attachment_data/file/213215/final-report.pdf [Accessed 20th October 2016].
7. National Advisory Group on the Safety of Patients in England. *A promise to learn – a commitment to act. Improving the safety of patients in England.* 2013. Available from: https://www.gov.uk/government/uploads/system/uploads/attachment_data/file/226703/Berwick_Report.pdf [Accessed 20th October 2016].
8. Keogh B. *Review into the quality of care and treatment provided by 14 trusts in England: overview report.* 2013. Available from: http://www.nhs.uk/nhsengland/bruce-keogh-review/documents/outcomes/keogh-review-final-report.pdf [Accessed 20th October 2016].
9. Nursing and Midwifery Council. The Code – professional standards of practice and behaviour for nurses and midwives. 2015. Available from: https://www.nmc.org.uk/globalassets/sitedocuments/nmc-publications/nmc-code.pdf [Accessed 20th October 2016].

10. Lilley R. Shelf warmer. *www.nhsManagers.net*. 7 September 2015. Available from: http://myemail.constantcontact.com/Shelf-warmer.html?soid=1102665899193&aid=mD-2ZY3kveY [Accessed 20th October 2016].

11. Cole-King A, Gilbert P. Compassionate care: the theory and the reality. *Journal of Holistic Healthcare* 2011; **8**(3): 29–37.

12. Youngson R. *Time to care*. Raglan: Rebelheart, 2012.

13. HEE (Health Education England). *Raising the bar: the shape of caring: a review of the future education and training of registered nurses and care assistants*. 2015. Available from: https://www.hee.nhs.uk/our-work/developing-our-workforce/nursing/shape-caring-review [Accessed 20th October 2016].

14. Jackson A, Irwin W. Dignity, humanity and equality: Principle of Nursing Practice A. *Nursing Standard* 2011; **25**(28): 35–7.

15. Goodrich J, Cornwell J. Seeing the person in the patient: the Point of Care Review Paper. 2008. Available from: www.kingsfund.org.uk/publications/the_point_of_care [Accessed 20th October 2016].

16. Chambers C, Ryder E. *Compassion and caring in nursing*. Oxford: Radcliffe, 2009.

17. Purtilo R. *Ethical dimensions in the health professions*, 4th edn. Elsevier, 2005.

18. Danielsen R, Cawley J. Compassion and integrity in health professions education. *Internet Journal of Allied Health Sciences and Practice* 2007; **5**(2).

19. National Quality Board. How to ensure the right people, with the right skills, are in the right place at the right time. 2013. Available from: https://www.england.nhs.uk/wp-content/uploads/2013/11/nqb-how-to-guid.pdf [Accessed 20th October 2016].

20. Mulholland H. Nursing chief: 'Nurse shortages are life threatening'. *Guardian*. 2 September 2015. Available from: https://www.theguardian.com/society/2015/sep/02/nursing-chief-janet-davies-shortages-affect-patients-lives [Accessed 20th October 2016].

21. Department of Health. *Women's mental health: into the mainstream*. London: Department of Health, 2002.

22. Care Services Improvement Partnership. *Informed gender practice – mental health care that works for women*. London: Department of Health, 2008.

23. Gallop R. Caring about the client: the role of gender, empathy and power in the therapeutic process. In: Tilley S (ed.). *The mental health nurse – views of practice and education*. Oxford: Blackwell Science, 1997: 28–41.

24. HM Government. *A call to end violence against women and girls – progress report 2010–15*. London: HM Government, 2015.

25. Itzin C. *Tackling the health and mental health effects of domestic and sexual violence and abuse*. London: Department of Health, 2006.

26. Howard L, Trevillion K, Khalifeh H, Woodall A, Agnew-Davies R, Feder G. Domestic violence and severe psychiatric disorders: prevalence and interventions. *Psychological Medicine* 2010; **29**: 881–93.

27. Walby S. *The cost of domestic violence*. London: Women and Equality Unit, 2004

28. HM Government. *Together we can end violence against women and girls: a strategy*. London: HM Government, 2009.

29. Phillips L, Jackson A. gender-specific mental health care. In: Phillips P, Sanford T, Johnston C (eds). *Working in mental health – practice and policy in a changing environment*. Abingdon: Routledge, 2012: chapter 9.

30. National Mental Health Development Unit. *Working towards women's well-being: unfinished business*. London: National Mental Health Development Unit, 2009.

31. Howard L, Trevillion K, Agnew-Davies R. Domestic violence and mental health. *International Review of Psychiatry* 2010; **22**(5): 525–34.

32. NHS Confederation. *Implementing national policy on abuse and violence, briefing June*. London: NHS Confederation, 2008.

33. Department of Health. *Mainstreaming gender and women's mental health: implementation guidance*. London: Department of Health, 2003.

34. RCN (Royal College of Nursing). *8 principles for practice, nurses promoting women's mental health and wellbeing*. London: RCN, 2005.

35. Sandy P, Shaw D. Attitudes of mental health nurses to self-harm in secure forensic settings: a multi-method phenomenological investigation. *Online Journal of Medicine and Medical Science Research* 2012; **1**(4): 63–75.

36. Woodtli M. Nurses' attitudes toward survivors and perpetrators of domestic violence. *Journal of Holistic Nursing* 2001; **19**(4): 340–59.

37. Spandler H, Stickley T. No hope without compassion: the importance of compassion in recovery-focused mental health services. *Journal of Mental Health* 2011; **20**(6): 555–66.

38. Department of Health. *Responding to violence against women and children – the role of the NHS*. London: Department of Health, 2010.

39. Department of Health. *The five year forward view for mental health*. London: Department of Health, 2016. Available from: https://www.england.nhs.uk/wp-content/uploads/2016/02/Mental-Health-Taskforce-FYFV-final.pdf [Accessed 28th October 2016].

40. Repper J, Perkins R. A journey of discovery for individuals and services. In: Phillips P, Sanford T, Johnston C (eds). *Working in mental health – practice and policy in a changing environment*. Abingdon: Routledge, 2012: chapter 7.

41. Mead S, Hilton D. Crisis and connection, speaking out. *Psychiatric Rehabilitation Journal* 2003; 87–94.

Further reading

Crawford P, Gilbert P, Gilbert J, Gale C. The language of compassion. *Taiwan International ESP Journal* 2011; **3**(1): 1–16

Itzin C. Tackling the health and mental health effects of domestic and sexual violence and abuse. Department of Health, 2006.

Available from: http://eprints.lincoln.ac.uk/605/1/uoa12ki02.pdf [Accessed 12th October 2016].

Relevant web pages

EVAW (End Violence against Women). Where are we now? 10 year review of Westminster government action to end violence against women and girls. EVAW, 2015. Available from: http://www.endviolenceagainstwomen.org.uk/data/files/resources/75/EVAW-Where-Are-We-Now-Nov-2015.pdf [Accessed 12th October 2016].

WHO (World Health Organization). Violence against women, intimate partner and sexual violence against women, fact sheet no. 239. Updated January 2016. Available from: http://www.who.int/mediacentre/factsheets/fs239/en/ [Accessed 12th October 2016].

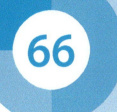

66 Services and supports for refugees and asylum seekers

NICHOLAS PROCTER, MONIKA FERGUSON, AMY BAKER AND ASMA BABAKARKHIL

LEARNING OUTCOMES

- To understand the mental health experiences and needs of people from refugee and asylum seeker backgrounds.

- To be able to identify the importance of cultural explanatory models in mental health, and explain how cultural competency can be achieved.

- To be aware of the complexities associated with the processes surrounding claims for asylum and the importance of working alongside migration support services.

- To recognize the general principles for providing community mental health support to people of asylum seeker and refugee backgrounds.

- To be able to identify appropriate emergency mental health strategies and supports.

- To understand the importance of refugees and asylum seekers participating in mental health research.

SUMMARY OF KEY POINTS

- Nurses play an important role in providing collaborative mental health care to people from refugee and asylum seeker backgrounds.

- Refugees and asylum seekers experience unique risk and protective factors which can influence their mental health.

- Mental health services offered to refugees and asylum seekers should be culturally appropriate; this can be facilitated through the development of cultural competence, aided by service user consultation, and efforts to understand and incorporate different explanatory models of mental health.

- Sensitivity should be given towards understanding and responding to the particular circumstances of refugees and asylum seekers – such as processes surrounding claims for asylum and visa reviews – which can exacerbate the experience of poor mental health.

INTRODUCTION

This chapter describes practical steps in meeting the mental health needs of refugees and asylum seekers. In providing such services, nurses may work with people at the very point of their distress – often during the processes attendant upon gaining asylum or, depending upon the outcome of the claim, a permanent protection visa. Although services may be provided external to immigration detention facilities, there is scope for mental health nurses to craft a caring response by acting as consultants to the multidisciplinary team working directly with asylum seekers. In this chapter, practical strategies are presented for generating trust and supportive counselling. Implications are drawn for nurses working across a range of practice settings, such as in accident and emergency departments, psychiatric clinics and community health. Continuity and integration of care is achieved by bridging discrete elements in the asylum seeker journey, such as legal reviews, news from home and ongoing psychosocial stressors in the context of different episodes, interventions by different providers or changes in illness status. Also important are therapeutic actions that build resilience intrinsically over time, such as refugee and asylum seekers, values, sustained supportive interpersonal relationships and therapeutic care plans. The central argument of this chapter is that no single organization or individual can improve mental health care and prevent mental illness for refugees and asylum seekers. Rather, the craft of caring is made possible through an interactive and collaborative approach.

JOHN'S STORY

My name is John. I am 24 years old and the eldest son in a family of 14. I was working for the government in Afghanistan when my parents and I started to receive death threats from the Taliban who were targeting government employees. Our lives were in danger.

Life in Afghanistan was difficult and, although I was enrolled in a journalism course, I was unable to study due to the adverse situation. Four of my best friends died one day on their way to work during a suicide bomb attack. Later, the school that my parents and I were establishing was attacked with a rocket-propelled grenade. I received death threats for being involved in establishing the school. We lived with the constant fear of death. The mental pressure this placed on me was severe – I was constantly hyper-alert; the fear and stress left me emotionally exhausted. I was afraid of going to work. This was very stressful because, as the eldest son, I was responsible for my family.

In 2009, I was told that I had been accepted as a genuine refugee and was sent on an aeroplane to Australia, alone. My family's case was still being processed. When I arrived, immigration representatives took me to my accommodation. It was the first time in my life that I was separated from my family. I was afraid. I was completely alone in a foreign, unfamiliar country where I did not speak the language and had no one from my country to assist me. Added to this was my concern and frustration for my family, whose lives were at high risk in Afghanistan.

I am still adjusting since 2009. My mental health problems often result in me feeling disoriented and distracted. I have a lot of pressure on my mind. I quickly forget things, get distracted easily and cannot complete my studies. I get bored easily and leave things half completed. I recall being like this as a child. I was often impatient and had difficulty completing work tasks, games or even sports. I believe this lack of cognitive focus was as a result of the rough and dangerous environment I grew up in.

REFUGEES, ASYLUM SEEKERS AND GLOBALIZATION

As of December 2015, almost 64 million people were registered globally with the United Nations High Commission for Refugees (UNHCR)[1] as 'Persons of Concern', which includes people of both refugee and asylum seeker backgrounds. The UNHCR defines a refugee as a person who:

owing to a well-founded fear of being persecuted for reasons of race, religion, nationality,

membership of a particular social group or political opinion, is outside the country of his nationality and is unable or, owing to such fear, is unwilling to avail himself of the protection of that country; or who, not having a nationality and being outside the country of his former habitual residence as a result of such events, is unable or, owing to such fear, is unwilling to return to it.[2]

At some point, every person who has been a refugee has been an asylum seeker. An asylum seeker is a person seeking protection under the 1951 Refugee Convention.[2] Usually, an asylum seeker is someone who has left his or her country of origin and formally applied for asylum in another country but has not yet had their application assessed.

Annually, the UNHCR provides a global report on the number and location of refugees, asylum seekers and displaced persons. The UNHCR estimates record that 2 million applications were received for asylum or refugee status in 2015.[3] Germany was the world's largest recipient of new individual applications (441,900), followed by the United States of America (172,700), Sweden (156,400) and the Russian Federation (152,500).[3] These claims were submitted by people seeking asylum from a large number of countries or territories, particularly the Syrian Arab Republic, Afghanistan, Iraq and Ukraine.

Many people seeking asylum originate from countries with histories of war, conflict and persecution. At the time of writing, several regions, such as Syria and Nigeria, are receiving extensive news coverage, with fierce and explosive fighting, unstable law and order and kidnapping being commonplace. In addition to people's lives being distanced from what is happening in their homeland, mental health and well-being and a fear of being forced to return are blended in the wake of expanding electronic communication, regulated and non-regulated people movements and the increasing global influences on personal and social life.[4]

With industrialized countries being home to asylum seekers, there is an increasing diversity of connections among phenomena once thought disparate and worlds apart. These connections involve ideas and ideologies, people and futures, images and messages, information technologies and techniques that are inevitably interrelated but not homogeneous.[5]

This chapter has been developed with this global context in mind, simultaneously incorporating the fundamental beliefs that prevention of mental health issues, mental illness and suicide should:

- understand the factors that heighten the risk of these occurring and the factors that are protective against them;
- involve inclusive decision making and collaborative partnerships between relevant organizations;
- identify the groups and individuals likely to benefit from interventions;
- develop, implement, evaluate and disseminate effective interventions that are culturally and linguistically appropriate.[6]

REFUGEE AND ASYLUM SEEKER MENTAL HEALTH

Global estimates of the prevalence of mental illness experienced by refugees and asylum seekers are difficult to determine; however, commonly reported conditions include depression, post-traumatic stress and anxiety.[7–9] As demonstrated in John's story, there is increasing acknowledgement of the role that previous (e.g. past trauma) and current (e.g. resettlement) experiences play in placing these individuals at greater risk of developing mental illness.[10] Among adult refugees and asylum seekers, various risk factors for mental illness are well-known: low English-language proficiency; loss of close family bonds and confidants; racism, discrimination and feelings of marginalization; limited understanding of the health system; and prior exposure to trauma.[11,12] Factors which may protect against mental illness include: positive family and peer relationships; ability to self-express; problem-solving and cognitive abilities; assertiveness; having confidants; having a clear cultural and linguistic identity; and satisfaction with family success and acculturation.[11] Similar risk and protective factors have been identified for children. A recent review of the mental health of displaced and refugee children found that, although stable settlement and social support could be protective, exposure to trauma and violence is a key risk factor.[13] This is particularly concerning considering the well-established link between childhood adversity and mental health problems in adulthood.[14,15] Unaccompanied minors, asylum seekers and former child soldiers are also at increased risk of mental health problems and mental illnesses.[16]

AMIR'S STORY

My name is Amir. I am in my third year of a Mechanical Engineering degree. I left Iraq with my family in 1996. I was 7 years old when the fishing vessel we were travelling on to Australia was stopped by a Norwegian ship. We were transferred to a warship where we spent 1 month circling in the ocean. During this time, the asylum seekers on the ship were taken up to the hot, metal deck and made to stay there for several hours with the sun blazing down. This happened daily. Many people fainted due to being unaccustomed to such heat.

We were kept in detention for 3 years. Since then, I have continued to have nightmares. I don't remember my dreams, but I always wake with a feeling of fear which lingers until I fall asleep again. I have insomnia and take a nerve relaxant medication (not sleeping pills) to help me sleep and reduce the active racing of my mind. I find

I think about all my problems at night. My nightmares have become routine, despite ongoing psychologist sessions since arriving in Australia. I have learned to live with it.

Friends and family often come to me with their problems and want me to listen, especially my mother. I find it stressful and burdensome to listen to negative stories but I don't wish to let my friends and family down so I don't complain, despite feeling down afterwards. I also find myself in the middle of my parents' arguments. My tolerance for quarrelling is very low. I hear it all the time; it's like a razor slowly cutting into my head every time I hear them fight. It ruins the rest of my day. The responsibility of being forced into the middle of my parents' fight and the expectation to intervene is highly stressful. I fear that, if I make the wrong decisions, my family will be angry.

After being released from detention, I would describe the ordeal over the last decade as being under constant mental attack. This feeling has never gone away despite some progress in settling in Australia. I believe that the damage to my mental state will be something I have to live with for the rest of my life, especially not being able to trust people because of the things that happened in the past. I'm always feeling uncertain and I believe it's from the years of uncertainty spent in detention. It's a lifelong struggle to keep pushing back the anger over what we've been through and I have to constantly make myself mentally positive. I also have to do positive things with my life to make me feel good about myself and stop me from falling back into anxiety, fear and sadness.

Self-harm and suicide

Amir's story highlights the impact that a mental health condition can have on one's daily life. In addition, there are also instances when the mental health experiences of refugees and asylum seekers reach crisis point, often expressed through self-harming and suicidal behaviours. There have been some high-profile suicides of asylum seekers in Europe and Australia, often following claims for permanent protection being refused. On Friday 18 May 2004, Zekria Ghulam Salem Mohammed died by suicide in Glasgow just days after he had been told by the British Home Office that his claims for asylum had been rejected and he must return to Afghanistan. Electronic and print media reports surrounding the death indicate that, after exhausting all legal attempts to stay in Britain, he was told that he would have to leave his flat, and his £38 per week allowance for food and other essentials was stopped. Informal, non-government supports failed to arrive and he was 'too proud to beg and scavenge for food in bins'.[17] Forbidden to work or study, starving, ashamed and broken, he felt there was no hope left and decided to end his life. As one of his close friends, who found his body, told Scottish television, 'They first killed his heart and drove him to such a condition that he took his own life'[18,19] (p.287).

Such anecdotal reports are not uncommon, as revealed by a recent study which explored the use of one emergency department by immigration detainees in Darwin, Australia.[20] For the duration of 2011, there were 770 attendances by 519 individual detainees, representing over half of the estimated population of immigration detainees in Darwin at the time. The most common primary diagnosis was 'psychiatric problems' (in 187 cases, or 24 per cent of attendances), of which 138 attendances were associated with self-harm. Although psychiatric attendances were less common in children than adults, 20 of the total attendances for psychiatric problems were by children aged 9 to 17 years (15 of which were related to self-harm). Chapters 22 and 23 have information on self-harm and suicide.

REFLECTION

Imagine that you were required to leave your homeland, fleeing persecution or other intolerable living conditions. What kind of experiences would you have had and how might these affect your everyday life?

CULTURAL CONSIDERATIONS OF MENTAL HEALTH

With awareness of how we live in a globalizing culture, we can look more deeply at how different cultures have different views of what constitutes mental health and mental illness, i.e. different cultural explanatory models. A person's explanatory model can include their beliefs regarding the cause, onset, nature and duration of the mental health/illness experience, as well as the treatment, healing and recovery process.[21] This is largely dependent upon what each particular culture and individual regards as 'normal' or 'abnormal' thought, feeling and/or behaviour, and the influence of other factors such as the immediate social environment, gender, socioeconomic status, education, religion or spiritual beliefs. In many cultures, the Western view of mental illness is a foreign concept. If it is understood at all, it may be seen through explanatory models of spiritual ancestry. It may also be heavily stigmatized and the

Western idea of recovery is almost unknown. As an example, individuals of diverse cultures and religions may consider mental illness to result from reasons such as karma, spiritual possession or mind–body imbalance.[22] Further, in some languages, there may not be words to describe mental illness such as depression.

For some, the Western notion of mental illness may be rejected. This may influence a range of factors, including how mental illness is understood and whether treatment is adhered to. In the craft of caring, openness to and understanding of these issues in practice helps develop cultural competence. Cultural competence is, in this sense, a set of behaviours, attributes and policy infrastructure that come together in a system or organization or among professionals to enable that system, organization or those professions to work effectively in cross-cultural situations.[23]

Cultural competency for assessment and treatment of mental health issues requires services to understand the concept of culture, its impact on human behaviour, and the interpretation and evaluation of thought, actions and behaviour. Cultural competency also implies recognition of other issues that are sometimes associated with working with people from different cultures (see chapter 38 on culturally safe care). These include stigma, isolation, communication and language difficulties, and sensitivity to specific problems experienced by people from diverse cultural backgrounds, clinicians and service providers when working with interpreters in the health setting. In health service delivery, cultural competency also includes the practitioner's ability to understand the emphasis many cultures place on the involvement of family in the service user's care and the role of family more widely, particularly in relation to confidentiality and gaining trust.

Based upon the work of Kleinman and Seeman,[24] this means examining the way in which symptoms of mental distress are understood and presented, the way help is sought and the way care is interpreted and evaluated by those who receive it. This process links the mental health experiences of relocation and settlement as they are held by refugees and asylum seekers, their leaders, healers and other concerned people, with health professionals' interpretation of them. The clinical work of mental health nurses – no matter how willing or keen to help – will be compromised if it does not take into account the person's understanding of health difficulties and what practitioners themselves see as different perceived causes of ill-health, optimal care and culturally appropriate support and treatment.[25]

Achievement of cultural competency will depend upon the practitioner's openness and flexibility related to cultural awareness. The cultural awareness questions listed below, adapted from Procter et al.,[11] are designed to help practitioners better understand the context of the person's mental health concerns, and to become more informed in their approach to that individual.

- Can you talk to me about how you came to be here? What do you usually call this problem that you're experiencing? (Once established, use the person's words for the problem.)
- Can you recall when _____ started, and why do you think it started then?
- Can you describe the main problems _____ has been causing you?
- Have you done anything to try to stop/manage _____ to make it go away or make it better? Did this work?
- In your culture, what would you or other people usually do to make _____ go away or make it better?
- So far, how have you been coping with _____?
- In your culture, is what you are experiencing considered 'severe'? What is the worst problem _____ could cause you?
- What type of help would you be expecting from me/our service?
- Are there people in your community who are aware that you are experiencing _____?
- What do they think caused you to experience _____? Are they doing anything to help you?

When providing services to people from culturally and linguistically diverse backgrounds, it is important to communicate clearly. Wherever possible, service users should be able to communicate in their preferred language, especially in stressful situations. If the service user requests an interpreter or has inadequate language skills, a professional interpreter should be used. The following tips will help discover how well and to what extent a service user speaks and understands English.[26]

- Ask questions the person has to answer in a sentence. Avoid questions that can be answered by 'yes' or 'no'. 'What'/'why'/'how'/'when' questions are best.
- Ask the person to repeat in their own words some information you have just given them.

If the person cannot answer the questions easily, or cannot repeat back information accurately, use a professional interpreter. When working across cultures, it is important to remember the following point:

- Asking people their name, address, date of birth and other predicable information is not an adequate test of English language skills.
- Having social conversation skills in English does not always mean a person understands complex information in spoken or written English.
- Verbal skills do not always equate with reading and writing skills. Remember the need to tell people their rights and get informed consent.
- People often lose their second language skills in stressful situations, e.g. when talking about mental health problems or seeking help.

- Due to the increased stigma of mental illness in some cultures, some service users may prefer an interpreter who is based outside their community (e.g. a phone interpreter from another area). For new and emerging communities, professional interpreters may not be established, in which case an informal interpreter from the community may be preferable to not having an interpreter.

Trauma-informed care

With past trauma (e.g. torture, violence) being a common experience for many refugees and asylum seekers, cultural competency on the part of mental health clinicians can benefit from the incorporation of trauma-informed care. This approach involves recognizing the presence of trauma symptoms and acknowledging the role that trauma has played in the person's life. Underlying trauma-informed care is a 'do no harm' approach, with the purpose of ameliorating, not exacerbating, the negative impacts of trauma.[27] To ensure that services are accessible and effective for individuals who have experienced trauma, Elliot and colleagues[28] suggest the following:

1. Recognize the impact of trauma on the development and coping strategies of the individual.
2. Set recovery from trauma as a key goal.
3. Incorporate an empowerment model, to facilitate the individual taking control of their life.

4. Work towards maximizing the individual's choice and control over their recovery.
5. Strive for therapeutic relationships that develop safety and trust[29] in the individual (i.e. non-traumatizing relationships).
6. Demonstrate respect for the individual's need for safety, respect and acceptance.
7. Emphasize the individual's strengths (focus on adaptations rather than symptoms, resilience rather than pathology).
8. Strive to minimize the possibilities of re-traumatization.
9. Demonstrate cultural competence, understanding the individual in the context of their life and background.
10. Encourage service user input when designing and evaluating services.

Many individuals may experience barriers to discussing trauma[30] and overcoming these barriers is important if the potential for trauma-informed care is to be maximized.

REFLECTION

Imagine that you are interviewing a refugee or an asylum seeker who appears to have some significant 'mental health problems'. Apart from the questions suggested above, what would you want to ask this person?

MIGRATION AGENT AND/OR LAWYER CONSULTATION

An important aspect of providing mental health services to refugees and asylum seekers relates to processes surrounding claims for asylum. The structure of individual mental health support should be built around the processes of seeking asylum and coping with rejections and setbacks during lengthy and, at times, complex legal processes. Similarly, supportive mental health counselling during migration agent/lawyer consultation has the potential to help asylum seekers prepare for the 'next stage' of their (application) journey, helping to build resilience and understand personal reactions to experiences and feelings (e.g. rejection, fear, frustration and disappointment).

Background issues for migration law support

Asylum seekers' suffering can become increasingly intolerable at times of re-interviewing and rejection of refugee claims by immigration officials. Asylum applications are considered in light of the information supplied and any facts known about the country the person is fleeing. Some people in immigration detention, at times of re-applying for permanent protection, suffer a denial of credibility because of inconsistencies in their story; this may lead to claims being dismissed on grounds of minor discrepancies.

Sometimes, this can have a flow-on effect whereby it is difficult for therapeutic trust to develop between the mental health provider and the individual.

People value and connect with organizations they trust, and this is critical in a system that is known to push people back into the community without adequate support. From this perspective, the craft of caring must embrace valuing human connectedness between organizations and asylum seekers who seek support. This approach is consistent with an extensive review of literature about treating possible suicide and life-threatening behaviour. The reviewers concluded that it is the trust inherent in the therapeutic relationship (chapter 3) that allows the person to take the necessary risks, do things differently, reach out during periods of acute and excruciating vulnerability and experiment with new skills, all essential for progress and recovery.[31]

It should also be acknowledged that mental distress and emotional problems can impact on the quality of information people can remember. There may be important differences between traumatic and non-traumatic memories. For example, initial recall of traumatic events by people with post-traumatic stress often does not involve typical narrative memory and the story of what happened may be fragmented, therefore appearing inconsistent. Chapter 67 is concerned with mental health, the law and human rights. This situation may be compounded by the fast track refugee assessment process. After an investigation into the fast track process, the UK parliament's Joint Committee on Human Rights found that:

> It is self-evident that some asylum seekers – most obviously torture victims and those who have been sexually abused – are unlikely to reveal the full extent of experiences to the authorities in such a short time period, and that this problem will be exacerbated where they are not able to access legal advice and representation and the support of organisations able to help them come to terms with their experiences.[32] (p.74)

Additional research in the UK has found that people seeking asylum who have post-traumatic stress at the time of their interviews are systematically more likely to have their claims rejected the longer their application takes.[33]

To make clinical mental health matters worse, not all countries and jurisdictions provide advance notice of review procedures. In some settings, there is no way of knowing well in advance the precise date and time when interviews to assess claims, invitations to interview or rejection letters will arrive, or what questions will be asked and what primary data source will be used to determine whether a homeland country is safe to return to. The level of distress reported among asylum seekers as a result of this uncertainty is significant.

Also significant as a background issue is the knowledge that suicide by people born overseas represents 25 per cent of all suicides in Australia.[34] Of these, 60 per cent are by people from non-English-speaking backgrounds.[35] Although suicide (chapter 23) is a behaviour, it is strongly associated with mental illness, and the risk factors pertinent to both mental illness and suicide for refugees and asylum seekers are overlapping and interrelated. Thus, the issue of mental health support and suicide prevention necessarily requires an integrated prevention response that acknowledges both the separateness of mental illness and suicide, and the association between the two.

Visa reviews for refugees and asylum seekers are handled by immigration authorities. Procedural delays and the fragmented way in which some reviews are undertaken leave many asylum seekers disillusioned and suspicious of the processes and sceptical of the outcome. It is important for both mental health professionals and migration agents/lawyers to be aware of these and other stressors that might impact upon refugees and asylum seekers.

Mental health supports with migration agent/lawyer consultation

With the nexus between mental health need and migration support so apparent, advocacy is an increasing feature of a carefully crafted caring response to assist asylum seekers.

It is recommended that asylum seekers who are given mental health services have them provided in conjunction with their migration agent/lawyer consultation. Indirect questioning and more attention being given to an asylum seeker's expression and explanation of personal narrative, metaphor and symbolism will help feelings to be articulated and promote a caring, supportive framework. This framework can provide an important backdrop for feelings to be received, lives revealed and cultural injunctions towards building resilience in order to continue moving forward through legal processes.

Mental health support with migration agent/lawyer consultation will help in a variety of ways:

- providing asylum seekers with a confidential relationship within which they are able to disclose personal circumstances in privacy, without fear that others may use such information to their detriment;
- providing opportunities for a closer relationship to develop between the mental health professional, migration agent/lawyer and asylum seeker;
- providing an important forum for discussing how relationships with others (such as volunteer support workers during application and review processes) can be strengthened, strategically focused and, as appropriate, sustained with the intensity they sometimes require over a lengthy, indefinite period of time.[36]

In addition, individual mental health support and migration agent/lawyer consultation can be conducted to match the asylum seeker's pace of learning what practical help is needed to advance legal processes. This is particularly suited to asylum seekers who, due to their length of time since being released from immigration detention, cope poorly with re-interviewing by immigration authorities and struggle to attain new ways of coping; such issues can be difficult for both the mental health clinician and migration agent/lawyer. This is especially important for asylum seekers who are contemplating suicide, who are suffering from poor concentration or who may be distracted by the complexity of interactions that can take place in group settings.

Finally, individual mental health support and migration agent/lawyer consultation may be useful for individuals who feel they need to differentiate themselves from others in group situations in order to feel they can be understood and helped – for example, those who have different political views or whose English-language skills are better than those of other asylum seekers.

What effect has the information contained so far in this chapter had on your feelings about asylum seekers and refugees?

COMMUNITY MENTAL HEALTH SUPPORT: OVERVIEW OF GENERAL PRINCIPLES

This section uses the term 'social intervention' for interventions that primarily aim to have positive social effects, and the term 'mental health intervention' is used for interventions that primarily aim to have positive mental health effects. The Constitution of the World Health Organization (1946) defines health as 'a state of complete physical, mental and social well-being, and not merely the absence of disease or infirmity'.[37] This chapter uses this definition as an anchor point and, at the same time, acknowledges that social interventions have secondary mental health effects and that mental health interventions have social effects, as the term 'psychosocial' suggests.

Community mental health should involve the following elements:

1. Preparation beforehand, including: (i) development of a system of coordination with specific focal persons responsible within each relevant organization; (ii) design of detailed plans to prepare for adequate social and mental health response; and (iii) education and training of relevant personnel in indicated social and psychological interventions.

2. Assessment and planning for the local context (i.e. cultural beliefs, setting, history and nature of mental health problems, family perceptions of distress and illness, ways of coping, resources within the community network, etc.). Planning should include quantitative assessment of disability and/or daily functioning as well as qualitative dimensions of context. When assessment uncovers a broad range of needs that are unlikely to be met, assessment reports should specify urgency of needs, local community resources and potential external resources.

3. Collaborative interventions, involving consultations and engagement between migration agents and/or lawyers, mental health workers and immigration officials and their contractors, non-government organizations and supporters working in the area, are essential to ensure sustainability. A multitude of agencies operating in a synchronized fashion will prevent wastage of valuable resources and help bring benefit to the asylum seeker.

Managing inter-agency conflict

An important consideration regarding mental health services for refugees and asylum seekers is potential conflict concerning assessment and care planning. This makes breakdown of communication and deadlock between people and organizations a very real possibility. The implications of this can be catastrophic – especially when the issue (e.g. admission to hospital) is time-sensitive. However, resolving the problem early on is ultimately more desirable in a health service where many issues have significant implications for interrelated parts of service provision.

When people collaborate more freely and openly, they are more likely to trust each other. When people trust their organizations, they are more likely to give of themselves in anticipation of future change and reward.[38] Knowledge of these and other interventions for people released from immigration detention are important for human service and health professionals because they are fundamental to the delivery of clinically relevant integrated services.

Emergency mental health strategies when application for asylum is rejected

In the event of a claim for asylum being rejected, evidence of previous behaviour may indicate that the impact on individuals or the family will be negative and place them at risk. The choice of intervention will vary with the phase and personal impact/severity of the rejection. The acute emergency phase is defined here as the period where the crude morbidity rate is elevated and the risk of self-injurious behaviour or harm to others is extreme. This period is followed by a reconsolidation phase when fundamental needs are again at a level comparable to that prior to the emergency.[39] There are a number of valuable early mental health interventions in the acute phase:

1. Establish and maintain contact with an interpreter and emergency mental health worker to manage urgent psychiatric crises (i.e. dangerousness to self or others, psychoses, severe depression, mania). If an individual has any pre-existing mental illness, sudden discontinuation of medication should be avoided (see chapter 47).

2. Acute interventions due to exposure to extreme stressors may be best managed without medication by following the principles of 'mental health first aid' in order to preserve life where a person may be a danger to themselves and/or others; to prevent major or permanent damage to a person's emotional health and well-being; and to prevent deterioration and promote recovery.[40] These principles involve: listening, conveying compassion, assessing needs, ensuring basic physical needs are met, not forcing talking, providing or mobilizing company from significant trusted others, encouraging but not forcing social support, and protecting from further harm.

3. Be cautious in the approach to an individual or family, particularly if the person is not known to the worker or interpreter, or the situation or environment is unfamiliar. Speak in a calm voice, saying that you are not here to hurt anyone and your actions are to help this person. Ask yourself the following questions:[40]
   'Am I in immediate danger?'
   'Is the person in any immediate danger?' (e.g. standing near a road or a dangerous object – actual or potential).
   'Is anyone else in immediate danger – especially children or other vulnerable people?'

'Can I safely remove a third person from danger?'
'Can I safely communicate with this person in his/her preferred language?'[40]

Valuable early social interventions may include establishing and disseminating an ongoing reliable flow of credible, accurate written and verbal information on: (i) the application process; (ii) efforts to establish the physical safety of self and family (if a family situation); and (iii) information on efforts being made by each organization or individual to help and support the person. Information should be disseminated in an uncomplicated manner and in a language most familiar to the individual and their family (i.e. understandable to a local 12-year-old) and empathic (showing understanding of the situation).

Assuming the availability of trusted others, it may be useful to organize non-intrusive emotional support and personal safety built around the above principles of mental health first aid. Due to the possible negative effects, it is not advisable to organize forms of single-session psychological debriefing that push people to share personal experiences beyond what they would naturally share.[41]

RESEARCH WITH REFUGEES AND ASYLUM SEEKERS

An important consideration when providing services to refugees and asylum seekers is research and evaluation of clinical effectiveness. Research that adopts an iterative consent process[42] is recommended, as it is participatory in nature. This means that at each point of the research and evaluation process, refugees and asylum seekers as community participants are active in reviewing the aims and objectives of the project and consent to participation is confirmed or rejected. Where possible, this should involve those refugees and asylum seekers who have a lived experience of mental illness and/or of being a mental health service user. Revising the aims, purposes and permissions of a research project with service users from refugee and asylum seeker backgrounds provides an additional opportunity to discuss and clarify information in an incremental and participative way as required. This open and participatory approach keeps the 'door open' for community participants to make informed choices about whether or not to continue with the project, decline to participate further or withdraw altogether. To enable meaningful engagement in research, it is important that refugees and asylum seekers are provided with sufficient time to consider being involved in, and becoming involved in, a project. Other considerations include issues related to accessibility, such as ensuring an interpreter is available (if required), and the importance of building rapport with community leaders to establish trust in the particular project.

It is also important to take into account the way in which past experiences can have a profound impact on how services are perceived now and in the future. For this reason, a non-probing, gentle and supportive inquiry[43] is the preferred method for engaging service users. For service users who have first-hand experience of system interaction with family or significant others, there may also be particular needs and considerations, such as feeling marginalized or let down.[44] Care should be taken by the researcher to prevent distressing symptoms or experiences (e.g. previous trauma) from resurfacing. Support and advocacy should be given as required (e.g. making a referral to a collaborating transcultural and/or community mental health centre).

REFLECTION

- What specific skills or qualities do you think people who work with refugees or asylum seekers need?

- Which of these skills or qualities do you currently have?

- To what extent do you have these skills and qualities?

- How might you develop them further? For those skills or qualities that you could develop further, what are some strategies or experiences that might help you to do this?

CONCLUSION

Globalization and the mass movement of people worldwide is an unavoidable side effect of war, trauma and regional dislocation. The provision of adequate resources through delivery of clinically relevant, integrated mental health support services is fundamental to prevent risk to refugees and asylum seekers. Continuity and integration of mental health care involving key stakeholders is best achieved by bridging the separate elements in the asylum seeker journey through preparing for visa appeals, visa reviews, news from home and ongoing psychosocial stressors – in the context of different episodes, interventions by different providers, and changes in mental health and well-being. Input from supportive networks that build resilience intrinsically over time is crucial as it sustains, for example, supportive interpersonal relationships and therapeutic care plans. To help strengthen continuity and integration of mental health supports for refugees and asylum seekers, well-resourced care must be experienced as culturally competent and appropriate. This will help provide refugees and asylum seekers with a sense of mental health care as connected and coherent. A fundamental aspect of the craft of caring for refugees and asylum seekers is the ability to synthesize different viewpoints to create culturally appropriate workable solutions.

References

1. UNHCR (United Nations High Commission for Refugees). *Populations of concern to UNHCR. UNHCR Global Report 2015*. Available from: http://www.unhcr.org/publications/fundraising/574ed5234/unhcr-global-report-2015-populations-concern-unhcr.html?query=populations of concern 2015 [Accessed 2nd August 2016].

2. International Refugee Rights Initiative. *The 1951 Convention relating to the status of refugees and its 1967 protocol.* 1951. Available from: http://www.refugeelegalaidinformation.org/1951-convention [Accessed 3rd August 2016].

3. UNHCR (United Nations High Commission for Refugees). Global trends: forced displacement in 2015 UNHCR asylum trends 2013: levels and trends in industrialized countries. 2014. Available from: http://www.unhcr.org/statistics/unhcrstats/576408cd7/unhcr-global-trends-2015.html [Accessed 2nd August 2016].

4. Giddens A. *Runaway world: how globalisation is reshaping our lives*. London: Profile Books, 1999.

5. Apparduari A. Globalisation and the research imagination. *International Social Science Journal* 1999; **51**: 229–38.

6. Australian Health Ministers. *Australian Health Ministers National Mental Health Plan 2003–2008*. Canberra: Australian Government, 2003.

7. Steel Z, Chey T, Silove D, Marnane C, Bryant RA, van Ommeren M. Association of torture and other potentially traumatic events with mental health outcomes among populations exposed to mass conflict and displacement: a systematic review and meta-analysis. *Journal of the American Medical Association* 2009; **302**: 537–49.

8. Lindencrona F, Ekblad S, Hauff E. Mental health of recently resettled refugees from the Middle East in Sweden: the impact of pre-resettlement trauma, resettlement stress and capacity to handle stress. *Social Psychiatry and Psychiatric Epidemiology* 2008; **43**: 121–31.

9. Fazel M, Wheeler J, Danesh J. Prevalence of serious mental disorder in 7000 refugees in western countries: a systematic review. *Lancet* 2005; **365** (9467); 1309–14.

10. Procter NG, Williamson P, Gordon A, McDonough D. Refugee and asylum seeker self harm with implications for transition to employment participation: a review. *Suicidologi* 2011; **16**(3): 30–8.

11. Procter NG, Babakarkhil A, Baker A, Ferguson M. Mental health of people of migrant and refugee background. In: Procter NG, Hamer H, McGarry D, Wilson R, Froggatt T (eds). *Mental health: a person centred approach*. Melbourne: Cambridge University Press, 2014: 197–216.

12. Minas H, Kakuma R, Too LS, Vayani H, Orapeleng S, Prasad-Ildes P, Turner G, Procter NG, Oehm D. Mental health research and evaluation in multicultural Australia: developing a culture of inclusion. *International Journal of Mental Health Systems* 2013; **7**(23): 1–25.

13. Fazel M, Reed RV, Panter-Brick C, Stein A. Mental health of displaced and refugee children resettled in high-income countries: risk and protective factors. *Lancet* 2012; **379**(9812): 266–82.

14. Kessler RC, McLaughlin KA, Green JG, Gruber MJ, Sampson NA, Zaslavsky AM, Aguilar-Gaxiola S, Alhamzawi AO, Alonso J, Angermeyer M, Benjet C, Bromet E, Chatterji S, de Girolamo G, Demyttenaere K, Fayyad J, Florescu S, Gal G, Gureje O, Haro JM, Hu CY, Karam EG, Kawakami N, Lee S, Lépine JP, Ormel J, Posada-Villa J, Sagar R, Tsang A, Üstün TB, Vassilev S, Viana MC, Williams DR. Childhood adversities and adult psychopathology in the WHO World Mental Health Surveys. *British Journal of Psychiatry* 2010; **197**(5): 378–85.

15. Fryers T, Brugha T. Childhod determinants of adult psychiatric disorder. *Clinical Practice & Epidemiology in Mental Health* 2013; **9**: 1–50.

16. Lustig SL, Kia-Keating M, Knight WG, Geltman P, Ellis H, Kinzie JD, Keane T, Saxe GN. Review of child and adolescent refugee mental health. *Journal of the American Academy of Child and Adolescent Psychiatry* 2004; **43**: 24–36.

17. Kelbie P. The life and death of an asylum seeker. *Independent* 2004; 29 May: 1–2.

18. Procter NG. They first killed his heart (then) he took his own life. Part 1: a review of the context and literature on mental health issues for refugees and asylum seekers. *International Journal of Nursing Practice* 2005; **11**: 286–91.

19. Procter NG. They first killed his heart (then) he took his own life. Part 2: practice implications. *International Journal of Nursing Practice* 2006; **12**(1): 42–8.

20. Deans AK, Boerma CJ, Fordyce J, De Souza M, Palmer DJ, Davis JS. Use of Royal Darwin Hospital emergency department by immigration detainees in 2011. *Medical Journal of Australia* 2013; **199**(11); 776–8.

21. Mental Health in Multicultural Australia 2014. *Framework for mental health in* multicultural Australia: towards culturally inclusive service delivery. 2014. Available from: http://framework.mhima.org.au/framework/index.htm [Accessed 4th June 2016].

22. Nguyen HT, Yamada AM, Dinh TQ. Religious leaders' assessment and attribution of the causes of mental illness: an in-depth exploration of Vietnamese American Buddhist leaders. *Mental Health Religion & Culture* 2012; **15**: 511–27.

23. Eisenbruch M. *The lens of culture, the lens of health: toward a framework and toolkit for cultural competence*. Sydney, Australia: Centre for Ethnicity and Health, University of New South Wales, 2004.

24. Kleinman A, Seeman D. Personal experience and illness. In: Albrecht GL, Fitzpatrick R, Scrimshaw SC (eds). *Handbook of social studies in health and medicine*. London: Sage, 2000: 230–43.

25. Procter NG. Mental health and human connectedness for all Australians. Paper presented at the 55th Annual Oration, The Great Hall, University of Sydney: Sydney, Australia: College of Nursing Australia, 2007.

26. Multicultural Mental Health in Australia 2004. *Cultural awareness questions and language competency tips*. 2004. Available from: http://www.mhima.org.au/Default.aspx?PageID=6320437&A=SearchResult&SearchID=33179040&ObjectID=6320437&ObjectType=1 [Accessed 4th June 2016].

27. Brown SM, Baker CN, Wilcox P. Risking connection trauma training: a pathway toward trauma-informed care in child congregate care settings. *Psychological Trauma: Theory, Research, Practice, and Policy* 2012; **4**: 507–15.

28. Elliot DE, Bjelajac P, Fallot RD, Markoff LS, Reed BD. Trauma-informed or trauma-denied: principles and implementation of trauma-informed services for women. *Journal of Community Psychology* 2005; **33**: 461–77.

29. Procter NG. Paper plates and throw away cutlery. 2014. Available from: http://www.safecom.org.au/procter1.htm [Accessed 3rd August 2016].

30. Shannon P, O'Dougherty M, Mehta E. Refugees' perspectives on barriers to communication about trauma histories in primary care. *Mental Health in Family Medicine* 2012; **9**: 47–55.

31. Rudd MD, Joiner TE, Rajab MH. *Treating suicidal behaviour: an effective, time limited approach*. London: Guilford Press, 2001.

32. Great Britain, Parliament, Joint Committee on Human Rights, Dismore A. *The treatment of asylum seekers: tenth report of session 2006–07*. London: Stationery Office, 2007. Available from:

http://www.publications.parliament.uk/pa/jt200607/jtselect/jtrights/81/81i.pdf [Accessed 3rd August 2016].

33. Herlihy J, Scragg P, Turner S. Discrepancies in autobiographical memory – implications for the assessment of asylum seekers: repeated interviews study. *British Medical Journal* 2002; **324**: 324–7.

34. Cantor CH, Neulinger K, Roth J, Spinks D. The epidemiology of suicide and attempted suicide among young Australians. In: Commonwealth Department of Health and Aged Care (ed.). *Setting the evidence-based research agenda for Australia: a literature review. National youth suicide prevention strategy.* Canberra: Commonwealth of Australia, 2000: 1–112.

35. Hassan R. *Suicide explained: the Australian experience.* Melbourne: Melbourne University Press, 1995.

36. Procter NG. Support for temporary protection visa holders: partnering individual mental health support with migration law consultation. *Psychiatry, Psychology and Law* 2004; **11**: 110–12.

37. WHO (World Health Organization). Health. 2014. Available from: http://www.who.int/trade/glossary/story046/en/ [Accessed 4th June 2016].

38. Weiss J, Hughes J. Want collaboration? Accept and actively manage conflict. *Harvard Business Review* 2005; March: 92–101.

39. WHO (World Health Organization). *Mental health in emergencies, mental and social aspects of health of populations exposed to extreme stressors.* Geneva: Department of Mental Health and Substance Dependence, World Health Organization, 2003.

40. Myhill K, Tobin M. *Mental health first aid for South Australians.* Adelaide, Australia: Mental Health Unit, Department of Human Services, 2001.

41. McFarlane AC. Debriefing: care and sympathy are not enough (Editorial). *Medical Journal of Australia* 2003; **178**: 533–4.

42. Procter NG. *Speaking of sadness and the heart of acceptance: reciprocity in education.* Sydney, Australia: Multicultural Mental Health Australia, 2004.

43. Mitchell TL, Radford JL. Rethinking research relationships in qualitative research. *Canadian Journal of Community Mental Health* 1996; **15**: 49–60.

44. Marshall SL, While AE. Interviewing respondents who have English as a second language: challenges encountered and suggestions for other researchers. *Journal of Advanced Nursing* 1994; **19**: 566–71.

Further reading

Baker A, Procter NG, Ferguson M. Engaging with culturally and linguistically diverse communities to reduce the impact of depression and anxiety: a review of current evidence. *Health and Social Care in the Community.* 2016; **24**: 386–398.

Kenny M, Procter NG. The fast track refugee assessment process and mental health of vulnerable asylum seekers. *Psychiatry, Psychology and Law* 2015; **23**: 62–68.

Posselt M, Procter NG, Galletly C, de Crespigny C. Merging perspectives: obstacles to recovery for youth from refugee backgrounds with comorbidity. *Australasian Psychiatry* 2015; **23**: 293–9.

Posselt M, Procter NG, Galletly C, de Crespigny C. Aetiology of coexisting mental health and alcohol and other drug disorders: perspectives of refugees and service providers. *Australian Psychologist* 2015; **50**: 130–40.

Procter NG, De Leo D, Newman, L. Suicide and self-harm prevention for detainees in immigration detention. *Medical Journal of Australia* 2013; **199**(11): 730–2.

Relevant web pages

Australasian Society for Traumatic Stress Studies. http://www.astss.org.au/

Canadian Council for Refugees. http://ccrweb.ca/

Multicultural Mental Health Resource Centre. http://www.multiculturalmentalhealth.ca/

Scottish Refugee Council. http://www.scottishrefugeecouncil.org.uk/

UK Refugee Council. http://www.refugeecouncil.org.uk/

Victorian Transcultural Mental Health (VTMH). http://www.vtmh.org.au/

Working with Interpreters. http://www.multicultural.sa.gov.au/new-migrants/language-support

Section 6

Opportunities and challenges for mental health nursing in the twenty-first century

Mental health, the law and human rights

MICHAEL HAZELTON AND PETER MORRALL

LEARNING OUTCOMES

- To be aware of the impact of human rights legislation on changes in mental health policy and practice locally and internationally.

- To understand the ways in which mental health legislation is designed to protect public safety.

- To have an overview of the changes in the relationship between mental illness and personal liberty over time.

- To understand the reasons why it can be difficult to achieve the aims of mental health reforms.

- To be aware of similarities and differences in how mental health and human rights policy and legislation operate in different countries.

SUMMARY OF KEY POINTS

- Human rights continue to be a complex and unsettled issue in mental health nationally and internationally.

- Human rights and legislation are intertwined with regard to mental health.

- An understanding of the historical and cultural background to human rights and the law can strengthen significantly the craft of care, and a comparison between England and Australia serves as a useful exposition of that significance.

INTRODUCTION

It is difficult to escape concluding that the single most pathogenic factor in the causation of mental illness is how we as humans mistreat each other.[1] (p.23)

This chapter focuses on mental health human and legal rights as well as related policies. It begins with an overview of the worldwide situation. Then it provides an account of the historical and present situation in England and that in Australia. England has been selected as a nation state with origins in the 'old world', while Australia is included for its 'new world' or postcolonial status. Importantly, both countries have placed considerable political emphasis on mental health reform in recent decades. Knowledge of historical, contemporary and cross-societal conditions and contexts of mental health law and its connection with human rights is crucial to the crafting of care.

OVERVIEW

Psychological predicaments, whether construed as disorders (also illnesses and diseases), problems with living, social deviances or phenomenological events, affect a huge number of people throughout the world. If such difficulties are understood as disorders, then collectively they have become one of the most, if not the most, serious health issue globally.

Take the example of schizophrenia, (chapter 24) only one of the mental disorders from the hundreds listed in the two formal medical classification schemas (see chapter 12). These are the fifth edition of the American Psychiatric Association's *Diagnostic and statistical manual of mental disorders* (DSM-V)[2] and the tenth revision of the World Health Organization's (WHO) *International statistical classification of diseases and related health problems* (ICD-10).[3] On annual World Mental Health Day in 2014, in a 'fact sheet' entitled 'Living with schizophrenia', the WHO made available to the media statistics about this disorder's incidence, morbidity and mortality, as well as the associated discrimination and human rights abuse:

- Schizophrenia is a severe mental disorder affecting more than 21 million people worldwide…
- Worldwide, schizophrenia is associated with considerable disability and may affect educational and occupational performance.
- People with schizophrenia are 2–2.5 times more likely to die early than the general population. This is often due to physical illnesses, such as cardiovascular, metabolic and infectious diseases…
- Stigma, discrimination and violation of human rights of people with schizophrenia is common.[4]

An international congress held in 2014 and organized by the World Federation for Mental Health (WFMH) and the Hellenic Psychiatric Association focused on the theme of that year's Mental Health Day. Professor George Christodoulou,[5] president of the WFMH, observed in his preface to the congress that improvements in care for people with schizophrenia have been halted or reversed in many countries due to the consequences of the economic crisis of 2007/08. Christodoulou mentions specifically the continued 'psychological pain' experienced by people diagnosed with schizophrenia: 'The pain is coupled with a perception of social isolation produced by the stigma attached to persons with schizophrenia and the resulting institutional way of treatment that still prevails in many parts of the world'[5] (p.3).

Aside from schizophrenia, anxiety (chapter 20) and depression (chapter 21) appear to be reaching epidemic proportions in countries which are economically developed and emerging. The Anxiety and Depression Association of America[6] points out that anxiety disorders are the most common form of mental disorder in the USA. At any one time 40 million adults are suffering from one form or other of anxiety. That is 18 per cent of the US population. Fifteen million USA citizens suffer from a major depressive disorder. That is nearly 7 per cent of the USA population. Furthermore, more than 800,000 people globally commit suicide. Twenty times more are estimated to have attempted suicide.[7] In China approximately 260 million people have been estimated as suffering from either a mild or major depressive disorder, with about a quarter-of-a-million suicides occurring annually. Each year depression/suicide costs the Chinese economy approximately US$8.35 billion.[8] Chinese economist Mao Yushi, in his book *Where does Chinese people's anxiety come from?*, published in 2013, claims that half the people of China feel more anxious than they did 5 years ago.[9] He suggests that this is due to social injustices such as the gap between the rich and the poor, an increasingly difficult job market and employment conditions, corruption, and the existence of a powerful and privileged dominant class.

Therefore, hundreds of millions of people worldwide at any given point in time are affected by mental difficulties which are diagnosed as a mental disorder or are experienced as disruptive to everyday functioning but without medical intervention being available, requested or enforced.[10] Moreover, many mental disorders continue to result in personal and social stigma, and the neglect of personal care and legal entitlements. Legal and human rights violations of people with mental and psychosocial disability are routinely reported in many if not most countries. These vary from minor to major infringements, including unmitigated cruelty and abandonment, sexual exploitation, authorized physical restraint and seclusion, inadequate and inappropriate medical treatment and inattention to basic needs regarding nutrition, privacy and hygiene.[11] Unless a country or region is subjected to dictatorial and undemocratic rule affecting all of the population, there are expected and routine social, cultural, civil and political entitlements, such as access to education, housing and employment, and the opportunity to marry, to have children and to vote. These entitlements have been ratified by various international treaties including the Convention on the Rights of Persons with Disabilities.[12] For people suffering from mental disorders, these entitlements are routinely inaccessible.[10]

Few countries have fully fledged and fully operative mental health policies, let alone a legal/rights framework or a suitable supply of medical and nursing staff.[13,10,11] Furthermore, warfare, civil strife and ecological disasters are increasingly recognized as undermining the mental health status of the affected populations, including the combatants involved directly in armed conflict, and emergency services personnel who deal with the aftermath of environmental disasters. Rates of mental disorder are likely to double following such conflicts and disasters.[11]

Referring to the WHO's long-term international plan, inaugurated in 2013, to remedy prejudice and malice towards mentally disordered people, Margaret Chan, director-general of the WHO has stated:

> *In the light of widespread human rights violations and discrimination experienced by people with mental disorders, a human rights perspective is essential in responding to the global burden of mental disorders. The action plan emphasizes the need for services, policies, legislation, plans, strategies and programmes to protect, promote and respect the rights of persons with mental disorders*

> *in line with the International Covenant on Civil and Political Rights, the International Covenant on Economic, Social and Cultural Rights, the Convention on the Rights of Persons with Disabilities, the Convention on the Rights of the Child and other relevant international and regional human rights instruments.*[10] *(p.7)*

There is, therefore, an admission by the WHO and the WFMH that well into the twenty-first century mental health policies and legislation to ameliorate human rights have failed to be generated, or, where generated and implemented, have failed to be effective.

ENGLAND

Humans have settled in various parts of the British Isles for tens of thousands of years, and various waves of immigration have continued up to the present time. However, it was not until the arrival in the fifth century of what became and remains its core tribe(s) – the Anglo-Saxons – that an 'English nation' began to emerge. The influence of the Anglo-Saxons was to spread beyond the boundaries of England's geopolitical area and into the east of Scotland.[14] Centuries later, the influence of England was to spread throughout the world. It became a major imperial power, the first industrialized nation, and the driving force of the British Empire on which 'the sun never set'.[15,16] Today England, as a constituent country of the UK, and notwithstanding likely exit from the European Union, is fully embedded in the global capitalist trade, its capital London is a key international financial services centre, it has the sixth-largest economy in the world, its language has become the international language for business and commerce, and dozens of countries continue to use its core tenets of jurisprudence in their legal systems.

The influence of England on the management of madness has also been significant. England's management of the mad (both care and control) was transported (literally and conceptually) to many parts of the world, as was its mental health legislation. Moreover, the signing of Magna Carta at Runnymede in England by King John 800 years ago signalled the beginning of political change which would increasingly enshrine more and more human rights for more and more people. This influence was to spread throughout the English-speaking world and was to impact on the formulation of the American Constitution.[17] However, England's prowess politically, economically, culturally and in relation to the law and human rights generally has not been replicated in the field of mental health.

History

The management of madness has a long history. Protecting the human rights of the mad has a relatively short history.

Whether by 'amateurs' (in families and communities) or 'professionals' (in institutions and the community) the mentally deviant have been admonished, denigrated, restrained, secluded, excluded and medicalized. Troublesome and troubled people (the disturbed, dangerous and disruptive) have succumbed to all manner of management, involving a fantastic array of implements and impositions aimed at, but only rarely achieving, changes to their human performance (their thoughts, behaviours and emotions). Examples include whips, shackles, cold water, rotating machines, bloodletting, purges, emetics, exercise, 'moral' labour, electricity, an ever-expanding range of pharmaceuticals and latterly a plethora of psychotherapies.[18,19] The realities of having to control the most disturbed, disruptive and dangerous of the mad were to affect the nature of policies and practices of the 'professionals', and were the main reason for their creation. That is, without a society being troubled by madness, the amateurs would have remained in charge of the management of madness.

Medical management of madness has been in existence, either bubbling in the background or fermenting in the foreground, for thousands of years.[18] In the Greco-Roman Empires, madness was considered a disease and thereby the province of those practising medicine. During medieval times in Europe and in the Middle East, medical opinion existed alongside, although dominated by, religious and folk notions of madness. But by the end of the nineteenth century in the West, medical domination of madness had become virtually absolute. Notwithstanding challenges from other disciplines and epistemologies purporting to deviate from the medicalized management of madness, this remains the case today. Furthermore, advances in medical diagnostic technology, psychopharmacology and psychosurgery, the embracing by psychiatry of talking therapies, together with the *de facto* if resentful compliance of psychiatric–mental health nursing, and the capitulation of clinical psychologists and psychotherapists to the 'power of psychiatry' (because they do not offer radical alternatives), medical control over madness and the mad business is once again in the ascendancy.

Compared with medicine, the law has been a relative latecomer to the management of madness. Indeed, it has been medical involvement in madness that has necessitated the expansion of legalized control. Moreover, it was the surge in the formal and institutionalized segregation of the mad during the nineteenth century that necessitated an expansion of medical and legal collusion to control this form of social deviance. Specific legislation was then enacted, rather than relying on local convention or criminal law.

Although most mad people were cared for by families if they were not troublesome, or simply roamed from place to place, community-based segregation had been advocated for troublesome mad people in ancient society. For example, Plato advised that 'if a man is mad' (no mention is made of mad women), his family must prevent injury to himself, to others and to property by keeping him at home.[20]

European laws in the Middle Ages were not consistent within each country and were influenced substantially by religious beliefs and decrees. This meant that madness was vulnerable to being perceived as witchcraft.[21] Such a label could have far worse consequences for the accused (torture, damnation and execution) than being left to roam or being confined.

Before the seventeenth century in England the troublesome mad, if not controlled by their families, were sent to bridewells (Tudor 'houses of correction'), common gaols and workhouses. The legislation that impelled this type of incarceration was not designed to deal with madness, but to punish the 'indolent' sections of the working class and serve as a warning to others that life would be hard if work was not found.[22] The building of workhouses began in the 1630s. The Poor Law Act of 1601 gave the responsibility to every English parish for the elderly, the sick, idiots and lunatics within its borders. The Act of Settlement of 1662 restricted what was already very limited support for only those who were bona fide residents. If such social deviants could not be encouraged to leave a parish, then they were sent to the workhouses along with the unemployed.

Institutional segregation began in England in the thirteenth century, when the religious order St Mary of Bethlehem of London ('Bedlam'), which was already providing care for the physically sick, began to accept the mad.[23] Other institutions were set up in continental Europe by the beginning of the Renaissance in the fifteenth century. For Michel Foucault, the seventeenth century was the age of the 'Great Confinement'.[24] For example, 6,000 mad people were incarcerated in the Hôpital Général de Paris, and incarceration of the mad was then to spread throughout France.

But the 'Great Confinement' came later in England. Apart from Bedlam, there were commercially run madhouses in the seventeenth century, but these were in the main for the 'wealthy mad'. By the eighteenth century the 'poor mad' might enter one of the newly created charitable voluntary asylums. John Perceval, son of the only British prime minister to be assassinated (Spencer Perceval), was incarcerated in a private asylum near Bristol from 1830 to 1832, having been diagnosed with what would now be considered schizophrenia. He wrote a remarkable account of his loss of liberty in a book entitled *Perceval's narrative*:

Now with regard to my treatment, I have to make at first two general observations ... First, the suspicion and the fact of being incapable of reasoning correctly, or deranged in understanding, justified apparently every person who came near me, in dealing with me also in a manner contrary to reason and contrary to nature ... Secondly, my being likely to attack the rights of others gave these individuals license, in every respect, to trample upon mine ... Instead of great scrupulousness being observed in depriving me of any liberty or privilege ... on the just ground, that for the safety of society my valuable rights were already taken away, on every occasion, in every dispute, in every argument, the assumed premise immediately acted upon was, that I was to yield, my desires to be aside, my few remaining privileges to be infringed upon for the convenience of others.[25]

REFLECTION

Describe the ways in which John Perceval's liberty would have been restricted within this nineteenth-century asylum. How is the liberty of patients residing in a twenty-first-century mental health ward/unit restricted?

It was, however, not until the nineteenth century that confinement ('asylumdom'),[26] not just of the troublesome mad but as a potential option for anyone troubled by psychological distress, became widespread. The Lunacy Act 1845 in England forced local authorities to provide for the mad through a massive public building programme. Asylums were to house more than 100,000 inmates by 1900. Moreover, these public asylums were given wide legal powers to compulsorily detain the mad.[22]

The designation of insanity had, ever since the Middle Ages, caused a dilemma for the law. The notion that the mad were not 'human', but essentially 'beasts', was common. As such, it was thought that they should logically be treated differently by the courts from other social deviants (for example, criminals). But for much of the period prior to asylumdom, there was no or little specialist mental health policy, let alone legislation.[27]

In England asylumdom was not instigated by the medical profession.[20,28] Doctors were not regarded as having effective remedies for madness. They were, as local notables, invited by the local authorities to act as administrators. Incarceration was perhaps for years, if not life, and inmates were exposed to horrendously callous treatments.[18] Today such lengthy confinement and bizarre management of the mad seems to be an inexcusable abuse of human rights. But the asylums had been built not only to separate the mad from the 'normals' but also to provide what was considered at the time humane care. In comparison with how the majority of the population lived in the nineteenth century, those in the asylum (usually) received food, shelter and medical attention (albeit rather primitive). Philanthropy and kindness co-existed with eugenics and cruelty.

The Victorian asylums, and those of the twentieth century, were an enormous financial investment, which could not be replicated today (see also chapter 4). They reflected high ideals. The mad could partake of fresh air in rural surroundings, in the extensive grounds and gardens that most of the asylums had procured.[29] Food and water were comparatively fresh, clean and nutritious. Recreation and rest were encouraged.

The profession of medicine had by the end of the nineteenth century monopolized the market in madness, having successfully neutralized the challenge from the Quakers who had set up alternative institutions based on 'moral therapy'.[20] Psychiatry was well established as a medical arena of expertise, and madness had become as much an 'illness' or 'disorder' as pneumonia or malaria. Legislation for the control of the mad had become highly specialized to authenticate the mass segregation of the mad. Institutional segregation and the law provided a captive audience on whom doctors could experiment and thereby develop their subspecialty of psychiatry.

Present

By the middle of the twentieth century, various social, technological and economic changes were affecting where and how the mad were to live. The discovery of antipsychotic drugs, the unsustainable financial burden of running what were now 'mental hospitals', along with a general shift in Western culture towards greater tolerance and liberty, and a score of reports about cruelty inflicted on the residents of these institutions, heralded widespread decarceration.[26,30] While not articulated as such, mental health law was supporting the human rights of the mad to live in mainstream society, and this trend for legislation to emphasize respect for the mad was occurring throughout Europe, North America and Australasia. Psychiatry's dominant position in the management of madness was undermined at this stage. The anti-psychiatry movement, social work, psychology, psychotherapy and psychiatric nursing were all vying for the top position in the hierarchy of disciplines managing madness. However, the power of psychiatry has since been boosted considerably by the arrival of new psycho-pharmacological products, the development of sophisticated diagnostic technology, improved dexterity in wielding the scalpel within the cerebral cortex, and the accomplishment of the genome map. Moreover, psychiatry was able to manoeuvre the management of madness to its benefit by replicating in the community its professional dominance founded in the asylums.[31] By embracing the regular scientific outpourings from genetics and neurology and new therapies and theories such as neo-Darwinism and cognitive-behaviourism, and authoring comprehensive and systematized diagnostic schemata (the latest of which is the DSM-V[2] of 2013), the status of psychiatry appears more assured than emasculated wherever it operates.

However, community care as a policy in England developed into a disaster with regard to the basic human rights of people diagnosed as mentally disordered. The failings of community care can largely be attributed to the failure of government to adhere to its financial obligation to use the funds previously used to support the operation of large institutions, so that local authorities could provide smaller forms of accommodation and appropriate staffing levels.[32] By the 1990s this failure had turned into a crisis in England and other countries where mass-scale decarceration had occurred.[31,33,13] Beyond the lack of funds to offer effective care in the community, inpatient facilities were also not adequately prepared or available to offer care for those mentally disordered people who needed intensive treatment and supervision. This resulted in seriously mentally disordered people living on the streets or in run-down bed-and-breakfast lodgings, or being admitted to prison. The crisis then became one of public and political confidence in mental health staff (principally psychiatrists and psychiatric–mental health nurses) to provide a competent service, particularly in relation to those who either were or were perceived to be dangerous.

The result of this crisis was a change in mental health law. The 2007 Mental Health Act (England and Wales) brought about measures intended to make it easier for staff to monitor people suffering from serious mental disorder living in the community, especially those considered dangerous. It also made it easier to forcibly remove from the community those in this group who were unable or unwilling to succumb to supervision and place them in secure accommodation. The mechanisms for dealing with dangerousness became 'community treatment orders', extra secure facilities and an increased use of compulsory admission and detention.

In 2014 the long-standing crisis in mental health care provision and practice was again being highlighted by politicians and practitioners. Between 2012 and 2104 in England seven people committed suicide and one homicide following difficulties accessing psychiatric inpatient care beds for mental health patients in crisis.[34,35] Pauline Binch was one of those who died:

Pauline Binch waited nine days for a bed – her husband John said 'she'd still be alive today if they'd found her a bed' … Following the fourth attempt to take her life, on 24 September [2013] her psychiatrist said that an inpatient admission was required and a request was sent to a bed manager. No bed was available between 24 and 29 September. On 30 September a bed did become available but the trust could not contact Pauline and that evening the bed was given to another patient. A bed was not found on 1, 2 or 3 October. At 20:45 BST on 3 October, Pauline's body was discovered at her home.[36]

Nearly 20,000 beds have been cut since 2011. This prompted the British government in 2014 to request health service agencies and clinicians' organizations to sign a 'Mental Health Crisis Care Concordat' which committed them to improving provision, intended to ensure that anyone in 'crisis' who needed care (particularly inpatient care) would have it supplied.[37] By that time, average inpatient occupancy was above 100 per cent.[34,35]

The Chief Medical Officer, in her 2014 annual report on public mental health priorities, pointed out the dire state of affairs in England regarding the 'gap' in care:

- There is a very significant overall treatment gap in mental healthcare in England, with about 75% of people with mental illness receiving no treatment at all.
- There has been a real-terms fall in investment of resources in mental health services in England since 2011.[38]

The Chief Executive and General Secretary of the Royal College of Nursing, Peter Carter, warned that mental health services were experiencing 'unprecedented strain' due to staff cuts and a shortage of inpatient accommodation, coinciding with a rise in demand for mental health services.[39]

During the year 2013/14, the new mental health act was used on more than 53,000 occasions to detain patients in NHS mental health inpatient care for longer than 72 hours. This represents more than a 10 per cent rise in detentions beyond 72 hours compared with the figure 10 years previously. A substantial rise in compulsory admissions to private hospitals has also taken place. In the year 2013/14 over 5,000 people were detained in non-NHS facilities. A further 4,500 were placed on community treatment orders during 2013/14, although this was lower than the previous year.[34,35]

In the year 2015 a general election took place in Britain. Mental health was high on the political agendas of many political parties. High-profile battles with mental health problems, such as those experienced by celebrities Stephen Fry and Ruby Wax, footballer Tony Adams, boxer Frank Bruno, journalist Alastair Campbell, and actor Catherine Zeta Jones, were prominent in media headlines. The deputy prime minister of the outgoing government, Nick Clegg, made a commitment to end the discrimination against mental health.[40] The introduction of access and waiting time targets for people with mental health problems in England was scheduled to start in April 2015 and was seen as the first step of reforming mental health services so that they share the same priority as physical health problems.

Yet despite the growth of empowerment and advocacy movements, 'consumer' representation within mental health services, publicity about the statistics indicating major deficiencies in mental health care, and the regular and escalating promises made by politicians, inpatient care and care in the community remain inadequate, inefficient and inexplicable.[41] Moreover, the chaos in care is connected to care-less control. The large number of mad people who have ended up in prison during the era of community care should be considered a major human rights imperfection. In a paradoxical reversal of history more and more mentally disordered people nowadays are becoming inadvertently criminalized, not only in England but in other Western countries as well.[42] These are the very countries that embarked on what was ostensibly a more humane approach to care than locking people away in 'human warehouses'.[26] An estimated 360,000 prisoners with serious mental illness reside in US jails at any one time.[42] Those not in prison may fare far worse: 'With no money, no place to live, and no treatment, people with mental illness ended up homeless, in the criminal justice system or dead'.[42]

This lack of choice other than prison has been attributed mainly to the de-institutionalization (or more accurately non-incarceration) of the mentally disordered, without comparative services becoming available in the community, along with a public response of 'not in my backyard'.

The Prisons and Probation Ombudsman's 2016 report for England and Wales comments that a high proportion of prisoners have a mental health problem, including personality disorder, psychosis, anxiety and depression, and drug/alcohol dependence.[43] Moreover, in England and Wales the suicide rate among prisoners, although it has been on a downward trend since the 1990s, remains significantly higher than that of the general population.[44]

Moving from basic human rights, such as having shelter other than prison, enough money to buy food and access to effective (mental) health provision, there are specific legal obligations to protect more than mere survival. It was 50 years after the passing of the Universal Declaration of Human Rights by the United Nations and the European Convention on Human Rights by the Council of Europe that England (and the rest of the UK) compiled its own human rights legislation,[45] therein providing qualified human rights for people with mental disorder.

First, the Act contains a principle of 'limited rights', meaning that 'persons of unsound mind' can be detained as long as the procedures used are legal. Second, there is a principle in the Act of 'qualified rights'. This determines that a person's private life can be interfered with 'for the protection of the rights and freedoms of others'. Compulsorily removing an individual from his or her home to enforce psychiatric treatment is therefore a possibility if he or she was deemed to be a risk to others or him-/herself. Third is the principle of 'proportionality'. This principle allows human rights to be interfered with, provided such interference is not arbitrary or unfair. That could result in the use of restraint and seclusion where this is viewed as necessary by the psychiatric staff. A fourth principle of the Act is that of 'incompatibility'. All present and future legislation has to be in accord with the Human Rights Act 1998.[46]

Furthermore, the Human Rights Act states that, before an individual can be compulsorily detained, a 'true' mental disorder must be established by 'objective' medical experts (Article 5). However, the Act omits to define mental disorder in any detail, and the inadequate defining of mental disorder also occurs in previous, present and impending mental health legislation. Moreover, it tautologically posits that the mental disorder must be of a kind or degree warranting compulsory confinement and that the validity of continued confinement depends on the persistence of such a mental disorder. There are also a number of exceptions to these specific conditions. For example, compulsory admission can occur in emergencies, and discharge may be deferred where there is 'public danger'.

But under Article 3 of the Human Rights Act there are no exclusions relating to mental disorder. This Article states that there must be 'freedom from torture and inhuman or degrading treatment or punishment'. It remains contentious whether or not compulsory detention, restraint, seclusion, enforced treatment and electroconvulsive therapy are inhuman and degrading or therapeutically necessary.

The Mental Health Act 2007 in particular impacts on the operation of the human rights legislation (and vice versa), along with concomitant local procedures, clinical practices

and technologies such as 'risk assessment', enforced treatment and electronic surveillance. Although mental health law has long been associated with control (of the mentally disordered for the protection of themselves and society), the 2007 Act is specifically attempting to resolve the tension between liberty and such control. On the control side is the increased surveillance of the mentally disordered living in the community, enabled by the introduction of community treatment orders and increased powers to admit compulsorily and enforce treatment. On the liberty side are the reasserted powers of the Mental Health Review Tribunals; the introduction of independent advocates; and the employment of the Mental Capacity Act of 2005 and its code of practice, and the Court of Protection,[47] to attempt to ensure that any deprivation of liberty is humane, proportional and necessary. Case law related to this balance is reported in periodic government updates on the Human Rights Act, by mental health lobby groups such MIND, and by websites such as Mental Health Law Online which primarily provide a resource for mental health practitioners working in England and Wales. One case on Mental Health Law Online refers to mistakes made by one of the agencies set up to monitor the balance between liberty and control:

[The Mental Health] tribunal's reasoning was inadequate. The tribunal stated that all the evidence was to the effect that MM's mental disorder 'warrants his treatment in hospital' … but it was only (part of) the medical evidence in which there was any confusion as to the criteria. The findings of fact (that the condition was chronic and relapsing etc.) did not show that the mental disorder warranted detention (or made it appropriate). The only finding that could support the tribunal's decision was the medical evidence, which was affected by reference to the wrong legal test …[48]

There has been government action to introduce legislation that furthers the rights of mentally disordered people, for example by ensuring parity between the legal rights of patients with physical disorders and those who have mental disorders. Again, however, these legal rights are tempered by exclusions which relate to those who are affected by the Mental Health Act 2007.[49] Moreover, since 2014 successive British Governments have pledged to ditch the Human Rights Act of 1998 and the 2016 'Brexit' vote has added weight to this undertaking.[50]

AUSTRALIA

The political and institutional arrangements that were the antecedents of the modern Australian state were transported from the UK along with the convicts during the early colonial period. Present-day Australia is an advanced industrialized nation with a culturally diverse population

of approximately 24 million.[51] Average life expectancy is in the mid-80s for women and the late 70s for men. Indigenous Australians constitute about 2 per cent of the population and have much lower life expectancy: on average, approximately 10 years less than their non-indigenous counterparts.[52] Recent research has shown that people with severe, prolonged mental illness also have a greatly reduced life expectancy,[53] a circumstance that, as we will see, raises human rights concerns similar to those for Indigenous Australians. The Australian political system is federated, with a national government and eight state/territory governments.

History

European colonization commenced in 1788 and almost immediately it became necessary to provide for those requiring treatment for insanity. Initially, this might be provided in a local gaol or other 'safe place'. Later, special asylums were established.[54] The asylums of the colonial period were usually located away from main population centres, and concentrated on providing a controlled and sheltered life for the residents.[55–57] The second half of the nineteenth century was a period of considerable development in mental health care, especially in New South Wales. Visits by mental health experts from the UK resulted in the introduction of moral treatment and the building of new asylums.[58]

The first half of the twentieth century, which included the two world wars and the Great Depression, was characterized by a severe shortage of funds, which seriously hampered the development of mental health services. In the mid-1950s a national inquiry into mental health services reported that local services compared unfavourably with other countries.[56] However, post-war optimism contributed to an increase in social pressure for reform, including in the mental health field. Throughout the 1960s and 1970s the now renamed psychiatric hospitals came under increasing public scrutiny as a mental health community care movement emerged, and new developments in social psychiatry and psychopharmacology suggested a treatment revolution.[56] By the late 1970s, community mental health services were developing as the old psychiatric institutions were being allowed to run down. While such developments were poorly coordinated and uneven across the country, they nevertheless contributed to a steady decline in the numbers of patients in psychiatric hospitals throughout the country – a trend that was referred to as de-institutionalization. It has been suggested that initially de-institutionalization occurred in a non-systematic way, often in response to increasing clinical optimism and changing social attitudes on the one hand, and economic imperatives and political scandal on the other hand.[54] The ad hoc nature of mental service development during the decades of non-systematic de-institutionalization led to situations such as that in New South Wales, in which by the mid-1980s about 90 per cent of people with severe mental illness were living in the community, whereas about 90 per cent of public mental health staff and funding were retained in the hospitals.[54] It was not until the late

1980s and 1990s that a more systematic and coordinated approach to de-institutionalization was formally integrated into mental health policy.[54,59]

The history of Australian mental health services indicates that significant reforms have almost always been accompanied by concerns surrounding the neglect and abuse of patients. In New South Wales alone, about 40 inquiries were conducted into psychiatric services between the early colonial period and the late 1980s.[57] This combination of controversies and official inquiries into mental health care has continued into the present day.[60,61]

Present

While Australia has a modern, comprehensive mental health system, there is nevertheless a high level of unmet need for treatment among many Australians who have a mental health problem or disorder.[62] Since the early 1990s a range of mental health-related issues and service shortcomings have been addressed through a national mental health strategy, implemented through successive 5-year plans.[63] A number of key policy expectations have evolved over the decades, including: that those who use mental health services ought to be able to do so close to where they live; that services should be responsive to the needs of patients; that effective care ought to be delivered continuously across a range of inpatient and ambulatory services; and that persons with mental illness ought not to have to endure reduced citizenship entitlements and human rights abuses. By the time of the fourth plan (2009–14), greater emphasis was being placed on social inclusion and recovery, prevention and early intervention, quality improvement and innovation, and accountability.[63]

While the reforms have undoubtedly brought increased resources and operational improvements,[64] there has been little evidence of beneficial impacts on citizenship participation and human rights protections for those with mental illness and their families.[62] Indeed, the findings of recent studies such as the Survey of High Impact Psychosis (SHIP) in Australia indicate that people with severe psychotic illness continue to face multiple challenges, including low educational achievement, high unemployment and high levels of alcohol or drug use.[65] In addition, 66.1 per cent of the participants in the SHIP study were current smokers and about half had metabolic syndrome. When SHIP participants were asked to identify the most important challenges facing them in the year ahead, they indicated the following (ranked from highest to lowest): financial matters, loneliness/social isolation, lack of employment, poor physical health/physical health issues, uncontrolled symptoms of mental illness and lack of stable/suitable housing.[66] Accordingly, concerns remain regarding the extent to which the policy aspirations of recent decades can be realized in practice, and the extent to which the onus for claiming rights set down in policy falls on the vulnerable individuals concerned – the users of mental health services.[67,68] Indeed, even holding membership in one of the 'caring' professions seems insufficient to safeguard against the likelihood of discrimination in the workplace on the basis of mental illness.[69] While people living with psychosis identify financial concerns, loneliness and secure accommodation among their most pressing challenges, the rehabilitation, housing and support services necessary for life in the community remain seriously underdeveloped.[66]

REFLECTION

Despite being a focus of Australia's National Mental Health Strategy for two decades, non-clinical needs such as financial concerns, loneliness/ social isolation, lack of stable/suitable housing and stigma and discrimination remain significant among the many challenges faced by people living with psychosis. Can you think of six reasons that make it very difficult for reforms set out in mental health policy to be enforced in practice?

Over the last few decades there have been numerous reports pointing to underdeveloped services and human rights violations affecting people with mental illness and their families throughout Australia. Perhaps the most prominent of these, the Human Rights and Equal Opportunity Commission Report,[57] found that people with mental illness were exposed to widespread systemic discrimination and were frequently denied access to rights and services to which they were entitled; that governments needed to assertively address and redress negative community attitudes toward people with mental illness; that savings accrued through de-institutionalization had not been redirected into the development of mental health and social care services in the community; and that services to support community living were seriously underdeveloped. More recent reports have raised similar concerns.[60,61] It is ironic that, in an era in which the policy aim is to liberalize mental health services, the experience of 'being in care' may be more restrictive than in the past. Inpatient mental health facilities have become much more risk-averse.[70,71] Risk management often seems to take precedence over therapeutic concerns – often in response to workplace health and safety requirements. Closed-circuit television monitoring, locked windows and doors, the use of 'high dependency' (i.e. seclusion) rooms, staff duress alarms and the use of security guards remain widespread in Australian inpatient mental health facilities. Importantly, such practices remain widespread despite a policy focus on reducing and where possible eliminating restraint and seclusion in mental health services[72] and evidence that such reductions

are possible.[73] There has also been heavy reliance on 'no tolerance' polices in dealing with patient aggression and violence. This development has been criticized for taking the therapeutic initiative away from health care providers, thus removing opportunities for building client engagement with care.[74,75]

One important aspect of the Australian mental health reforms has been the revision of mental health legislation. At the most basic level, mental health law is concerned with finding a balance between safeguarding the rights of individuals with mental illness and the public's right to safety. As part of the National Mental Health Strategy, a number of initiatives have sought to review and redirect Australian mental health legislation, which operates within separate state and territory jurisdictions.[76] An example of revised Australian mental health legislation is the Mental Health Act 2007 (New South Wales),[77] an outline of which is provided in Table 67.1.

The 2007 Act continued many of the features of the previous (1990) Act, but it also included important new features, such as: a focus on providing care and treatment in the community; assistance of those affected by mental illness to live and work as active citizens; increased emphasis on involving patients in treatment planning; and acknowledgement and support of the role of carers of people with mental health problems and disorders. In 2008 Australia ratified the United Nations Convention on the Rights of People with Disabilities,[78] creating a legally binding requirement to bring all Australian mental health legislation in line with the principles set out in that international agreement. Similar to legislative changes elsewhere in Australia and internationally,[76,79] the Mental Health Amendment (Statutory Review) Act 2014 (New South Wales)[80] initiates a process of bringing mental health legislation in New South Wales into accordance with the standards set out in the UN Convention. Important adjustments to the 2007 Act include: adding a requirement to consider consumer views and expressed wishes in the development of treatment and recovery plans and, where reasonably practicable, to gain consumer consent for such plans; extending an existing requirement to consult with and inform carers of people detained under the Act and to nominate one such carer as a principal care provider; enabling voluntary patients to be detained in a mental health facility for up to 2 hours to enable a medical officer to determine if further detention in the facility for assessment is warranted; and to tighten the requirements to be met for administering electroconvulsive therapy to people under 16 years of age. The provisions of the Mental Health Act 2007 (New South Wales) as amended by the Mental Health Amendment (Statutory Review) Act 2014 (New South Wales) are broadly similar to those found in other Australian states and territories and also overseas; for example, the Mental Health Act 2007 (England and Wales).

Table 67.1 Mental Health Act 2007 (New South Wales)

Chapter 2: Preliminary	Outlines the name of the Act, specifies the date of commencement and defines key terms.
Chapter 2: Voluntary admission to facilities	Outlines types of voluntary admission to mental health facilities, including children and persons under guardianship. Outlines procedures for discharge, review and detention. Specifies procedures pertaining to refusal of voluntary admission.
Chapter 3: Involuntary admission and treatment in and outside facilities	Outlines procedures for involuntary detention and treatment in mental health facilities, including admission to and initial treatment; continuing detention; and leave of absence. Specifies procedures for involuntary treatment in the community using community treatment orders.
Chapter 4: Care and treatment	Outlines principles and procedures pertaining to the care and treatment of persons under the Act and the use of mental health treatments, including pharmacological and electroconvulsive treatments. Provides for consideration of the rights of patients detained under the Act and their primary carers, including requirements for notification and information sharing regarding medication and rights surrounding detention. Specifies procedures for the transfer of patients to or from mental health facilities and/or other health facilities.
Chapter 5: Administration	Outlines administrative procedures for the governance of public and private mental health facilities. Specifies procedures governing responsibilities and powers of official visitors, accredited persons and powers of inspection.
Chapter 6: Mental Health Review Tribunal	Outlines the constitution, membership, responsibilities and procedures of the Mental Health Review Tribunal, including the use of legal representation, determination of whether a person is a 'mentally ill person' or a 'mentally disordered person' and the use of interpreters.
Chapter 7: Jurisdiction of Supreme Court	Outlines rights of appeal to the Supreme Court, including considerations of jurisdiction.
Chapter 8: Interstate application of mental health laws	Outlines procedures for the transfer of patients between New South Wales and other Australian states and territories. Specifies procedures for interstate implementation of New South Wales community treatment orders; the recognition of and provision of services in respect of interstate orders; and the apprehension of persons under the powers of the Act.
Chapter 9: Miscellaneous	Outlines restrictions, limitations and regulations pertaining to the Act.

An important feature of the 2007 Act was that formal consideration must be given to the role that carers play in providing ongoing emotional and material support for people with mental illness. The amendments introduced via the 2014 Act extended an earlier requirement that a 'primary carer' be appointed for each patient detained in a mental health facility, to enable the nomination of more than one carer (renamed designated carer) and the identification of a principal care provider. This may be a guardian, where one has been appointed, or a parent, if the patient is under 18 years of age. Most often, however, a spouse or other person primarily responsible for providing care and support for the patient will be nominated. Principal care providers now have rights to certain types of information in respect of a patient,

such as notification within 24 hours that a person has been involuntarily detained in a mental health facility; they now also have the right to appear at mental health inquiries involving the person under their care, and the right to apply to have that person discharged from a mental health facility. Other important reforms introduced via the 2014 amendments include: the addition of recovery from mental illness and the removal of references to the control of patients within the objects of the Act; insertion of a requirement to support people with mental illness to pursue their own recovery; the introduction of a principle requiring reasonable efforts to obtain consumer consent to treatment plans and recovery plans; and the monitoring of capacity to consent, and support for persons who lack capacity to understand such plans.

- Look up the mental health act or similar legislation that operates in your state or country and compare it with the Mental Health Act 2007 (New South Wales). In what important ways is your local mental health legislation similar to or different from the New South Wales Act?

- What provisions exist within your local mental health legislation to protect the rights of people who are involuntarily detained in a mental health facility?

While the 2007 Act and the 2014 amendments undoubtedly reflect the ongoing liberalization of mental health legislation in Australia and overseas, research such as the SHIP study[65,66] highlight the ongoing serious vulnerabilities of people with mental health problems and disorders. At the same time the finding of reports nationally[60,61] and internationally[10] continue to highlight the extent to which widespread public perceptions in this area continue to be influenced by age-old fears surrounding madness. Following Turner,[81] we can note the ontological vulnerabilities and social precariousness associated with mental illness and question the extent to which the policy and legislative reforms of recent decades have made real progress in addressing these. Moreover, emerging mental health issues, such as the psychological sequelae of exposure to cyberbullying and other forms of personal and institutionalized violence, are adding substantially to the quantum of human distress.[82,83,1]

A key aspect of current mental health reform in many countries has been attempts to transform the mental health patient into the mental health consumer. While the aim has been to elevate the status of those with mental illness to citizens and to shift therapeutic discourse towards a focus on recovery, such reforms have not gone unchallenged. For instance, it has been suggested that if (mental health) 'consumerism' implies choice, there are any number of circumstances in which patients might face very limited choice or may even be denied choice.[62] The life experiences of many people with mental illness are difficult to reconcile with the idea of 'consumer choice'. We need only think of what it might be like to face involuntary admission to a mental health facility, or to be the subject of a community treatment order requiring treatment with powerful psychiatric drugs. Even 'voluntary' patients can find it difficult to manage the structures and procedures found in mental health services.

Similarly, it has been suggested that, while the recovery movement was instigated by the actions of patients and their advocates, it has long since been co-opted by policy makers, academics, managers and health care practitioners; in effect the progressive potential in recovery has to some extent been neutralized through processes of professionalization and bureaucratization.[84] Undoubtedly, mental health nursing, both in Australia and internationally, has invested heavily in the notions of (mental) health consumerism and recovery – the terms have become part of our everyday professional discourse. In Australia we may talk about recovery, and note its formal inclusion as a principle in recent amendments to mental health legislation. However, we should also note that: over 50 per cent of people with psychosis in Australia meet criteria for metabolic syndrome, which in part reflects the iatrogenic effects of psychiatric pharmacotherapy;[65] measurable improvements in the mental health of Indigenous Australians remain elusive;[85] the physical health of Australians with mental illness is among the poorest in the community;[66] and concerns continue to be raised regarding the influence of the pharmaceutical industry on the conduct of medical science and health professional practice.[86] It seems important to ask how such trends and issues might be reconciled with the notion of recovery. How might recovery-focused services be developed in a mental health system characterized by power imbalances and competing demands?

In the end, it may be that the notion of mental health consumerism is contrary to other forms of citizenship that operate more on the basis of 'grass roots' activism. Many users of mental health services prefer to be thought of as survivors, or activists, rather than consumers. Increasingly, such people are entering into social and political alliances that seek to challenge and reshape the institutional structures and arrangements that govern mental health care.[62] While there have undoubtedly been significant changes in mental health policy and mental health legislation in recent decades, it is not yet apparent that the new directions have brought clear improvements to the lives of those who are the users of mental health services.

CONCLUSION

The relationships among mental health, the law and human rights have been and remain characterized by complex tension. In both 'old world' England and 'new world' Australia, issues of fear and control co-exist with structural and attitudinal changes regarding, for example, recovery, citizenship and consumer choice. To understand this complex tension, what has to be appreciated is the historical background to the management of 'madness' in both countries *and* the present seismic social transformations originating from economic and cultural globalization that are affecting every country. This understanding underpins substantially the craft of mental health care because it allows decisions and attitudes to be based on relevant background knowledge.

For readers who would like to follow up the circumstances surrounding mental health law and human rights in other countries, we have provided a list of relevant websites containing information about the tense complexity of balancing such factors as the liberty of, and understanding of, people with mental disorder, the legitimate requirement to protect society, and the abuse of mentally disordered people by society and psychiatry.

SERVICE USER COMMENTARY

Simon Swinson

Living as I do with schizophrenia, I am aware of my human rights to some extent. However, I don't recall human rights concerns or legal issues being raised in a service context, except for complaints procedures. The right to complain about services (especially those provided by non-governmental organizations) has been emphasized by mental health service managers and clinical staff on numerous occasions. When I have been involved in discussions regarding the Mental Health Act, it has been as a consumer representative sitting on departmental committees. In many ways I feel poorly informed regarding my legal rights and responsibilities. I have not been subjected to mandatory hospitalization under the Mental Health Act, and if this were to occur (which is possible given the nature of my illness) I am not sure I would know where to turn. I have participated in numerous meetings, briefings and conferences over the years, and feel I have a good understanding of the workings of the mental health system. However, on reading this chapter I realized I am poorly informed regarding mental health law. Indeed, I wondered whether the main opportunity to learn about the legal mechanisms surrounding mandatory detention under the Mental Health Act is to find oneself the subject of it. Reading this chapter has had a powerful instructional impact; it aligns with much of my own experience of mental health services over several decades. Perhaps even more importantly, reading the chapter has caused me to reflect on what I don't know and why that might be.

Simon Swinson is a service user living with schizophrenia.

ACKNOWLEDGEMENT

Our thanks go to Simon Swinson for his very candid service user commentary on the chapter.

References

1. Middleton W, Stavropoulos P, Dorahy M, Kruger C, Lewis-Fernandez R, Martinez-Taboas A, Sar V, Brand B. Institutional abuse and social silence: an emerging global problem. *Australian and New Zealand Journal of Psychiatry* 2014; **48**(1): 22–5.
2. American Psychiatric Association. *Diagnostic and statistical manual of mental disorders, fifth edition (DSM-5)*. Arlington, VA: American Psychiatric Association, 2013.
3. WHO (World Health Organization). *International statistical classification of diseases and related health problems 10th revision (ICD-10). Version for 2010*. Geneva: WHO, 2010. Available from: http://apps.who.int/classifications/icd10/browse/2010/en#/F60.8 [Accessed 5th June 2016].
4. WHO (World Health Organization).. *Schizophrenia: fact sheet no. 397*. 2014. Available from: http://www.who.int/mediacentre/factsheets/fs397/en/ [Accessed 5th June 2016].
5. Christodoulou G. Living with schizophrenia: World Mental Health Day 2014 – foreword. Occoquan, Vancouver, Canada: World Mental Health Foundation, 2014.
6. Anxiety and Depression Association of America. Facts & statistics. 2014. Available from: http://www.adaa.org/about-adaa/press-room/facts-statistics [Accessed 5th June 2016].
7. WHO (World Health Organization). *Preventing suicide: a global initiative*. Geneva: WHO 2014.
8. Cheng W, Xin Z. The heavy toll of depression in China. Beijing: Caixin Online, 2012. Available from: http://www.marketwatch.com/story/the-heavy-toll-of-depression-in-china-2012-11-15 [Accessed 5th June 2016].
9. Mao Y. *Where does Chinese people's anxiety come from?* Beijing: Qunyan Press, 2013.
10. WHO (World Health Organization). *Mental health action plan 2013–2020*. Geneva: WHO, 2013.
11. WHO (World Health Organization). *Facts on mental health 1-10 [wars and disasters]*. 2014. Available from: http://www.who.int/features/factfiles/mental_health/mental_health_facts/en/ [Accessed 5th June 2016].
12. United Nations. *The Convention on the Rights of Persons with Disabilities*. New York: United Nations, 2006.
13. Morrall P, Hazelton M (eds). *Mental health: global policies and human rights*. London: Whurr, 2004.
14. Kumar K. *The making of English national identity*. Cambridge: Cambridge University Press, 2003.
15. Paxman J. *The English*. London: Penguin Books, 1999.
16. Paxman J. *Empire: what ruling the world did to the British*. London: Viking Australia, 2012.
17. Black C. *A new birth of freedom: human rights, named and unnamed*. New Haven, CT: Yale University Press, 1999.
18. Porter R. *A social history of madness: stories of the insane*. London: Weidenfeld & Nicolson, 1987.
19. Morrall P. *The trouble with therapy: sociology and psychotherapy*. Chichester: Open University Press/McGraw-Hill, 2008.
20. Porter R. *Madness: a brief history*. Oxford: Oxford University Press, 2003.
21. Gibson M. *Reading witchcraft: stories of early English witches*. London: Routledge, 1999.
22. Busfield J. (ed.). *Rethinking the sociology of mental health*. Oxford: Blackwell, 2001.
23. Andrews J, Porter R, Tucker P, Waddington K. *The history of Bethlem*. London: Routledge, 1997.

24. Foucault M. *Histoire de la folie à l'âge classique* [translated as *Madness and civilization*]. Paris: Plon, 1961.

25. Perceval J. *Perceval's narrative* (ed. G Bateson). London: Hogarth, 1962 (original 1840): 119–20.

26. Scull A. *Decarceration: community treatment and the deviant: a radical view*, 2nd edn. Cambridge: Polity, 1984.

27. Robinson DN. *Wild beasts and idle humours: the insanity defense from antiquity to the present*. Cambridge, MA: Harvard University Press, 1996.

28. Scull A. *Madness: a very short introduction*. Oxford: Oxford University Press, 2011.

29. Gittins D. *Madness in its place. Narratives of Severalls Hospital 1913–1997*. London: Routledge, 1998.

30. Miller P, Rose N. (eds). *The power of psychiatry*. Cambridge: Polity, 1986.

31. Morrall P. *Mental health nursing and social control*. London: Whurr, 1998.

32. Busfield J. *Mental illness*. Cambridge: Polity, 2011.

33. Morrall P. *Madness & murder*. London: Whurr, 2000.

34. McNicoll A. Deaths linked to mental health beds crisis as cuts leave little slack in system. *Community Care: Inspiring Excellence in Community Care*. 2014a. Available from: http://www.community care.co.uk/2014/11/28/deaths-linked-mental-health-beds-crisis-cuts-leave-little-slack-system/ [Accessed 5th June 2016].

35. McNicoll A. Rise in Mental Health Act detentions as NHS bed availability drops. *Community Care: Inspiring Excellence in Community Care*. 2014b. Available from: http://www.communitycare.co.uk/2014/10/31/rise-mental-health-act-detentions-nhs-bed-availability-drops/ [Accessed 5th June 2016].

36. Buchanan M. Seven mental health patients died waiting for beds. *BBC News*. 28th November 2014. Available from: http://www.bbc.co.uk/news/uk-30236927 [Accessed 5th June 2016].

37. Department of Health. *Mental health crisis care agreement*. London: Department of Health, 2014. Available from: https://www.gov.uk/government/publications/mental-health-crisis-care-agreement [Accessed 5th June 2016].

38. Davies S. *Annual Report [England] of the Chief Medical Officer 2013, public mental health priorities: investing in the evidence*. London: Department of Health, 2014.

39. Carter P. quoted in: Nurses warn of mental health services strain. *BBC News*. 23rd November 2014. Available from: http://www.bbc.co.uk/news/health-30150747 [Accessed 5th June 2016].

40. Clegg N. Making mental health a priority. 2014. Available from: https://www.gov.uk/government/speeches/nick-clegg-making-mental-health-a-priority [Accessed 5th June 2016].

41. King's fund. *Bringing together physical and mental health: A new frontier for integrated care*. London: King's Fund, 2016.

42. Slate R, Buffington-Vollum J, Johnson W. *The criminalisation of mental illness*. Durham, NC: Carolina Academic Press, 2013.

43. Prisons and Probation Ombudsman. *Prisoner mental health*. London: Office of the Prisons and Probation Ombudsman, 2016.

44. Senior J, Appleby L, Shaw J. The management of mental health problems among prisoners in England and Wales. *International Psychiatry* 2014; **11**(3): 56–8.

45. European Court of Human Rights. *European Convention on Human Rights*. Strasbourg: Council of Europe, 1998 – first adopted 1953. Available from: http://www.echr.coe.int/Documents/Convention_ENG.pdf [Accessed 5th June 2016].

46. Home Office. *Human Rights Act 1998*. London: Stationery Office, 2000.

47. Lord Chancellor. *Mental Capacity Act 2005: Code of Practice*. London: Department for Constitutional Affairs, 2007.

48. Mental Health Law Online. *Re MM (2013) MHLO 150 (UT)*. 2014. Available from: http://www.mentalhealthlaw.co.uk/Re_MM_(2013)_MHLO_150_(UT) [Accessed 5th June 2016].

49. Department of Health. *Closing the gap: priorities for essential change in mental health [England]*. London: Social Care, Local Government and Care Partnership Directorate, 2014.

50. Wilkinson M. Quoted 'Human Rights Act will be scrapped in favour of British Bill of Rights, Liz Trust [Justice Minister] pledges'. Daily Telegraph, 22nd August, 2016.

51. Australian Bureau of Statistics. *Australian demographic statistics (3101.0)*. 2014. Available from: http://www.healthinfonet.ecu.au/health-facts/overviews

52. Australian Indigenous Health*InfoNet*. *Overview of Aboriginal and Torres Strait Islander health status 2015*. 2016. Available from: http://www.healthinfonet.ecu.edu.au/health-facts/overviews [Accessed 12th December 2016].

53. Galletly C, Foley D, Waterreus G, Castle D, McGrath J, Mackinnon A, Morgan V. Cardiometabolic risk factors in people with psychotic disorders: the second Australian National Survey of Psychosis. *Australian and New Zealand Journal of Psychiatry* 2012; **46** (8): 753–61.

54. Rosen A. The Australian experience of deinstitutionalisation: interaction of Australian culture with the development and reform of its mental health services. *Acta Psychiatrica Scandinavica* 2006; **113** (Suppl. 429): 81–9.

55. McDonald D. Hospitals for the insane in the young colony. In: Pern J, O'Carrigan J (eds). *Australia's quest for colonial health. Some influences on early health and medicine in Australia*. Brisbane, Australia: Department of Child Health, Royal Children's Hospital Brisbane, 1983: 183–90.

56. Lewis M. *Managing madness: psychiatry and society in Australia 1788–1980*. Canberra, Australia: Australian Government Publishing Service, 1988.

57. Human Rights and Equal Opportunity Commission. *Human rights and mental illness. Report of the National Inquiry into the Human Rights of People with Mental Illness*. Canberra, Australia: Australian Government Publishing Service, 1993: 5.

58. Crichton A. *Slowly taking control?* Sydney, Australia: Allen and Unwin, 1990.

59. Doessel D, Scheurer R, Chant D, Whiteford H. Australia's National Mental Health Strategy and deinstitutionalisation: some empirical results. *Australian and New Zealand Journal of Psychiatry* 2005; **39**(11/12): 989–94.

60. Mental Health Council of Australia, Brain and Mind Institute, Human Rights and Equal Opportunity Commission. *Not for service: experiences of injustice and despair in mental health care in Australia*. Canberra: Mental Health Council of Australia, 2005.

61. Australian Parliament Senate Select Committee on Mental Health. *A national approach to mental health – from crisis to community. First report*. Canberra: Commonwealth of Australia, 2006.

62. Hazelton M. Mental health, citizenship and human rights in four countries. *Health Sociology Review* 2005; **14**: 230–41.

63. Commonwealth of Australia. *Fourth National Mental Health Plan: an agenda for collaborative government action in mental health 2009–2014*. Canberra: Commonwealth of Australia, 2009.

64. Whiteford H, Buckingham B, Manderscheid R. Australia's national mental health strategy. *British Journal of Psychiatry* 2002; **80**: 210–15.

65. Morgan V, Waterreus A, Jablensky A, Mackinnon A, McGrath J, Carr V, Bush R, Castel D, Cohen M, Harvey C, Galletly C, Stain H, Neil A, McGorry P, Hocking B, Shah S, Saw S. People living with psychotic illness in 2010: the second Australian National Survey of Psychosis. *Australian and New Zealand Journal of Psychiatry* 2012; **46**(8): 735–52.

66. Carr V, Whiteford H, Groves A, McGorry P, Shepherd A. Policy and service development implications of the second Australian National Survey of High Impact Psychosis (SHIP). *Australian and New Zealand Journal of Psychiatry* 2012; **46**(8): 708–18.

67. Watchirs H. *Application of rights analysis instrument to Australian mental health legislation. Report to the Australian Health Ministers Advisory Council National Mental Health Working Group*. Canberra, Australia: Commonwealth Department of Health and Aged Care, 2000.

68. Johnstone M. Stigma, social justice and the rights of the mentally ill: challenging the status quo. *Australian and New Zealand Journal of Mental Health Nursing* 2001; **10**(4): 200–9.

69. Joyce T, McMillan M, Hazelton M. The workplace and nurses with a mental illness. *International Journal of Mental Health Nursing* 2009; **18**: 391–7.

70. Hazelton M, Rossiter R, Sinclair E, Morrall P. Encounters with the 'dark side': new graduate nurses' experiences in a mental health service. *Health Sociology Review* 2011; **20**(2): 172–86.

71. Clancy L, Happell B, Moxham L. The language of risk: common understanding or diverse perspectives? *Issues in Mental Health Nursing* 2014; **35**: 551–7.

72. National Mental Health Working Group. *National safety priorities in mental health: a national plan for reducing harm*, Canberra: Health Priorities and Suicide Prevention Branch, Department of Health and Ageing, Commonwealth of Australia, 2005.

73. Gaskin C, Elsom S, Happell B. Interventions for reducing the use of seclusion in psychiatric facilities. *British Journal of Psychiatry* 2007; **191**: 298–303.

74. Wand T, Coulson K. Zero tolerance: a policy in conflict with current opinion on aggression and violence management in health care. *Australian Emergency Nursing Journal* 2006; **9**: 163–70.

75. Stone T, Hazelton M. An overview of swearing and its impact on mental health nursing practice. *International Journal of Mental Health Nursing* 2008; **17**: 206–12.

76. Callaghan S, Ryan C. Rising to human rights challenge in compulsory treatment – new approaches to mental health law in Australia. *Australian and New Zealand Journal of Psychiatry* 2012; **46**(7): 611–20.

77. Mental Health Act 2007 (New South Wales). Available from: http://www.austlii.edu.au/au/legis/nsw/consol_act/mha2007128/ [Accessed 12th December 2016].

78. United Nations. *Convention on the Rights of Persons with Disabilities. 'Additional harm' and compulsory orders*. Geneva: United Nations, 2006.

79. Anand S, Pennington-Smitgh P. Compulsory treatment: rights, reforms and the role of realism. *Australian and New Zealand Journal of Psychiatry* 2013; **47**(10): 895–8.

80. Mental Health Amendment (Statutory Review) Act 2014 (NSW). Available from: http://www.austlii.edu.au/au/legis/nsw/num_act/mhara2014n85461.pdf [Accessed 12th December 2016].

81. Turner B. Outline of a theory of human rights. In: Turner B (ed.). *Citizenship and social theory*. London: Sage, 1993: 162–90.

82. Kozlowska K, Durheim E. Is bullying in children and adolescents a modifiable risk factor for mental illness? *Australian and New Zealand Journal of Psychiatry* 2013; **48**(3): 288–9.

83. Scott J, Moore S, Sly P, Norman R. Bullying in children and adolescents: a modifiable risk factor for mental illness. *Australian and New Zealand Journal of Psychiatry* 2009; **48**(3): 209–12.

84. Hamer H, Finlayson M, Warren H. Insiders or outsiders? Mental health service users' journey's towards full citizenship. *International Journal of Mental Health Nursing* 2014; **23**(3): 203–1.

85. Parker P. Mental illness in Aboriginal and Torres Strait Islander Peoples. In: Purdie N, Dudgeon P, Walker R (eds). *Working together: Aboriginal and Torres Strait Islander mental health and wellbeing principles and practice*. Canberra: Commonwealth Department of Health and Ageing, 2010: 65–74.

86. Boyce P, Malhi G. Supping with the devil? The dangers of liaisons between pharma and our profession. *Australian and New Zealand Journal of Psychiatry* 2012; **46**(6): 493–4.

Further reading and relevant web pages

General

Dudley M, Silove D, Gale F (eds). *Mental health and human rights: vision, praxis, and courage*. Oxford: Oxford University Press, 2012.

Kelly B. *Dignity, mental health and human rights*. Farnham: Ashgate, 2015.

Mfoafo-M'Carthy M, Huls S. Human rights violations and mental illness: implications for engagement and adherence. *Sage Open* 2014; January–March: 1–18. Available from: http://sgo.sagepub.com/content/spsgo/4/1/2158244014526209.full.pdf [Accessed 5th June 2016].

Morrall P, Hazelton M (eds). *Mental health: global policies and human rights*. London: Whurr, 2004.

Chile

CINTRAS: Center for Psychological Health and Human Rights in Chile. http://dieschwelle.de/en/project-partners/southamerica.html

Human Rights Watch. Chile. https://www.hrw.org/americas/chile

China

Amnesty International. Six months after mental health law took effect, involuntary psychiatric commitment continues. 2013. Available from: http://www.amnesty.org.uk/blogs/countdown-china/chrb-six-months-after-mental-health-law-took-effect-involuntary-psychiatric [Accessed 20th September 2016].

China Law and Policy. Mental health law. http://chinalawandpolicy.com/tag/mental-health-law/

India

Anjali. Mental Health Rights Organization. http://www.anjalimentalhealth.org/

Human Rights Watch. 'Treated worse than animals': abuses against women and girls with psychosocial or intellectual disabilities in institutions in India. 2014. Available from: http://www.hrw.org/sites/default/files/reports/india_forUpload.pdf [Accessed 20th September 2016].

Russia

European Court of Human Rights. Case of Lashin v. Russia. 2013. Available from: http://hudoc.echr.coe.int/sites/fra/pages/search.aspx?i=001-116020#{"itemid":["001-116020"]} [Accessed 20th September 2016].

Independent Psychiatric Association of Russia. http://humanrightshouse.org/Articles/5385.html

South Africa

Burns JK. The mental health gap in South Africa – a human rights issue. 2011. Available from: http://www.equalrightstrust.org/ertdocumentbank/ERR06_special_Jonathan.pdf [Accessed 20th September 2016].

South African Federation of Mental Health. www.charitysa.co.za/sa-federation-for-mental-health.html

USA

Dart T. Mentally ill Texas inmate's execution stayed by federal appeals court. *Guardian*, 3 December 2013. Available from: http://www.theguardian.com/us-news/2014/dec/03/mentally-ill-texas-inmate-execution-stayed-scott-panetti [Accessed 20th September 2016].

Center for the Human Rights of Users and Survivors of Psychiatry. http://www.chrusp.org/home/about_us

Vietnam

Melbourne School of Population and Global Health (University of Melbourne). *National Taskforce for Mental Health System Development in Vietnam.* 2014. Available from: www.cimh. unimelb.edu.au/research_and_publications/imhr/national_ taskforce_vietnam [Accessed 20th September 2016].

Amnesty International. *Annual Report: Vietnam.* 2013. Available from: https://www.amnesty.org/en/countries/asia-and-the-pacific/viet-nam [Accessed 20th September 2016].

Zimbabwe

In2mental health. *Global Mental Health Inside Stories: Ignicious Murambidzi, Harare, Zimbabwe.* 2013. Available from: www. in2mentalhealth.com/2013/08/31/global-mental-health-inside-stories-ignicious-murambidzi-harare-zimbabwe/ [Accessed 5th June 2016].

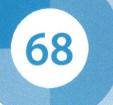

68 The political landscape of mental health care

DAWN FRESHWATER

LEARNING OUTCOMES

- To have a clearer understanding of the political discourses that drive notions of professional identity and the rhetoric of collaboration.

- To have a broader knowledge of the implications of the politics of performance, especially those that privilege 'algorithmic thinking' in the shape of metrics and over-regulation.

- To be able to define and describe how formulaic approaches to contemporary mental health care constitute algorithmic thinking.

- To recognize how algorithmic thinking and political understandings of collaboration impact on service delivery and experiences of care.

SUMMARY OF KEY POINTS

- This chapter focuses on and scrutinizes the political landscape of mental health care.
- In interrogating the relationships and discourses that concern professional identity, it also highlights the inherent rhetoric of collaboration.
- It is argued that much of the contemporary political landscape of mental health care constitutes 'algorithmic thinking'[1] rather than a dialogic approach to caregiving.

- It is argued that the politics of performance, especially those that privilege algorithmic thinking in the shape of metrics and over-regulation, directly impact on service delivery and the experience of care.
- The human mode of being, articulated through aesthetic rationality, is proposed as an alternative approach to caregiving.

INTRODUCTION

This chapter is situated within the contemporary political debates and changing socio-economic environments of the twenty-first century, in particular those that originate in economic capitalism and global competitiveness. It is interested in a strong evaluation of the construction and deconstruction of caring, specifically collaborative practices, professional identity and regulatory discourses, created in and through mental health care.[2] There is a wealth of literature

765

available, which continues to theorize about collaborative practices in mental health care and which has scrutinized the practice of mental health nursing per se. Chapter 1 of this book deals more fully with the development, theory and practice of mental health nursing and as such these issues will not be explicitly addressed in this chapter. Nevertheless, this current chapter aligns closely with much of the analysis drawn through chapter 1, chapter 71 on nursing metrics and chapter 6 on evidence-based practice, all of which have relevance and connections to both the political and collaborative identities of mental health nursing explicated here.

Practice is often differentiated from theory; that is, doing something as opposed to thinking about something.

However, this distinction is overdrawn. Action and thought are interactive. Practices are grounded in understandings people have about the world, and these understandings are in turn influenced by the effect of their practices and actions on the world. In other words, there is an interactive and collaborative exchange between theory and practice in the practice of mental health care, which in turn constructs and is constructed by both the prevailing external 'economies of performance' and internal 'ecologies of practice'.[3] As persons are the practitioners of both theories and practices of care, it could be argued that the professionals and the professions such as mental health nursing perform themselves into being.

BACKGROUND

Contemporary discourses of caring and clinical practices in mental health emphasize regulation, safety and managed care. Financial and political drivers constrain practices and practitioners to task-focused care and depersonalized care, rather than the preferred model of many nursing theorists, that of evidence-based, personalized, relational care. It is true to say that all professional practices, including those related to health care, are shaped by discourses that privilege critical thinking and yet also militate against it, resulting in self-justification, and unhealthy ways of reducing cognitive dissonance (for example, see Stronach et al.[3]). Caring has consistently avoided being subjected to a deconstruction, despite challenges to the taken-for-granted assumptions that underpin such a concept. 'Caring' and 'nursing' have been, and continue to be, used interchangeably, creating an interesting nexus. The word 'care', for example, refers to affective components of the concept of caring.[4] This is in contrast to nursing, which Nightingale referred to as a call of duty, and one which carried spiritual connotations.[5]

These concepts have been iterated and developed over time, until we have what we now work with in the twenty-first century: concepts that are owned and contested by, and indeed used to define, a multiplicity of nursing and related allied health disciplines, supporting, as it does, the discourse of collaboration and partnership working.

> ## REFLECTION
>
> - Spend a few minutes on your own, or with a colleague, identifying what makes nursing unique, and how it differs from caring in its broadest sense.
>
> - Following this, deepen your reflection by identifying what makes mental health nursing unique and how you might describe this distinctiveness to a funder or policy maker.

COLLABORATION AND PARTNERSHIPS IN MENTAL HEALTH NURSING

Collaboration is politically and economically driven, at least in part, even where the fundamental premise is that of improved care. Mental health nurses collaborate and work in partnership with consumers and carers, clinically with national and international partners; interprofessionally to foster improvements in mental health care; with policy makers in order to inform priorities and policy agendas; and with academics and researchers to bridge the theory–practice gap. They also work collaboratively across an increasing spectrum of clinical areas with government and non-government organizations. Collaboration and partnerships have also allowed nurses to work outside the acute health care silo, as they strive to improve quality of life for consumers and carers living in the community.

An analysis of the abstracts presented at a recent international conference for mental health nurses and practitioners, for which the theme was 'Collaboration and

partnerships in mental health nursing',[6] indicates the depth with which the mantra of collaboration and partnership is now *theoretically* rooted in the discourse of the profession.

While collaborative practice and partnership working are generally viewed by mental health practitioners as positive, they are also, in part, experienced as a threat to the profession.

The growing global trend favouring the funding of health care research that is explicitly driven by and committed to interdisciplinary research is mirrored by national and international health systems' prioritization of transdisciplinary education and training.[7,8] There is little doubt that collaboration and collaborative relationships are central to the success of this approach, and, as has been argued, are taken unquestioningly to be the key to effective clinical and interdisciplinary health care practices.[7,9,10] This recent obsession with collaboration in health care, which reflects the changing practice domain and the importance of partnerships to the profession, is particularly relevant to this book. Psychiatric practices and mental health care rely heavily on interactions between and across a number of related disciplines, each with its own uniquely constructed discourse, which contributes to the composite discourse of interdisciplinary collaboration in mental health care.[7]

In their comprehensive review of the core concepts and theories informing interprofessional collaboration, D'Amour and colleagues[10] were able to discern five core themes being attributed varying degrees of significance throughout the material they examined, namely sharing, partnership, power, interdependency and process.

From an overall perspective, collaboration can be described as a dynamic and evolving process of communicative interaction through which participants are able to breach their usual professional boundaries, in order to accommodate multiple levels of collegiate sharing (of values, information, responsibility and action), to such a degree of interdependency as to render team members equitable in influencing team business and for mutual respect towards individual specialist knowledge, expertise and experience to exist.[7]

The discourse of collaboration and partnership working is well rehearsed within the mental health care literature and is now being subjected to a more critical reading. As Freshwater, Cahill and Essen[7] note, theorists usually locate interprofessional collaboration somewhere on a continuum between the apparently autonomous actions of co-located individuals and this integrated ideal. The most frequent terms that D'Amour et al.[10] found being used to describe the context for collaboration (albeit inconsistently and without clear definition) are *multidisciplinary*, *interdisciplinary* and *transdisciplinary*.

It would be easy to conflate this group of related words, which at root suggest degrees of convergence between practice disciplines, with shades of the communicative process outlined above. But the very idea of a 'discipline' suggests compliance with a set of established rules for conduct, and the deliberate exclusion of other less compatible pursuits. So it is perhaps not the case that distinct practice disciplines can themselves be said to converge, but rather that there are a set of co-existing social expectations which dictate that those who follow a particular discipline should do so while working cooperatively with colleagues who adhere to the same, similar or different disciplines. Conventional depictions of professionalism usually include a moral rubric along the lines of it being professionally virtuous to work cooperatively with others, even if doing so sometimes requires a degree of personal stoicism.[11]

However, the feature that most clearly defines a profession is perhaps inevitably the boundary it manages in territorializing a particular set of skills and attributes constitutive of its practice discipline.[12] This can bring it into conflict with other professions and groups, particularly those who would stake a similar territorial claim.

Cameron[13] identified what she believed were naïve assumptions underlying prevalent managerial discourse pertaining to interprofessional practice, namely that professionals will have the ability, willingness and capacity to move beyond their respective professional boundaries without facing significant challenges. She researched the question of whether there are in fact impenetrable boundaries between professions working within the UK National Health Service, finding that boundary disputes often occur when increased collaborative demands appear alongside a policy agenda that is perceived by members of one or more professions to be to their detriment and to the possible advantage of another. References to boundary disputes can be found elsewhere in the literature, often expressed as 'professional jealousy' and 'rivalry'. Such territorialism has led to examples of horizontal violence and exemplifies the antithesis of collaboration and teamwork.[14]

This willingness on the part of professionals to collectively protect their shared territorial interests led Cameron to suggest that the very existence of different professional disciplines, which she describes as fragmented fields of knowledge, presents a fundamental source of resistance to service, and thereby, practice reforms.

Excessive idealization of notions of collaborative practice risks overlooking both an unavoidable tension between countervailing strands of disciplinary and cooperative experience (depending on the degree of paradigmatic resonance that already exists between proximate disciplines) *and* the socio-political context in which interprofessional practice occurs. Threats to job security, which increasingly surface alongside appeals for collaboration linked to fiscal austerity measures,[13] are bound to have an impact upon professional judgement. Yet the primary discourse of interprofessional collaboration usually appears to disregard such influences by emphasizing individuation and personal agency, portraying collaborative acts as having a purely professional onus and necessitating individual personal compromise.

Examining the situational aspects of this everyday co-production and maintenance of professional boundaries gives us an important and perhaps more realistic picture of interprofessional collaboration than abstract depictions of formal professional relations are often able to provide.

REFLECTION

- Describe or reflect on an incident where you believe you behaved in a particularly collaborative manner.

- How would you define the attributes, attitude and actions that constituted this experience?

- How would you expect an expert collaborator to behave?

PROFESSIONS, PROFESSIONAL DISCOURSE AND PROFESSIONAL PRACTICE IN MENTAL HEALTH

Before getting into the debate on the thorny issue of what constitutes a profession, I would first like to clarify how I am applying the term 'discourse' within the context of this chapter. Discourse is defined as a set of rules and assumptions for organizing and interpreting the subject matter of an academic or practice discipline, or a field of study.[7] Williams[15] noted the complex discourse and narrative that abound in the literature around academe and what constitutes a profession. In his challenging and thought-provoking sociological analysis of the relationship between the academic and the professional, he reminds us that traditional conceptualizations of academics' sense of professionalism are simply social constructions. That is to say, they are always in the process of becoming; they are dynamic, contingent, iterative, partial and unstable. Nevertheless, professions adhere to and attempt to define themselves, at least in part, by shared minimum understandings and expectations, many of which form the basis of codes of professional conduct, and indeed underpin professional curricula and training schema. Williams[15] argues that 'professions and academe have developed a symbiotic relationship, although which is "tenant" and which "host", and which derives benefit from which, is characteristically contested' (p.536).

Professional practices and their regulation, and collaboration among disciplines, cannot be presented as apolitical. As Fisher and Freshwater[16] argue, mental health and social functioning are significantly shaped by social and political issues, including the exercise of power. All present a challenge to the conceptualization and identity of what it is to be a professional and the identity of a profession. This is a debate that has been well rehearsed by and about mental health nurses. Health care and health care policy, like higher education, are challenged and influenced by a range of changing socio-economic and environmental factors,[1] not least increasing pressure, most often neoliberal in origin, for greater and more transparent accountability, audit and metric-ization – that is, economies of performance.[1,3,17]

This overemphasis on audit and regulation is focused on the 'being' of the profession (auditing its current state), rather than the 'becoming' of the profession (appreciation of the movement and fluency).[18] This overemphasis treats identity and professions as if they are static and unchanging, while what is captured and measured is a snapshot of a moment in time – a moment that does not capture everything, but may of course capture an essence. It has long been held that definitional certainty of the term 'profession', at least within the sociology of the professions, is unlikely.[19] Friedson notes, with reference to the difficulty of defining professions, that there must be some shared minimum understanding present in order to enable the referent to be discriminated in the world.[20] In the context of mental health nursing, questions and debates that perpetuate stories that the profession cannot define itself or what it does, or identify its unique contribution to health care practice (its 'value proposition', so to speak), continue to frame mental health nursing as being in a state of flux.

However, such stories are prefaced on the notion of identity as continuous, failing to recognize that the referent to which the definition of 'professional' points is context-dependent and historically changing. Such reports seek to define professionalism removed from the context of its practice and offer limited insights into its meaning. The economic and political demands of the twenty-first century require mental health nursing to define and identify its value proposition, but it is equally important to place that value proposition in the context of one of the fundamental values of mental health care itself. Roughly translated, this value proposition speaks to the dichotomy of delivering personalized professional care, while meeting the needs of external governance, within the frame of the prevailing business model. The underlying considerations of occupational autonomy and control and the moral values of integrity and trust may well be taken into account by those seeking to professionalize, but the ideological agendas of state, managerial and even intraprofessional hierarchies cannot be denied or ignored.

Stronach et al.[3] write lucidly of the state of dissonance in which many nursing professionals find themselves. Gannon,[21] referring to Stronach,[17] proposes that 'Professional identities are worked in the gap between the increasing neoliberal pressures for accountability and audit, or "economies of performance" and individual and collective "ecologies of practice"' (p.868), confirming the contention that the professional is framed as an implementer of policy.[3] Williams,[15] drawing on the work of Stronach et al.,[3] suggests that 'Professions exist, it would appear, in "inside-out/outside-in" negotiating space between the two competing agendas of the "ecologies of practice" (linked to intra-professional hierarchies) and the "economies of performance" (linked to state and managerial agendas)' (p.535). In this sense, professions and professionals, inhabit two competing discourses: the inside-out, and the outside-in.

Ecologies of performance

Williams[15] and Stronach[17] observe that ecologies of performance are a combination of shared and personal experience, are inside-out and emerge from interactions within the profession and are signalled to those outside the profession. It could be argued that much of the knowledge that underpins the ecology of performance is tacit and experiential, as for example many nursing theorists have argued (including Benner and Polanyi). Examples of the ecology

Mental health nursing narratives in the twenty-first century: distinctive or extinct?

68

of performance include the Scope of Professional Practice, the Scope of Practice 2013 and Australian Standards of Practice 2010.[6]

Economies of performance

Economies of performance are described as *ways of construing a profession from outside the profession*. Such external depictions are closely linked to performative and managerialist ways of measuring what constitutes professional practice, often referred to as the audit culture, or measurement by metric. Examples of economies of performance include Health Education England health care commissioners and regulators. The Francis report[22] is one example of how external regulatory bodies work, in this case through peer review, to highlight areas where internal regulatory mechanisms are deemed to have failed.

> ## REFLECTION
>
> Turning your attention to your own area of practice, focus on the implicit signals and tacit and explicit rules and discourses that are used to strengthen the ecology of performance.

In February 2012, the final report of the Mid Staffordshire NHS Foundation Trust Public Inquiry was published. This inquiry had investigated complaints regarding standards of care in the Stafford Hospital. The report revealed that, while the Trust ostensibly appeared to be compliant with the standards set by official regulating bodies, 'appalling conditions of care were able to flourish'. This was partially attributed to a culture that prioritized targets over care, resulting in a particular neglect of older patients. The regulatory mechanisms had clearly failed to ensure 'compassionate care', a value

that was subordinated to the pressures of complying with managerial targets.[16,23] The dangers of poor care will always be present in contexts where the values of care are forced to cede in the face of instrumental rationality.[16] Fisher and Freshwater[16] welcome the view represented in the Francis report that 'blaming individuals for systematic failures is generally fruitless', but note that the report advocates a route towards compassionate care through the enforcement of professional values associated with 'strong leadership' and 'the rigorous policing of fundamental standards' (p.768).

The Francis report may now be regarded as a 'critical moment' that exposed a 'crisis of care', but the warning signs that something has gone awry have been around for some time. Fisher and Freshwater[16] note that Phillips and Benner's 1995 book *The crisis of care* highlighted how the moral obligation for compassion and goodness was being eclipsed by depersonalized procedures and market imperatives in the USA.[24] It is important to point out that these two apparently competing discourses are not set up as a binary, at least not here. Nursing, including mental health nursing, has lived with many binaries, including the theory–practice gap, psychological versus physical care, art and science, etc. The last thing mental health care needs is to be defined by another binary! So what should we do, then, when the professionalism and integrity of health care practices, specifically those within the sphere of ecologies of mental health practice, are being viewed so critically in the light of 'economies of performance'?

That the identity of nursing is being challenged cannot be contested. For the most part, the response has been to produce, or at least attempt to explicate more transparently, the ecologies of performance. But is this the answer, to set ecologies of performance against the economies of performance? Both discourses are made up of complex and unavoidably political drivers.

MENTAL HEALTH NURSING NARRATIVES IN THE TWENTY-FIRST CENTURY: DISTINCTIVE OR EXTINCT?

There continues to be an ongoing tension between stories and science; people in organizations are storytellers and their stories constitute valid empirical materials for research and evidence of performance, representing as they do ecologies of practice. (See chapters 71 and 6 for further exposition of measurement and evidence of effective mental health nursing.) Narratives are fundamental diagnostic tools that foster the spread of common understandings within communities of workers. In telling stories, people seek to make sense, not of events themselves, but of accounts of them. The question is not so much 'What is mental health nursing?', but 'What purpose does asking the question serve?' We may find ourselves asking the question in order to keep the story alive, dynamic; to remind ourselves of our identity, who we are; to remind

ourselves of the meaning we inscribed in nursing and being a nurse.

Storying mental health nursing is both an act of creating truth and finding it. This notion of storytelling in mental health practices is fundamental, as it speaks not only to the professional identity of a specified nursing discipline, but also to the very performance of mental health practice itself. Narratives of self and identity, stories of personhood and construction and deconstruction of self through storying are at the heart of much mental health nursing care. In this sense mental health nursing is a social intervention, which involves the actions of people, and so understanding human intentions and motivations is essential to understanding its implementation and subsequent evaluation. At each stage of any social intervention, the intervention could work as expected or misfire, but that misfiring is also part of the process of healing and caring. Thus mental health nursing is an iterative process and involves feedback and negotiation, based on pragmatism and circumscribed indeterminacy.

Mental health interventions are embedded in social systems, and how they work is shaped by context, meaning that they have to be modified as they are implemented. The intervention is a product of its context, and is situated within an open system that feeds back on itself (using internal and external feedback data). Successful titration and delivery of these intervention chains reflect the skills and

talents of mental health professionals. Attempts to describe or measure whether intervention chains work using a conventional measure, such as a systematic review or audit, is difficult although not impossible, with the answer likely to be 'to an extent', which is not really of use to policy makers or funders!

In this sense we have a collective responsibility to question assumptions and to stimulate inquiry into the nature and consequences of social power relations within seemingly competing systems and competing paradigms, those of ecologies and economies of performance. In essence, these are not truly competing, but complementary.

MENTAL HEALTH NURSING AS CARING

Caring science is a term proposed by Gage,[25] who described nurses as *creating* their art and *practising* their science. As previously mentioned, caring has consistently avoided being subjected to deconstruction, despite challenges to taken-for-granted assumptions, i.e. that nurses feel compassion and act with integrity. Moving between the universal (caring) and the particular (nursing) is not easy, for of course there are a plurality of fictions of caring and of nursing that we live with and within, and which feel reasonably comfortable at some level. Australian ethicist Stan Van Hooft,[26] in his essay on caring, describes caring as a model of human agency and motivation. It is seen as part of human structure and, he argues, it takes at least two forms, namely caring for self and caring for others. This dual form of caring is expressed in a variety of ways and functions at four levels:

- the biological level, in which caring is expressed as instincts for surviving and nurturing;
- the perceptual level, in which caring is expressed as emotion and has cultural constructions of the world;
- the evaluative level, in which caring is expressed as pragmatic projects and social solidarity;
- the spiritual level, in which caring is expressed as ethics and morality.

All of these, I am sure you would agree, contribute to the formulation of an integrated and continuous holistic systems theory that underpins mental health nursing.

The level of instability of our systems – and by that I mean the inner and the outer political and economic

systems – means that continuity and integrated caregiving are fragmented, within what is perceived as a fragmented system and a fragmented world. The discourse of care is even further tested when practitioners challenge the received wisdom that is generally held, that nurses and health professionals do not engage in non-caring events, or criminal or deviant activities, especially those that inflict harm on someone in their charge under a fiduciary relationship, as was found in the Francis report,[22] and in the Canadian report entitled *Risky business*[27] which was essentially a report on the death of a mental health patient in custody in the presence of mental health nurses.

Stability is, of course, an illusion. Broken continuity or continuous fragmentation of care is really what we can hope for at best: we are all broken and human; we are all inconsistent, complex, incongruent and ambiguous. This is the paradox of the human condition, and it is an important realization for both the carers and the cared for. Easy to state, hard to enact. We only need to look at the level of professional jealousy and professional terrorism that takes place in health-related professions; the literature on nursing is replete with examples of behaviours such as overt and covert non-physical hostility such as sabotage, scapegoating, backstabbing and negative criticism, failure to respect privacy and keep confidences, non-verbal innuendo and lack of openness – essentially a lack of humanity and humility. This is in direct contrast to this chapter's reflection from a service user, who experienced collaboration and benefited from the 'broken continuity' of care.

SERVICE USER'S PERSPECTIVE

As a general adult nurse of many clinical and academic years, the concepts of holistic care that encompass physical and mental well-being and absence of ill-health are not unfamiliar – in other words, the interdependence of

psycho-socio-emotio-politico-spiritual being that makes us who we are as humans. The concepts of care and respect in terms of a nursing philosophy are, again, part of the familiar terrain and core to the landscape of life. Until, I became a patient, and experienced the personal nature of and, dare I say, realization that the dependence on health care services takes hold.

It's not just about becoming ill – in my case, being affected by burnout, anxiety attacks, severe depression and suicidal thoughts – but it's also about the overwhelming feelings of guilt and shame. Guilt and shame that I was not able to function any more in my work environment, that I only felt 'safe' indoors with the blinds closed, and the overwhelming paralysis of the shame that I wasn't able to cope, that the 'strong' me that 'everyone' respected was a plaster cast rather than the purest marble I'd led myself to believe. And that, as I had convinced myself, was the way that others viewed me.

A series of personal coaches, the occupational health medic, the psychotherapists, the psychiatrists, the general practitioner and other assorted health care professionals all attempted to help me in their own ways, and from their own professional perspective, by helping me to see where I was in relation to where I'd come from, both as a person and as a professional. This experience resulted in a bizarre and conflicting intersection between the searching personal vulnerability and the determinedly stoic professional. I understood this to be a mammoth task for those treating me and I could see their continual risk assessment regarding my personal safety. This was another source of guilt, and my years of people pleasing would surface during and after each session. I wanted them to succeed in treating me, not for me, but for them. I found myself giving the 'right' responses so that I would leave them 'convinced' of my safety, but all the while considering ways to end it all. Making it look like an accident was important, as I wanted no one to feel the guilt of failure that I was feeling at that point in my existence. And it was an existence; life was no joy. All I seemed to face was an endless void, all that I had done or achieved was worthless – in fact I'd only succeeded in damaging people on the way and I was convinced that I had only brought heartache and disappointment to those who held me dear. More guilt.

Only retrospectively do I understand and appreciate that the health care providers could read me like a book. It has become apparent to me, in the years following the crisis I was then in, that they had dealt me trump cards. They played my professional cards, my feelings of responsibility, and had shown that they believed in me and trusted what I said and did. I realize now that in doing this they gave me the self-worth and responsibility that I'd lost en route. It was the perception of being in partnership, of giving me some degree of control over my destiny, and their belief in me that helped me come through the crisis. It was the openness of the service providers in discussing what they needed to communicate with each other and asking my permission that helped me understand that what I wanted was important, that I was worth listening to and I was worth respecting. The dialogue and the subliminal communication was, for me, the intervention that helped me regain a grip on my life.

I am still in recovery from what I now understand to be the violent and destructive work environment that I was in. I 'am allowed' to initiate ongoing consultation regarding my medication dosage and support needs. I am now able to look forward in anticipation. It remains a fragile balance, but I'm getting there thanks to the health care professionals who are in partnership with me and support me to see the value of myself, and who have allowed me to believe in myself.

I have experienced what it means to have patient/client-centred care and it has been empowering.

At this point I would like to return to what Roach[28] defines as the human mode of being, which she constructs as:

- compassion;
- competence;
- confidence;
- conscience;
- commitment;
- comportment.

Roach's[28] human mode of being is of import to this chapter, and specifically those modes of being that capture human caring. In the Francis report,[22] for example, compassion, the ability to suffer with and to have sensitivity to suffering, was sadly lacking. Compassion in caring is not a new characterization; however, I might call on mental health practitioners to revisit the notion of compassion and to develop a new lens on clinical intimacy, an intersubjectivity of being in which the silence of knowing each other's experience is as profound as touch.

The application of competence is critical and in my view relates to the ever-present tension between power and caring, the evidence for which is seen in the volume of literature related to power in the helping professions. Once again, how can we approach the notion of competence differently? Sellman[29] argues that the term competence has been misappropriated, referring as it does now to ritualized prescriptive protocols and pathways, what I might call formulaic and mechanistic approaches to care, a type of machine consciousness required to appear competent.[1] Caring from a machine consciousness does not lend itself well to compassionate interventions.

Fisher and Freshwater[16] consider this tension between compassionate care and a sociability of care through managerialism and argue for a renewed approach to thinking about the delivery of care. Highlighting the value of Roslyn Bologh's feminist understanding of aesthetic rationality in fostering a sociability of care within caring contexts, they argue that dominant organizational understandings of rationality need to be extended in ways that acknowledge that compassionate care is enacted within social relationships. They go on to say that this requires a degree of authentic emotional engagement on the part of formal caregivers that is more typically associated with relationships in the private sphere. This then suggests that

compassionate care requires an enlarged understanding of rationality, one that prioritizes the importance of relationships. The model that often prevails is one of the lone practitioner isolated from colleagues, alienated from the organization and subjugated by a disciplinary culture driven by targets.

Bologh[30] sees aesthetic rationality as a mainly unacknowledged female form of rationality (in the sense that it is associated with domestic and communal relations) that is in the broadest sense appreciative of and responsive to beauty. This is not a reference merely to visual beauty but encompasses anything that *attracts our feelings in a way that we deem desirable*. Aesthetic rationality brings together mind, body, feelings and senses and seeks to create a world that enriches and empowers people, and in this respect it is concerned with recognition. This would include tending to the body in physically sensitive ways, or invoking well-being through the organization of playful or social activities, or simply listening attentively and responding in ways that foster a person's sense of belonging.

CONCLUSION

In conclusion, and to return to the theme of this section, that of nursing in the twenty-first century, I propose a dialogical approach to understanding how best we might lever the contribution that mental health nursing might make to the financial, political and economic contexts of health. Rather than seeing economies of performance and ecologies of practice as colliding and competing, I propose a dialogue between what I might refer to as wisdom and courage.

Dialogue is something of a common participation in which we are playing a game not against each other but with each other. The object of the dialogue is not to analyse or win an argument or even to exchange opinions. Rather, it is to suspend our own opinions and to look at and listen to the opinions of others; to suspend them all and to see what they all mean.

Thus, in an age of algorithms of care, we should not rail against algorithms. Rather, we need to be asking: what sort of model of care do we need? Fisher and Freshwater[16] respond to this question with the proposal of a sociability

of care, one that is based on dialogue and aesthetic rationality, a model that encapsulates both the cowardice and the bravery of the profession, one that encourages heart and wisdom to speak powerfully for and against the profession. A 'sociability of care' cannot be conjured up or enforced through the imposition of authority; it requires a deeply embedded change of culture that is achieved through collective dialogue and commitment. Is this a model of caring that mental health professionals and practitioners would feel ownership of? Can it be tested? Can we live it? Will it make a difference?

In the search for a definition of mental health nursing in the twenty-first century, a socio-political economic model of integrated care might at first seem to be the wrong place to look. However, rather than concentrating on the individual practitioner, or a dichotomized view of people and their motivations, or viewing experiences from within a specific lens, it does indeed seem more appropriate to define and describe the practices of mental health nursing within that much wider context.

References

1. Freshwater D. (Con)fusing commerce and science: mixed methods research and the production of contextualized knowledge. *Journal of Mixed Methods Research* 2014; **8**(2): 111–14.
2. Fisher P, Freshwater D. An emancipatory approach to practice and qualitative inquiry in mental health: finding 'voice' in Charles Taylor's ethics of identity. *Ethics and Social Welfare* 2014; **9**(1): 2–17.
3. Stronach I, Corbin B, McNamara O, Stark S, Warne T. Towards an uncertain politics of professionalism: teacher and nurse identities in flux. *Journal of Education Policy* 2010; **17**(1): 109–38.
4. Freshwater D, Cahill J. Care and compromise: developing a conceptual framework for work-related stress. *Journal of Research in Nursing* 2010; **15**(2): 173–83.
5. Nightingale F. *Notes on nursing: what it is and what it is not.* Edinburgh: Wadman, 1859.
6. Australian College of Mental Health Nurses Inc. *Mental health nurses in Australia. Scope of practice 2013 & standards of practice 2010.* Canberra: ACMHN, 2010 and 2013.
7. Freshwater D, Cahill J, Essen C. Discourses of collaborative failure: identity, role and discourse in an interdisciplinary world. *Nursing Inquiry* 2014; **21**(1): 59–68.

8. Essen C, Freshwater D, and Cahill J. Towards an understanding of the dynamic socio-material embodiment of interprofessional collaboration. *Nursing Inquiry* 2015; **22**(3): 210–20.

9. Hornby S, Atkins J. *Collaborative care: interprofessional, interagency and interpersonal.* Oxford: Blackwell Science, 2000.

10. D'Amour D, Ferrada-Videla M, San Martin Rodriguez L, Beaulieu M. The conceptual basis for interprofessional collaboration: Core concepts and theoretical frameworks. *Journal of Interprofessional Care* 2005; **19**(s1): 116–31.

11. Molyneux J. Interprofessional teamworking: what makes teams work well? *Journal of Interprofessional Care* 2001; **15**(1): 29–35.

12. Hall P. Inter-professional teamwork: professional cultures as barriers. *Journal of Interprofessional Care* 2005; **19**(Suppl. 1): 188–96.

13. Cameron AM. Impermeable boundaries? Developments in professional and interprofessional practice. *Journal of Interprofessional Care* 2011; **25**(1): 53–8.

14. Freshwater D. Crosscurrents: against cultural narration in nursing. *Journal of Advanced Nursing* 2000; **32**(2): 481–4.

15. Williams K. Troubling the concept of the 'academic profession' in 21st century higher education. *Higher Education* 2008; **56**(5): 533–44.

16. Fisher P, Freshwater D. Towards compassionate care through aesthetic rationality. *Scandinavian Journal of Caring Sciences* 2014; **28**(4): 767–74.

17. Stronach I. *Globalizing education, educating the local.* London: Routledge, 2010.

18. Freshwater D. *Forging identity through collaboration: ecologies and economies of performance in MHN.* Perth: ANZMHN Conference, 2013.

19. Evetts J. Short note: the sociology of professional groups: new directions. *Current Sociology* 2006; **54**(1): 133–43.

20. Freidson E. *Professional powers.* Chicago: University of Chicago Press, 1986.

21. Gannon S. Globalizing education, educating the local: how method made us mad. *Journal of Education Policy* 2012; **27**(6): 867–9.

22. Francis R. *The Mid Staffordshire NHS Foundation Trust Public Inquiry.* London: Stationery Office, 2013.

23. Berwick D. *A promise to learn – a commitment to act: improving the safety of patients in England.* London: NHS, 2013.

24. Philips SS, Benner PE (eds) *The Crisis of Care: Affirming and Restoring Caring Practices in the Helping Professions.* Washington DC: Georgetown Press, 1995.

25. Gage J. Embracing the art and science of nursing. *Kai Tiaki Nursing New Zealand* 2003; **9**(10): 18–19.

26. Van Hooft S. *Caring: an essay in the philosophy of ethics.* Boulder, CO: University Press of Colorado, 1995.

27. Office of the Correctional Investigator, Canada. *Risky business: an investigation of the treatment and management of chronic self-injury among federally sentenced women – final report.* Ottawa: Office of the Correctional Investigator, 2013.

28. Roach S. *Caring: the human mode of being.* Toronto, ON: University of Toronto Press, 1984.

29. Sellman D. *What makes a good nurse.* London: Jessica Kingsley, 2010.

30. Bologh RW. *Love or greatness: Max Weber and masculine thinking – a feminist inquiry.* London: Taylor & Francis, 2009.

Further reading

Australian Human Rights Commission. Mental health for all: what's the vision? 1997. Available from: https://www.humanrights.gov.au/news/speeches/mental-health-all-whats-vision [Accessed 13th September 2016].

Beck J, Young MFD. The assault on the professions and the restructuring of academic and professional identities: a Bernsteinian analysis. *British Journal of Sociology of Education* 2015; **26**(2): 183–97.

Fisher P, Freshwater D. An emancipatory approach to practice and qualitative inquiry into mental health: finding 'voice' in Charles Taylor's ethics of identity. *Ethics and Social Welfare* 2014; **9**(1): 2–7.

Fisher P, Freshwater D. Methodology and mental illness: resistance and restorying. *Journal of Psychiatric and Mental Health Nursing* 2014; **21**(3): 197–205.

Kennedy P, Lieberman J. Politics of psychiatry and mental health care. 2014. Available from: http://www.patrickjkennedy.net/articles/politics-psychiatry-and-mental-health-care [Accessed 13th September 2016].

Stronach I. *Globalizing education, educating the local. How method made us mad.* London: Routledge, 2010.

Wheatley MJ. *Leadership and the new science.* San Francisco: Berrett-Koehler, 1999.

Relevant web pages

Beresford P. Mental health is in no fit state, whatever the politicians say. *The Conversation.* 2013. Available from: http://theconversation.com/mental-health-is-in-no-fit-state-whatever-the-politicians-say-15743 [Accessed 13th September 2016].

69 Physical health care

LOUISE E. HOWARD AND NADA MUSSA

LEARNING OUTCOMES

- To be able to recognize the important role that mental health nurses have in promoting the physical health and well-being of people with severe mental illness.

- To be able to identify prevalent physical health conditions experienced by people with severe mental illness.

- To be aware of the factors contributing to poor physical health.

- To be aware of areas for assessment of physical health needs and available tools and resources.

- To be familiar with interventions to promote physical health and well-being.

SUMMARY OF KEY POINTS

- The Department of Health[1] identifies that the priority of mental health care should be to enable those with mental health problems to live healthier and longer lives. Mental health nurses play an important role in helping individuals to achieve this.

- Mental health nurses need an understanding of the range of factors that influence health, how to systematically assess physical health needs and risk, and how to deliver effective health promotion.

- Development of collaborative and empowering relationships with service users enables them to have a sense of control over their health and overall well-being.

- Physical health and well-being are essential in the journey to recovery from severe mental illness.

INTRODUCTION

This chapter offers an overview of the physical health needs of people with severe mental illness (SMI) and outlines the important role that mental health nurses (MHNs) can play in supporting individuals to improve their physical health and well-being.

It is well documented that people with SMI experience increased levels of morbidity and mortality in comparison with the general population.[2] Despite the fact that this has been recognized for some time, research during the last decade has continued to identify that people with SMI are experiencing poor physical health and are dying prematurely.[3] The Schizophrenia Commission[4] found that people with SMI still have a life expectancy that is 15 to 20 years lower than that of the general population. Evidence appears to show a widening health divide between those who have a SMI and those who do not.[5] While the health and life expectancy of the general population has improved over the past 50 years, those with SMI have been 'left behind'.[6]

Inherent to the professional values of all MHNs should be the provision of holistic, person-centred and recovery-focused care. The impact that poor physical health has on people and their recovery from SMI is significant. Good physical health is important to people with SMI, and they do want to receive physical health care.[7] Therefore consideration of the physical health needs of the people with whom we work should be integral to our role and to the craft of caring.

REFLECTION

- Do you think that consideration of physical health needs is an integral part of your role as an MHN, or is this someone else's role?

- How confident are you in assessing physical health and providing physical health care?

- Do you regularly consider physical health needs in your care plans?

WHAT ARE THE PHYSICAL HEALTH NEEDS OF PEOPLE WITH SMI?

As stated, people with SMI experience higher morbidity rates than the general population, particularly in relation to diabetes, cardiovascular disease (CVD) and respiratory disease. Diabetes alone is two to four times more prevalent than in the general population.[8] Worryingly, figures from the new Health and Social Care Information Centre show that overall mortality among mental health service users aged 19 and over in England is 3.6 times the rate of the general population[9] (see Table 69.1). Specifically higher rates were identified for respiratory disease, diseases of the digestive system (primarily liver disease) and circulatory diseases (in particular ischemic heart disease).

Metabolic syndrome refers to a cluster of risk factors which together significantly increase the risk of developing CVD (see Box 69.1). This has become a particular concern for people with SMI. A high prevalence has been identified particularly in those taking atypical antipsychotics.[11] Central obesity and insulin resistance are key risk factors.

By examining each of the risk factors individually, it can be readily understood why people with schizophrenia are at particular risk of metabolic syndrome.[11] Obesity is a real concern for people with SMI, with excess weight gain being up to three times more prevalent in people with schizophrenia than in the general population.[12,13] Fifty-eight per cent of those with severe depression have also been found to be overweight or obese.[14] Obesity itself increases the risk of developing hypertension. Despite high rates of metabolic syndrome, screening for mental health services users is poor.[15]

There is a mixed picture for the prevalence of difference cancers in people with SMI. DeHert et al.[16] provide a succinct review of the research in this area. The Disability Rights Commission[3] identified that women with schizophrenia are 42 per cent more likely to die from breast cancer. Increased levels of prolactin (a side effect of some atypical antipsychotics) and low uptake of breast screening may contribute to this figure. Additionally, people with schizophrenia are 90 per cent more likely to develop bowel cancer. Risk factors for bowel cancers include poor dietary intake and high alcohol intake, which are common in those with SMI.[17]

Sexually transmitted diseases such as HIV and hepatitis B and C are also more prevalent. One study by Blank et al.[18]

Table 69.1 Overall mortality among mental health service users aged 19 and over in England

Respiratory disease	Nearly 4 x general population death rates
Diseases of digestive system	Just over 4 x general population death rates
Diseases of circulatory system	2.5 x general population death rates

BOX 69.1: METABOLIC SYNDROME

For a person to be defined as having metabolic syndrome they must have:
Central obesity (defined as waist circumference ≥ 94 cm for European men and ≥ 80 cm for European women, with ethnicity-specific values for other groups).
Plus any two of the following four factors:

- raised triglyceride level
- reduced HDL (high density lipo-protein) cholesterol
- raised blood pressure, or treatment of previously diagnosed hypertension
- raised fasting plasma glucose or previously diagnosed type 2 diabetes

Source: International Diabetes Federation.[10]

observed that people with schizophrenia were 1.8 times more likely to have a diagnosis of HIV, and patients with a mood disorder were 3.8 times more likely to have such a diagnosis, compared with the general population.

Other common health issues experienced by people with SMI, which can have serious consequences, include constipation, poor oral health and eye conditions.[19] Skin conditions and foot problems often secondary to poor self-care are also common.

> **REFLECTION**
>
> - Think about the service users with whom you work.
> - What physical health needs or risks are you aware of?
> - What impact do any physical health needs have on their overall well-being?

WHY DO PEOPLE WITH SMI EXPERIENCE POOR PHYSICAL HEALTH?

Understanding why people with SMI experience poor physical health is essential if strategies to intervene and improve health are going to be effective. MHNs need to be knowledgeable about the multiple factors that interplay to increase the risk to physical health, and must be confident about helping service users avoid or reduce modifiable risks.[19]

Lifestyle factors

The influence of lifestyle factors is important, not just for those with SMI. Scott and Happell[5] present a clear picture of a range of factors that impact negatively on the health of individuals with SMI, including increased rates of smoking, poor dietary intake, low physical activity levels and increased use of illicit substances and alcohol. An overview of these factors and others is now provided.

DIETARY INTAKE

People with SMI tend to have less nutritious diets than the general population. In general such individuals have a lower intake of fruit and vegetables, higher levels of saturated fat consumption, lower levels of dietary fibre and often a high consumption of sugar-laden fizzy drinks.[17,20,21] People with schizophrenia have also been found to have lower intake of vitamins A and C and beta-carotene.[22,23] Poor dietary intake can lead to malnutrition and service users can experience both over- and undernutrition, with resulting weight increase and possible obesity, or weight loss. Both over- and undernutrition have a significant impact on morbidity and risk of mortality, and good nutrition is important for maintaining both good physical and mental health. BAPEN[24] found that 1 in 5 people admitted to a mental health unit were malnourished. Undernutrition is of particular concern for older people, with 10 per cent of all older people being affected,[25] but it is not exclusive to this age group. People of all ages with varying mental health conditions can experience undernutrition.

SMOKING

Smoking prevalence among people with mental illness is substantially higher than the general population. There are three million smokers in UK with a mental health diagnosis, and there has been no change in smoking prevalence in the last 20 to 30 years.[26] Prevalence varies across different mental health diagnoses, with studies finding that 40 to 50 per cent of people with depressive and anxiety disorders smoke, as do up to 75 per cent of people with schizophrenia.[27] This compares with approximately 21 per cent of the general population.[9] People with SMI are also more likely to smoke heavily and are more nicotine-dependent, which increases the risk of smoking-related harms such as lung disease and cancers.[8,28]

A number of reasons for increased smoking rates have been identified. These include genetic and environmental factors influencing vulnerability, neurobiological associations between tobacco and various mental health conditions, and individual factors. Those living in institutional settings report that it helps combat feelings of boredom and isolation.[28,29] A significant issue has also been a culture of acceptance of smoking in mental health services, despite an emphasis upon smoke-free environments and the provision of specialist smoking cessation services.[30] Professionals' beliefs and attitudes towards smoking and smoking cessation for people with SMI have a significant impact on the interventions and support provided.[30,31]

> **REFLECTION**
>
> - Consider the belief statements in Box 69.2.
> - Do you share these beliefs? Are they based on experience or fact?
> - How do your attitudes and beliefs impact on how you approach the issue of smoking cessation?
> - How would you argue against each statement and what evidence is there available to support your counterargument?

BOX 69.2: BELIEF STATEMENTS WITH REGARD TO SMOKING IN PEOPLE WITH SMI

- Smoking is their only pleasure in life, and I don't want to be the one taking it away.

- Challenging smoking means risking the therapeutic relationship and I'm not going to do that.

- Smoking is the smallest thing these people have to deal with.

- It's the only thing they have control over; it's unethical to remove it.

- Mental health patients who are not allowed to smoke become more aggressive and hard to manage.

- Smoking helps people with mental illness self-medicate.

- People with mental illness are not interested in quitting smoking.

- It is too difficult for people with mental illness to quit smoking.

- Quitting smoking will interfere with recovery from mental illness.

- Dealing with their mental illness is the priority; addressing smoking is not my responsibility.

Source: Adapted from Ratschen et al.[31] and Hehir et al.[32]

PHYSICAL ACTIVITY

A sedentary lifestyle is a contributory risk factor for CVD, particularly because of its association with obesity. Regular physical activity can have significant benefits for both physical health (for example, reduction of risk of CVD and diabetes) and mental health.[33,34] However, people with SMI often struggle with this. Research[35] has indicated that people with SMI are interested in physical activity and enjoy it, yet such individuals often report low levels of confidence in being able to undertake exercise when feeling sad or stressed and that they receive little or no support from family and friends. In addition, mental health professionals do not regularly promote or support increased physical activity.

The current health recommendation from the Department of Health[36] with regard to physical activity is that adults (aged 19 to 64 years) and older people (aged 65+) should undertake 150 minutes each week of moderate- to vigorous-intensity physical activity (and adults should aim to do some physical activity every day). It is recommended that muscle strengthening activity should also be included twice a week.[36] However, a report from the British Heart Foundation[37] stated that less than half of all adults in the UK are meeting these recommended aims, with the proportion declining with age. With an established link between socio-economic status and levels of physical activity[38] and additional potential challenges for people with SMI, it is not surprising that levels of physical activity are low.

SUBSTANCE AND ALCOHOL USE

In the UK it is thought that the number of people with a co-existing mental illness and either substance or alcohol dependence is high and may be increasing.[39] The prevalence of co-existing mental health and substance use problems may affect between 30 and 70 per cent of those presenting to health and social care settings.[40] These individuals are likely to be experiencing a complex array of mental health, psychological and social needs, but also significant physical health needs. Harmful alcohol and substance use (chapter 31) can lead to hypertension, liver disease, reduced fertility and gynaecological problems in women, heart disease stroke and cancer, and substance use in particular can increase the risk of contracting blood-borne viruses such as hepatitis B and C and HIV.[41]

SEXUAL HEALTH

It is suggested that those with SMI are more likely to engage in high-risk behaviour in relation to their sexual health. Higher rates of alcohol and substance use may in part contribute to sexual risk taking.[42] Behaviours may include casual sexual encounters, less regular use of condoms, and using sex for some material gain. People with SMI may also be at risk of sexual exploitation and may struggle to negotiate safe sex with partners. Their risk of poor sexual health and sexually transmitted infections is therefore increased.[43] Compounding this is the poor consideration paid to sexual health by mental health professionals, who often find the subject difficult to discuss and address, and who may have poor knowledge and awareness of risks.[44]

Psychotropic medication

While psychotropic medications may be efficacious for many in helping to manage symptoms of mental illness, they may have potentially health-damaging side effects (chapter 47). Atypical antipsychotics can result in weight gain, hyper-prolactinaemia, hyperlipidaemia, sedation, cardiovascular issues, postural hypotension, altered glucose metabolism and increased risk of diabetes.[45] Although there are differences in side effect profiles among the drugs available, all have potential consequences for physical health, with the risk of CVD causing most concern. Further details about side effects and monitoring can be found in chapters 47 and 48.

The impact of side effects such as weight gain can be significant to a person's self-esteem, confidence and emotional well-being, as illustrated in the following 'Service user's perspective', provided by a young woman who took antipsychotic medication.

Indirect consequences of mental illness

Factors related to the mental illness itself are also significant. Ongoing symptoms, such as suspiciousness, low mood, cognitive difficulties and lack of motivation, can make it difficult for individuals to spontaneously report physical health concerns or to engage in activities to improve physical well-being. Experience of stigma can also make people mistrust health professionals. Socio-economic issues may also compound difficulties in accessing health-supporting services in addition to making lifestyle changes.

Barriers to adequate care

The National Audit of Schizophrenia[4] found inconsistencies in care provision by Mental Health Trusts across the country. The audit revealed that on average only 29 per cent of people with schizophrenia had received a full health check (body mass index, smoking, blood pressure, blood glucose and lipids). These are basic checks which could all be undertaken by MHNs and which could all indicate a health risk requiring intervention.

Chadwick et al.[46] undertook a review of studies from the last decade from the service user perspective in relation to physical health. Studies revealed issues around inaccessibility of physical health care and a mistrust

SERVICE USER'S PERSPECTIVE

As the weeks went by, my body weight began to become more of an issue that caused me further emotional stress. Unfortunately with the majority of antipsychotic medication come side effects and one of them is weight gain. After being on a depot for just 2 weeks I started to gain weight and my family and friends started to notice the drastic change in my weight. I tried everything to help reduce my weight, I joined the gym, I did a few intense Zumba classes a few times a week. I closely monitored my diet, I cut out all fats and reduced my portion sizes significantly but the weight just wouldn't drop. I knew that this weight gain was not normal weight gain, but the effect of the meds, as at times I looked and felt quite swollen.

My mum would try to reassure me, however. She'd say I was still beautiful even though I had gained a bit of weight, and that it was also better than spending all my life in and out of hospital; and my siblings seemed equally supportive. But unfortunately, in the real world, not everyone is as emotionally delicate with you as your family. As my weight increased, I found myself isolated at work, my colleagues would no longer engage with me socially, and at times I'd overhear some of them talking about me and my weight gain – and not in a nice way. It was all a really hard time for me, especially as I had good memories of how things were before my illness and the medication.

SERVICE USER'S PERSPECTIVE

My physical health problems began when I was pregnant 7 years ago. I started having pains in my knees and legs so I went to the doctors. I went several times. Each time I felt the doctors fobbed me off. They didn't listen to me. Even when my support worker came with me I didn't think they listened to me. I thought ... am I explaining myself properly? I gave up hope ... I thought I'm never going to get to the bottom of this knee pain. I did have tests and X-rays but initially they didn't find anything. It's difficult to trust doctors; they don't explain things very well, in a way that I can understand. The problems went on for years. Even my parents and family didn't believe me. That upset me. My mental illness can make me mistrust people. I get lots of negative thoughts often around people not believing me.

My physical health was on my mind constantly. I became worried about cancer, blood clots ... I was really anxious all the time. I can get confused and have a lot of negative thoughts, often about my physical health. Once when I was admitted to a mental health hospital a junior doctor on the ward noticed me limping. He said to me that he could see that I was in pain. It felt good to know that I was believed. This was a mental health ward but they picked up on this. I had more tests and they did eventually show that there was a problem. I thought I wasn't mad after all. I am now waiting for an operation. It makes me sad that it took so long to get to this point.

of services, including practical difficulties such as long waiting times, hurried appointments and crowded waiting areas. Service users felt that professionals lacked information, education and knowledge of illness and treatment options. They reported poor physical assessments and experienced diagnostic overshadowing, which led to service users not disclosing concerns. Diagnostic overshadowing is when symptoms of physical illness are attributed to someone's mental illness and thus dismissed by health care professionals.

The following 'Service user's perspective' from a woman who has schizophrenia illustrates some of the issues that are identified far too frequently by those accessing services.

> **REFLECTION**
>
> - Do you regularly talk to your service users and carers about their experience of physical health care?
> - How can their experiences guide improvements in care within your teams and services?
> - What is your role in facilitating this?

WHAT PHYSICAL HEALTH CARE SHOULD BE PROVIDED?

It is clearly stated within the updated National Institute for Health and Care Excellence (NICE) guidelines on psychosis and schizophrenia[47] that both primary and secondary care services have key responsibilities in regard to the comprehensive assessment of medical and physical health needs and the provision of evidenced-based interventions. The NICE guidance for bipolar disorder[48] also refers to the importance of monitoring and physical assessment. The Royal College of Psychiatrists has also published its own standards for psychiatric services which can be used to support policies, service development and auditing of care provision.[49]

Assessment, monitoring and screening of physical health

Contact with a mental health team may provide the first opportunity for an individual with mental illness to have their physical health needs assessed. Research has demonstrated that, despite an emphasis of responsibility on primary care with regard to meeting physical health needs, in practice this is not consistently delivered and issues with accessibility to services are prevalent.[3] Mental health professionals need to work with primary care to provide this, and local policies and integrated care agreements need to be in place. Contact with mental health services may also mean the initiation of treatment that can increase physical health risks, and therefore there is a duty of care to ensure that effective health monitoring is provided.

With the nursing process in mind, assessment is the first step to identifying an individual's needs in order to enable the development of a collaborative care plan (see chapter 13 for more information on assessment, and chapter 50 for more on collaborative care planning). The assessment process does not need to be an overly complicated or onerous task, but MHNs do need to have a clear understanding of what is required and the resources available, and they need to possess the appropriate level of knowledge and skills. A comprehensive physical health check carried out by a competent practitioner such as a MHN can provide the opportunity to screen for cardiovascular risk, offer education regarding lifestyle and ask about other physical conditions.[50]

> **REFLECTION**
>
> In order to undertake a comprehensive physical health assessment:
>
> - What practical considerations should you consider beforehand?
> - How might you undertake and structure your assessment?
> - What would you want to assess and find out?

In order to carry out a systematic assessment of physical health, a structured approach is important. MHNs may be routinely collecting information about a person's health; however, if this is just merely recorded and not reviewed systematically, the potential significance of the information gathered may not be identified. A full physical assessment and review should be a multidisciplinary activity, with local policies indicating the key professional responsibilities and roles. The existing therapeutic relationship (chapter 3) between a MHN and a service user can offer the ideal opportunity to engage in a dialogue about physical health and well-being as well as health assessment and monitoring as part of day-to-day care.

Prior to undertaking any assessment, the service user's informed consent must be sought. The assessment process should be undertaken in a way that enables the service user to feel comfortable in sharing personal information. See chapters 13, 14 and 15 for more on assessment. Sensitivity, privacy and cultural awareness are required. If a service user is unable or unwilling to provide consent (chapter 18), then this should be documented and reviewed regularly. General observational information can still be gathered, and information obtained from the service user's GP, carers or family members, which can help indicate any immediate health concerns.

Monitoring of physiological observations and the NEWS

Undertaking physiological observations or taking vital signs can provide a useful indicator of current health status. The National Patient Safety Association has raised concerns about the lack of recognition of deterioration of patients' physical state within acute hospitals.[51] They reported a lack of recording of full observations throughout a patient's stay, a delay in recognizing when patients were becoming unwell and poor communication of risk between nurses and doctors. This issue has also been recognized in mental health wards, and as a consequence the introduction of a National Early Warning Score (NEWS) is recommended. The NEWS[52] is a track and trigger system which scores six physiological parameters; respiration rate, systolic blood pressure, heart rate, temperature, oxygen saturations and level of consciousness using the AVPU ('alert, voice, pain, unresponsive') system. The use of this tool is especially important following rapid tranquilization and sedation of patients.

Patient safety is dependent on accurate measurement of physiological vital signs and accurate documentation, with appropriate responses and escalation of intervention. MHNs need to be accountable for their skills and ensure they are following best practice in undertaking physical observations. It should also be recognized that, when delegating this responsibility to unqualified health care assistants, the MHN still maintains accountability for their practice. Training and supervision should be available and accessed.

Mental-health-specific physical assessment tools

In addition to the national and local guidance available, several tools have been developed to support physical health assessment and screening within a mental health setting which MHNs could readily utilize. These include the Physical Health Check Tool[53] and the Health Improvement Profile.[54] The Positive Cardiometabolic Health Resource[55] also provides an intervention framework for patients taking antipsychotic medication.

THE PHYSICAL HEALTH CHECK TOOL (PHC)

The PHC was first developed by a multidisciplinary research group based within a community mental health team who were aiming to improve the provision of physical health care.[56] The tool has recently been reviewed and updated by Rethink Mental Illness[53] in collaboration with service users, carers and practitioners from both primary and secondary care. It is designed to be used by mental health staff to assess physical health needs and stimulate a dialogue between the practitioner and the service user. This dialogue or conversation aims to identify unmet needs and to facilitate a collaboratively agreed action plan with the service user. The tool can be easily incorporated into the Care Programme Approach (chapter 37). The tool consists of four sections:

1. General health and lifestyle
2. Symptom checklist
3. Screening checks
4. Agreed action plan

Completing the PHC with service users may be the vital first step to raising awareness of physical health and to addressing unmet physical health needs. Examples of agreed actions following the check may include interventions such as smoking cessation support, referral for medical review or other supportive interventions such as referral to chiropody or dental care.

THE SERIOUS MENTAL ILLNESS HEALTH IMPROVEMENT PROFILE (HIP)

The HIP[54] is a physical risk assessment tool which aims to help MHNs profile the physical health of individuals with SMI. The tool also directs the user to the relevant evidence based interventions to address identified needs. Twenty-eight health parameters have been identified through research as shown in Box 69.3:

Research into the implementation of the tool has produced promising findings in relation to its feasibility, its effectiveness

BOX 69.3: HIP HEALTH PARAMETERS

Body mass index	Breast check (women and men)
Waist circumference	Menstrual cycle
Pulse	Smoking status
Blood pressure	Exercise
Temperature	Alcohol intake
Liver function tests	Diet: five portions of fruit and vegetables a day
Lipid levels	Diet: fat intake
Glucose	Fluid intake
Cervical smear	Caffeine intake
Prostate and testicles check	Cannabis use
Sleep	Safe sex
Teeth	Urine
Eyes	Bowels
Feet	Sex satisfaction

for detecting physical comorbidity and planning evidenced-based interventions, its acceptability to service users and clinicians and its potential to prevent further deterioration of health. However, further research is needed to demonstrate any significant impact on improving cardiovascular risk.[57,58]

THE POSITIVE CARDIOMETABOLIC HEALTH RESOURCE

With cardiovascular and metabolic disease presenting the largest risk for people with SMI, a focus on assessment of both non-modifiable and modifiable risk factors is pertinent, as previously discussed. NICE clearly identifies the assessment requirements of adults with schizophrenia and psychosis and specifically states that health professionals should 'Routinely monitor weight, and cardiovascular and metabolic indicators of morbidity in people with psychosis and schizophrenia'[47] (p.13).

The Positive Cardiometabolic Health Resource[55] is an intervention framework for people taking antipsychotic medication. However, it is applicable to those taking other psychotropic medication. It clearly sets out the essential components of a screening assessment of cardiometabolic risk (smoking, lifestyle and life skills, body mass index, blood pressure, glucose regulation and blood lipids) and outlines a range of evidence-based guidance and interventions. The key message of the resource is: 'Don't just screen, intervene'[55] (p.1). It provides a valuable guide for MHNs in the consideration of care provided to service users and can support practice development for multidisciplinary teams within clinical areas.

Approaches to promoting health and supporting lifestyle change

MHNs can promote health by identifying the physical health needs of individuals (as discussed above), by raising awareness of physical health issues and by supporting people to implement strategies for improving their physical health. It is essential that a collaborative approach is taken, with the service user and MHN jointly prioritizing need and any planned actions. Family or carer involvement may also be helpful.

The Schizophrenia Commission[4] advocates that tailored health promotion programmes should be provided to enable people to take more responsibility for their own health and that these should start in acute units. Key areas for health promotion should be dietary intake, physical activity and smoking. Weight management interventions – both as an early intervention, for example, on commencement of antipsychotic medication, and as an ongoing strategy – are essential. NICE[47] recommends that people with psychosis or schizophrenia, especially those taking antipsychotics, should be offered a combined healthy eating and physical activity programme by their mental health care provider. MHNs should incorporate health promotion into their care; however, low expectations of practitioners regarding the ability of service users to make

lifestyle changes can lead to therapeutic nihilism.[59] If we are to embrace the recovery approach, then we need to maintain an optimistic approach and deliver approaches that can motivate people to make and sustain changes.

De Hert et al.[60] identify that many individuals with SMI do not recognize the need to change a behaviour or do not have the knowledge and skills to make changes to their lifestyle to improve health, and therefore awareness raising is important. However, when attempting to provide health messages, practitioners often resort to an 'advice giving' role which is likely to be ineffective and can result in them being perceived as the 'health police' rather than a facilitator for change by the recipient. Instead, it is more useful to engage in a dialogue whereby an exchange of information occurs between service user and practitioner. Before providing health information it is helpful to ascertain what somebody already knows about the particular issue, what their particular concerns are and what they want to know so that health information can be individualized. There are lots of accessible resources to support discussions, such as those provided by the British Heart Foundation, Diabetes UK and other health promotion organizations. Co-produced information resources may be particularly useful, such as those provided by Rethink (see 'Relevant web pages' section).

Providing information alone rarely leads to sustained behaviour change. There are multiple factors influencing behaviour change, which include predisposing factors such as knowledge, beliefs, age, gender, culture and socioeconomic factors; enabling factors such as individual ability and skill and available resources; and reinforcing factors such as social and peer support.[61] Motivational interviewing is an evidenced-based approach to prompt and support behaviour change with its facilitative style of communication.[62] (See chapter 39 for further information about motivational interviewing.)

NICE[63] outlines key recommendations for professionals when seeking to promote behaviour change. They state that selected interventions should enable individuals to:

- understand the short-, medium- and longer-term consequences of their health-related behaviours;
- feel positive about the benefits of health-enhancing behaviours and changing their behaviour;
- plan their changes in easy steps over time;
- recognize that their social contexts and relationships may affect their behaviour, and identify and plan for situations that might undermine the changes they are trying to make;
- plan explicit 'if … then' coping strategies to prevent relapse;
- make a personal commitment to adopt health-enhancing behaviours by setting (and recording) goals to undertake clearly defined behaviours, in particular contexts, over a specified time;
- share their behaviour goals with others.

Any plan needs to be mutually agreed with the service user and tailored to their individual circumstances. It is important to recognize that sometimes things do not go as planned and change does not occur or is not maintained. This is normal, regardless of whether someone has a mental health issue or not. Any success or attempts should be positively acknowledged and lessons sought from the situation. Continuing encouragement and support should be provided and an optimistic approach for future change maintained.

DeHert et al.[60] provide some practical suggestions/behavioural interventions to help support healthy eating behaviours and encourage physical activity for people with SMI. When sharing these suggestions, it is important to include and discuss with any family members or carers who live with or support someone (Table 69.2).

> ### REFLECTION
>
> - What health advice have you been given by a health professional?
> - Have you managed to change health behaviour or make a lifestyle change?
> - What helped and enabled you to do this?
> - How does your experience inform how you might support someone else to change their behaviour?

The hospital environment

The following 'Service user's perspective', provided by a young woman who had several admissions to hospital, illustrates the impact the ward environment can have on someone's physical well-being.

> ### REFLECTION
>
> - Consider the 'Service user's perspective' above. Could the MHNs on the ward have provided more support to manage any potential weight gain during her stay?
> - What opportunities are there within hospital wards to promote physical activity and help avoid prolonged periods of inactivity?
> - Do hospital wards provide healthy living activities or groups for service users?

MHNs need to be proactive in seeking opportunities to promote health and take a lead in improving access to hospital environments and services that support overall well-being. Within inpatient settings, consideration should be given to how the ward environment supports healthy behaviours such as nutrition and physical activity. How accessible is a healthy diet? Are there opportunities for physical activity? Is health information readily available? Do wards offer opportunities to develop peer support, self-management

Table 69.2 Strategies to promote healthy eating and physical activity

Strategies to promote healthy eating	*Healthy eating behaviour* Reducing fast food/takeaways
	Increasing healthy food items (fruits, vegetables, fish); decreasing high glycaemic index food items and mono-unsaturated fats
	Reducing processed fat-free food
	Making healthy snack choices
	Controlling portion size
	Eating four to six small meals
	Eating more slowly
	Minimizing intake of soft drinks with sugar and with artificial sweeteners
	Education Reading food labels
	Learning to discern differences between physiological and psychological appetite and eating
	Keeping food diaries/plans/exchange tables
	Learning cooking skills
	Healthy food shopping
Strategies to promote physical activity	Keeping activity diaries, daily activity list
	Increasing physical activity such as moderate intensity walking
	Reduce sedentary behaviours (TV watching, video/computer games, etc.)
	Treating/reducing sedation and motor side effects of medications

SERVICE USER'S PERSPECTIVE

SERVICE USER'S PERSPECTIVE

Throughout my year-long stay in hospital from the time of my diagnosis, my physical health began to deteriorate. The times at which I had been admitted as an inpatient would often lead me to gain several pounds due to the lack of activity available. Unfortunately, the hospital had not invested in other forms of therapeutic activity for patients and I often felt like a fish in a tank with little to occupy my mind; and my body was physically restricted to the ward and a few other areas. I would be in a very sedentary state. Despite the enclosed size of the ward(s), I would generally be given a high dose of oral medication which would normally sedate me and I would spend most of the day asleep in bed and then wake for dinner at 5pm, and then after dinner go back to my dorm and sleep until nightly meds. So of course my mind was getting the mental rest it needed due to the sedative and tranquil atmosphere, but my physical health was suffering as I was slowly becoming more and more inactive.

SERVICE USER'S PERSPECTIVE

Although I was told by health professionals and friends alike not to worry too much about my physical state or appearance but to focus on my mental well-being, I knew back then that it was something that was important to me and in fact to society in general. I found that staying physically well was a great motivator and allowed me to physically and mentally put myself back into society and engage in the social interactions I would have taken for granted before be coming unwell. My journey in particular has been very difficult; as my mental health symptoms fluctuated, so did the levels to which I would take care of my physical health too. But I know now, from my 5 years of living with a mental health condition, that taking care of one's physical health and avoiding neglecting it can make the overall journey to recovery a lot more accomplishable and perhaps faster.

and community engagement? Can patients access dental and screening services? Is information on health issues accessible and signposted? Similarly, we should ask: how are people living in the community accessing community resources and opportunities to promote and improve health? Practical support, which considers the range of factors influencing health and health behaviour, is important, and approaches should be tailored to meet the additional challenges faced by people experiencing SMI. Dieticians, physical therapists and smoking cessation advisors are all likely to be accessible either within the Mental Health Trust or through mainstream public health/health promotion services. Opportunities to co-work and collaborate with these professionals will enhance the care offered by MHNs to individuals and will help develop MHNs' own skills. Peer support can also be particularly valuable in enabling and empowering service users.

Advocacy and liaison

Finally, a key role for MHNs is advocacy. The accessibility of health services and the possibility of stigma can impede the provision of appropriate care, and can lead individuals to feel distrustful of health professionals and their intervention. People who have received previously unhelpful responses from services may need practical support to access information, treatment and care. Those with long-term conditions should be supported to access primary care and specialist services. Even within one's own multidisciplinary team the MHN may need to advocate for the service user – for example, by supporting collaborative decision making with regard to medication prescribing. In order to work effectively within a multidisciplinary and integrated care framework, MHNs need to be competent and confident in their role and to be able to communicate and liaise effectively with other health professionals. Establishing good relationships between local practitioners and services can also enhance the care provided.

CONCLUSION

Good physical health is an important contributor to a sense of well-being and can support recovery for those experiencing SMI. The avoidable premature morbidity and mortality experienced by many people with SMI cannot be ignored.

Meeting physical health needs and promoting physical well-being are integral to the overall craft of caring, and MHNs have a responsibility to ensure they have the knowledge, skills and attitude required to do this.

ACKNOWLEDGEMENTS

The author would like to express her sincere thanks to the two service users who kindly shared their experiences and reflections for this chapter.

References

1. Department of Health. *Closing the gap: priorities for essential change in mental health.* London: Stationery Office, 2014.

2. Brown S, Kim M, Mitchell C, Inskip H. Twenty-five year mortality of a community cohort with schizophrenia. *British Journal of Psychiatry* 2010; **196**: 116–21.

3. DRC (Disability Rights Commission). *Equal treatment: closing the gap: a formal investigation into the physical health inequalities experienced by people with learning disabilities and/or mental health problems.* London: DRC, 2006.

4. Schizophrenia Commission. *The abandoned Illness, a report by the Schizophrenia Commission.* London: Rethink Mental Illness, 2012.

5. Scott D, Happell B. The high prevalence of poor physical health and unhealthy lifestyle behaviours in individuals with severe mental illness. *Issues in Mental Health Nursing* 2011; **32**: 589–97.

6. Chang C-K, Hayes R, Perera G, Broadbent M, Fernandes A, Lee W, Hotopf M, Stewart R. Life expectancy at birth for people with serious mental illness and other major disorders from a secondary mental health care case register in London. *PLoS One* 2001; **6**(5): e19590. Available from: http://www.plosone.org/article/info:doi/10.1371/journal.pone.0019590 [Accessed 8th December 2016].

7. Osborn DPJ, King MB, Nazareth I. Participation in cardiovascular risk screening by people with schizophrenia or similar mental illnesses; a cross sectional study in general Practice. *British Medical Journal* 2003; **326**: 1122–3.

8. Busche B, Holt R. Prevalence of diabetes and impaired glucose tolerance in patients with schizophrenia. *British Journal of Psychiatry* 2004; **184**: 67–71.

9. Health and Social Care Information Centre. *Mental Health Bulletin: annual report from MHMDS returns – England, 2011–12, further analysis and organisation-level data.* London: Health and Social Care Information Centre, 2012.

10. IDF (International Diabetes Federation). *The IDF Consensus worldwide definition of metabolic syndrome.* Belgium: IDF, 2006.

11. Usher K, Foster K, Park T. The metabolic syndrome and schizophrenia: the latest evidence and nursing guidelines for management. *Journal of Psychiatric and Mental Health Nursing* 2006; **13**: 730–4.

12. Allison D, Casey D. Anti-psychotic induced weight gain; a review of the literature. *Journal of Clinical Psychiatry* 2001; **62** (suppl. 7): 22–31.

13. Citrome L, Vreeland B. Obesity and mental illness. *Modern Trends in Pharmacopsychiatry* 2009; **26**: 25–46.

14. Simon G, Von Korff M, Saunders K, Miglioretti D, Crane P, Van Belle G, Kessler R. Association between obesity and psychiatric disorders in the US adult population. *Archives of General Psychiatry* 2006; **63**(7): 824–30.

15. Barnes T, Paton C, Cavanagh M, Hancock E, Taylor D. A UK audit of screening for the metabolic side effects of antipsychotics in community patients. *Schizophrenia Bulletin* 2007; **33**: 1397–401.

16. De Hert M, Correll C, Bobes J, Cetkovich-Bakmas M, Cohen D, Asai I, Detraux J, Gautam S, Moller H, Ndetei D, Newcomer J, Uwakwe R, Leucht S. Physical illness in patients with severe mental disorders. I. Prevalence, impact of medications and disparities in health care. *World Psychiatry* 2011; **10**: 52–77.

17. McCreadie R. Diet, smoking and cardiovascular risk in people with schizophrenia. *British Journal of Psychiatry* 2003; **183**: 534–9.

18. Blank M, Mandell D, Aiken L, Hadley T. Co-occurrence of HIV and serious mental illness among Medicaid Recipients. *Psychiatric Services* 2002; **53**(7): 868–73.

19. Robson D, Gray R. Serious mental illness and physical health problems: a discussion paper. *International Journal of Nursing Studies* 2007; **44**: 457–66.

20. Peet M. Diet, diabetes and schizophrenia. *British Journal of Psychiatry* 2004; **184** (suppl. 47): 102–5.

21. Amani R. Is dietary pattern of schizophrenia patients different from healthy subjects? *BMC Psychiatry* 2007; **7**: 15.

22. Brown S, Inskip H, Barraclough B. Causes of excess mortality in schizophrenia. *British Journal of Psychiatry* 2000; **177**: 212–17.

23. McCreadie R. Scottish Schizophrenia Lifestyle Group. Diet, smoking, and cardiovascular risk in people with schizophrenia: descriptive study. *British Journal of Psychiatry* 2003; **183**: 534–9.

24. Russell CA, Elia M. *Nutrition Screening Survey in the UK and Republic of Ireland in 2010. A report by BAPEN.* London: BAPEN, 2011.

25. European Nutrition for Health Alliance and BAPEN. *Malnutrition among older people in the community: policy recommendations for change.* London: European Nutrition for Health Alliance, 2006.

26. Royal College of Psychiatrists. *Smoking and mental health: a joint report by the Royal College of Physicians and the Royal College of Psychiatrists.* London: RCP, 2013.

27. Diaz F, James D, Botts S, Maw L, Susce M. Tobacco smoking behaviours in popular disorder: a comparison of the general population, schizophrenia and major depression. *Bipolar Disorders* 2009; **1**(2): 154–65.

28. Campion J, Checinski K, Nurse J, McNeill A. Smoking by people with mental illness and benefits of smoke-free mental health services. *Advances in Psychiatric Treatment* 2008; **14**: 217–28.

29. Mental Health Foundation. *Taking a deep breath; the mental health implications of anti-smoking legislation.* London: Mental Health Foundation, 2007.

30. Ratschen E, Britton J, McNeill A. The smoking culture in psychiatry: time for change. *British Journal of Psychiatry* 2011; **198**: 6–7.

31. Ratschen E, Britton J, Doody G, Leonardi-Bee J, McNeill A. Tobacco dependence, treatment and smoke-free policies: a survey of mental health professionals' knowledge and attitudes. *General Hospital Psychiatry* 2009; **31**: 576–82.

32. Hehir A, Indig D, Prosser S, Archer V. Implementation of a smoke-free policy in a high secure mental health inpatient facility: staff survey to describe experience and attitudes. *BMC Public Health* 2013; **3**: 315.

33. Press V, Freestone I, George C. Physical activity: the evidence of benefit in the prevention of coronary heart disease. *QJM: an International Journal of Medicine* 2003; **96**(4): 245–51.

34. Acil A, Dogan S, Dogan, O. The effects of physical exercises to mental state and quality of life in patients with schizophrenia. *Journal of Psychiatric and Mental Health Nursing* 2008; **15**(10): 808–15.

35. Ussher M, Stanbury L, Cheeseman V, Faulkner G. Physical activity preferences and perceived barriers to activity among persons with severe mental illness in the United Kingdom. *Psychiatric Services* 2007; **58**(3): 405–8.

36. Department of Health. *Physical activity guidelines in the UK: review and recommendations.* London: Stationery Office, 2011.

37. BHF (British Heart Foundation). *Physical Activity Statistics 2012*. London: BHF, 2012.

38. Giles-Corti B, Donovan R. Socioeconomic status differences in recreational physical activity levels and real and perceived access to a supportive physical environment. *Preventative Medicine* 2002; **35**(6): 601–11.

39. Phillips P, McKeown O, Sandford T. *Dual diagnosis – practice in context*. Oxford: Wiley-Blackwell, 2010.

40. Crome I, Chambers P, Frisher M, Bloor R, Roberts D. *The relationship between dual diagnosis: substance misuse and dealing with mental health issues*. London: Social Care Institute for Excellence, 2009.

41. NTA (National Treatment Agency for Substance Misuse). *Why invest? How drug treatment and recovery services work for individuals, communities and society*. London: NTA, 2012.

42. Susser E, Mille M, Valenci E, Colson P, Roche B, Conove S. Injection drug use and risk of HIV transmission among homeless men with mental illness. *American Journal of Psychiatry* 1996; **1153**: 794–8.

43. Cournos, F, McKinnon M, Sullivan G. Schizophrenia and comorbid Human Immunodeficiency Virus or Hepatitis C Virus. *Journal of Clinical Psychiatry* 2005; **66** (suppl. 6): 27–33.

44. Hughes E, Gray R. HIV prevention for people with serious mental illness: a survey of mental healthworkers' attitudes, knowledge and practice. *Journal of Clinical Nursing* 2009; **18**(4): 591–600.

45. Ucok A, Gaebel W. Side effects of atypical antipsychotics: a brief overview. *World Psychiatry* 2008; **7**: 58–62.

46. Chadwick A, Street C, McAndrew S, Deacon M. Minding our own bodies: reviewing the literature regarding the perceptions of service users diagnosed with serious mental illness on barriers to accessing physical health care. *International Journal of Mental Health Nursing* 2012; **3**: 211–19.

47. NICE (National Institute for Health and Care Excellence). *Clinical Guideline 178: Schizophrenia and psychosis in adults; treatment and management*. London: NICE, 2014.

48. NICE (National Institute for Health and Care Excellence) *Bipolar disorder: the management of bipolar disorder in adults, children and adolescents, in primary and secondary care*. London: NICE, 2006.

49. Royal College of Psychiatrists. *Physical health in mental health OP 67*. London: Royal College of Psychiatrists, 2009.

50. Hardy S. Maintaining physical health in severe mental illness. *Independent Nurse* 2009; 2 Feb: 26–7.

51. National Patient Safety Agency. *Recognising and responding appropriately to early signs of deterioration in hospitalised patients*. London: National Patient Safety Agency, 2007.

52. Royal College of Physicians. *National Early Warning Scores: standardising the assessment of acute-illness severity in the NHS*. London: Royal College of Physicians, 2012.

53. Rethink. *A physical health check for mental health service users*. London: Rethink, 2011.

54. White J, Gray R, Jones M. The development of the serious mental illness physical Health Improvement Profile. *Journal of Psychiatric and Mental Health Nursing* 2009; **16**: 493–8.

55. Lester H, Shiers D, Rafi I, Cooper S, Holt R. *Positive Cardiometabolic Health Resource: an intervention framework for patients with psychosis on antipsychotic medication*. London: Royal College of Psychiatrists, 2012.

56. Phelan M, Stradins L, Amin D, Isadore R, Hitrov C, Doyle A, Inglis R. The Physical Health Check: a tool for mental health workers. *Journal of Mental Health* 2004; **13**(3): 277–84.

57. Shuel F, White J, Jones M, Gray R. Using the serious mental illness health improvement profile (HIP) to identify physical problems in a cohort of community patients: a pragmatic case series evaluation. *International Journal of Nursing Studies* 2010; **47**: 136–45.

58. Bressington D, Mui J, Hulbert S, Cheung E, Bradford S, Gray R. Enhanced physical health screening for people with severe mental illness in Hong Kong: results from a one-year prospective case series study. *BMC Psychiatry* 2014; **14**: 57.

59. Holt R, Peveler R. Diabetes and cardiovascular risk in severe mental illness: a missed opportunity and challenge for the future. *Practical Diabetes International* 2010; **27**: 79–84.

60. De Hert M, Cohen D, Bobes J, Cetkovich-Bakmas M, Leucht S, Ndetei D, Newcomer J, Uwakwe R, Asai I, Moller HJ, Gautam S, Detraux J, Correll CU. Physical illness in patients with severe mental disorders. II. Barriers to care, monitoring and treatment guidelines, plus recommendations at the system and individual level. *World Psychiatry* 2011; **10**(2): 138–51.

61. Davies L, Donatelle R. *Access to health*, 9th edn. San Francisco: Benjamin Cummings Publishing Company, 2006.

62. Miller W, Rollnick S. *Motivational interviewing; helping people change*, 3rd edn. New York: Guilford Press, 2013.

63. NICE (National Institute for Health and Care Excellence). *Behaviour change: the principles of effective practice. Clinical Guideline PH6*. London: NICE, 2007.

Further reading

Collins E, Drake M, Deacon M. *The physical care of people with mental health problems: a guide for best practice*. London: Sage, 2013.

Cormac I, Gray D (eds). *Essentials of physical health in psychiatry*. London: Royal College of Psychiatrists, 2012.

Nash M. *Physical health and wellbeing in mental health nursing: clinical skills for practice*, 2nd edn. Maidenhead: Open University Press, 2014.

Relevant web pages

BAPEN (malnutrition and nutritional care in the UK). www.Bapen.org.uk

British Heart Foundation. www.BHF.org.uk

Diabetes UK. www.diabetes.org.uk

National Obesity Forum. www.nationalobesityforum.org.uk

Rethink. Physical health check tool (and other resources). http://www.rethink.org/about-us/health-professionals/physical-health-resources

Royal College of Psychiatrists. Improving physical and mental health. http://www.rcpsych.ac.uk/mentalhealthinfo/improvingphysicalandmh.aspx
This provides links to resources for supporting the physical health of people with mental health problems and learning difficulties and the mental health of people with physical health problems.

70 Mental health promotion

THOMAS J. CURRID AND CARL CHANDRA

LEARNING OUTCOMES

- To be able to define the concept of mental health and describe how it differs from mental illness.
- To understand core concepts in psychological and social well-being and how they relate to mental health promotion.
- To be aware of how the Ottawa Charter relates to mental health promotion.
- To be able to outline a comprehensive rationale for mental health promotion.
- To understand the interdisciplinary and inter-sectoral nature of mental health promotion.
- To be able to discuss the role of the mental health nurse, with reference to evidence-based approaches.

SUMMARY OF KEY POINTS

- Mental health is a fundamental component of our overall health and well-being and can be considered as a matter of social justice.
- There are a diverse number of factors that determine our mental health; these range from how we feel about ourselves to the value that our community places on us.
- Mental health promotion and mental illness prevention overlap, but they are two distinct approaches.

- Mental health promotion tends to focus on efforts that will enhance positive mental health, while mental illness prevention focuses on the causes of the illness or what can be done to avoid the illness.
- Mental health promotion is a key activity that requires input from macro, meso and micro levels of intervention, and it should reflect an intersectoral approach.
- The evidence base for effective mental health interventions is increasing and takes a lifespan approach.

INTRODUCTION

Our health status is an important aspect of our lives and is central to our personal well-being. As we co-exist with fellow human beings at varying levels, health impacts at individual, societal and geographical levels. The health of an individual can have many influences and effects. Broadly speaking, these may be considered as micro, meso and macro effects. For example, the recent outbreak of the Ebola virus in Africa had severe impacts on the individual (micro), their community (meso) and internationally (macro). Health also has more interdependent implications for areas including personal growth and accomplishment, human rights, economic growth and sustainability.

These interdependent variables are referred to in the first three principles of the World Health Organization's (WHO) constitution.[1] The constitution states that:

1. Health is a state of complete physical, mental and social well-being and not merely the absence of disease or infirmity.
2. The enjoyment of the highest attainable standard of health is one of the fundamental rights of every human being without distinction of race, religion, political belief, economic or social condition.
3. The health of all peoples is fundamental to the attainment of peace and security and is dependent upon the fullest co-operation of individuals and States. (p.1)

The role that health plays in our daily lives is becoming more visible, along with the ways it contributes significantly to all of the developments and maintenance of our evolving world. Additionally, the importance of promoting health as a generic unequivocal intervention for nurses is also beginning to be recognized. It may be argued that all nurses have a duty to promulgate health promotion concepts and practices. Health promotion is an integral part of a nurse's role and can be considered as the foundation upon which nursing endeavours are built. Further, health promotion is an ongoing process in the art and craft of caring, as may be seen throughout this chapter.

However, health promotion can be a varied and complex nursing intervention which combines and draws upon differing philosophies, ideologies, professional orientations, personal values and resources. For nurses who are in training or those at an early career stage, health promotion concepts and practices may be challenging and confusing, especially when set in the context of conceptual frameworks or other roles that nurses undertake. For example, while concepts such as mental health and mental illness are used interchangeably, practices such as health promotion and disease prevention can be misunderstood as being the same thing. For this reason, it may be helpful at this stage to offer some explanations of concepts and definitions, in order to delineate differences. To support this approach, it may be argued that if we are to promote and engage in the craft of caring in mental health, we need to understand what it is that we are targeting or hoping to promote.

MENTAL HEALTH

As we can see in the first principle of the WHO constitution, health status includes physical, mental and social well-being and does not just refer to the absence of illness. Similarly, mental health is much broader than the absence of psychopathologies and has many facets that are important to psychological well-being. One definition offered by the WHO[2] is that: 'Mental health is a state of well-being in which an individual realizes his or her own abilities, can cope with the normal stresses of life, can work productively and is able to make a contribution to his or her community'. While this definition offers a move towards understanding mental health, it does not explicate terms very well, nor does it particularly focus on the psychological dimensions related to self-appraisal or esteem. Other areas and processes that are known to impact on positive mental health are also omitted. These include autonomy, choice, resilience, self-worth and respect for individualism.[3]

Hedonic and eudemonic concepts

Drawing from both psychological and social research, others[4,5] have offered a more operational definition of positive mental health, based on concepts of hedonic and eudemonic well-being. Hedonic well-being relates to feelings of pleasure, happiness, satisfaction and interest in life. It originates from social research into the quality of life of Americans, which was aimed at increasing knowledge of well-being which could then be incorporated into policies that sought to improve quality of life.[4] However, opponents to the hedonic movement argued that well-being was much more than seeking pleasure and happiness and argued that living a life of virtue and actualizing one's potential was also an important pathway to mental well-being.[5] For example, proponents of humanistic psychology focused on self-actualization and personal growth, rather than focusing on the compensation of weakness and deficits which was dominant at that time in the field of psychology.[6] As a result, research into eudemonic well-being which focused on achievements and realizing one's potential was carried out, and these concepts are now universally accepted as forming part of the definition and as being essential for mental health.[4]

Operationalization of concepts

Arguing that prior research into psychological well-being has failed to define its essential features, and that purported conceptions of psychological well-being had little theoretical rationale, Ryff[7] undertook a study to operationalize, converge and define core dimensions of psychological well-being. These dimensions have been operationalized as follows.

- *Self-acceptance.* This is considered to be a central feature of mental health in which a person holds positive attitudes towards themselves and their past life.
- *Positive relations with others.* Having the ability to love is a central component of mental health. An ability to form and maintain relationships with others while being able to express affection and empathy is key to experiencing deeper relationships for psychological well-being.
- *Autonomy.* The ability to commit to one's own personal values rather than having to seek approval of others offers a sense of freedom of choice and norms governing everyday life.
- *Environmental mastery.* The ability to manage a complex environment to meet one's needs and which is suitable for personal development is characteristic of positive mental health. Active participation in and mastery of the environment is considered an indication of maturity through which the person can advance in the world.
- *Purpose in life.* Having goals and feeling that there is a purpose and meaning to life creates a sense of direction and offers hope to individuals. In turn this can influence proactive positive behaviours that add to achievements and affirmations of self-efficacy.
- *Personal growth.* Self-development and achievement enable the individual to realize their potential and ability. Further, it can contribute to resilience, so that the individual continues to develop rather than becoming static or fixed when difficult situations occur. Challenges are considered as openness to experience rather than threats to one's existence.

The above list refers primarily to psychological well-being and personal fulfilment, but it is acknowledged that these dimensions also contribute to social well-being. Keyes[4,8] asserts that, in the context of mental health, it is also important to include the social existence of the individual as they remain embedded in social structures and communities. Similar to Ryff's[7] approach, Keyes[8] has proposed an operational definition and indicators of social well-being. While social well-being is operationalized as the appraisal of the individual's circumstances and functioning in society, other constituents and indicators include:

- *Social integration.* This refers to the appraisal of the quality of one's relationship to society. Those with good mental health feel they are connected with society and integrate with others in a cohesive and inclusive manner.
- *Social acceptance.* Those who demonstrate social acceptance have favourable views of others, trust them, think others are capable of kindness, feel comfortable with

them and can be considered as the social comparable or analogue to personal acceptance.
- *Social contribution.* This is the belief in one's own role in society. This may encompass aspects such as engaging in behaviours that contribute positively to society, and understanding and believing in the vital role and obligations that they have in the world.
- *Social actualization.* This is the belief that society has potential which is being realized through the participation of its members. It involves a belief that the growth trajectory of society is evolving in a manner from which they can benefit.
- *Social coherence.* This refers to the ability to understand and make meaning of what is happening in society. Healthier individuals are considered to be those who can see their personal lives as meaningful, logical and consistent.

There is a strong argument to be made that the craft of caring involves a number of the above dimensions, which are reflected in contemporary recovery-focused frameworks (see chapters 35 and 36).

REFLECTION

- Having read the above operational constructs of psychological and social well-being, and set in context with your own mental health, do you consider that these constructs are more representative of mentally healthy behaviours?

- Do you see any overlaps or interdependence between psychological well-being and social well-being? If so, what are they?

- If you were to critique these, what points might you raise? For example, would these operational definitions apply to all cultures? Might some of them conflict with the moral or spiritual beliefs of individuals?

Flourishing and languishing

Previously, mental health and mental illness were seen as opposite ends of the spectrum. It was considered that lower levels of mental illness or severity of illness gave rise to higher levels of mental health.

More recently, alongside the introduction of the positive psychology and sociology movement, there has been a move to view mental health as a syndrome of symptoms of positive feelings and positive functioning in life.[9] The terms 'flourishing' and 'languishing' are now often used within the literature to refer to states of positive or negative experiences of mental health. Corey Keyes, a positive sociologist, was the first to introduce the contemporary terms flourishing and languishing.[10] Flourishing is considered to be a state in which the individual experiences positive emotions, prospers, thrives and functions well psychologically and with emotional vitality. On the other hand, languishing is considered to be having low levels of well-being, including feeling emptiness, stagnation and hollowness.[9,11] Languishing is not to be confused with mental illness, nor should the absence of mental illness be considered as being mentally healthy. Even when people are free of mental illness, they can experience many challenges in daily functioning.

Two continua model

Keyes[12] proposes a two continua model of mental health and illness. This two continua model asserts that, although mental health and illness are related, one continuum identifies the presence or absence of mental health, while the other identifies the presence or absence of mental illness. Complete mental health is seen as a complete state and not the absence of mental illness. In this model, Keyes asserts that mental health must consist of symptoms of positive functioning. The three diagnostic elements of positive mental health are: flourishing, moderate and languishing mental health.

Individuals with flourishing mental health report experiencing at least one measure of hedonic well-being (for example, in the last 30 days regularly feeling cheerful, happy, calm and peaceful), plus six or more elements of positive functioning (such as self-acceptance, social acceptance). Those with languishing mental health report experiencing at least one measure of hedonic well-being and reporting that they never or seldom (once or twice a month) experience feelings of positive functioning. For example, they feel life lacks interest and engagement. Those who report neither flourishing nor languishing are considered as having moderate mental health.[13] While a more in-depth explanation of the model is beyond the scope of this chapter, there is an ever-increasing support base for this model that is based on initial studies and replication studies, which can be accessed from electronic library databases.

REFLECTION

- Above it states that 'Languishing is not to be confused with mental illness, nor should the absence of mental illness be considered

as being mentally healthy.' What are your thoughts on this? Can one have feelings of emptiness and not be described as mentally ill? Many carers who find the role of caring as challenging, yet are functioning well and feel valued, may report feelings of 'being stuck' or not flourishing – would you consider them to be mentally ill?

- Now consider those service users who may have mental illness but who may be prospering and experiencing emotional vitality. Would you consider them to have good mental health? Lastly, consider this question: are all those people without a diagnosis of mental illness leading more healthy and productive lives than the mentally ill?

Developments of constructs

To conclude and summarize this section, there are a number of points that may be helpful in increasing and gaining a more in-depth critical perspective of mental health which may be useful and applicable to mental health promotion. Health promotion is central to the craft of caring. The construct of mental health is contested and subject to debate. Issues that can influence these constructs include culture (chapter 38), socio-economic and political influences (chapter 68), age and gender.[14] Historically, while health was considered as the absence of illness, it has now been developed to include constructs that take account of social and mental dimensions. As outlined in this section, this development is mirrored in mental health constructs and recovery-orientated frameworks. Historically, the de facto construct whereby individuals along a continuum were seen as either mentally ill or mentally well prevailed. Much of the research and theories focused on perceived weakness and deficits. Over the years this has been changing to take account of bio-psychosocial models and other psychological dimensions, such as personal growth and self-actualization, being incorporated into mental health constructs. With the introduction of the positive psychology movement, mental health constructs now reflect a much more informed[14] and multidimensional approach that builds on earlier psychosocial theories and reflects the evolving nature of the individual, society and relationships.

THE CONCEPT OF MENTAL HEALTH PROMOTION

Now that mental health constructs have been explored, it would seem logical to progress by identifying what is meant by mental health promotion and the rationale for undertaking this activity. However, before doing so, it may be useful to reflect at this point and consider your own concepts and ideas of what mental health promotion is. This reflection may challenge or indeed confirm your perspectives.

REFLECTION

- How would you define mental health promotion?
- What do you think are the key factors to consider when implementing mental health promotion activities?

Wills and Jackson[15] posit that, within the UK, the term 'health promotion' is not always used, but instead the term 'public health' is sometimes used to describe the nurse's role. In part this may be due to the traditional view of public health as interventions and efforts to improve the health of communities by providing protection from environmental hazards and responding to health needs. More recently, however, the UK's Faculty of Public Health[16] has incorporated the role of health promotion into its definition of public health as: 'The science and art of promoting and protecting health and well-being, preventing ill-health and prolonging life through the organised efforts of society'.

Mental health promotion is also sometimes confused with mental illness prevention. As they sit alongside one another, there is an overlap in many areas, and many mental health promotion activities impact positively on mental illness prevention. For example, someone who is lonely and who attends a social group as part of their recovery journey from depression may be doing so to reduce the likelihood of their depression reoccurring, while simultaneously increasing positive mental health – for example, increasing social relationships.[17,18] However, mental health promotion and mental illness prevention are two distinct approaches. As alluded to earlier, mental health promotion tends to focus on efforts that will enhance positive mental health, while mental illness prevention focuses on the causes of the illness or what can be done to avoid the illness.[17,18] Prevention can be thought of as reducing incidence and prevalence.

The WHO[2] offers the following as a definition of mental health promotion:

Mental health promotion involves actions to create living conditions and environments that support mental health and allow people to adopt and maintain healthy lifestyles. These include a range of actions to increase the chances of more people experiencing better mental health.

The definition above implies that mental health promotion involves efforts and interventions that support well-being, while also creating environments that will enhance mental health. At the simplest level, it could be argued that mental health promotion involves any activity that aims to promote mental health. However, not all activities that people choose or engage in to promote their mental health have long-term positive effects. For example, someone who has low self-esteem could engage in drinking alcohol to help them to go out and socialize. It may be that over a long period the person then begins to use this strategy to help cope, and thus over the longer term they may become dependent on the use of alcohol to interact with others. While mental health promotion strategies can be very personal to the individual, it is also important that the person understands the potential benefits as well as risks that may arise from engaging in unhelpful activities that may have longer-term negative consequences.

Mental health promotion has a strong personal developmental aim, as it endeavours to build strengths and resilience and maximize personal resources. Others emphasize the role of mental health promotion at different levels: enhancing individual, familial and community mental health,[19,20] in an attempt to situate the scope of this valuable resource within a trajectory that spans from the micro to the macro level. In doing so it highlights the global context which demonstrates that mental health promotion can be an interdependent collective action of society and governments. If people are to be encouraged to adopt healthy lifestyles, then modifiable factors such as unsupportive communities or poor health literacy need to be addressed. There needs to be a broad support approach from a range of community organisations upwards to governmental departments both at national and international level.

Mental health promotion can be a political and a contentious issue often due to the wide-ranging competing perspectives, structures, values and attitudes that prevail across countries and continents.[21] This is further complicated and factious when issues such as the determinants of positive mental health are absent within the society. These range from employment to housing, and include issues such as racism, sexism, homophobia, stigmatisation and other negative attitudes expressed. As rates of mental illness increase and the burden that people experience from distress become more widely known, governments worldwide are increasing their engagement in this particular field of health promotion. The scope of mental health promotion is continuously broadening and now involves interventions that aim to reduce health inequalities, improve the quality of life and significantly reduce social disadvantage. Though initially one may think of mental health promotion as a role for health and social care professionals, when set in context to the determinants of health, one can see that it is as much the responsibility of community leaders and politicians as it is of health and social care professionals. Mental health promotion is a topic that is gaining momentum across spectrums and settings. These range from the perinatal period to old age and from schools to workplaces. As the evidence base for mental health promotion increases, few can ignore the imperative necessity in enhancing and strengthening this emerging field.

Principles and rationale of mental health promotion

The principles and rationale of mental health promotion can be traced from a number of sources which have developed over the years on the basis of observations, strategies, research and reports.[4,18,22–26] Alongside this, people who had experience of mental illness began to voice their dissatisfaction about services they were receiving, particularly as many wanted to reintegrate into society and realize their potential. They wanted more than just symptom relief and wanted to enjoy life just like the other people around them.[24] Rather than accept a deficits model of mental health, people wanted to build on their capacity, capabilities and strengths and engage in meaningful activities that would enable them to live more fulfilling lives. Simultaneously, others from various professional and lay backgrounds began to question the status quo that existed at the time, including the severe stigma that was attached to mental illness, and ideologies that portrayed the mentally ill as unable to contribute much to society. Just like many other emancipatory movements that seek to bring about social justice, voices were heard and people began to comprehend the underlying arguments for mental health promotion.

Ottawa Charter

On 21 November 1986, the first international conference on health promotion was held as part of a new international public health movement. The Ottawa Charter was then established and its logo was created (see Figure 70.1). While it did not focus specifically on mental health promotion, it has served as a vehicle by which mental health promotion could flourish. Though now it is some time since it was introduced, it is still widely respected and referred to as a key international document for thinking about health promotion and taking health promotion action.[27] As will

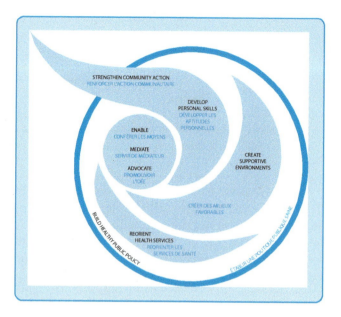

Figure 70.1 Ottawa Charter logo. (*Source: Ottawa Charter for Health Promotion.*[22])

be seen later, both the action areas and the strategies relate closely to what are now considered the principles of mental health promotion.

The logo (Figure 70.1) is intended to convey that health promotion is a comprehensive and multi-level strategy. The logo identifies five key action areas and three health promotion strategies. The five key action areas are:

1. *Build healthy public policy.* This includes and places responsibility on policies that may impact on the health of the population, such as work-related policies or environmental policies. In the logo, this action area is placed at the circumference of the circle to illustrate that building healthy policies is the key to encompassing other action areas.

2. *Create supportive environments for health.* Environments are constantly changing and can impact adversely on the individual's health. Therefore policies must constantly be updated so that they continue to improve health.

3. *Strengthen community action for health.* Communities need to be empowered to make decisions and implement local interventions that reflect the needs of their local community, rather than following directives that can sometimes be set by central governments. Individuals within the communities have expertise in being able to inform what their local community needs and what is best suited to them.

4. *Develop personal skills.* Personal skills development can range widely and may include employment skills, assertiveness, education, emotional intelligence, problem solving and reflective skills. These skills equip the individual with a more informed and enhanced ability to plan, manage and control issues that pertain to their personal health.

5. *Re-orient health services.* Health services are not the only organizations that can promote and deliver health care. For example, many people attend educational institutions to help them learn about a particular illness and deal with it more effectively. Health services need to work together in a collaborative manner to promote health (see chapter 69 for more information on physical health care).

The three basic strategies for health promotion are:[22]

1. *Advocate.* Good health is a major resource for social, economic and personal development and an important dimension of quality of life. Political, economic, social, cultural, environmental, behavioural and biological factors can all favour health or be harmful to it. Health promotion action aims at making these conditions favourable through advocacy for health.

2. *Enable.* Health promotion focuses on achieving equity in health. Health promotion action aims at reducing differences in current health status and ensuring equal opportunities and resources to enable all people to achieve their fullest health potential. This includes a secure foundation in a supportive environment, access to information, life skills and opportunities for making healthy choices. People cannot achieve their fullest health potential unless they are able to take control of those things that determine their health. This must apply equally to women and men.

3. *Mediate.* The prerequisites and prospects for health cannot be ensured by the health sector alone. More importantly, health promotion demands coordinated action by all concerned: by governments, by health and other social and economic sectors, by nongovernmental and voluntary organizations, by local authorities, by industry and by the media. People in all walks of life are involved, as individuals, families and communities. Professional and social groups and health personnel have a major responsibility to mediate between differing interests in society for the pursuit of health.

Based on the Ottawa Charter's action areas and strategies, mental health is considered an integral part of health. Several years ago the WHO proposed that there is 'no health without mental health'. Since then, this proposition has been adopted by individuals, governments, mental health services at international and European level, professional bodies and policy makers.[28] Perhaps this may be considered one of the foundational principles and logical rationale for mental health promotion. When you consider the inextricable links between mental and physical health, the comorbidities to be found and the bi-directional relationships between the two,[29] the proposition becomes even more apparent. If we are to achieve a healthier society, then we need to ensure that mental health is central to this aim.

Health is a fundamental right and has been enshrined in international and regional human rights treaties.[30] For example, Article 12:1 of the International Covenant on Economic, Social and Cultural Rights[31] states that: 'The States Parties to the present Covenant recognize the right of everyone to the enjoyment of the highest attainable standard of physical and mental health.' There is a strong case to argue that mental health is a matter of social justice. Social justice refers to opportunity within society, support of human rights and enabling society to function better. The right to good mental health and well-being can be considered a matter of justice, insofar as it is necessary for optimum living and therefore an entitlement. However, that is not to say that people have the right not to be unhealthy. Everyone deserves a good state of mental health.

Though the cost–benefit ratio of mental health promotion is not as well established as those associated with mental illness prevention, nevertheless there is a strong economic case for mental health promotion. Keyes[32] found that those who were flourishing and considered as having complete mental health reported having fewer days away from work due to illness, lower risk of cardiovascular disease and other chronic physical illness with age, fewer health limitations, less health care utilization and greater psychosocial functioning, such as high resilience and lower levels of helplessness. Friedli and Parsonage[33] assert that mental health promotion and prevention can be extremely beneficial when compared with the costs of treatment across the lifespan. Knapp et al.,[34] in their analysis of the economic case for mental health promotion and prevention, concluded that many interventions showed value for money, had a range of positive impacts, such as better educational performance, improved employment/earnings and reduced crime, and were of low cost to deliver.

While the above principles and rationale may have more pertinence to ethical and economic principles, Barry[35] offers principles that pertain to the delivery of mental health promotion. Barry points out that mental health promotion involves populations as well as individuals, and that when implementing socio-ecological programmes (interaction between people and their environment), one needs to be aware of socio-environmental influences that may impact on the individual's behaviour and attitude. Therefore it is important to understand the multiple interacting system influences on their everyday lives and address the social, physical and socio-economic environments that determine the mental health of individuals and populations. Programmes to enhance mental health promotion need to be multi-level and intersectoral in nature, and also need to address systems change. For example, issues such as social inclusion, stigma and discrimination need to be addressed. As the pathways to mental health involve a range of interventions that lie within and outside health care services – such as schools and workplaces – it follows that mental health promotion needs to be intersectoral in nature. Mental health is everyone's business.

Deciding which mental health promotion intervention to use

If we are to improve mental health promotion, it is useful to identify interventions that are known to be effective. However, before doing so, it is also important to consider factors that impact on positive mental health. Resources are likely to be scarce relative to the demands for them, and also relative to the population.[36] Therefore it is important to take a critical analytical approach to the presentation of need and also to have clear outcomes in mind. It is important to be able to formulate the presentation in a rigorous manner that takes account of maintenance factors, individual attributes or attitudes, as well as the meaning that the intervention may have. For example, someone who experiences poverty, associated hardships and emotional distress may be considered as someone who would benefit from some form of financial assistance. However, when exploring the presentation in more depth, it may transpire that the person does have a good living wage, but perhaps their ability to manage resources

REFLECTION

If you were caring for a person who had a learning disability and who was also depressed, based on the principles, action areas and strategies mentioned earlier in this chapter, how would you begin to implement a programme to promote that person's mental health?

is poor. In view of this, it is likely to be of greater benefit if the person was assisted in improving their skills in managing resources.

Another relevant factor is the evidence base for mental promotion. It is still only emerging, and given that mental health promotion is multi-faceted, there are many studies that could be considered relevant. Alongside this, of the studies to date, many would benefit from a more rigorous methodology to enable the measurement of more robust outcomes.[18,21] Despite this, Barry[14] argues that mental health promotion programmes have been found to result in long-lasting positive effects on health and social functioning with the additional effect of reducing mental disorders.

EVIDENCE-BASED INTERVENTIONS

The perinatal period is a time when women may be more at risk of mental illness and psychological distress, and those who have a pre-existing mental illness may be at increased risk of relapse or recurrence of the condition. As a consequence, mothers may find it difficult to take care of their baby's emotional, cognitive and other development needs which may have an adverse impact on the infant later.[37] The Family Nurse Partnership is a preventive approach for vulnerable first-time young mothers (during pregnancy and until the infant is 2 years old) based on intensive and structured home visiting delivered by specially trained nurses. Randomized controlled trials[38,39] have demonstrated short-, medium- and long-term benefits for both infants and mothers, many of whom had low incomes, were unmarried and had lower intelligence quotient. These benefits included improved prenatal heath, improved emotional and behavioural development in children, fewer childhood injuries, increased maternal employment and increased school readiness.[38–40]

Many school-attending children face social and emotional development difficulties which can escalate into behavioural difficulties that impact on their education. Consequently, difficulties at school can have adverse impacts on career and job opportunities. In a meta-analysis of school-based universal interventions which involved social and emotional learning programmes (these programmes aim to promote students' self-awareness, social

awareness, relationships and decision making, while also aiming to improve student attitudes and beliefs about self, others and school), Durlak and Wells[41] found that, compared to controls, participants demonstrated significantly improved social and emotional skills, attitudes, behaviours and an 11 percentage point gain in academic achievement.

Stress reduction is an important health promotion endeavour from both a physical (see chapter 69) and mental health perspective. While the adverse effects of stress can have serious negative impacts on a person's health, it can also adversely impact on significant others, occupation and other daily activities of living such as socializing. In a meta-analysis of studies that focused on mindfulness-based stress reduction (MBSR) (chapter 44), Grossman et al.[42] concluded that results suggested that MBSR may help a broad range of individuals to cope with clinical and non-clinical problems. Since this study, Chiesa and Serretti[43] have undertaken a meta-analysis of MBSR in healthy subjects. Results showed that MBSR is able to reduce stress in healthy individuals, while also decreasing ruminative thinking and trait anxiety as well as increasing empathy and self-compassion.

Peer support is mutual exchange of help between service users. This may be in the form of social, emotional or practical support. It focuses on individual strengths and not weaknesses and works towards the well-being of the individuals.[44] There is not a strong body of evidence to support this initiative, but the research that has been published is very positive and promising. Benefits include feeling empowered, greater confidence and self-esteem, less stigmatization, a greater sense of identity and feeling more valued.[45]

Employment can have many benefits that can impact positively on mental health. Employment can be satisfying, build self-esteem and self-worth, be rewarding and lead to the acquisition of further life skills.[46] However, other employment issues may detract from the benefits of work for mental health. These include stress, bullying, exclusion, relationships with peers and managers and lack of support networks.[46] Butterworth et al.[47] investigated whether the benefits of employment depended on its psychosocial quality (levels of control, demands, complexity, job security and pay) and whether poor quality jobs are associated with better mental health than unemployment. Results indicate that unemployed respondents had poorer mental health than those who were in employment, but the mental health of those who were unemployed was comparable to those in jobs of the poorest psychosocial quality. Therefore, if we are to reap the benefits of employment for mental health, factors that contribute to poor psychosocial quality must be improved.

The social inclusion and prevention of loneliness of older people is an important facet of general and mental health promotion. Loneliness and depression (chapter 21) can act in a synergistic manner to diminish well-being.[48] Loneliness is a risk factor in Alzheimer's disease (chapter 33) and over the years can accelerate physiological ageing, leading to increased morbidity and mortality.[49,50] However, educational and social activity have proven to be effective in combating loneliness[51] as well as addressing maladaptive social cognitions[52] and performance anxiety in social situations.[53]

THE ROLE OF THE NURSE

As you may have already gleaned, many of the principles, strategies and principles of mental health promotion reflect the values and philosophy of recovery-oriented mental health practice (see chapters 3, 35 and 36 for more information on developing and maintaining therapeutic relationships and recovery). As the philosophy and process of recovery is already covered in other chapters of this book, there is little value in repeating it here. Suffice to say, recovery involves a great deal of mental health promotion.

The Nursing and Midwifery Council[54] states in its *Standards for pre-registration nursing education* that:

All nurses must understand public health principles, priorities and practice in order to recognise and respond to the major causes and social determinants of health, illness and health inequalities. They must use a range of information and data to assess the needs of people, groups, communities and populations, and work to improve health, wellbeing and experiences of healthcare; secure equal access to health screening, health promotion and healthcare; and promote social inclusion. 5.1 Mental health nurses must work to promote mental health, help prevent mental health problems in at-risk groups, and enhance the health and wellbeing of people with mental health problems.

As stated earlier, mental health promotion is everyone's business. Perhaps the first place to begin is with yourself. As a mental health nurse, you are a role model for mental health promotion and therefore must convey its importance to service users, carers, peers and others. This begins with the therapeutic use of self (see chapter 3). This will require reflection on your own values and beliefs and seeking to uncover any unconscious bias that you may have towards the people that you care for. Unconscious bias may be thought of as an immediate judgement based on our past background, cultural environment and personal experiences.[55] Unconscious bias can have effects such as exclusion, withdrawing our support or being discriminatory. If, for example, we hold beliefs that certain groups do not want to work or are not interested in a particular mental health promotion intervention, then, without being aware of it, we may not even approach them to offer them the information or support. Most people with mental illness want to work,[56] yet rates of unemployment among the mentally ill are high.[57] It may be that the stigma that surrounds mental illness is an implicit stigma.[58]

Stigma towards the mentally ill still prevails and it can be a barrier to recovery, as it significantly reduces self-esteem and self-worth and reduces life opportunities and independent functioning over and above the impairments related to mental disorders.[59] However, it is important to understand that stigma is not only an attitude and behaviour demonstrated by those who have no mental illness; those with mental illness may also internalize negative stereotypes, resulting in self-stigma.[60] Additionally, staff who work in mental health services can also stigmatize.[61,62] In view of this, one needs to be reflective and challenge one's own prejudices and negative stereotypes.

While mental health nurses have a leading role to play in mental health promotion, one needs to be cognizant that it cannot be carried out in isolation and, as mentioned earlier, needs an interprofessional and intersectoral approach. Undoubtedly, this will also require input from service users, who have much expertise and experience to offer. Determinants of health extend way beyond health care systems, so it is important that these are taken into consideration and reflected in mental health promotion approaches.

Nurses are privileged to hear life stories and many very personal accounts of the difficulties that people experience. They are therefore very well placed to influence and write policy and should be encouraged to participate in consultation and discussion of frameworks and policies. Moreover, they are in a pivotal position to promote mental health by delivering policy content, creating awareness of it and also undertaking research to further this emerging sphere.

CONCLUSION

Mental health promotion is an integral and imperative part of the nurse's caring role, and it is therefore important for all nurses to have a thorough understanding of this sphere. Having knowledge of the differences between concepts of mental illness and mental health will guide nurses in understanding what their role entails and the outcomes that they hope to achieve. As health promotion can be a complex area, and can be delivered at different levels, nurses must work with others to make it a reality. The various delivery levels do bring challenges, particularly when resources are limited. However, it must be remembered that as the determinants of poor mental health are many, implementation must be intersectoral, and this can help with increasing resources. Though there may be resistance, or little interest, shown from fields that may have little knowledge of their role in promoting mental health, this can be an opportunity for nurses to use their leadership skills of influencing, enlightening and communicating their passion and commitment for a better and fairer society.

References

1. WHO (World Health Organization). *Constitution of the World Health Organization*. 2006. Available from: http://www.who.int/governance/eb/who_constitution_en.pdf [Accessed 1st September 2016].
2. WHO (World Health Organization). Mental health: strengthening our response. Fact sheet no. 220. 2014. Available from: http://www.who.int/mediacentre/factsheets/fs220/en/ [Accessed 1st September 2016].
3. Fischer R, Boer D. What is more important for national well-being: money or autonomy? A meta-analysis of well-being, burnout, and anxiety across 63 societies. *Journal of Personality and Social Psychology* 2011; **101**(1): 164.
4. Westerhof GJ, Keyes CL. Mental illness and mental health: the two continua model across the lifespan. *Journal of adult development* 2010; **17**(2): 110–19.
5. Henderson LW, Knight T. Integrating the hedonic and eudaimonic perspectives to more comprehensively understand wellbeing and pathways to wellbeing. *International Journal of Wellbeing* 2012; **2**(3): 196–221.
6. Delle Fave A, Massimini F, Bassi M. Hedonism and eudaimonism in positive psychology. In: Fave A, Massimini F, Basi M (eds). *Psychological selection and optimal experience across cultures*. Dordrecht: Springer, 2011: 3–18.
7. Ryff CD. Happiness is everything, or is it? Explorations on the meaning of psychological well-being. *Journal of Personality and Social Psychology* 1989; **57**(6): 1069.
8. Keyes CLM. Social well-being. *Social Psychology Quarterly* 1998; **61**(2); 121–40.
9. Keyes CL. The mental health continuum: from languishing to flourishing in life. *Journal of Health and Social Behaviour* 2002; **43**(3): 207–22.
10. Hone LC, Jarden A, Schofield GM, Duncan S. Measuring flourishing: the impact of operational definitions on the prevalence of high levels of wellbeing. *International Journal of Wellbeing* 2014; **4**(1): 62-90..
11. Hefferon K, Boniwell I. Introduction to positive psychology. In: Hefferon K, Boniwell I. *Positive psychology: theory, research and applications*. McGraw-Hill Education (UK), 2011: chapter 1.
12. Keyes CL. Mental illness and/or mental health? Investigating axioms of the complete state model of health. *Journal of Consulting and Clinical Psychology* 2005; **73**(3): 539.
13. Keyes CL, Cartwright K. Well-being in the West: Hygieia before and after the demographic transition. In: Morandi A, Nambi ANN (eds). *An integrated view of health and well-being*. Dordrecht: Springer, 2013: 3–23.
14. Barry MM. Addressing the determinants of positive mental health: concepts, evidence and practice. *International Journal of Mental Health Promotion* 2009; **11**(3): 4–17.
15. Wills J. Jackson L. Health and health promotion. In: Wills J (ed.). *Fundamentals of health promotion for nurses*. Chichester: Wiley, 2014: chapter 1.
16. UK's Faculty of Public Health. What is public health? Available from: http://www.fph.org.uk/what_is_public_health [Accessed 1st September 2016].
17. Kalra G, Christodoulou G, Jenkins R, Tsipas V, Christodoulou N, Lecic-Tosevski D, Bhugra D. Mental health promotion: guidance and strategies. *European Psychiatry* 2012; **27**(2): 81–6.
18. Herrman H, Saxena S, Moodie R. *Promoting mental health: concepts, emerging evidence, practice: a report of the World Health Organization, Department of Mental Health and Substance Abuse in collaboration with the Victorian Health Promotion Foundation and the University of Melbourne*. Geneva: World Health Organization, 2005.
19. Currid TJ. Health promotion and people with mental health issues. In: Wills J (ed.). *Fundamentals of health promotion for nurses*. Chichester: Wiley, 2014: chapter 15.
20. Pollett H. *Mental health promotion: a literature review*. Ottawa, Ontario: Canadian Mental Health Association, 2007.
21. Keleher H, Armstrong R. *Evidence-based mental health promotion resource*. Report for the Department of Human Services and VicHealth, Melbourne, Australia, 2005.
22. *Ottawa Charter for Health Promotion: (1986) First International Conference on Health Promotion: Ottawa, 21 November 1986*. Geneva: WHO, 1986.
23. WHO (World Health Organization). *Alma Ata Declaration*. Geneva: WHO, 1978.
24. Anthony WA. Recovery from mental illness: the guiding vision of the mental health service system in the 1990s. *Psychosocial Rehabilitation Journal* 1993; **16**(4): 11.
25. Barry MM, Jenkins R. *Implementing mental health promotion*. Elsevier Health Sciences, 2007.
26. Friedli L. *Mental health, resilience and inequalities*. Geneva: WHO, 2009.

27. Lahtinen E, Joubert N, Raeburn J, Jenkins R. Strategies for promoting the mental health of populations. In: Herrman H, Saxena S, Moodie R. *Promoting mental health: concepts, emerging evidence, practice: a report of the World Health Organization, Department of Mental Health and Substance Abuse in collaboration with the Victorian Health Promotion Foundation and the University of Melbourne.* Geneva: WHO, 2005.

28. Churchill R. No health without mental health: a role for the Cochrane Collaboration [editorial]. *Cochrane Database of Systematic Reviews* 2010; 10.

29. Currid T J, Turner A, Bellefontaine N, Spada, MM. (2012). Mental health issues in primary care: implementing policies in practice. *British Journal of Community Nursing*, **17**(1): 21–6.

30. WHO (World Health Organization). Health and human rights. Fact sheet no. 323. 2013. Available from: http://www.who.int/mediacentre/factsheets/fs323/en/ [Accessed 1st September 2016].

31. United Nations. International Covenant on Economic, Social, and Cultural Rights. 1966. Available from: http://www.ohchr.org/EN/ProfessionalInterest/Pages/CESCR.aspx [Accessed 1st September 2016].

32. Keyes C. Promoting and protecting mental health as flourishing: a complementary strategy for improving national mental health. *American Psychologist* 2007; **62**(2): 95–108.

33. Friedli L, Parsonage M. *Promoting mental health and preventing mental illness: the economic case for investment in Wales.* Cardiff: Mental Health Promotion Network, 2009.

34. Knapp M, McDaid D, Parsonage M. Mental health promotion and mental illness prevention: the economic case. 2011. Available from: http://www.crisiscareconcordat.org.uk/wp-content/uploads/2014/11/Knapp_et_al__MHPP_The_Economic_Case.pdf [Accessed 1st September 2016].

35. Barry MM. Generic principles of effective mental health promotion. *International Journal of Mental Health Promotion* 2007; **9**(2): 4–16.

36. Knapp M, McDaid D. Making an economic case for prevention and promotion. *International Journal of Mental Health Promotion* 2009; **11**(3): 49–56.

37. Murray L, Cooper PJ. Effects of postnatal depression on infant development. *Archives of Disease in Childhood* 1997; **77**(2): 99–101.

38. Olds DL. The nurse–family partnership: an evidence-based preventive intervention. *Infant Mental Health Journal* 2006; **27**(1): 5–25.

39. Olds D, Henderson CR Jr, Cole R, Eckenrode J, Kitzman H, Luckey D, Pettitt L, Sidora K, Morris P, Powers J. Long-term effects of nurse home visitation on children's criminal and anti-social behavior: 15-year follow-up of a randomized controlled trial. *JAMA: The Journal of the American Medical Association* 1998; **280**(14): 1238–44.

40. Department of Health. *FNP summary evidence leaflet.* London: Department of Health, 2011.

41. Durlak JA, Wells AM. Primary prevention mental health programs for children and adolescents: a metaanalytic review. *American Journal of Community Psychology* 1997; **25**(2): 115–52.

42. Grossman P, Niemann L, Schmidt S, Walach H. Mindfulness-based stress reduction and health benefits: a meta-analysis. *Journal of Psychosomatic Research* 2004; **57**(1): 35–43.

43. Chiesa A, Serretti A. Mindfulness-based stress reduction for stress management in healthy people: a review and meta-analysis. *Journal of Alternative and Complementary Medicine* 2009; **15**(5): 593–600.

44. Mental Health Foundation. Peer support in mental health and learning disability. 2012. Available from: http://social-welfare.bl.uk/subject-areas/services-client-groups/adults-mental-health/mentalhealthfoundation/peer12.aspx [Accessed 11th September 2016].

45. Repper J, Aldridge B, Gilfoyle S, Gillard S, Perkins R, Rennison J. *Peer support workers: theory and practice.* London: Centre for Mental Health and Mental Health Network, NHS Confederation, 2013.

46. Black DC. *Working for a healthier tomorrow.* London: The Stationery Office, 2008.

47. Butterworth P, Leach LS, Strazdins L, Olesen SC, Rodgers B, Broom DH. The psychosocial quality of work determines whether employment has benefits for mental health: results from a longitudinal national household panel survey. *Occupational and Environmental Medicine* 2011; doi:10.1136/oem.2010.059030.

48. Cacioppo JT, Hughes ME, Waite LJ, Hawkley LC, Thisted RA. Loneliness as a specific risk factor for depressive symptoms: cross-sectional and longitudinal analyses. *Psychology and Aging* 2006; **21**(1): 140.

49. Wilson RS, Krueger KR, Arnold SE, Schneider JA, Kelly JF, Barnes LL, Tang Y, Bennett DA. Loneliness and risk of Alzheimer disease. *Archives of General Psychiatry* 2007; **64**(2): 234–40.

50. Hawkley LC, Cacioppo JT. Loneliness matters: a theoretical and empirical review of consequences and mechanisms. *Annals of Behavioral Medicine* 2010; **40**(2): 218–27.

51. Cattan M, White M, Bond J, Learmouth A. Preventing social isolation and loneliness among older people: a systematic review of health promotion interventions. *Ageing and Society* 2005; **25**(1): 41–67.

52. Masi CM, Chen HY, Hawkley LC, Cacioppo JT. A meta-analysis of interventions to reduce loneliness. *Personality and Social Psychology Review* 2010; doi: 10.1177/1088868310377394.

53. Knowles ML, Lucas GM, Baumeister RF, Gardner WL. Choking under social pressure: social monitoring among the lonely. *Personality and Social Psychology Bulletin* 2015; **41**(6): 805–21.

54. Nursing and Midwifery Council. *Standards for pre-registration nursing education.* 2010. Available from: http://www.nmc.org.uk/globalassets/sitedocuments/nmc-publications/standards-for-pre-registration-nursing-education-16082010.pdf [Accessed 1st September 2016].

55. Equality Challenge Unit. Unconscious bias. 2015. Available from: http://www.ecu.ac.uk/guidance-resources/employment-and-careers/staff-recruitment/unconscious-bias/ [Accessed 1st September 2016].

56. Borg M, Kristiansen K. Working on the edge: the meaning of work for people recovering from severe mental distress in Norway. *Disability and Society* 2008; **23**(5): 511–23.

57. Singh S. Mental health and work: United Kingdom. 2014. Available from: http://www.keepeek.com/Digital-Asset-Management/oecd/employment/mental-health-and-work-united-kingdom_9789264204997-en#page12 [Accessed 1st September 2016].

58. Stier A, Hinshaw SP. Explicit and implicit stigma against individuals with mental illness. *Australian Psychologist* 2007; **42**(2): 106–17.

59. Hinshaw SP, Stier A. Stigma as related to mental disorders. *Annual Review of Clinical Psychology* 2008; **4**: 367–93.

60. Rüsch N, Corrigan PW, Todd AR, Bodenhausen GV. Implicit self-stigma in people with mental illness. *Journal of Nervous and Mental Disease* 2010; **198**(2): 150–3.

61. Ross CA, Goldner EM. Stigma, negative attitudes and discrimination towards mental illness within the nursing profession: a review of the literature. *Journal of Psychiatric and Mental Health Nursing* 2009; **16**(6): 558–67.

62. Schulze B. Stigma and mental health professionals: a review of the evidence on an intricate relationship. *International Review of Psychiatry* 2007; **19**(2): 137–55.

Further reading

Barry MM, Clarke AM, Jenkins R, Patel V. A systematic review of the effectiveness of mental health promotion interventions for young people in low and middle income countries. *BMC Public Health* 2013; **13**(1): 835.

Barry MM, Jenkins R. *Implementing mental health promotion*. Oxford: Elsevier Health Sciences, 2007.

Clarke AM, Kuosmanen T, Barry MM. A systematic review of online youth mental health promotion and prevention interventions. *Journal of Youth and Adolescence* 2015; **44**(1): 90–113.

Herrman H, Moodie R, Saxena S. Mental health promotion. In: Patel V, Woodward A, Feigin V, Heggenhougen HK, Quah SR (eds). *Mental and neurological public health: a global perspective* Amsterdam: Elsevier, 2010; 450.

Knapp M, McDaid D, Parsonage M. *Mental health promotion and mental illness prevention: the economic case*. London: Department of Health, 2011.

Kobau R, Zack MM. Mental health promotion in public health: perspectives and strategies from positive psychology. *American Journal of Public Health* 2011; **101**(8): E1.

Relevant web pages

All Wales, Mental Health Promotion Network. http://www.publicmentalhealth.org/

European Network for Mental Health Promotion. http://www.mentalhealthpromotion.net/?i=handbook.en.home

Scottish Government. Promoting good mental health. http://www.gov.scot/Topics/Health/Services/Mental-Health/Strategy/Promoting

UK Faculty of Public Health. Examples of interventions. http://www.fph.org.uk/examples_of_interventions

Well London. Mental well-being. http://www.welllondon.org.uk/788/policy-and-guidance-for-mental-well-being.html

WHO (World Health Organization). Mental health: strengthening our response. http://www.who.int/mediacentre/factsheets/fs220/en/

71 Nursing metrics and mental health nursing

MARY CHAMBERS AND SARAH MARKHAM

LEARNING OUTCOMES

- To appreciate the importance of making the contribution of mental health nursing to service user recovery visible.

- To recognize that working in partnership with mental health service users will make the process of measuring the contribution of mental health nurses to recovery more authentic, realistic and meaningful.

- To be aware that nursing does not happen in a vacuum but as part of a multidisciplinary team; it is impossible to measure everything and therefore there is a need for purposeful, directed focus or foci.

- To understand that not all measurement has to detract from the core values of mental health nursing and can inform quality improvement.

SUMMARY OF KEY POINTS

- Before attempting to measure mental health nursing, it is necessary to understand what service users want and how this can vary among individual service users.

- Service users and mental health nurses working in partnership makes for a more authentic, informed, realistic assessment of the contribution of nursing to recovery.

- Measuring mental health nursing outcomes is possible using simple, easy-to-use, validated tools.

- Measurement in mental health nursing is challenging but necessary to inform and improve practice and to make nursing's contribution to recovery visible.

INTRODUCTION

Over the last few decades, increasing attention has been given to the nature and quality of health care services, including the services available to people with mental health problems. Some of the drivers for this emphasis are the increasing demands for health care, rising expectations among mental health service users, advances in medical technology and the increasing costs of health care. Other influencing factors are the advances and variation in clinical practice, concerns for patient safety, changing work environments, accountability of health care providers and limited resources.

To have an indication of the overall quality of care, it is important to examine nursing performance, as nurses are the largest group of health professionals and the group with the highest level of service user contact. Understanding the quality of nursing care is critical to gauging the overall performance of health care organizations, as was highlighted in the Francis Report.[1] This report indicated the need for a methodology to measure nursing performance so that good and less than good practice could be identified and monitored. It has been previously pointed out that the systematic measurement of quality in nursing performance has become important in the drive to document nursing's influence on patient safety and outcomes and the quality of health care delivered by institutions.[2] Indicators of nursing performance are important not only to institutions; they are also important for enabling nursing to gain greater professional respect, in both the health care sector and the academic scientific community.

In England the importance of quality assessment and improvement in health care, including mental health, has been outlined in a range of policy documents and guidelines.[3-6] With respect to nursing, the most important of these was the Next Stage Review of the National Health Service (NHS), chaired by Lord Darzi. This report[6] recommended the identification of evidence-based metrics to measure the outcomes of nursing interventions and patients' experiences, as part of improving the quality of health care. Around the same time the report by Griffiths et al.[7] focused on the state of the art of nursing metrics. It stressed that the development and implementation of sound quality indicators in all nursing disciplines is an important step in the integration of nursing into overall NHS governance processes. It also pointed out that for mental health nursing this was more challenging.

DEFINING QUALITY OF CARE

To assess the quality of health care accurately, it is essential to have clearly defined concepts of what quality consists of, and to convert these concepts into concrete, measurable criteria; that is, the predefined standards of structure, process and/or outcome.[8] There are several interpretations of quality, many of which capture the complex nature of care.[9] The Darzi report[6] defined quality care as that which is clinically effective, safe and a positive personal experience. With respect to nursing care, these parameters have been refined as effectiveness (pertaining to the positive benefits of care), safety (pertaining to the potentially adverse effects of care) and compassion (pertaining to care delivered with dignity and respect, with an emphasis on good communication).[7]

To facilitate measurement, quality and its related concepts must be translated into assessable standards. One way of doing this is to formulate the chosen quality concepts into standardized (performance and/or clinical) indicators. A (performance and/or clinical) indicator is a measurable statement that captures the important characteristics of an aspect of clinical care. (In the context of this chapter we are concerned with mental health nurse and service user interaction.) An indicator acts as a 'flag' to audit the extent to which actual practice adheres to predetermined standards of care, to promote continuous quality enhancement.[10] Indicators first and foremost work to help understand and improve a given part of the health care system. This is achieved by monitoring performance against agreed standards or benchmarks and providing a mechanism by which care providers, from point of care to senior management, can be held accountable for the quality of their services.[7]

Assessment and reporting against agreed benchmarks are important to help identify appropriate standards of, and approaches to, organizational structures. Such organizational structures include staffing levels, gaps in quality, further research, and education and training.[11] Through the use of agreed standards, nurses will also be able to evaluate and compare the quality of their own clinical practice and that of their colleagues.[10]

MEASURING QUALITY IN NURSING

Examining nursing performance is a vital part of assessing overall health care standards. As previously stated, nurses are the largest group of health professionals and the group with the highest level of service user contact; their performance is therefore critical to the quality of patient care and the overall performance of health care organizations. Systematic measurement of quality in nursing performance has thus become important in the drive to document nursing's influence on patient safety and outcomes and the quality of health care delivered by institutions.[2] Measurable nursing indicators are also an important means for nursing to gain professional respect, in the health care sector as well as the scientific community, in accordance with current drivers towards evidenced-based practice.[12]

To this end, nursing as a discipline must justify its effectiveness within the health care team, be more adept and sophisticated at articulating its contribution to patient outcomes, thus making clear its value to multi-professional teams and the overall business of health care organizations.[13] This point was made more recently by Maben et al.,[14] who stated that 'nursing metrics are needed to show how nurses contribute to the overall architecture for healthcare quality in the NHS' (p.21).

This is especially important in the current UK environment of austerity, an emphasis on patient choice and payment by results. All of these drivers impact heavily on the nature of health care provision, including mental health services.[15]

Over the past decade, a number of national and regional nurse-sensitive indicators and benchmarking measures have been developed, especially in the USA, largely driven by the financing of the US health care system.[2] These measures include the American Nurses Association's National Database of Nursing Quality Indicators and the California Nursing Outcomes Database.[11]

Widespread adoption of such measures among health care organizations has, however, been lacking, as has any subsequent public reporting. Nursing's performance and contribution to quality health care delivery remains significantly less transparent than that of medical staff and health care institutions as a whole.[2]

There has been recent progress with respect to measuring the quality of nursing care in the UK. Some of this has occurred at a local level – for example, the work of McCance et al.[16] who, through the use of a consensus approach, identified eight indicators considered core to nursing and midwifery and situated within a person-centred care approach.

An example of a more national approach is the NHS Safety Thermometer in England. This thermometer aims for 'harm free care' and mainly focuses on the measurement of pressure sores, venous thromboembolism (VTE) prevention, falls, catheters and urinary tract infections. While this is a step in the right direction, like all other attempts at measuring nursing quality it does not include anything specific to mental health. The focus of the thermometer is on hospital acute care, with the level of reporting at a high level rather than at clinical/ward level, and therefore it is difficult to see the connection between the 'bedside and the board'.

Most of the work assessing care quality and performance in nursing has focused on quantifiable activities, those that are easily defined, observed and counted, to the detriment of any real measure of the quality of nurses' activities.[12] They are mainly concerned with aspects of care relating to safety, nutrition, pain and patient experience.[7] A literature review identified the most common indicators of nursing-sensitive outcomes as pressure ulcers, failure to rescue, falls, and health care associated infection.[7] Other structural indicators were staff-related, including staffing levels, skill mix and staff satisfaction and well-being.[7] Very similar findings have been noted by Idvall et al.,[17] Bostick et al.[18] and Needleman et al.[11] The most commonly investigated issue in studies of nursing performance is the link between service user outcomes and structural variables such as nurse hours per patient, nurse staffing mix, absenteeism, turnover and education.[11]

Some have warned that the overwhelming focus on outcome measures fails to reflect the more complex nature of nursing. These include, for example, the wider structural and procedural factors that impact on the delivery of care and consequent patient outcomes.[12] The relationship between patient outcomes and structural and procedural aspects of health care need to be validated by clinical evidence, an approach that is currently lacking within nursing.[11,7]

A focus on patient outcomes is also problematic due to the multi-professional nature of contemporary health care. There is considerable difficulty associated with distinguishing individual professional groups' contributions to patient outcomes,[15,11] something that is particularly relevant to mental health nursing care.

It has therefore been suggested that, if one is interested in the influence of a single discipline only, one should measure process indicators.[15] This leads to the next section of this chapter, on measuring quality in mental health nursing – a specialist area.

REFLECTION

Thinking of interactions you have had with service users, what do you think they might like to see included in a tool that would measure the nature of your interactions, and why?

MEASURING QUALITY IN MENTAL HEALTH NURSING

The above discussion has focused on nursing in general and has highlighted that none of the above attempts to measure quality in nursing care has concentrated on mental health nursing. However, this has been attempted outside the UK; for example, in Australia, using a large Delphi study, Skews at al.[19] identified eight validated, clinical indicators for use in Australia and New Zealand. However, it would appear that this study did not involve any mental health service users. In New Zealand other work has taken place, as outlined by O'Brien et al.,[10] which focused on the development and validation of bicultural clinical indicators. Following validation, the study identified five factors with good internal consistency. One strength of this study was that consumers/service users were involved throughout.

Before considering the issues and challenges relating to metrics in mental health nursing, it is important to consider the core concepts that underpin mental health nursing. The key concept is therapeutic engagement, as indicated by Peplau,[20,21] which is the main focus for the remainder of this chapter. Our reasons for deciding to concentrate on therapeutic engagement will become evident later. Therapeutic engagement, according to McAndrews et al.,[22] is structured, uninterrupted, meaningful time, whereby the service user has the opportunity to discuss concerns with a nurse who is respectful and sensitive to their needs. For more on therapeutic relationships, see chapter 3.

Embedded within the relationship surrounding therapeutic engagement are the values of dignity and respect, empathy and understanding, openness and honesty, partnership and reciprocity, growth and development resulting in shared learning. Given that so many of these are nebulous concepts, and therefore difficult to measure, it is not surprising that until recently little attention has been given to the development of a metric for mental health nursing. However, it has become imperative that this forms an important part of the research agenda for mental health nursing if it is to secure its future. More detail on the future of mental health nursing can be found in chapters 1 and 68.

> ### REFLECTION
>
> Think of a therapeutic relationship you had with a service user. What for you were the important aspects of that relationship and what did you learn about yourself personally and professionally? If you had to measure how you felt during and after the interaction with that service user, how would you go about it?

CAN THE INVISIBLE BE MADE VISIBLE?

Metrics are a derivative of psychometrics and are concerned with objective measurement of behavioural and mental processes, as indicated by Callaghan.[23] In a keynote presentation, Callaghan refers to the writings of Thorndike, who stated that 'If a thing exists, it exists in some amount; if it exists in some amount, it is capable of being measured'[23] (p.2). According to Callaghan, this is the guiding philosophy behind metrics. As indicated above, the nature of mental health nursing is complex due to the invisibility of its core components: interpersonal relationships and therapeutic engagement. What takes place between the nurse and the service user in that 'interactional space' is hard to capture and difficult to quantify but does 'count' in terms of service user recovery. This corresponds to the view of Albert Einstein, who has been credited with saying: 'Not everything that can be counted counts, and not everything that counts can be counted.' So already we have a tension about what counts and what can be counted, which highlights a dilemma that has surrounded mental health nursing. It is well recognized that the vast majority of mental health nurses' essential skills are either invisible or difficult to define and/or measure in meaningful ways.[24–26] It is therefore not unreasonable to suggest that this explains why so little attention has been given to making the core skills of mental health nursing visible and quantifiable. This lack of clarity, in terms of the concreteness surrounding mental health nursing, means that the value of mental health nursing has been difficult to articulate, due to the range and nature of roles and functions performed,[26] as well as the roles played by mental health nurses in multidisciplinary teams.[27]

Mental health nursing as a discipline has thus had a hard time negotiating its identity, finding itself between the two very different epistemological foundations of medicine and interpersonal relationships.[28]

> ### REFLECTION
>
> - How would you best capture patients' levels of satisfaction with nursing interactions in a manner that would inform further interaction?
>
> - How might you control for confounding factors, such as the patients' mental state, need for support and desire to engage?

WHY NOW THE INTEREST IN MENTAL HEALTH NURSING METRICS?

As previously stated, the political climate is constantly changing. Today in the UK there is an emphasis on determining the quality of care as experienced by those who use health and social care services. To some extent this emphasis has been driven by the recent enquiries resulting in reports that highlighted failings in care delivery, such as the Francis Report[1] (acute care) and the Winterbourne View (Gloucestershire Council) enquiry (learning disability).[29] Neither of these episodes of uncompassionate care was directly related to mental health nursing, but they do have implications for it, as illustrated below.

A second driver is the current government emphasis on austerity and ensuring value for money. This places an onus on all health care services to rationalize their spending and provide evidence-based outcomes to show that the money has been well spent. Metrics are a standard means of measuring the outcomes and effects of processes, and therefore trusted markers of the quality of spending options. The third driver, and the most important one with respect to mental health nursing, is the commissioned enquiries on nursing as a result of the Francis Report.[1] As with many such episodes of poor quality care, the nursing profession tends to come under scrutiny, whether deservingly or not; not infrequently the role of nurse education is called into question, and the Francis Report was no exception. The Royal College of Nursing commissioned Lord Willis to lead an independent inquiry into what excellent preregistration nursing education in the UK should look like and how it should be delivered – the Willis Commission.[30]

After taking evidence from a number of key stakeholders, the report *Quality with compassion: the future of nursing education*[30] was published. The report stated that there were no major shortcomings in nursing education and that it could not be held directly responsible for poor practice or the perceived decline in standards of care. The outcomes of this report could have been better disseminated and highlighted; perhaps this was politically motivated on the part of those who did not want to hear the message.

Following on from the Francis Report, there was also the Berwick Report[31] and the independent report *Winterbourne View – time for change*.[32] All of these reports indicated the need for patient-centred, safe care that was compassionate and well-informed and where patients had a voice – something that was not new in mental health nursing. As a result of these reports, Health Education England commissioned Lord Wills to carry out an independent inquiry – the Shape of Caring review. This inquiry was to focus on both care staff and registered nurses to determine if current education and training was fit for purpose. The subsequent report, *Raising the bar: shape of caring. A review of the future of education and training of registered nurses and care assistants*,[33] has generated much debate among academic mental health nurses. This debate has been fuelled by a key recommendation of the report which challenged the current four-branch (general, children, mental health and learning disability) model of training; it advocates for a more flexible approach, with greater parity between physical and mental health. The discomfort generated by this suggestion motivated some senior mental health nurse academics, for example Coffey et al.,[34] to have a commentary published in the *Journal of Psychiatric and Mental Health Nursing*. The authors consider that it is

the potential loss of the knowledge and skills of the mental health nursing workforce that is of concern. They use the 'evidence' of the National Confidential Inquiry into Suicide and Homicide by People with Mental Illness,[35] which observed that, in services with fewer mental health nurses, suicide rates appear to increase. In a second commentary in the same issue of the journal, McKeown and White[36] present further argument, suggesting that it is the systems in which nurses work that are the cause of poor care, rather than the model of nurse education, and that therefore changing the education approach will not eliminate the problem. Nevertheless, this report and the earlier report by the Willis Commission raise issues around nurse education with implications for mental health nursing. As previously mentioned, neither of the last two enquiries into lack of compassionate care involved mental health nurses. However, regardless, mental health nursing could be the end-loser unless we can make explicit what we do and the impact of our interventions on service user recovery. Therefore, there is an urgent need for the development of reliable methods of assessing the impact of mental health nursing interventions.

Measurement is not new to mental health nurses, and many use a variety of standardized measures in daily practice, but unfortunately such use is not widespread. Therefore, whatever measure or measures are introduced to assess the nature and outcomes of mental health nurses' interventions, they need to be simple, easy to use, reliable and valid; they must fit easily into daily clinical practice; and developed in partnership with service users.

REFLECTION

What would be the benefit to you, and to the service users with whom you interact, of using a tool that measures the impact of your interactions on service user recovery?

DEVELOPING A METRIC FOR USE IN MENTAL HEALTH NURSING

The development of a valid and reliable instrument to measure therapeutic engagement is not straightforward. As pointed out by Callaghan,[23] certain criteria need to be considered, such as establishing an operational definition, which is the classification of a concept in terms of how it is measured. In terms of mental health nursing many definitions exist but they all have some reference to a partnership relationship between nurse and service user, based on integrity and respect for dignity, and in which the service user is facilitated to achieve their personal goals through developing a range of coping strategies.

The fundamental aspect of this process is therapeutic engagement,[22] and therefore this is the focus for developing a metric for mental health nursing. It is important to

have a focus for measuring the impact of mental health nursing as it is impossible to measure all that mental health nurses do. In 1952, when Peplau[20] wrote her seminal work on therapeutic relationships, she was of the view that mental health nurses carried out a number of roles and functions, such as mother (*in loco parentis*), technical (assistant), socializing (agent) and environmental (officer). This diversity of roles reflects the multidimensional nature of mental health/nursing care and mental health service user needs. It emphasizes the requirement for a holistic model of practice, promoting service user recovery. Similarly, nursing metrics need to reflect this multidimensionality and be comprehensive in the features of nursing practice that they capture and measure.

To produce a metric for mental health nursing it is important to ensure that whatever tool is used, it must be reliable and valid and developed using psychometric principles. It must have a sufficient number of items, a means of scoring responses and data that are subjected to different statistical tests. This process can be time consuming, which provides a further explanation for the limited attention given to metrics in mental health nursing.

WHAT DO SERVICE USERS WANT?

Considering that mental health nursing is a partnership relationship between nurse and service user, any tool developed to measure therapeutic engagement must have service user involvement. That involvement needs to begin by asking service users what they want from nurses and the treatment and care they provide. Once that is established, it will also be important to know how services might be measured, so that the measurement captures what is meaningful to service users and their recovery. There are several ways in which this information can be obtained; for example, by using focus groups, the nominal group technique or the Delphi method, as outlined by O'Brien et al.[10] Considerable commitment is required on the part of both service users and mental health nurses in the development of such instruments, as they require test–retest reliability, and therefore the process involves asking individuals to repeat the same test at two different intervals. For service users, this can be difficult for a variety of reasons, depending on the context.

REFLECTION

- Put yourself in a service user's shoes; imagine you were a service user in a mental health setting. In what aspects of your daily living and planning for the future would you need support?

- Now imagine yourself as a nurse involved in the care of such a service user. How would you determine how well you had engaged with and supported this service user, and how could you capture this using a metric-based approach?

DEVELOPING A TOOL TO MEASURE THERAPEUTIC ENGAGEMENT

The following is a very brief outline of the approach taken to develop a therapeutic engagement tool (TEQ) for use by registered mental health nurses (RMHNs) and service users on acute mental health inpatient units. The tool was developed using psychometric principles in keeping with those indicated by Callaghan.[23] This approach aimed to develop a valid, reliable and easy-to-use tool for integration into daily clinical practice.

Stage 1: Finding out what service users want and statement generation
This was achieved by individual interviews with 19 detained service users and a therapeutic engagement workshop attended by service users and clinical and nurse academics ($n = 70$). Following analysis, the data from these two activities were combined, generating the statements for the first draft questionnaires. The result was two 25-item questionnaires – one for RMHNs, the other for service users. Each questionnaire had five sections, resulting from the thematic analysis of the above datasets, and used a five-point Likert scale.[37,38]

Following review by an expert panel, revisions were made to the questionnaires in preparation for the pre-testing phase. This was necessary in order to identify any problems with the tool at an early stage.[39]

For the pre-testing, service user members of an education and research group ($n = 12$) were invited to give feedback on the questionnaires. This was achieved through the use of a focus group. Feedback from both service users and nurses was positive, but changes were suggested. Following the revision, the questionnaires to be used at the next stage consisted of 20 statements and a four-point Likert scale.

Stage 2: Item reduction
For this stage of the study, four mental health trusts were involved, with 86 service users and 68 registered nurses participating. The data generated were subjected to factor analysis to determine if the scale had internal consistency and more than one factor. It was determined that both questionnaires had good internal consistency, and two factors – care delivery and care interactions.

Stage 3: Validation
This was an essential stage to demonstrate whether or not the questionnaires measured what they were supposed to measure. To do this, the questionnaires in the study were measured against two other well-established tools. For this stage, 565 nurses and 558 service users completed all three questionnaires. The result was that the two developed questionnaires were as valid as the already standardized measures.

CONCLUSION

In this chapter we have explored the concept, relevance, applicability and construction of nursing metrics. Health care and clinical practice are becoming increasingly driven by the need for quality assurance and improvement, and for this to be evidence-based, formally measured and audited. There is therefore pressure on nursing education and practice to reflect this. Another important trend is increasing public and patient involvement in health care and recognition of the benefit of 'lived experience' informing the further development of all areas of modern nursing, including the creation and deployment of nursing metrics. Given that nurses work as part of the wider multidisciplinary team and that their practice reflects this, any nursing metric must be developed with this dynamic in mind; hence the importance of focusing on a specific aspect of mental health nursing, namely nurse–service user interaction. As with any form of nursing intervention, the use of nursing

metrics offers an opportunity for nurses to reflect on their practice, both with fellow professional and service users. This aims to enhance the quality of engagement, mutual learning and the actualization of better outcomes for all.

One of the most problematic features of the service user–nurse relationship is that what is intended (by the nurse) as care is not necessarily experienced as such by the service user. Both nurse and service user may have the same goals – for example, recovery, self-reliance and a better quality of life – but differ in how they think these goals should be attained. Adaptive engagement is a means of nurse and service user developing a shared understanding of needs and means of satisfying them. It is important that nursing metrics capture the quality of this process in a manner which subsequently informs and facilitates the resolution of such differences of opinion. In doing so, nursing metrics become a key tool in embedding quality improvement into daily practice.

References

1. *Francis Report of the Mid Staffordshire NHS Foundation Trust Public Inquiry.* 6 February 2013. Available from: http://webarchive. nationalarchives.gov.uk/20150407084003/http://www. midstaffspublicinquiry.com/report [Accessed 21st May 2016].
2. Kurtzman ET, Jennings BM. Capturing the imagination of nurse executives in tracking the quality of nursing care. *Nursing Administration Quarterly* 2008; **32**(3): 235–46.
3. DH (Department of Health). *Improving health and care: the role of the outcomes frameworks.* London: DH, 2012.
4. DH (Department of Health). *Essence of care: benchmarks for the fundamental aspects of care.* London: DH, 2010.
5. DH (Department of Health). *National standards, local action: health and social care standards and planning framework 2005/06–2007/08.* London: DH, 2004.
6. Professor the Lord Darzi of Denham KBE. High quality care for all – NHS Next Stage Review Final Report. DH, 17 July 2008.
7. Griffiths P, Jones S, Maben J, Murrells T. *State of the art metrics for nursing: a rapid appraisal.* London: National Nursing Research Unit, King's College London, 2008.
8. Donabedian A. The quality of care: how can it be assessed? *Archives of Pathology & Laboratory Medicine* 1997; **121**(11): 1145–50.
9. Campbell MK, Mollison J, Steen N, Grimshaw JM, Eccles M. Analysis of cluster randomized trials in primary care: a practical approach. *Family Practice* 2000; **17**(2): 192–6.
10. O'Brien AP, O'Brien AJ, Hardy DJ, Morrison-Ngatai E, Gaskin JC, Boddy JM, McNulty N, Ryan T, Skews G. The development and validation of clinical indicators for mental health nursing standards of practice in Aotearoa/New Zealand. *International Journal of Nursing Studies* 2003; **40**: 853–61.
11. Needleman J, Kurtzman ET, Kizer KW. Performance measurement of nursing care: state of the science and the current consensus. *Medical Care Research and Review* 2007; **64**(suppl. 2): 10S–43S.
12. Stevens KR. The impact of evidence-based practice in nursing and the next big ideas. *Online Journal of Issues in Nursing* 2013; **18**(2).
13. Spilsbury K, Meyer J. Defining the nursing contribution to patient outcome: lessons from a review of the literature examining nursing outcomes, skill mix and changing roles. *Journal of Clinical Nursing* 2001; **10**(1): 3–14.
14. Maben J, Morrow E, Ball J, Robert G, Griffiths P. *High quality care metrics for nursing.* London: National Nursing Research Unit, King's College London, 2012.
15. Crow SM, Hartman SJ, Mahesh S, McLendon CL, Henson SW, Jacques P. Strategic analyses in nursing schools: attracting, educating, and graduating more nursing students: part I – strengths, weaknesses, opportunities, and threats analysis. *Health Care Manager* 2008; **27**(3): 234–44.
16. McCance T, Telford L, Wilson J, Macleod O, Dowd A. Identifying key performance indicators for nursing and midwifery care using a consensus approach. *Journal of Clinical Nursing* 2012; **21**(7–8): 1145–54.
17. Idvall E, Rooke L, Hamrin E. Quality indicators in clinical nursing (a review of the literature). *Journal of Advanced Nursing* 1997; **25**: 6–17.
18. Bostick JE, Rantz MJ, Flesner MK, Riggs CJ. Systematic review of studies of staffing and quality in nursing homes. *Journal of the American Medical Directors Association* 2006; **7**(6): 366–76.
19. Skews G, Meehan T, Hunt G, Hoot S, Armitage P. Development and validation of clinical indicators for mental health nursing practice. *Australian and New Zealand Journal of Mental Health Nursing* 2000; **9**(1): 11–18.
20. Peplau HE. *Interpersonal relations in nursing – a conceptual frame of reference for psychodynamic nursing.* New York. Springer Publishing Company, 1952.
21. Peplau HE. *Interpersonal relations in nursing – a conceptual frame of reference for psychodynamic nursing,* 2nd edn. London: Palgrave, 1988.
22. McAndrews S, Chambers M, Nolan F, Thomas B, Watts P. Measuring the evidence: reviewing the literature on the measurement of therapeutic engagement in acute mental health inpatient wards. *International Journal of Mental Health Nursing* 2013; **23**(3): 2–9.
23. Callaghan P. Measuring up: the use of measurement scales in mental health nursing. Paper presented at 'From knowledge comes nursing; from nursing comes knowledge: psychiatric nursing as practice and as scholarship', Vienna, 18–20 October 2006.
24. Brown M, Fowler G. *Psycho-dynamic nursing: a biosocial orientation.* Philadelphia: BB Saunders Co., 1979.
25. Michael JP. Invisible skills: how recognition and value need to be given to the 'invisible skills' frequently used by mental health nurses, but often unrecognized by those unfamiliar with mental health nursing. *Journal of Psychiatric and Mental Health Nursing* 1994; **1**(1): 56–7.

26. Chambers M. Mental health nursing: the challenge of evidence based practice. *Mental Health Practice* 1998; **1**(8): 18–22.
27. Atwal A, Caldwell K. Nurses' perceptions of multidisciplinary team work in acute health-care. *International Journal of Nursing Practice* 2006; **12**(6): 359–65.
28. MacCabe C. Nurse–patient communication: an exploration of patients' experiences. *Journal of Clinical Nursing* 2004; **13**(1): 41–9.
29. Flynn M. *Winterbourne View Hospital – a serious case review*. South Gloucestershire Safeguarding Adults Board, 2012. Available from: http://hosted.southglos.gov.uk/wv/report.pdf [Accessed 2nd August 2016].
30. Willis Commission. *Quality with compassion: the future of nursing education* 2012. Available from: http://www.williscommission.org.uk/__data/assets/pdf_file/0007/495115/Willis_commission_report_Jan_2013.pdf [Accessed 2nd August 2016].
31. Berwick D. *A promise to learn – a commitment to act: improving the safety of patients in England*. London: National Advisory Group on the Safety of Patients in England, 2013.
32. Bubb S. *Winterbourne View – time for change*. Independent report, 26 November 2014.
33. HEE (Health Education England). *Raising the bar: shape of caring. A review of the future of education and training of registered nurses and care assistants*. London: HEE, 2015.
34. Coffey M, Duxbury J, Pryjmachuk S. The shape of caring review: what does it mean for mental health nursing? *Journal of Psychiatric and Mental Health Nursing* 2015; **22**: 736–9.
35. *The National Confidential Inquiry into Suicide and Homicide by People with Mental Illness Annual Report 2015: England, Northern Ireland, Scotland and Wales July 2015*. Manchester: University of Manchester, 2015. Available from: http://www.hqip.org.uk/public/cms/253/625/19/208/NCISH-Annual-Report-2015.pdf?realName=BKDG5c.pdf [Accessed 2nd August 2016].
36. McKeown M, White J. The future of mental health nursing: are we barking up the wrong tree? *Journal of Psychiatric and Mental Health Nursing* 2015; **22**: 722–8.
37. Likert R. A technique for the measurement of attitudes. *Archives of Psychology* 1932; **140**: 1–55.
38. Allen E, Seaman C. Likert scales and data analyses. *Quality Progress* 2007; **40**(7): 64–5.
39. Nunnally JC, Bernstein IH. *Psychometric theory*, 3rd edn. New York: McGraw-Hill, 1994.

Further reading

Burton R, Ormrod G. *Nursing: transition to professional practice*. Oxford: Oxford University Press, 2011.

Foulkes M. Nursing metrics: measuring quality in patient care. *Nursing Standard* 2011; **25**(42): 40–5.

Griffiths PD, Jones S, Maben J, Murrells T. *State of the art metrics for nurses: a rapid appraisal*. London: National Nursing Research Unit at King's College London, 2008.

Hannah KJ, Hussey P, Kennedy MA, Ball M (eds). *Introduction to nursing metrics*. London: Springer, 2014.

Harris JL, Roussel LA, Thomas T, Dearman C. *Project planning & management: a guide for nurses and interprofessional teams*. Burlington, MA: Jones & Bartlett, 2015.

Relevant web pages

Heart of England NHS Foundation Trust. Nursing work flow – metrics. http://www.heartofengland.nhs.uk/nursing-workflow-metrics/

King's College London. High quality care metrics for nursing. http://eprints.soton.ac.uk/346019/1/High-Quality-Care-Metrics-for-Nursing----Nov-2012.pdf

NHS Institute for Innovation and Improvement. Nursing quality metrics: measuring and improving what matters to patients.

http://www.institute.nhs.uk/hia_-_other_submissions/other_submissions/nursing-quality-metrics-measuring-and-improving-what-matters-to-patients.html

Nursing Dashboards – Measuring Quality RCN. https://www2.rcn.org.uk/__data/assets/pdf_file/0004/428440/004198.pdf

Royal College of Physicians. Increased research and patient participation. https://www.rcplondon.ac.uk/projects/outputs/increased-research-and-patient-participation

72 Health care technology and mental health nursing

MARITTA VÄLIMÄKI

LEARNING OUTCOMES

- To be aware of a large number of technology users.
- To be aware of various definitions of health care technology.
- To be aware of health technology solutions used in the field of mental health.
- To be familiar with the benefits and problems of, barriers to and prerequisites for health technology use.
- To be aware of the necessity of involving different partners in designing, developing and evaluating health technology for mental health nursing.
- To be able to reflect on the real opportunities for health technology use in mental health nursing.

SUMMARY OF KEY POINTS

- The use of technological applications has increased globally.
- Technology is one of the most rapidly developing areas in health care services.
- Health care technology has been used widely in various user groups, but its effectiveness has been less systematically evaluated.
- Health care technology may have potential in mental health nursing but requires careful planning in clinical practice.
- The role of different partners in implementing health technology in mental health nursing is crucial.

INTRODUCTION

Barker[1] proposed a definition of nursing almost 60 years ago, describing it as: 'a significant, therapeutic, interpersonal process. It functions cooperatively with other human processes that make health possible for individuals in communities … Nursing is an educative instrument, a maturing force, that aims to promote forward movement of personality in the direction of creative, constructive, personal and community living' (p.5). In the same book, Barker[1] also uses a definition first proposed by Peplau, stating that 'nursing can take as its unique focus the reactions of patient or client to the circumstances of his illness or health problem' (p.5). Both of these definitions are still relevant today. They also offer a description of the basic elements of nursing.

If nurses have a fundamental role in mental health care what role may, in the future involve more and more information technology as technology becomes an integral part of mental health care?

The fact is that the availability of computer technology and the internet has made it possible to deliver interventions via the web.[2] According to December 2013 data, wireless broadband penetration has grown to 72.4 per cent in the OECD (Organisation for Economic Co-operation and Development) area, which means that there are almost three wireless subscriptions for every four inhabitants. The development is driven by strong demand for smartphones and tablets. For example, seven countries (Finland, Australia, Japan, Sweden, Denmark, Korea and the USA) exceed the 100 per cent penetration threshold.[3] The use of mobile phones has also increased globally. An average of 83 per cent of adults own a mobile telephone and 73 per cent send text messages. Young adults are the most active in sending text messages: 95 per cent of people aged 18–29 years sent and received about 88 text messages daily.[4]

At the same time, not all people have computers, access to the internet or opportunities to use sophisticated applications. Among the different regions, technology-enabled programmes are less systematically used in the Middle East and in African countries.[5] Yet the potential benefits of technology are particularly promising, given the critical shortage of health workers and poor distribution of service providers in many low- and middle-income countries,[6,7] and technology has already been used to facilitate patient communications, for example in cases of HIV/AIDS, tuberculosis, family planning and reproductive health programmes.[8]

Many people still choose not to use the internet and not to make use of online resources, as has been stated in the 2014 Global Internet Report:

> *As a result, when considering how to bridge the digital divide, it is important to differentiate those who could afford to go online, but choose not to, from those who do not have access or could not afford it anyway. It is also important to consider the issues that impact those already online, such as improved security and privacy measures. Addressing those concerns will not just impact those already online, but improve the experience for those considering going online.[9] (p.12)*

DEFINITIONS OF HEALTH TECHNOLOGY

There are various definitions of health technology. According to the World Health Organization,[10] health technology 'refers to the application of organized knowledge and skills in the form of devices, medicines, vaccines, procedures and systems developed to solve a health problem and improve quality of lives'.

The National Information Center on Health Services Research and Health Care Technology[11] defines health

In this chapter my aim is to discuss the role of health technology in mental health nursing, in light of some real examples. The chapter begins with an overview of how health technology has been defined in the literature. Second, it describes health technology solutions which have been used in mental health care. Third, it describes the benefits, problems, barriers and prerequisites in the use of health technology, in light of examples found in the literature and my own experience of conducting research in this field. Fourth, the necessity for users' involvement in designing, developing and evaluating health technology in mental health nursing is also identified. Throughout the chapter, readers will be prompted to reflect on the opportunities for health technology use in mental health nursing in relation to different topics.

In order to achieve my goals, I will first recount one case: a fictional study, which is a combination of real-life people living with us in the community.

CASE STUDY 1

A 25-year-old girl, Katie, has been suffering from depression for about 3 years. She has a scheduled appointment at an outpatient clinic once a month, but she is sometimes too tired to keep her appointment with a mental health nurse. She has also medication for her depression. She is living with her parents and spends most of her time at home with her computer. She is unemployed and dreams of an opportunity to apply to study at university. However, she has never done so. She uses Facebook and writes there daily. She also posts pictures on the internet in order to share with others how her image will change due to her weight loss. She has been bullied for years at school because of being overweight. She is occasionally active in social media, sometimes sitting at the computer at night as well. After staying up late and communicating with other people, she is sometimes too tired to get out of bed. Her mother is worried about her friends on the internet and tries to limit her computer use at home.

technology as the practical application of knowledge to improve or maintain individual and population health. It identifies three ways to describe health technology:[11]

- its physical nature;
- its purpose;
- its stage of diffusion.

We will now take a closer look at each of these in turn.

First, health technologies can be grouped on the basis of their physical nature; for example, they can be drugs, biologics (such as vaccines), devices, equipment and supplies, procedures, public health programmes, support systems, or organizational and managerial systems.

Second, technologies can be grouped according to their health care purpose. These different purposes may be prevention (e.g. protecting people against disease by preventing it from occurring), screening (e.g. detecting a disease or abnormality), diagnosis (e.g. identifying the cause and nature or extent of disease in a person with clinical signs or symptoms), treatment, rehabilitation (e.g. restoring, maintaining or improving a physically or mentally disabled person's functioning and well-being) or palliation (e.g. improving the quality of life of patients, alleviating pain, symptom management, etc.).

Third, technologies may be assessed at different stages of diffusion and maturity. The categories may be as follows: future (e.g. undergoing bench or laboratory testing), experimental (e.g. using animals or other models), investigative (i.e. undergoing testing on humans), established (i.e. considered by clinicians to be a standard approach to a particular condition or indication and diffused into general use) or abandoned (e.g. demonstrated to be ineffective or harmful).

Health technology assessment (HTA) is a means of assessing different ways in which science and technology are used in health care and disease prevention. It covers medical, social, economic and ethical issues. HTA provides policy makers with objective information about technology use and its benefits. With this information, policy makers can formulate health policies that are safe, effective, patient-focused and cost-effective. In order to do this, HTA should be transparent, unbiased, robust and

systematic – firmly rooted in research and scientific methods. Examples of health technologies include diagnostic and treatment methods, medical equipment, pharmaceuticals, rehabilitation and preventive methods, but also organizational and support systems used to deliver health care.[12]

The term 'health technology' often refers to eHealth. However, eHealth is the use of information and communication technologies (ICT) for health[13] and its focus is more limited than that of health technology in general. There is still a lack of consensus on the meaning of different concepts, such as eHealth. This may lead to uncertainty among academics, policy makers, providers and consumers.[14] It is important to recognize that definitions of 'health technology' are wide-ranging, and differences between these definitions can also be found. When the concept of health technology is used, it is therefore important to identify what type of technology is being referred to.

To prevent confusion and to avoid being overly technical, when we are discussing health technology in this chapter, we are simply referring to technological devices or solutions that are aimed at supporting the mental health of individuals or groups.

REFLECTION

- Carry out an online search for other definitions for health technology on websites, in electronic databases, etc.

- Did you find alternative definitions for the concept of health techology? If so, what were the differences between these and the definitions given in this chapter?

HEALTH TECHNOLOGY SOLUTIONS FOR DIFFERENT USER GROUPS

Different interventions have been designed to support people of different ages with social communication difficulties. Telephones, emails and online technologies can deliver education and engage individuals in symptom management and self-care.[15] The use of interactive voice-response telephone systems and text messaging to monitor symptoms and side effects for individuals under treatment for mental health problems in primary care have also been tested.[16,17] Various therapies, such as cognitive behavioural therapy, have been computerized.[18] Technologies can also deliver training in mental health treatment and communication skills to primary care staff.[19]

One example involving children is a collaborative computer game, which the children played with an adult. In the study by Murphy et al.,[20] with children aged 5 to 6 years ($n = 32$), the children's performance was observed as they played the game with a classmate. The children who had received the intervention, in contrast to the control group

who had not, showed significant gains in their pragmatic skills, an improvement in their performance on the computer game, and greater use of high-quality questioning during collaboration. In addition, the children who played the game made significantly more positive statements about the game and about their partners. The findings suggest that the intervention increased confidence and enjoyment among children.

Internet-based programmes have been developed for the prevention or care of depression, anxiety or stress, emotional distress, eating disorders, alcohol and drug abuse and smoking cessation.[21,22] For adolescents, an essential part of communication and information seeking includes sensitive health issues such as sexuality.[23] The internet is also used to seek information about mental health problems. This is the case regardless of whether young students have a problem themselves. According to Burns and colleagues,[24] 20 per cent of young people ($N = 1990$) had personally experienced a mental health problem in the previous 5 years and 31 per cent had used the internet as a source of health information for this problem.[24]

The stresses caused by the transition to university can make this a demanding time for many young people.[25] It has been demonstrated that mental disorders are one reason for the high level of disability in university students.[26,27] Mental disorders may also have a negative impact on academic participation and outcomes. This was found by Eisenberg et al.,[28] who conducted a survey in a large public university (response rate 56.6 per cent, $N = 2,843$). The survey showed that the estimated prevalence of any depressive or anxiety disorder was 15.6 per cent for undergraduates and 13.0 per cent for graduates, while suicidal ideation was reported by 2 per cent of students. Those with financial difficulties were reportedly at higher risk for mental health problems.

Various internet interventions have also been developed and tested on students. The literature has focused, for example, on substance misuse:[29] it shows that web-based brief alcohol interventions have been found to be effective in reducing the quantity and frequency of alcohol consumption among heavy-drinking young adults and students.[30–34] A telephone survey in Canada showed that current drinkers are generally more likely to have access to the internet than abstainers.[35] Especially heavy drinkers have been shown to benefit from a PC Windows-based behavioural treatment programme.[36] Reavley and Jorm[37] also conducted a review of interventions to prevent or intervene early in alcohol misuse. The evidence of effectiveness was found to be strongest for brief motivational interventions and for personalized normative interventions, which were delivered using computers or in individual face-to-face sessions. Some interventions to prevent or intervene early in depression or anxiety in students were also identified. These were mostly face-to-face, cognitive behavioural/skill-based interventions. In addition, one social marketing intervention to raise awareness of depression and treatments showed some evidence of effectiveness. The authors concluded that, although the web has been proposed as an ideal method to deliver interventions to higher education students, there is still very limited evidence that interventions are effective in preventing or intervening early in depression and anxiety disorders in this group.[37]

The use of social media technology is an emerging trend for patients seeking health information. Its use appears to be on the increase among patients across the health care spectrum. This was found in a review of 12 articles by Househ et al.[38] According to the review, a promising future was envisaged for patients' use of social media. However, the evidence related to the efficacy and effectiveness of social media is currently limited. Various challenges were also identified. These were related to privacy and security concerns, usability, the manipulation of identity, and misinformation.[38]

E-therapies have been developed for various devices, such as mobile phones, web portals and the internet.

Rozbroj et al.[39] reviewed 24 web- and mobile phone-based e-therapies according to their performance in eight key areas, such as the use of inclusive language and content; and whether they addressed mental health stressors for lesbians and gay men, such as experiences of stigma related to their sexual orientation, coming out, and relationship issues that are specific to lesbians and gay men. The analysis revealed that e-therapies seldom addressed the stressors from the areas identified. About half of the therapies (58 per cent; 14 out of 24) contained instances that assumed or suggested the user was heterosexual, with instances especially prevalent among better-evidenced programmes.

Serious problems in health technology interventions are related to participants' willingness to use those new technologies. In research, the literature uses the term 'attrition'. Attrition is the loss of randomly assigned participants or participants' data in effectiveness studies where patients have been randomized, for example to two groups (intervention and control groups). As well as giving an indication of the methodological quality of the study, it may also tell the researchers how acceptable the intervention is to the specific patient groups. In Box 72.1, you can find

BOX 72.1: ASSESSING THE ACCEPTABILITY OF AN INTERVENTION FOR USERS

If a researcher wants to ascertain the effectiveness of a telephone intervention for patients with depression, patients ($N = 400$) can be randomized into two study groups, i.e. study arms: (1) one group of patients ($n = 200$) will receive a telephone call every day for 2 weeks (and participate in their usual care at an outpatient clinic); and (2) one group of patients ($n = 200$) will receive only regular care at an outpatient clinic.

Patients are monitored every second day with specific instruments. If it emerges that the patients in the telephone call group do not 'participate' in the telephone intervention (i.e. do not answer the calls) and do not appear in follow-up, leading to a greater amount of missing data, we may ask: 'Why are patients not willing to participate?' or 'What are the consequences for our study?'

One reason for patients disappearing from a telephone study may be that patients dislike the telephone intervention. If attrition rates exceed 30 or 40 per cent in either study arm, either in the intervention or the control group, this may be considered indicative of flaws in the study.[40] In any case, the higher the attrition rate, the lower the quality of the study.

an example of how acceptance of an intervention can be assessed in outcome studies.

Eysenbach[41] discusses the problem of a substantial proportion of users dropping out of eHealth trials before completion, or stopping using the application. He offers two examples. The first is an internet-based evaluation of a panic disorder self-help web programme, where only 12 out of 1,161 (about 1 per cent) of participants completed the 12-week programme.[42] His second example is the evaluation of the MoodGym programme, which has five modules targeting people with depression. It was found that only 97 out of 19,607 participants completed all five modules in an 'open' setting, while 41 out of 182 completed all of them in a trial setting.[43,44]

On the contrary, Pratt et al.[45] examined the feasibility and potential effectiveness of an automated telehealth intervention, supported by nursing health care management, among adults with serious mental illnesses and chronic medical conditions. They conducted a study with 70 individuals with serious mental illnesses and chronic medical conditions. The telehealth intervention was delivered for 6 months. Most participants (89 per cent) were involved in at least 70 per cent of the telehealth sessions; participation was associated with improvements in self-efficacy for managing depression and diastolic blood pressure. Almost all participants reported that their understanding of their medical condition was 'much better' or 'somewhat better' after the intervention. The authors concluded that the results demonstrated the feasibility and acceptability of automated telehealth supported by a nurse care manager. Similar experiences were also reported for the MieliNet study, where patients with schizophrenia dropped out of patient education sessions less often than expected. One reason for this success was that the intervention was integrated into daily activities on the psychiatric ward and there was a group of nurses who were actively engaged in this new intervention.[46]

> **REFLECTION**
>
> Look back at the case study presented in the introduction. Consider what type of health technology might be suitable for Katie. What is the rationale for your opinion?

BENEFITS AND DRAWBACKS OF USING HEALTH TECHNOLOGY

We are now aware that there are a large number of different health technological solutions available in the field of mental health. We have also seen that it is not always easy to use or implement new technological solutions in clinical practice. Implementing a new intervention is easier if staff members are aware of its benefits to patients, to themselves, to the health care organization and so on. In Table 72.1, the benefits and possible problems of health technology-based interventions are identified.

> **REFLECTION**
>
> Consider what types of benefits and problems might result if Katie were to start to use a health technology intervention to handle her bad feelings and signs of depressions. What is the rationale for your opinion? What kind of evidence do you have?

Table 72.1 Benefits and problems of health technology use in mental health services

Benefits	Problems
Anonymity – reduces stigma between users	Collaboration between people is not real
Freedom from time and space	Unlimited use may cause problems in daily routines
Self-engagement and self-management	Requires motivation and engagement
Easy access	Users may drop out of services due to a lack of monitoring and support
Less expensive treatment	Costs may be transferred to other partners
No travel costs	Isolation
Variety of communications	Lack of face-to-face communication

BARRIERS AND SUPPORTIVE FACTORS IN ADOPTING HEALTH TECHNOLOGY

In the literature, a number of barriers to the adoption of health technology have been identified. First, problems related to a lack of interoperability among various systems have been found in different countries.[47] For example, a technology may be fragmented and its implementation in practice may vary. This problem can be very challenging, especially for the management of people with multiple health problems, in cases where a large number of actors are managing the individual patient's situation[48] and the information flow between partners should be smooth.

Second, concerns about the protection of privacy and data security are crucial issues in the use of health technology in health care.[49] Young et al.[50] examined adults' perceptions of and attitudes to home-based health information technology with personal electronic health records. In-depth interviews with 35 American 46- to 72-year-old adults revealed concerns related to technological discomfort, privacy or security concerns and lack of relative advantage.[50]

Third, the reluctance of health care professionals to undertake interventions that include information technology has been reported in many studies. Nurses in mental health who are in a key position to deliver such interventions may not do so because of both lack of skills and fear of potential adverse effects on relationships with their patients.[46] Nurses' attitudes may also be associated with their job satisfaction. This was found in Koivunen's[51] study, in which nurses with very positive attitudes towards internet use reported less stress and more job satisfaction than nurses with neutral attitudes towards internet use. Thus, user acceptance has been seen as an important factor in explaining the success or failure of information system implementation.[52]

Fourth, organizational culture has been reported to be connected with the acceptance and use of health technology.[53] Close administrative cooperation during the implementation process supports the acceptance of health technology.[54] Conversely, a lack of communication and information may impair staff's acceptance and use of an application, whereas an IT-friendly environment and substantial communication have a positive influence on system adoption.[55]

In general, the provision of staff resources and the allocation of specific time for organizing new interventions using information technology would support the implementation of computer use. Nurses have also emphasized that patient-centred nursing practices can facilitate the implementation of information technology in clinical practice. In addition, nurses' on-the-job training can support them in using technology, help to familiarize them with new methods and, further, give them self-confidence to implement an intervention in daily practice.[56]

REFLECTION

- Consider what type of barriers you might face in supporting health technology use for Katie. What is the rationale for your opinion?

- What are your personal experiences of using health technology for people with depression, or other mental problems?

- What are your personal attitudes toward technology use in mental health nursing and how would they affect your practice?

PREREQUISITES FOR THE USE OF HEALTH TECHNOLOGY

Koivunen[57] has developed recommendations for best practice, for improving the acceptance and use of information technology among nurses working in psychiatric hospitals. These recommendations have been modified here in this book for use in those areas of mental health where there are plans to implement health technology in clinical practice.

Resource allocation

- *Steering the process.* The IT implementation process needs a steering group. It should consist of a representative of the application producer, an administrative member of the organization, technical staff, nurses and patients.
- *Equipment and rooms.* Functional and usable equipment for the use of the application in the organization must be ensured before the implementation of the new application. Adequate rooms and spaces for use of the application must be ensured.
- *Time.* Sufficient time for the implementation process and use of the new application should be guaranteed.
- *Staff resources.* Sufficient resources for nurses should be ensured.
- *Technical support.* Technical support should be ensured during the implementation process, and it should also be available to meet nurses' and patients' individual needs.

Collaboration

- *Meetings.* Realization of collaboration can be ensured by regular informative meetings with multidisciplinary groups.
- *Team working.* Collaboration and systematic communication among representatives of the application producer, an administrative member of the organization, technical staff, nurses and especially patients should be ensured.

Computer skills

- *Evaluating computer skills.* If the level of the users' computer skills is not known, this should be assessed using surveys or interviews before the implementation of the new IT application.

Education and training

- *Content of the curriculum.* The content of the IT education curriculum needs to be based on computer skills and individual educational needs. The results of the computer skills evaluation should be used when creating the curriculum.

- *Pedagogical methods.* The pedagogical methods used in IT education must be based on individual needs. Depending on these needs, individual training or small-group instruction should be offered. Use of time should also be based on individual needs. The guidance of computer experts or mentors is advisable.

Patient–nurse relationship

- *Nurses' patient education competence.* Nurses' competence for patient education with IT needs to be ensured by evaluations or discussions.
- *Patient-oriented operations.* Possible changes in the patient–nurse relationship must be taken into account; patients are seen as active collaborators with nurses, not as objects of care. Therefore, patients' own perspectives and mental status should be taken into account.

Instructions for application use

- *Written instructions.* Written instructions to improve the use of the new application must be produced before its implementation.
- *Usability of the written instructions.* An evaluation of the written instructions for the application must be carried out before and also during the implementation. The participation of nurses, technical staff and patients in the evaluation of the understandability of written instructions should be ensured.

Usability and impact of the application

- *Technical functionality of the application.* The user-friendliness and usefulness of the application must be ensured by evaluating technical functionality. The participation of nurses, technical staff and patients in the evaluation should be ensured.
- *Content of the application.* The relevance and comprehensibility of the content of the application should be ensured by an evaluation of the content. The participation of nurses and patients in the evaluation process should be guaranteed.
- *Benefits of the application.* The possible benefits and possible negative effects of the new application should be analysed by patients, nurses and administrative personnel in the organization.
- *Systematic evaluation process.* Systematic feedback on the impact of the application must be provided.
- *Ethical issues.* Ethical issues in using technology should be considered from different points of view.

> ### REFLECTION
>
> Consider what different steps would be needed to implement health technology safely in Katie's treatment.

CONCLUSION

The use of health technology is still a controversial issue in mental health care. Some people think that health care technology cannot have a prominent role in nursing because it takes time away from direct patient care.[58] Research has also shown that nurses may have doubts about how technology may restrict people's social communication. This can be seen in nurses' responses which emphasize the importance of having social contact with a supportive person whom the patient can meet regularly, meaning that information technology is not the only means of maintaining social contacts.[59] In light of the experiences of a research group in which I participate at the University of Turku, it seems that nurses see themselves as a key tool for patient recovery and they express concerns that technology may disrupt the important therapeutic relationship between the nurse and the patient.

On the other hand, as Barker[1] has emphasized, nurses do 'not make' people develop, far less 'change' them; neither do they 'teach' them anything directly. Instead, nurses provide the conditions necessary for the person to experience growth, development and change, and to learn something significant from their own experience. Could health technology then be one possible means to support people's growth?

On the contrary, the younger generation may see technology as a more natural way of communicating. This was seen in a study by Maijala et al.,[60] in which the use of a question–answer column for patients with schizophrenia ($N = 100$) was analysed. It showed that the most common age of users was 18 to 24 years and that column use was heaviest among students (44 per cent). Out of 85 questions or comments sent to the column, 31 per cent were related to medication, 25 per cent to illness and medical examinations, 4 per cent to daily life and coping with it and 2 per cent to places to receive treatment. In general, health technology interventions may be applicable for young people already using the internet to connect with other young people.[24] Wider acceptance of health technology may be advantageous for young adults, because it allows them to access information at a self-selected time and place while remaining anonymous.[34]

In any case, the use of health technology in mental health care requires a new type of education in order to enable nurses to provide nursing via the internet or computer.

A 32-YEAR-OLD MALE SERVICE USER'S PERSPECTIVE

Today technology plays a significant role in many fields. I believe that it comes more naturally to some people than to others that technology is used as a part of health in mental health issues. On the other hand, it does not suit some people at all. I myself have had a great deal to do with health care professionals, and I can understand that technology undoubtedly makes many things easier and that it can support treatment. For example, when things have been written down they can be checked later. When nowadays everyone is in a greater hurry, technology can facilitate information transfer. It can ensure that information concerning the patient can be located more easily. Another advantage is that if one wants to obtain information on one's own illness, health or treatment, things can be made easier to understand, because the information can be further illustrated using the means technology affords. It makes it easier to assimilate the information. One can refer to the information again later and make one's own use of it.

On the contrary, some may have concerns about whether the information in databases remains confidential. I have sometimes noticed that information entered in documents by staff does not always correspond to my own thoughts about the situation. Sometimes professionals place emphasis on things which are not so significant. On looking back at some past situation together, or reflecting what has occurred earlier, the old issues are still listed there in the paperwork. Also, the replacement of personal communications with text message reminders, or other technology, may suggest, for example, for a depressed person, that he is cared about even less.

Different generations use technology in different ways. Not everyone has access to a computer; some may only access them in libraries. Therefore, it should be remembered that when something new is produced which is not available to all, earlier forms of treatment should not be abandoned. Examples of this are face-to-face meetings and providing information in person. Not everyone has the same skills or command of technology. For technology to really work, people should listen to service users and consider who benefits most from the technology. Although in principle using technology is normal, it is still little used in the field of care. Before it starts to be used more widely, its possible benefits and drawbacks should be ascertained through research. It is also necessary to consider people's experiences of using technology. Although studies of efficacy may report that technology is easy to use and helps in everyday matters or in understanding one's illness, people's actual experiences of using it should not be overlooked. Technology should be evaluated according to what it feels like for the user, and not just its ability to reduce the number of treatment sessions that are needed.

At its best, technology can work alongside other treatments, but not replace them. Finland is a country where people often live a long distance from places for treatment. In this environment, technology can support people. It is important that when a person needs help, he or she can access it at that exact moment. Technology could bring help close to people, at least until they can access help in person. Nowadays it cannot be taken for granted that a person can get treatment exactly when they need it. Therefore, technology can be a good aid in addition to conventional treatment, which can help people cope and increase the efficacy of treatment. But it should be borne in mind that each person is an individual. In mental health problems, it is always also a matter of a person's life. Thus technology cannot be used in the same way with everyone. Each person is an individual, and each person needs individual help.

References

1. Barker P (ed.). *Psychiatric and mental health nursing. The craft of caring*, 2nd edn. Boca Raton: CRC Press, 2008.
2. White A, Kavanagh D, Stallman H, Klein B, Kay-Lambkin F, Proudfoot J, Drennan J, Connor J, Baker A, Hines E, Young R. Online alcohol interventions: a systematic review. *Journal of Medical Internet Research* 2010; **12**(5): e62.
3. OECD (Organisation for Economic Co-operation and Development). OECD broadband statistics update. 2014. Available from: http://www.oecd.org/sti/broadband/broadband-statistics-update.htm [Accessed 9th June 2016].
4. Smith A. Americans and text messaging; 31% of text message users prefer texting to voice calls, and young adults stand out in their use of text messaging. *Pew Internet and American Life Project*, 2011.
5. CHMI (Center for Health Market Innovations). *Programs.* Washington: CHMI, 2010. Available from: http://healthmarketinnovations.org/programs [Accessed 9th June 2016].
6. WHO (World Health Organization). *The World Health Report 2006: working together for health*. Geneva: WHO, 2006.
7. WHO (World Health Organization) and Global Health Workforce Alliance. *The Kampala Declaration and agenda for global action*. Geneva: WHO, 2008.

8. Lewis T, Synowiec C, Lagomarsino G, Schweitzer J. E-health in low- and middle-income countries: findings from the Center for Health Market Innovations. *Bulletin of the World Health Organization* 2012; **90**: 332–40.

9. Internet Society. *Global internet report 2014*. Geneva: Internet Society, 2014. Available from: http://www.internetsociety. org/sites/default/files/Global_Internet_Report_2014_0.pdf [Accessed 9th June 2016].

10. WHO (World Health Organization). Technology, health. 2016. Available from: http://www.who.int/topics/technology_medical/ en/ [Accessed 18th August 2016].

11. NICHSR (National Information Center on Health Services Research and Health Care Technology). HTA 101: II. Fundamental concepts. 2014. Available from: http://www.nlm.nih.gov/nichsr/ hta101/ta10104.html#Heading10 [Accessed 9th June 2016].

12. European Commission. Health technology assessment. 2014. Available from: http://ec.europa.eu/health/technology_ assessment/policy/index_en.htm [Accessed 9th June 2016].

13. WHO (World Health Organization). eHealth. Available from: http://www.who.int/ehealth/en/. 2014. [Accessed 9th June 2016].

14. Pagliari C, Sloan D, Gregor P, Sullivan F, Detmer D, Kahan JP, Oortwijn W, MacGillivray S. What is eHealth (4): a scoping exercise to map the field. *Journal of Medicine Internet Research* 2005; **7**(1): e9.

15. Gerstle RS. E-mail communication between pediatricians and their patients. *Pediatrics* 2004; **114**: 317–21.

16. Gardner W, Kelleher KJ, Pajer KA. Multidimensional adaptive testing for mental health problems in primary care. *Medical Care* 2002; **40**(9): 812–23.

17. Kelleher KJ, Stevens J. Evolution of child mental health services in primary care. *Academic Pediatric* 2009; **9**: 7–14.

18. NICE (National Institute for Health and Care Excellence). Computerised cognitive behavioural therapy for depression and anxiety, 2013. NICE technology appraisal guidance [TA97]. 2013. Available from: https://www.nice.org.uk/guidance/ta97 [Accessed 18th August 2016].

19. Kemper KJ, Foy JM, Wissow LS, Shore S. Enhancing communication skills for pediatric visits through online training using video demonstrations. *BMC Medical Education* 2008; **8**: 8.

20. Murphy SM, Faulkner DM, Reynolds LR. A randomised controlled trial of a computerised intervention for children with social communication difficulties to support peer collaboration. *Research in Developmental Disabilities* 2014; **35**(11): 2821–39.

21. Griffiths K, Christensen H. Review of randomised controlled trials of internet interventions for mental disorders and related conditions. *Clinical Psychologist* 2006; **10**: 16–29.

22. Spek V, Cuijpers P, Nyklicek I, Riper H, Keyzer J, Pop V. Internet-based cognitive behaviour therapy for symptoms of depression and anxiety: a meta-analysis. *Psychological Medicine* 2007; **37**: 319–28.

23. Mitchell KJ, Ybarra ML, Korchmaros JD, Kosciw JG. Accessing sexual health information online: use, motivations and consequences for youth with different sexual orientations. *Health Education Research* 2013; **29**: 147–57.

24. Burns JM, Davenport TA, Durkin LA, Luscombe GM, Hickie IB. The internet as a setting for mental health service utilisation by young people. *Medical Journal of Australia* 2010; **7**(192) (11 Suppl): S22–S26.

25. Buchanan JL. Prevention of depression in the college student population: a review of the literature. *Archives of Psychiatric Nursing* 2012; **26**(1): 21–42.

26. Mowbray CT, Megivern D, Mandiberg JM, Strauss S, Stein CH, Collins K, Lett R. Campus mental health services: recommendations for change. *American Journal of Orthopsychiatry* 2006; **76**(2): 226–37.

27. Hunt J, Eisenberg D. Mental health problems and help-seeking behavior among college students. *Journal of Adolescent Health* 2010; **46**(1): 3–10.

28. Eisenberg D, Gollust SE, Golberstein E, Hefner JL. Prevalence and correlates of depression, anxiety, and suicidality among university students. *American Journal of Orthopsychiatry* 2007; **77**(4): 534–42.

29. Elliott JC, Carey KB, Bolles JR. Computer-based interventions for college drinking: a qualitative review. *Addictive Behaviors* 2008; **33**(8): 994–1005.

30. Bewick BM, Trusler K, Barkham M, Hill AJ, Cahill J, Mulhern B. The effectiveness of Web-based interventions designed to decrease alcohol consumption – a systematic review. *Preventive Medicine* 2008; **47**(1): 17–26.

31. Kypri K, Hallett J, Howat P, McManus A, Maycock B, Bowe S, Horton NJ. Randomized controlled trial of proactive Web-based alcohol screening and brief intervention for university students. *Archives of Internal Medicine* 2009; **169**(16): 1508–14.

32. Hustad JT, Barnett NP, Borsari B, Jackson KM. Web-based alcohol prevention for incoming college students: a randomized controlled trial. *Addictive Behaviors* 2010; **35**(3): 183–9.

33. Kypri K, McCambridge J, Vater T, Bowe SJ, Saunders JB, Cunningham JA, Horton NJ. Web-based alcohol intervention for Māori university students: double-blind, multi-site randomized controlled trial. *Addiction* 2013; **108**(2): 331–8.

34. Voogt CV, Poelen EA, Kleinjan M, Lemmers LA, Engels RC. The effectiveness of the 'what do you drink' Web-based brief alcohol intervention in reducing heavy drinking among students: a two-arm parallel group randomized controlled trial. *Alcohol* 2013; **48**(3): 312–21.

35. Cunningham JA, Selby PL, Kypri K, Humphreys KN. Access to the internet among drinkers, smokers and illicit drug users: is it a barrier to the provision of interventions on the world wide web? *Medical Informatics and the Internet in Medicine* 2006; **31**(1): 53–8.

36. Squires DD, Hester RK. Using technical innovations in clinical practice: the Drinker's Check-Up software program. *Journal of Clinical Psychology* 2004; **60**(2): 159–69.

37. Reavley N, Jorm AF. Prevention and early intervention to improve mental health in higher education students: a review. *Early Intervention in Psychiatry* 2010; **4**(2): 132–42.

38. Househ M, Borycki E, Kushniruk A. Empowering patients through social media: the benefits and challenges. *Health Informatics Journal* 2014; **20**: 50–8.

39. Rozbroj T, Lyons A, Pitts M, Mitchell A, Christensen H. Assessing the applicability of e-therapies for depression, anxiety, and other mood disorders among lesbians and gay men: analysis of 24 web- and mobile phone-based self-help interventions. *Journal of Medical Internet Research* 2014; **16**(7): e166.

40. Amico RA. Percent total attrition: a poor metric for study rigor in hosted intervention designs. *American Journal of Public Health* 2009; **99**(9): 1567–75.

41. Eysenbach G. The law of attrition. *Journal of Medicine Internet Research* 2005; **7**(1): e11.

42. Farvolden P, Denisoff E, Selby P, Bagby RM, Rudy L. Usage and longitudinal effectiveness of a Web-based self-help cognitive behavioral therapy program for panic disorder. *Journal of Medicine Internet Research* 2005; **7**(1): e7.

43. Christensen H, Griffiths KM, Korten AE, Brittliffe K, Groves C. A comparison of changes in anxiety and depression symptoms of spontaneous users and trial participants of a cognitive behavior therapy website. *Journal of Medicine Internet Research* 2004a; **6**(4): e46.

44. Christensen H, Griffiths KM, Jorm AF. Delivering interventions for depression by using the internet: randomised controlled trial. *British Medical Journal* 2004; **328**(7434): 265.

45. Pratt SI, Bartels SJ, Mueser KT, Naslund JA, Wolfe R, Pixley HS, Josephson L. Feasibility and effectiveness of an automated telehealth intervention to improve illness self-management in people with serious psychiatric and medical disorders. *Psychiatric Rehabilitation Journal* 2013; **36**(4): 297–305.

46. Anttila M, Välimäki M, Hätönen H, Luukkala T, Kaila M. Use of web-based patient education sessions on psychiatric wards. *International Journal of Medical Informatics* 2012; **81**(6): 423–33.

47. Anderson GF, Frogner BK, Johns RA, Reinhardt UE. Health care spending and use of information technology in OECD countries. *Health Affairs* 2006; **25**(3): 819–31.

48. Reinhardt UE. Does the aging of the population really drive the demand for health care? *Health Affairs* 2003; **22**(6): 27–39.

49. Schoenberg R, Safran C. Internet based repository of medical records that retains patient confidentiality. *British Medical Journal* 2000; **321**(7270): 1199–203.

50. Young R, Willis E, Cameron G, Geana M. 'Willing but unwilling': attitudinal barriers to adoption of home-based health information technology among older adults. *Health Informatics Journal* 2014; **20**: 127–35.

51. Koivunen M, Kontio R, Pitkänen A, Katajisto J, Välimäki M. Occupational stress and implementation of information technology among nurses working on acute psychiatric wards. *Perspectives in Psychiatric Care* 2013; **41**(1): 41–9.

52. Khalifa M, Liu V. The state of research on information system satisfaction. *Journal of Information Technology Theory and Applications* 2004; **5**(4): 37–49.

53. Lorenzi MN, Riley RT. Organizational issues = change. *International Journal of Medical Informatics* 2003; **69**(2–3): 197–203.

54. Lium J-T, Tjora A, Faxvaag A. No paper, but the same routines: a qualitative exploration of experiences in two Norwegian hospitals deprived of the paper based medical record. *BMC Medical Informatics and Decision Making* 2008; **8**: 2.

55. Yusof MM, Kuljis J, Papazafeiropoulou A, Stergioulas LK. An evaluation framework for Health Information Systems: human, organization and technology-fit factors (HOT-fit). *International Journal of Medical Informatics* 2007; **77**(6): 386–98.

56. Koivunen M, Hätönen H, Välimäki M. Barriers and facilitators influencing the implementation of an interactive internet-portal application for patient education in psychiatric hospitals. *Patient Education and Counseling* 2008; **70**: 412–19.

57. Koivunen M. The impacts of information technology on staff's abilities and practice in psychiatric hospitals. *Annales Universitatis Turkuensis, Medica Odontologica* 2009, Ser D 837. University of Turku, Finland.

58. Office of the National Coordinator for Health Information Technology. *Important facts about EHR adoption and the EHR incentive program: recent survey findings.* Washington, DC: US Department of Health and Human Services, 2011.

59. Anttila M, Koivunen M, Välimäki M. Information technology-based standardized patient education in psychiatric inpatient care. *Journal of Advanced Nursing* 2008; **64**(2): 147–56.

60. Maijala R, Anttila M, Koivunen M, Pitkänen A, Kuosmanen L, Välimäki M. Internet delivered question and answer column for patients with schizophrenia. *Informatics for Health and Social Care* 2014; **24**: 1–12. [Epub ahead of print]

Further reading

Alvarez-Jimenez M, Alcazar-Corcoles MA, Gonzalez-Blanch C, Bendall S, McGorry PD, Gleeson JF. Online, social media and mobile technologies for psychosis treatment: a systematic review on novel user-led interventions. *Schizophrenia Research* 2015; **156**: 96–106.

Athanasopoulou C, Suni S, Hätönen H, Apostolakis I, Lionis C, Välimäki M. Attitudes towards schizophrenia on YouTube: a content analysis of Finnish and Greek videos. *Informatics for Health and Social Care* 2015; **41**(3): 1–18.

Athanasopoulou C, Hätönen H, Suni, S, Lionis C, Griffiths KM, Välimäki M. An analysis of online health information on schizophrenia or related conditions: a cross-sectional survey. *BMC Medical Informatics and Decision Making* 2013; **815**(13): 98.

Kalckreuth S, Trefflich F, Rummel-Kluge C. Mental health related internet use among psychiatric patients: a cross-sectional analysis. *BMC Psychiatry* 2014; **14**: 368.

Khazaal Y, Chatton A, Cochand S, Hoch A, Khankarli MB, Khan R, Zullino DF. Internet use by patients with psychiatric disorders in search for general and medical informations. *Psychiatric Quarterly* 2008; **79**: 301–9.

Miller BJ, Stewart A, Schrimsher J, Peeples D, Buckley PF. How connected are people with schizophrenia? Cell phone, computer, email, and social media use. *Psychiatry Research* 2015; **225**(3): 458–63.

Schrank B, Sibitz I, Unger A, Amering M. How patients with schizophrenia use the internet: qualitative study. *Journal of Medical Internet Research* 2010; **12**(5): e70.

Torous J, Friedman R, Keshavan M. Smartphone ownership and interest in mobile applications to monitor symptoms of mental health conditions. *JMIR mHealth and uHealth* 2014; **2**(1): e2.

Välimäki M, Hätönen H, Lahti M, Kuosmanen L, Adams CE. Information and communication technology in patient education and support for people with schizophrenia. *Cochrane Database of Systematic Reviews* 2012; **10**: CD007198.

Younes N, Chollet A, Menard E, Melchior M. E-mental health care among young adults and help-seeking behaviors: a transversal study in a community sample. *Journal of Medical Internet Research* 2015; **17**(5): e123.

Unützer J, Choi Y, Cook I, Oishi S. A web-based data management system to improve care for depression in a multicenter clinical trial. *Psychiatric Services* 2002; **53**(6): 671–8.

Relevant web pages

Australian National University. Beacon 2.0. https://beacon.anu.edu.au/

Beating the Blues. http://www.beatingtheblues.co.uk/

BluePages. http://www.bluepages.anu.edu.au/

Changeways Clinic and the Centre for Applied Research in Mental Health and Addiction. *Self-care depression program: antidepressants skills workbook.* http://www.sfu.ca/carmha/publications.html

Mood Gym. https://moodgym.anu.edu.au/welcome

MoodHelper. https://www.kpchr.org/moodhelper/default.aspx

MyMind. Centre for Mental Wellbeing. http://mymind.org/

Orygen Youth Health, University of Melbourne. MoodMemos. http://www.moodmemos.com/

PatientsLikeMe. http://www.patientslikeme.com/

Stress and Mood Management. http://www.centerforworkforcehealth.com/

Youth Mental Health: A Parent's Guide. http://ymhonline.com/loginpage.asp

73 Mental health nursing in the twenty-first century

PATRICK CALLAGHAN AND DEBBIE BUTLER

LEARNING OUTCOMES

- To understand the context of mental health nursing in the twenty-first century.
- To be aware of contemporary issues concerning mental health nursing.
- To understand the experience of mental health nursing from the perspective of a mental health service user.
- To describe a vision for mental health nursing.

SUMMARY OF KEY POINTS

- Mental health nursing in the twenty-first century is an art, a science and a craft.
- It is a fundamental human right and it enables individuals and communities to transform their health and well-being.
- It is a complex intervention that adopts a recovery-focused co-production approach.
- Mental health nursing education articulates the knowledge and performance criteria necessary for effective practice.
- Mental health nursing research adopts a pragmatic evidence-based approach.
- Mental health nursing leadership is evident at the point of care delivery and all layers of the systems within which it operates.
- Leaders must inspire, support and secure mental health nursing and help create the conditions under which it will flourish.

INTRODUCTION

This chapter examines the status of mental health nursing in the twenty-first century from the authors' own and others' experiences, observations and evidence. We consider the context of mental health nursing; critique contemporary issues in practice, education, research and leadership; and present a vision for mental health nursing.

THE CONTEXT OF MENTAL HEALTH NURSING IN THE TWENTY-FIRST CENTURY

The international context

Mental health problems affect people in all parts of the world, accounting for 13 per cent of the global burden of disease, yet only 6 per cent of financial resources for health are given to mental health.[1] The consequences of these disorders are estimated to incur a worldwide cost of approximately US$16.1 trillion in loss of productivity, severe impacts on quality of life, arrested social development, increased risk of suicide, stigma, discrimination, inequity and medical problems such as diabetes and cardiovascular disorders.[2,3]

The WHO Mental Health Action Plan for 2013–2020[4] aims to promote mental well-being, prevent mental disorders and reduce mortality and morbidity, under six principles with related targets (see Table 73.1).

Nurses account for the highest number of professionals providing mental health care; the median average number of nurses per 100,000 of the population working in mental health is 5.8, more than all other professionals combined,[5] making mental health nurses pivotal to the delivery of the WHO Action Plan.

The national context

Mental health nursing is influenced by the international direction of travel, as described in the WHO Action Plan and national strategies and policies. In the UK, where we now have devolved government, each country has its own mental health strategy. There are similarities in each strategy around improving mental health and well-being, preventing and reducing ill-health, improving access to services, reducing stigma, discrimination and inequalities, and addressing physical as well as mental health. Working in partnership with those using services, their friends and primary caregivers is a feature in all plans, and is captured neatly by the phrase 'no decision about me without me' taken from the title of an NHS strategy document.[6]

Within the UK, strategic visions for nursing have been published; two of these relate to mental health nursing, and two have relevance for all nurses. These are shown in Table 73.2.

> ### REFLECTION
>
> Consider the visions described in Table 73.2. Reflect on the contribution you can make to the delivery of these strategies.

Following on from the English Chief Nursing Officer's vision for nursing and midwifery, the national director of mental health and learning disability nursing published his vision for the nursing and midwifery

Table 73.1 The WHO Mental Health Action Plan 2013–2020: key principles and targets[4]

Principle	Target
Universal access and equity	All people with mental illness should have access to services that help them achieve or recover the highest possible standard of living irrespective of standing or status in society.
Human rights	All mental health strategies and services must be compliant with human rights conventions and agreements.
Evidence-based practice	All services provided must be based on scientific evidence and good practice.
Life course approach	Policies, plans and services need to take account of health and social care needs at all stages of life.
Multisectoral approach	A comprehensive and coordinated response is advocated that utilizes health, social care, education, employment, housing and other relevant sectors.
Empowerment of persons	All people with mental health problems should be involved in planning, policy, legislation, service provision and evaluation.

Table 73.2 Visions for nursing in the twenty-first century

The Chief Nursing Officer's Review of Mental Health Nursing in England (2006)[7]	Scottish Government. rights, relationships and recovery: the report of the National Review of Mental Health Nursing in Scotland[8]	Department of Health. Compassion in practice: a vision and strategy for nurses, midwives and care staff[9]	The US Institute of Medicine's (IOM) report: The future of nursing (2010)[10]	Australian College of Mental Health Nurses, Standards for practice for Australian mental health nurses (2010)[11] (p.6)
Putting values into practice *Values* Promote a culture that values and respects the diversity of individuals, and enables their recovery. **Improving outcomes for service users** *Communication* Use a range of communication skills to establish, maintain and manage relationships with individuals who have mental health problems, their carers and key people involved in their care. *Physical care* Promote physical health and well-being for people with mental health problems. *Psychosocial care* Promote mental health and well-being, enabling people to recover from debilitating mental health experiences and/ or achieve their full potential, supporting them to develop and maintain social networks and relationships.	**Culture and values: strengthening the climate of care** Mental health nursing is about caring for people and their significant others, spending time with them and developing sound interpersonal relationships. Mental health nursing is rights-based, with a person-centred focus, promoting values and principles-based practice. **The adoption of recovery principles** Adoption of models of care that are relationships-based and use contact time to foster recovery. **Practice and services** Prioritizing the focus of care towards acute inpatient, crisis care and home treatment services.	*Care*: putting care at the heart of nursing and all health and social care organizations. It is argued that care is the essence of mental health nursing. Mental health nurses can care by 'mobilising hope, confidence and trust between themselves and the persons for whom they care'[12] (p.44). *Compassion*: showing a profound awareness and understanding of suffering and taking steps to relieve it.[13] *Competence*: delivering effective care based upon the best available and best possible evidence. *Communication*: using the most effective communication skills. *Courage*: having the personal strength and vision to defend and uphold the best care.	Four key messages: *Nurses should practise to the full extent of their education and training*: a recognition that although nurses are trained to the highest educational and practice level, their licence to practise is determined by varying state legislations, many of which do not permit nurses to practise to the level for which they are educated. *Nurses should achieve higher levels of education and training through an improved education system that promotes seamless academic progression*: a recognition of the importance of nurses achieving higher levels of education to ensure they can deliver safe, patient-centred care.	*Standard 1*: The mental health nurse acknowledges diversity in culture, values and belief systems and ensures his/her practice is non-discriminatory, and promotes dignity and self-determination. *Standard 2*: The mental health nurse establishes collaborative partnerships that facilitate and support people with mental health issues to participate in all aspects of their care. *Standard 3*: The mental health nurse develops a therapeutic relationship that is respectful of the individual's choices, experiences and circumstances. This involves building on strengths, holding hope and enhancing resilience to promote recovery. *Standard 4*: The mental health nurse collaboratively plans and provides ethically based care consistent with the mental, physical, spiritual, emotional, social and cultural needs of the individual. *Standard 5*: The mental health nurse values the contributions of other agencies and stakeholders in the collaborative provision of holistic, evidence-based care and in ensuring comprehensive service provision for people with mental health issues.

(Continued)

Table 73.2 (continued)

The Chief Nursing Officer's Review of Mental Health Nursing in England (2006)[7]	Scottish Government. rights, relationships and recovery: the report of the National Review of Mental Health Nursing in Scotland[8]	Department of Health. Compassion in practice: a vision and strategy for nurses, midwives and care staff[9]	The US Institute of Medicine's (IOM) report: The future of nursing (2010)[10]	Australian College of Mental Health Nurses, Standards for practice for Australian mental health nurses (2010)[11] (p.6)
Psychosocial care Promote mental health and well-being, enabling people to recover from debilitating mental health experiences and/or achieve their full potential, supporting them to develop and maintain social networks and relationships. *Risk and risk management* Work with individuals with mental health needs in order to maintain health, safety and well-being. **A positive, modern profession** *Multidisciplinary and multi-agency working* Work collaboratively with other disciplines and agencies to support individuals to develop and maintain social networks and relationships. *Personal and professional development* Demonstrate a commitment to the need for continuing professional development and personal supervision activities, in order to enhance knowledge, skills, values and attitudes needed for safe and effective nursing practice.	Adopting the strengths-based approach to recovery. Preparing mental health nurses to work effectively with older adults. Enhancing the role of mental health nurses in early intervention and risk assessment. Developing the role of mental health nurses in health promotion, health improvement and reducing inequalities. **Education and development** Developing a national framework to attract the right people into the profession. Emphasizing continuing professional development. Involving service users and carers in all aspects of mental health nursing. The development of mental health support workers. Developing and embedding strong leadership. Strengthening mental health nursing education.	*Commitment:* a pledge to provide the most effective care at all times and in all circumstances.	*Nurses should be full partners, with physicians and other health care professionals in redesigning health care in the United States:* being a full partner in all aspects of care requires enhanced leadership training and education to equip nurses with the necessary skills to identify system problems and effective solutions, implement changes and evaluate the impact of these changes. *Effective workforce planning and policy making require better data collection and an improved information infrastructure:* implementing better systems to identify and meet workforce needs to deliver the required level of care.	*Standard 6:* The mental health nurse actively pursues opportunities to reduce stigma and promotes social inclusion and community participation for all people with mental health issues. *Standard 7:* The mental health nurse demonstrates evidence-based practice and actively promotes practice innovation through lifelong education, research, professional development, clinical supervision and reflective practice. *Standard 8:* The mental health nurse's practice incorporates and reflects common law requirements, relevant statutes and the nursing profession's code of conduct and ethics. The mental health nurse integrates international, national, local and state policies and guidelines with professional standards and competencies. *Standard 9:* The mental health nurse holds specialist qualifications and demonstrates advanced specialist knowledge, skills and practice, integrating all the standards competently and modelling leadership in the practice setting.

contribution to *No health without mental health* with a vision for public mental health nursing which consists of three levels:

1. promoting mental health and well-being through reducing stigma and discrimination;
2. early interventions to prevent physical ill health;
3. working in partnership with other public health practitioners.[14]

Given that nurses are the largest group of health care providers in developed, emerging and developing countries, it is not surprising to find in some countries particular strategies providing a steer for nursing practice and education. The focus on mental health nursing in England and Scotland may be a reflection of the increasing burden of disease of mental health problems and the fact that mental health is increasingly a national health priority. These strategies acknowledge that nurses are central to the delivery of high quality health care. The link between how nurses are educated and how they practise is addressed in each of these strategies, but the Institute of Medicine report[10] makes a stronger case for why nurses need higher levels of education. In the UK, the nature of nursing education is subject to (polarized) debate; on one side are those who argue that nurses have little need of degree-level university-provided education, and on the other are those arguing the opposite. In Australia the challenge is to ensure a minimal level of performance for registered nurses working in mental health settings in the absence of specific mental health nursing undergraduate curricula.

Common among the visions for mental health nursing is the recognition that mental health nursing does not take place in a vacuum and that nurses must work in partnership with other health care professionals, as well with people using services, and their respective carers. The vision for mental health nursing set out in this chapter has been shaped by the strategic visions reported above; by the first author's experience of providing mental health care, education, conducting research and leading a large university school; by the second author's experiences of using mental health services and working collaboratively with educators, clinicians and researchers; and by a review of evidence assessing the role of mental health nurses in shaping people's health and well-being.

THE ROLE OF MENTAL HEALTH NURSES IN HELPING INDIVIDUALS AND COMMUNITIES SHAPE THEIR HEALTH AND WELL-BEING

Mental health nursing practice

Mental health nurses spend around 50 per cent of their time in direct contact with service users. The amount of time spent on therapeutic activities ranges from 4 to 20 per cent. Encounters are more often initiated by service users. Contact time decreases with seniority and experience and contact time diminishes over time.[15,16] Yet there is significant evidence showing how therapeutic engagement leads to improved outcomes for mental health service users.[17] Also, many routine mental health nursing interventions, especially those that happen on acute mental health wards, appear invisible in that they often occur 'under the radar', they may lack a systematic approach and the work appears to be subsumed within the wider team approach in acute wards.[18,19] This work is seldom published to bring it to wider attention and recognition[20] and, despite therapeutic engagement being a key component of mental health nursing, this element is seldom used as a metric for mental health nursing.[21]

Mental health nurses have been criticized for failing to adopt a recovery-focused approach to their practice (chapters 35 and 36),[22-24] and this has led to the development of roles such as that of peer support worker (PSW). A PSW is invariably a person with lived experience of mental health issues who is employed to provide a more recovery-focused approach to care, based on the principles of shared understanding, respect and mutual empowerment.[25,26] The role of PSWs is now being systematically researched, with early results[27,28] from mental health nursing researchers showing their promise in delivering care that *may* be promoting service users' recovery better than standard approaches to care.

People living with mental health problems have a shortened life expectancy by up to 20 years on account of physical health problems (chapter 69) that are often untreated.[29-31] Mental health nurses have been initially slow to rise to this challenge, but momentum is gathering and improvements are starting to occur.[32-34]

Mental health nursing education

In response to various reports that questioned whether nursing education improved care, a strategic review of nursing education was commissioned by Health Education England and the Nursing and Midwifery Council. This was the Shape of Caring Review, chaired by Lord Willis, who chaired a similar review in 2012 that the Royal College of Nursing commissioned. In its 2012 review report, the Willis Commission[35] wrote: 'The commission found no major shortcomings in nursing education that could be held responsible for poor practice or the decline in standards of care.' *Raising the bar*,[36] the report arising from the Shape of Caring Review, made

34 recommendations within 8 themes. Notable among the recommendations is the call for consideration of the development of a 'flexible' model of nursing education: a 2 + 1 + 1 approach – 2 years general, 1 year field-specific and a 1-year preceptorship period – that eschews the current approach of four fields of practice.

Twenty-first-century concerns about mental health nursing education are also focused on commissioned reviews of curricula content and delivery, delineating the required knowledge and performance criteria necessary for practice.[7] A report by the Australian Mental Health Nurse Education Taskforce[37] reviewed mental health input to generic pre-registration nursing courses in Australia, and recommended that course accreditation bodies ensure mental health nursing benchmarked content is incorporated into courses they approve; that federal government, states and territories develop consumers and carers' capacity to be involved in all aspects of mental health education; and that universities be provided with funding to enable them to establish a centre housing mental health teaching resources that others can access.

The experiences and effects of service user and carer involvement in teaching and learning have been examined at length.[38,39] This has been shown to improve the quality of teaching and learning, so that it is almost routine – a welcome development that has really taken off this century.

Debate about alternative methods of providing students with clinical experience while in education emerged from the English *Chief Nursing Officer's Review of Mental Health Nursing* in 2005,[7] which was influenced by a scoping review that the first author and others conducted on behalf of Mental Health Nurse Academics UK,[40] as well as his pilot study with colleagues at City University, London.[41] What emerged from this work was a proposal for a hybrid model that included using location-based placements for longer periods, during which students would have the opportunity to work with senior staff to develop leadership skills, in a host trust, with a named mentor/supervisor throughout training and exposure to client attachment in the final year of their programme. Some of these ideas are now evident in curricula, although the latter, which is popular among service users and students, has not really taken off.

Undergraduate and graduate mental health nursing education is delivered exclusively in universities. As a result, it is not immune to the arguments and debates about universities first discussed by Newman in *The idea of a university*[42] and Collini's *What are universities for?*,[43] in which the expansion of the university sector to include vocational subjects such as nursing has prompted Collini to reconsider the role of universities in the twenty-first century.

Critiques of nursing's role in universities[44–46] have revisited some of the ideas of these texts, particularly Newman's work, with little agreement emerging on the nature, position and place of nursing, and the proper role and focus of members of the nursing academy in the university sector. On the one hand, Thompson and Watson[45] argue for nursing to embody the ideal view of the university as a place for enlightened, liberal, free-thinking ideas, eschewing the value of certain 'applied' elements and using practice development as an example. In contrast, Rolfe[47] has challenged these authors' reading of Newman, and their acceptance of his ideas. He argues the case for practice development being part of the solution to the problems of academic nursing – the unbridled acquiescence to practice demands, for example, that Thompson and Watson cite. To the disinterested onlooker, this may appear as an irrelevant spat between self-regarding academics that has little to do with the 'real' world of nursing. But this would be to miss an important point. In light of the Willis Review of nursing education, debates around the role and purpose of university education for nurses will be fundamental to the future shape of nursing care.

Mental health nursing research and scholarship

In relation to research, issues of interest tend to coalesce around views that research without scholarship will stifle the development of robust theories of (mental health) nursing[47] and render it a technical exercise devoid necessarily of scholarship, the lack of an agreed approach for the focus of mental health nursing research[48,49] and the lack of impact of mental health nursing research on health and social care policy, practice, and individuals and communities' health and well-being.

Mental health nurses are leading research programmes that are helping to transform people's recovery from debilitating mental health problems such as anxiety and depression,[50,51] improving nurses' practice in, and service users' experiences of, acute mental health wards;[52] leading projects that are improving the physical health needs of people living with mental health issues;[53–56] leading national and international work on recovery-focused practice and the development of Recovery Colleges;[57] driving collaborative mental health nursing,[58] steering national initiatives to reduce restrictive practices; and seeking to prevent and manage violence in mental health settings.[59–62] These studies are underpinned by significant, competitive research grants, and this attests to the importance of the work being reported.

Zauszniewski[62] and colleagues published a review of 10 years of empirical work on psychiatric and mental health nursing published between 2000 and 2012 in five US-based mental health nursing journals. This paper shows that mental health nurses published 553 papers, 71 per cent of which were intervention studies, among which 38 per cent tested psychological interventions, 17 per cent social interventions and 1 per cent biological interventions; 17 per cent tested all three of these domains. Of the published studies, 54 per cent were conducted in the US; the remaining were published in Korea, Australia, the UK, Taiwan, Canada, the Netherlands, Singapore, Turkey, Norway, Jordan, Finland, Thailand, Switzerland and Portugal. Eighty-five per cent focused on mentally ill or mentally healthy individuals. Only 15 per cent had as their focus mental health nurses, students or other staff. The review also reported an increase over the 10 years in studies directed towards people living with mental health issues and a decrease in studies focused on nurses, students and other staff. This shift in focus is to be welcomed, as it suggests that there is more research focused on direct service user benefit. However, only 28 per cent of the intervention studies used random samples and had a control group, and this may impede the translation of the findings into practice. Ten per cent of studies used qualitative approaches, suggesting that less attention has been given to understanding and exploring people's experiences of health, ill-health and health care.

Through work funded by the European Union, Dave Richards, a mental health nurse and Professor of Mental Health Services Research at Exeter University, and colleagues across Europe have trained many nurses in using complex intervention designs to enhance rigorous testing of the effect of nursing interventions. This initiative has led to the development of the REFLECTION[63] network of researchers, which seeks to improve the evidence base underpinning nursing interventions.

On the face of the evidence, mental health nursing research, or research that mental health nurses conduct, is thriving, tackling important issues, working collaboratively with many stakeholders including people using services and their carers, who are helping to steer decisions about what gets researched, and how, and beginning to show impact where it matters for people's health and well-being, for national and global agendas and for organizations providing mental health services.

Recovery-focused mental health nursing theories, including Barker's Tidal Model, appear to have contemporary currency, judging by the increasing attention given to these in the anecdotal, empirical and policy literature,[64] where they are showing promise in enabling people living with mental health issues to transform their health and well-being and lead lives that are more meaningful and satisfying to them. They also appear to be popular and acceptable to most people, although they have their critics.[65] Unlike previous models of mental health nursing, the Tidal Model has been developed with people who use mental health services, is person-centred and acknowledges the role of reclamation, a situation whereby people rediscover their sense of self through sharing personal stories. Whether recovery approaches outlast previous models remains to be seen. If they fail in their adoption, it is hard to know what will succeed.

Mental health nursing writers in the twenty-first century appear more concerned with 'theories *for* mental health nursing'[66] that propose an approach that includes psychological, sociological, biological, humanistic and ethical models. Inherent in this approach is the view that mental health nurses must use eclectic approaches to understand their practice and the experiences of the people for whom they care.

Mental health nursing leadership

Finally, in relation to mental health nursing leadership, some of the pertinent issues in the twenty-first century concern top-down approaches, clarifying role expectations, using evidence to implement decisions and employing effective communication skills in meeting the challenges of supporting, nurturing and empowering others.[67,68] Other issues being examined include the subjugation of a specific mental nursing agenda at the expense of a general corporate agenda when mental health nurses achieve leadership positions, and people's general perceptions of leadership being out of touch with the reality of frontline care and the rightful role of mental health nursing leaders in applying situational and transformative leadership.[69]

A VISION FOR MENTAL HEALTH NURSING IN THE TWENTY-FIRST CENTURY

In this section, we will revisit ideas that Callaghan and Owen[70] first reported in the early part of the century. We have expanded upon these ideas to account for concepts of mental health nursing that have emerged since their editorial was published. We have summarized this vision in Table 73.3.

REFLECTION

Examine the vision described in Table 73.3. Describe how you might embrace this vision in your day-to-day practice as a mental health nurse.

Table 73.3 A vision for mental health nursing in the twenty-first century

Vision	Description
Mental health nursing is a complex, collaborative, person-centred, recovery-focused art, science and craft.	Mental health nurses must work in partnership not only with service users and their carers but also with the wider communities and agencies with whom service users and their carers interact. It is rooted in people's experiences, and it recognizes people's expertise and ability to manage their lives. Mental health nursing encompasses hope, opportunity, control and optimism. The capable mental health nurse will: • adopt a recovery-based approach using co-production methods; • encourage advocacy; • form good human relationships; • work in psychosocial ways and combat discrimination; • practice in an evidence-based way.[71] Mental health nursing is a fundamental human right to which people living with incapacitating distress have access. The goals to which most of us aspire, and which are fundamental to our own quality of life – health; paid, productive occupation; social support; safe, secure shelter; and freedom from fear, discrimination and prejudice – are central to the lives of people with mental health issues. The art of mental health nursing is expressed by the application of person-centred *values* in practice; the science is evident through the use of sound clinical judgement underpinned by the best possible *evidence* where available, or inferred evidence where evidence is absent; the craft of mental health nursing is apparent from the demonstrable use of mental health nursing *skills* in practice. We accept a more contemporary view of evidence-based health[72] that prioritizes ethical care and shared decision-making with service users and their representative agents, and emphasizes human aspects of care with strong service user choice based upon sound interpersonal skills. Mental health nursing contains several interacting components that generate an array of possible, variable and demonstrable outcomes. Such outcomes will be recognized and/or defined by those seeking mental health nursing care as crucial to leading lives that are meaningful and satisfying to them, as defined by them. The mental health nursing process comprises: • *engagement:* developing a robust therapeutic relationship; • *explaining:* providing sufficient information as to the purpose of all mental health nursing interactions; • *involving:* ensuring that service users, their carers and friends are involved; where desired adopting the Triangle of Care;[73] • *assessing:* carrying out a person-centred assessment of needs; • *planning:* developing a plan of care to address agreed needs and enable achievement of aspirational goals; • *implementing:* the application of the art, science and craft of mental health nursing; • *reviewing:* regular formal and informal review to ensure that mental health nursing care is having the planned effect. For mental health nurses working in acute wards we recommend adopting the Safewards approach to mental health nursing in acute wards (see: http://www.safewards.net/model-diagram).

(Continued)

Table 73.3 *(continued)*

Vision	Description
Mental health nursing education articulates the values, knowledge and performance criteria necessary for the *routine* practice that inspires students to help people transform their health and well-being.	Teaching focuses on: • articulating values and applying them to practice; • improving the process and outcome of mental health nursing; • a positive modern profession: improving, upholding and projecting a positive image of mental health nursing.
Mental health nursing research is based on a pragmatic evidenced-based approach.	The pragmatic evidence-based approach is characterized by: • methodological rigour coupled with high clinical need and relevance; • working collaboratively with service users and other stakeholders at all stages of the research process; • structure, process and outcome evaluations; • using the most appropriate and innovative methods to address research questions that service users and carers also recognize as important to their needs that will also appeal to funders; • translatable – showing impact on practice, people's health and well-being, policy, macro and micro economics, culture and organizations.
Mental health nursing leaders inspire, support and secure mental health nursing and help create the conditions under which it will flourish.	We recommend that mental health nursing leaders: • apply situational, transformative leadership; • act with integrity and honesty; • engage staff in decision-making; • clarify their own and others' role expectations; • use actual and inferred evidence to implement decisions; • employ sound communication skills using a variety of methods; • inspire, support, nurture and empower others; • promote the profession and project a positive image with influence and gravitas locally, nationally and internationally.

SERVICE USER'S PERSPECTIVE

Walking down the dark corridor smelling of urine with patients sitting in door wells seems a long time ago. 1986 saw my first encounter with a psychiatrist. I think, on reflection, that this was the worst day of my life. My generation was bought up to worship doctors and nurses and adhere to what they said. The psychiatrist I had turned out to be very supportive. At this time mental ill-health had (I believe) more bad press than now. So much so that the hospital I referred to earlier was known as 'Mapperley Mad House'. Patients who were allowed out were seen walking through the local shopping area in their pyjamas. Alongside the negative attitudes of mental health nursing staff, this reinforced the stigma that was attached to the patients.

I remember seeing a film a few years ago that looked at patient experience in what I will call the old days, showing wards that were overcrowded and basically left the patients to get on with it. Reflecting on that and my experience over many years using mental health services, I do feel nursing in the twenty-first century is vastly different.

Walking down that corridor I mentioned earlier was frightening. I had not been given any information about what would happen to me. I was told where and when to go but nothing else.

I saw a junior doctor who asked lots and lots of questions, most of which I don't remember, partly because it was a long time ago but mostly because I was so distressed. I had recently had a premature baby and suffered with post-natal depression with psychosis. I do remember one thing, however – a friend told me, and I have told others, that having a baby doesn't come with an instruction booklet.

My first CPN from the mother and baby unit told me things would get much worse before they got better. I thought this inappropriate and made sure I didn't see her again. It was after this I made my first walk down that long corridor.

Over the next few years I had both good and bad experiences. I believe because of these I took on and learned the role of a mental health patient, or the sick role.

My outlook on mental health nursing changed once I was referred to a day centre, most of which are now closed. I became a service user rep at the centre and was asked if I wanted to sit on an interview panel for an assertive outreach team. I did, and following this a while later I became one of the first service users employed by my local trust to advise on the service user and carer perspective. The good practice was there, ticking many boxes. But having spoken to friends and colleagues, and from personal experience, we did in fact tick those rather small and insignificant boxes. A colleague told a cohort of Masters students that it's all good to go out to dinner on your reputation, but really asking those on the receiving end of care how they felt is more important. Life continued and things began to change. My diagnosis of personality disorder became more recognized by government after several high-profile media stories. As part of the government's commission of PD services, I worked with some senior managers and clinicians from around 25 different stakeholders.

I have to say being involved in these large projects changed my views of the clinical staff and I believe they reciprocated that view.

As time has gone on, the relationship between staff and patient has relaxed. People are involved more in their care, not always according to the proper policies, but at least it has been discussed openly. Some service users, however, have taken on the role of a patient and are quite happy to be nursed. Government policy promotes 'recovery' but due to financial cutbacks, nurses do experience great pressure to move people through the system. So there is a dichotomy for both service users and nurses as to how patients progress in short periods of care.

Although those nurses that I have seen and worked with feel pressured because of this way of working, I have had many a discussion with mental health nurses who said they weren't happy in their work because of the pressure put on them and having to work with some high-need patients. This often results in services imposing an unnecessary care pathway on service users who are told abruptly to do it. Social workers working with nurses will have to be supporting those patients.

Debbie Butler is a mental health service user and consultant of 28 years' experience.

REFLECTION

Consider how you would address the concerns that are raised in the account reported by the service user.

CONCLUSION

Mental health nursing is an art, a science and a craft. It excels when mental health nurses work in collaboration with people using mental health services, their caregivers and representative agencies, as well as other mental health workers. Mental health nursing is driven by a values, culture and evidence-based, personalized care that embeds an expectation of mental health nursing as a fundamental human right. Mental health nursing is helping individuals and communities transform their health and well-being. Mental health nursing is also a complex intervention, containing several interacting components, that generates an array of possible, variable and demonstrable outcomes. For mental health nursing to succeed, it must adopt a recovery-focused co-production approach that those seeking mental health nursing care recognize as crucial to leading lives that are meaningful and satisfying to them, *as defined by them*. Mental health nursing education must articulate the knowledge and performance criteria that will deliver *routinely* core competencies in the application of sound interpersonal skills, collaborative assessment of needs with service users and their carers, interventions that have been shown evidentially to meet these needs and will be widely acceptable to people with whom mental health nurses care, evaluation that needs have been met and the keeping of defensible practice records – these things constitute the process of mental health nursing.

Mental health nursing research should adopt a pragmatic evidence-based approach that shows clear clinical relevance and need, coupled with methodological rigour, whatever the methods, translatable to practice.

Mental health nursing leadership should be evident at the point of care delivery and all layers of the systems within which it operates. Leaders must inspire, support and secure mental health nursing and help create the conditions under which it will flourish.

There is an increasing body of evidence that suggests mental health nursing is thriving in the twenty-first century, although formidable challenges remain. The vision described here should help mental health nurses rise to these challenges.

References

1. WHO (World Health Organization). The *mental health atlas.* Geneva: WHO, 2011.
2. Ganju V. Non-communicable diseases and the mental health gap: what is to be done? *International Journal of Psychiatry* 2012; **9**(4): 79–80.
3. Bass JK., Borneman TH, Burkey M, Chehil S, Chen L, Copeland JR, Eaton WW, Ganju V, Hayward E, Hock RS, Kidwai R, Kolappa K, Lee PT, Minas H, Or F, Raviola GJ, Saraceno B, Patel V. A United Nations General Assembly special session for mental, neurological and substance use disorder: the time has come. *PLOS Medicine* 2012; **9**(1): e1001159, doi:10.1371)/journal bmed/1001159.
4. WHO (World Health Organization). *Global Mental Health Action Plan.* Geneva: WHO, 2013.
5. WHO (World Health Organization). *The mental health atlas 2014.* Geneva: WHO, 2015.
6. Department of Health. *Liberating the NHS: no decision about me, without me.* London: Department of Health, 2012.
7. Department of Health. *Values into action: the Chief Nursing Officer's Review of Mental Health Nursing in England.* London: DH, 2006.
8. Scottish Government. *Rights, relationships and recovery: the report of the National Review of Mental Health Nursing in Scotland.* Edinburgh: NHS Scotland, 2006.
9. Department of Health. *Compassion in practice: a vision and strategy for nurses, midwives and care staff.* London: DH, 2013.
10. IOM (Institute of Medicine). *The future of nursing: leading change, advancing health.* Washington, DC: IOM, 2010.
11. ACMHN (Australian College of Mental Health Nurses). *Standards for practice for Australian mental health nurses 2010.* Canberra: ACMHN, 2010.
12. Stickley T, Stacy G. Caring: the essence of mental health nursing. In: Callaghan P, Playle J, Cooper L (eds). *Mental health nursing skills.* Oxford: Oxford University Press, 2006: 44–55.
13. Gilbert P. *The compassionate mind.* London: Constable, 2010.
14. Thomas B. *Vision and strategy: the nursing contribution to the health and well-being of people with learning disabilities.* Leeds: NHS England, 2013.
15. Bee PE, Richards DA, Loftus S, Lovell K, Baker JA, Cox D. Mapping nursing activity in acute inpatient mental healthcare settings. *Journal of Mental Health* 2006; **15**(2): 217–26.
16. Sharac J, McCrone P, Clement S, Thornicroft G. The economic impact of mental health stigma and discrimination: a systematic review. *Epidemiologia e Psichiatria Sociale* 2010; **19**(3): 223–32.
17. Bentall RP, Lewis S, Tarrier G, Haddock DR, Day J. Relationships matter: the impact of the therapeutic alliance on outcome in schizophrenia. *International Congress on Schizophrenia Research* 2003; **20**: 319.
18. Bowers L, Simpson A, Alexander J, Hackney D, Nijman H, Grange A, Warren J. The nature and purpose of acute psychiatric wards: the Tompkins acute ward study. *Journal of Mental Health* 2005; **14**: 625–35.
19. Cleary M. The realities of mental health nursing in acute inpatient environments. *International Journal of Mental Health Nursing* 2004; **13**(1): 53–60.
20. Delaney KR, Johnson ME. Meta-synthesis of research on the role of psychiatric inpatient nurses: what is important to staff? *Journal of the American Psychiatric Nurses Association* 2014; **20**(2): 1–13.
21. McAndrew S, Chambers M, Nolan F, Thomas B, Watts, P. Measuring the evidence: reviewing the literature of the measurement of therapeutic engagement in acute mental health inpatient wards. *International Journal of Mental Health Nursing* 2014; **23**(23): 212–20.
22. Bassett T, Repper J. Travelling hopefully. *Mental Health Today* 2005; November: 16–18.
23. Barker P, Buchannan-Barker P. Myth of mental health nursing and the challenge of recovery. *International Journal of Mental Health Nursing* 2011; **20**: 337–44.
24. Stickley T, Bassett T (eds). *Learning about mental health practice.* London: Wiley, 2008.
25. Mead S, MacNeil C. Peer support: what makes it unique? *International Journal of Psychosocial Rehabilitation* 1996; **10**(2): 29–37.
26. Repper J, Perkins R. *Social inclusion and recovery.* London: Bailliere Tindall, 2003.
27. Repper J. *Final report for Closing the Gap through Changing Relationships Project – introducing peer support workers in mental health services.* London: Health Foundation, 2013.
28. Simpson A, Flood C, Rowe J, Quigley J, Henry S, Hall C, Evans R, Sherman P, Bowers L. Results of a pilot randomised controlled trial to measure the clinical and cost effectiveness of peer support in increasing hope and quality of life in mental health patients discharged from hospital in the UK. *BMC Psychiatry* 2014; **14**: doi: 10.1186/1471-244X-14-30.
29. Robson D, Gray R. Serious mental illness and physical health problems: a discussion paper. *International Journal of Nursing Studies* 2007; **44**: 457–66.
30. Tosh G, Clifton A, Bachner M. General physical health advice for people with serious mental illness. *Cochrane Database of Systematic Reviews* 2011; **2**: CD008567.
31. Naylor C, Parsonage M, McDaid D, Knapp M, Fossey M, Galea A. *Long term conditions and mental health: the cost of co-morbidities.* London: Kings Fund & Centre for Mental Health, 2012.
32. Mairs H, Bradshaw T. Early recognition and screening for psychosis. In: Fleming M, Martin C (eds). *Mental health and wellbeing.* Hampshire: Swan & Horn, 2014: 119–29.
33. Bradshaw T, Mairs H. Obesity and serious mental ill health: a critical review of the literature. *Healthcare* 2014; **2**: 1–19.
34. Lovell K Wearden A, Bradshaw T, Tomenson B, Pedley R, Davies L, Hussain N, Warburton J, Woodham A, Escott D, Swarbrick C, Femi-Ajao O, Marshall M. An exploratory randomized controlled study of a healthy living intervention in early intervention services for psychosis: the INTERvention to encourage ACTivity, improve diet, and reduce weight gain (INTERACT) study. *Journal of Clinical Psychiatry* 2014; **75**(5): 498–505.
35. Willis P. Report of the Willis Commission 2002: executive summary. 2010. Available from: http://www.williscommission.org.uk/__data/assets/pdf_file/0007/495115/Willis_commission_report_Jan_2013.pdf [Accessed 2nd September 2016].

36. HEE (Health Education England), NMC (Nursing and Midwifery Council). *Raising the bar: shape of caring: a review of the future education and training of registered nurses and care assistants*. London: HEE & NMC, 2015. Available from: http://hee.nhs.uk/wp-content/blogs.dir/321/files/2015/03/2348-Shape-of-caring-review-FINAL.pdf [Accessed 2nd September 2016].

37. Mental Health Nurse Education Taskforce. *Final report: mental health in pre-registration nursing courses*. Melbourne: Mental Health Workforce Advisory Committee, 2008.

38. Simpson A, Reynolds L, Light I, Attenborough J. Talking with the experts: evaluation of an online discussion forum involving mental health service users in the education of mental health nursing students. *Nurse Education Today* 2008; **28**(5): 633–40.

39. Stickley T, Stacey G, Pollock K, Smith A, Betinis J, Fairbank S. The practice assessment of student nurses by people who use mental health services. *Nurse Education Today* 2010; **30**(1): 20–5.

40. Callaghan P, Cooper L, Gray R. Rethinking clinical placements for mental health nursing students. *Mental Health Practice* 2007; **10**(5): 18–20.

41. Turner L, Callaghan P, Eales S, Park A. An evaluation of the introduction of a pilot client attachment scheme in mental health nursing education. *Journal of Psychiatric and Mental Health Nursing* 2004; **11**: 414–21.

42. Newman JH. *The idea of a university*. New Haven: Yale University Press, 1899.

43. Collini S. *What are universities for?* London: Penguin, 2012.

44. Rolfe G. Cardinal John Henry Newman and 'the ideal state and purpose of a university': nurse education, research and practice development for the twenty-first century. *Nursing Inquiry* 2012; **19**: 28–106.

45. Thompson DR, Watson R. Editorial – professors of nursing: what do they profess? *Nurse Education in Practice* 2006; **6**: 123–6.

46. Thompson DR. Is nursing viable as an academic discipline? *Nurse Education Today* 2009; **29**: 694–7.

47. Rolfe G. Writing-up and writing-as: rediscovering nursing scholarship. *Nurse Education Today* 2009; **29**: 816–20.

48. Stevenson C. Qualifying psychiatric/mental health nursing research. In: Cutcliffe JR, Ward MF (eds). *Key debates in psychiatric/mental health nursing*. London: Churchill Livingstone, 2006: 314–22.

49. Wellman N. 'Pro' quantitative methods (on being a good craftsperson). In: Cutcliffe JR, Ward MF (eds). *Key debates in psychiatric/mental health nursing*. London: Churchill Livingstone, 2006: 323–35.

50. Lovell K, Lamb J, Gask L, Bower P, Waheed W, Chew-Graham C, Lamb J, Aseem S, Beatty S, Burroughs H, Clarke P, Dowrick A, Edwards S, Gabbay M, Lloyd-Williams M, Dowrick C. Development and evaluation of culturally sensitive psychosocial interventions for under-served people in primary care. *BMC Psychiatry* 2014; **14**(1): 217.

51. Richards DA, Bower P, Pagel C, Weaver A, Utley M, Cape J, Pilling S, Lovell K, Gilbody S, Leibowitz J, Owens L, Paxton R, Hennessy S, Simpson A, Gallivan S, Tomson D, Vasilakis C. Delivering stepped care: an analysis of implementation in routine practice. *Implementation Science* 2012; **7**: 3.

52. Bowers L, James K, Quick A, Simpson A, SUGAR, Stewart, D, Hodsoll J. Reducing conflict and containment rates on acute psychiatric wards: the Safewards cluster randomised controlled trial. *International Journal of Nursing Studies* 2015; **52**(9): 1412–22.

53. Callaghan P, Phillips P, Khalil E, Carter T. Meeting the physical health-care needs of people with substance misuse problems: evaluation of a nurse-led blood-borne virus programme. *International Journal of Mental Health Nursing* 2012; **21**: 248–58.

54. Hardy S, Hinks P, Gray R. Screening for cardiovascular risk in patients with severe mental illness in primary care: a comparison with patients with diabetes. *Journal of Mental Health* 2013; **22**(1): 42–50.

55. Bradshaw T, Davies E, Stronach M, Richardson K, Hermann L. Helping people with serious mental illness to cut down or stop smoking. *Mental Health Practice* 2014; **17**(6): 14–20.

56. Happell B, Scott D, Platania-Phung C. Provision of preventive services for cancer and infectious diseases among individuals with serious mental illness. *Archives of Psychiatric Nursing* 2012; **26**: 192–201.

57. Repper J, Grant G, Nolan M, Enderby P. Carer's experiences of mental health services and views about assessments: lessons from the Partnership in Carer Assessments Project (PICAP). In: Stickley T, Bassett T (eds). *Learning about mental health practice*. Chichester: John Wiley & Sons, 2007: 419–38.

58. Cox LG, Simpson A. Cultural safety, diversity and the servicer user and carer movement in mental health research. *Nursing Inquiry* 2015; doi: 10.1111/nin.12096.

59. Duxbury J. Minimizing the use of coercive practices in mental health: the perfect storm. *Journal of Psychiatric and Mental Health Nursing* 2015; **22**(2): 89–91.

60. Steinert T, Whittington R. A bio-psycho-social model of violence related to mental health problems. *International Journal of Law and Psychiatry* 2013; **36**: 168–75.

61. Abderhalden C, Nedham I, Dassen T, Halfens R, Haug HJ, Fischer J. Structured risk assessment and violence in acute psychiatric wards: randomised controlled trial. *British Journal of Psychiatry* 2008; **193**: 44–50.

62. Zausniewski JA, Bekhet A, Haberlein S. A decade of published evidence for psychiatric and mental health nursing interventions. *Online Journal of Issues in Nursing* 2012; **17**(3): DOI: 10.3912/OJIN.Vol17No03HirshPsy01.

63. REFLECTION Network. Available from: http://www.reflection-network.eu/ [Accessed 2nd September 2016].

64. Barker P. The Tidal Model: the healing potential of metaphor within a patient's narrative. *Psychosocial Nursing and Mental Health Services* 2002; **40**(7): 42–50.

65. Edgley A, Stickley T, Wright N, Repper J. The politics of recovery in mental health: a left libertarian policy analysis. *Social Theory and Health* 2012; **10**(2): 121–40.

66. Stickley T, Wright N (eds). *Theories for mental health nursing: a guide for practice*. London: Sage, 2014.

67. Callaghan P, Repper J, Clifton A, Stacey G, Carter T. Evaluation of the Chief Nursing Officer's Review of Mental Health Nursing in England: case studies from selected Mental Health Trusts. *Journal of Psychiatric and Mental Health Nursing* 2011; **19**(5): 455–65.

68. Holm AL, Severinsson E. The role of mental health nursing leadership. *Journal of Nursing Management* 2010; **18**: 463–71.

69. Hughes F. Leadership in mental health nursing. *Journal of Psychosocial Nursing* 2008; **46**(9): 1–9.

70. Callaghan P, Owen S. Editorial: psychiatric and mental health nursing: past, present and future. *Journal of Psychiatric and Mental Health Nursing* 2005; **12**: 639–41.

71. Stickley T, Bassett T. (eds). *Learning about mental health practice*, 1st edn. Chichester: John Wiley & Sons Ltd, 2008.

72. Greenhalgh T, Howick J, Maskrey N. Evidence-based medicine: a movement in crisis. *British Medical Journal* 2014; **348**: g3725.

73. Carers Trust. *The Triangle of Care: carers included: a guide to best practice in mental health care in England*. London: Carers Trust, 2013.

Further reading

ACMHN (Australian College of Mental Health Nurses). *Standards for practice for Australian mental health nurses 2010*. ACMHN, Canberra, 2010.

Department of Health. *Values into action: the Chief Nursing Officer's Review of Mental Health Nursing in England*. London: DH, 2006.

Department of Health. *Compassion in practice: a vision and strategy for nurses, midwives and care staff.* London: DH, 2013.

HEE (Health Education England), NMC (Nursing and Midwifery Council). *Raising the bar: shape of caring: a review of the future education and training of registered nurses and care assistants.* London: HEE & NMC. 2015. Available from: http://hee.nhs.uk/wp-content/

blogs.dir/321/files/2015/03/2348-Shape-of-caring-review-FINAL.pdf on 28 July 2015 [Accessed 2nd September 2016].

IOM (Institute of Medicine). *The future of nursing: leading change, advancing health.* Washington, DC: IOM, 2010.

Scottish Government. *Rights, relationships and recovery: the report of the National Review of Mental Health Nursing in Scotland.* Edinburgh, NHS Scotland, 2006.

Relevant web pages

Centre for Mental Health. http://www.centreformentalhealth.org.uk/

European Academy of Nursing Science. http://www.european-academy-of-nursing-science.com/

Horatio: European Psychiatric Nurses. http://www.horatio-web.eu/

International Journal of Mental Health Nursing. http://onlinelibrary.wiley.com/journal/10.1111/(ISSN)1447-0349/issues

Journal of Psychiatric and Mental Health Nursing. http://onlinelibrary.wiley.com/journal/10.1111/(ISSN)1365-2850

Mental Health Nurse Academics UK. http://chhs-web.swan.ac.uk/mhnauk/

Mental Health Foundation. http://www.mentalhealth.org.uk/

Mental Health Nurses Association. http://www.unitetheunion.org/how-we-help/list-of-sectors/healthsector/healthsectoryourprofession/mhna/

Rethink Mental Illness. http://www.rethink.org/living-with-mental-illness/recovery

Royal College of Psychiatrists. http://www.rcpsych.ac.uk/

Safewards. http://www.safewards.net/

Star Wards. http://www.starwards.org.uk/

Tidal Model. http://www.tidal-model.com/

Index

Note: Page numbers in *italic* refer to figures, tables or boxes